European Surgical Orthopaedics
and Traumatology

European Federation of National Associations of Orthopaedics and Traumatology

Committees and Task Forces

EFORT Executive Committee

Executive Board
Dr. Manuel Cassiano Neves *President*
Ass. Prof. Dr. Per Kjaersgaard-Andersen, *Secretary General*
Prof. Dr. Pierre Hoffmeyer, *Immediate Past President*
Mr. Stephen R. Cannon, *1st Vice President*
Prof. Dr. Enric Cáceres Palou, *2nd Vice President*
Prof. Dr. Maurilio Marcacci, *Treasurer*
Prof. Dr. Klaus-Peter Günther, *Member at Large*
Dr. George Macheras, *Member at Large*
Prof. Dr. Philippe Neyret, *Member at Large*

Co-Opted Members
Mr. John Albert
Mr. Michael Benson
Prof. Dr. Thierry Bégué
Prof. Dr. George Bentley, *Past President*
Prof. Dr. Nikolaus Böhler, *Past President*
Dr. Matteo Denti
Prof. Dr. Karsten Dreinhöfer
Prof. Dr. Pavel Dungl
Prof. Dr. Norbert Haas
Prof. Dr. Karl Knahr
Prof. Dr. Wolfhart Puhl, *Past President*
Prof. Dr. Nejat Hakki Sur
Prof. Dr. Karl-Göran Thorngren, *Past President*

Scientific Coordination 15th EFORT Congress, London 2014

Chairman
Mr. Stephen Cannon

Standing Committees

EAR Committee
Prof. Dr. Nikolaus Böhler

Education Committee
Prof. Dr. Klaus-Peter Günther

Ethics Committee
Mr. Michael Benson

EA & L Committee
Prof. Dr. Wolfhart Puhl

Finance Committee
Prof. Dr. Maurilio Marcacci

Health Service Research Committee
Prof. Dr. Karsten Dreinhöfer

Portal Steering Committee
Prof. Elke Viehweger

Publications Committee
Prof. Dr. George Bentley

Scientific Congress Committee
Prof. Dr. Enric Cáceres Palou

Speciality Society Standing Committee
Dr. Matteo Denti

Task Forces and Ad Hoc Committees

Awards & Prizes Committee
Prof. Dr. George Bentley

Fora
Prof. Dr. Thierry Bégué

Travelling & Visiting Fellowships
Prof. Dr. Philippe Neyret

Musculoskeletal Trauma Task Force
Prof. Dr. Norbert Haas

EFORT Foundation Committee
Prof. Dr. Karl-Göran Thorngren

George Bentley

Editor

European Surgical Orthopaedics and Traumatology

The EFORT Textbook

Volume 2

With 3294 Figures and 278 Tables

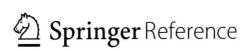 Springer Reference

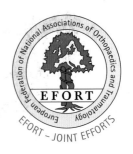

Editor
George Bentley
University College London
London, UK

Royal National Orthopaedic Hospital
Stanmore, Middlesex, UK

ISBN 978-3-642-34745-0   ISBN 978-3-642-34746-7 (eBook)
ISBN 978-3-642-34747-4 (print and electronic bundle)
DOI 10.1007/978-3-642-34746-7
Springer Heidelberg New York Dordrecht London

Library of Congress Control Number: 2014932431

Printed on acid-free paper

Springer is part of Springer Science+Business Media (www.springer.com)

Foreword

In recent years, we have seen Europe going through major changes in different fields, and education is no exception. The search for the best practice in order to meet the increasing expectations of the patients becomes obligatory in our daily activities, and education plays a major role in achieving this goal.

EFORT is also conscious that even in well-developed orthopaedic resident programmes in Europe, there can be considerable inconsistencies in the level of knowledge that is required to proceed to consultant practice, and we are also aware that in terms of assessment at the end of training there is also a wide variation.

A decade ago, Jacques Duparc took the first initiative of providing a European view in the orthopaedic speciality by publishing *Surgical Techniques in Orthopaedics and Traumatology*. Presently, we are witnessing constant changes in many aspects of our lives in Europe and especially in orthopaedics and traumatology. During the last years, we have seen major improvements in our field; so we thought it was the time to provide an updated comprehensive textbook covering the major fields of current importance. This book will provide a major source for all trainees in the preparation for their end-of-training examinations and assessments but also to all others involved in the practice of our speciality. The launch of the textbook *European Surgical Orthopaedics and Traumatology* offers a new perspective in terms of Orthopaedic education and will contribute to the minimizing of the variations still seen throughout Europe.

The European flavour provided by the most prominent orthopaedic and traumatology surgeons from different countries will allow for the development of the best current practice across Europe and enhance the process of harmonization of orthopaedic education. The standardization of the minimal requirements for the training in orthopaedics and traumatology has been one of the major goals of EFORT, and this textbook will provide important guidance in this sense.

It would have been impossible to launch this textbook/encyclopaedia without the participation of a multitude of anonymous people that have contributed to it in a disinterested way, but I have to thank especially the Editor, George Bentley, for his tremendous work. Without his tenacity, commitment, vision and most of all his expertise and hard work, it would have been impossible to arrive at the stage of publication. Also a special thanks to our publisher Springer and their team for their professionalism.

As President of EFORT, I am very proud of this major achievement and I trust that this book will be useful for both trainees and specialists in their current practice as well as in expanding their knowledge and surgical horizons.

Manuel Cassiano Neves/Lisbon, 2014
EFORT President 2013–2014

Preface

This EFORT textbook was developed by the Executive Committee following the excellent *Surgical Techniques in Orthopaedics and Traumatology* edited by Prof. Jacques Duparc a decade ago.

Following discussions with two major publishers, we were assured that a hard copy textbook/encyclopedia would fill an important niche in the surgical literature.

Our aim was to produce a text which would act as a surgical techniques guide, but also embrace the total management of the patients which, it is now realised, is vital to best surgical practice and maximal patient outcomes.

I was very enthusiastic because, as an Englishman with some exposure to European literature and practice, I realised this book would present an exciting opportunity to bring together and publicise the rich variety and quality of clinical practice, research, and literature available in Europe, which was not fully appreciated by much of the English-speaking world.

The layout of the book is traditional in some ways, but I was anxious that all the authors should present their views in their own personal style. Therefore the book is arranged in 10 sections and the chapters have a common overall format. Each chapter has a contents section for easy checking and keywords, but the "flavour" of the authors' professional approach to the topic is apparent from reading each individual chapter.

Hence, this book is a unique collection of chapters on all the major conditions we deal with in orthopaedics and traumatology, presented in a lively way and embracing many well-tested techniques and management protocols.

The overall aim was to produce a source (major reference work) which will be equally valuable to trainees, all those involved in education and training, and those whose profession is in a general rather than super-specialised practice. Hence each chapter has sub-sections on, literature, relevant basic sciences, clinical assessment, indications for surgery, pre-operative planning, surgical techniques, post-operative management, rehabilitation, complications and outcomes.

I must pay tribute to the Section Editors who have been excellent and without whom the book would not have been started, let alone written. Here I must mention particularly Franz Langlais, who was tragically taken from us early on. Their expertise and enthusiasm have been invaluable. Nevertheless, because of the requirement to have a common approach and theme, and conscious that many authors are not primary English speakers, I thought it essential to edit and review the whole text personally. Therefore, any defects are mine.

Throughout I have had unqualified support from all my colleagues on the Executive Committee, in particular the supervising Presidents, Karl-Göran Thorngren, Miklos Szendroi, Pierre Hoffmeyer and Manuel Cassiano Neves, together with an abundance of useful advice. Per Kjaersgaard-Anderson has been a tower of strength as my adviser especially in our final preparation and negotiations.

The actual process of producing such a book is sometimes challenging. It would not have been possible without my secretary/PA, Rosemary Radband. Her rapid and expert way of handling data, and some authors, made it possible. The Springer team – Gabriele Schroeder, Sylvia Blago and particularly Simone Giesler – has been excellent, expert, completely professional, and a pleasure to work with. Latterly Susan Davenport of EFORT has given unstinting support.

This task has been a great privilege and pleasure for me. I have come to appreciate and sometimes wonder at the works of my author colleagues. My thanks are not sufficient to express my gratitude to you all.

This book may never be published again in hard copy but the E-copy will be easy to update in future. We now have an authoritative and unique European base for our future educational programmes which will, I hope, enrich all our surgical lives.

George Bentley   London, 2014

About the Editor

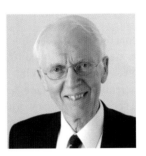

Professor George Bentley D.Sc., MB, ChB, E.C.F.M.G. (USA), ChM, FRCS (Eng.), FRCS (Ed.), F.Med.Sci.

Professor Bentley is Emeritus Professor of Orthopaedics at University College London and Honorary Consultant Orthopaedic Surgeon at the Royal National Orthopaedic Hospital NHS Trust, London.

From 1991 he was Director and Professor of Orthopaedics, in the Institute of Orthopaedics and Musculo-Skeletal Science, University College London (UCL), and Director of Clinical Studies at the Royal National Orthopaedic Hospital, Stanmore.

His training in Orthopaedics and Traumatology was in the University Hospitals of Sheffield, Birmingham, Manchester, Pittsburgh (USA) and Oxford, where he was University Reader in Orthopaedics, before spending 6 years as Professor of Orthopaedic and Accident Surgery in the University of Liverpool and the Royal Liverpool and Children's Hospitals.

From 1982 he took up the only Chair of Orthopaedics in the University of London, based at the Royal National Orthopaedic and Middlesex Hospitals.

His pioneering research in cell-engineering, on successful transplantation of articular and growth-plate chondrocytes in both normal and arthritic knee joints, published in *Nature* in 1971, laid the foundation of present-day human cell-engineering, now a worldwide clinical field.

Clinically, he established major units for hip and knee joint replacement and the first cartilage cell transplantation unit in the UK. He has completed 10 randomised controlled clinical trials in scoliosis, hip and knee joint replacement and cartilage cell transplantation.

He is a renowned surgical educator, having won the "Golden Stethoscope" awarded to the best clinical teacher, in the University of Oxford. In London, at

RNOH, he established the largest postgraduate training programme in the UK, which trains 25 % of orthopaedic and trauma surgeons in Britain. During his time as elected Fellow and Vice-President on the Council of the Royal College of Surgeons of England, he chaired the Training Board, responsible for supervision of all surgical training in the England and Wales. Simultaneously he was Chairman of the Intercollegiate Examinations Board for the UK qualifying diploma of F.R.C.S. (Tr. and Orth.), from 1996 to1999.

He founded an orthopaedic educational programme at RNOH and associated hospitals which, over 3 years, covers all aspects of Orthopaedics and Traumatology, and an M.Sc. degree course of London University.

Undergraduate teaching and examination has been a continuing lifelong commitment in Sheffield, Birmingham, Manchester, Oxford, Liverpool and UCL Medical Schools.

The Institute of Orthopaedics and Musculo-Skeletal Science employs 100+ scientific and clinical staff and is funded by the research councils and charitable institutions. Professor Bentley and his colleagues have published over 500 peer-reviewed scientific papers and he has presented over 500 lectures at universities and specialist centres worldwide.

He has written three major textbooks and contributed chapters to many other orthopaedic and trauma texts.

In 1985 he was elected President of the British Orthopaedic Research Society, and in 1990 Vice-President and President of the British Orthopaedic Association. In 1995 he was elected Chairman of the Scientific Committee of EFORT and was responsible for developing the scientific programmes of the Barcelona Congress and subsequent congresses and instructional courses across Europe.

Through 2002 to 2005 he served as Vice-President and President of EFORT.

Currently, as Chairman of the Scientific Publications Committee of EFORT, he has developed educational programmes and a curriculum for trainees, especially those who wish to sit the European Board of Orthopaedics and Traumatology (EBOT) examination. Additionally, he has edited the EFORT Instructional Course Lecture Books for the last 5 years.

As well as being a member and reviewer for many scientific journals – *JBJS*, *BJJ*, *BJr*, *Journal of Orthopaedic Research*, *British Medical Journal*, *Lancet*, *Journal of Rheumatology*, *Biomaterials*, *The Knee* etc. – he has been European Editor-in-Chief of the *Journal of Arthroplasty* since 2001.

In 1999 he was elected Honorary Fellow "Membre d'Honneur" of the Société Francaise de Chirurgie Orthopédique et Traumatologique (S.O.F.C.O.T.) and of the Royal College of Surgeons of Edinburgh. He was the first orthopaedic surgeon to be elected to the prestigious Fellowship of the Medical Academy of Science, London, and, in 2009, to the Honorary fellowship of the Royal Society of Medicine.

He is married to Ann and they have one daughter, Sarah, and two sons, Paul and Stephen.

Section Editors

General Orthopaedics and Traumatology

George Bentley University College London, London, UK

Royal National Orthopaedic Hospital, Stanmore, Middlesex, UK

Karl-Göran Thorngren Department of Orthopaedics, Lund University Hospital, Lund, Sweden

Spine

George Bentley University College London, London, UK

Royal National Orthopaedic Hospital, Stanmore, Middlesex, UK

Björn Strömqvist Department of Orthopedics, Skåne University Hospital, Malmö, Sweden

Shoulder

Pierre Hoffmeyer University Hospitals of Geneva, Geneva, Switzerland

George Bentley University College London, London, UK

Royal National Orthopaedic Hospital, Stanmore, Middlesex, UK

Arm, Elbow and Forearm

Konrad Mader Section Trauma Surgery, Hand and Upper Extremity Reconstructive Surgery, Department of Orthopaedic Surgery, Førde Sentralsjukehus, Førde, Norway

George Bentley University College London, London, UK

Royal National Orthopaedic Hospital, Stanmore, Middlesex, UK

Hand and Wrist

Frank Burke The Pulvertaft Hand Centre, Derbyshire Royal Hospital, Derby, UK

George Bentley University College London, London, UK

Royal National Orthopaedic Hospital, Stanmore, Middlesex, UK

Pelvis and Hip

Klaus-Peter Günther Department of Orthopaedic Surgery, University Hospital Carl Gustav Carus Dresden, Medical Faculty of the Technical University Dresden, Dresden, Germany

George Bentley University College London, London, UK

Royal National Orthopaedic Hospital, Stanmore, Middlesex, UK

Thigh, Knee and Shin

Nikolaus Böhler Orthopädische Abteilung, Allgemeines Krankhaus Linz, Linz, Austria

George Bentley University College London, London, UK

Royal National Orthopaedic Hospital, Stanmore, Middlesex, UK

Ankle and Foot

Dishan Singh Royal National Orthopaedic Hospital, Stanmore, Middlesex, UK

George Bentley University College London, London, UK

Royal National Orthopaedic Hospital, Stanmore, Middlesex, UK

Musculo-Skeletal Tumours

Stephen Cannon Clementine Churchill Hospital, Harrow, Middlesex, UK

Sarcoma Unit, Royal National Orthopaedic Hospital, Stanmore, Middlesex, UK

George Bentley Royal National Orthopaedic Hospital, Stanmore, Middlesex, UK

Paediatric Orthopaedics and Traumatology

Aresh Hashemi-Nejad Royal National Orthopaedic Hospital, Stanmore, Middlesex, UK

George Bentley University College London, London, UK

Royal National Orthopaedic Hospital, Stanmore, Middlesex, UK

Manuel Cassiano Neves Orthopaedic Department, Hospital Cuf Descobertas, Parque das Nações, Lisboa, Portugal

Contents

Volume 3

Volume 6

—

Contributors

Ali Abbasian Guys and St Thomas' Hospital, London, UK

Antonio Abramo Hand and Upper Extremity Unit, Department of Orthopedics, Lund University Hospital, Lund, Sweden

Lars Adolfsson Department of Orthopaedics, Linköping University Hospital, Linköping, Sweden

Max Aebi MEM Research Center, University of Bern and Orthopaedic Department, Hirslanden-Salem Hospital, Bern, Switzerland

Faik K. Afifi Department of Orthopaedic Surgery and Traumatology, Kantonsspital Baselland, Bruderholz, Switzerland

Per-Henrik Ågren Stockholms Fotkirurgklinik, Sophiahemmet, Stockholm, Sweden

Ahmet Alanay Department of Orthopaedics and Traumatology, Comprehensive Spine Center, Acibadem Maslak Hospital, Istanbul, Turkey

Firas Al-Dabouby Orthopedic Division, Hashemite University, Prince Hamza Teaching Hospital, Amman, Jordan

Hesham Al-Khateeb Royal National Orthopaedic Hospital, NHS, Stanmore, Middlesex, UK

Robin Allum Heatherwood and Wexham Park Hospitals NHS Trust, Berkshire, UK

Karl Fredrik Almqvist Department of Orthopaedic Surgery and Traumatology, Ghent State University, Ghent, Belgium

Giulio Altadonna Clinic of Orthopaedic and Sports Traumatology, Biomechanics Laboratory, Rizzoli Orthopaedic Institute, Bologna University, Bologna, Italy

Amit Amin St George's Hospital, Tooting, London, UK

R. Amirfeyz Bristol Royal Infirmary, Bristol, UK

John C. Angel Royal National Orthopaedic Hospital, London, UK

Samuel A. Antuña Shoulder and Elbow Unit, La Paz University Hospital, Universidad Autónoma de Madrid, Madrid, Spain

Imran Anwar Kadoorie Centre for Critical Care Research and Education, Trauma Unit, John Radcliffe Hospital, University of Oxford, Oxford, UK

Alessandro Aprato Orthopaedic Department, University of Turin, Turin, Italy

Pooler Archbold Royal Victoria Hospital, Belfast, Northern Ireland, UK

Jean-Noel Argenson Institute for Motion and Locomotion, Center for Osteoarthritis Surgery, Université de la Méditerranée, Assistance Publique des Hôpitaux de Marseille, CHU Sainte Marguerite, Marseille, France

Dan Armstrong Pulvertaft Hand Centre, Derby, UK

Mathieu Assal Clinique La Colline, Geneva, Switzerland

J. M. Aubaniac Institute for Motion and Locomotion, Center for Osteoarthritis Surgery, Université de la Méditerranée, Assistance Publique des Hôpitaux de Marseille, CHU Sainte Marguerite, Marseille, France

David Backstein Mount Sinai Hospital, University of Toronto, Toronto, ON, Canada

Thanos Badekas Foot and Ankle Clinic Metropolitan Hospital, Athens, Greece

Eleni Balabanidou University Hospital Southampton, Southampton, UK

José Ballesteros Orthopedic Department, Hospital Clínico Barcelona, Barcelona, Spain

Stefano Bandiera Department of Oncologic and Degenerative Spine Surgery, Istituto Rizzoli, Bologna, Italy

Olivier Barbier Service d'Orthopédie et de Traumatologie, Cliniques Universitaires St-Luc, Université Catholique de Louvain, Bruxelles, Belgium

Raúl Barco Shoulder and Elbow Unit, La Paz University Hospital, Universidad Autónoma de Madrid, Madrid, Spain

R. Barker Princess Elizabeth Orthopaedic Unit, Royal Devon and Exeter Hospital, Devon, UK

A. Barnard Pulvertaft Hand Centre, Derby, UK

Louis Samuel Barouk Yvrac, France

Pierre Barouk Clinique du Sport, Merginac, France

Matthew Barry The Royal London Hospital, Whitechapel, London, UK

Philippe Beaufils Orthopaedic Department, Centre Hospitalier de Versailles, Le Chesnay, France

M. G. Benedetti Movement Analysis Laboratory, Istituto Ortopedico Rizzoli, University of Bologna, Bologna, Italy

George Bentley University College London, London, UK

Royal National Orthopaedic Hospital, Stanmore, Middlesex, UK

A. Benzi Sports Traumatolgy Department, Rizzoli Othopaedic Institute, University of Bologna, Bologna, Italy

Arne Berner Queensland University of Technology, Brisbane, Australia

Peter Bernstein Department of Orthopaedic Surgery, University Hospital Carl Gustav Carus Dresden, Dresden, Germany

Ágnes Berta Department of Orthopaedics, Uzsoki Hospital, Budapest, Hungary

Jean-Luc Besse Université Lyon 1, IFSTTAR, LBMC UMR–T 9406 – Laboratoire de Biomécanique et Mécanique des Chocs, Bron, France

Hospices Civils de Lyon, Centre Hospitalier Lyon–Sud, Service de Chirurgie Orthopédique et Traumatologique, Pierre–Bénite, France

Jagmeet S. Bhamra The London Sarcoma Service, Royal National Orthopaedic Hospital, Stanmore, Middlesex, UK

Giuseppe Bianchi Istituti Ortopedici Rizzoli, 5th Division, Bologna, Italy

Elcil Kaya Bicer Centre Albert Trillat, Groupe Hospitalier Nord, Hospices Civils de Lyon, Lyon-Caluire, France

Caroline Bijnen-Girardot Hong Kong, Hong Kong SAR

Roberto Binazzi Department of Orthopedic Surgery, Villa Erbosa Hospital, University of Bologna, Bologna, Italy

Rolfe Birch War Nerve Injury Clinic at Defence Medical Rehabilitation Centre, Epsom, Surrey, UK

Martin Bircher Department of Trauma and Orthopaedics, St. George's Hospital, London, UK

Alessandro Bistolfi Department of Orthopaedics, Traumatology and Rehabilitation, CTO/M Adelaide Hospital, Turin, Italy

B. Bittersohl Department of Orthopedic Surgery, University Hospital of Düsseldorf, Düsseldorf, Germany

B. Blondel Orthopedic Pediatric Department, Timone Children Hospital, Marseille, France

Hospital for Joint Diseases, New York University, New York, NY, USA

Gordon Blunn John Scales Centre for Biomedical Engineering, Institute of Orthopaedics and Musculo-Skeletal Science, University College London, Royal National Orthopaedic Hospital, Stanmore, Middlesex, UK

Matteo Bo Expert Consultant in Industrial Installations, Prodim srl, Turin, Italy

Nikolaus Böhler Orthopädische Abteilung, Allgemeines Krankhaus Linz, Linz, Austria

Philippe Boisrenoult Orthopaedic Department, Versailles Hospital, Le Chesnay, France

Jens G. Boldt Siloah Hospital Guemligen, Orthopaedic Centre, Muri/Bern, Switzerland

Gerard Bollini Orthopedic Pediatric Department, Timone Children Hospital, Marseille, France

T. Bonanzinga Sports Traumatolgy Department, Rizzoli Othopaedic Institute, University of Bologna, Bologna, Italy

Stefano Boriani Department of Oncologic and Degenerative Spine Surgery, Istituto Rizzoli, Bologna, Italy

Gráinne Bourke Leeds Teaching Hospitals Trust, Leeds, UK

Judith V. M. G. Bovée Leiden University Medical Centre, Leiden, The Netherlands

Elena Maria Brach del Prever Department of Orthopaedics, Traumatology and Rehabilitation, University of the Studies of Turin, Turin, Italy

Christopher Bradish Great Ormond Street Hospital, London, UK

Timothy W. R. Briggs The London Sarcoma Service, Royal National Orthopaedic Hospital, Stanmore, Middlesex, UK

M. J. Brito Infectious Disease Department, Hospital Dona Estefania, Lisbon, Portugal

Matthew T. Brown The London Sarcoma Service, Royal National Orthopaedic Hospital, Stanmore, Middlesex, UK

Colin Bruce Department Children's Orthopaedic Surgery, Alder Hey Children's Hospital, Liverpool, UK

D. Bruni Sports Traumatolgy Department, Rizzoli Orthopaedic Institute, University of Bologna, Bologna, Italy

Tymoteusz Budny Zentrum für Orthopädie, Klinik für Allgemeine Orthopädie, Münster, Germany

P. Buma Department of Orthopedics, Radboud University Nijmegen Medical Centre, Nijmegen, The Netherlands

Tim Bunker Princess Elizabeth Orthopaedic Centre, Exeter, UK

Frank Burke The Pulvertaft Hand Centre, Derbyshire Royal Hospital, Derby, UK

Klaus Burkhart Department of Orthopaedic and Trauma Surgery, University of Cologne, Cologne, Germany

Dan Butler Kadoorie Centre for Critical Care Research and Education, Trauma Unit, John Radcliffe Hospital, University of Oxford, Oxford, UK

Enric Cáceres Palou Department Hospital Vall d'Hebron, Autonomous University of Barcelona, Barcelona, Spain

M. Cadossi Department of Orthopaedic and Trauma Surgery, Istituto Ortopedico Rizzoli, Bologna, Italy

Peter Calder The Royal National Orthopaedic Hospital, Stanmore, Middlesex, UK

J. L. Campagnolo Orthopaedic Department, Hospital Dona Estefania, Lisbon, Portugal

Doug Campbell Leeds General Infirmary, Leeds, UK

Sara Camurri Orthopaedic and Trauma Department, Orthopaedic Pediatrics and Neuro-Orthopedic Unit, Humanitas Research Hospital, Rozzano Milano, Italy

Federico Canavese Department of Pediatric Surgery, University Hospital Estaing, Clermont Ferrand, France

Stephen Cannon Clementine Churchill Hospital, Harrow, Middlesex, UK

Sarcoma Unit, Royal National Orthopaedic Hospital, Stanmore, Middlesex, UK

Rodolfo Capanna Centro Traumatologico Ortopedico (CTO), Policlinico di Careggi, Firenze, Italy

Antonio Cartucho Orthopaedic Department, Hospital Cuf Descobertas, Lisbon, Portugal

Manuel Cassiano Neves Orthopaedic Department, Hospital Cuf Descobertas, Parque das Nações, Lisboa, Portugal

Pierre-Paul Casteleyn Department of Orthopaedics and Traumatology, University Hospital, Brussels, Belgium

Fabio Catani Movement Analysis Laboratory, Istituto Ortopedico Rizzoli, University of Bologna, Bologna, Italy

Dimitri Ceroni Department of Paediatric Orthopaedics, Children's Hospital and University Hospital Geneva, Geneva, Switzerland

Panteleimon Chan Barts and The London NHS Trust and The London Children's Hospital, Whitechapel, London, UK

Bertrand Cherrier Saint Antoine Hospital, Pierre et Marie Curie University, Paris, France

E. Choufani Orthopedic Pediatric Department, Timone Children Hospital, Marseille, France

Grégoire Ciais Service de Chirurgie Orthopédique, Hôpital Universitaire de Bicetre, Le Kremlin-Bicetre, France

Andrew W. Clarke Royal National Orthopaedic Hospital NHS Trust, Stanmore, Middlesex, UK

Philippe Clavert Centre de Chirurgie Orthopedique et de la Main, Illkirch-Graffenstaden, France

Marina Clement-Rigolet Service de Chirurgie Orthopédique, Hôpital Universitaire de Bicetre, Le Kremlin-Bicetre, France

David Cloke Department of Orthopaedics, Freeman Hospital, High Heaton, Newcastle-upon-Tyne, UK

Melanie Coathup John Scales Centre for Biomedical Engineering, Institute of Orthopaedics and Musculo-Skeletal Science, University College London, Royal National Orthopaedic Hospital, Stanmore, Middlesex, UK

Simone Colangeli Department of Oncologic and Degenerative Spine Surgery, Istituto Rizzoli, Bologna, Italy

Paul H. Cooke Nuffield Orthopaedic Centre, Headington, Oxford, UK

Stephen A. Copeland The Reading Shoulder Surgery Unit, Capio Reading Hospital, Reading, UK

Tony Corner West Hertfordshire Hospitals NHS Trust, Watford and St. Albans Hospitals, Watford, UK

Olivier Cornu Service d'Orthopédie et de Traumatologie, Cliniques Universitaires St-Luc, Université Catholique de Louvain, Bruxelles, Belgium

Tim A. Coughlin Pulvertaft Hand Centre, Royal Derby Hospital, Derby, UK

Charles Court Spine Unit, Orthopaedic Department, Bicetre University Hospital, AP-HP Paris, Université Paris-Sud ORSAY, Le Kremlin Bicêtre, France

Timothy Cresswell Pulvertaft Hand Centre, Royal Derby Hospital, Derby, UK

U. Culemann Celle General Hospital, Celle, Germany

Nicholas Cullen The Royal National Orthopaedic Hospital, Stanmore, Middlesex, UK

C. Cuocolo Department of Orthopaedics, Traumatology and Occupational Medicine, University of Turin, Turin, Italy

Zoe H. Dailiana Department of Orthopaedic Surgery, Faculty of Medicine, School of Health Sciences, University of Thessalia, Biopolis, Larissa, Greece

Jens Dargel Department of Orthopaedic and Trauma Surgery, University of Cologne, Cologne, Germany

Lieven De Wilde Department of Orthopaedic Surgery and Traumatology, Ghent University Hospital, Ghent, Belgium

Ralf Decking Department of Orthopaedics, St. Remigius Krankenhaus Opladen, Germany

Paul-André Deleu Foot and Ankle Institute, Parc Leopold Clinic, Brussels, Belgium

Christian Delloye Service d'Orthopédie et de Traumatologie, Cliniques Universitaires St-Luc, Université Catholique de Louvain, Bruxelles, Belgium

J. Demakakos Hospital for Joint Diseases, New York University, New York, NY, USA

Guillaume Demey Centre Albert Trillât Hôpital de le Croix-Rousse, Lyon, France

Lyon Ortho Clinic – Clinique de la Sauvegarde, Lyon, France

K. Deogaonkar Northern Ireland Higher Surgical Training Programme for Trauma and Orthopaedics, Musgrave Park Hospital, Belfast, UK

Bernhard Devos Bevernage Foot and Ankle Institute, Parc Leopold Clinic, Brussels, Belgium

Berardo Di Matteo Clinic of Orthopaedic and Sports Traumatology, Biomechanics Laboratory, Rizzoli Orthopaedic Institute, Bologna University, Bologna, Italy

Joseph J. Dias University Hospitals of Leicester NHS Trust, Leicester General Hospital, Leicester, UK

P. D. S. Dijkstra Leiden University Medical Centre, Leiden, The Netherlands

Rozalia Dimitriou Academic Department of Trauma and Orthopaedics, School of Medicine, University of Leeds, Leeds, UK

Davide Donati Istituti Ortopedici Rizzoli, 5th Division, Bologna, Italy

Simon Donell Norfolk and Norwich University Hospital, Norfolk, UK

George Dowd Royal Free Hospital/Wellington Hospital, London, UK

Cameron Downs Princess Alexandra Hospital, Queensland University of Technology, Brisbane, Australia

Thomas Dreher Paediatric Orthopaedics and Foot Surgery, Department for Orthopaedic and Trauma Surgery, Heidelberg University Clinics, Heidelberg, Germany

Tomas K. Drobny Reconstructive Knee Surgery, Schulthess Klinik, Zürich, Switzerland

Denis Dufrane Banque de tissus de l'Appareil locomoteur, Cliniques Universitaires St-Luc, Université Catholique de Louvain, Bruxelles, Belgium

Christian Dumontier Hôpital Saint Antoine, Paris, France

Deborah M. Eastwood Royal National Orthopaedic Hospital, Stanmore, Middlesex, UK

David Elliot Hand Surgery Department, St Andrew's Centre for Plastic Surgery, Broomfield Hospital, Chelmsford, Essex, UK

Roger J. H. Emery St. Mary's Hospital, Imperial College NHS Trust, London, UK

Department of Mechanical Engineering, Imperial College, London, UK

European Hospital Georges Pompidou, APHP, University Paris Descartes, Paris, France

João Espregueira-Mendes Clínica Saúde Atlântica –Porto, Minho University, Braga, Portugal

Richard Eyb Orthopädische Abteilung, Sozialmedizinisches Zentrum Ost Donauspital, Wien, Austria

Denise Eygendaal Department of Orthopaedics, Upper Limb Unit, Amphia Hospital, Breda, The Netherlands

J. Fabry Department of Orthopaedics and Traumatology, University Hospital, Brussels, Belgium

Mark Farndon Harrogate District Hospital, Harrogate, North Yorkshire, UK

Pasquale Farsetti Department of Orthopaedic Surgery, University of Rome "Tor Vergata", Rome, Italy

Camdon Fary Western Health, Footscray, VIC, Australia

Antonio A. Faundez Department of Surgery, Service de Chirurgie Orthopédique et Traumatologie de l'Appareil Moteur, University of Geneva Hospitals and Faculty of Medicine, Geneva, Switzerland

Jean-Marc Féron Orthopaedic and Trauma Surgery Department, Saint Antoine Hospital, Pierre et Marie Curie University, Paris, France

Michel-Henri Fessy Centre Hospitalier Lyon Sud, Chirurgie Orthopédique et Traumatologique, Pierre Benite, France

Giuseppe Filardo Clinic of Orthopaedic and Sports Traumatology, Biomechanics Laboratory, Rizzoli Orthopaedic Institute, Bologna University, Bologna, Italy

John Fisher Institute of Medical and Biological Engineering, School of Mechanical Engineering, University of Leeds, Leeds, UK

John A. Fixsen Hospital for Sick Children, London, UK

Xavier Flecher Institute for Motion and Locomotion, Center for Osteoarthritis Surgery, Université de la Méditerranée, Assistance Publique des Hôpitaux de Marseille, CHU Sainte Marguerite, Marseille, France

P. A. Fleming The John Charnley Research Institute, Wrightington Hospital, Wigan, Lancashire, UK

Jonas Franke Nottingham Shoulder and Elbow Unit, Nottingham University Hospitals, Nottingham, UK

F. Frenos Centro Traumatologico Ortopedico (CTO), Policlinico di Careggi, Firenze, Italy

Niklaus F. Friederich Department of Orthopaedic Surgery and Traumatology, Kantonsspital Baselland, Bruderholz, Switzerland

Daniel Fritschy Hôpital de La Tour, Meyrin, Switzerland

Olivier Gagey Orthopaedic Department, Paris-South University, Paris, France

Paolo Gallinaro Department of Orthopaedics, Traumatology and Rehabilitation, University of the Studies of Turin, Turin, Italy

Reinhold Ganz Faculty of Medicine, University of Bern, Bern, Switzerland

Shawn Garbedian Mount Sinai Hospital, University of Toronto, Toronto, ON, Canada

J. W. M. Gardeniers Department of Orthopedics, Radboud University Nijmegen Medical Centre, Nijmegen, The Netherlands

Christos Garnavos Glyfada, Athens, Greece

Alessandro Gasbarrini Department of Oncologic and Degenerative Spine Surgery, Istituto Rizzoli, Bologna, Italy

Czar Louie Gaston Oncology Unit, Royal Orthopaedic Hospital NHS Foundation Trust, Birmingham, UK

Thomas Gausepohl Klinik für Unfallchirurgie, Hand- und Wiederherstellungschirurgie, Klinikum Vest GmbH, Marl, Germany

Nicholas Geary Wirral University NHS Trust, Upton, Wirral, UK

Thorsten Gehrke Orthopaedic Surgery, ENDO-Klinik Hamburg, Hamburg, Germany

Pablo E. Gelber Hospital de la Santa Creu i Sant Pau, Universitat Autònoma de Barcelona (UAB), Barcelona, Spain

Hans A. J. Gelderblom Leiden University Medical Centre, Leiden, The Netherlands

A. Ghassemi University College Hospital, London, UK

Antoine de Gheldere The Newcastle upon Tyne Hospitals - NHS Foundation Trust, Newcastle upon Tyne, UK

Riccardo Ghermandi Department of Oncologic and Degenerative Spine Surgery, Istituto Rizzoli, Bologna, Italy

Roberto Giacometti Ceroni Hip Department, IRCCS Istituto Ortopedico Galeazzi, Milan, Italy

Sandro Giannini Movement Analysis Laboratory, Istituto Ortopedico Rizzoli, University of Bologna, Bologna, Italy

Department of Orthopaedic and Trauma Surgery, Istituto Ortopedico Rizzoli, Bologna, Italy

Peter V. Giannoudis Academic Department of Trauma and Orthopaedics, School of Medicine, University of Leeds, Leeds, UK

Henk Giele Oxford Radcliffe Hospitals, Oxford, UK

Panagiotis D. Gikas The London Sarcoma Service, Royal National Orthopaedic Hospital, Stanmore, Middlesex, UK

West Hertfordshire Hospitals NHS Trust, Watford and St. Albans Hospitals, Watford, UK

Paul Gillespie Department of Trauma and Orthopaedics, St. George's Hospital, London, UK

Philippe Gillet Centre Hospitalier Universitaire, Liège, Belgium

Andy J. Goldberg UCL Institute of Orthopaedics & Musculoskeletal Science, Royal National Orthopaedic Hospital NHS Trust, Stanmore, Middlesex, UK

Hans Gollwitzer ATOS Klinik München, and Klinik für Orthopädie und Sportorthopädie am Klinikum rechts der Isar, Technische Universität München, München, Germany

Vincent Gombault Foot and Ankle Institute, Parc Leopold Clinic, Brussels, Belgium

David Gordon Luton and Dunstable University Hospital, Luton, UK

Taco Gosens St. Elisabeth Hospital Tilburg, Tilburg, The Netherlands

Georg Gosheger Zentrum für Orthopädie, Klinik für Allgemeine Orthopädie, Münster, Germany

Martin Gough Evelina Children's Hospital/One Small Step Gait Laboratory, Guy's and St Thomas' NHS Foundation Trust, London, UK

Nikolaos Gougoulias Frimley Park Hospital, Frimley, Frimley, UK

C. F. Gouveia Infectious Disease Department, Hospital Dona Estefania, Lisbon, Portugal

G. Grabmeier Orthopädische Abteilung, Sozialmedizinisches Zentrum Ost Donauspital, Wien, Austria

Reiner Gradinger Klinik für Orthopädie und Sportorthopädie am Klinikum rechts der Isar, Technische Universität München, München, Germany

A. Grassi Sports Traumatolgy Department, Rizzoli Othopaedic Institute, University of Bologna, Bologna, Italy

Andrew J. Graydon Starship Hospital, Auckland, New Zealand

Thomas M. Gregory St. Mary's Hospital, Imperial College NHS Trust, London, UK

Department of Mechanical Engineering, Imperial College, London, UK

European Hospital Georges Pompidou, APHP, University Paris Descartes, Paris, France

Franz Grill Pediatric Orthopaedic Department, Orthopaedic Hospital, Speising, Vienna, Austria

Robert J. Grimer Royal Orthopaedic Hospital, Birmingham, UK

Allan E. Gross Mount Sinai Hospital, Toronto, ON, Canada

C. Guardia Orthopedic Pediatric Department, Timone Children Hospital, Marseille, France

José Guimarães Consciência Orthopaedic Department, FCM-Lisbon New University, Lisbon, Portugal

Klaus-Peter Günther Department of Orthopaedic Surgery, University Hospital Carl Gustav Carus Dresden, Medical Faculty of the Technical University Dresden, Dresden, Germany

Norbert P. Haas Center for Musculoskeletal Surgery, Charité – Universitätsmedizin Berlin, Berlin, Germany

Peter Habermeyer Section for Shoulder and Elbow Surgery, ATOS Clinic, Munich, Germany

Fares Sami Haddad University College London Hospitals, NHS Trust, London, UK

Moussah Hamadouche Department of Orthopaedic and Reconstructive Surgery, Centre Hospitalo-Universitaire Cochin-Port Royal, Paris, France

Paul Hamilton Cambridge University Hospitals, NHS Foundation Trust, Cambridge, UK

László Hangody Department of Orthopaedics, Uzsoki Hospital, Budapest, Hungary

Sammy A. Hanna Royal National Orthopaedic Hospital, Stanmore, Middlesex, UK

Aristote Hans-Moevi Centre de Chirurgie Orthopedique et de la Main, Illkirch-Graffenstaden, France

J. Hardes Zentrum für Orthopädie, Klinik für Allgemeine Orthopädie, Münster, Germany

Albrecht Hartmann Department of Orthopaedic Surgery, University Hospital Carl Gustav Carus Dresden, Medical Faculty of the Technical University Dresden, Dresden, Germany

Aresh Hashemi-Nejad Royal National Orthopaedic Hospital, Stanmore, Middlesex, UK

Russell Hawkins Royal National Orthopaedic Hospital, NHS, Stanmore, Middlesex, UK

Tim Hems The Hand Clinic, Department of Orthopaedic Surgery, The Victoria Infirmary, Glasgow, UK

Simon A. Henderson Musgrave Park Hospital, Belfast, UK

Carlos Heras-Palou Pulvertaft Hand Centre, Derby, UK

Deborah Higgs Royal National Orthopaedic Hospital, Stanmore, Middlesex, UK

Michael T. Hirschmann Department of Orthopaedic Surgery and Traumatology, Kantonsspital Baselland, Bruderholz, Switzerland

Pierre Hoffmeyer University Hospitals of Geneva, Geneva, Switzerland

Joerg H. Holstein Department of Trauma, Hand and Reconstructive Surgery, University of Saarland, Homburg/Saar, Germany

Samantha Hook Princess Elizabeth Orthopaedic Centre, Exeter, Devon, UK

Monika Horisberger Orthopaedic Department, University Hospital Basel, Basel, Switzerland

Tracy Horton Pulvertaft Hand Centre, Royal Derby Hospital, Derby, UK

Jonathan R. Howell Princess Elizabeth Orthopaedic Unit, Royal Devon and Exeter Hospital, Devon, UK

Ernesto Ippolito Department of Orthopaedic Surgery, University of Rome "Tor Vergata", Rome, Italy

Kaywan Izadpanah Department for Orthopedic Surgery and Traumatology, Freiburg University Hospital, Freiburg, Germany

Matthias Jacobi Orthopaedic Department, Hôpital Cantonal Fribourg, Fribourg, Switzerland

Roland P. Jakob Orthopaedic Department, Hôpital Cantonal Fribourg, Fribourg, Switzerland

Prakash Jayakumar Barts Health NHS Trust, Whitechapel, London, UK

Zhongmin Jin State Key Laboratory for Manufacturing System Engineering, Xian Jiaotong University, Xian, China

Institute of Medical and Biological Engineering, School of Mechanical Engineering, University of Leeds, Leeds, UK

Elizabeth O. Johnson School of Medicine, University of Athens, Athens, Greece

R. Jose University Hospitals Birmingham, Birmingham, UK

Jean-Luc Jouve Orthopedic Pediatric Department, Timone Children Hospital, Marseille, France

André Kaelin Clinique des Grangettes, Chêne-Bougeries, Switzerland

Nikolaos K. Kanakaris Academic Department of Trauma and Orthopaedics, School of Medicine, Leeds General Infirmary, Leeds, West Yorkshire, UK

John F. Keating Department of Orthopaedic Trauma, Royal Infirmary, Little France, Edinburgh, Scotland, UK

Johnny Keller Department of Orthopaedic Surgery, University Hospital of Aarhus, Aarhus, Denmark

Jean-François Kempf Centre de Chirurgie Orthopedique et de la Main, Illkirch-Graffenstaden, France

Luc Kerboull Marcel Kerboull Institute, Paris, France

Marcel Kerboull Marcel Kerboull Institute, Paris, France

L. A. Kashif Khan The Edinburgh Shoulder Clinic, Royal Infirmary of Edinburgh, Edinburgh, UK

Young-Jo Kim Harvard Medical School, Adolescent and Young Adult Hip Unit, Children's Hospital Boston, Boston, MA, USA

Jörn Kircher Shoulder and Elbow Surgery, Klinik Fleetinsel Hamburg, Hamburg, Germany

Department of Orthopaedics, Medical Faculty, Heinrich–Heine–University, Düsseldorf, Germany

Stephan Kirschner Department of Orthopaedic Surgery, University Hospital Carl Gustav Carus Dresden, Medical Faculty of the Technical University Dresden, Dresden, Germany

Per Kjærsgaard-Andersen Section for Hip and Knee Replacement, Department of Orthopaedics, Vejle Hospital, University of South Denmark, Vejle, Denmark

Christian Kleber Center for Musculoskeletal Surgery, Charité – Universitätsmedizin Berlin, Berlin, Germany

Zdenek Klezl Department of Trauma and Orthopaedics, Spinal Unit, Royal Derby Hospital, Derby, UK

Peter Kloen Department of Orthopaedic Surgery, Academic Medical Center, Amsterdam, The Netherlands

Karl Knahr Surgical Orthopaedics and Traumatology, Vienna, Austria

Izaak F. Kodde Department of Orthopaedics, Upper Limb Unit, Amphia Hospital, Breda, The Netherlands

D. Koehler University of Saarland, Homburg/Saar, Germany

Zinon T. Kokkalis School of Medicine, University of Athens, Haidari, Athens, Greece

Elizaveta Kon Clinic of Orthopaedic and Sports Traumatology, Biomechanics Laboratory, Rizzoli Orthopaedic Institute, Bologna University, Bologna, Italy

Sujith Konan Orthopaedic Trainee NE(UCH) Thames Rotation, London, UK

George Kontakis Academic Department of Trauma and Orthopaedics, School of Medicine, University of Crete, Crete, Greece

Philippe Kopylov Hand and Upper Extremity Unit, Department of Orthopedics, Lund University Hospital, Lund, Sweden

Thomas Christian Koslowsky Department of Surgery, St. Elisabeth Hospital, Cologne, Germany

Rainer I. Kotz Department of Orthopaedics, Medical University Vienna, Vienna, Austria

Rüdiger Krauspe Department of Orthopedic Surgery, University Hospital of Düsseldorf, Düsseldorf, Germany

Martin Krismer Department of Orthopaedics, Innsbruck Medical University, Innsbruck, Austria

Raul A. Kuchinad Health Sciences Centre, University of Calgary, Calgary, AB, Canada

Timo Laine ORTON Orthopaedic Hospital, Helsinki, Finland

Patrick Laing Department of Orthopaedics, Wrexham Maelor Hospital, Wrexham, North Wales, UK

Simon M. Lambert The Shoulder and Elbow Service, Royal National Orthopaedic Hospital, Stanmore, Middlesex, UK

Mikko Larsen Department of Plastic, Reconstructive and Hand Surgery, Launceston General Hospital, Launceston, TAS, Australia

Pierre Lascombes Pediatric Orthopedics, University of Geneva – HUG, Geneva, Switzerland

Thibaut Leemrijse Foot and Ankle Institute, Parc Leopold Clinic, Brussels, Belgium

R. Legre Plastic and Reconstructive Surgery Department, Conception Hospital, Marseille, France

Michael Leunig Department of Orthopedics, Schulthess Clinic, Zürich, Switzerland

Surjit Lidder Barts and The London NHS Trust and The London Children's Hospital, Whitechapel, London, UK

David Limb Chapel Allerton Hospital, Leeds, UK

Tommy Lindau Pulvertaft Hand Centre, Derby, UK

University of Derby, Derby, UK

University of Bergen, Bergen, Norway

European Wrist Arthroscopy Society (EWAS)

Alberto Lluch Institut Kaplan, Barcelona, Spain

Manuel Llusa Orthopedic Department, Valle Hebrón Hospital, University of Barcelona, Barcelona, Spain

Claus Löcherbach University of Lausanne, Lausanne, Switzerland

P. M. Longis Faculté de Médecine, Nantes, France

Jan W. Louwerens Sint Maartenskliniek, Nijmegen, The Netherlands

David Loveday Norfolk and Norwich University Hospital, Norwich, UK

D. Luciani Department of Orthopaedic and Trauma Surgery, Istituto Ortopedico Rizzoli, Bologna, Italy

Teija Lund ORTON Orthopaedic Hospital, Helsinki, Finland

Sebastien Lustig Centre Albert Trillat, Groupe Hospitalier Nord, Hospices Civils de Lyon, Lyon-Caluire, France

Konrad Mader Section Trauma Surgery, Hand and Upper Extremity Reconstructive Surgery, Department of Orthopaedic Surgery, Førde Sentralsjukehus, Førde, Norway

Robert A. Magnussen Department of Orthopaedics, Sports Health and Performance Institute, The Ohio State University, Columbus, OH, USA

Pierre Maldague Foot and Ankle Institute, Parc Leopold Clinic, Brussels, Belgium

Maurilio Marcacci Clinic of Orthopaedic and Sports Traumatology, Biomechanics Laboratory, Rizzoli Orthopaedic Institute, Bologna University, Bologna, Italy

G. M. Marcheggiani Muccioli Sports Traumatolgy Department, Rizzoli Othopaedic Institute, University of Bologna, Bologna, Italy

Robert W. Marshall Department of Orthopaedic Surgery, Royal Berkshire Hospital, Reading, UK

Carlo Marco Masoero Department of Energetics, Polytechnic School of Engineering of Turin, Turin, Italy

Alessandro Massè Department of Orthopaedics, Traumatology and Occupational Medicine, University of Turin, Turin, Italy

Thomas Mattes Department of Orthopaedics and Traumatology, Klinik am Eichert, Göppingen, Germany

Georg Matziolis Department of Orthopaedics, Center for Musculoskeletal Surgery, Charité-Universitätsmedizin Berlin, Berlin, Germany

H. Michael Mayer Spine Centre Munich, Schön Klinik München Harlaching, München, Germany

Mario Mercuri Istituti Ortopedici Rizzoli, 5th Division, Bologna, Italy

Jonathan Miles Royal National Orthopaedic Hospital, Stanmore, Middlesex, UK

Michael B. Millis Harvard Medical School, Adolescent and Young Adult Hip Unit, Children's Hospital Boston, Boston, MA, USA

Ash Moaveni Pulvertaft Hand Centre, Derby, UK

Joan C. Monllau Hospital de la Santa Creu i Sant Pau, Universitat Autónoma de Barcelona (UAB), Barcelona, Spain

Alberto Monteiro Clínica Espregueira-Mendes F.C. Porto Stadium – FIFA Medical Centre of Excellence, Porto, Portugal

J. R. Morley Princess Elizabeth Orthopaedic Unit, Royal Devon and Exeter Hospital, Devon, UK

Ante Mrkonjic Hand and Upper Extremity Unit, Department of Orthopedics, Lund University Hospital, Lund, Sweden

Lars P. Müller Department of Orthopaedic and Trauma Surgery, University of Cologne, Cologne, Germany

Michael Müller Department of Orthopaedics and Department of Accident and Reconstructive Surgery, Centre for Musculoskeletal Surgery, Charité – University Medicine, Berlin, Germany

Urs K. Munzinger Orthopädie am Zürichberg, Zurich, Switzerland

Iain R. Murray Department of Trauma and Orthopaedics, The University of Edinburgh, Edinburgh, UK

Danyal H. Nawabi Chelsea and Westminster Hospital, London, UK

Hospital for Special Surgery, New York, NY, USA

Royal National Orthopaedic Hospital, Stanmore, Middlesex, UK

Lars Neumann Nottingham Shoulder and Elbow Unit, Nottingham University Hospitals, Nottingham, UK

John Newman Litfield House Medical Centre, Bristol, UK

Philippe Neyret Centre Albert Trillat, Groupe Hospitalier Nord, Hospices Civils de Lyon, Lyon-Caluire, France

Nick Nicolaou Maidstone & Tunbridge Wells NHS Trust, Maidstone, UK

Iris M. Noebauer-Huhmann Department of Biomedical Imaging and Image-guided Therapy, Medical University Vienna, Vienna, Austria

Michael Nogler Department of Orthopaedics, Innsbruck Medical University, Innsbruck, Austria

Mary O'Brien Pulvertaft Hand Centre, Derby, UK

Antonio Odasso Health Medicine, Turin, Italy

Paul O'Donnell Department of Radiology, Royal National Orthopaedic Hospital, Middlesex, Stanmore, UK

G. A. Odri Faculté de Médecine, Nantes, France

Acke Ohlin Lund University, Sweden, Malmö, Sweden

Deniz Olgun Department of Orthopaedics and Traumatology, Hacettepe University, Ankara, Turkey

A. Olivier The London Sarcoma Service, Royal National Orthopaedic Hospital, Middlesex, Stanmore, UK

Heikki Österman ORTON Orthopaedic Hospital, Helsinki, Finland

Alistair M. Pace York Teaching Hospital NHS Foundation Trust, York, UK

Chris Paliobeis The Wellington Hospital, London, UK

J. Palmer The London Sarcoma Service, Royal National Orthopaedic Hospital, Stanmore, Middlesex, UK

Adam Pandit The Shoulder and Elbow Service, Royal National Orthopaedic, Stanmore, Middlesex, UK

Joannis Panotopoulos Department of Orthopaedics, Medical University Vienna, Vienna, Austria

Artemisia Panou Orthopaedic and Trauma Department, Orthopaedic Pediatrics and Neuro-Orthopedic Unit, Humanitas Research Hospital, Rozzano Milano, Italy

Costas Papakostidis Department of Trauma and Orthopaedic Surgery, Hatzikosta General Hospital, Ioannina, Greece

Derek H. Park Royal National Orthopaedic Hospital, Stanmore, Middlesex, UK

Lee Parker Royal National Orthopaedic Hospital, Stanmore, Middlesex, UK

S. Parratte Institute for Motion and Locomotion, Center for Osteoarthritis Surgery, Université de la Méditerranée, Assistance Publique des Hôpitaux de Marseille, CHU Sainte Marguerite, Marseille, France

Steve Parsons Royal Cornwall Hospitals, Cornwall, UK

Norbert Passuti Faculté de Médecine, Nantes, France

Dietmar Pennig Klinik für Unfallchirurgie/Orthopädie, Hand- und Wiederherstellungschirurgie, St. Vinzenz- Hospital Köln, Köln, Germany

Hélder Pereira Centro Hospitalar Pòvoa de Varzim-Vila do Conde, Clínica Espregueira-Mendes F.C. Porto Stadium – FIFA Medical Centre of Excellence, Porto, Portugal

Carsten Perka Department of Orthopaedics and Department of Accident and Reconstructive Surgery, Centre for Musculoskeletal Surgery, Charité – University Medicine, Berlin, Germany

Daniel Perry School of Population, Community and Behavioural Sciences, University of Liverpool, Liverpool, UK

Department Children's Orthopaedic Surgery, Alder Hey Children's Hospital, Liverpool, UK

Rui Pinto Orthopaedic Department, S. JoĀo Hospital, Porto, Portugal

Spiros G. Pneumaticos 3rd Department of Orthopaedic Surgery, School of Medicine, University of Athens, Athens, Greece

Tim Pohlemann University of Saarland, Homburg/Saar, Germany

Eva Pontén Department of Pediatric Orthopaedic Surgery, Astrid Lindgren Children's Hospital, Karolinska University Hospital, Stockholm, Sweden

Lorenzo Ponziani Orthopedic Unit at the Ceccarini Hospital, Riccione, Italy

Nicola Portinaro Orthopaedic and Trauma Department, Orthopaedic Pediatrics and Neuro-Orthopedic Unit, Humanitas Research Hospital, Rozzano Milano, Italy

Franco Postacchini Department of Orthopaedic Surgery, University "Sapienza", Rome, Italy

Roberto Postacchini Department Orthopaedic Surgery Israelitic Hospital, IUSM, Rome, Italy

Delio Pramhas Surgical Orthopaedics and Traumatology, Vienna, Austria

Bernd Preininger Department of Orthopaedics, Center for Musculoskeletal Surgery, Charité-Universitätsmedizin Berlin, Berlin, Germany

Nicolas Pujol Orthopaedic Department, Versailles Hospital, Le Chesnay, France

N. Pujol-Cervini Orthopaedic Department, Centre Hospitalier de Versailles, Le Chesnay, France

Frank T. G. Rahusen Department of Orthopaedics, St. Jans Gasthuis, Weert, The Netherlands

Trichy S. Rajagopal Department of Orthopaedic Surgery, Royal Berkshire Hospital, Reading, UK

Manoj Ramachandran Barts and The London NHS Trust and The London Children's Hospital, Whitechapel, London, UK

Stefan Rammelt Clinic for Trauma and Reconstructive Surgery, University Hospital Carl-Gustav Carus, Dresden, Germany

Neta Raz Department of Orthopaedic Surgery, Royal Berkshire Hospital, Reading, UK

Bnai Zion Medical Center, Haifa, Israel

Jai G. Relwani East Kent University Hospital, Ashford, Kent, UK

Nikolaos Rigopoulos Department of Orthopaedic Surgery, Faculty of Medicine, School of Health Sciences, University of Thessalia, Biopolis, Larissa, Greece

W. H. C. Rijnen Department of Orthopedics, Radboud University Nijmegen Medical Centre, Nijmegen, The Netherlands

Carla S. P. van Rijswijk Leiden University Medical Centre, Leiden, The Netherlands

Peter Ritschl Orthopaedic Clinic Gersthof, Vienna, Austria

Marco J. P. F. Ritt Department of Plastic, Reconstructive and Hand Surgery, VU Medical Centre, Amsterdam, The Netherlands

Andrew H. N. Robinson Cambridge University Hospitals, NHS Foundation Trust, Cambridge, UK

C. Michael Robinson The Edinburgh Shoulder Clinic, Royal Infirmary of Edinburgh, Edinburgh, UK

Thierry Rod Fleury Division of Orthopaedics and Trauma Surgery, University Hospitals of Geneva, Geneva, Switzerland

Benedict A. Rogers Mount Sinai Hospital, University of Toronto, Toronto, ON, Canada

Andreas Roposch Great Ormond Street Hospital for Children, Institute of Child Health, University College London, London, UK

Oleg Safir Mount Sinai Hospital, University of Toronto, Toronto, ON, Canada

Asif Saifuddin Royal National Orthopaedic Hospital NHS Trust, Stanmore, Middlesex, UK

Anthony Sakellariou Frimley Park Hospital, Frimley, Frimley, UK

Tiago Saldanha Giology Department, EGAS Moniz Hospital - CHLO, Lisboa, Portugal

Guillem Saló Orthopaedic Department, Spine Unit, Universitat Autònoma de Barcelona, Barcelona, Spain

Jari Salo Helsinki University Hospital, Töölö Hospital, HUS, Helsinki, Finland

Mikel San-Julian Department of Orthopaedic Surgery, University of Navarra, Pamplona, Spain

Dietrich Schlenzka ORTON Orthopaedic Hospital, Helsinki, Finland

B. W. Schreurs Department of Orthopedics, Radboud University Nijmegen Medical Centre, Nijmegen, The Netherlands

J. C. M. Schrier Orthopedics and Traumatology, Isala Clinics, Zwolle, The Netherlands

Reinhard Schuh Foot and Ankle Center Vienna, Vienna, Austria

Department of Orthopaedics, Medical University of Vienna, Vienna, Austria

Michael Schütz Princess Alexandra Hospital, Queensland University of Technology, Brisbane, Australia

Joseph Schwab Department of Orthopedic Surgery, Massachusetts General Hospital, Boston, MA, USA

Wolfgang Schwägerl Wien, Austria

Laurent Sedel Orthopaedic Department, University of Paris Denis Diderot, Hopital Lariboisière (APHP), Paris, France

Raphaël Seringe Hôpital Cochin APHP, Université Paris-Descartes, Paris, France

Elvire Servien Centre Albert Trillat, Groupe Hospitalier Nord, Hospices Civils de Lyon, Lyon-Caluire, France

Roger Sevi Hille Yafe Hospital, Hadera, Israel

Nuno Sevivas Hospital de Braga, Clínica Espregueira-Mendes F.C. Porto Stadium – FIFA Medical Centre of Excellence, Porto, Portugal

S. Shetty Department of Radiology, Royal National Orthopaedic Hospital, Stanmore, Middlesex, UK

Haim Shtarker Department of Orthopaedic Surgery and Traumatology, Western Galilee Hospital, Nahariya, Israel

Rafael J. Sierra Mayo Clinic, Rochester, MN, USA

L. Sierrasesúmaga University of Navarra, Pamplona, Spain

François Signoret Saint Antoine Hospital, Pierre et Marie Curie University, Paris, France

P. D. Siney The John Charnley Research Institute, Wrightington Hospital, Wigan, Lancashire, UK

Dishan Singh Royal National Orthopaedic Hospital, Stanmore, Middlesex, UK

Harvinder Singh University Hospitals of Leicester NHS Trust, Leicester General Hospital, Leicester, UK

Marco Sinisi Peripheral Nerve Injury Unit, Royal National Orthopaedic Hospital, Stanmore, Middlesex, UK

Chris Smith Princess Elizabeth Orthopaedic Centre, Exeter, UK

Marc Soubeyrand Service de Chirurgie Orthopédique, Hôpital du Kremlin-Bicêtre, Le Kremlin-Bicêtre, France

Panayotis N. Soucacos School of Medicine, University of Athens, Athens, Greece

Kirsten Specht Section for Hip and Knee Replacement, Department of Orthopaedics, Vejle Hospital, University of South Denmark, Vejle, Denmark

Eric L. Staals Istituti Ortopedici Rizzoli, 5th Division, Bologna, Italy

David Stanley Sheffield Teaching Hospitals NHS Foundation Trust, Sheffield, UK

James C. Stanley York Teaching Hospital, NHS Foundation Trust, York, UK

Petros Z. Stavrou Academic Department of Trauma and Orthopaedics, School of Medicine, Leeds General Infirmary, Clarendon Wing, Leeds, UK

Evangelismos Hospital, Athens, Greece

Zois P. Stavrou Henry Dunant Hospital, Athens, Greece

Michael M. Stephens Mater Private Hospital, Dublin, Ireland

Richard Stern Division of Orthopaedics and Trauma Surgery, University Hospitals of Geneva, Geneva, Switzerland

Maik Stiehler University Centre for Orthopaedics and Traumatology, University Hospital Carl Gustav Carus, Dresden, Germany

Walter Michael Strobl Clinic for Pediatric Orthopaedic and Neuroorthopaedic Surgery, Orthopaedic Hospital Rummelsberg, Schwarzenbruck, Nuremberg, Germany

Jan Stulik Spine Surgery Department, University Hospital Motol, Praha, Czech Republic

Norbert Suedkamp Department for Orthopedic Surgery and Traumatology, Freiburg University Hospital, Freiburg, Germany

Mark G. Swindells Pulvertaft Hand Centre, Derby, UK

Panagiotis Symeonidis 2nd Orthopedic Clinic University of Thessaloniki, Thessaloniki, Greece

Miklós Szendrői Department of Orthopaedics, Semmelweis University, Budapest, Hungary

George Szőke Department of Orthopaedics, Semmelweis University, Budapest, Hungary

Magnus Tägil Hand and Upper Extremity Unit, Department of Orthopedics, Lund University Hospital, Lund, Sweden

Antonie H. M. Taminiau Department of Orthopaedics, Leiden University Medical Centre, Leiden, The Netherlands

Chanan Tauber Kaplan Hospital Rehovot, Rehovot, Israel

Mark Tauber Section for Shoulder and Elbow Surgery, ATOS Clinic, Munich, Germany

Sally Tennant Royal National Orthopaedic Hospital, Stanmore, Middlesex, UK

Karl-Göran Thorngren Department of Orthopaedics, Lund University Hospital, Lund, Sweden

Roger M. Tillman Oncology Unit, Royal Orthopaedic Hospital NHS Foundation Trust, Birmingham, UK

Michael Alan Tonkin Royal North Shore Hospital, University of Sydney, Sydney, Australia

Carlos Torrens Orthopedic Department, Hospital Universitario del Mar de Barcelona, Barcelona, Spain

Alexandros Touliatos Department of the First Orthopaedic Department, General Hospital of Athens, Athens, Greece

Ian A. Trail Hand and Upper Limb Surgery, Wrightington Hospital, Wigan, Lancashire, UK

Georgios K. Triantafyllopoulos 3rd Department of Orthopaedic Surgery, School of Medicine, University of Athens, Athens, Greece

Hans-Jörg Trnka Foot and Ankle Center Vienna, Vienna, Austria

Francois Tudor British Orthopaedic Trainees Association, Stanmore, Middlesex, UK

Philippa Tyler The Royal National Orthopaedic Hospital, Stanmore, Middlesex, London, UK

Maite Ubierna Spine Unit, Hospital Germas Trias i Pujol Badalona, Barcelona, Spain

Victor Valderrabano Orthopaedic Department, University Hospital Basel, Basel, Switzerland

Angiola Valente Department of Orthopaedic and Traumatology, San Luigi Gonzaga Hospital, University of Turin, Turin, Italy

Matteo Benedetti Valentini Department of Orthopaedic Surgery, University of Rome "Tor Vergata", Rome, Italy

H. van Dam Hand Surgery Department, St Andrew's Centre for Plastic Surgery, Broomfield Hospital, Chelmsford, Essex, UK

Michiel A. J. van de Sande Leiden University Medical Centre, Leiden, The Netherlands

C. N. van Dijk Department of Orthopaedic Surgery, Academic Medical Center, University of Amsterdam, Amsterdam, The Netherlands

Tom Van Isacker Service d'Orthopédie et de Traumatologie, Cliniques Universitaires St-Luc, Université Catholique de Louvain, Bruxelles, Belgium

Marie Van Laer Department of Orthopaedic Surgery and Traumatology, Ghent University Hospital, Ghent, Belgium

Alexander Van Tongel Department of Orthopaedic Surgery and Traumatology, Ghent University Hospital, Ghent, Belgium

F. Vannini Department of Orthopaedic and Trauma Surgery, Istituto Ortopedico Rizzoli, Bologna, Italy

Pedro Varanda Hospital de Braga, Clínica Espregueira-Mendes F.C. Porto Stadium – FIFA Medical Centre of Excellence, Porto, Portugal

B. L. Vázquez-García University of Navarra, Pamplona, Spain

Peter Verdonk Department of Orthopaedic Surgery and Traumatology, Monica Ziekenhuizen, Antwerpen, Belgium

René Verdonk Department of Orthopaedic Surgery and Traumatology, Ghent University Hospital, Ghent, Belgium

Richard Villar The Wellington Hospital, London, UK

César Vincent Spine Unit, Orthopaedic Department, Bicetre University Hospital, AP-HP Paris, Université Paris-Sud ORSAY, Le Kremlin Bicêtre, France

Mihai Vioreanu Royal College of Surgeons Ireland, Ballinteer, Ireland

A. J. H. Vochteloo Leiden University Medical Centre, Leiden, The Netherlands

Gershon Volpin Departments of Orthopaedic Surgery and Traumatology, Western Galilee Hospital, Nahariya, Israel

Rüdiger von Eisenhart-Rothe Klinik für Orthopädie und Sportorthopädie am Klinikum rechts der Isar, Technische Universität München, München, Germany

Richard Wallensten Department of Orthopaedics, Karolinska University Hospital, Stockholm, Sweden

David Warwick Hand Surgery, University Hospital Southampton, Southampton, UK

Vincent Wasserman Service de Chirurgie Orthopédique, Hôpital Universitaire de Bicetre, Le Kremlin-Bicetre, France

Wolfram Wenz Paediatric Orthopaedics and Foot Surgery, Department for Orthopaedic and Trauma Surgery, Heidelberg University Clinics, Heidelberg, Germany

Florent Weppe Centre Albert Trillât Hôpital de le Croix-Rousse, Lyon, France

Philippe Wicart Hôpital Necker – Enfants malades AP-HP, Université Paris-Descartes, Paris, France

Johannes I. Wiegerinck Department of Orthopaedic Surgery, Academic Medical Center, University of Amsterdam, Amsterdam, The Netherlands

Keith Willett Kadoorie Centre for Critical Care Research and Education, Trauma Unit, John Radcliffe Hospital, University of Oxford, Oxford, UK

Andy M. Williams Chelsea and Westminster Hospital, London, UK

Timothy Huw David Williams Royal National Orthopaedic Hospital, Stanmore, Middlesex, UK

J. Brad Williamson Division of Neurosciences, Salford Royal Hospital, Salford, UK

W. Winkelmann Department of Orthopedics, University Hospital and Medical School, Münster, Germany

Eivind Witso St. Olav's University Hospital, Norwegian University of Science Trondheim, Trondheim, Norway

B. M. Wroblewski The John Charnley Research Institute, Wrightington Hospital, Wigan, Lancashire, UK

Timo Yrjönen ORTON Orthopaedic Hospital, Helsinki, Finland

S. Zaffagnini Sports Traumatolgy Department, Rizzoli Othopaedic Institute, University of Bologna, Bologna, Italy

Luigi Zagra Hip Department, IRCCS Istituto Ortopedico Galeazzi, Milan, Italy

Peter Zenz Orthopädisches Zentrum Otto Wagner Spital, Wien, Austria

Christoph Zilkens Department of Orthopedic Surgery, University Hospital of Düsseldorf, Düsseldorf, Germany

Gianfranco Zinghi Rizzoli Orthopedic Institute, University of Bologna, Bologna, Italy

Hans Zwipp Clinic for Trauma and Reconstructive Surgery, University Hospital Carl-Gustav Carus, Dresden, Germany

Part II

Spine

Applications of Prostheses and Fusion in the Cervical Spine

Robert W. Marshall and Neta Raz

Contents

Abstract

Cervical and lumbar fusions are well-established procedures for the treatment of a wide range of spinal disorders. Whilst both have a good record of success, there are concerns about the impact of spinal fusion on movement and the biomechanical effects upon the remainder of the spine, particularly the levels adjacent to the fusion.

Although many indications for spinal fusion would be contra-indications for intervertebral disc arthroplasty, the particular indication of degenerative disc disease allows for both forms of treatment. Intervertebral disc replacement is relatively new and as yet unproven in the long term, but there has been a great trend towards arthroplasty in the last 15–20 years.

The history of spinal fusion is considered, the design and development of the prosthetic disc replacements described, and the current evidence for both procedures outlined. The success rates, complications and impact upon the spine as a whole will be compared.

The anterior surgical procedures for fusion and arthroplasty are almost identical, but fusion can also be performed through posterior and posterolateral approaches. For the purposes of this chapter only the anterior surgical approaches will be covered.

R.W. Marshall (✉) • N. Raz
Department of Orthopaedic Surgery, Royal Berkshire
Hospital, Reading, UK
e-mail: robmarshall100@hotmail.com

Keywords

Adjacent Level Disease • Cervical • Complications • Fusion • History • Myelopathy • Prosthesis • Prosthetic Design • Root Compression

G. Bentley (ed.), *European Surgical Orthopaedics and Traumatology*,
DOI 10.1007/978-3-642-34746-7_215, © EFORT 2014

and Radiculography • Spine • Surgical Indications and Contra-Indications • Surgical Technique

History of Spinal Fusion and Intervertebral Disc Replacement in the Cervical Spine

The limitations of posterior cervical surgery in treating the axial neck pain, nerve root and spinal cord compression syndromes resulting from degenerative disc disease in the cervical spine led to the development of anterior surgery in the 1950s.

Using the anterior cervical spine approach described by Southwick and Robinson in 1957 [1], Smith and Robinson [2] developed an effective decompression and fusion technique and reported good results, but warned about the potential for some specific complications such as oesophageal perforation, recurrent laryngeal nerve damage and Horner's syndrome. At late follow-up the reproducibility of this technique was proven [3]. Other authors have reported excellent results using this technique. [4–6] There was a reported incidence of pseudarthrosis of 7 % per level with the technique and this was sometimes responsible for failure.

Other techniques for anterior grafting and fusion of the cervical spine were developed by Cloward [7] in 1958 with a dowel grafting technique and Bailey and Badgeley [8] in 1960 with an intervertebral trench and shaped autograft. The Cloward technique became highly popular, but the late results were disappointing due to graft collapse and failure of fusion.

Cervical plating was introduced to support the autograft and immobilise the motion segment and there were reports suggesting that the fusion rate improved considerably [9, 10].

However, others have not found much advantage in using a cervical plate [11, 12].

Hankinson and Wilson introduced the treatment of microscope-assisted discectomy without anterior cervical fusion and good results were reported [13]. Others have also shown that decompression without fusion can produce

equivalent results and as many as 75 % go on to spontaneous fusion [14–20]. Laing [19] found that over 50 % of anterior cervical discectomies developed loss of the normal cervical lordosis and a third had a segmental kyphus, but the clinical results were not compromised in the short term.

Long-term outcome after anterior cervical decompression alone revealed excellent results initially (90 %), dropping to 67 % at follow-up (3–18 years) mainly due to neck pain and degenerative change at other cervical levels [20].

A prospective randomised controlled study from Finland found equivalent results at a minimum of 4-year follow-up for anterior cervical discectomy alone, autograft without plating and autograft with plating. It was concluded that fusion was unnecessary [12].

However, Yamamoto found that cervical decompression with fusion provided more reliable relief of neck pain [21]. Cases of pseudarthrosis were associated with neck pain in other publications [22, 23]. Re-operation to ensure firm fusion can improve the outcome of cases where pseudarthrosis was responsible for continued neck pain [24]. In another study, late results of cervical discectomy alone were found to be inferior to anterior cervical fusion [25].

Many alternatives to iliac crest bone graft fusion have been tried and they have been reviewed very well by Chau and Mobbs [26]. Despite the drawback of donor site complications for iliac crest autograft nothing else has produced better results. Xenografts (usually bovine) have produced worse fusion rates. Allograft is expensive, carries a small risk of disease transmission and gives an acceptable fusion rate, but fusion rates are still inferior to autograft. Ceramics have been shown to be a very reasonable alternative to iliac crest autograft. Whilst bone morphogenic protein (BMP) has powerful osteo-inductive properties, it is expensive and has yet to be proven as a worthwhile alternative.

Based upon Bagby's stainless steel fusion cage [27] invented to treat "wobbler syndrome" in race-horses, stand-alone cages were introduced for both lumbar spine and cervical fusions to avoid the need for iliac crest autografts, which

Fig. 1 Evolution of the Prestige intervertebral disc (Medtronic Sofamor Danek)

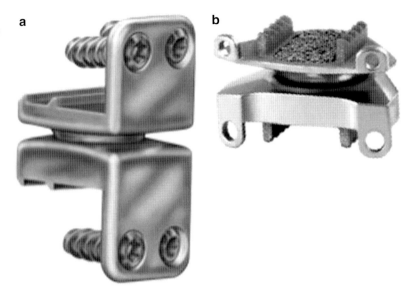

carried the disadvantages of donor site pain and lateral cutaneous nerve damage. Good results were achieved with a variety of cages made of synthetic materials such as Titanium and polyetherether ketone. Two prospective, randomised controlled trials showed results of cage fusions were equivalent to autogenous, iliac crest tricortical grafts [28, 29].

The first attempt to maintain cervical mobility by any form of arthroplasty was reported in 1966 by Fernstrom using a metal ball-bearing spacer, but no late outcome or experience with other cases was ever published [30].

No other attempts at disc arthroplasty were published until the work of Cummins et al. from Bristol, who reported 20 cases treated by the Prestige disc with maintenance of movement in the majority and satisfactory clinical outcome [31]. The device consisted of two stainless steel plates which were fixed to the vertebral bodies by anterior screws. This design made the device incompatible with MRI and also meant that two adjacent discs could not be treated. Modifications of the device included changing from a ball and socket to a ball and trough design, changing from a stainless steel to a composite of titanium and ceramic (thus MRI compatible), and from screw fixation to the insertion of two serrated rails into prepared grooves within the bony end-plates (Fig. 1).

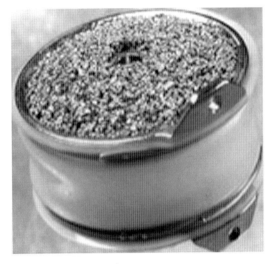

Fig. 2 The Bryan disc (Medtronic Sofamor Danek)

The Bryan Cervical Disc prosthesis (Fig. 2) is a low-friction polyurethane nucleus surrounded by a polyurethane covering, placed between two titanium alloy shells. There is a milling device for preparation of the end-plates to stabilize the prosthesis.

Since its first description [32] this has become one of the most popular disc prostheses.

It has been shown in multi-centre randomized trials to produce clinical outcomes comparable to anterior cervical decompression and fusion (ACDF) (see below).

Prosthetic Design

There are many different cervical arthroplasty designs emerging with short-term evidence for some of them [32–41]. The true place of arthroplasty, the ideal disc design and the salvage procedures to deal with failures have yet to be established.

Some are modular, others non-modular, some are constrained whilst others are unconstrained. Fixation can be by means of screws or by press-fit designs. There are metal end-plates made of cobalt chrome, stainless steel or titanium. Others are ceramic or made of materials like polyetherether ketone. Some have metal-on-metal articulation, others employ polyethylene or polyurethane. Prostheses can be porous- coated or coated with hydroxyapatite or calcium phosphate [42] (Fig. 3).

The use of cobalt chrome or stainless steel prostheses makes interpretation of M.R.I. scans difficult post-operatively because of the metal artefact interfering with the image quality [43]. Others have shown that the artefact is dependent upon the strength of the magnet and is variable [44] (Fig. 4).

Despite emphatic claims by the manufacturers, no one design has been proven to be superior to any other and short term results are very satisfactory, irrespective of the design or materials used. This is not at all surprising when one considers the excellent results achieved by anterior cervical discectomy alone, i.e. without fusion or insertion of any prosthesis! [12–20].

We must keep in mind that the real benefits of anterior cervical fusion or disc replacement come from the spinal cord and nerve decompression, the fundamental aim of any such procedure.

Indications for Surgery in Cervical Syndromes

The consequences of cervical disc degeneration are the commonest reasons for surgical treatment in the cervical spine – the degenerative process can lead to cervical disc herniation with acute onset of neck pain, radicular pain radiating down the upper limb and the neurological syndromes of radiculopathy or myelopathy, but usually there is more insidious development of

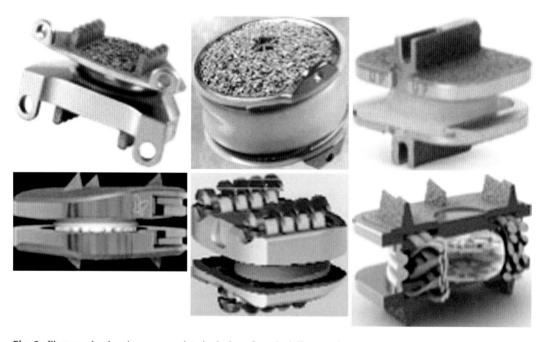

Fig. 3 Photographs showing some variety in design of cervical disc prostheses

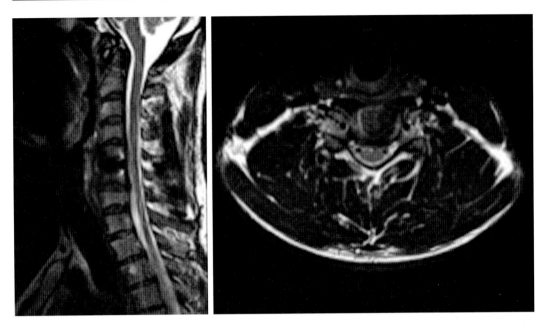

Fig. 4 MRI – T2 sagittal and axial images showing minimal artefact after decompression and M6 (C.4-5) disc replacement

similar syndromes due to uncovertebral joint and facet joint hypertrophy together with disc degeneration and a circumferential rim of osteophyte around the disc space.

Remember that cervical disc and facet joint degeneration are extremely common and are often found incidentally on radiographs or magnetic resonance imaging carried out for other purposes. Boden et al. showed that cervical degeneration was present in 60 % of *asymptomatic* patients over the age of 40 years, 5 % had disc herniation and 20 % appeared to have foraminal stenosis. In patients under 40 years of age degenerative disc disease was seen in 20 % and incidental disc herniation was found in 10 % [45] (Fig. 5).

This means that cervical degeneration is a benign part of the natural ageing process, so it is essential for the clinician to correlate clinical features accurately with imaging information before embarking upon any invasive forms of treatment.

Treatment of acute neck pain and cervical nerve compression syndromes consists of temporary use of a soft collar, physiotherapy and x-ray-guided steroid injections.

In a randomised controlled trial Kuijper et al. showed no difference in treated and untreated groups of brachialgia at 6 months, but there were some early benefits in the treated group [46].

Surgery is only indicated for the intractable cases of brachialgia and persistent focal neurological deficit or for the much more serious condition of spinal cord compression with myelopathic features.

Single or double level disease can be treated by anterior cervical decompression and fusion or by decompression and insertion of a prosthetic disc replacement.

Evidence for Cervical Arthroplasty as an Alternative to Anterior Cervical Fusion

Cervical Nerve Root Compression and Radiculopathy

In randomised controlled trials for three different intervertebral disc replacements, the disc replacement option has been found to be at least equivalent to anterior cervical fusion at a follow-up of

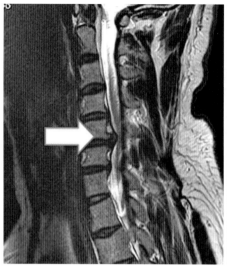
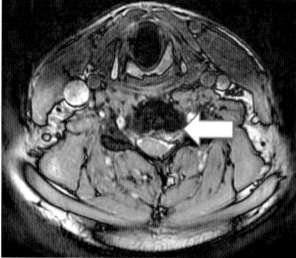

Fig. 5 MRI T2 Sagittal and T2 axial images showing a left sided C5-6 intervertebral disc prolapse with C6 nerve compression (*arrowed*)

at least 2 years and in one study up to 5 years [33–38].

The arthroplasty patients had better clinical outcome at 2 years. Device-related complications were also lower in this group.

The favourable clinical and angular motion outcomes that were previously noted at 1- and 2-years' follow-up after cervical disc replacement with the Bryan Cervical Disc Prosthesis appear to persist after 4 and 6 years of follow-up [37].

In assessing the Prestige II disc (Medtronic) – Burkus et al. started a randomised controlled multicentre trial in 2002 of single level total disc replacement or anterior cervical decompression and fusion with allograft and plate fixation in 541 patients.

Five patients in the fusion group had re-operations and the disc arthroplasty group had better clinical and neurological outcome at 24 months and this difference was maintained at 5 years. Re-operation was less common in the total disc replacement group [41].

In the United States, Food and Drug Administration investigational device exemption study of the ProDisc-C prosthesis, Murrey et al. found that the Prodisc C was equal to or superior to ACDF. The two-year prospective, randomised, controlled multi-centre study compared the use

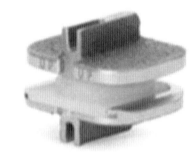

Fig. 6 The Prodisc C prosthesis (Synthes)

of the ProDisc-C cervical disc replacement with anterior discectomy and fusion with allograft for single-level symptomatic disease. There was a statistically significant difference in the number of revision procedures in the two groups, 8.5 % (9 of 106) of the anterior discectomy and fusion group and 1.9 % (2 of 103) of the disc replacement group. The ProDisc-C was successful in 73.5 % (76 of 103) and anterior discectomy and fusion and plating in 60.5 % (64 of 106) at follow-up of 24 months [39] (Fig. 6).

From the above evidence it can be concluded that the three most commonly used artificial discs are producing similar results for treatment of cervical radiculopathy. They are no worse than anterior cervical fusion and there are some perceived benefits in terms of early return to work and initial clinical scores. No single device has any clear advantage at this stage.

Cervical Myelopathy

Brain et al. first described the syndrome of myelopathy in 1952 [47].

Multiple factors play a critical role in the development of cervical spondylosis and subsequent cord compression and its consequences of cervical myelopathy. The progression of spondylotic changes begins with cervical disc degeneration. With aging, dehydration and disorganisation of the disc leads to disc height collapse. Increased mechanical stress on the end-plates initiates osteophyte formation along the end-plates. These osteophytes serve to increase the load-bearing surface of the end-plates to compensate for spine hypermobility secondary to the loss of disc material. Compensatory bone growth due to uncinate process hypertrophy may also occur. Ossification of the posterior longitudinal ligament (OPLL) can develop and is a particular problem amongst Asians [48].

This condition is usually painless although some have neck pain. There is a variable rate of neurological deterioration with the development of upper motor neurone dysfunctional changes in all four limbs. Patients may complain of numbness of the fingers, loss of dexterity with impairment of fine tasks such as fastening buttons, writing or playing musical instruments. Later, they may develop poor lower limb control, with walking difficulty and an obvious spastic paraparesis.

Physical signs include sensory impairment, weakness, brisk reflexes commensurate with the level of the pathology, Hoffmann's sign and dysdiadochokinesia in the upper limbs, Romberg's sign, abnormal plantar responses and ankle clonus. The tandem walking test is often a good way of observing impaired function in more subtle cases of myelopathy.

The natural history of cervical myelopathy is not fully understood. Some of the early papers suggest that after initial neurological deterioration the condition can stabilise and be followed by a long period of clinical stability, especially if the myelopathy is mild on presentation [49].

Nurick later confirmed this pattern [50]. However, both studies noted that patients who were older or had significant progressive disability had a worse prognosis.

Other studies that the myelopathy may deteriorate at a variable rate and even if the neurological condition stabilises for some time, there is often a late deterioration [51–53].

In a series of 1,355 patients with cervical spondylotic myelopathy treated conservatively, Epstein et al. found that 64 % showed no improvement and 26 % deteriorated [52]. Clark and Robinson, found that approximately 50 % of patients with cervical spondylotic myelopathy treated medically deteriorated neurologically [53].

Syman and Lavender found that 67 % of their patients with cervical spondylotic myelopathy experienced functional deterioration [54].

Some argue that patients do badly with conservative medical management, and that surgery is preferable, even in mild cases. They suggest that early surgical intervention can lead to improved neurological outcomes [55–57].

Prognosis after surgery was better for patients with less than 1 year of symptoms, younger age, fewer levels of involvement, and unilateral motor deficit.

Phillips examined 65 patients treated surgically and found that symptoms of less than 1 year's duration significantly correlated with benefit from treatment [57].

Although patients seldom have complete resolution of their myelopathy and any improvement after surgery can be modest, surgery usually prevents any further cord deterioration. The outcome after surgery is superior to procrastination and further neurological deterioration.

Surgical treatment of cervical myelopathy has historically been by anterior cervical decompression and fusion for one or two levels of cervical stenosis or posteriorly by cervical laminectomy, laminoplasty or laminectomy with lateral mass fusion for three or more affected levels.

Surgical treatment should decompress the spinal cord adequately and prevent the development of a cervical kyphosis. The decompression should be carried out anteriorly in cases of kyphosis and where the main compressing force lies anteriorly due to disc and osteophyte prominences, but posterior surgery is preferable for multi-level disease, posterior compression or ossification of the posterior longitudinal ligament.

The anterior decompression and fusion as described by Smith and Robinson or Cloward has a proven record for this condition and many consider that it is important to fuse the spine to prevent the repeated irritation of the myelomalacic section of spinal cord that could result from disc replacement and the preservation of movement at the diseased level [2–8].

However, when the cohorts of myelopathic patients in the multi-centre trials of the Bryan disc and Prestige discs in the U.S.A. were analysed, the outcome of treating myelopathy by disc replacement was equivalent to the fusion cases with improved neurological status in approximately 90 % of cases. This suggests that concerns of treating myelopathy by disc replacement are not justified in the case of single level disease with anterior cord compression [58].

However, in cases with multi-level disease, kyphosis or ossification of the posterior longitudinal ligament, cervical disc arthroplasty remains contra-indicated.

The Evidence for Adjacent Level Disease After Anterior Cervical Fusion

One of the prime motivations for the development of cervical disc replacement has been the desire to prevent the alteration of the spinal biomechanics that would result from spinal fusion and have been blamed for causing accelerated degeneration of adjacent spinal segments. The influential paper by Hillibrand et al. [59], reported the incidence of symptomatic adjacent segment disease as 2.9 % per year after anterior cervical fusion and extrapolation suggested that

25.6 % of the fusion patients would develop symptomatic adjacent segment disease within 10 years. The chances were even higher at the C5-6 and C6-7 levels. However, longer constructs were found to have a lower incidence of adjacent level degeneration, this surprise finding has fuelled the debate about whether adjacent level disease was caused by deleterious biomechanical effects or was simply the progression of the natural history of degenerative disc disease.

Goffin et al. [37] also found a 92 % incidence of radiographic changes at adjacent segments 5 years after anterior cervical decompression and fusion.

Robertson et al. studied radiological changes and symptomatic adjacent-level cervical disc disease after single-level discectomy and subsequent cervical fusion versus arthroplasty using the Bryan disc. New radiographic changes were seen in 34.6 % of the fusion cases and in 17.5 % of the arthroplasty group at 24 months. Symptoms related to these changes only developed in 7 % of the fusion cases with none in the arthroplasty cases [60].

Although controversy still exists regarding the role of natural progression of degeneration versus the effects of spinal fusion, there does seem to be an undesirable alteration of biomechanics after fusion that arthroplasty may avoid. Cervical arthroplasty has not yet been proven to reduce the rate of adjacent segment deterioration and longer term follow up is necessary. However, it does seem as if cervical arthroplasty can restore relatively normal biomechanical function [61].

Indications for cervical disc replacement or anterior cervical discectomy and fusion:

1. Decompression of one or two level cervical degeneration between C3 and T1 with nerve root compression without instability or cervical kyphosis.
2. Single level cervical degeneration causing myelopathy due to anterior pathology between C3 and T1.
3. Adjacent level symptomatic disc degeneration after previous cervical fusion.
4. Axial neck pain – but this is not well supported by the literature.

Indications for anterior cervical fusion where disc arthroplasty is contra-indicated:

1. Cervical nerve root compression at three levels of the cervical spine
2. Cervical myelopathy at more than one level – better suited to anterior corpectomy and fusion
3. Cervical kyphosis requiring neural decompression
4. Cervical instability (demonstrated on flexion and extension lateral radiographs)
5. Any situation with loss of structural integrity of the anterior column – e.g. infection or tumour damage
6. Indications for decompression in cases with severe facet joint degeneration
7. Osteoporosis
8. Previous laminectomy
9. Rheumatoid disease
10. Conditions leading to ankylosis of the spine such as ankylosing spondylitis, ossification of the posterior longitudinal ligament (OPPL) and diffuse idiopathic skeletal hyperostosis (DISH) [42].

Surgical Management

Decompression and Disc Arthroplasty

During patient preparation the surgeon must ensure that the clinical picture is carefully correlated with the imaging findings (e.g. Fig. 5) so that the surgeon is clear about the level and extent of the nerve or cord compression. Sufficient time should have elapsed to ensure that conservative treatment has failed.

Patient consent should be obtained after full explanation about the risks and potential benefits of the procedure.

Prophylactic antibiotics are administered intravenously.

Under general anaesthesia via endotracheal intubation, the patient should be placed supine over the radiolucent end of the operating table with a support behind the neck and the head in a neutral position to facilitate good imaging and

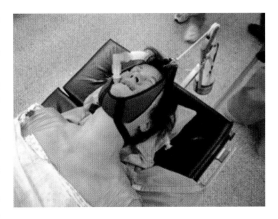

Fig. 7 Photograph of traction applied to a harness. Careful alignment of head and neck with head support. Shoulders are taped down to improve x-ray access

thus accurate mid-line placement of the prosthesis.

Intermittent calf compression is continued throughout the procedure for prophylaxis against thrombo-embolism.

Some favour external traction with a Mayfield support or a head harness to which varying weights can be attached at different stages of the procedure to allow different degrees of intervertebral distraction.

Taping of the shoulders to keep them down during the operation enables better access for intra-operative imaging (Fig. 7).

Prior to commencement of the operation the surgeon should ensure that good lateral and anteroposterior imaging can be obtained using the biplanar image intensifier.

A left-sided approach is favoured to reduce the risk of recurrent laryngeal nerve damage [1].

The level of the intended operation can be marked on the skin so that the skin incision can be placed in an ideal position. Infiltration of the skin and subcutaneous tissues with Bupivicaine 0.5 % and Adrenaline in a solution of 1 in 200,000 units can cut down bleeding and reduce the post-operative analgesic requirements.

After antiseptic preparation of the skin and application of sterile drapes, a transverse skin crease incision is made extending from the anterior border of the left sternocleidomastoid muscle to a point just across the mid-line. Haemostasis is

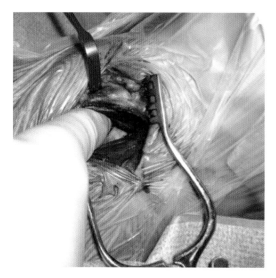

Fig. 8 Blunt finger tip dissection to expose the vertebral column

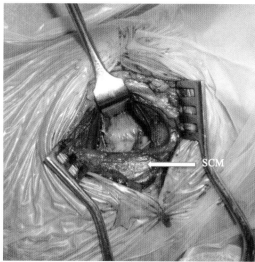

Fig. 9 Southwick-Robinson left-sided approach medial to the left sternocleidomastoid muscle (SCM)

achieved by a combination of monopolar and bipolar diathermy.

The approach is that described by Southwick and Robinson [1]. Dissection is medial to the medial border of the sternocleidomastoid muscle and medial to the carotid sheath.

A combination of fine scissor and blunt dissection with a finger tip opens up the fascial planes and allows direct access to the front of the vertebral column (Figs. 8–10).

The discs, vertebrae and longus colli muscles are thus exposed. The level of the disc is checked with a needle in the disc space and the image intensifier in the lateral position (Fig. 11).

The image intensifier is then placed in position for anteroposterior imaging and the mid-line of the disc is marked using diathermy on the vertebra on either side of the disc space (Fig. 12).

Although the external traction via the harness can suffice, we prefer to insert parallel Caspar distraction pins which are placed in the mid-line of the vertebra on either side of the disc space (Fig. 13). It is important that the pin in the vertebra above is placed in the superior part of the vertebra and the lower pin in the lower part of the inferior vertebra so that they are not in the way of the instruments for disc space preparation and the insertion of the artificial disc.

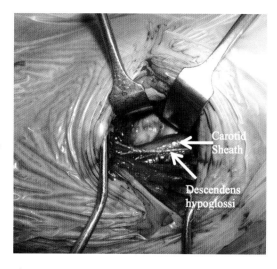

Fig. 10 Dissection continues medial to the carotid sheath. The descending branch of the hypoglossal nerve is seen overlying the carotid sheath

Once the disc space is distracted, the intervertebral disc is excised. A high speed burr and fine Kerrison cervical bone punches are used to remove posterior osteophyte. The posterior longitudinal ligament is exposed and removed with the fine punches until the spinal cord and cervical nerve roots have been fully decompressed.

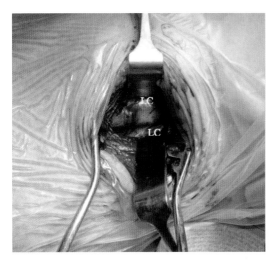

Fig. 11 Exposure of the vertebral column with the longus colli muscle (*L.C.*) on either side of the midline

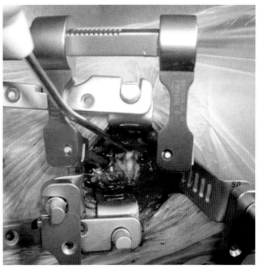

Fig. 13 Caspar distraction and retractors (Braun Aesculap) in place allowing excellent access for removal of cervical disc and posterior osteophyte. The spinal cord and cervical nerves are fully decompressed

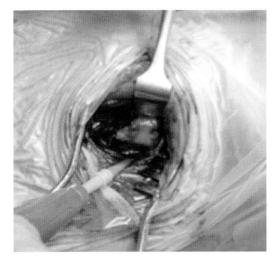

Fig. 12 Diathermy is used to mark the mid-line

Up to this stage, the operation of cervical discectomy and nerve decompression is the same, but from now on, there are differences depending upon whether the disc is to be replaced by a cervical disc prosthesis or anterior cervical fusion is planned.

Cervical Disc Replacement

For cervical disc replacement the end-plates of the vertebral bodies are prepared in the manner dictated by the choice of artificial disc. The Prestige disc (Medtronic Sofamor Danek) is used in the

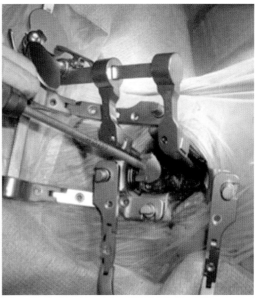

Fig. 14 Trial implant is used to obtain optimal implant size

procedure described below. The trial implants are used to obtain an optimally-sized device and the appearances checked on lateral fluoroscopy (Fig. 14). It is important to remove the distraction at this stage so that the tension in the disc space can

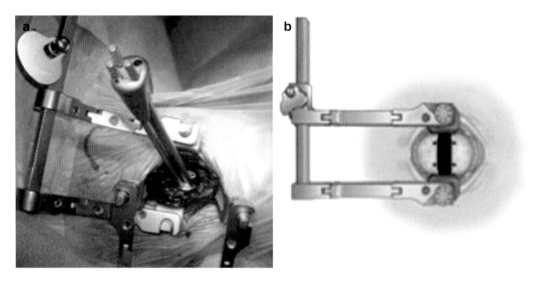

Fig. 15 (**a**) Photograph, (**b**) Diagram, showing pinning of guide and drilling of four holes to mark sites for rail slots for the prosthesis

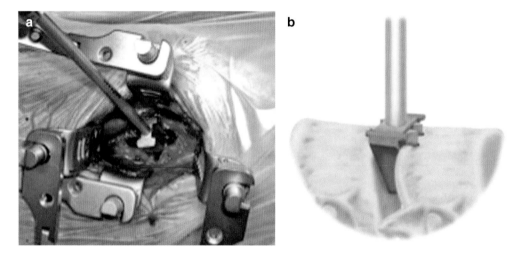

Fig. 16 (**a**) Photograph, and (**b**) diagram, showing the insertion of the rail cutter to create slots in the position dictated by the drill-holes

be judged. If the distraction were left in place, there would be a danger of using too large a prosthesis, which could impede movement and also interfere with facet joint function (Figs. 15–18).

The wound is closed with an absorbable continuous suture (Polyglycolic acid) – suturing the platysma muscle and then a subcuticular layer to minimise scarring. The authors advise a redivac drain for the first 24 h to deal with any postoperative bleeding. Discharge from hospital is allowed after 24–48 h.

A soft collar is recommended for 4 weeks to allow for soft tissue healing and to prevent extreme movement initially.

The patient is followed at 6 weeks, 3 months and then 6 months with dynamic lateral

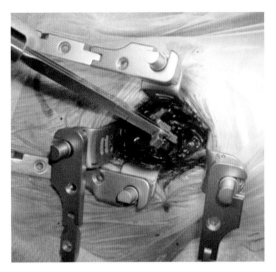

Fig. 17 Insertion of the Prestige prosthesis using the introducer

radiographs at the final visit to confirm good anchorage of the components and that the level has remained mobile as intended.

The Alternative Procedure of Anterior Cervical Decompression and Fusion

The approach is identical to that described above up until the completion of the decompression. Then, when fusion is preferred to disc replacement (See indications and contra-indications above) we favour decortication of the end-plates using a high speed burr, followed by insertion of a shaped tricalcium phosphate (TCP) block into the disc space, and application of an anterior cervical plate (Fig. 19).

Wound closure, drainage and post-operative care are the same as described for disc arthroplasty.

Complications of Anterior Cervical Surgery

Approach-Related Complications

Most complications are related to the surgical approach with possible damage to the soft tissues, vessels and nerves. They include: haemorrhage,

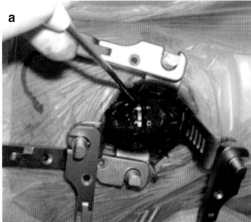

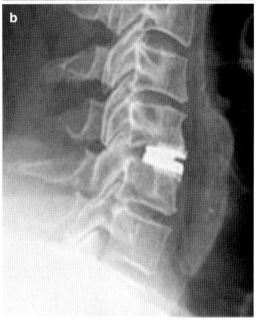

Fig. 18 (**a**) Photograph showing appearances after disc insertion and (**b**) x-ray checking of disc position

infection, dysphagia, hoarseness due to recurrent laryngeal nerve damage and Horner's syndrome due to disturbance of the cervical sympathetic nerves.

Complications Specific to Cervical Disc Replacement

Device related problems with the Bryan disc were very rare [36]. Prostheses that were well placed showed no tendency to migrate and

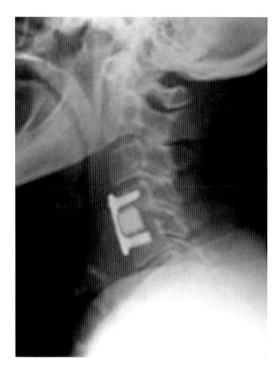

Fig. 19 Lateral radiograph of TCP block and overlying plate

no device had to be "explanted" at 2 years of follow-up.

An analysis of patients in the European multi-centre trial on the Bryan disc revealed that prevertebral ossification at the operated level occurred in 17.8 % of cases and 11 % of cases had negligible movement on dynamic radiographs (less than 2°) [62]. Heterotopic bone was especially likely in older males.

Ossification after inserting the Prodisc C device was reported by Bertagnoli et al. in patients with a 1 year follow-up without any appearance of fusion [63]. Later, Bertagnoli observed a 9.4 % incidence of heterotopic ossification among 117 patients treated with Prodisc C and followed for more than 2 years [64].

In a 4 year follow up, Suchomel et al. found heterotopic ossification (grade III) in 45 % of implants and segmental ankylosis (grade IV) in another 18 %. This finding had no clinical consequences and 92 % of patients were satisfied with their results [65].

At 5 year follow up after the Prestige disc implantation, complete ankylosis was only seen

in 3.2 % and an average of 6.5° of movement was retained at the operated level [41].

Longer follow up may be associated with prosthetic failure, but no reports exist at present.

Complications Specific to Anterior Cervical Fusion

• *Graft related*
Donor site: Pain, infection and damage to the lateral cutaneous nerve of the thigh with painful neuroma formation.

Neck graft site:

Failure of fusion can occur, especially where alternatives to autograft are used. If there is a painful pseudarthrosis, re-operation may be required with re-grafting.

When internal fixation is not used, migration of the graft can occur.

• *Internal fixation related*
Devices such as cages can subside through the vertebral end-plates.

Anterior plates can become displaced and screws may loosen.

Plates can also impinge upon neighbouring levels and lead to adjacent level disease.

• *Adjacent level degeneration*
Although fusions have been incriminated in the development of junctional changes at neighbouring levels, it is not definitely proven that the changes are in excess of those that would occur with the natural history of cervical degeneration [59].

Conclusions Regarding Anterior Cervical Surgery: Disc Replacement or Fusion

Current evidence suggests that cervical disc replacement is a safe and good alternative to anterior cervical fusion. Equivalent early results can be achieved and movement is preserved in the majority, but not in all cases.

Revision surgery for anterior cervical surgery is feasible and not particularly hazardous.

Disc replacement is a justifiable alternative to fusion, but the long-term results are not yet known.

The possibility of sparing the adjacent segment degeneration by restoring better biomechanical function is attractive, but it remains an unproven concept. The patients from the randomised controlled trials comparing fusion and disc arthroplasty will require longer follow-up before we can be convinced that disc replacement is capable of preventing adjacent level degeneration.

References

1. Southwick WO, Robinson RA. Surgical approaches to the vertebral bodies in the cervical and lumbar regions. J Bone Joint Surg Am. 1957;39-A(3):631–44.

2. Smith GW, Robinson RA. The treatment of certain cervical-spine disorders by anterior removal of the intervertebral disc and interbody fusion. J Bone Joint Surg Am. 1958;40-A:607–24.

3. Robinson R, Walker A, Ferlic D. The results of anterior interbody fusion of the cervical spine. J Bone Joint Surg Am. 1962;44:1569–87.

4. De Palma AF, Cooke AJ. Results of anterior interbody fusion of the cervical spine. Clin Orthop. 1968;60:169–85.

5. White 3rd AA, Southwick WO, Deponte RJ, Gainor JW, Hardy R. Relief of pain by anterior cervical-spine fusion for spondylosis. A report of sixty-five patients. J Bone Joint Surg Am. 1973;55(3):525–34.

6. Bohlman HH, Emery SE, Goodfellow DB, Jones PK. Robinson anterior cervical discectomy and arthrodesis for cervical radiculopathy. Long-term follow-up of one hundred and twenty-two patients. J Bone Joint Surg Am. 1993;75(9):1298–307.

7. Cloward RB. The anterior approach for removal of ruptured cervical disks. J Neurosurg. 1958;15:602–17.

8. Bailey RW, Badgley CE. Stabilization of the cervical spine by anterior fusion. J Bone Joint Surg Am. 1960;42-A:565–94.

9. Stoll A. Plating for ACDF. Surg Neurol. 2002;57(2):140.

10. Caspar W, Geisler FH, Pitzen T, Johnson TA. Anterior cervical plate stabilization in one- and two-level degenerative disease: overtreatment or benefit? J Spinal Disord. 1998;11:1–11.

11. Grob D, Peyer JV, Dvorak J. The use of plate fixation in anterior surgery of the degenerative cervical spine: a comparative prospective clinical study. Eur Spine J. 2001;10(5):408–13.

12. Savolainen S, Rinne J, Hernesniemi J. A prospective randomized study of anterior single-level cervical disc operations with long-term follow-up: surgical fusion is unnecessary. Neurosurgery. 1998;43(1):51–5.

13. Hankinson HI, Wilson CB. Use of the operating microscope in anterior cervical discectomy without fusion. J Neurosurg. 1975;43:452–6S.

14. Hirsch C, Wickbom I, Lidstrom A, Rosengren K. Cervical-disc resection: a follow-up of myelographic and surgical procedure. J Bone Joint Surg Am. 1964;46:1811–21.

15. Martins AN. Anterior cervical discectomy with and without interbody bone graft. J Neurosurg. 1976;44:290–5.

16. Rosenorn J, Hansen EB, Rosenorn MA. Anterior cervical discectomy with or without fusion: a prospective study. J Neurosurg. 1983;59(2):252–5.

17. Wilson DH, Campbell DD. Anterior cervical discectomy without bone graft. Report of 71 cases. J Neurosurg. 1977;47(4):551–5.

18. Watters 3rd WC, Levinthal R. Anterior cervical discectomy with and without fusion. Results, complications, and long-term follow-up. Spine. 1994;19(20):2343–7.

19. Laing RJ, Ng I, Seeley HM, Hutchinson PJ. Prospective study of clinical and radiological outcome after anterior cervical discectomy. Br J Neurosurg. 2001;15:319–23.

20. Nandoe Tewarie RD, Bartels RH, Peul WC. Long-term outcome after anterior cervical discectomy without fusion. Eur Spine J. 2007;16(9):1411–6.

21. Yamamoto I, Ikeda A, Shibuya N, Tsugane R, Sato O. Clinical long-term results of anterior discectomy without interbody fusion for cervical disc disease. Spine. 1991;16(3):272–9.

22. Newman M. The outcome of pseudarthrosis after cervical anteriorfusion. Spine. 1993;18(16):2380–2.

23. Brunton FJ, Wilkinson JA, Wise KS, Simonis RB. Cine radiography in cervical spondylosis as a means of determining the level for anterior fusion. J Bone Joint Surg Br. 1982;64(4):399–404.

24. Farey ID, McAfee PC, Davis RF, Long DM. Pseudarthrosis of the cervical spine after anterior arthrodesis. Treatment by posterior nerve-root decompression, stabilization, and arthrodesis. J Bone Joint Surg Am. 1990;72(8):1171–7.

25. Thorell W, Cooper J, Hellbusch L, Leibrock L. The long-term clinical outcome of patients undergoing anterior cervical discectomy with and without intervertebral bone graft placement. Neurosurgery. 1998;43(2):268–73; discussion 273–4.

26. Chau A, Mobbs R. Bone graft substitutes in anterior cervical discectomy and fusion. Eur Spine J. 2009;18:449–64.

27. Bagby GW. Arthrodesis by the distraction-compression method using a stainless steel implant. Orthopedics. 1988;11:931–4.

28. Hacker RJ, Cauthen JC, Gilbert TJ, Griffith SL. A prospective randomised multicenter clinical evaluation of an anterior cervical fusion cage. Spine. 2000;25:2646–54.

29. Siddiqui AJ. Cage versus tricortical graft for cervical interbody fusion. A prospective randomized trial. J Bone Joint Surg Br. 2003;85-B:1019–25.

30. Fernstrom U. Arthroplasty with intercorporal endoprosthesis in herniated disc and in painful disc. Acta Chir Scand Suppl. 1966;357:154–9.

31. Cummins BH, Robertson JT, Gill SS. Surgical experience with an implanted artificial cervical joint. J Neurosurg. 1998;88:943–8.

32. Bryan Jr VE. Cervical motion segment replacement. Eur Spine J. 2002;11 Suppl 2:92–7.

33. Hacker RJ. Cervical disc arthroplasty: a controlled randomized prospective study with intermediate follow-up results. J Neurosurg Spine. 2005;3(6):424–8.

34. Lafuente J, Casey A, Petzold A, Brew S. The Bryan cervical disc prosthesis as an alternative to arthrodesis in the treatment of cervical spondylosis. J Bone Joint Surg. 2005;87-B:508–12.

35. Sasso RC, Smucker JD, Hacker RJ, Heller JG. Artificial disc versus fusion: a prospective, randomized study with 2-year follow-up on 99 patients. Spine. 2007;32(26):2933–40.

36. Goffin J, Van Calenbergh V, van Loon J, et al. Intermediate follow-up after treatment of degenerative disc disease with the Bryan Cervical Disc Prosthesis: single-level and bi-level. Spine. 2003;28:2673–8.

37. Goffin J, van Loon J, Van Calenbergh F, Lipscomb B. A clinical analysis of 4- and 6-year follow-up results after cervical disc replacement surgery using the Bryan cervical disc prosthesis. J Neurosurg Spine. 2010;12(3):261–9.

38. Heller J, Sasso R, Papadopoulos S, Anderson P, Fessler R, Hacker R, Coric D, Cauthen J, Riew D. Comparison of Bryan cervical disc arthroplasty with anterior cervical decompression and fusion. Spine. 2009;34(2):101–7.

39. Murrey D, Janssen M, Delamarter R, Goldstein J, Zigler J, Tay B, Darden B. Results of the prospective, randomized, controlled multicenter Food and Drug Administration investigational device exemption study of the ProDisc-C total disc replacement versus anterior discectomy and fusion for the treatment of 1-level symptomatic cervical disc disease. Spine J. 2009;9(4):275–86.

40. Beaurain J, Bernard P, Dufour T, Fuentes JM, Hovorka I, Huppert J, Steib JP, Vital JM, Aubourg L, Vila T. Intermediate clinical and radiological results of cervical TDR (Mobi-C) with up to 2 years of follow-up. Eur Spine J. 2009;18(6):841–50.

41. Burkus JK, Haid RW, Traynelis VC, Mummaneni PV. Long-term clinical and radiographic outcomes of cervical disc replacement with the prestige disc: results from a prospective randomized controlled clinical trial. J Neurosurg Spine. 2010;13(3):308–18.

42. Jaramillo-de la Torre J, Grauer J, Yue J. Update on cervical disc arthroplasty: where are we and where are we going? Curr Rev Musculoskelet Med. 2008;1:124–30.

43. Sekhon LH, Duggal N, Lynch JJ, Haid RW, Heller JG, Riew KD, Seex K, Anderson PA. Magnetic resonance imaging clarity of the Bryan, Prodisc-C, Prestige LP, and PCM cervical arthroplasty devices. Spine. 2007;32(6):673–80.

44. Antosh IJ, DeVine JG, Carpenter CT, Woebkenberg BJ, Yoest SM. Magnetic resonance imaging evaluation of adjacent segments after cervical disc arthroplasty: magnet strength and its effect on image quality. J Neurosurg Spine. 2010;13(6):722–6.

45. Boden SD, McCowin PR, Davis DO, Dina TS, Mark AS, Wiesel S. Abnormal magnetic-resonance scans of the cervical spine in asymptomatic subjects. A prospective investigation. J Bone Joint Surg Am. 1990;72(8):1178–84.

46. Kuijper B, Tans JT, Beelen A, Nollet F, de Visser M. Cervical collar or physiotherapy versus wait and see policy for recent onset cervical radiculopathy: randomised trial. BMJ. 2009;339:b3883.

47. Brain WR, Northfield D, Wilkinson M. Neurological manifestations of cervical spondylosis. Brain. 1952;75:187–225.

48. Dorsi MJ, Witham TF. Surgical management of cervical spondylotic myelopathy. Neurosurg Q. 2009;19(4):302–7.

49. Lees F, Turner J. Natural history and prognosis of cervical spondylosis. Br Med J. 1963;2:1607–10.

50. Nurick S. The natural history and the results of surgical treatment of the spinal cord disorder associated with cervical spondylosis. Brain. 1972;95(1):101–8.

51. Roberts AH. Myelopathy due to cervical spondylosis treated by collar immobilization. Neurology. 1966;16:951–4.

52. Epstein JA, Epstein NE. The surgical management of cervical spinal stenosis, spondylosis, and myeloradiculopathy by means of the posteri- or approach. In: Sherk HH, Dunn EJ, Eismont FJ, et al., editors. The cervical spine. 2nd ed. Philadelphia: J.B. Lippincott; 1989. p. 625–43.

53. Clark E, Robinson PK. Cervical myelopathy: a complication of cervical spondylosis. Brain. 1956;79:483.

54. Syman L, Lavender P. The surgical treatment of cervical spondylotic myelopathy. Neurology. 1967;17:117–26.

55. McCormick WE, Steinmetz MP, Benzel EC. Cervical spondylotic myelopathy: make the difficult diagnosis, then refer for surgery. Cleve Clin J Med. 2003;70:899–904.

56. Montgomery DM, Brower RS. Cervical spondylotic myelopathy: clinical syndrome and natural history. Orthop Clin North Am. 1992;23:487–93.

57. Phillips DG. Surgical treatment of myelopathy with cervical spondylosis. J Neurol Neurosurg Psychiat. 1973;36:879–84.

58. Riew D, Buchowski J, Sasso R, Zdeblick T, Metcalf N, Anderson P. Cervical disc arthroplasty compared with arthrodesis for the treatment of myelopathy. J Bone Joint Surg Am. 2008;90:2354–64.

59. Hillibrand AS, Robbins M. Adjacent segment degeneration and adjacent segment disease: the consequences of spinal fusion? Spine J. 2004;4(6):190S–4.

60. Robertson JT, Papadopoulos SM, Traynelis VC. Assessment of adjacent-segment disease in patients treated with cervical fusion or arthroplasty: a prospective 2-year study. J Neurosurg Spine. 2005;3(6):417–23.

61. Pickett GE, Rouleau JP, Duggal N. Kinematic analysis of the cervical spine following implantation of an artificial cervical disc. Spine. 2005;30(17):1949–54.

62. Leung C, Casey AT, Goffin J, Kehr P, Liebig K, Lind B, Logroscino C, Pointillart V. Clinical significance of heterotopic ossification in cervical disc replacement: a prospective multicenter clinical trial. Neurosurgery. 2005;57(4):759–63.

63. Bertagnoli R, Yue JJ, Pfeiffer F, Fenk-Mayer A, Lawrence JP, Kershaw T, Nanieva R. Early results after ProDisc-C cervical disc replacement. J Neurosurg Spine. 2005;2(4):403–10.

64. Bertagnoli R. Heterotopic ossification at the index level after Prodisc-C surgery: what is the clinical relevance? Spine J. 2008;8:123S.

65. Suchomel P, Jurák L, Beneš III V, Brabec R, Bradáč O, Elgawhary S. Clinical results and development of heterotopic ossification in total cervical disc replacement during a 4-year follow-up. Eur Spine J. 2010;19:307–15.

Surgical Treatment of the Cervical Spine in Rheumatoid Arthritis

Zdenek Klezl and Jan Stulik

Contents

Z. Klezl (✉)
Department of Trauma and Orthopaedics, Spinal Unit,
Royal Derby Hospital, Derby, UK
e-mail: zklezl@aospine.org

J. Stulik
Spine Surgery Department, University Hospital Motol,
Praha, Czech Republic

Abstract

Cervical spine involvement in rheumatoid arthritis (RA) is common and can lead to severe pain, irreversible neurological deterioration and even death. It presents a challenge to the treating physician as the pain, neurological symptoms and instability cannot be equated with each other.

RA of the cervical spine follows the same pathophysiology as in the peripheral joints and leads to instability due to atlanto-axial subluxation, mid- and lower cervical spine instability and basilar invagination. The clinical presentation is variable and neurological assessment is difficult due to peripheral disease. Patients with minimal symptoms can have major life-threatening instability.

Treatment goals are to prevent irreversible neurological deficit, alleviate intractable pain and to avoid death due to cord compression.

Timing of surgical interventions is extremely important. It is generally recommended to address the instability (usually C1/C2) early in order to avoid more extensive fixation and fusion. Surgical stabilization is challenging because of suboptimal bone quality, increased risks of infection and difficult post-operative rehabilitation but generally leads to favourable outcomes. Referral of patients to specialist rheumatology centres and screening of cervical spine with flexion-extension radiographs and MRI scans seems optimal to avoid

G. Bentley (ed.), *European Surgical Orthopaedics and Traumatology*,
DOI 10.1007/978-3-642-34746-7_24, © EFORT 2014

patients presenting with major deformity, instability and advanced myelopathy. Surgical treatment of the rheumatoid cervical spine is very demanding and should therefore be performed at centres where cervical spine surgery is performed on a regular basis. In our experience, even advanced neurological deficit can significantly improve following well-executed surgery.

Keywords

Cervical spine • Classification • Diagnosis • Indications for surgery • Posterior • Rehabilitation • Rheumatiod arthritis • Techniques: fixation: -anterior, C1-2, occipito-cervical, sub-axial, upper thoracic

General Introduction and Classification

Rheumatoid arthritis (RA) is a progressive, immunologically-mediated disease with serious physical, psychological and economic consequences and the aetiology is unknown [25, 29]. RA affects about 1 % of the world population, more than 2.9 million Europeans and over 2 million patients in the United States. The clinical course of RA fluctuates and prognosis is unpredictable [14, 15]. 70 % of patients with recent onset of RA show evidence of radiographic changes within 3 years of diagnosis [39]. 50 % of RA patients are unable to work due to disability within 10 years of disease onset [1, 3, 32, 42].

The disease usually starts at metatarsophalangeal and metacarpophalangeal joints and is characterized by inflammation of the synovial membrane, destruction of hyaline cartilage and peri-articular inflammation resulting in bony erosions and formation of synovial cysts. [10, 20] These processes lead to joint laxity, instability, subluxation and deformity (Figs. 1 and 2).

RA is generally classified according to the American Rheumatologic Association functional capacity score.

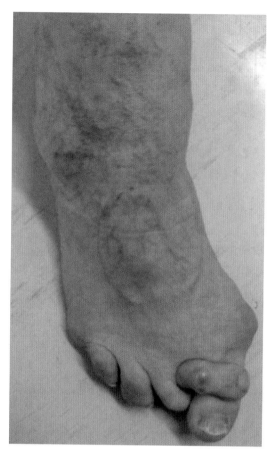

Fig. 1 Significant deformity of the ankle and foot

Class I	Complete ability to carry on all usual duties without handicap
Class II	Adequate for normal activities despite a handicap of discomfort or limited motion at one or more joints
Class III	Limited only to few or none of the duties of usual occupation or self- care.
Class IV	Incapacitated, largely or wholly bedridden or confined to a wheelchair; little or no self-care.

It was observed that in the last decade the incidence of the disease has dropped significantly with fewer total hip and knee replacements performed on rheumatoid patients compared with previous years [9, 17, 41]. The treatment has changed as well with the use of new disease-modifying anti-rheumatic drugs, (anti-tumour necrosis factor and anti-interleukin 1 agents)

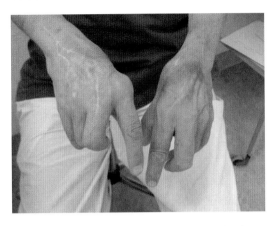

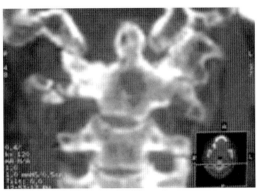

Fig. 3 Basilar invagination caused by destruction of C0-C1 and mainly C1-C2 joints

Fig. 2 Status post multiple surgeries for deformity, instability and pain in the area of both wrists and hands

which led to decrease in steroid use and better treatment results.

Cervical spine involvement is common in RA (up to 90 %) with neurological involvement occurring in 7–13 % of patients and the pathophysiology follows the same pattern as that of the small peripheral joints.

Involvement of the cervical spine was first described by British geneticist Sir Archibald Garrod in 1890 in his study of 500 patients, of whom 178 had the cervical spine affected [43]. The disease usually starts at the C1-C2 level as erosive synovitis affecting the ligaments around the dens and joint capsules in the area which leads to hypermobility of C0-C1 and C1-C2 joints and later mainly to atlano-axial anterior subluxations. C1-C2 joints may be affected by erosions and destruction of bone and cartilage resulting in lateral subluxation or, as the joints are symmetrically destroyed, the whole of C2 (including the dens) migrates proximally into the foramen magnum. This is also referred to as basilar invagination, vertical subluxations of the dens or cranial settling (Fig. 3).

Dens erosions are frequent and pannus may form around the dens, narrowing the spinal canal significantly. In case of significant destruction of the anterior arch of C1 or the dens [which can fracture once weakened] rare posterior subluxations of C1/C2 can occur (Figs. 4–6). Sub-axial spine, intervertebral discs and facet joints can be involved in one or more levels usually leading to

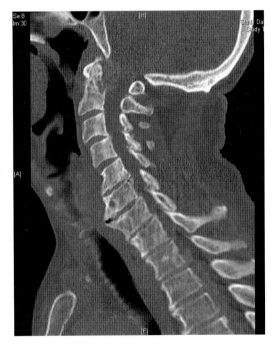

Fig. 4 Massive panus formation visible behind the dens, which is eroded at its base

"step" deformity due to subluxations (staircase or stepladder appearance of sub-axial spine).

Conlon et al [8] demonstrated that 50 % of patients with cervical spine involvement had radiological signs of instability. Anterior atlanto-axial subluxation represents two-thirds of rheumatoid cervical subluxations (65 %), 20 % are lateral and 10 % posterior [3, 10, 23].

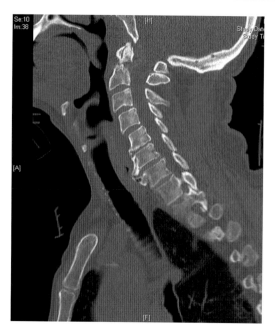

Fig. 5 Subsequent fracture of the eroded dens

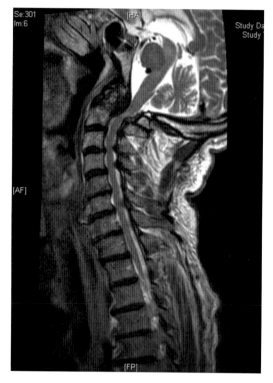

Fig. 6 Peridental panus causing cord compression at the C1 level with high signal in the spinal cord present

The incidence of lower cervical spine subluxation ranges between 20 % and 25 %. Basilar invagination with or without atlanto-axial subluxation occurs in approximately 20 % of patients. Neurological deficit varies from 11 % to 58 % [7, 13, 36], which is due to the difficulty in detecting subtle loss of strength from spinal cord compression in the presence of weakness and disuse atrophy arising from painful peripheral joints (Figs. 1 and 2).

Neurological deterioration can be irreversible and the presence of myelopathy is an indicator of significant cord compression. Patients with advanced myelopathy have poor prognosis. Typical signs and symptoms of myelopathy include weakness, spasticity, bowel and bladder dysfunctions, loss of proprioception, hyperreflexia, positive Hoffmann sign, gait disturbance, paraesthesia and loss of dexterity. In many older RA patients these signs and symptoms can be difficult to assess. Worsening neurological deficit is most frequently hidden in the patients' history in expressions like: "I cannot unbutton my shirt; I can no longer walk the usual distance; I can no longer walk; my gait is very unstable; whenever I bend my head I feel electric shocks in my arms and legs or I lose consciousness". A careful examiner should focus on this highly significant information. Electrophysiological examination is extremely helpful in diagnosis of early cord compression. It can be performed as dynamic examination in extension and flexion of the head. Pathological potentials are frequently recorded in flexion, when the cord compression occurs.

Up to 10 % of patients with RA die of unrecognized spinal cord or brain stem compression. It usually takes about 10 years for severe instability to develop but in patients with the mutilating form of the disease it can occur within 2 years of diagnosis. Various functional scoring systems have been used to classify and monitor neurological deficit.

The most frequent are the Frankel's classification grading system for acute spinal cord injuries (Table 1), Ranawat's classification of neurological deficit [34] (Table 2), Nurick's classification

Table 1 Acute spinal cord injury – Frankel Classification grading system

Grade A	Complete neurological injury – no motor or sensory function clinically detected below the level of the injury.
Grade B	Preserved sensation only – no motor function clinically detected below the level of the injury; sensory function remains below the level of the injurybut may include only partial function (sacral sparing qualifies as preserved sensation).
Grade C	Preserved motor non-functional – some motor function observed below the level of the injury, but is of no practical use to the patient.
Grade D	Preserved motor function – useful motor function below the level of the injury; patient can move lower limbs and walk with or without aid, but does not have a normal gait or strength in all motor groups.
Grade E	Normal motor – no clinically detected abnormality in motor or sensory function with normal sphincter function; abnormal reflexes and subjective sensory abnormalities may be present.

Table 2 Ranawat Classification of Neurologic Deficit

Class I	Pain, no neurologic deficit
Class II	Subjective weakness, hyperreflexia, dyesthesias
Class III	Objective weakness, long tract signs
Class IIIA	Class III, ambulatory
Class IIIB	Class III, nonambulatory

system for myelopathy on the basis of gait abnormalities [28] (Table 3) and JOA or modified JOA systems [21].

Diagnosis

Diagnosis of rheumatoid arthritis is by exclusion of other seronegative spondyloarthopathies such as ankylosing spondylitis, systemic lupus erythematosis, psoriatic arthritis, reactive arthritis (formerly Reiter's syndrome) and other poly-arthropathies associated with inflammatory bowel disease.

Laboratory tests include ESR which is elevated, rheumatoid factor is positive in 70–80 % of patients, anti-nuclear factor is positive in 30–70 % of patients. CRP is non-specific but can be used as a marker of the activity of the disease.

Cervical spine involvement is seen well on plain radiographs, which frequently show subtle signs of atlanto-axial instability. The full extent of instability can be appreciated on flexion and extension views. Plain radiographs provide little information on real space available for the spinal cord (SAC) and MRI scans are routinely used to determine the SAC which should ideally be more than 14 mm in the upper cervical spine. SAC less than 14 mm is considered to be pathological and if less than 10 mm is regarded as critical and usually with a poor prognosis. MRI is the examination of choice for demonstrating possible changes in the spinal cord, ligamentum transversum atlantis, intervertebral discs of the sub-axial spine or of the pannus, which may significantly narrow the spinal canal [11, 22].

Table 3 Nurick's classification system for myelopathy on the basis of gait abnormalities

Grade	Root signs	Cord involvement	Gait	Employment
0	Yes	No	Normal	Possible
I	Yes	Yes	Normal	Possible
II	Yes	Yes	Mild abnormality	Possible
III	Yes	Yes	Severe abnormality	Impossible
IV	Yes	Yes	Only with assistance	Impossible
V	Yes	Yes	Chair bound or bed ridden	Impossible

Fig. 7 Different measurements of cranial migration of the dens

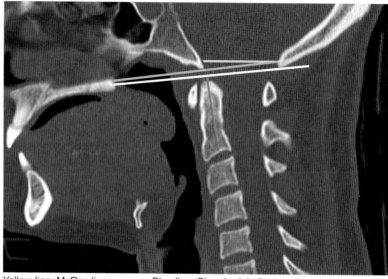

Yellow line: McRay line   Blue line: Chamberlain line
White line: McGregor line   Red line: Redlund-Johnell and Pettersson parameter

High resolution MRI scans may be useful in the future [40]. MRI is a static examination and although the SAC seems reasonable on scans taken in the supine position, dynamic compression may regularly occur with head flexion. CT scans are valuable in assessing bone loss, rotatory and lateral subluxation and play a major role in pre-operative planning, determining the course of the vertebral arteries and the dimension of structures where we plan to introduce screws in the C1 and C2 vertebrae.

Basilar invagination or cranial settling is measured using various methods and lines [35] (Figs. 7 and 8).

McGregor line: Caudal part of occiput to hard palate. When dens is 4.5 mm. above this line, it is a pathological finding.

McRay [method or lines]: Occiput to clivus (foramen magnum diameter), tip of the dens should not cross this line.

Redlund-Johnell and Pettersson parameter: Distance from middle of the bottom of C2 endplate to McGregor line which should be less than 34 mm. in men and less than 29 mm. in women.

Clark station of the atlas: The Odontoid process is divided into thirds; 1st third (upper) should correspond to the anterior ring of atlas.

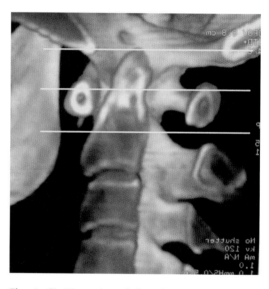

Fig. 8 Clark's station of the atlas evaluating cranial migration of the dens

Once the C1-C2 joints are destroyed, the middle third of the odontoid corresponds to the ring of atlas indicating mild to moderate cranial settling and when the bottom third of C2 corresponds to the ring of atlas, there is severe cranial settling [6].

Ranawat criterion: The distance between the centre of the second cervical pedicle and the transverse axis of the atlas is measured along the axis of the odontoid process. Once the distance between these two lines is less than 15 mm in males and less than 13 mm in females, cranial settling is present.

Riew et al [35] found that none of the currently published lines and parameters used alone can diagnose basilar invagination accurately. The highest accuracy was reached using a combination of criteria by Clark [6], Redlund-Johnell, Pettersson and Ranawat. If any of these suggest basilar invagination, CT or MRI should be performed. This also demonstrates the need for a low threshold for requesting MRI scans in relation to possible pannus formation as described by Dvorak [11].

Indications for Surgery

The major challenge is to have the right indications and to avoid unnecessary high risk surgery. As discussed previously, pain cannot be equated to instability, or instability to neurological symptoms. Careful detailed follow up of rheumatoid arthritis patients leads to correct indications for surgery which are:

1. Intractable pain
2. Increasing neurological deficit (even sub-clinical, documented on somatosensory or motor evoked potential or both)
3. Posterior atlanto-dental interval (SAC) less than 14 mm
4. Cervicomedullary angle of less than 135°
5. Lateral subluxation of more than 2 mm
6. Increasing instability (atlanto-axial or cranial settling).

Indications for surgery have changed in the recent years with surgeons being more pro-active, encouraged by the good results following surgery. Surgery for cervical myelopathy is no longer considered as waste of effort and resources, but has major role in treatment of this potentially lethal condition [17, 26]. There is currently no level-one evidence on surgical treatment of myelopathy in rheumatoid arthritis patients. The best available evidence is documented in the study by Matsunaga et al [26]. They have compared treatment results of a surgically-treated group of 19 patients and conservatively-treated group of 21 patients, who were treated in different hospital. Patients were observed until death. The survival rate in the surgical group was 84 % in 5 years and 37 % in 10 years, 68 % of them improved clinically. There was no improvement in the conservative group, 76 % worsened, all patients were bedridden by 3 years and none survived for longer than 8 years. Singh et al looked at 50 surgically-treated patients with myelopathy and compared this group to 34 patients who declined surgery or were not fit for it, by using the validated 30 m walking test. The test confirmed lasting improvement following surgery at 3 years. Unoperated patients continued to deteriorate. Interestingly, they noticed remarkable improvement of severe myelopathy in older patients [37, 38]. This was also our experience.

In the majority of cases, the disease manifests itself as atlanto-axial instability with clinical symptoms varying from very subtle to a severe myelopathic picture. If detected early it is best treated by atlanto-axial immobilization (fusion), which eliminates severe pain, further subluxation and progressive tissue destruction and cranial settling. We try to avoid fusion to the occiput because this leads to significant decrease of flexion of the head, which makes activities of daily living difficult e.g. eating or brushing teeth.

Pre-Operative Preparation and Planning

Pre-operative assessment should be elaborate, considering the systemic nature of the illness, increased incidence of anaemia in chronic disease, increased risk of both frequency and severity of post-surgical infections (especially associated with immunosuppressive agents) and significantly reduced bone quality.

Spinal instrumentation for the upper and lower cervical spine has made enormous progress since the time Gallie published his C1-C2 simple wiring technique in 1937 [12]. Double wiring technique was then introduced by Jenkins and Books. Sub-laminar wires have been used for

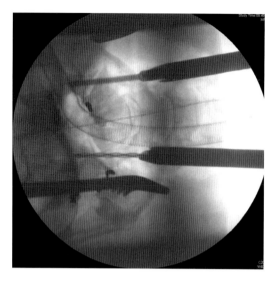

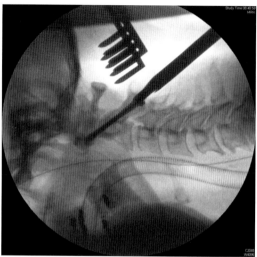

Fig. 9 AP intraoperative view of transarticular screw fixation (Magerl)

Fig. 10 Lateral intra-operative view of the same technique

many years to stabilize the spine together with structural bone graft harvested from the pelvis or later with Luque or Ransford loops.

Modern instrumentation started with first universal system combining plate-rod screw fixation developed by Jeanneret in 1992. Wiring techniques are no longer used except as part of transarticular screw fixation or in special circumstances. There is very little room for non-instrumented posterior decompressions in RA patients.

Some of the commonly used techniques are:

1. Transarticular C1-C2 screw fixation (Figs. 9 and 10) as described by Magerl [16]
2. Lateral mass C1-C2 fixation described by Goel [11] and Harms and Melcher [18]
3. Occipito-cervical stabilization
4. Occipito-thoracic stabilization
5. Anterior approach, placement of strut graft or cage and plate fixation.

All the posterior techniques carry the risk of injury to the vertebral artery and require pre-operative imaging to minimize the risk. Solanki and Crockard [27, 38] identified a frequent abnormal course of the vertebral artery in their extensive work (22 % vertebral artery groove anomalies noted). Currently careful planning using lateral and sagittal CT reconstructions of the C1-C2 is routinely performed.

The posterior approach dominates surgical treatment of rheumatoid patients. Indications for the trans-oral approach are extremely rare. The approach is no longer indicated for pannus resection as it resolves within a few months of an atlanto-axial fusion (Figs. 11 and 12) [16, 22]. Trans-oral decompression is indicated in severe cases of irreducible cranial migration of the dens into the foramen magnum and in cases of cervico-medullary compression.

Once the C1-C2 instability is combined with cranial migration of the dens, occipito-cervical fixation is used. Unfortunately atlanto-axial instability with cranial settling is frequently combined with sub-axial instability and subluxation. In these cases occipito-cervical fixation is extended down to the upper thoracic spine (C0-T1) to avoid junctional instability (Figs. 13 and 14).

Complex deformities (Figs. 15 and 16), which involve both upper and lower cervical spine, require a combination of both anterior and posterior stabilization (Figs. 16 and 17). This is also true for trans-oral surgery. Once the anterior resection of the C1 arch is performed, posterior stabilization is neccessary.

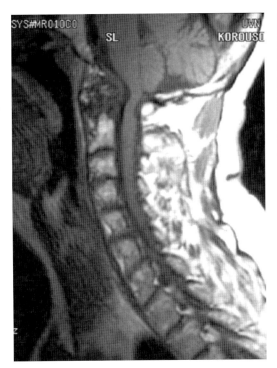

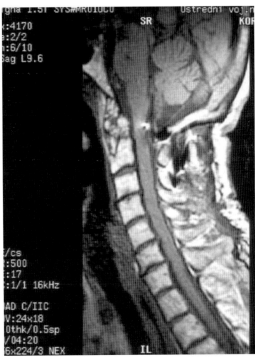

Fig. 11 Panus extent before surgery and after 5 months following C1-C2 fixation

Fig. 12 Panus extent before surgery and after 5 months following C1-C2 fixation

Operative Techniques

Posterior Approach

The patient is placed in prone position in reverse Trendelenbourg position (head up) with the head placed on a head-rest or in a Mayfield clamp. Positioning of the head is very important and should be done by the surgeon himself or a qualified assistant. Maximum care should be taken to avoid injury to the eyes, which is an infrequently reported, but potentially catastrophic complication. Hair should be shaved above the external occipital protuberance to facilitate sterile draping. A mid-line incision should be drawn on the skin to avoid oblique incisions. Identifying mid-line after the skin incision is not easy and is best done at the distal part of the incision, where the fibrous septum separating the muscles on each side is better developed. Dissection in this plane significantly reduces

bleeding at this stage. Bony landmarks are identified by palpation, the occiput, usually bifid and prominent spinous process of C2 and the highest spinous process of T1. The tubercule of C1 can be palpated proximally to the spinous process of C2. However, sometimes it cannot be palpated, because it lies right below the occipital bone especially in cases of cranial settling. Exposure of the bony elements in the occipito-cervical area should start in the mid-line and expand laterally, symmetrically on both sides. Subperiosteal dissection of muscle insertions leads to less muscle damage and facilitates later reinsertion to C2.

Lateral fluoroscopy is necessary, the C-arm is located opposite the surgeon.

Exposure of the occipital bone is not associated with any problems but exposure of C1 can be. Exposure is carried out from the tubercule of C1 which is in the midline out laterally. The safe zone is considered to be 1.5 cm to each side. Further exposure should be done with extreme

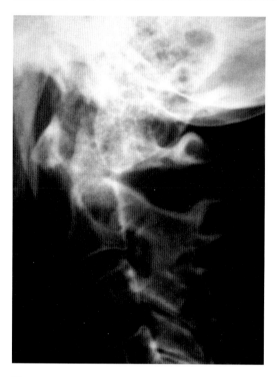

Fig. 13 Pre-operative films showing dens erosion, atlanto-axial instability and lateral subluxation

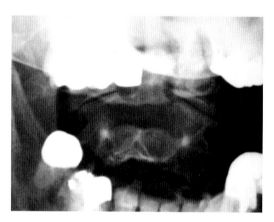

Fig. 14 Pre-operative films showing dens erosion, atlanto-axial instability and lateral subluxation

caution with a thin rasp or clamp-held peanut to avoid vertebral arteries as they emerge from the lateral masses of C1 and converge medially on the proximal surface of C1. In case of transarticular screw placement, wires,

cable-wires or a non-resorbable strong suture need to be passed under the arch of C1 (Magerl). This should be done carefully using a blunt needle or Dechamp suture-passer to avoid CSF leak or cord injury. In case of lateral mass screw insertion (Goel, Harms), the entry point of the screw is identified under the C1 arch by strict sub-periosteal dissection to avoid injury to the C2 nerve root and venous plexus which may lead to profuse bleeding. The lamina of C2 is exposed laterally to the edges of the lamina, the atlanto-axial membrane between the arch of C1 and C2 is exposed and the pedicle of C2 is identified by palpation from inside the canal using a Milligan dissector. Once all the anatomical landmarks are identified, screw insertion can be performed. A towel clip attached to the spinous process of C2 is helpful in stabilizing it during the exposure. Profuse bleeding is sometimes encountered even with very gentle dissection of the C1 lateral masses. Quick placement of the partially-threaded screw and tamponade of the venous plexuses by the screw head and Surgicel will help.

Transarticular Screw Fixation

Screws are inserted from the posterior aspect of C2 lamina parallel to the spinal canal across the joints of C1-C2 into the lateral masses of C1 (Figs. 17–20) [16]. The screws should avoid vertebral arteries. It is recommended to place the screws as medially and as proximally in the sagittal plane as possible. This technique includes graft insertion in between the arches of C1 and C2 which is secured in position by wire, cable-wire or suture. Well-positioned graft provides 3-point stable fixation. This technique requires reduced alignment of C1 and C2. Partial reduction of C1-C2 on the table can be performed by pulling on the cable wire or strong suture around the C1 arch, which is always introduced first. It is sometimes difficult to follow the trajectory of the screw in the lateral view because of the prominent back of the patient.

This requires:

1. enlarging the exposure to the upper thoracic spine,
2. using a cannulated screw technique,

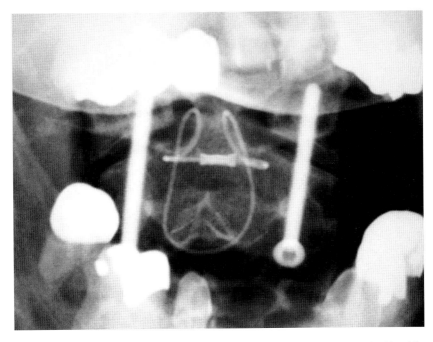

Fig. 15 Transarticular fixation with bonegraft held in place between the arches of C1 and C2 with cable wire

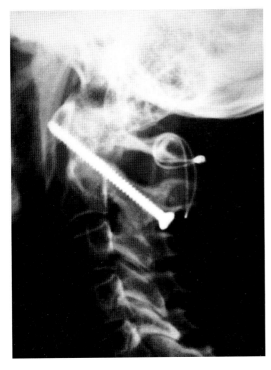

Fig. 16 Transarticular fixation with bonegraft held in place between the arches of C1 and C2 with cable wire

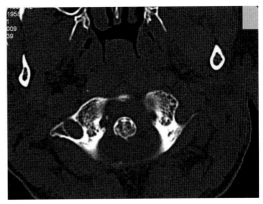

Fig. 17 Major atlanto-axial subluxation on axial CT and lateral X ray

3. using percutaneous screw placement through two stab incisions at the level of T2-T4 with normal exposure of C1 and C2 (preferred option).

From our experience as well as that of the technique's author, we do not advocate exposure and decortications of the C1-C2 joints as originally recommended.

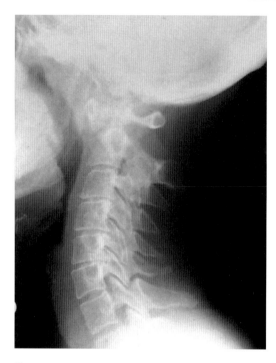

Fig. 18 Major atlanto-axial subluxation on axial CT and lateral X ray

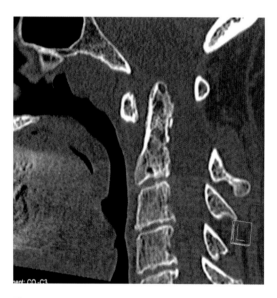

Fig. 19 CT sagittal and coronal view of the same patient

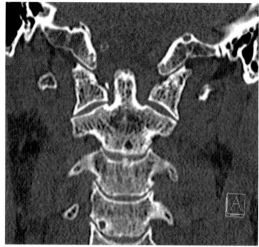

Fig. 20 CT sagittal and coronal view of the same patient

C1-C2 Fixation

Screws are placed into lateral masses of C1 either straight or slightly converging medially [13, 18]. Special screws with partially threaded shafts are available to avoid irritation of the C2 nerve root by the screw thread which is a well-recognized disadvantage of the method. C2 crews are transpedicular screws as described by Judet in 1962. The screws used have polyaxial heads and allow reduction of subluxation on the table, which is a well-recognized advantage of the method (Figs. 21–25).

The stability of the two constructs is the same, provided the Magerl technique is combined with the wiring. Sometimes the arch of C1 is missing and in that case the Goel/Harms technique would seem better. It has been considered that the pedicle screw fixation of the Goel/Harms technique had lower risk of intra-operative injury of the vertebral artery. However, in the study by Makoto et al, the risks were found to be the same [24].

Sometimes pedicle or transarticular screws cannot be used in C2 vertebra because of unfavourable vascular anatomy. Wright's technique is a good option [42]. Screws are placed into the lamina of C2 which is well-developed and are connected to the rest of the construct (Figs. 26–29).

In case of a complication at C1-C2 level, the Gallie's or Brook's and Jenkin's single or double wiring techniques or occipito-cervical instrumentation [30] can be used as a secondary option.

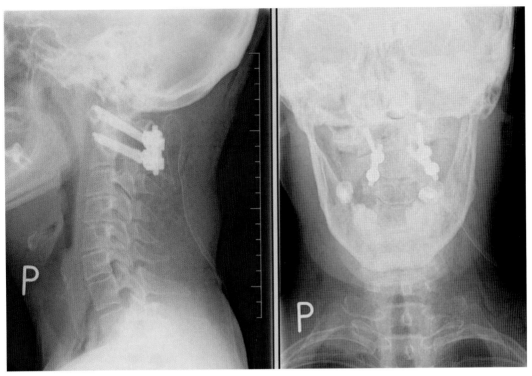

Fig. 21 Lateral and AP X ray of posterior C1-C2 fixation according to Goel-Harms with good reduction of the subluxation

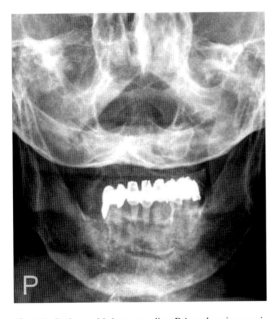

Fig. 22 Patient with long-standing RA and major cervical spine involvement

Occipito-Cervical Fixation

Occipito-cervical fixation is usually indicated in advanced stages of the disease which is associated with cranial settling. Sub-periosteal dissection of the rectus capitis posterior minor and major exposes the occipital bone. The bone is thicker in the mid-line. Screws should therefore be placed in this area and not above the inion, which could result in profuse bleeding from the intracranial sinus. All currently available instrumentations have special occipital plates which allow for independent placement and later connection with the rods attached to the upper or lower cervical spine. The thickness of occipital bone in the mid-line varies from 10-16 mm. Drilling the screw holes should at all times be done using a depth-restricting sleeve to avoid injuring the cerebellum. Sometimes a CSF leak is encountered, which is not a serious complication. It is sealed by screw placement in the hole. Three screws usually

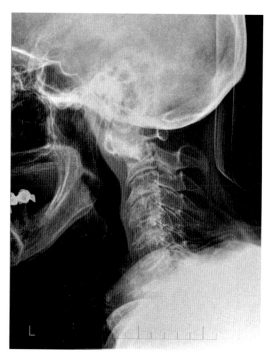

Fig. 23 Patient with long-standing RA and major cervical spine involvement

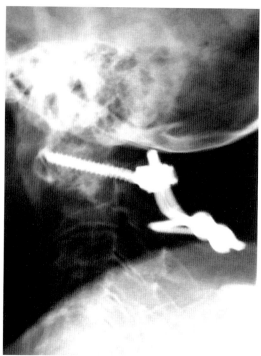

Fig. 25 Patient underwent surgery using the Wright technique of anchoring screws in the lamina of C2

provide enough stability. If the older plate – rod systems are used, the occipital plates should be contoured towards the midline and screw holes should be drilled aiming towards the mid-line of the occiput. Rod contouring is very important in extensive fixations extending to the thoracic spine. Post-operative position of the head should be discussed with the patient. The rods should be contoured to approximately 90°. A common mistake is excessive flexion (group of mushroom pickers) or rarely exaggerated extension (group of astrologers) (Figs. 30–34).

Sub-Axial Fixation

In cases where sub-axial fixation is necessary, lateral mass screw insertion is used in C3–C7. Two techniques were described by Roy-Camille and Magerl. The latter is used widely because it provides better screw purchase in the bone, the screw canal is longer and purchase is bi-cortical. The surgical technique was recently simplified by Bayley et al [2]. Their investigation was based on analysis of 80 digitized cervical spine CT scans.

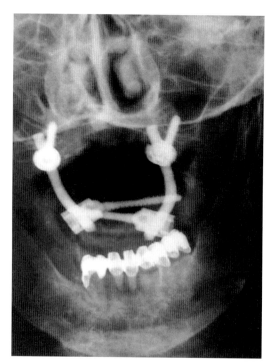

Fig. 24 Patient underwent surgery using the Wright technique of anchoring screws in the lamina of C2

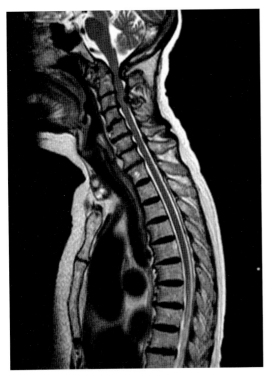

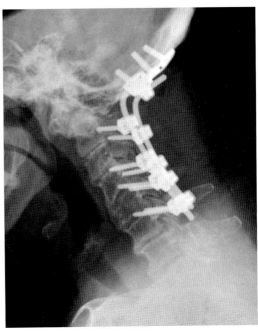

Fig. 28 Occipito-cervical fixation was performed following wide decompression of the cord using independent occipital plate in combination with top loading polyaxial screws

Fig. 26 74 year old female, Ranawat 3B with cord compression at foramen magnum and C3-C4 level

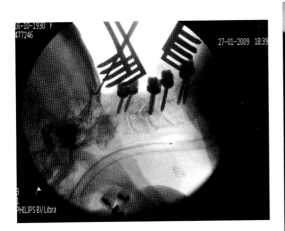

Fig. 27 Intra-operative confirmation of decompression of the foramen magnum with ball tip hook

A virtual screw trajectory, 2 mm from and parallel to the lamina was placed through the lateral mass of C3 to C7 vertebrae and potential violation of the transverse foramen was assessed and was not found. The authors have been using this

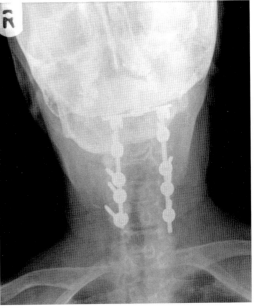

Fig. 29 Occipito-cervical fixation was performed following wide decompression of the cord using independent occipital plate in combination with top loading polyaxial screws

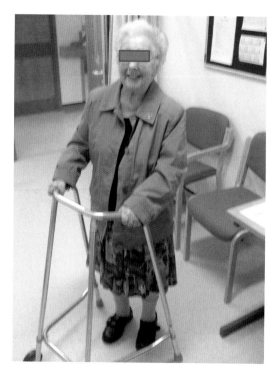

Fig. 30 Patient has regained sphincter control, self care and mobilizing with an aid

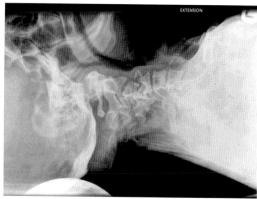

Fig. 32 Flexion-extension films demonstrating partial mobility at the area of destruction of subaxial spine and atlanto-axial subluxation as well

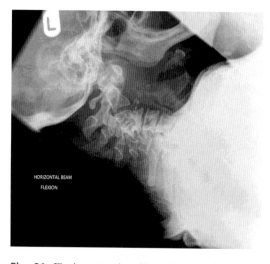

Fig. 31 Flexion-extension films demonstrating partial mobility at the area of destruction of subaxial spine and atlanto-axial subluxation as well

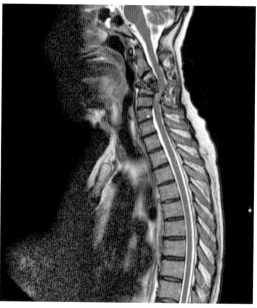

Fig. 33 MRI view of the critical spinal canal stenosis and myelopathy at C4 level

laminar guidance for the last 15 years without injury to the vertebral artery. The technique usually requires resection of the bifid spinous processes in order to aim the drill sufficiently

laterally [2]. Apart from lateral masses, pedicles may be used as anchoring points for screws. This especially applies to the C7 level where pedicle screw fixation is frequently superior to the lateral mass. Confirmation of the absence of the vertebral artery has to be done on preoperative imaging. The medial angulation of the C7 pedicles can be assessed. In case of any doubt,

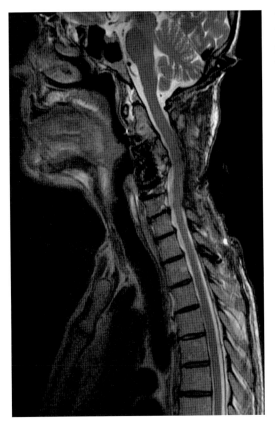

Fig. 34 MRI scan following 1st stage of anterior surgery which helped to improve the sagittal alignment of the cervical spine

small fenestration of the lamina enables direct palpation of the pedicle from inside the spinal canal. Pedicle screw technique is not used routinely in other than C7 segment. Intra-operative navigation makes the pedicle screw placement safer and will probably lead to more frequent use of the technique, especially in osteoporotic bone.

Upper Thoracic Spine Fixation

Fixation to the upper thoracic spine is done by inserting transpedicular screws into the T2, T3 or T4 pedicles. Another possibility is claw fixation using laminar hooks. Use of polyaxial screw heads significantly simplified the fixation in transition of cervical to thoracic spine because connection to the rods is much easier. Intra-operative imaging of the upper thoracic pedicles may be

very difficult and therefore key-hole opening of the spinal canal and palpation of the medial border of the pedicle from inside of the spinal canal with a Milligan dissector, as mentioned above, is an option.

Anchoring individual screws is critical, especially in osteoporotic bone and multi-point fixation is usually performed.

Performing posterior cervical fusion remains a controversial issue; based on our good experience with fusion we support fusion in rheumatoid patients. Meticulous decortication with a high-speed burr creates an ideal host bed for the autologous locally-harvested or iliac crest bone graft. Bone graft is carefully placed onto the decorticated areas and compressed to allow good contact as osteoblasts are very good "climbers" but very bad "jumpers". Use of BMP-2 is also a viable option. Bone graft harvesting is a separate surgical procedure with associated morbidity and complications in up to 15–20 % with frequently wound healing problems. Good results have been reported without fusion [27].

Anterior Approaches

The trans-oral approach was frequently used to decompress the spinal cord from peridental pannus. It has been found to be unnecessary because resolution occurs with immobilization. Trans-oral decompression is indicated in cases of fixed kyphotic deformity and brain stem compression. The decompression usually involves resection of the anterior arch of C1, sometimes also of the clivus. Stabilizaton by anterior C1-C2 transarticular screws is possible and usually posterior stabilization follows.

Although pre-operative traction is seldom used in RA patients, it is used in cases of major basilar invagination of the dens. Reduction of the invagination can be achieved thus eliminating need for trans-oral decompression.

The anterior approach to the sub-axial spine is same as for any other pathology. We must stress the presence of suboptimal bone quality. Preservation of intact bony end-plates is essential for force transmission to the bone graft or mesh cage. Cement screw augmentation is a viable option in cases of severe osteoporosis (Figs. 35–40).

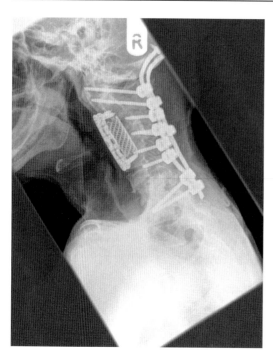

Fig. 35 AP and lateral X rays demostrating 2nd stage surgery from posterior approach, occipito-thoracic stabilization

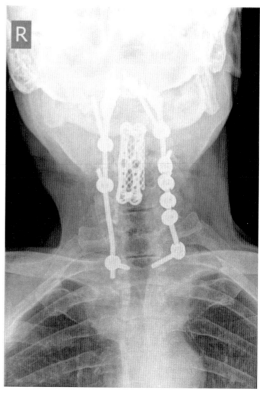

Fig. 36 AP and lateral X rays demostrating 2nd stage surgery from posterior approach, occipito-thoracic stabilization

Post-Operative Care and Rehabilitation

Stable fixation of the cervical spine facilitates post-operative care and subsequent rehabilitation. This is frequently very demanding especially due to the advanced peripheral joint involvement. Fixation should be stable enough to enable patients to sit and walk within a few days. Successful post-operative rehabilitation involves early mobilization, input from occupational therapists and provision of domestic aftercare. In general, activity and exercise provoke favourable responses in physical and psychological benefits. Dynamic (aerobic) exercises as well as hydrotherapy are used to enhance range of motion in joints, muscle power and co-ordination and to prevent contractures. Because hand function is frequently compromised in myelopathy patients, specific long-term exercises concentrating on fine movement of the hand and fingers are necessary. These focus on exercises which simulate activities of daily living like buttoning a shirt, locking-unlocking doors, opening a window, and handling cups and cutlery. Recently the use of electrical stimulation and exercise to increase muscle strength in patients after surgery for cervical spondylotic myelopathy was reported by Pastor [31].

Complications

Intra-Operative

Most serious complications with catastrophic consequences involve the spinal cord and the vertebral arteries. The spinal cord can be injured during positioning, so this has to be done in a very careful and controlled way. The spinal cord can be injured by inserting screws and wires into the spinal canal, and passing wires under the arch of C1 may be difficult when there is little space

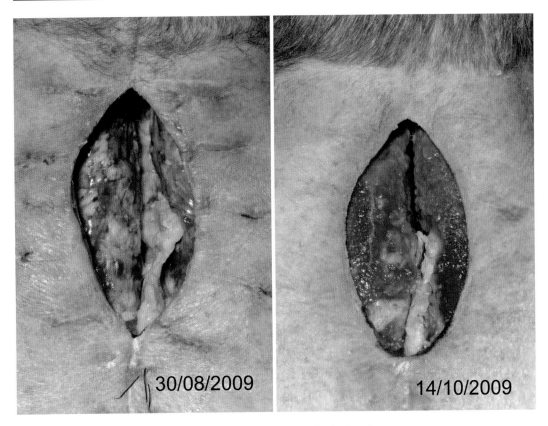

Fig. 37 Major improvement in wound appearance with VAC dressing in 6 weeks

left for the dorsally-displaced spinal cord. Spinal cord monitoring is extremely helpful when major instability or deformity is treated.

Even with adequate pre-operative planning, injury of the vertebral artery while drilling transarticular or C2 pedicle screws may happen. Wright and Lauryssen looked at risks of vertebral artery injury in 2492 patients. They concluded that the risk of injury per patient was 4.1 %, neurological deficit at 0.2 % and mortality of 0.1 % [43]. The best way to control the bleeding is to insert a shorter screw. The authors have experienced 2 such episodes and know of further 5 which all were treated in this way, luckily without any major neurological consequences. This experience was confirmed by retrospective evaluation of 15 patients who had one vertebral artery ligated during cervical spine tumour resection. All patients had pre-operative angiography which demonstrated equal or smaller size of the ligated artery [19]. It is important not to continue with drilling C2 on the other side once one artery is already injured. The other area where the artery can be injured is at the top of C1. Safe exposure of C1 arch is considered to be up to approximately 15 mm on each side of the arch from the mid-line. In general, the vertebral artery is difficult to ligate unless an adequate exposure is made. Therefore balloon occlusion in case of continuous bleeding is recommended [43].

Profuse bleeding from the venous plexuses can be encountered while preparing the entry point for the C1 lateral mass screws. It is best treated by using Gelfoam, Surgicel or Floseal and applying pressure on the area by the polyaxial screw head.

Post-operative early complications: wound dehiscence and infection are the most frequent

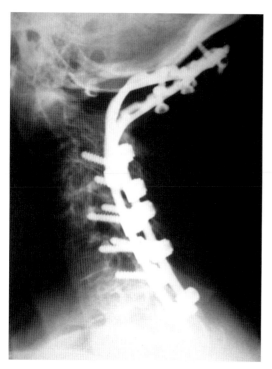

Fig. 38 Dislodgement of instrumentation following a fall from standing height

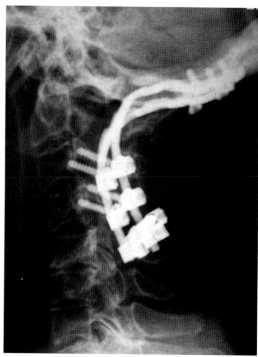

Fig. 39 Progressive junctional instability below the instrumentation

post-operative complications, which require revisions, re-drainage and re-suture. VAC dressing (Fig. 41) is a major help in this area. Wound healing problems may also occur at the occiput right at the top of the cervical collar. A collar should not be worn in the bed unless absolutely necessary.

Post-operative late complications include: dislodgement of instrumentation, non-union and adjacent segment instability. Dislodgement of instrumentation can be caused by sub-optimal anchoring of screws in the bone due to poor bone quality or surgical technique. Non-union with progressive instability and adjacent segment instability are late complications. Although spinal surgeons fight for every mobile segment, careful consideration has to be made in RA patients. If subtle signs of instability are detected at other levels on pre-operative imaging, extending fusion below these segments is recommended even if this represents extending the fixation down to the upper thoracic spine.

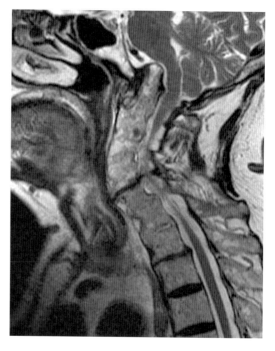

Fig. 40 Major extent of cranial migration of the dens and sub-axial involvement of the cervical spine, patient declined to have surgery

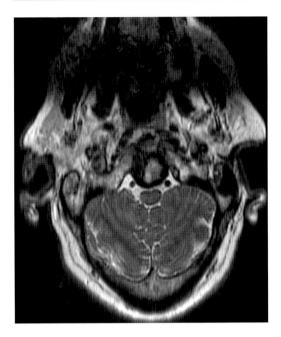

Fig. 41 Major extent of cranial migration of the dens and sub-axial involvement of the cervical spine, patient declined to have surgery

Summary

It is essential that the general medical Physicians and Rheumatologists are aware of the possible devastating effects RA may cause to upper and lower cervical spine. Regular follow- up and screening of RA patients using dynamic X rays and MRI in rheumatology centres is ideal to avoid presentation of patients with major instability, deformity and late stages of cervical myelopathy. Gradual worsening of patient's performance, hand function or walking should be warning clinical signs.

Although the majority of RA patients are managed conservatively, indications for surgical treatment are frequent. RA patients represent a major if not the biggest challenge to the spinal surgeon. Although it seems the disease is less aggressive as it used to be due to the availability of newer generation drugs, we still need to be aware of the major devastation it can cause when it is active. Significant progress has been made in development of spinal instrumentation, polyaxial screw-rod constructs, occipital plates etc, which facilitate more extensive fixation, ranging from C1-C2 to occipito-thoracic levels. The vast majority of interventions are by a posterior approach. Indication for a trans-oral approach for pannus resection no longer exists since the pannus resorbs well following stabilization of the C1-C2 segment. The current strategy is to address cervical instability rather earlier than later. Because it most frequently involves atlanto-axial area, C1-C2 fixation according to Magerl or Goel-Harms is logical. Careful pre-operative planning is essential when using both techniques because of the possible abnormal course of the vertebral arteries. C1-C2 fixation prevents further destruction of the atlanto-axial joints and progressive migration of the dens proximally. It also results in less restricted movement than occipito-cervical fixations. When dealing with more advanced stages of the disease more extensive surgery is necessary including the occiput. Adequate position of head should be maintained especially when the fixation extends to the upper thoracic spine. Minimal sub-axial subluxations should be considered when planning shorter occipito-cervical fixation, usually in young patients. All potentially unstable levels should be involved in the instrumentation eliminating the need for revision surgery for adjacent segment instability.

Surgical treatment of cervical spine involvement in patients with RA is associated with difficulties and complications but is equally rewarding to the patients and the treating surgeons.

References

1. Allaire SH, Prashker MJ, Meenan RF. The costs of rheumatoid arthritis. Pharmacoeconomics. 1994;6(6): 513–22.
2. Bayley E, Zia Z, Kerslake R, Klezl Z, Boszczyk BM. Lamina-guided lateral mass screw placement in the sub-axial cervical spine. Eur Spine J. 2010;19(4): 660–4.
3. Boden SD, Dodge LD, Bohlman HH, Rechtine GR. Rheumatoid arthritis of the cervical spine. A long-term analysis with predictors of paralysis and recovery. J Bone Joint Surg Am. 1993;75(9):1282–97.

4. Brattström H, Granholm L. Atlanto-axial fusion in rheumatoid arthritis. A new method of fixation with wire and bone cement. Acta Orthop Scand. 1976;47(6):619–28.

5. Casey ATH, Crockard AH, Pringle J, O'Brien MF, Stevens JM. Rheumatoid arthritis of the cervical spine: Current techniques for management. Orthop Clin North Am. 2002;33:291–309.

6. Clark CR, Goetz DD, Menzes AH. Athrodesis of the cervical spine in rheumatoid arthritis. J Bone Joint Surg Am. 1989;71:381–92.

7. Conaty JP, Mongan ES. Cervical fusion in rheumatoid arthritis. J Bone Joint Surg Am. 1981;63(8):1218–27.

8. Conlon PW, Isdale IC, Rose BS. Rheumatoid arthritis of the cervical spine. An analysis of 333 cases. Ann Rheum Dis. 1966;25(2):120–6.

9. Da Sylva D, Doran MF, Crowson CS, O'Fallon WM, Matteson EL. Declining use of orthopedic surgery in patients with rheumatoid arthritis? Results of long-term, population-based assessment. Arthritis Rheum. 2003;49:216–20.

10. Dreyer SJ, Boden SD. Natural history of rheumatoid arthritis of the cervical spine. Clin Orthop Relat Res. 1999;366:98–106.

11. Dvorak J, Grob D, Baumgartner H, Gschwend N, et al. Functional evaluation of the spinal cord by magnetic resonance imaging in patients with rheumatoid arthritis and instability of upper cervical spine. Spine. 1989;14(10):1057–64 (Phila Pa 1976).

12. Gallie WE. Fractures and dislocations of the spine. Am J Surg. 1939;46:495–9.

13. Goel A, Laheri V, Harms J, Melcher P. Posterior C1-C2 fusion with polyaxial screw and rod fixation. Spine. 2001;26:2467–71. Spine (Phila Pa 1976). 2002 Jul 15; 27(14): 1589–90.

14. Grassi W, De Angelis R, Cervini C. Corticosteroid prescribing in rheumatoid arthritis and psoriatic arthritis. Clin Rheumatol. 1998;17(3):223–6.

15. Grassi W, De Angelis R, Lamanna G, Cervini C. The clinical features of rheumatoid arthritis. Eur J Radiol. 1998;27(Suppl 1):S18–24.

16. Grob D, Magerl F, McGowan DP. Spinal pedicle fixation: reliability and validity of roentgenogram- based assessment and surgical factors on successful screw placement. Spine. 1990;15(3):251 (Phila Pa 1976).

17. Hamilton JD, Gordon M-M, McInnes IB, Johnston RA, Madhok R, Capell HA. Improved medical and surgical management of cervical spine disease in patients with rheumatoid arthritis over 10 years. Ann Rheum Dis. 2000;59:434–8.

18. Harms J, Posterior MRP. C1–C2 fusion with polyaxial screw and rod fixation. Spine. 2001;26(22):2467–71 (Phila Pa 1976).

19. Hoshino Y, Kurokawa T, Nakamura K, Seichi A, Miyoshi K. A report on the safety of unilateral vertebral artery ligation during cervical spine surgery. Spine. 1996;21(12):1454–7.

20. Katz WA, Bland JH. Shoulder, neck and thorax. In: Diagnosis and management of rheumatoid disease. 2nd ed. Philadelphia: JB Lippincott Co, 1988, p. 88–120.

21. Uchida K, Nakajima H, Sato R, Baba H. Multivariate analysis of the neurological outcome of surgery for cervical compressive myelopathy. J Orthop Sci. 2005;10(6):564–73.

22. Larson E-M, Holtas S, Zygmunt S. Pre and postoperative MR imaging of the craniocervical junction in rheumatoid arthritis. Am J Roentgenol. 1989;152:561–6.

23. Lipson SJ. Rheumatoid arthritis in the cervical spine. Clin Orthop Relat Res. 1989;239:121–7.

24. Makoto Y, Masashi N, Shunsuke F, Takashi N. Comparison of the Anatomical Risk for Vertebral Artery Injury Associated With the C2-Pedicle Screw and Atlantoaxial Transarticular Screw. Spine. 2006;31(15):E513–7.

25. Markenson JA. Worldwide trends in the socioeconomic impact and long-term prognosis of rheumatoid arthritis. Semin Arthritis Rheum. 1991;21(2 Suppl 1):4–12.

26. Matsunaga S, Ijiri K, Koga H. Results of a longer than 10-year follow-up of patients with rheumatoid arthritis treated by occipitocervical fusion. Spine. 2000;25(14):1749–53 (Phila Pa 1976).

27. Moskovich R, Crockard HA, Shott S. Occipitocervical stabilization for myelopathy in patiens with rheumatoid arthritis. J Bone Joint Surg Am. 2000;82A:349–65.

28. Nurick S. The pathogenesis of the spinal cord disorder associated with cervical spondylosis. Brain. 1972;95(1):87–100.

29. Oda T, Fujiwara K, Yonenobu K, Azuma B, Ochi T. Natural course of cervical spine lesions in rheumatoid arthritis. Spine. 1995;20(10):1128–35 (Phila Pa 1976).

30. Omura K, Hukuda S, Katsuura A, Saruhashi Y, Imanaka T, Imai S. Evaluation of posterior long fusion versus conservative treatment for the progressive rheumatoid cervical spine. Spine. 2002;27(12):1336–45 (Phila Pa 1976).

31. Pastor D. The use of electrical stimulation and exercise to increase muscle strength in a patient after surgery for cervical spondylotic myelopathy. Physiother Theory Pract. 2010;26(2):134–42.

32. Pincus T. Long-term outcomes in rheumatoid arthritis. Br J Rheumatol. 1995;34(2):59–73.

33. Rana NA. Natural history of atlanto-axial subluxation in rheumatoid arthritis. Spine. 1989;14(10):1054–6 (Phila Pa 1976).

34. Ranawat CS, O'Leary P, Pellicci P. Tsairis P Cervical spine fusion in rheumatoid arthritis. J Bone Joint Surg Am. 1979;61(7):1003–10.

35. Riew KD, Hilibrand A, Palumbo MA. Diagnosing basilar invagination in the rheumatoid patient. J Bone Joint Surg Am. 2001;83:194–200.

36. Sherk HH. Atlantoaxial instability and acquired basilar invagination in rheumatoid arthritis. Orthop Clin North Am. 1978 Oct;9(4):1053–63.

37. Singh A, Choi D, Crockard A. Use of walking data in assessing operative results for cervical spondylotic myelopathy: long-term follow-up and comparison with controls. Spine. 2009;34(12):1296–300 (Phila Pa 1976).

38. Solanki GA, Crockard HA. Peroperative determination of safe superior transarticular screw trajectory through the lateral mass. Spine. 1999;24(14):1477–82 (Phila Pa 1976).

39. Van der Heijde DM, van Riel PL, van Rijswijk MH, et al. Influence of prognostic features on the final outcome in rheumatoid arthritis: a review of the literature. Semin Arthritis Rheum. 1988;17(4):284–92.

40. Vetti N, Alsing R, Kråkenes J, Rørvik J, Gilhus NE, Brun JG, Espeland A. MRI of the transverse and alar ligaments in rheumatoid arthritis: feasibility and relations to atlantoaxial subluxation and disease aktivity. Neuroradiology. 2010;52:215–23.

41. Ward MM. Decreases in rates of hospitalization for manifestations of severe rheumatoit arthritis. Arthritis Rheum. 2004;50:1122–31.

42. Weinblatt ME. Rheumatoid arthritis: treat now, not later! Ann Intern Med. 1996;124(8):773–4.

43. Wright NM, Lauryssen C. Vertebral artery injury in C1–2 transarticular screw fixation. J Neurosurg. 1998;88:634–40.

44. Zeidman SM, Ducker TB, Raycroft J. Trends and complications in cervical spine surgery: 1989–1993. J Spinal Disord. 1997;10(6):523–6.

Thoracic Outlet Syndrome

Henk Giele

Contents

H. Giele
Oxford Radcliffe Hospitals, Oxford, UK
e-mail: henk.giele@mac.com

Abstract

Thoracic outlet syndrome (TOS) in its simplest form is postural compression of the subclavian artery causing relative ischaemia of the upper limb presenting as fatigue, claudication and pallor usually with overhead activity or caudal depression of the shoulder. The compression may become constant rather than postural, and the compression may involve the nerves of the brachial plexus rather than the artery. The classic neurological presentation is of compression of the lower roots or lower trunk of the brachial plexus presenting with severe ulnar neuropathy but including wasting of abductor pollicis brevis (the median nerve T1 innervated muscle) and including sensory disturbance of the medial forearm (the medial cutaneous nerve of the forearm arises proximally from the medial cord). However such obvious signs of severe neuropathy are very rare and usually the compression or irritation is mild, intermittent, postural, and proximal leading to ill-defined symptoms and signs. In these cases thoracic outlet syndrome is a frustrating condition to diagnose, leading many to ignore it or even refute its existence.

This chapter aims to assist in the diagnosis and treatment of thoracic outlet syndrome by explaining both the classic and difficult presentations of the syndrome, the examination manoeuvres, investigative techniques, the indications for surgery, the operative approach, outcomes and complications.

G. Bentley (ed.), *European Surgical Orthopaedics and Traumatology*,
DOI 10.1007/978-3-642-34746-7_23, © EFORT 2014

Keywords
Aetiology • Anatomy and biomechanics • Clinical diagnosis and tests • Complications • Non-operative treatment • Operative technique • Operative treatment • Results • Thoracic outlet

Box 1 Synonyms for Thoracic Outlet Syndrome
Thoracic Inlet syndrome
Scalenus Anticus syndrome
Costo-clavicular compression
Cervical rib syndrome
Nafzigger syndrome

General Introduction

Thoracic outlet syndrome like all syndromes is a constellation of symptoms and signs that allow clinical diagnosis and treatment. However unlike other syndromes the constellation of symptoms and signs in thoracic outlet syndrome are so ill-defined, that there are many doctors who doubt the existence of the condition.

The name of the condition [1, 2] refers to the symptoms and pathology arising from compression or irritation of the vessels and nerves as they pass from the chest into the neck. However only the sympathetic trunk, T1 nerve root and subclavian vessels pass through the thoracic outlet or inlet (as some prefer to name it), and as such the name is a misnomer, as the actual syndrome includes compression or irritation of all the longitudinal structures as they pass along the neck and into the arm. For example, thoracic outlet syndrome encompasses compression or other pathology except tumours, at any point along the path of the brachial plexus from the exit of the nerves from their foramina to their entry into the arm at the distal limits of the axilla, clearly involving nerves that never pass through the thoracic outlet. Compression can occur to the vessels and nerves as they descend between the scalenes, pass through the thoracic outlet if they do so, or as they pass over the first rib, still between scaleneus anterior and scaleneus medius muscles, pass under the clavicle and under pectoralis minor and around the coracoid into the arm. Hence a large number of synonyms for thoracic outlet syndrome exists (Box 1).

Apart from these normal anatomical structures the region is rich in anatomical variations, the best known being the cervical rib. The cervical rib represents the easily visualized bony evidence of an anomaly but the presence of which indicates potential for enormous variation in unseen soft tissue anomaly. To add further complexity the pathology in thoracic outlet syndrome may be positional and intermittent. The pathology can effect artery or vein or both, or the pathology may effect any or part of the nerves of the brachial plexus. Nerve compression causes symptoms by ischaemia, and proximal peripheral nerve lesions can be difficult to diagnose due to the large quantity of neural cross-over between nerve branches and fascicles. Complete inactivity of a brachial plexus root may not manifest as weakness, palsy, altered sensibility or numbness but by pain, lack of endurance, fatigue or by no symptoms at all. Indeed in most cases thoracic outlet syndrome presents as a pain syndrome. To best understand this difficult syndrome, we should examine and diagnose those discrete cases of vascular occlusion, or definite neurological loss that can be localised to the neck gaining experience before tackling the more difficult more common cases presenting with poorly defined symptoms and signs.

Aetiology and Classification

Thoracic outlet syndrome can be classified as vascular or neurogenic. Vascular cases are generally arterial but rare cases of venous compression are reported. Neurogenic cases can be true neurogenic with clearly demonstrable neural "lesions" localizable to the brachial plexus or presumed neurogenic as lesions cannot be clearly demonstrable but are suggested to arise from the plexus.

There are of course cases of involvement of both vessels and nerves complicating things further. The pathology and symptoms can be static/ constant or positional. Most commonly it is a pain syndrome but can present as a sensory or motor palsy, weakness or with claudication or loss of endurance. Thoracic outlet syndrome can also be classified according to the site of presumed pathology. Three levels of TOS exist; inter-scalene, costo-clavicular and infra-clavicular (also known as retro-pectoral).

The incidence of thoracic outlet syndrome is unknown, hardly surprising given the variation in pathology and the difficulty in diagnosis. How-ever it has been reported to occur as commonly as 1 per 1,000 people. Thoracic outlet syndrome is more common in females, perhaps as much as fivefold. It generally presents in the early twenties but can present in children and at older ages. Up to 25 % can be bilateral. Most cases are neurogenic, with 10 % being vascular and 5 % being both.

The cause of thoracic outlet syndrome is an anatomical arrangement that compresses or irri-tates passing neurological or vascular structures. The cause may often remain unknown. Why, if the cause is an anatomical arrangement or variation, do symptoms only arise later in life? If the anatom-ical arrangement partially compresses or just irri-tates the vessels then prolonged repetitive insults must occur before intimal and structural changes become apparent in the vessel wall [3]. With increasing age the tolerance of the peripheral nerves to ischaemia and irritation diminishes and the adaptations and postural mechanisms to avoid compression become more difficult. The descent of the scapula is more common and marked in women and, associated with age, increases the tension in the plexus and reduces the costo-clavicular space. These patients frequently have a slumped posture, steep supra-clavicular slopes, a less concave supra-clavicular fossa, apparently long necks and protracted shoulders. There is an association with large breasts perhaps as these contribute to poor posture or by traction on the shoulders producing acromio-clavicular descent. There may have been a recent increase in weight as there is a weak association with being over

weight. Frequently there has been a preceding history of carpal and/or cubital tunnel release. There is an association with occupations that involve working with the arms elevated such as hair dressers, teachers, brick layers and plas-terers, swimmers and weight-lifters, either due to the provocative postures these occupa-tions adopt or because these postures cause functional changes to the scalenes or other structures provoking thoracic outlet syndrome. Finally it may be that an element of trauma either acute or cumulative may be necessary in some cases in order to create fibrosis or muscu-lar spasm or inflammation before the symptoms arise. Contraction or spasm of the scalene mus-cles resulting from irritation of their nerve supply from the brachial plexus or other rea-sons, causes elevation of the first rib, causing greater irritation and the establishment of a vicious cycle [4].

Relevant Applied Anatomy, Pathology and Basic Science: Biomechanics

The anatomy of the region is the anatomy of the posterior triangle of the neck. The bony land-marks are the first rib extending from the trans-verse process to the manubrium, the cervical vertebrae especially the foramen of the C5-8 and T1 nerves and the lateral processes, the clavicle and in the infra-clavicular fossa, the coracoid. The roots of the brachial plexus emerge from the foramina lying anterior to the scalenus medius, which runs from origins on the transverse processes to insertions on the middle and posterior portions of the cranial and lateral aspects of the first and second rib. The long thoracic nerve arising from C5, 6 and 7 merges within the scalenus medius and travels through it. Anterior to the plexus and the sub-clavian artery lies the scalenius anterior inserting onto the anterior portion of the first rib. Anterior to this muscle lies the phrenic nerve, which is seldom involved in TOS, and the subclavian vein. The subclavian artery and plexus to a lesser extent cause a shallow groove in the cranial surface of the first rib called the

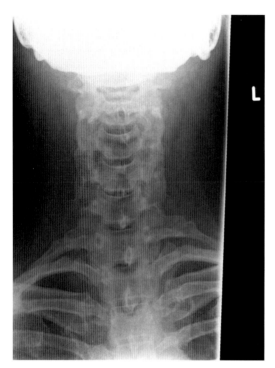

Fig. 1 Anatomy of the thoracic outlet

inter-scalene groove. The plexus is stacked vertically as it passes between the scalenes over the first rib, so that the lower trunk has most contact and deviation, hence the predominance of symptoms in this distribution. The plexus and artery as they pass over the rib emerging from behind scalenus anterior are confined posteriorly and inferiorly by the scalenus medius-covered ribs, and anteriorly by the fat pad, and the clavicle. Depression of the clavicle or abduction of the shoulder reduces this space and can lead to compression of the structures. Hence the exacerbation of symptoms when working with the arms overhead or when carrying heavy objects. The structures then pass under the clavicle medial to the coracoid under the insertion of pectoralis minor to enter the arm. Here too, they can get compressed or irritated in the relatively uncommon infra-clavicular TOS (Fig. 1).

Common bone anatomical anomalies associated with thoracic outlet syndrome are cervical ribs, and long transverse processes of the C7 vertebrae. Cervical ribs occur in 0.2–0.5 % of the population but are over-represented in thoracic outlet syndrome sufferers (10 %), either because cervical ribs cause thoracic outlet syndrome or because the presence of the cervical rib re-inforces the diagnosis. The cervical rib can be complete articulating with the manubrium, complete by articulating with the first rib (usually by a large tubercle at the level of the interscalene groove), or partial whereby it does not articulate but the anterior end of the rib but is attached by fibrous bands extending to to the first rib or sternum. An over-long C7 transverse process may represent a vestigial attempt to develop a cervical rib or be associated with soft tissue anomalies that may compromise the passage of the nerves and vessels into the arm. An elongated C7 transverse process, one which extends beyond the lateral limits of the T1 process, may be associated with a scalenus intermedius muscle. Clavicle distortion from osteoma or non- or mal-union can reduce the costo-clavicular space producing symptoms particularly on depression of the shoulder. Bone tumours affecting the first rib or clavicle such as exostoses or fibrous dysplasia can compromise the space for transit of the structures.

The soft tissue anomalies are more varied, harder to identify and difficult to detect preoperatively. The scalenes may hypertrophy in response to exercise, especially in weight-lifters and swimmers. The scalenes may have a common origin and only split late in their descent down the neck reducing the interscalene space. The scalenes may have well-developed aponeuroses that present sharp edges or hard surfaces with which to compress components of the plexus or vessels. The scalenes may have anomalous insertions on to the first rib such that the inter-scalene groove is obliterated or narrowed. Roos described and classified 9 different anomalous scalene bands that could cause TOS [5]. Anomalous muscles such as the scalene intermedius or minimus-that arises from the transverse processes and inserts onto the dome of the pleura, may occur and compromise the T1 root [6].

The pathomechanics of nerve compression are oedema, ischaemia, demyelination,

Schwann- cell necrosis and axonal injury, the degree of which correlates with the severity and chronicity of the compression. The peripheral axons can be severely affected whilst those in the centre or located away from the stimulus can be unaffected. This particularly relative to the size of the nerves, and the large number and variety of inter-connections between nerves at the brachial plexus level explain the vagueness of symptoms and signs.

Diagnosis

Thoracic outlet syndrome is often said to be a diagnosis of exclusion and indeed one has to exclude other peripheral nerve compression disorders and radiculopathy. Unfortunately carpal tunnel syndrome can on occasions present with thoracic outlet syndrome-like symptoms. One must have an awareness of thoracic outlet syndrome in order to consider it as part of the differential diagnosis of a patient presenting with upper limb pain, paraesthesia, numbness, weakness, or other vague symptoms. If you do not look for TOS, you will never diagnose it.

History

Pain

The common presentation is of arm pain. Classic vascular thoracic outlet syndrome presents with claudication type aching associated with activity especially with arm elevation. Classic neurological thoracic outlet syndrome affecting the lower trunk presents with dull aching pain in the ulnar nerve distribution but including the medial forearm, often when carrying heavy objects or on arm elevation. However the arm pain can be in any distribution depending on which part of the plexus is involved. Upper trunk TOS may present with shoulder and lateral arm pain, and middle trunk or posterior cord involvement with pain experienced at the back of the arm, elbow or forearm. The pain or sensory symptoms may not be in a known peripheral nerve distribution or dermatome. The pain could be described as

constant or intermittent, burning or aching, sharp or dull, provokable or unchanging. There may be associated pain affecting the neck, shoulder, para-scapular region, back, face and descriptions of headache. Some of these secondary pain symptoms may be related to mechanisms employed to avoid vascular or neural compression such as elevating the clavicles and protracting the shoulders to enlarge the costo-clavicular space.

Vasomotor Symptoms

These symptoms are generally not the main presenting complaint but can often be elicited. They reflect either the involvement of the sympathetic nerves or disturbance of the neural pathways of sweating, temperature regulation, vascularity and permeability of vessels. Either hypo- or hyperhidrosis may occur, exaggerated cutaneous colour change in response to ambient temperature or emotion and the hands may be described as being constantly cold or hot; there may be a complaint of swelling. Other vascular symptoms are end-stage presentations of digital gangrene, evidence of emboli, or of venous congestion.

Motor Symptoms

Weakness or lack of endurance are common features of thoracic outlet syndrome particularly with activities overhead or carrying weights. Dropping objects and clumsiness are recalled similar to carpal and cubital tunnel syndromes.

Examination

Musculoskeletal

Examination of the upper limb should ensure normal passive range of motion of the joints, absence of injuries that might explain neurological lesions, and exclude disorders such as a frozen shoulder, medial epicondylitis, or pisi-triquetral arthritis.

Vascular

Examine for venous distention particularly in postures such as arm elevation or depression.

Venous engorgement, cyanosis and swelling may indicate venous obstruction. In severe cases this may indicate subclavian or axillary vein thrombosis known as Paget-Schroetter syndrome. Feel and compare the pulses between arms, and at different sites of the upper limb. Embolic phenomena such as nail bed infarcts, Raynaud's phenomenon and gangrene may rarely be present. Bruits should be excluded by careful auscultation.

Neurological

Examination should include a complete upper limb neurological examination. In classic TOS there may be sensory disturbance in the ulnar nerve distribution but in addition involvement of the medial cutaneous nerve of forearm indicating a proximal lesion (as this branch arises from the medial cord of the plexus and indicates thoracic outlet syndrome rather than ulnar neuropathy). Sensory disturbance can occur in any distribution depending on the elements of the plexus involved. There may be no sensory disturbance present. In classic TOS, motor signs may include intrinsic weakness or wasting involving both ulnar and median-innervated intrinsics indicating a T1 or lower trunk lesion, but more commonly there are no such signs. Fatigue and reduced endurance are difficult to assess. Carpal and cubital tunnel syndrome should be excluded using standard examination techniques for these conditions and their provocative tests.

Neck

The range of neck motion should be checked to elicit any evidence of cervical arthropathy.

Provocative Tests

The provocative tests for thoracic outlet syndrome are less sensitive and specific than those for carpal tunnel and cubital tunnel syndrome but are presented here for completeness.

Adson's test [7] involves adducting the arm, extending the neck and rotating it towards the affected side thereby stretching the scalenes. The arm is gently retracted downwards depressing the clavicle as the patient is requested to inspire deeply and hold their breath. This elevates the first rib and contracts the scalenes. A positive test is one that elicits a reduction or cessation of the radial pulse or provocation of the pain or sensory symptoms. The pathogenesis of the positive test is thought to be stretching of the scalenes and their aponeuroses or anomalous associated bands compressing the artery or plexus.

Reverse Adson's test [8] involves the same arm position, breath holding and downward retraction but the head and neck are held flexed and rotated away from the affected side thereby allowing the scalenes to contract and bulge compressing the plexus.

Wright's hyper-abduction test [9] assesses the radial pulse when the arm is abducted. Loss of the pulse is a positive test but occurs in 25 % of asymptomatic people. The mechanism is thought to be compression of the subclavian artery as it courses around the coracoid and may indicate an infra-clavicular thoracic outlet syndrome. However, imaging studies show that the costo-clavicular space and the retro-pectoralis space are both decreased with arm elevation.

Falconer's test [10] or the military brace position or costo-clavicular compression test, also sometimes called Halstead's test, places the shoulders in an extended retropulsed position with slight downward traction of the arms whilst feeling the radial pulses. A positive test is a diminution or obliteration of the pulse or provocation of the neurological symptoms. This position probably exaggerates costo-clavicular compression. Narakas's test abducts the arm to 90° with traction and provokes symptoms.

Spurling's test differentiates radiculopathy from brachial plexopathy by provoking symptoms with compression on the vertex either when the neck is laterally flexed towards the affected side or away from the affected side respectively.

The cervical rotation lateral flexion test [11] is positive when there is reduced neck flexion when the head is turned away from the affected side compared to when it is turned towards the affected side. The mechanism of this test is suggested to be that subluxation of the first rib attachment to the transverse process reduces flexion on rotation and displaces the brachial plexus anteriorly thus reducing the space for it's passage through the neck.

Roos' elevated arm stress test (EAST) [12] is non -specific with provocation of symptoms in patients with carpal tunnel and cubital tunnel syndrome as well as in thoracic outlet syndrome. The Roos test is performed by abducting and elevating the arms in external rotation with the elbows flexed and then flexing and extending the digits for 2 min and observing for pallor of the hand and provocation of symptoms including claudication of the forearm muscles.

Gage's test [13] detects tenderness of the scalenes which are thought to be inflamed in cases of thoracic outlet syndrome. Gage went further in then injecting local anaesthetic into the scalenes which he considered indicative of thoracic outlet syndrome if it resulted in temporary resolution of symptoms.

Morley's compression test [14] is provocation of the neurological symptoms when gently compressing the plexus in the supra-clavicular fossa. This test is the most compelling clinical sign of thoracic outlet syndrome in my experience. The plexus may also be tender and Tinel's test may provoke pain or paraesthesia.

Though each test independently may be of limited value due to low sensitivity and specificity, we have found that if a patient has three or more positive clinical signs they are more likely to benefit from surgery. I perform all the provocative tests other than the injection of local anesthesia.

Investigations

Neurophysiology

When thoracic outlet syndrome is suspected nerve conduction studies including EMG should be requested asking the neurophysiologist to investigate for carpal and cubital tunnel syndrome as well as for any evidence of brachioplexopathy. In the classic true neurologic thoracic outlet syndrome the neurophysiology may demonstrate denervation changes on electromyography, and more rarely with increased severity and duration of "compression" there may be changes in F-latency and SEP. Reduced nerve conduction is a late neurophysiological sign usually correlating to easily detected clinical signs [15]. Localization of the lesion can be helpful if nerve conduction studies detect involvement of the medial cutaneous nerve of forearm in cases presenting as ulnar neuropathy. However the main usefulness in TOS for neurophysiological studies is to exclude carpal and cubital tunnel syndromes.

Imaging

Part of the difficulty in imaging this syndrome is that it is a dynamic syndrome and that posture pays a large component. Imaging is generally static and performed supine. MRI is the main imaging technique in TOS [16]. MRI should be arranged for the cervical vertebrae to exclude cervical causes of the symptoms such as disc prolapse with root compression. MRI of the brachial plexus may demonstrate deviation of the plexus over or around anomalous structures, but rarely shows the anomalous structures themselves. The MRI may show compression of the subclavian vessels and post-stenotic dilatation. However, a negative MRI does not exclude TOS, importantly though it will exclude a tumour such as a Pancoast-Tobias tumour of the apex of the lung as the cause of symptoms. Plain radiographs of the chest and neck should be requested as MRI may not detect cervical ribs, elongated transverse processes or other bony abnormalities. MRA may be necessary if vessel occlusion or partial obstruction are considered. CTA may allow comparison between different postures of the arm. MRA and CTA in this region should obviate the need for angiography. Both can detect occlusion but find it harder to discriminate normal and abnormal compression with postural changes. Ultrasound can be helpful as a dynamic imaging technique as the plexus can be viewed in differing arm positions.

Treatment and Indications for Surgery

Non-Operative

The initial treatment of thoracic outlet syndrome is always non-operative. This comprises analgesia, relaxants, and physiotherapy. The therapy is aimed at relaxing and stretching the scalenes, strengthening the scapula muscles to increase shoulder support, increase shoulder and scapula mobility, increase the costo-clavicular space by improvement of posture, elevation of the shoulder acromio-clavicular joint and implementation of strategies to avoid provocative postures [17, 18]. These strategies may show response within 3 weeks but if not, should continue to be trialled for 3 months. Analgesics are usually NSAID's, and neuropathic pain medications such as gabapentin or pregabalin, coupled with anti-depressants such as amitriptylene to aid sleep if required. Recently botulinum toxin denervation of the scalenes has been reported to provide symptomatic relief for those waiting for surgery [19].

Operative

The indications for operative treatment are failure of conservative non-operative management, the absence or exclusion of other peripheral neuropathies or failure of resolution of symptoms following surgical release of the carpal tunnel and cubital tunnel, and continuing symptoms and signs diagnostic for thoracic outlet syndrome. The operation offered is an exploration of the brachial plexus and subclavian artery, and decompression and neurolysis depending on intra-operative findings. As such the patients should be informed that the chance of improvement is only 50 %, though in reality with good patient selection the outcomes are much better.

Operative Technique

Various approaches described for thoracic outlet syndrome, the supra-clavicular, the infra-clavicular, the posterior and the axillary, along with combined approaches. The supra-clavicular approach is the preferred approach to thoracic outlet syndrome, and will be described in detail below. The axillary approach involves an axillary incision with the patient in the lateral position and extra-thoracically removing the cervical or first rib. This axillary approach does not directly explore or release the vessels or plexus. Though this approach delivers an increased costo-clavicular space, this approach fails to address the possible suspension of the plexus by anomalous bands between the scalenes or a scalenus minimus or allow for a neurolysis and so is less useful for neurogenic thoracic outlet syndrome. The posterior approach incises through the trapezius, levator scapulae and scalenus medius to expose the plexus from behind.

Supra-Clavicular Exploration Technique

The procedure involves a general anaesthetic. The patient is positioned supine, with the head turned away from the affected side, and the neck extended with a bolster in the ipsi-lateral trapezius region. The neck, axilla and arm is prepped leaving the sternal notch and upper sternum exposed as well as the clavicle, axilla, whole upper limb including shoulder. After infiltration with local anesthesia with adrenaline, a 5–7 cm. long supra-clavicular incision is made above the mid-point of the clavicle. This is deepened through platysma. The lateral clavicular insertion of sternomastoid is divided, leaving a cuff on the clavicle to facilitate later repair. The lateral border of sternomastoid is released from the fascia. The fascia is incised just above and parallel to the clavicle, exposing the supraclavicular nerves and external jugular vein which are retracted laterally. Omohyoid is identified lying a little more cranially and medially. The medial belly of omohyoid points to the level of the C5 root. Omohyoid is retracted superiorly and held there with a small self-retainer. The deep fascia is incised and the pre-plexural fat pad is swept cranially exposing the plexus. The transverse cervical and dorsal scapular vessels may be within this fat pad and need to be divided but can sometimes be retracted intact. The divisions of the upper trunk of the brachial plexus lie most superficially and are the first exposed and, following this, the middle and lower trunk. Scalenus anterior is identified medially, as is the phrenic nerve lying superficially upon it, running from lateral to medial as it courses towards the chest. The lateral border of the anterior scalene is incised freeing it from the thin fascial sheet covering it and the plexus. Scalenus anterior is retracted medially exposing the roots and the subclavian artery. The relationship of the scalenes, artery and plexus is explored. For example a frequent cause of thoracic outlet syndrome is an anomalous insertion of scaleneus medius onto the first rib extending too far anteriorly inter-digitating with the anterior scalene thus obliterating the inter-scalene groove, and causing the plexus to have to cross this part of the scalenus medius as well as the first rib as it traverses inferiorly. These anomalies are frequently fibrous or aponeurotic and have been described as bands.

The lower insertion of scaleneus anterior to the first rib is divided and the distal 1–2 cm of muscle excised to prevent it's re-attachment, protecting the phrenic nerve (superficial) and the subclavian artery (deep) from injury. The artery is released and the plexus is neurolysed. If a cervical rib is present this is exposed superior and inferior to the plexus and removed at this stage. The costo-clavicular space is assessed by placing a finger under the clavicle over the plexus and then abducting the arm. A tight space will pinch the finger preventing full abduction, indicating that first rib excision is necessary. The first rib is dissected by releasing the attachment of scalenus medius superiorly and the intercostals inferiorly. A Cloward's punch is used to nibble across the neck of the first rib and then across the body as far anterior as possible. The rib is then removed, and the costo-clavicular space checked again. If the finger is no longer squeezed between clavicle and the second rib on abduction of the arm then sufficient space has been created for the safe passage of the plexus and vessels. The cavity is filled with saline and a Valsalva manoeuvre requested from the anesthetist to check for a pneumothorax and air leak. There is commonly a parietal pleural hole allowing fluid and air to enter the thorax, but a true air leak from a visceral pleural injury is uncommon. If an air leak is present a chest tube with an underwater seal is inserted through the lateral fourth intercostal space. The fat pad is replaced over the plexus, and the omohyoid restored. The sternomastoid is repaired as well as the platysma and skin. No drain is inserted as the wound is usually dry. The arm is placed in a "broad-arm"sling.

Post-Operative Care and Rehabilitation

Regular analgesia is prescribed. The patient is encouraged to mobilise the shoulder and arm as comfort allows and to remove the sling as soon as possible. As in other nerve decompressions, immediate mobilization of the joints prevents adhesions of the nerve and joint stiffness. Deep breathing exercises are encouraged especially if there is pleuritic pain. The wound is reviewed at 2 weeks by which time the sling should be discarded. Discomfort around the operation site is common for a few weeks but should not prevent full range of motion of the shoulder and arm.

Outcomes

Outcomes of operative exploration vary according to the indication. If definite neurological or vascular thoracic outlet syndrome are present then relief of symptoms is predictable; however in the majority of indefinite cases symptomatic relief is less predictable. Similarly if identifiable anatomical anomalies are detected pre-operatively there is a greater chance of a successful outcome. Reported outcomes are extremely variable, ranging from 37 % to 90 % improvement [20, 21]. The large variation in reported outcomes reflects the difficulty in diagnosis, assessment and measuring symptoms, the variation in patient selection and surgical procedure, and the variation in outcome measures. It is most simple to report improvement of symptoms on a grade as excellent to poor; a few report measures such as DASH or SF-12. Study numbers range from 700 or more to less than 20 [22]. For example, Scali [23] reported an average 8 year follow-up on 26 patients with neurogenic thoracic outlet syndrome diagnosed by a positive Roos test or postive response to scalene block, treated by scalenotomy alone (2), scalenectomy plus cervical rib excision (6), scalenectomy plus first rib excision (18), eight cases were done by the axillary approach and the rest by the supra-clavicular. Two cases (9 %) required further operations. Of the 26 patients 22 were followed up, 72 % returned to work, and 68 % reported their outcomes as good or excellent. 27 % still used narcotics post-operatively.

Outcomes are reported to be much worse if symptoms have persisted for greater then 24 months [24], or if the patients are involved in compensation [25]. Poorer outcomes were also associated with acute ischaemia, sensory or motor deficit, poorly systematized neurological symptoms as presenting complaints, extended resection of the first rib, and severe post-operative complications [26]. The importance of complete posterior resection of the first rib was emphasized by correlation of outcomes with length of posterior stump of first rib [27].

Recurrent thoracic outlet syndrome occurs in up to 50 % of indefinite cases usually within 2 years [28]. These may warrant re-exploration, but the outcomes are even less predictable, but can be excellent.

Complications

The commonest complication is failure of resolution of all the symptoms. The patients frequently report improvement but less commonly complete cure. In most cases the symptoms recede to a level at which no further intervention is necessary. However, if symptoms fail to resolve then the diagnosis should be re-examined and efforts made to re-investigate and again confirm or refute other potential diagnoses. If there has been little or no improvement with the operation then the diagnosis is incorrect, the nerves intrinsically injured beyond recovery (though this state should be identifiable preoperatively by neurophysiology), or incomplete decompression performed.

The second commonest complication is recurrence of symptoms. If this occurs the history and examination and investigation of the patient should be repeated. Symptoms may recur due to scarring, progressive neural changes from the previous insult, recurrence of the compression due to further descent of the shoulder or loss of ability to compensate or accommodate for the compression. If other diagnoses are excluded and the diagnosis of thoracic outlet syndrome is secure then re-exploration of the plexus and vessels may be indicated. This is particularly indicated if the initial procedure involved either scalenus anterior release, or cervical rib excision alone preserving the first rib. It is for this reason that a complete release comprising the above *and* first rib excision is recommended by some surgeons. Some surgeons excise only a small middle segment of the first rib but then the remaining anterior or posterior segments under the traction of the scalenes can migrate superiorly causing recurrent compression. First rib excision should be complete posteriorly and extend sufficiently anterior such that upward migration of any remaining rib would be medial to the passage of the plexus and artery. Supra-clavicular and retro-clavicular decompression will not be effective for infra-clavicular thoracic outlet syndrome for which an infra-clavicular exploration and pectoralis minor release is required. The possibility of infra-clavicular thoracic outlet syndrome should be considered.

In recalcitrant thoracic outlet syndrome with notable fibrosis around or within the plexus, there may be benefit in wrapping the plexus in a well vascularised layer of fat in order to protect it from further injury and provide a gliding layer under the clavicle. This fat can be transferred from the deltopectoral region obtained through the same supra-clavicular incision, or as a free tissue transfer of omentum or groin fat. Alternatively the superficial fascia from pectoralis major can be transferred.

Operative complications are bleeding, chyle leak and seroma, pneumothorax, haemothorax or pleural effusion, numbness of the operative site extending onto the anterior chest, injury to the phrenic nerve, brachial plexus, sympathetic chain or recurrent laryngeal nerve, shoulder stiffness, neural adhesions and recurrence.

Bleeding is usually minor but can be more worrying wih rupture of the subclavian artery from atheromatous plaques and post-stenotic aneurysmal dilation associated with compression of the artery. Deaths have been reported from catastrophic hemorrhage. Prevent catastrophic bleeding by gentle retraction of the artery only if necessary. Be prepared to split the chest to expose the origin of the subclavian artery if uncontrolled bleeding occurs. Chyle leak and seroma result from injury to the thoracic duct as it enters the subclavian vein at the root of the neck. If injury to the thoracic duct or its branches are seen at time of operation then the leak must be ligated or clipped, as diathermy is not effective. If a chyloma appears post-operatively then the patient should be placed on a low fat diet until the leak stops and the swelling or drainage diminishes. Injury to the phrenic nerve may result in respiratory difficulties requiring intensive care support for some days post-operatively or leading to basal lung collapse and infection. Longer term shortness of breath from diaphragm palsy can result, necessitating diaphragmatic plication. Pleural effusion or haemothorax results from usually small quantities of blood or fluid tracking from the operative site into the pleural space causing pleuritic pain. Very rarely the pleural defect is made in the parenchymal pleura leading to an air leak and requiring the placement of a chest drain. Injury to the brachial plexus from traction on retracting, is usually at worst a temporary neurapraxia causing some discomfort and weakness, that recovers within a couple of months. Injury to the sympathetic chain results in a Horner's syndrome for which no intervention is necessary other than reassurance as it usually resolves. Injury to the recurrent laryngeal nerve is mainly a theoretical possibility due to its proximity to the operative site. The numbness of the operative site can extend onto the anterior chest wall down as far as the nipples due to injury to the supraclavicular nerves that traverse the incision. Despite the best attempts to preserve these supraclavicular nerves, they frequently get stretched or divided. The patient should be encouraged to desensitize the area to reduce the hypersensitivity as neural ingrowth from surrounding areas occurs.

Summary

Thoracic Outlet syndrome is a complicated nebulous syndrome as it encompasses a diverse array of pathologies affecting the subclavian artery, vein and brachial plexus causing perplexing symptoms and signs and only corralled together by virtue of their anatomical arrangement as they depart the axial skeleton for the upper limb. There are those surgeons who doubt the existence of such a nebulous condition, and others who diagnose every hand complaint as thoracic outlet syndrome. The truth must lie between the two camps. If one is not aware of the possibility of thoracic outlet syndrome and how to diagnose it, then one will never consider its diagnosis. Careful diagnosis and patient selection can result in excellent resolution of symptoms either from physiotherapy or following surgical intervention. The surgery is challenging but rewarding technically and on outcomes.

Box 2 Differential Diagnoses for Symptoms of Thoracic Outlet Syndrome
Carpal tunnel syndrome
Cubital tunnel syndrome
Radial tunnel syndrome
Parsonage Turner or Amyotrophy
Raynaud's phenomenon
Vibration white finger
Reflex sympathetic dystrophy or chronic regional pain syndrome
Supra-scapular nerve compression
Sub-acromial bursitis
Rotator cuff injuries
Cervical arthritis

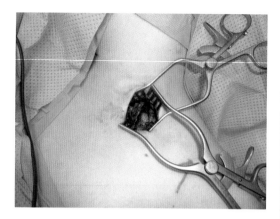

Fig. 2 The incision and exposure from the supraclavicular approach. Note the mass in the wound

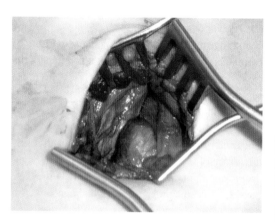

Fig. 3 The mass is bony (dome-shaped protruding from the bottom of the wound) and displaces the upper trunk of the plexus anterior and superior (on the right of the wound) and the middle trunk cranially. Scalenus anterior lies medial. Unseen, the subcavian artery is compressed between the mass and the posterior edge of scalenus anterior

Box 3 Complications of Brachial Plexus Exploration, Artery and Neurolysis and Excision of Cervical and First Rib
Immediate
- Bleeding
- Pleural hole leading to haemothorax
- Pneumothorax
- Injury to nerves-brachial plexus, phrenic, sympathetic, recurrent laryngeal, long thoracic, resulting in palsy, numbness, raised diaphragm, chest infection, dyspnoea,

sympathetic changes to the limb and a Horner's syndrome, hoarseness, change in voice, scapula winging.
Early
- Pleuritic pain
- Chest infection
- Hematoma and wound infection
- Shoulder stiffness
- Weakness
- Chyle leak

Late
- Numbness or allodynia in supraclavicular nerve distribution
- Recurrence
- Shoulder stiffness

Box 4 An Illustrative Case
A 16 year-old girl presented with a 12-month history of left arm fatigue, and left para-scapular and shoulder pain and ache extending down the lateral aspect of the arm, into the dorsum of the forearm. There was associated positional global hand paraesthesia. Her symptoms were exacerbated by arm elevation performed as part of her training as a hairdresser.

On examination, she had no sensory loss, no motor weakness, but fatigue on repetitive testing. Examination showed loss of her radial pulse on arm abduction, and some reduction in pulse volume with Adson's test. Palpation of her neck revealed a palpable mass in the left supraclavicular fossa, gentle pressure on which provoked her symptoms. Roos test also provoked her symptoms.

Her cervical radiograph showed the cervical rib. The MRI showed the cervical rib but no anomaly to the plexus. The neurophysiological studies were normal.

She had no improvement with 3 months of therapy and was offered surgery. After

(continued)

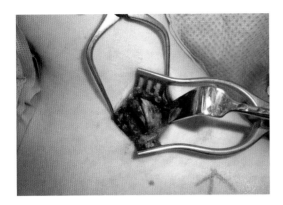

Fig. 4 The scalenus anterior, cervical and first rib having been excised, the subclavian artery and the plexus can now be seen passing unimpeded through the thoracic outlet

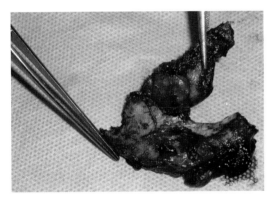

Fig. 5 The excised specimen showing the cervical rib superiorly, descending anteriorly to form a nodular articulation with the first rib, which was the mass viewed in Figs. 2 and 3. Orientation is vertebrae to the right of the picture and sternum to the left

Box 4 An Illustrative Case (continued)

incision and exposure the prominent mass was confirmed to be the articulation between the cervical and first rib at the level of the scalene groove (Fig. 2). Closer examination showed (Fig. 3) that the mass was causing deviation of the plexus and compression of the subclavian artery. The scalenus anterior was released with excision of the distal few centimetres. The cervical rib was excised. Assessment of the costo-clavicular space showed this was

still tight and hence the first rib was also excised. The resulting defect (Fig. 4) allowed tension free passage of the brachial plexus through the thoracic outlet, and released the subclavian artery, which had a post-stenotic dilatation. Reconstruction of the cervical rib and first rib articulation on the table demonstrates the space this mass occupied (Fig. 5).

Post-operatively there were no complications and complete resolution of her symptoms.

References

1. Peet RM, et al. Thoracic-outlet syndrome: evaluation of a therapeutic exercise program. Proc Staff Meet Mayo Clin. 1956;31(9):281–7.
2. Roos DB. Historical perspectives and anatomic considerations. Thoracic outlet syndrome. Semin Thorac Cardiovasc Surg. 1996;8(2):183–9.
3. Eden K. The vascular complications of cervical ribs and first thoracic rib abnormalities. Br J Surg. 1939;27(105):111–39.
4. Ochsner A, Gage M, DeBakey M. Scalenus anticus (Naffziger) syndrome. Am J Surg. 1935;28:669–71.
5. Roos DB. Congenital anomalies associated with thoracic outlet syndrome. Anatomy, symptoms, diagnosis, and treatment. Am J Surg. 1976;132(6):771–8.
6. Lawson FL, Mc KK. The scalenus minimus muscle. Can Med Assoc J. 1951;65(4):358–61.
7. Adson AW, Coffey JR. Cervical ribs:a method of anterior approach for relief of symptoms by division of scalenus anticus. Ann Surg. 1927;85:839–57.
8. Adson AW. Surgical treatment for symptoms produced by cervical ribs and the scalenus anticus muscle. Surg Gynecol Obstet. 1947;85(6):687–700.
9. Wright IS. The neurovascular syndrome produced by hyperabduction of the arms. Am Heart J. 1945;29(1):1–19.
10. Falconer MA, Weddell G. Costoclavicular compression of the subclavian artery and vein: relation to the scalenus anticus syndrome. Lancet. 1943;242(6270):539–44.
11. Lindgren KA. Conservative treatment of thoracic outlet syndrome: a 2-year follow-up. Arch Phys Med Rehabil. 1997;78(4):373–8.
12. Roos DB. Transaxillary approach for first rib resection to relieve thoracic outlet syndrome. Ann Surg. 1966;163(3):354–8.

13. Gage M, Parnell H. Scalenus anticus syndrome. Am J Surg. 1947;73(2):252–68.
14. Morley J. Brachial pressure neuritis due to a normal first thoracic rib: its diagnosis and treatment by excision of rib. Clin J. 1913;XLII(29):461–3.
15. Passero S, Paradiso C, Giannini F, Cioni R, Burgalassi L, Battistini N. Diagnosis of thoracic outlet syndrome Relative value of electrophysiological studies. Acta Neurol Scand. 1994;90:179–85.
16. Demondion X, et al. Imaging assessment of thoracic outlet syndrome. Radiographics. 2006;26(6):1735–50.
17. Aligne C, Barral X. Rehabilitation of patients with thoracic outlet syndrome. Ann Vasc Surg. 1992;6(4):381–9.
18. Kenny RA, et al. Thoracic outlet syndrome: a useful exercise treatment option. Am J Surg. 1993;165(2):282–4.
19. Jordan SE, et al. Selective botulinum chemodenervation of the scalene muscles for treatment of neurogenic thoracic outlet syndrome. Ann Vasc Surg. 2000;14(4):365–9.
20. Lepantalo M, et al. Long term outcome after resection of the first rib for thoracic outlet syndrome. Br J Surg. 1989;76(12):1255–6.
21. Bhattacharya V, et al. Outcome following surgery for thoracic outlet syndrome. Eur J Vasc Endovasc Surg. 2003;26(2):170–5.
22. Hempel GK, et al. 770 consecutive supraclavicular first rib resections for thoracic outlet syndrome. Ann Vasc Surg. 1996;10(5):456–63.
23. Scali S, et al. Long-term functional results for the surgical management of neurogenic thoracic outlet syndrome. Vasc Endovascular Surg. 2010;44(7):550–5.
24. Cheng SW, et al. Neurogenic thoracic outlet decompression: rationale for sparing the first rib. Cardiovasc Surg. 1995;3(6):617–23. discussion: 624.
25. Franklin GM, et al. Outcome of surgery for thoracic outlet syndrome in Washington state workers' compensation. Neurology. 2000;54(6):1252–7.
26. Degeorges R, Reynaud C, Becquemin JP. Thoracic outlet syndrome surgery: long-term functional results. Ann Vasc Surg. 2004;18(5):558–65.
27. Mingoli A, et al. Long-term outcome after transaxillary approach for thoracic outlet syndrome. Surgery. 1995;118(5):840–4.
28. Altobelli GG, et al. Thoracic outlet syndrome: pattern of clinical success after operative decompression. J Vasc Surg. 2005;42(1):122–8.

Conservative Management of Spinal Deformity in Childhood

Federico Canavese, Dimitri Ceroni, and André Kaelin

Contents

Federico Canavese is the author of the section
"Conservative Treatment of Idiopathic Scoliosis" and
Dimitri Ceroni is the author of the section "Conservative
Management of Kyphosis"

F. Canavese
Department of Pediatric Surgery, University Hospital
Estaing, Clermont Ferrand, France
e-mail: canavese_federico@yahoo.fr

D. Ceroni
Department of Paediatric Orthopaedics, Children's
Hospital and University Hospital Geneva, Geneva,
Switzerland
e-mail: dimitri.ceroni@hcuge.ch

A. Kaelin (✉)
Clinique des Grangettes, Chêne-Bougeries, Switzerland
e-mail: andre.kaelin@grangettes.ch

Abstract

Casting and bracing for spinal deformities are very traditional ways of stabilizing or correcting spinal deformities during growth. There is still open debate about their influence in positive outcome.

Indications for bracing for scoliosis and kyphosis in the growing period depend on accurate history and clinical examination, as well as imaging and documentation of progression. Bracing systems must be effective and tolerable for the patients. The team conducting the treatment must be convinced of its effectiveness and transmit this conviction to the patient and his family. These are the basic conditions for a successful treatment. In the following paper, scoliosis treatment and kyphosis treatment are discussed.

Keywords

Conservative Orthopaedic treatment • Idiopathic scoliosis • Kyphosis • Physical therapy • Scoliosis • Spinal braces • Spine • Spine deformities • Spine growth • Unbalanced spine

Conservative Treatment of Idiopathic Scoliosis

Introduction

The strategy for the treatment of idiopathic scoliosis depends upon the size and pattern of the deformity, and its potential for progression.

During the past decade, several studies have confirmed that the natural history of adolescent idiopathic scoliosis can be positively affected by non-operative treatment, particularly bracing [1–6]. The primary objective of non-operative treatment is to successfully arrest progressive curves or correct curves that cause or may likely cause disability. Orthotic device selection is based on the type and level of the curve and the anticipated tolerance of the patient. Avoidance of unnecessary surgery, cosmetic improvement, and an increase of vital capacity as well as pain control, are also of major importance [7–14].

In 1985, the Scoliosis Research Society (SRS) initiated a controlled clinical trial study to investigate the effectiveness of bracing as treatment for scoliosis. Patients of the same age, curve pattern and curve severity were divided into two groups, one treated with bracing and one untreated. Results published in 1993 demonstrated that brace treatment was effective compared with natural history [2]. In another study [3], the records and radiographs of more than 1,000 scoliotic patients treated by bracing were reviewed and compared with unbraced patients [15]. This retrospective study confirmed that bracing was an effective treatment to slow or arrest the progression of most spinal curvatures in skeletally-immature patients compared with those untreated by this method. Furthermore, a meta-analysis of 20 studies showed that bracing 23 h per day was significantly more successful than any other non-operative treatment [4, 6]. Nevertheless, there are some patients for whom brace treatment is not effective [16].

Other forms of non-surgical treatment, such as chiropractic or osteopathic manipulation, acupuncture, exercise or other manual treatments, or diet and nutrition, have not yet been proven to be effective in controlling spinal deformities.

The purpose of this review is to summarize the available knowledge related to the conservative treatment of adolescent idiopathic scoliosis.

When to Start Treatment

Observation is appropriate treatment for small curves, curves that are at low risk of progression, and those with a natural history that is favourable at the completion of growth. Indications for brace treatment are a growing child presenting with a curve of 25°–40° or with a curve less than 25° that has shown documented progression. Curves of 20°–25° in those with pronounced skeletal immaturity (Risser 0, Tanner 1 or 2) should also be treated immediately. By contrast, contra-indications for bracing are children who has completed growth, or growing children with a curve of over 45°, or under 25° without documented progression [2, 3, 6, 17]. True thoracic lordosis is also a contra-indication for orthotic treatment due to the effect of orthoses on the thoracic spine. A child with a non-supportive home situation or who refuses to wear a brace should not be considered for brace treatment.

Body habitus has been found to be a predictive factor of poor outcome in the orthotic treatment of adolescent idiopathic scoliosis. Overweight adolescent patients will have greater curve progression and be less successful with bracing. In addition, the ability of a brace to transmit corrective forces to the spine through the ribs and soft tissue may be compromised in these patients and this factor should be taken into account when making treatment decisions [18].

A prospective, multi-centre study conducted by Nachemson et al. in several countries showed that the success rate of bracing was significantly higher compared to observation and surface electrical stimulation [2]. A meta-analysis of 20 studies further supported this finding and showed that the weighted mean proportion of success was low for lateral electrical surface stimulation and for observation, and progressively higher for bracing at 8, 16, or 23 h per day. The study concluded that bracing 23 h per day was significantly more successful than any other treatment [4]. Furthermore, a recently published systematic review concluded that bracing adolescent idiopathic scoliosis is effective in the long-term [19]. However, it remains controversial as to whether or not a bracing program can decrease the frequency of surgery [20, 21]. A recently published systematic review used the number of surgically-treated patients as an indicator of failure of bracing and reported a broad spectrum ranging from 1 % to 43 % [22, 23].

Method of Treatment

When patients are first fitted with a brace, there is an initial adjustment period of usually 1–2 weeks. Initially, the patient is prescribed to wear the brace for a specific number of hours per day and the orthosis is left slightly loose to allow the patient to gradually adjust to it. The brace is increasingly tightened daily until the appropriate level of snugness is reached. If any areas of tenderness or skin irritation develop, the brace is adjusted for optimal fit. Roentgenograms are performed after 4 weeks with the brace in place to verify the fit and determine the degree of curve reduction. Repeated roentgenograms should be performed approximately every 4–6 months with the brace removed to follow the progression of the curve. No further roentgenograms are required with the brace in place as all reduction is achieved at the time of the initial fitting. If any major adjustments are made to the brace, a roentgenogram is necessary to verify position.

Hours Per Day

Studies conducted on the number of hours per day of brace wearing show that the more hours per day the brace is worn, the better the result. The brace is usually prescribed for full-time wear with time out for bathing, swimming, physical education and sport. The child should be encouraged to be active in sporting activities while continuing to wear the brace if possible. Contact sports are not allowed with the brace to protect other participants. These activities generally represent an average of 2–4 h a day to ensure brace-wearing of 21–23 h daily.

Use of the brace part-time or only at night has been advocated by some physicians and is widely used in some institutions. However, there is a paucity of long-term follow-up data to prove the effectiveness of this wearing regimen in adolescents, and all series on effective orthotic treatment were with full-time wear.

Wiley et al. analysed the results of bracing according to the wearing regimen. Patients were divided into non-compliant (less than 12 h per day), part-time (between 12 and 18 h per day), and full-time brace wearing (between 18 and 23 h per day). The initial curves were similar in the three groups. Patients who wore the brace less than 12 h per day had an average curve progression from 41.3° to 56.3°, and those who wore the brace part-time progressed from 37.6° to 41.2°. Significant curve improvement was noted in the full-time patient group and curves measured 35.7° at final follow-up compared to 39.3° at brace fitting. In addition, the surgical rate also depended on brace compliance with 73 % in non-compliant patients compared to 9 % in the fully compliant group [24].

Green [25] reported that 16 h per day of bracing was effective in slowing curve progression. He studied a heterogeneous group of patients with curves between 23° and 49° and found that only 9 % curves progressed 5° or more. However, both Boston and Milwaukee braces were used for treatment and follow-up was limited. Similarly, Emans et al. [26] found part-time brace wear to be as effective as full-time wear for smaller curves. Allington and Bowen [27] reported no difference in the efficacy of full-time versus part-time wear using the Wilmington brace for curves of 30°–40°, but observed that 58 % of patients progressed more than 5° in the brace. Peltonen et al. [28] also noted that the results of 12 h per day of bracing were similar to the results of 23 h per day.

When to Stop Treatment

Brace-weaning stops when the patient reaches skeletal maturity, determined as the finding of

a Risser sign of 4, i.e., more than 12 months post-
menarche and lack of growth in height. Over
a period of 2–3 months, the time of brace wear
is decreased progressively and a roentgenogram
is then performed of the patient without the brace.
If the spine remains stable, brace weaning continues over another 2–3 months with a further
progressive decrease in brace wear. After the
second phase of weaning, another roentgenogram
without the brace is performed to verify the stability of the spine. If stability is maintained, the
weaning programme continues until the patient is
completely independent of the brace. If at any
time during the weaning process the stability of
the spine is in question, the bracing regime is
continued.

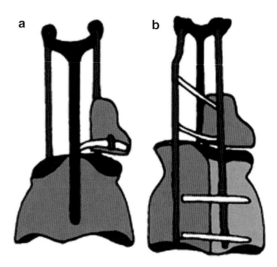

Fig. 1 Milwaukee brace. (**a**) Front view, (**b**) back view

Complications of Brace Treatment

Problems encountered due to brace treatment
include skin irritation, a temporary decrease in
vital capacity, and mild chest wall and inferior rib
deformation. Skin irritation is a common problem
and more frequent in warm climates and during
the summer months due to the increase in heat
and sweat. To reduce the likelihood or occurrence
of skin irritation, frequent changing of the cotton
undergarment is recommended, but discontinuation of brace treatment due to skin irritation is
uncommon. The vital capacity may be temporarily reduced in patients treated with thoraco-
lumbo-sacral orthosis and mild chest wall and
inferior rib deformation can appear during treatment. However, when brace use is discontinued,
the mild rib cage deformity disappears. No severe
permanent chest wall deformities have been
described following brace treatment [7–14].

Brace Types

Cervico-Thoraco-Lumbo-Sacral Orthosis (Milwaukee Brace)

The Milwaukee brace (Fig. 1), also named
cervico-thoraco-lumbo-sacral orthosis (CTLSO),
is a full torso brace extending from the pelvis to
the base of the skull. It was originally designed by

Blount and Schmidt in 1946 for post-operative
care when surgery required long periods of immobilization and it has subsequently been used for
thoracic and double curves. Milwaukee braces are
often custom-made from a mould of the patient's
torso. One anterior and two posterior bars are
attached to a pelvic girdle made of leather or
plastic, as well as a neck ring. The ring has an
anterior throat mould and two posterior occipital
pads, which fit behind the patient's head. Lateral
pads are strapped to the bars and adjustment of
these straps holds the spine in alignment.

Curve patterns that should be treated in
a Milwaukee brace are thoracic curves that have
an apex at or above T8, double thoracic, and other
double curves when the apex of the thoracic component is above T8, i.e., double thoracic and lumbar, or double thoracic and thoracolumbar patterns.

Success rate. Curves between 20° and 29°
with a Risser sign between 0 and 1 progressed
28 % less than untreated curves of similar magnitude (40 % vs. 68 %, respectively). Treated
curves of similar magnitude, but a Risser sign of
2 or more, progressed 10 % less than untreated
curves (10 % vs. 23 %, respectively). Similarly,
curves between 30° and 39° with a Risser sign
between 0 and 1 progressed 14 % less than
untreated curves of similar magnitude (43 % vs.
57 %, respectively). Treated curves of similar

magnitude, but a Risser sign of 2 or more, progressed 21 % less than untreated curves (22 % vs. 43 %, respectively) [3, 15].

Thoraco-Lumbo-Sacral Orthosis

To improve patient compliance, substantially less bulky and lightweight thoraco-lumbo-sacral orthoses (TLSO) were developed. TLSO is the generic name for a group of orthoses characterized by a pelvic portion similar to the pelvic section of the Milwaukee brace and an upper portion extending up to one or both axillae or only to the lower thoracic area. Although there are many variations in their design, generally named after the city or centre of origin, they all function on the same principle. This type of brace is generally prescribed for lumbar and thoracolumbar curves, and thoracic curves with an apex at or below T8.

Boston Brace

Watson, Hall and Stanish first introduced the Boston brace in the mid-1970s and reported on its efficacy on 1977 [29]. The brace (Fig. 2) opens at the back and corrects curvatures by pushing the spine with small pads placed against the ribs, which are also used for partial rotational correction. These pads are usually placed in the back corners of the brace so that the body is thrust forward against the front of the brace, which acts to hold the body upright. Areas of relief are

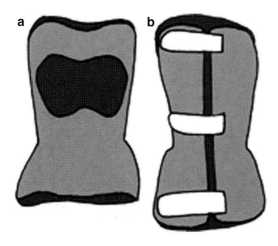

Fig. 2   Three-point Boston brace. (**a**) Front view, (**b**) back view

provided opposite the sites of corrective force to allow the patient to pull the spine away by active muscular effort [26]. The brace also has a 15° lumbar lordosis built into it. The brace runs from just above the seat of a chair (when a person is seated) to around shoulder blade height and is not particularly useful in correcting very high curves [5, 23, 24, 26, 29].

Success rate. The brace has been shown to be particularly effective for curves ranging from 20° to 59° between T8 and L2. At the beginning of treatment, brace correction is about 50 % (Fig. 3), decreasing to 15 % by the time of brace discontinuance. With Boston brace treatment, approximately half of the curves (49 %) remain unchanged, 39 % are stabilized with a final correction of 5°–15°, 4 % are stabilized with a correction superior to 15°, 4 % lose between 5° and 15°, and 3 % progress more than 15°. A study by Emans et al. reported that 11 % of patients underwent surgery during the period of bracing [26].

Wilmington Brace

In the early 1970s, Dean MacEwen developed the Wilmington brace, also known as the duPont Brace. The Wilmington brace is a custom-made, plastic, underarm thoraco-lumbo-sacral orthosis. The brace is a total contact orthosis and is designed as a body jacket, which opens in the front for easy removal and is held closed by adjustable straps. Similar to the Boston brace, it is not useful in correcting very high curves [27].

Success rate. Progression of the deformity by 5° or more is generally observed in 36 % of patients treated with full-time bracing for a curve of less than 30° compared to 41 % of patients managed with part-time bracing. Failure rates are higher in patients with curves between 30° and 40° managed with both full-time (58 %) and part-time bracing (59 %) [27].

Lyon Brace

The Lyon brace (Fig. 4) was designed by Stagnara in 1947. It is composed of a pelvic section with axillary, thoracic and lumbar plates connected in units by two vertical aluminium rods, one anterior and one posterior. The pelvic section is composed of two lateral valves, one for each hemipelvis. The valves

Fig. 3 Right thoracic
scoliosis. (**a**) Anteroposterior full spine
radiograph without brace,
(**b**) immediately post first
brace fitting

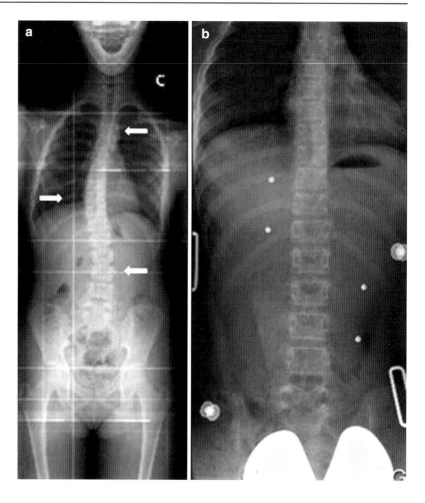

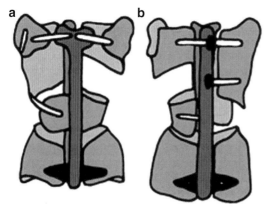

Fig. 4 Lyon brace. (**a**) Front view, (**b**) back view

are connected by metal pieces to the vertical aluminium rods. Forces are applied at the two neutral
vertebrae and a counterforce is applied at the apex of
the curve. It is usually prescribed for progressive
scoliosis with lumbar or low thoracolumbar curves
between 30° and 50° [30, 31].

Success rate. The overall efficacy of the Lyon
brace is 95 %. However, it drops to 87 % for thoracic
curves and to 80 % in patients with Risser sign 0.

Chêneau Brace

Jacques Chêneau designed the original Chêneau
brace in 1979. The brace is commonly used
for the treatment of scoliosis and thoracic

hypokyphosis in many European countries, Israel and Russia. However, it is not commonly prescribed in North America and the United Kingdom. The Chêneau brace utilizes large, sweeping pads to push the body against its curve and into blown out spaces and is usually coupled with the Schroth physical therapy method. The Schroth theory holds that the deformity can be corrected through retraining muscles and nerves to learn what a straight spine feels like, and by breathing deeply into areas crushed by the curvature to help gain flexibility and to expand [32, 33]. The brace helps patients to perform their exercises throughout the day. It is asymmetrical and used for patients of all degrees of severity and maturity, and often worn 20–23 h daily. The brace principally contracts to allow for lateral and longitudinal rotation and movement [34].

Rigo-Chêneau System (RCS Brace)

Rigo et al. have further developed the original Chêneau brace by designing the Rigo-Chêneau System (RCS) brace. The main indication are curves up to 60° (first grade scoliosis: angle up to 40°, and second grade scoliosis, between 40° and 60°, according to the Rigo classification [35]).

Malaga Brace

The Malaga brace is a custom-made TLSO, commonly prescribed in Southern Spain, but relatively unknown outside that country. It is a corrective spinal orthosis used in the treatment of coronal plane curves, but with no derotation element incorporated in the brace.

The brace is of monovalve construction with a posterior opening that closes with metal fasteners. The patient wears the brace for approximately 23 h per day and it is indicated for progressive curves between 20° and 30°.

SPoRT Brace (also known as "Sforzesco" Brace)

The SPoRT (Symmetric, Patient-oriented, Rigid, Three-Dimensional active) brace is symmetrical and built with a plastic frame re-inforced with aluminium rods. It has two lateral elements that cover the back from the pelvis to the armpits, and the abdomen. These are linked to a posterior, centrally-located, aluminium rod, and the brace closes anteriorly with straps on the abdomen and another transverse bar at the level of the manubrium sterni. The brace corrects hip misalignments through padding. Large, sweeping, thick pads push the spine to a corrected position. To prevent overcorrection, however, the brace also has "stop" pads to hold the spine from moving too far in the other direction. This brace is used for all curve patterns and types, even for those ones considered as too late for brace treatment by other schools. It is typically worn 22 h a day and often coupled with a physical therapy program [36, 37].

Success rate. In terms of Cobb's angle, most curves have been shown to remain stable or to slightly improve. The SPoRT brace developing team found that it is possible to obtain scoliosis correction similar to cast in the corrective phase of adolescent idiopathic scoliosis treatment [37].

Night Braces
Charleston Brace

The Charleston bending brace (Fig. 5) was designed with the idea that compliance would increase if the brace was worn only at night.

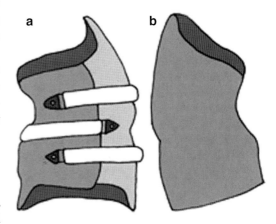

Fig. 5 Charleston brace. (**a**) Front view, (**b**) back view

Hooper and Reed collaborated in 1978 on the early development of this new side-bending brace for nocturnal wear. The orthosis is asymmetrical and fights against the body's curve by overcorrecting the deformity. It grips the hips much like the Boston brace and rises to approximately the same height, but pushes the patient's body to the side. It is used in single, thoracolumbar curves in patients 12–14 years of age (before structural maturity) who have flexible curves in the range of 25–35° [38–40].

Success rate. Patients with a curve over 25° and a Risser sign between 0 and 2 showed a rate of surgery between 12 % and 17 % [38, 39, 41]. In a 2002 study, it has been shown to be equally effective as the Boston brace [41].

Providence Brace

The Providence brace was developed by D'Amato, Griggs and McCoy in the mid-1990s. The brace works by the application of controlled, direct, lateral and rotational forces on the trunk to move the spine toward the midline or beyond the mid-line. It does not bend the spine as with the Charleston bending brace. The goal is to use the centreline as a reference and bring the apices of the scoliotic curve to that line or beyond through the application of lateral forces. This involves the use of three-point-pressure systems and void areas that are located opposite these pressures. Compared with natural history and the prospective study data of Nachemson et al. [2], the Providence brace is effective in preventing curve progression of deformities less than 35° and low apex curves of over 35°. It is more successful in curves with apex curves at or below T9 compared to curves with apex cephalad to T8 [42, 43].

Success rate. Recent studies showed that the Providence night brace generally achieves an average of about 90 % for brace correction of the primary curve and during follow-up, progression of the curve of more than 5° should be expected in about 25 % of cases. The night brace may be recommended for the treatment of adolescent idiopathic scoliosis with curves less than 35° in lumbar and thoracolumbar cases [42, 43].

Soft Brace
SpineCor Brace

The SpineCor brace was developed by Coillard and Rivard in the mid-1990s. The brace has a pelvic unit made of plastic, from which strong elastic bands wrap around the body, pulling against curves, rotations, and imbalances. It is most successful when patients have relatively small and simple curvatures and are structurally young and compliant. The SpineCor bracing method is an adjustable, flexible, and non-invasive technique providing correction that continues as a child moves and grows. The brace is usually worn 20 h a day and the patient can remove it for no more than 2 h a day.

Success rate. A 2003 study reported that after 2 years, the SpineCor brace is able to correct scoliotic curves by 5° in 55 % of patients. The remaining 45 % were stabilized (38 %) or worsened by more than 5° (7 %). However, recent studies demonstrated a trend different from the findings of the SpineCor developing team and reported a lower success rate than rigid spinal orthosis [44–46].

Other Conservative Treatments

Opinions differ in the international literature on the efficacy of conservative approaches to scoliosis treatment. Alternative forms of non-surgical treatment, such as chiropractic or osteopathic manipulation, acupuncture, exercise or other manual treatments, or diet and nutrition, have not yet been proven to be effective in controlling spinal deformities.

Although a subject of debate, most experts agree that physiotherapy alone will not affect the progression of a structural scoliosis. However, there is agreement that a selective physical therapy program in conjunction with brace treatment is beneficial. The triad of out-patient physiotherapy, intensive in-patient rehabilitation, and bracing has proven effective in conservative scoliosis treatment in central Europe [32, 33].

Acupuncture involves penetration of the skin by thin, solid, metallic needles that are stimulated either manually or electrically and it is commonly used for pain control throughout the world, although the putative mechanisms are still unclear. To date, only one study has been published and the effects of acupuncture in the treatment of patients with scoliosis require further investigation [47].

Electrotherapy was hailed as a promising therapy, but failed to alter the natural history of idiopathic scoliosis. With electrotherapy, the lateral muscles on the convexity of the curve are stimulated electrically. It has been shown that no benefit was observed in approximately half of the patients treated by night- time electrotherapy and that the difference in progression between bracing programs and electrical stimulation was not significantly different [27, 48].

Conclusions

Brace treatment is the only method that has been proven to alter the natural history of idiopathic scoliosis. However, different orthosis and many bracing regimens exist. Observation is appropriate for small curves, whereas bracing is generally indicated for progressive curves or for curves over 29° in a skeletally immature child. Braces are generally prescribed for more than 20 h a day and the results of brace treatment correlates to treatment compliance. Problems encountered with bracing are limited.

Conservative Management of Kyphosis

Introduction

Kyphosis is an exaggerated outward curvature of the spine in the flexion/extension axis, producing a "humpback" appearance. Excessive kyphosis can be associated with a variety of conditions, such as congenital spinal anomalies, neuromuscular disease, bone dysplasia, trauma, infection, neoplasm, irradiation therapy, surgical laminectomy, and metabolic disorders [49]. Most of these kyphotic deformities require usually surgical treatment. In adolescents, many conditions present with kyphotic curves such as postural

kyphosis, idiopathic kyphosis, osteochondral dystrophies and, above all, Scheuermann's kyphosis. The main purpose of this review is to summarize the available knowledge related to the kyphotic deformities and to their conservative treatment in the teenage population.

Scheuermann's Kyphosis

Scheuermann's kyphosis is the most common cause of hyperkyphosis in adolescence; its reported prevalence ranges from 0.4 % to 8 % of the general population, but its true prevalence is probably understated since it is either missed or attributed to poor posture [50–53] (Fig. 6).

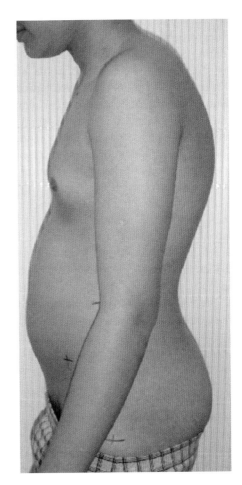

Fig. 6 A fourteen-year-old male teenager presented to our consultation with an unaesthetic Scheuermann's kyphosis. He complained about occasional low back pain

This affection has no specific gender prevalence [53–56]. The onset of Scheuermann's kyphosis usually starts just before puberty, after ossification of the ring apophysis, as a structural kyphotic deformity of thoracic or thoracolumbar spine. The typical patient is between the late juvenile to age 16 years, commonly between 12 and 15 years [55].

The thoracic pattern is the most common and is associated, most of the time, with compensatory non-structural hyperlordosis of the cervical and lumbar spine [57]. The apex of the deformity localized between T7 and T9. The thoracolumbar pattern, whose apex localized between T10 and T12, is less frequently encountered but it has the poor reputation being the most likely to progress after the end of skeletal growth [58]. The natural history of Scheuermann's in adolescents shows that progression is faster when curves are large, and during peak growth velocity [49]; however, curves are generally considered to be stable after maturity [49]. In the majority of patients, thoracic kyphosis is painless and partially flexible [56]; when symptomatic, pain may be aggravated by physical exertion [55]. At clinical examination, the most common findings are forward protruded position of the head, round anteriorly-positioned shoulders, anterior flexion contractures of the shoulder joint, flexion contracture of the hip joint, and hamstrings tightness. In the Adam's forward bend-test, the patients with Scheuermann's disease demonstrate an area of angulation in a fixed or relatively fixed kyphotic curve [55].

At present, the aetiology of Scheuermann's kyphosis remains unknown, but several factors seem important in the pathogenesis of this affection, such as a genetic contribution [59, 60] or an abnormal mechanical loading of the growing spine [54, 56]. Scheuermann's disease is considered hereditary, although the hereditary pattern has not been clearly defined [55]. The mode of inheritance may be autosomal dominant, with a high degree of penetrance and variable expressivity [59]. Reports suggest heritability of identical radiological changes in monozygotic twins, sibling recurrence, and transmission through generations [60]. An interesting new theory of pathogenesis has recently been described by Fotiadis and al. According to these authors, a smaller length of sternum than the normal may be correlated with the appearance of thoracic Scheuermann's kyphosis, since a smaller length of this bone could increase the compressive forces on the vertebral end-plates anterioly, allowing uneven growth of the vertebral bodies with wedging [61].

Disorganized enchondral ossification similar to Blount's disease, a reduction in collagen, or an increase in mucopolysaccharides in the end-plate, are common histopathological findings noted in adolescents with Scheuermann's kyphosis [62, 63]. It is readily differentiated from postural roundback radiographically because of the presence of vertebral bony wedging, vertebral end-plate irregularity, diminished anterior vertebral growth, and premature disc degeneration [53]. Other pathological entities that must be differentiated include idiopathic kyphosis, osteochondral dystrophies, congenital kyphosis, and spondylo-epiphyseal dysplasias [55]. Currently, Scheuermann's kyphosis is the more frequent affection requiring a brace treatment in skeletally-immature patients.

Radiographic Evaluation

How to do a Good Radiograph

Initial evaluation for kyphosis should include anteroposterior (AP) and lateral standing radiographs, including the entire spine, the cranium and the femoral heads. Careful attention should be paid to patient positioning and radiologic technique in order to achieve correct visualization of the upper thoracic spine. The optimal lateral radiograph should be taken in the standing position with the arms anteriorly flexed at 90°, and resting on a support [64, 65] or in the clavicular position [66, 67]. The kyphosis can then be measured from the uppermost tilted vertebra to the lowermost tilted vertebra, whatever these may be [65]. Nevertheless, some radiographs may be somewhat indistinct in the upper thoracic area and the end-plates cannot be adequately seen for a good measurement [65]. This problem can be often be overcome by re-creating the contour by drawing a line along the anterior vertebral body cortices [65]. Once this "best-fit line" has been drawn, perpendiculars to that line can be used to measure the kyphosis (unpublished data by F. Takeuchi & F. Denis).

What is Normal

The measurement of thoracic kyphosis is confusing, as some authors routinely measure T2–T12, T4–T12, or T5–T12, even if these are not the maximally tilted vertebrae [65]. When the kyphosis is measured between the first and the twelfth thoracic vertebrae, the mean thoracic kyphosis in children and adolescents ranges from 33° [64] to 43° [68], with very large ranges and standard deviations. There is still a controversy as to what is the normal range of thoracic kyphosis. The old statement found in many text, that normal is from 20° to 40° is no more justifiable. Currently, curves ranging from 15° to 55° can be considered as "physiologic kyphosis" [65]. Beyond this limit, kyphosis becomes abnormal, which is confirmed by the fact that postural roundback rarely exceeds 60° while Scheuermann's typically does [49].

Radiologic Criteria of Scheuermann's Disease

The radiographic diagnosis of Scheuermann's disease requires anterior vertebral wedging more than 5° in at least three contiguous vertebrae, as defined by Sorensen [69] (Fig. 7). Secondary radiographic findings included irregular apical vertebral end-plates, anterior narrowing of disc spaces, and Schmorl's nodes [49]. The anteroposterior view of the spine may show mild scoliosis, typically less than 20° and nonprogressive [56, 70]. However, most of the time, these curves are not real scoliotic curves; in fact, vertebral rotation is often absent and apparent scoliotic curves have to be attributed to non-orthogonal view on the AP radiograph of the thoracic kyphotic or lumbar lordotic curves. Thoracic Scheuermann's kyphosis is usually compensated either by lumbar hyperlordosis (>50 %) or by thrusting the lumbar spine backwards. These compensatory phenomenon's are

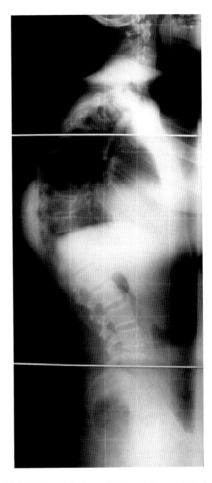

Fig. 7 Radiographic investigations demonstrated a 75° Scheuermann's thoracic curve, which was partially reducible

thought to result in increased stresses on the pars interarticularis that may account for the increased incidence of spondylolisthesis reported in adolescents with Scheuermann's disease [55].

Description of Sagittal Spinal Imbalance

Radiographic evaluation does not have to limit itself to measure the kyphotic deformation: studying the global sagittal balance has to be conducted taking into consideration the position of the spine, and that of the pelvis and the hips. Legaye et al. have demonstrated the key importance of the anatomical parameter of "pelvic incidence" in the regulation of the sagittal curves of the spine and in the individual variability of the sacral slope and the lordosis curve [71, 72]. The pelvic incidence is formed by the line connecting the centre of the upper end-plate of S1 to the centre of the axis of the hips and by the line perpendicular to the tangent to the centre of the upper end-plate of S1. Pelvic incidence is a fixed anatomical value for each individual and corresponds to the sum of two postural parameters called sacral tilt (ST) and pelvic tilt (PT) [71, 72]. Therefore any change in sacral tilt produces a change in pelvic tilt, and vice versa. In children and adolescents with thoracic Scheuermann's kyphosis, two mechanisms may be implemented to compensate the sagittal imbalance. First, pelvic tilt can increase by rotation of the pelvis around the line passing through the femoral heads. Rotating the pelvis forwards (classically called pelvic anteversion) displaces the S1 end-plate anteriorly and increases the sacral inclination (sacral tilt). If the lumbar spine is mobile, the sagittal balance will be ensured by increasing lumbar lordosis (picture). When the pelvis appears backwards rotated (pelvic retroversion due to tight hamstrings), sacral inclination appears weak and, as a result, a second mechanism is called into play: in this situation, the sagittal balance is ensured by thrusting the lumbar spine backwards without using the natural lumbar lordosis. This lumbar postural inversion is recognized to increase the facet joint pressure especially at the level of L4–L5 and L5–S1, and to concentrate sagittal shear-force at the level of the pars interarticularis, with the spondylolysis risk which results from this.

Additional Investigations

Additional imaging studies should include radiographs of the left hand and wrist (bone age), passive hyperextension views, and in many cases magnetic resonance. Lateral hyperextension views give interesting information about the flexibility of the kyphotic curves. Magnetic resonance imaging is used in the evaluation of neurological deficits, intervertebral disc degeneration and disc herniation, for atypical forms of Scheuermann's disease with non-diagnostic findings in conventional radiographs [55].

Natural History

Before implementing any treatment, the Orthopaedic surgeon should be aware of the natural history of the disease, specific criteria for initiating therapy and, above all, must weigh the benefits against the complications of the prescribed treatment. The natural history of Scheuermann's in teenagers shows that progression is faster during peak growth velocity, especially when the curves are important [49]. After the end of the puberty, the curves will generally not increase [49]. Particular attention should be paid to thoracolumbar kyphosis, since these curves have the poor reputation to be the most likely to progress after the end of the growth [58]. Most of the patients with Scheuermann's report greater back pain, embarrassment about their physical appearance which can progress to psychological distress, but do not appear to be disabled by their symptoms [54]. Nevertheless, patients with Scheuermann's hyperkyphosis work usually in lighter jobs and announce interference with daily activities [54]. Most of the patients with the lumbar or thoraco-lumbar form of the disease present usually with more important and permanent low back pain [59]. Neurologic complications secondary to severe kyphosis, dural cysts, or thoracic disc herniation have been described in a small number of patients with untreated Scheuermann's kyphosis [73–75]. The consequences of kyphotic deformity on pulmonary function remain unclear since no correlation is found with cardiopulmonary insufficiency, except for the curves of more than to $100°–110°$ [54]. Unfortunately, there is still a lack of literature regarding the natural history of Scheuermann's kyphosis and there are therefore a few questions that still need to be answered in order to establish guidelines for treatment.

Non-Operative Treatment

Indications

During the past decade, several studies have confirmed that the natural history of adolescent kyphosis can be positively affected by non-operative treatment, particularly bracing [76–80]. Indications for conservative treatment include pain, progression of deformity, neuropathy, but also cosmesis, in Scheuermann's curves measuring 55°–75°. For curves measuring beyond 75°, it seems legitimate to consider spinal fusion even if brace treatment may be successful in several cases [79]. Braces are useful for Scheuermann's kyphosis measuring 55°–75°, provided the patients still have significant growth remaining. As spinal growth continues until the end of the puberty, it seems consistent to start with brace treatment even after the pubertal growth peak. On this subject, teenagers with Risser's score less or equal to two require bracing (unpublished data by Richards B.S. and Katz D.E. Texas Scottish Rite Hospital). By contrast, contra-indications for bracing are an adolescent who has completed growth, or a growing child with curve of over 80°, especially if these are located in the upper part of the thoracic spine. Teenagers with non-supportive home situations or who refuse to wear a brace should not be considered for bracing. Finally, angular structural kyphosis due to an anterior vertebral wedging has to be considered as predictive factor of poor outcome in the orthotic treatment of Scheuermann's kyphosis.

Types of Braces

Currently, only bracing has demonstrated to be effective in decreasing or in stabilizing progression of kyphotic curves. The goal of the bracing is not only to arrest progression but also to achieve permanent improvement in the thoracic kyphosis. This can result only if the anterior vertebral height is restored by application of hyperextension forces (unpublished data by Richards B.S. and Katz D.E. Texas Scottish Rite Hospital). Without reconstitution of the anterior vertebral height, the deformity will inevitably recur following bracing's removal. In the past, many braces have been described in the treatment of Scheuermann's kyphosis. For many years, the most commonly-used brace was the Milwaukee brace [56, 76, 79], which acts as a three-point orthosis promoting dynamic extension of the thoracic spine; this brace effectively applies a 3-point corrective force to the mid-thoracic spine and simultaneously decreases the excessive lumbar lordosis. The Milwaukee brace is the primary orthosis recommended for kyphosis located to the thoracic spine, especially if the apex of the deformity is located at or cephalad to T6 and T8. Consecutively, other types of bracing have been manufactured to relieve the psychological problems associated with the Milwaukee brace's occipital-chin ring to the patient, and therefore to improve patient's compliance to wear the brace. The polypropylene thoracolumbosacral orthosis (TLSO) is a popular 3-point orthosis with an anterior sternal extension or padded anterior shoulder outriggers and a posterior spinal pad. Like the Milwaukee brace, TLSO also diminishes the lumbar lordosis. TLSO is indicated above all for kyphotic deformities whose apex below the eighth or ninth thoracic vertebra. Other braces, such as polypropylene lumbosacral orthosis (LSO) (Fig. 8) or the active-passive Gschwend erection corset, reduce the lumbar lordosis severely, and by doing so, force the patient to actively right himself out of the kyphotic thoracic posture. These devices are efficient for curves with an apex below T8–T9, and the indications for using these braces are partially flexible kyphotic curves. More recently, Weiss and al. suggested that braces using only transverse corrective forces may achieve reduction rates similar to those obtained by Milwaukee brace. In the same way, Riddle and al felt that TLSO results were comparable to those with the Milwaukee brace. Currently, computer-aided design/computer-aided manufacture (CAD/CAM) and other computer technology had been introduced in order to eliminate uncomfortable physical contact for the teenagers, as well as the orthotist's skills. The first results suggest that CAD/CAM braces are more comfortable and therefore better tolerated by patients with equivalent correction if not superior.

Treatment Modalities

At the beginning of the brace treatment, there is an initial adjustment period of a few weeks. Initially, the patient is prescribed to wear the brace for a specific number of hours per day,

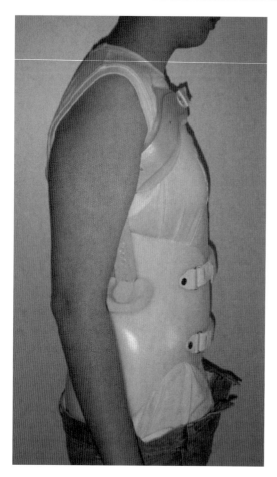

Fig. 8 The patient was prescribed to wear a polypropylene thoracolumbosacral orthosis (TLSO) with padded anterior shoulder outriggers and a posterior spinal pad

with the orthosis adjusted. When the patient is accustomed to the brace-wearing, the brace may be tightened until the appropriate level of snugness. Roentgengrams are performed during the first fitting with the brace correctly tightened, in order to check the degree of curve correction. To be effective, the brace should correct instantaneously the deformity at least 50 %. Thereafter, the compliant patient should wear the cast on a full-time basis (22–24 h daily) or at least 20 h per day for an average of 12–18 months. Areas of skin irritation are treated with local application of medical alcohol or bepanthen lotion. Ideally, bracing should be continued until skeletal maturity to provide the best outcome. Males should be

especially encouraged to wear the chosen orthosis until later adolescence (Risser grade 5). Unfortunately, this is difficult to achieve as the adolescents tend to become less compliant with bracewear over time. Repeated roentgenograms should be performed approximately every 4–6 months with the brace removed during the preceding 24 h to follow the improvement of the curve. In the most severe or stiff deformities, "preparative" cast treatment may be considered to improve the curve's flexibility before switching to a brace [52, 55]. This effect has been well demonstrated using the methods of Ponte & Stagnara.

Expectable Results of Bracing

Whilst unlikely in idiopathic scoliosis, brace treatment often results in some permanent reduction of spinal deformity in Scheuermann's kyphosis. In most series, the results of bracing are very interesting in compliant patients, with approximately 40–50 % of correction (Fig. 9). In absolute values, final mean improvement range between 6° and more than 20°. In our hospital, we analyzed the results in 20 patients who had used a polypropylene thoracolumbosacral orthosis and had been followed for 45 months. The average age of the patients at the initiation of treatment was 13 years and 6 months, the average duration of the brace-wearing was 21 months, the mean improvement of kyphosis was 22°, whereas the mean improvement of the posterior lumbar inversion was 15 mm. In our experience also, a 1° of angular improvement of the kyphosis per month of brace-wearing was noted.

Parallel to the reduction of the thoracic kyphosis, curve response to Orthopaedic treatment was noted in the form of a decrease of the vertebral body wedging (Fig. 10). Some studies also demonstrated that correction of kyphosis was due to a realistic partial reconstitution of the anterior vertebral height by the application of extension forces [77, 81]. Flexible deformities seem to predict best results after brace treatment [78]. However, some authors consider that initial maximal wedging or initial assessment of curve flexibility do not influence the degree of improvement in the angular deformity [82]. As for scoliosis, bracing is less successful in overweight teenagers, since

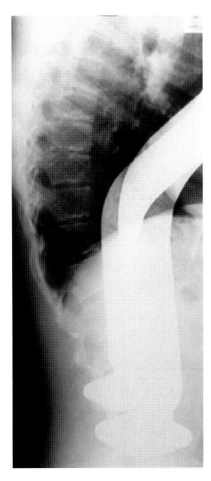

Fig. 9 Radiograph performed after the first brace wearing demonstrated that the brace was effective as it corrected instantaneously 50 % of the deformity

the ability of the brace to transmit correctives forces to the spine through bony surfaces and soft tissues may be compromised in these patients. Following brace discontinuation, some loss of correction may occur, but in the majority of cases, the deformity is improved and the curve correction is maintained [53, 77–79]. Usually, larger deformities at the onset of the treatment show greater losses of correction after bracing is discontinued. On the other hand, correction achieved in smaller deformities seems better maintained following brace discontinuation. This potential loss of correction occurring after brace's removal is the reason why some authors recommend that the patient continue the brace treatment full time or at least part-time, usually

at night, until maturity [56]. For patients presenting at the post-pubertal stage with little or no growth remaining, it is illogical and therefore not acceptable to undertake brace treatment [52, 55]. In fact, after skeletal maturity, casting or bracing cannot correct the anterior vertebral wedging and attempts to use either technique are probably not warranted. Progression of the deformity, requiring other type of treatment, is more likely observed in patients with poor bracewear compliance, in kyphotic curves of more than 75°, in patients with severe and rigid curves and in atypical forms of the disease [56, 79].

Other Conservative Treatments

As for scoliose, there is no consensus in the international literature on the efficacy of conservative approaches to kyphosis treatment. Other forms of conservative treatment, such as chiropractic or osteopathic manipulation, acupuncture, superficial electric stimulation, exercise or other manual treatments, or diet and nutrition, have not yet been proven to be effective in controlling spinal deformities. In the same way, practice of extension sports such as gymnastics, swimming and basketball are usually advised but these recommendations raise more of belief than of true scientifically established results [55]. Intensive physiotherapy exercise programs for postural improvement have been tried for many years but without any conclusive data that physical therapy alone can benefit kyphotic improvement [56]. Nevertheless, long-term physical therapy, osteopathy, manual therapy, exercise program, and psychological therapy may be an interesting alternative to control the pain, even if no correction is expectable on the deformity [83].

Conclusion

Brace treatment for Scheuermann's hyperkyphosis is currently regarded as the only effective treatment approach that may modify the natural history of the affection. Evidence about other forms of conservative treatment is scanty. Different orthosis and many bracing regimens exist; the current belief among the orthopedic surgeons is that

Fig. 10 The final radiograph realized 24 months after the end of treatment demonstrated that a good correction persisted even after stopping bracewearing

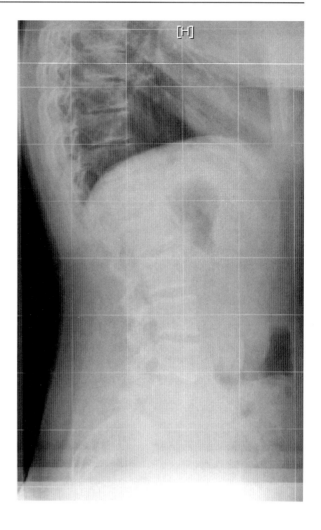

results obtained with actual more comfortable orthosis are comparable to those with the Milwaukee brace. The brace should be worn ideally at least 20 h per day until skeletal maturity to provide the best outcome. Bracing is generally indicated for curves between 55° and 75° in skeletally immature teenagers. As for scoliosis, results of brace treatment are correlated to patient's compliance and problems encountered with it are limited.

References

1. Fernandez-Filiberti R, Flynn J, Ramirez N, Trautmann M, Alegria M. Effectiveness of TLSO bracing in the conservative treatment of idiopathic scoliosis. J Pediatr Orthop. 1995;15:176–81.

2. Nachemson A, Peterson L, Members of the Brace Study Group of the Scoliosis Research Society. Effectiveness of treatment with a brace in girls who have adolescent idiopathic scoliosis. J Bone Joint Surg Am. 1995;77:815–22.

3. Lonstein JE, Winter RB. The Milwaukee brace for the treatment of adolescent idiopathic scoliosis: a review of 1020 patients. J Bone Joint Surg Am. 1994;76:1207–21.

4. Rowe DE, Bernstein SM, Riddick MF, Adler F, Emans JB, Gardner-Bonneau E. A meta-analysis of the efficacy of non-operative treatments for idiopathic scoliosis. J Bone Joint Surg Am. 1997;79:664–74.

5. Olafsson Y, Saraste H, Soderlund V, Hoffsten M. Boston brace in the treatment of idiopathic scoliosis. J Pediatr Orthop. 1995;15:524–7.

6. Asher MA, Burton DC. Adolescent idiopathic scoliosis: natural history and long term treatment effects. Scoliosis. 2006;1:2.

7. Noonan KJ, Dolan LA, Jacobson WC, Weinstein SL. Long-term psychosocial characteristics of patients

treated for idiopathic scoliosis. J Pediatr Orthop. 1997;17:712–7.

8. Götze C, Liljenqvist UR, Slomka A, Götze HG, Steinbeck J. Quality of life and back pain: outcome 16.7 years after Harrington instrumentation. Spine. 2002;27:1456–64.

9. Betz RR, Bunnell WP, Lamrecht-Mulier E, et al. Scoliosis and pregnancy. J Bone Joint Surg Am. 1987;69:90–6.

10. Danielsson AJ, Nachemson AL. Childbearing, curve progression, and sexual function in women 22 years after treatment for adolescent idiopathic scoliosis. A case–control study. Spine. 2001;26:1449–56.

11. Barrios C, Pérez-Encinas C, Maruenda JI, Laguía M. Significant ventilatory functional restriction in adolescents with mild or moderate scoliosis during maximal exercise tolerance test. Spine. 2005;30:1610–5.

12. Chong K, Letts R, Cumming G. Influence of spinal curvature on exercise capacity. J Pediatr Orthop. 1981;1:251–4.

13. Jackson RP, Simmons EH, Stripinis D. Incidence and severity of back pain in adult idiopathic scoliosis. Spine. 1983;8:749–56.

14. Pehrsson K, Danielsson A, Nachemson A. Pulmonary function in patients with adolescent idiopathic scoliosis: a 25 year follow-up after surgery or start of brace treatment. Thorax. 2001;56:388–93.

15. Lonstein JE, Carlson JM. The prediction of curve progression in untreated idiopathic scoliosis during growth. J Bone Joint Surg Am. 1984;66:1061–71.

16. Noonan KJ, Weinstein SL, Jacobson WC, Dolan LA. Use of the Milwaukee brace for progressive idiopathic scoliosis. J Bone Joint Surg Am. 1996;78:557–67.

17. Carr WA, Moe JH, Winter RB, Lonstein JE. Treatment of idiopathic scoliosis in the Milwaukee brace. J Bone Joint Surg Am. 1980;62:599–612.

18. O'Neill PJ, Karol LA, Shindle MK, Elerson EE, BrintzenhofeSzoc KM, Katz DE, Farmer KW, Sponseller PD. Decreased orthotic effectiveness in overweight patients with adolescent idiopathic scoliosis. J Bone Joint Surg Am. 2005;87:1069–74. javascript: AL_get(this, 'jour', 'J Bone Joint Surg Am'.).

19. Maruyama T. Bracing adolescent idiopathic scoliosis: a systematic review of the literature of effective conservative treatment looking for end results 5 years after weaning. Disabil Rehabil. 2008;30:786–91.

20. Weiss HR, Weiss G, Schaar HJ. Incidence of surgery in conservatively treated patients with scoliosis. Pediatr Rehabil. 2003;6:111–8.

21. Rigo M, Reiter CH, Weiss HR. Effect of conservative management on the prevalence of surgery in patients with adolescent idiopathic scoliosis. Pediatr Rehabil. 2003;6:209–14.

22. Dolan LA, Weinstein SL. Surgical rates after observation and bracing for adolescent idiopathic scoliosis: an evidence-based review. Spine. 2007;32:S91–100.

23. Lange JE, Steen H, Brox JN. Long-term results after Boston brace treatment in adolescent idiopathic scoliosis. Scoliosis. 2009;4:17.

24. Wiley JW, Thomson JD, Mitchell TM, Smith BG, Banta JV. Effectiveness of the Boston brace in treatment of large curves in adolescent idiopathic scoliosis. Spine. 2000;25:2326–32.

25. Green NE. Part-time bracing of adolescent idiopathic scoliosis. J Bone Joint Surg Am. 1986;68:738–43.

26. Emans JB, Kaelin A, Bancel P, Hall JE, Miller ME. The Boston bracing system for idiopathic scoliosis: follow-up results in 295 patients. Spine. 1986;11:792–801.

27. Allington NJ, Bowen JR. Adolescent idiopathic scoliosis: treatment with the Wilmington brace. J Bone Joint Surg Am. 1996;78:1056–62.

28. Peltonen J, Poussa M, Ylikoski M. Three year results of bracing in scoliosis. Acta Orthop Scand. 1988; 59:487–90.

29. Watts HG, Hall JE, Stanish W. The Boston brace system for the treatment of low thoracic and lumbar scoliosis by the use of a girdle without superstructure. Clin Orthop. 1977;126:87–92.

30. Stagnara P, de Mauroy JC. Résultats à long terme du traitement orthopédique lyonnais. In: Stagnara P, editor. Actualités en rééducation fonctionnelle et réadaptation. 2ème série. Paris, Ed. Masson; 1977. p. 33–6.

31. Stagnara P, Desbrosses J. Scolioses essentielles pendant l'enfance et l'adolescence: résultats des traitements orthopédiques et chirurgicaux. Rev Chir Orthop. 1960;46:562–75.

32. Weiss HR. Conservative treatment of idiopathic scoliosis with physical therapy and orthoses. Orthopade. 2003;32:146–56.

33. Weiss HR. Rehabilitation of adolescent patients with scoliosis – what do we know? A review of the literature. Pediatr Rehabil. 2003;6:183–94.

34. Chêneau J. Orthese de scoliose, 1ère Edition. Chêneau, J., Saint Orensm; 1990

35. Rigo M. Intra-observer reliability of a new classification correlating with brace treatment. Pediatr Rehabil. 2004;7:63.

36. Negrini S, Marchini G. Efficacy of the symmetric, patient-oriented, rigid, three-dimensional, active (SPoRT) concept of bracing for scoliosis: a prospective study of the Sforzesco versus Lyon brace. Eura Medicophys. 2007;43:171–81.

37. Negrini S, Marchini G, Tomaello L. The Sforzesco brace and SPoRT concept (symmetric, patient-oriented, rigid, three-dimensional) versus the Lyon brace and 3-point systems for bracing idiopathic scoliosis. Stud Health Technol Inform. 2006;123:245–9.

38. Price CT, Scott DS, Reed FEJ, Riddick MF. Nighttime bracing for adolescent idiopathic scoliosis with the Charleston bending brace. Preliminary report. Spine. 1990;15:1294–9.

39. Price CT, Scott DS, Reed FEJ, Sproul JT, Riddick MF. Nighttime bracing for adolescent idiopathic scoliosis with the Charleston bending brace: long-term follow-up. J Pediatr Orthop. 1997;17:703–7.

40. Federico DJ, Renshaw TS. Results of treatment of idiopathic scoliosis with the Charleston bending brace. Spine. 1990;15:886–7.

41. Gepstein R, Leitner Y, Zohar E, Angel I, Shabat S, Pekarsky I, Friesem T, Folman Y, Katz A, Fredman B. Effectiveness of the Charleston bending brace in the treatment of single-curve idiopathic scoliosis. J Pediatr Orthop. 2002;22:84–7.

42. D'Amato CR, Griggs S, McCoy B. Nighttime bracing with the providence brace in adolescent girls with idiopathic scoliosis. Spine. 2001;26:2006–12.

43. Yrjönen T, Ylikoski M, Schlenzka D, Kinnunen R, Poussa M. Effectiveness of the providence nighttime bracing in adolescent idiopathic scoliosis: a comparative study of 36 female patients. Eur Spine J. 2006;15:1139–43.

44. Wong MS, Cheng JC, Lam TP, Ng BK, Sin SW, Lee-Shum SL, Chow DH, Tam SY. The effect of rigid versus flexible spinal orthosis on the clinical efficacy and acceptance of the patients with adolescent idiopathic scoliosis. Spine. 2008;33:1360–5.

45. Coillard C, Vachon V, Circo AB, et al. Effectiveness of the SpineCor brace based on the new standardized criteria proposed by the scoliosis research society for adolescent idiopathic scoliosis. J Pediatr Orthop. 2007;27:375–9.

46. Coillard C, Leroux MA, Zabjek KF, et al. SpineCor – a non-rigid brace for the treatment of idiopathic scoliosis: post-treatment results. Eur Spine J. 2003;12:141–8.

47. Weiss HR, Bohr S, Jahnke A, Pleines S. Acupuncture in the treatment of scoliosis – a single blind controlled pilot study. Scoliosis. 2008;3:4.

48. Cassella MC, Hall JE. Current treatment approaches in the nonoperative and operative management of adolescent idiopathic scoliosis. Phys Ther. 1991;71:897–909.

49. Stricker SJ. The malaligned adolescent spine-part 2: Scheuermann's kyphosis and spondylolisthesis. Int Pediatr. 2002;17:135–42.

50. Damborg F, Engell V, Andersen M, Kyvik KO, Thomsen K. Prevalence, concordance, and heritability of Scheuermann kyphosis based on a study of twins. J Bone Joint Surg. 2006;88:2133–6.

51. Lings S, Mikkelsen L. Scheuermann's disease with low localization. A problem of under-diagnosis. Scand J Rehabil Med. 1982;14:77–9.

52. Lowe TG, Kasten MD. An analysis of sagittal curves and balance after Cotrel-Dubousset instrumentation for kyphosis secondary to Scheuermann's disease. A review of 32 patients. Spine. 1994;19:1680–5.

53. Lowe TG, Line BG. Evidence based medicine: analysis of Scheuermann kyphosis. Spine. 2007;32:S115–9.

54. Murray PM, Weinstein SL, Spratt KF. The natural history and long-term follow-up of Scheuermann kyphosis. J Bone Joint Surg. 1993;75:236–48.

55. Papagelopoulos PJ, Mavrogenis AF, Savvidou OD, Mitsiokapa EA, Themistocleous GS, Soucacos PN. Current concepts in Scheuermann's kyphosis. Orthopedics. 2008;31:52–8. quiz 9–60.

56. Wenger DR, Frick SL. Scheuermann kyphosis. Spine. 1999;24:2630–9.

57. Jansen RC, van Rhijn LW, Duinkerke E, van Ooij A. Predictability of the spontaneous lumbar curve correction after selective thoracic fusion in idiopathic scoliosis. Eur Spine J. 2007;16:1335–42.

58. Lowe TG. Scheuermann disease. J Bone Joint Surg. 1990;72:940–5.

59. Lowe TG. Scheuermann's disease. Orthop Clin North Am. 1999;30:475–87, ix.

60. McKenzie L, Sillence D. Familial Scheuermann disease: a genetic and linkage study. J Med Genet. 1992;29:41–5.

61. Fotiadis E, Grigoriadou A, Kapetanos G, Kenanidis E, Pigadas A, Akritopoulos P, et al. The role of sternum in the etiopathogenesis of Scheuermann disease of the thoracic spine. Spine. 2008;33:E21–4.

62. Ippolito E, Bellocci M, Montanaro A, Ascani E, Ponseti IV. Juvenile kyphosis: an ultrastructural study. J Pediatr Orthop. 1985;5:315–22.

63. Scoles PV, Latimer BM, DigIovanni BF, Vargo E, Bauza S, Jellema LM. Vertebral alterations in Scheuermann's kyphosis. Spine. 1991;16:509–15.

64. Boseker EH, Moe JH, Winter RB, Koop SE. Determination of "normal" thoracic kyphosis: a roentgenographic study of 121 "normal" children. J Pediatr Orthop. 2000;20:796–8.

65. Winter RB, Lonstein JE, Denis F. Sagittal spinal alignment: the true measurement, norms, and description of correction for thoracic kyphosis. J Spinal Disord Tech. 2009;22:311–4.

66. Faro FD, Marks MC, Pawelek J, Newton PO. Evaluation of a functional position for lateral radiograph acquisition in adolescent idiopathic scoliosis. Spine. 2004;29:2284–9.

67. Horton WC, Brown CW, Bridwell KH, Glassman SD, Suk SI, Cha CW. Is there an optimal patient stance for obtaining a lateral 36″ radiograph? A critical comparison of three techniques. Spine. 2005;30:427–33.

68. Mac-Thiong JM, Berthonnaud E, Dimar 2nd JR, Betz RR, Labelle H. Sagittal alignment of the spine and pelvis during growth. Spine. 2004;29:1642–7.

69. Sorensen KH. Scheuermann's juvenile kyphosis. Clinical appearances, radiography, aetiology, and prognosis. Copenhagen: Munksgaard; 1964.

70. Bradford DS. Juvenile kyphosis. Clin Orthop Relat Res. 1977;128:45–55.

71. Legaye J. Unfavorable influence of the dynamic neutralization system on sagittal balance of the spine. Rev Chir Orthop Reparatrice Appar Mot. 2005;91:542–50.

72. Legaye J, Duval-Beaupere G, Hecquet J, Marty C. Pelvic incidence: a fundamental pelvic parameter for three-dimensional regulation of spinal sagittal curves. Eur Spine J. 1998;7:99–103.

73. Bradford DS, Garcia A. Herniations of the lumbar intervertebral disk in children and adolescents. A review of 30 surgically treated cases. JAMA. 1969;210:2045–51.

74. Chiu KY, Luk KD. Cord compression caused by multiple disc herniations and intraspinal cyst in Scheuermann's disease. Spine. 1995;20:1075–9.

75. Yablon JS, Kasdon DL, Levine H. Thoracic cord compression in Scheuermann's disease. Spine. 1988; 13:896–8.

76. Bradford DS, Moe JH, Montalvo FJ, Winter RB. Scheuermann's kyphosis and roundback deformity. Results of Milwaukee brace treatment. J Bone Joint Surg. 1974;56:740–58.

77. Montgomery SP, Erwin WE. Scheuermann's kyphosis – long-term results of Milwaukee braces treatment. Spine. 1981;6:5–8.

78. Riddle EC, Bowen JR, Shah SA, Moran EF, Lawall Jr H. The duPont kyphosis brace for the treatment of adolescent Scheuermann kyphosis. J South Orthop Assoc. 2003;12:135–40.

79. Sachs B, Bradford D, Winter R, Lonstein J, Moe J, Willson S. Scheuermann kyphosis. Follow-up of Milwaukee-brace treatment. J Bone Joint Surg. 1987;69:50–7.

80. Weiss HR, Turnbull D, Bohr S. Brace treatment for patients with Scheuermann's disease – a review of the literature and first experiences with a new brace design. Scoliosis. 2009;4:22.

81. Pola E, Lupparelli S, Aulisa AG, Mastantuoni G, Mazza O, De Santis V. Study of vertebral morphology in Scheuermann's kyphosis before and after treatment. Stud Health Technol Inform. 2002;91: 405–11.

82. Platero D, Luna JD, Pedraza V. Juvenile kyphosis: effects of different variables on conservative treatment outcome. Acta Orthopaed Belgica. 1997;63: 194–201.

83. Weiss HR, Dieckmann J, Gerner HJ. Effect of intensive rehabilitation on pain in patients with Scheuermann's disease. Stud Health Technol Inform. 2002;88:254–7.

New Surgical Techniques in Scoliosis

Acke Ohlin

Contents

A. Ohlin
Lund University, Sweden, Malmö, Sweden
e-mail: acke.ohlin@med.lu.se

Keywords

Scoliosis history • New techniques-contoured rods, anterior and posterior approaches • Pedicle screws • Screw design • Endoscopic techniques • Growing rods • Distraction systems • Guided-growth systems • Titanium implants

A Brief Historical Review

About 50 years ago Harrington introduced a distraction system for scoliosis with one hook at top and one at bottom of the spinal curvature [1]. The principal diagnosis of his primary patient cohort was post-polio-myelitis deformity. It was the first instrumentation for scoliosis and it was used worldwide for at least three decades.

Almost 10 years later Dwyer employed an anterior system with a cable connecting vertebral bodies with anterior body screws made from titanium which, after removal of the intervertebral discs, enabled major correction. He reported on the technique and his early experience with the eight first cases in 1969 [2]. Zielke from Germany refined this system and presented in 1976 an anterior system with a thin threaded rod [3]. These two anterior systems were however kyphogenic. Cable and rod breakage were both common. In the early 1990s Kaneda from Japan introduced an anterior double rod system with which the surgeons also could manage the sagittal plane deformity. With this technique an excellent correction was frequently achieved, when performing correction in the thoracolumbar and thoracic regions [4]. However a non-reversible reduction of pulmonary function was regularly observed after surgery in the middle and upper thoracic spine [5, 6]. This impairment is most often not clinically important when the patient still is young, but eventually when the patient is old, this reduction of pulmonary function may affect the general body function.

In the late1970s Luque reported a method of posterior spinal segmental instrumentation for deformities. This was based on rods connected to the spine by multiple sublaminar wires [7]. Using this technique, patients with neurological disorders other than poliomyelitis, also could be effectively instrumented.

In the mid 1980s Cotrel and Dubousset introduced a multi-segmental double rod posterior system (CD) with hooks. This method addressed also the sagittal plane [8]. By the advent of the transpedicular screw technique, introduced to the non-French- speaking world in the early 1980s, the CD technique was further developed with screws in the lumbar spine and combined with wires and hooks in the thoracic region, creating the hybrid technique.

Later Innovation in Techniques

A new approach, representing further development of the CD system and the hybrid techniques was presented by Suk from South Korea in 1994 [9]. Initially he was considered unorthodox because he introduced screws into hypoplastic pedicles on the concave side of a scoliotic curve very close to the spinal cord. A few surgeons made study visits to Seoul and introduced this technique to USA in the late 1990s. This method has gained great recognition and is today accepted at many institutions.

Technique

After a standard posterior exposure, entry points of the screws are identified. Guide pins are inserted at expected entry points and checked by X-ray or fluoroscopy before preparing the screw tracts by different means – a drill and/or a probe [10]. Some surgeons prefer a direct technique using a curette or burr to create a wider entry and then observe the wall of the pedicle before making the channel for the screw [11]. In difficult circumstances, a small fenestration to the epidural space can be very helpful, with the dural sac under direct observation. These fenestrations are also very useful in rigid cases to create a "posterior release", removing the ligamenta flava and capsular structures and sometimes the whole joint especially on the concave side. In our experience screws are inserted at every level on the concave side of the curve, and at almost all levels on the convexity.

The current generally-accepted technique for scoliosis correction was originally developed by Suk and is as follows:

A contoured rod is applied into the screw heads on the concavity, bent or, preferably, overbent depending on the existing scoliotic curve (Fig. 1a–f). The next step is the simple rod de-rotation. The rod is rotated 90° [10]. By this means a virtually straight spine may be created (Fig. 1a–f). However the vertebral rotation may seem not to be much affected if not increased during this phase. Therefore a de-rotational manoeuvre has been developed – DVR-direct vertebral rotation [12]. By applying de-rotational forces on screw handles attached to screw heads on both sides in the apical region, the rotation of the scoliotic deformity can be reduced significantly. Before inserting the stabilising rod on the convexity, the joints and all posterior cortical surfaces are decorticated to induce a fusion. With this multiple-fixation technique, the use of bone grafts from iliac crest seems to be unnecessary thus avoiding donor site pain problems [13]. Pain problems from iliac crest have been recorded in up to 25 % of 2-year post-operative follow-ups [14]. The use of transverse bars between rods are probably not necessary since the vertebral bodies work as connectors between screws [15].

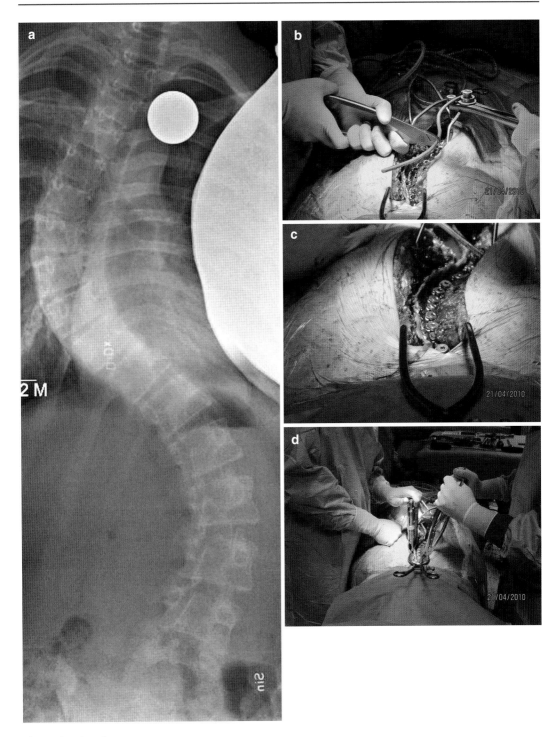

Fig. 1 (continued)

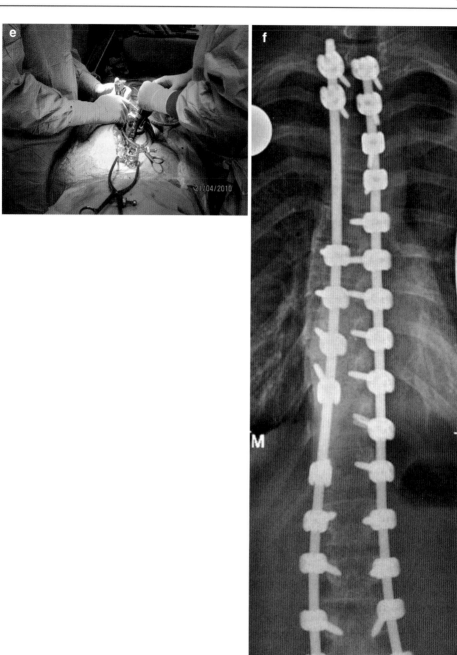

Fig. 1 (**a**) A postmenarchial girl, 14 years of age with AIS, preop PA. (**b**) Peroperatively, all screws are inserted, the concave rod is overbent. (**c**) The first rod is inserted. (**d**) Simple rod derotation, the assistants push at the convex side to inhibit further rotation. (**e**) Postoperatively, PA, at 6 months. (**f**) Direct Vertebral Rotation (DVR) by means of screw handles attached to the screw heads in the apical area

Transverse connectors at the top of a construct can even be harmful – in rare cases of progressive proximal junctional kyphosis a pull-out of upper screws may occur. There are reports of late compression of the spinal cord by ploughing screws and the use of transverse connectors may play a role [16].

Cantilever reduction techniques followed by DVR can also be made to obtain correction in all planes. With this technique two rods, pre-bent for the estimated sagittal profile, are simultaneously inserted into sequential screws heads on both sides, either in a caudo-cranial or opposite direction. Different methods to push the rods into the screw heads can be used. This correction technique is especially useful in cases with neuromuscular C-shaped scoliosis where the simple rod rotation technique as described above, does not easily result in a good correction.

Fixation of the pelvis has been a matter of continuous debate. In neuromuscular scoliosis with a pelvic tilt exceeding 20° there is a general acceptance to also include pelvis in the instrumentation and fusion. The pelvis may however be considered as a part of the scoliotic deformity and the necessity to include it in the fusion construct may not be quite obvious. Some surgeons stop at L5, bearing in mind the well developed ilio-lumbar ligamentous apparatus [17]. Multiple observations show that there is a high incidence of loss of pelvic fixation (windscreen-wiper sign). This is believed to be due to the long lever arms in combination with a poor bone stock. Previously the pelvic fixation was most often achieved by the Galveston [18] technique, which is time-consuming and may be difficult to achieve. The distal part of the longitudinal rod had to be bent and inserted in to the ilium. Today, almost all manufacturers of spinal implants provide the surgeon with connectors to attach the long rods to iliac screws making this ilio-lumbar fixation easier and faster. These connections are however sometimes prominent and may be painful. There is also a higher risk of deep infection when undertaking surgery in the pelvic area.

Adult Scoliosis

In adult scoliosis the same instrumentation methods are used as in adolescents. A more aggressive posterior release is frequently needed and sometimes also osteotomies may be necessary to achieve the intended correction. Problems with sagittal decompensation are however frequent; Cho et al. recently reported that up to 40 % of an adult cohort operated upon experienced these problems, especially in the lower lumbar area [19].

One probable reason for this is a poor sagittal balance pre-operatively and this must be corrected at the time of scoliosis correction. Screw loosening is another problem evident in this group of older patients. Solutions suggested are techniques to introduce bone cement into the screw channel, either directly with a syringe prior to inserting the screw or by means of a delivery system with special screws with a cement canal and perforations at the shaft and tip. No published results are yet available for the latter technique. One series from Belgium exists utilising this technique with poor results–and remains unpublished [20]. Trials with hydroxyapatite screws are in progress and promising results in human and animal studies have been published [21, 22]. Another line of development has been expandable pedicle screws. Data from biomechanical laboratories have provided positive results, however no convincing clinical success has yet been presented [23, 24].

Screw Head Development

During the last 10 years a significant development of screw head technology in spine instrumentation has occurred. Initially mono-axial as well as poly-axial screws were marketed. With mon-axial screws a perfect perpendicular fit between rod and screw is not always possible to obtain. This is because the screw trajectory in the thoracic spine is more caudally-oriented due to anatomical reasons. Some few of our early patients when using the Suk technique and

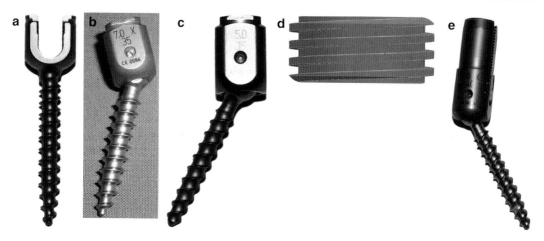

Fig. 2 (**a**) Mono-axial screw. (**b**) Uni-axial screw, permitting motion of the screw head in one plane. It gives probably a better correction in the coronal plane. (**c**) Polyaxial screw, the screw head permits a motion of about 25° to facilitate rod insertion. When the inner screw is fixed there is no more motion. (**d**) "Innie screw" – the thread design reduces "head spread" forces, which occurred with earlier screw designs. (**e**) Polyaxial reduction screw, enabling gradual correction, especially useful in severe deformities. Multiple subsequential screws are used simultaneously to diffuse forces when the rod is attached

titanium alloy implants reported noise from the back early post-operatively. Clinically, the backs became silent about 6 months post-operatively but the reason was obvious – an imperfect fit permitted some motion between screw heads and rods. For deformity correction, the poly-axial screw does not transmit the applied force to the spine but a great deal is lost in changing the screw head position. This means that extent of the correction is somewhat lost [25]. One way to solve this problem was the development of uni-axial screws, permitting a motion of the screw head in the cranio-caudal direction thus improving the fit of the rod in screw head (Fig. 2a–d). Clinically, the reporting of "noisy backs" is today very rare. The configuration of threads within the screw head has also undergone a further development from wedge-shaped to right-angle threads reducing the risk of having a "head-spread". This means that the tulip-formed head wings were spread due to force vectors with the former configuration of threads with subsequent poor fitting and long-term reduction in stability. Poly-axial screws are still used in the ends of a construct where stabilisation is the goal and not correction. Another development is the temporary extensions of the screw head, by flanges or "tabs" which are removed at the end of the procedure. This creates the possibility of a cantilever correction manoeuvre by having a row of screws of this type thus enabling delivery of the rod into multiple screw heads by means of working on the inner screws more evenly. This way of rod insertion or pushing with more evenly-distributed forces reduces the risk of screw pull-out. This is particularly useful in rigid neuromuscular cases with an associated poor bone stock.

We still observe that the inner screws become loose but today it is a rare occurrence. The reason is metallurgical – one cannot apply more force between the screw driver tip and the inner screw – otherwise screws can deform.

Recently a new low-profile system with an unconventional screw-rod locking mechanism has been developed – The Range Spinal System-by the K2M company. Until now no clinical results have been presented.

Spinal Cord Monitoring

Spinal cord monitoring is today considered mandatory during deformity surgery, in Scandinavia at least. At present, motor evoked potential monitoring (MEP's), which record the function of the spinal cord motor tract in real time, is to be preferred to the older and less reliable somato-sensory evoked potentials (SSEP) [26]. Most units employ both. The Scoliosis Research Society now advises that spinal cord monitoring is its preferred method of intra-operative spinal cord functional assessment [27].

Results

Since scoliosis is a deformity, not only in the coronal plane, but also involves rotation and associated change in the sagittal profile; the radiographic assessment of correction cannot be estimated only as a change of the Cobb angle.

Several reports indicate a correction in the coronal plane (Cobb), when using Suk's method, in the range of 65–75 % [21, 28, 29]. All-screw construct were superior to hybrid instrumentation in adolescent idiopathic scoliosis, with reported values of 70 % correction with screws versus 56 % with a hybrid construct when measuring the Cobb angle [28].

The corrective effect in an adult population was also significantly better in all-screw than in hybrid instrumentation, 56 % versus 41 % Cobb correction was reported by Rose et al. [30]. The true degree of pre- and post-operative rotation can only be assessed by means of CT (or MRI) and measuring the most rotated vertebra [29, 31]. This vertebra is most often located at the apex of the curve or one segment above or below [29, 32]. The reported de-rotational effect is in the range from 30 % to 60 % [12, 29, 33, 34].

Correction of the lower end vertebral tilt (LEVT) is of interest to reduce the risk of progression in the lumbar area in the long term. The Suk technique is effective in reducing LEVT in 70 % of cases [12, 29].

With respect to ability to correct the often hypokyphotic or even lordotic thoracic spine the literature is confusing. There are reports indicating that the Suk technique is inferior to hybrid constructs [33]. When using more rigid rods however, a re-creation of the thoracic kyfosis can actually be made with correction values in the range 5–7° [12, 29].

Another issue is that of economy. How many screws are needed to achieve a satisfactory correction? Clementz et al. have shown, that for a series of both hybrid and all-screw constructs, the number of anchors significantly improve the coronal correction when assessed by means of conventional radiography [35]. We have recently observed, by means of low-dose CT, that in all-screw constructs, the density of screws significantly affects the de-rotation as well as the re-creation of the thoracic sagittal profile [36]. With respect to coronal correction and LEVT, there was however, no statistically significant association between screw density and the result.

The use of screws is not without risk for neurological compromise and it is, based on the Scoliosis Research Society Morbidity and Mortality Committee's data, reported to occur in 1.75 % of cases operated on for adolescent idiopathic scoliosis posteriorly; no data on type of anchors was however mentioned [37].

The rate of mis-placed thoracic pedicle screws, evaluated with CT, varies widely from 6 % to 50 % [38–40]. Different definitions of mis-placements probably contribute to this variability in reported figures [41]. There is also a significant learning curve to achieve a low mis-placement rate [42].

Computer-assisted Orthopaedic surgery (CAOS), has been shown to improve the positioning of pedicle screws, at least in the lumbar spine [43]. A newer technique (the O-Arm) utilising a CT-like imaging intra-operatively together with a navigation system (Stealth Station) can hopefully be of benefit and reduce the number of misplaced screws. The radiation dose, when following the manufacturers' recommendation, is at present too high for young patients in our opinion. Recent studies indicate the radiation dose can be reduced by 10 times when using the O-Arm without compromising the required image quality for optimal spinal surgery [44].

Trials with rods made from memory metals have been completed in Beijing, China, in the 1980s. A recent report has been published in the English literature. Wang et al. used such rods temporarily for the correction and subsequently replaced them with conventional rods. They reported corrections of a mean 71 % Cobb, which was similar to many following the Suk technique [45].

Endoscopic Techniques

Jacobeus, a Swedish doctor of internal medicine, published his early-experience of thoracoscopy as well as laparoscopy in 1910 [46]. In the early 1990s, Regan from USA re-introduced this approach, for spinal surgery [47]. Blackman, Newton and Picetti, respectively, further developed this approach, for endoscopic correction of thoracic scoliotic curves. By means of this technique, a very good correction of moderate thoracic scoliotic curves could be obtained without any significant respiratory deterioration, which is one of the drawbacks of the open anterior technique [6]. These procedures are however very time-consuming and therefore this technique is not widespread today (Fig. 2a–d).

In the 1950s trials with stapling over discs on the convexity of a thoracic curve were performed but it was abandoned due to poor results [48]. By the turn of the millennium, Betz from Philadelphia presented endoscopically-inserted staples made from memory metal, over the convex discs in the thoracic as well as the lumbar regions [49]. From the positioning on the operating table, no significant corrective forces could be applied to the deformed spine. The presented results are comparable with these of brace treatment – 30 % need a further surgical treatment and 70 %were apparently effective [49, 50]. The results of stapling are not based on a prospective study and no controls for comparison between groups exists. Therefore no conclusion can be drawn. The limited Malmö experience of Betz staples consists of 12 cases that were stapled for idiopathic scoliosis with similar inclusion criteria as Betz's [49]. Of these more than six have undergone further and definite surgery [51]. Lenke has presented a similar technique, "The Tether"–connecting endoscopically-inserted vertebral body screws with a polymeric band under compression. He has reported promising results, the number of which is unfortunately very low [52]. Legislative policies have however stopped further trials in human beings, at least in the USA.

Growing-Rod Systems

VEPTR

In the late 1980s Campbell in the USA, was presented with a child patient a little more than 1 year of age, with aplasia of five ribs on one side. This malformation resulted in a severe scoliosis and the child needed a ventilator. The patient was operated on with a thoracotomy incision and the contracted soft tissue in the dysplastic region was divided. After distraction of the chest wall this was stabilised by two Steinmann pins turned around the second and tenth rib and the soft tissues of the chest wall were reconstructed. Soon the child was off the ventilator. Today after repeated surgical operations, the boy is able to play football.

Further development of this approach has resulted in a new approach to spine deformity surgery in children. This is the extra-spinal technique for the management of the deformed spine by VEPTR (Vertical Expandable Prosthetic Titanium Rib). Much research in the field of respiratory disturbance due to spine and chest wall deformities has been stimulated due to the dramatic effect of this particular case, and Campbell has then coined the term "Thoracic Insufficiency Syndrome", TIS [53].

The VEPTR technique is at present popularised worldwide and used in cases of primary thoracic wall disorders as well as in cases of congenital scoliosis. This includes several syndromes with respiratory compromise due to spinal deformities such as myelodysplasia and many others. It has also been used in cases of early onset idiopathic scoliosis. The patient has to be operated on repeatedly and with lengthening – usually every 6 months. Three fixation methods can be used. From the proximal ribs at the top, instrumentation may be made to more distal ribs, or the vertebral arches/pedicles or to the pelvis (Fig. 3a, b).

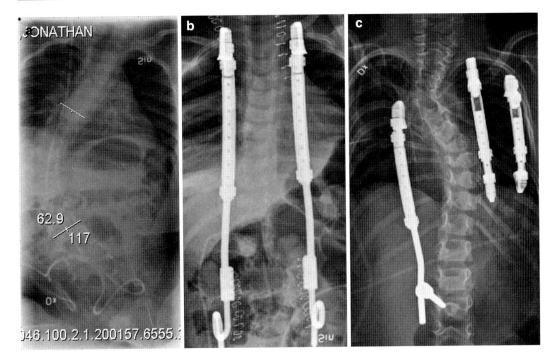

Fig. 3 (a) A boy 4 years of age with collapsing spine due to myelodysplasia, preop PA. (b) Surgery with subcutaneous insertion of VEPTR rods, rib to pelvis. Peroperative blood loss was 20 ml, postop PA. (c) A 5 year old girl with congenital scoliosis, three VEPTR devices were inserted

Further developments with bilateral rods, one on the corrective side and one on the stabilising side have been presented. Many problems have been observed, e.g., migration of anchor sites and therefore a further development has been presented – (VEPTR 2) –this new version has multiple cranial rib anchors. In cases of kyphosis it must be used with great caution since severe deterioration of this curvature has been observed repeatedly when using VEPTR.

The expected effect of VEPTR on long-term respiratory improvement assessed by pulmonary function test is still unclear. However impressive clinical and radiographic results have been presented [54, 55]. With this technique we can today provide many of our present patients a therapy, for which we previously had no good management to offer. By means of this indirect spine corrective surgery, one hasn't "burnt one's bridges."

Skaggs has recently presented a technique similar to VEPTR where you can use conventional modern spinal instruments. By means of this you can create a distraction between the lower spine to the chest wall and there is no need for special instruments during primary surgery or lengthenings [56].

Other Growing-Rod Systems

In children with little or no remaining growth potential left; correction and fusion has been and still is the "gold standard" in the operative treatment of scoliosis expected to exceed 50° or more Cobb angle at skeletal maturity.

Recent advances in the understanding of spine and thoracic cage development have shown that fusing a spine too early, not only results in a shorter stature but also result in a reduced volume of the thoracic cage with detrimental effects on respiration for the rest of the life. At the age of 10 years, the remaining growth of lung volume has been considered to be 50 % [57]. Growth arrest of the spine affects the growth of the ribs and the thoracic cage [58]. These new insights have resulted in the development and popularisation of growing-rod systems, enabling a straightened spine to grow further.

Growing-rod systems can be divided into those based on distraction or those based on guided growth.

The VEPTR technique, presented above can also be considered as a growing rod system but not principally necessarily anchored to the spine.

Distraction Systems

In the immature scoliotic spine one can create a cranial and distal anchor connected by rods, which can be lengthened at different periods, usually, a 6 month interval being preferred. The anchors to the spine at either end can be hooks, screws and sublaminar wires or combination of these. There has been a discussion whether to use a single or double-rod system. At present there is evidence for the double-rod construct being superior [59].

The place where distraction is applied can be at the ends of the rod, but the preference is the middle where domino connectors are used or specially made boxes containing parts of the rods.

Experience has shown that the distractive effect of lengthening procedures often disappear after 6 lengthenings or more. Histological examinations of specimens from facet joint in such cases have revealed degenerative changes in cartilage [60].

Guided-Growth System

A system based on multiple sublaminar wires connecting contoured rods to the spine (the Luque-trolley technique), but too long to permit growth was introduced in the early 1990s. With this technique, exposure of periosteal tissue was unavoidable which made spontaneous fusion frequent. The results of this correction technique have not been as good as expected and at present this technique is used infrequently [61].

A less invasive technique has recently been presented – the Shilla technique [62]. It was proposed by Richard McCarty who, according to the legend, had his idea when waking up at a luxurious Shilla hotel in South Korea (Shilla was one of the longest sustained dynasties in Korean history – 650–918 A.D.). It is based on an upper and a lower foundation by screw fixation. In the apical region of the deformity, two to four pairs of screws are inserted where a deformity correction is performed locally. With a temporary rod holding the apical correction, a long rod on the opposite side is inserted from below, tunnelled to the "middle region" where the rod is loosely fixed to these screws and further tunnelled in the sub-fascial muscle layer to the upper foundation. A stabilising rod is then inserted on the opposite side. Both rods are "too" long at both ends. The inner-screws in the middle are full fixed and here a formal fusion is performed; at the ends a special screw construct makes the inner screw fixation not firmly fixed, permitting the "too long" rods to slide in the end screws (Fig. 4). Guided growth technique can also be performed by the use of dual rods, i.e., implanting a fully fixed thicker rod at the bottom and having the thinner end of the "too long" rod passing screw heads with the larger diameter at top, enabling growth.

Problems identified are many, e.g., loosening of end screws due to long lever arms. In systems used for Shilla and when utilising Titanium implants, wear in the interface of screws and rods may occur at the end foundations due to motion of Titanium implants against each other, giving rise to a foreign body reaction with synovial-like fluid accumulation.

All these new growing rod systems are accompanied by many problems. The foundations at both ends are exposed to great mechanical forces because of long lever arms and therefore they are at an increased risk of mechanical loosening. The repeated lengthening operations are all an infection and soft tissue healing risk. An infection can, in many cases, be managed by temporary removal of the implants at the infection site, which after

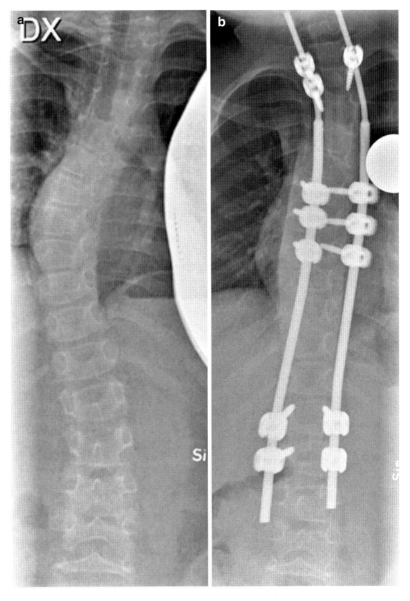

Fig. 4 (**a**) Shilla procedure in a 4 year old girl with syndromic scoliosis. Three pairs of screws in the apical area are locked, in either end the screws are not fully locked and the rods are intentionally too long, permitting growth. (**b**) PA postoperatively

antibiotic therapy and after some time, can be re-inserted with success. The whole process is in most cases favourable in spite of these complications [63].

Titanium

Titanium-alloy (Ti4V6Al) implants were popularised in spine surgery primarily due to their relative compatibility to MR-scanning.

Even pure titanium always contains traces of iron, which creates disturbances in imaging.

There have been some retrospective studies showing significantly lower incidence of implant associated infections when using Ti or Ti-alloy implants [64, 65]. Also Muscik et al. showed that it was possible to revise late infected stainless steel implants to titanium implants without recurrence of infection in 10 consecutive cases [66].

Interestingly there is a basic atomic/molecular explanation for this. In the sphere of researchers around Brånemark, who coined the term of osseointegration and successfully introduced Ti jaw screws in odontology, there have been reports published explaining why Ti implants not are subjected to infection in such a mileau as the mouth [67].

These laboratory investigations are not easy to comprehend – even by the well-read Orthopaedic surgeon! A brief explanation of the process is as follows:

All Ti implants, pure Ti as well as its alloys, are covered by a layer of TiO_2 as soon as they are exposed to the atmosphere. The inflammatory processes in the operative site induce inflammatory cells, e.g., leukocytes and macrophages, to release peroxidase enzymes (a more detailed explanation can be found in the literature of ROS, reactive oxidative specimen, which are out of the scope of the present presentation). In this environment a Ti-hydroxy-peroxide gel is formed. This gel will cover the whole implant. It is subsequently degraded to TiO_2 and during that process H_2O_2 as well as oxygen radicals are released. No bacteria will survive in this particular environment. The host cells are also at risk for the toxic influence and go necrotic, however they are soon replaced by new host cells in the vicinity. In cases of

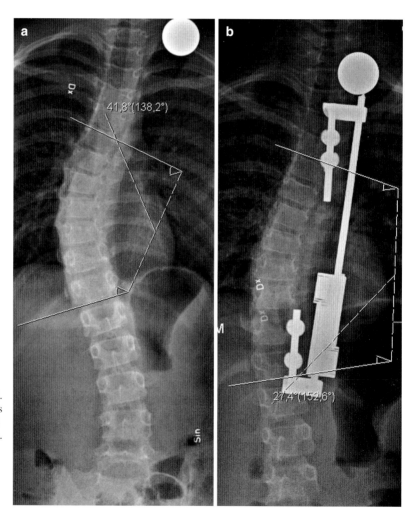

Fig. 5 (**a**) Magnetic rod (the French Phenix design). The patient is a boy 9 years of age, not tolerating brace treatment, preoperative PA. (**b**) Postoperative PA, the caregiver apply and rotate a magnet externally, with an estimated extension of 0.1 mm every morning

hematogenous deposition of bacteria in the vicinity of implants, these are protected by a similar chain of events.

There is, as mentioned, a scarce literature on the benefit of Ti implants for posterior implant instrumentation. In our own experience in Malmö, after having made more than 700 posterior Ti-alloy constructs, we have observed only two cases of late infection [51]. This is in contrast to our experience of a late infection rate of up to 5 % when using stainless steel implants in posterior spine surgery. The latter figures are in accordance with other reports [68].

The Future

Regarding spinal instrumentation for Paediatric scoliosis we can expect that further development of the endoscopic techniques in early progressive cases will be a reality.

For growing techniques there are lines of developments of implantable devices whereby one can distract rod systems by means of energy transferred magnetically from an external source [69]. Hopefully this will reduce the number of open distraction procedures all of which are expensive, time consuming and, of course, carry a potential risk of infection (Fig. 5a, b).

In general, further genetic and biomedical research will hopefully increase our understanding of underlying mechanism for spine deformity development. Furthermore, we can expect to predict when progression will occur, ensuring that the timing of interventions will be more precise.

References

1. Harrington PR. Treatment of scoliosis. Correction and internal fixation by spine instrumentation. J Bone Joint Surg Am. 1962;44-A:591–611.
2. Dwyer AF, Newton NC, Sherwood AA. An anterior approach to scoliosis. A preliminary report. Clin Orthop Relat Res. 1969;62:192–202.
3. Zielke K, Stunkat R, Beaujean F. Ventrale derotation-spondylodese. Arch Orthop Unfallchir. 1976;85(3): 257–77.
4. Kaneda K, Shono Y, Satoh S, Abumi K. New anterior instrumentation for the management of thoracolumbar and lumbar scoliosis. Application of the Kaneda two-rod system. Spine. 1996;21:1250–61.
5. Kim YJ, Lenke LG, Bridwell KII, Kim KL, Steger-May K. Pulmonary function in adolescent idiopathic scoliosis relative to the surgical procedure. J Bone Joint Surg Am. 2005;87:1534–41.
6. Kishan S, Bastrom T, Betz RR, Lenke LG, Lowe TG, Clements D, D'Andrea L, Sucato DJ, Newton PO. Thoracoscopic scoliosis surgery affects pulmonary function less than thoracotomy at 2 years postsurgery. Spine. 2007;32(4):453–8.
7. Luque E. The anatomic basis and development of segmental spinal instrumentation. Spine. 1982;7:257–9.
8. Cotrel Y, Dubousset J. Nouvelle technique d'ostéosynthèse rachidienne segmentaire par voie postérieure. Rev Chir Orthopédique. 1984;70:489–94.
9. Suk SI, Lee CK, Min HJ, CHO KH, Oh JH. Comparison of Cotrel-Dubousset pedicle screws and hooks in the treatment of idiopathic scoliosis. Int Orthop. 1994;18(6):341–6.
10. Suk SI, Kim WJ, Lee SM, Kim JH, Chung ER. Thoracic screw fixation in spinal deformities. Are they really safe? Spine. 2001;26(18):2049–57.
11. Kim YJ, Lenke LG, Bridwell KH, Cho YS, Riew KD. Free hand pedicle screw placement in the thoracic spine: is it safe? Spine. 2004;29(3):333–42.
12. Lee SM, Suk SI, Chung ER. Direct vertebral rotation: a new technique of the three dimensional deformity correction with segmental pedicle screw fixation in adolescent idiopathic scoliosis. Spine. 2004;29(3):343–9.
13. Betz RR, Lavelle WF, Samdani AF. Bone grafting options in children. Spine. 2010;35(17):1648–54.
14. Skaggs DL, Samuelson MA, Hale JM, Kay R, Tolo VT. Iliac crest bone grafting in spine surgery in children. Spine. 2000;25(18):2400–2.
15. Jeszinsky D. Personal Communication; 2008.
16. Alanay A, Cil A, Acaroglu E, Caglar O, Akgun R, Marangoz S, Yazici M, Surat A. Late spinal cord compression caused by pull-out thoracic pedicle screws: a case report. Spine. 2003;28(24):E 506–10.
17. Leong JC, Luk KD, Chow DH, Woo CW. The biomechanical function of the iliolumbar ligament in maintaining stability of the lumbosacral junction. Spine. 1987;12(7):669–70.
18. Allen Jr BL, Ferguson RL. The Galveston technique for L-rod instrumentation of the scoliotic spine. Spine. 1982;7(3):276–84.
19. Cho KJ, Suk SI, Park SR, Kim JH, Kang SB, Kim HS, Oh SJ. Risk factors of sagittal decompensation after long posterior instrumentation and fusion for degenerative scoliosis. Spine. 2010;35(17):1595–601.
20. Sörensen R. Personal Communication; 2009.
21. Sanden B, Olerud C, Petrén-Mallmin M, Larsson S. Hydroxyapatite coating improves fixation of pedicle screws. A clinical study. J Bone Joint Surg Br. 2002;84(3):387–9.

22. Upsani WW, Farusworth CL, Tomlinson T, Chambers RC, Tsutsui S, Slivka MA, Mahar AT, Newton PO. Pedicle screw surface coatings improve fixation in nonfusion spinal constructs. Spine. 2009;34(4):335–43.

23. Cook SD, Barbera J, Rubi M, Salkeld SL, Whitecloud TS. Lumbosacral fixation using expandable pedicle screws: an alternative in reoperation and osteoporosis. Spine J. 2001;1:109–14.

24. Lei W, Wu X. Biomechanical evaluation of expansive pedicle screw in calf vertebrae. Eur Spine J. 2006;15:321–6.

25. Lonner BS, Auerbach JD, Estreicher MB, Kean KE. Thoracic pedicle screw instrumentation: the learning curve and evolution in technique in the treatment of adolescent idiopathic scoliosis. Spine. 2009;34(20):2158–64.

26. Andersson G, Ohlin A. Spatial facilitation of motor evoked responses in spinal cord during spine surgery. Clin Neurophysiol. 1999;100(4):720–4.

27. Dormans JP. Establishing a standard of care for neuromonitoring during spinal deformity surgery. Spine. 2010;35(25):2180–5.

28. Kim YJ, Lenke LG, Kim J, Bridwell KH, Cho SK, Cheh G, Sides B. Comparative analysis of pedicle screw versus hybrid instrumentation in posterior fusion of adolescent idiopathic scoliosis. Spine. 2006;31(3):291–8.

29. Abul-Kasim K, Karlsson MK, Ohlin A. Increased rod stiffness improves the degree of deformity correction in adolescent idiopathic scoliosis. Scoliosis 2011;6:13.

30. Rose PS, Lenke LG, Bridwell KH, Mulconrey DS, Cronen GA, Buchowski JM, Schwend RM, Sides BA. Pedicle screw instrumentation for adult idiopathic scoliosis. An improvement over hook/hybrid fixation. Spine. 2009;34(8):852–7.

31. Aaro S, Dahlborn M, Svensson L. Estimation of vertebral rotation in structural scoliosis by computer tomography. Acta Radiol Diagn. 1978;19(6):990–2.

32. Acaroglu E, Yazici M, Deviren V, Alanay A, Cila A, Surat A. Does transverse apex coincidence with coronal apex level (regional or global) in adolescent idiopathic scoliosis. Spine. 2001;26(10):1143–6.

33. Newton PO, Yaszay B, Upsani VV, Pawelek JB, Bastrom TP, Lenke LG, Lowe T, Crawford A, Betz R, Lonner B. Preservation of thoracic kyphosis is critical to maintain lumbar lordosis in the surgical treatment of adolescent idiopathic scoliosis. Spine. 2010;35(14):1365–70.

34. Asghar J, Samdani AF, Pathys JM, D'andrea LP, Guille JT, Clementz DH, Betz RR. Computed tomography evaluation of rotation correction in adolescent idiopathic scoliosis: a comparison of an all pedicle screw construct versus a hook-rod system. Spine. 2009;34(8):804–7.

35. Clementz DH, Betz RR, Newton PO, Rohmiller M, Marks MC, Bastrom T. Correlation of scoliosis curve correction with number and type of fixation anchors. Spine. 2009;34(20):2147–50.

36. Abul-Kasim K, Ohlin A. A high screw density improves the degree of correction in the management of adolescent idiopathic scoliosis by segmental screw fixation. 2011; in manuscript 2010.

37. Coe JD, Arlet V, Donaldson W, Berven S, Hanson DS, Mudiyam R, Perra JH, Shaffrey CI. Complications in spinal fusion for adolescent idiopathic scoliosis in the new millennium. A report of the Scoliosis Research Society Morbidity and Mortality Committee. Spine. 2006;31(3):345–9.

38. Di Silvestre M, Parisini P, Lolli F. Complications of thoracic pedicle screws in scoliosis treatment. Spine. 2007;32(15):1655–61.

39. Upendra BN, Meena D, Chowdhury B, Ahmad A, Jayaswal A. Outcome-based classification for assessment of thoracic pedicular screw placement. Spine. 2008;33(4):384–90.

40. Abul-Kasim K, Ohlin A, Strömbeck A, Maly P, Sundgren PC. Radiological and clinical outcome of screw placement in adolescent idiopathic scoliosis: evaluation with low-dose computed tomography. Eur Spine J. 2010;19(1):96–104.

41. Abul-Kasim K, Strömbeck A, Ohlin A, Maly P, Sundgren PC. Reliability of low radiation dose CT in the assessment of screw placement after posterior scoliosis surgery, evaluated with a new grading system. Spine. 2009;34(9):941–8.

42. Abul-Kasim K, Ohlin A. The rate of screw misplacement in segmental pedicle screw fixation in adolescent idiopathic scoliosis; The effect of learning curve and cumulative experience. Acta Orthop. 2011;82(1):50–5; Epub 2010.

43. Laine T, Lund T, Ylikoski M, Lohikoski J, Sclenzka D. Accuracy of pedicle screw insertion with and without computer assistance: a randomized controlled clinical study in 100 consecutive patients. Eur Spine J. 2000;9(3):235–40.

44. Abul-Kasim K, Söderberg M, Ohlin A. Optimization of radiation exposure and image quality of the cone-beam O-arm intraoperative imaging system in spinal surgery. J Spine Disord Techn. 2012;25(1):52–58.

45. Wang Y, et al. Temporary use of shape memory spinal rod in the treatment of scoliosis. Eur Spine J. 2010. doi:10.1007/s 00586-010-1514-7; On line publ.

46. Jacobeaus HC. Ueber die Möglichkeit die Zystoskopie bei Untersuchung seröser Höhlungen anzuwenden. Muench Med Wochenschrift. 1910;57:2090–2.

47. Regan JJ, Mack MJ, Picetti GD. A technical report on video-assisted thoracoscopy in thoracic spinal surgery. Spine. 1995;20(7):831–7.

48. Smith AP, von Lackum WH, Wylie R. An operation for stapling vertebral bodies in congenital scoliosis. J Bone Joint Surg Am. 1954;36:342–8.

49. Betz RR, Ranade A, Samdani AF, Chafetz R, D'Andrea LP, Gaughan JP, Asghar J, Grewal H,

Mulcahey MJ. Vertebral body stapling: a fusionless treatment option for a growing child with moderate idiopathic scoliosis. Spine. 2010;35(2):169–76.

50. Danielsson AJ, Hasserius R, Ohlin A, Nachemson AL. A prospective study of brace treatment versus observation alone in adolescent idiopathic scoliosis: a follow-up mean of 16 years after maturity. Spine. 2007;32(20):2198–207.

51. Ohlin A. Personal Observation; 2010.

52. Lenke LG. Personal Communication; 2009.

53. Campbell RM, Smith MD. Thoracic insufficiency syndrome and exotic scoliosis. J Bone Joint Surg Am. 2007;89-A(Suppl1):108–22.

54. Skaggs DL. Hybrid distraction-based growing rods. In: Akbarnia BA, Yazici M, Thompson GH, editors. The growing spine. Berlin/Heidelberg: Springer; 2010. p. 601–11.

55. Emans JB, Caubet JF, Ordonez CL, Lee EY, Ciarlo M. The treatment of spine and chest wall deformities with fused ribs by expansion thoracostomy and insertion of vertical expandable prosthetic titanium rib. Spine. 2005;30:S58–68.

56. Motoyama EK, Deeney VF, Fine GF, Yang CI, Mutich RL, Walczak SA, Moreland MS. Effects of lung function of multiple expansion thoracoplasty in children with thoracic insufficiency syndrome: a longitudinal study. Spine. 2006;31(3):284–90.

57. Dimeglio A, Bonnel F, Canavese F. Normal growth of the spine and thorax. In: Akbarnia BA, Yazici M, Thompson GH, editors. The growing spine. Berlin/Heidelberg: Springer; 2010. p. 13–42.

58. Karol LA, Johnston C, Mladenov K, Schochet P, Walters P, Browne RH. Pulmonary function following early thoracic fusion in non-neuromuscular scoliosis. J Bone Joint Surg Am. 2008;90:1272–81.

59. Akbarnia BA, Marks DS, Boachie-Adjei O, Thompson AG, Asher MA. Dual growing rod technique for the treatment of progressive early onset scoliosis: a multi-center study. Spine. 2005;30(17 Suppl):S46–57.

60. Marks DS. Personal Communication; 2006.

61. Pratt RK, Webb JK, Burwell RG, Cummings SL. Luque trolley and convex epiphysiodesis in the management of infantile and juvenile idiopathic scolisis. Spine. 1999;24(15):1538–47.

62. McCarty R. Growth guided instrumentation: Shilla procedure. In: Akbarnia BA, Yazici M, Thompson GH, editors. The growing spine. Berlin/Heidelberg: Springer; 2010. p. 593–600.

63. Bess S, Akbarnia BA, Thompson GH, Sponseller PD, Shah SS, Sebaie HE, Boachie-Adjei O, Karlin LI, Canale S, Poe-Kochert C, Skaggs DL. Complications of growing-rod treatment for early-onset scoliosis. Analysis of one hundred and forty patients. J Bone Joint Surg Am. 2010;92:2533–43.

64. Soultanis KC, Pyrovolou N, Zahos KA, Karaliotas GI, Lenti A, Liveris I, Babis GC, Soucacos PN. Late postoperative infection following spinal instrumentation: stainless steel versus titanium implants. J Surg Orthop Adv. 2008;17(3):193–9.

65. Mueller FJ, Gluch H. Adolescent idiopathic scoliosis (AIS) treated with arthrodesis and posterior titanium instrumentation: 8–12 years follow up without late infection. Scoliosis. 2009;12:4–16.

66. Muschik M, Lück W, Schlenzka D. Implant removal for late-developing infection after instrumented spinal fusion for scoliosis: reinstrumentation reduces loss of correction. A retrospective analysis of 45 cases. Eur Spine J. 2004;13(7):645–51.

67. Tengvall P, Hörnsten EG, Elwing H, Lundström I. Bactericidal properties of a titanium-peroxy gel obtained from metallic titanium and hydrogen peroxide. J Biomed Mater Res. 1990;24(3):319–30.

68. Ho C, Sucato DJ, Richards BS. Risk factors for the development of delayed infections following posterior spinal fusion and instrumentation in adolescent idiopathic scoliosis patients. Spine. 2007;32(20):2272–7.

69. Miladi L, Dubousset JF. Magnetic powered extensible rod for thorax or spine. In: Akbarnia B, Yazici M, Thompson GH, editors. The growing spine. Berlin/Heidelberg: Springer; 2010. p. 585–92.

Surgical Management of Neuromuscular Scoliosis

J. Brad Williamson

Contents

Abstract

This chapter will discuss the problems associated with neuromuscular scoliosis in general, consider the more common diseases in which scoliosis occurs, and mention the problems associated with outcome measurement in this group of conditions.

Spinal deformity is a consequence of many neuromuscular conditions and is the result of lack of muscular control and muscular weakness.

Although there are similarities between curve patterns in different neuromuscular diseases, each disease is unique and each brings its own set of challenges. To speak of "neuromuscular scoliosis" as a single condition or disease is to grossly oversimplify the situation and to underestimate the consideration which needs to be given in establishing a treatment path.

Keywords

Anaesthesia • Blood loss • Cardio-respiratory assessment • Classification • Complications • Conservative treatment • Neuromuscular-Duchenne dysystrophy, spinal muscular atrophy, cerebral palsy • Operative techniques • Outcomes • Radiology • Scoliosis • Surgical treatment

J.B. Williamson
Division of Neurosciences, Salford Royal Hospital,
Salford, UK
e-mail: brad.williamson@srft.nhs.uk

G. Bentley (ed.), *European Surgical Orthopaedics and Traumatology*,
DOI 10.1007/978-3-642-34746-7_32, © EFORT 2014

Classification

The Scoliosis Research Society classification is the most commonly used (Fig. 1). This divides neuromuscular scoliosis according to diagnosis, the main division being into those caused by disorders of the nerves –neuropathic- and those caused by disorders of the muscle –myopathic. This classification is widely used, particularly in the United States, but is imperfect and does not reflect contemporary knowledge of neuromuscular conditions- for example Charcot Marie Tooth Disease is a disorder of peripheral nerve, rather than a spinocerebellar condition as classified [1]. It does not serve to inform the surgeon about management, as the grouping does not contain any commonality of surgical pathology, or indication of associated problems. European neurologists and surgeons only regard curves caused by diseases with progressive neurological deterioration as being truly neuromuscular, with those caused by static neurological lesions such as cerebral palsy not being classified as neuromuscular. This chapter recognizes the European point of view, but also considers the problems of cerebral palsy scoliosis as it is numerically the most common.

General Considerations

Neuromuscular scoliosis is generally of earlier onset and has a greater propensity to deteriorate than idiopathic scoliosis due to the underlying neuromuscular mechanism.

The functional reserve of the neuromuscular patient is less, and the effects of the scoliosis may be to impair the capacity for independent ambulation or precipitate dependence on aids. Functional considerations are thus more important than in idiopathic scoliosis. In those already confined to a wheelchair increasing pelvic obliquity may make seating difficult. Severe pelvic obliquity may remove the use of one hand, the arm being required to prop the child up in the chair in the face of a severe trunkal imbalance. The child

I   NEUROPATHIC

   A.   Upper motor neuron
      1.   Cerebral palsy
      2.   Spinocerebellar degeneration
         a.   Friedreich's ataxia
         b.   Charcot-Marie-Tooth disease
         c.   Roussy-Levy disease.
      3.   Syringomyelia
      4.   Spinal cord tumour.
      5.   Spinal cord trauma.

   B.   Lower motor neuron
      1.   Poliomyelitis
      2.   Other viral myelitides
      3.   Traumatic
      4.   Spinal muscular atrophy
         a.   Wernig-Hoffman disease.
         b.   Kugelberg-Welander disease.
      5.   Dysautonomic (Riley-Day syndrome).

II   MYOPATHIC

   A.   Arthrogryposis.

   B.   Muscular dystrophy
      1.   Duchenne's muscular dystrophy
      2.   Limb-girdle dystrophy
      3.   Fascioscapulohumeral dystrophy

   C.   Fiber-type disproportion.

   D.   Congenital hypotonia.

   E.   Myotonia dystrophica.

Fig. 1 Scoliosis Research Society – classification of neuromuscular scoliosis

thus becomes a "functional quadriplegic", with only one useful hand (Fig. 2).

The systemic nature of some neuromuscular diseases means that co-morbidities are common and often severe. Respiratory function is affected not only by the mechanical effects of the scoliosis, but also by the muscular weakness and poor co-ordination of the respiratory muscles. Myopathies also affect the cardiac and respiratory muscles. These factors need to be considered when making a treatment plan.

The risks of surgical intervention are greater than in a non-neuromuscular population. Prolonged peri-operative intubation in those with poor lung function makes respiratory infection more likely. Long operative times and malnutrition increase the chance of wound infection and pressure area problems. Cardiomyopathy and huge fluid shifts mean that patients are often haemodynamically unstable in the peri-operative period, mandating the involvement of skilled

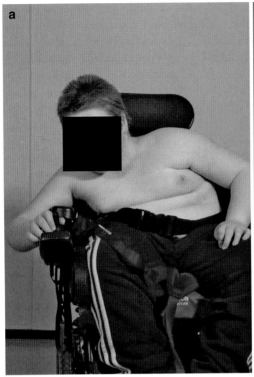 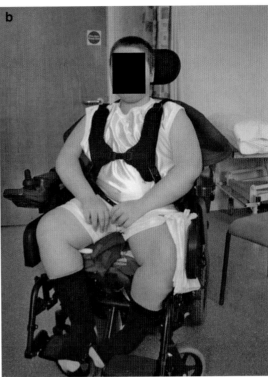

Fig. 2 Pre and post operative sitting posture of a boy with Duchenne Muscular Dystrophy (case of Mr NJ Oxborow) (**a**) Pre-operative, (**b**) Post-operative

anaesthetists and intensivists Disuse osteoporosis means that meticulous attention to fixation techniques and acknowledgment of the need for load-sharing is required.

Treatment

Conservative Treatment

Conservative treatment of neuromuscular spinal disorders is difficult.

Orthotic management, usually in the form of a custom moulded thoracolumbosacral orthosis (TLSO), is often employed. It is suggested that a TLSO may prevent or slow curve progression, but the evidence for this is poor. In those with flexible curves, a moulded orthosis may increase functional capability by allowing a more upright posture. In those with more severe or rigid curves this form of management produces little functional benefit, and is beset by skin problems.

Wheelchair fitting may also be regarded as an aspect of conservative treatment especially in those for whom surgical treatment is inappropriate. Seating a child with a severe curve is a task not to be underestimated. "Off the peg" chairs may be modified by the use of inserts and pads in those with relatively minor deformity, but those with severe deformity will require a custom moulded seat.

Tightly fitting lycra suits – "sleep suits", said to work by enabling greater proprioceptive feedback by increasing input from the skin, are often prescribed by physiotherapists, but there is little high quality evidence of their efficacy.

Surgical Treatment

Pre-Operative Evaluation
Radiology
The radiological assessment of neuromuscular scoliosis is more difficult than the assessment of

idiopathic scoliosis. Consistent positioning of the paralysed patient is difficult, and erect x-rays are often impossible to take. If standing x-rays are not feasible then it is sometimes possible to take seated x-rays in the wheelchair, but this requires skilled technical staff. Often it is impossible to get the whole spine on such films and detail of the pelvis is obscured by the shadow of the thighs. The use of a highly moulded wheelchair or matrix seat precludes taking x-rays in the chair and we must then use supine x-rays. Error may be introduced by faulty or inconsistent positioning in those with a flaccid paralysis, and it is of course impossible to assess the sagittal plane deformity from radiographs taken in the lying position.

There are a number of different ways of measuring the frontal plane spinal deformity, but measurement of the Cobb angle has been shown to have the smallest inter-observer error, with measurements being taken by multiple observers on the same radiograph [2]. Similarly a variety of methods of measurement of pelvic obliquity exist, but comparison of the intercristal line with the horizontal yields the most consistent measurements.

Patients with severe deformities may require imaging with CT scanning pre-operatively to assess the extent of secondary bony dysplasia and assess the pedicles or other anchor sites for competency. Patients with intra-spinal problems at the root of their diagnosis will need MR scanning pre-operatively.

Cardiorespiratory Assessment

Most patients being considered for corrective surgery are already under the care of a paediatric neurological team. The importance of their input into the planning of surgery, pre-operative assessment and peri-operative management cannot be overestimated. Many children will already be having respiratory support, and some will be on treatment and monitoring for their cardiomyopathy. Multi-disciplinary input into the planning of peri-operative management can result in a smoother passage for the patient, and fewer unforeseen problems. A history regarding respiratory problems, infections and management can be obtained from the parents or specialist nurse or physiotherapist who accompanies the patient. Physical examination may reveal signs of respiratory failure.

There are a number of pathological processes at the root of respiratory insufficiency in neuromuscular scoliosis;

Firstly, chest wall deformity and diaphragmatic restriction by thoracolumbar curvature and pelvic obliquity increase the work of breathing. This latter is particularly important given the diaphragm's major role in quiet respiration.

Secondly, muscular weakness secondary to the underlying pathology hampers the ability to breath. In patients with some neuropathic conditions bulbar problems lead to incoordination of swallowing and aspiration, with frequent respiratory infections lessening the respiratory reserve. The cough is often weak, due to a combination of coordination and muscle strength problems.

The assessment of cardiorespiratory status is fundamental to the performance of safe surgery in neuromuscular scoliosis. Spinal corrective surgery is a huge physiological stress, in a patient who is already compromised because of neuromuscular disease. Even in a heterogeneous group of patients – 38 % neuromuscular – lung function declined by up to 60 % in the immediate postoperative period, recovering only 2 months after surgery [3] It can be seen that an adequate respiratory reserve is required for safe surgery.

It is clear that assessment of respiratory function is important in the assessment of fitness for surgery. Spirometry is often performed, but in some conditions there are technical issues which limit its usefulness. In cerebral palsy poor coordination may give a falsely pessimistic outlook, whereas in paralytic conditions weakness of this orbicularis oris may impair the ability to make a seal around the mouthpiece, resulting in an inaccurate assessment. Respiratory volume is indicated by the Forced Vital Capacity (FVC) which is usually reported as a percentage of that predicted from the height (arm span is often used in the wheelchair bound or scoliotic). The ability to generate an explosive expulsion – as in coughing – is indicated by the Forced Expiratory Volume in 1 s (FEV1). Sniff nasal inspiratory pressure (SNIP) may give a good indication of this latter, and is technically easier in this population [4].

Percentage of predicted FVC gives a good indication of the respiratory risk in a given procedure. Generally an FVC of less than 30 % predicted gives cause for concern [5] but with adequate cardiac function need not preclude surgery by an experienced team. In our centre we have safely operated upon a boy with Duchenne's muscular dystrophy with only 17 % of the predicted FVC.

Many patients nowadays have active respiratory management as part of their neurology treatment. It is not uncommon for children to have home oxygen or home respiratory support. Oxygen dependency or the use of nocturnal BIPAP need not disqualify the patient from spinal surgery. Many of our patients with Spinal Muscular Atrophy are treated with nocturnal BIPAP. After surgery they are usually extubated in the recovery area, and re-established on BIPAP before discharge to the high- dependency unit.

Some neuromuscular conditions such as Duchenne's Muscular Dystrophy and Friedreich's Ataxia are complicated by a progressive cardiomyopathy. In these patients a detailed assessment of cardiac function is required pre-operatively. Electrocardiographic abnormalities are common, especially in myotonic dystrophy and Duchenne, but hard to quantify. All such patients should undergo echocardiography to obtain a quantification of left ventricular function. This is sometimes technically difficult because of chest wall deformity secondary to the scoliosis. In these circumstances trans-oesophageal echocardiography or even an isotope MUGA scan may be required. Generally speaking, those with a left ventricular ejection fraction of less than 50 % require medical assessment/treatment before consideration of surgery.

In spite of these acknowledged respiratory difficulties there is ample evidence that with suitably skilled peri-operative care surgery in children with neuromuscular scoliosis can be undertaken safely (Bentley et al. [64]).

Almenrada and Patel [5] found that of their population of patients with non-idiopathic scoliosis only 25 % needed ventilatory support post-operatively. Of this 25 %, no attempt was made to extubate in the immediate post-operative period in half, ventilatory support being elective for patients with prolonged surgery or very high blood loss. Of the boys with Duchenne Muscular Dystrophy 40 % were ventilated post-operatively. Bach and Sabharwal [6] presented five patients with poor lung function and a diagnosis of Duchenne Muscular Dystrophy or spinal muscle atrophy, all of whom were extubated to non-invasive positive pressure ventilation post-operatively. However Yuan et al. found that boys with neuromuscular scoliosis and poor FEV1 were most likely to require post-operative ventilation [7].

Anaesthetic Considerations

The peri-operative management of children with neuromuscular scoliosis is not a matter for the occasional anaesthetist. As well as the general requirement for familiarity with the problems of the various neuromuscular diseases, some diseases are associated with specific susceptibility to anaesthetic agents. For example Central Core Disease shares an allele with malignant hyperpyrexia, and cross- reactions are sometimes seen in Duchenne muscular dystrophy.

Patients with myotonic dystrophy are sensitive to suxamethonium, which can cause ventricular tachycardia or fibrillation with cardiac arrest. It is wise to avoid the use of suxamethonium in all cases of progressive muscle weakness.

Nutritional Status

There is a well-documented relationship between nutritional status and peri-operative complications in those undergoing Orthopaedic surgery [8]. Protein depletion correlates well with increased mortality, impaired wound healing, and increased wound infection rates. Given that the metabolic stresses of spinal reconstructive surgery are perhaps greater than any other form of Orthopaedic surgery it is sensible to optimize nutritional status before surgery. Nutritional assessment can take the form of BMI measurement (bearing in mind that obesity as well as low BMI can be an indicator of poor nutrition), assessment of serum protein and albumen levels. It has been shown that patients with a serum albumin level of less than 3.5 g%. or a lymphocyte count of less than 1,500 per cubic ml. have greater infection rates, periods of intubation and length of stay [8].

There are many reasons for nutritional impairment in this group of patients. Incoordination of the muscles of mastication and swallowing may make eating difficult. Gastro-oesphageal reflux is common, leading to oesophagitis, vomiting and aspiration. Ideally surgically-remediable factors should be addressed prior to the consideration of spinal surgery, but one may find oneself in the situation of balancing the sub-optimal nutritional state against delaying surgery in a curve which is progressing relentlessly. Laparoscopic fundoplication will provide an answer to reflux related problems, whilst mechanical problems with eating can be addressed by the insertion of a PEG gastrostomy. A co-ordinated, multi-disciplinary approach to children with neuromuscular scoliosis will enable the spinal surgeon to be presented with the patient in the best possible condition.

Operative Techniques

Although each neuromuscular diagnosis brings with it a unique set of challenges, there are a number of common problems which face the surgeon.

Pelvic Obliquity

The configuration of neuromuscular curves is different from that of non-neuromuscular curves. The curves are longer, more "C" shaped and frequently extend to the lumbar spine, involving the sacro-pelvis. Pelvic obliquity is thus a common feature. The problems which follow from pelvic obliquity are those of ischial pressure areas (especially in thin patients), difficulty in seating, toilet/hygiene difficulty, and sometimes hip subluxation. Correction of pelvic obliquity is therefore an important part of deformity correction.

Although the L5 vertebra is firmly anchored to the pelvis by the iliolumbar ligaments, only with the advent of the Galveston technique [9] was it possible to apply consistent corrective forces to the pelvis. The addition of pedicle screw fixation, either in the sacrum or L5 further increased the strength of the construct and allowed the application of greater corrective forces. The Galveston technique describes the passage of a bone anchor down a thick tube of iliac bone stretching from the region of the posterior inferior iliac spine, superior to the sciatic notch to the roof of the acetabulum (the "Galveston channel"). The anchor originally described was the end of a spinal rod. This necessitated the performance of a complex, three-dimensional rod-bending manoeuvre towards the end of a procedure which was often long and tiring. The technical difficulty of this procedure should not be underestimated.

More recently it has been usual to fix to the pelvis using pelvic screws or bolts. This is technically much more straightforward, and the resulting construct performs as well as Galveston rods in correction of obliquity [10, 11].

Such pelvic fixation is bulky, and the screw heads sit in the relatively superficial area of the posterior iliac crest. In the poorly-nourished neuromuscular population the screws can often be felt, and serious skin problems are not uncommon. These can be mitigated, but not abolished by meticulous attention to detail – countersinking the screw head, the use of as few bulky connectors as possible and careful approximation of the thoracolumbar fascia over the screw head.

Once a secure ilio-sacral foundation has been established correction of pelvic obliquity can be accomplished by the application of cantilever forces by means of reduction of the (usually convex) rod to the curve. This manoeuvre is aided by the application of a distraction force to the high side of the pelvis.

More severe pelvic obliquity can be addressed by the application of corrective forces by intra-operative halo femoral traction. In this technique a halo is applied to the patient's skull before prone positioning, and a supracondylar pin or wire applied to the femur ipsilateral to the high side of the pelvis. Traction is then applied to the femur, and counter traction to the halo. A little anti-Trendelenburg positioning is helpful. By this method a good postural correction of pelvic

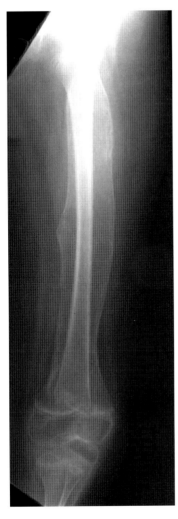

Fig. 3 Healing of supracondylar femoral fracture following intra-operative traction

In view of the significant complication rate associated with sacro-pelvic fixation, and the firm fixation of L5 to the sacro-pelvis, some authors have questioned the need for sacro-pelvic fixation, even in patients with marked pelvic obliquity. McCall and Hayes [14] compared patients fused to L5 with those fused to the sacro-pelvis. Although the groups were similar, the method of allocation was not stated. They found that in both groups the correction of pelvic obliquity was good, but slightly better and better maintained in the sacro-pelvic group.

Sacro-pelvic fixation has a high complication rate. Emami et al. [15] performed a retrospective review of 54 deformity patients fused to the sacro-pelvis. A variety of fixation techniques were used (11 Luque/Galveston, 36 Isola S1 and pelvic bolts, 12 Isola bi-cortical S1 screws) and there was a complication rate, mostly associated with sacro-pelvic fixation of almost 50 %. In addition 10 patients required further surgery for pseudarthrosis, and 9 required removal of iliac bolts.

Tsuchiya [16] also found a significant complication rate in patients having sacro-pelvic fixation – a 6 % lumbosacral pseudarthrosis rate and a significant rate of iliac fixation problems [14].

Edwards et al. [17] compared patients fused to L5 and the sacro-pelvis. The complication rate was high in both groups – of 27 fused to L5, 22 had complications, whereas the 12 fused to S1 experienced 75 complications. Those fused to the sacro-pelvis underwent significantly more procedures than those fused to L5 (1.7 procedures per patient in L5 group vs. 2.8 in the S1 group). There was no difference in the clinical outcomes.

Modi [18] examined 55 patients and examined the correction of pelvic obliquity and the relationship to pelvic fixation. He found that if there was more than 15° of pre-existing pelvic obliquity and pelvic fixation was not performed then there was a significantly greater loss of correction of pelvic obliquity with follow-up. The functional significance of this loss was not clear.

There is a trend to question the need for complex sacro-iliac fixation. Bilateral fixation may

obliquity can be achieved, which can be developed further by the use of the surgical techniques mentioned above. The utility of this technique in a group of 20 patients was reported by Takeshita et al. [12]. Vialle et al. [13] reported better results, and shorter operative times in patients who underwent intra-operative traction than those subjected to more traditional manoeuvres alone. Although intra-operative traction is a useful technique it is not without pitfalls. The insertion of traction pins in those with osteoporotic bone is a cause for concern – we have had one patient who suffered an ipsilateral supracondylar fracture of the femur (Fig. 3).

not be required, unilateral fixation may suffice. In view of the evidence above, the complication rate of sacro-iliac fixation may outweigh the potential benefits. Further work is required.

Severe Curves

Because neuromuscular scoliosis is of earlier onset than idiopathic scoliosis, and has a propensity to progress even after skeletal maturity, neuromuscular curves tend to be larger than idiopathic ones. This tendency is exacerbated by having a higher threshold for intervention in children with such co-morbidities. Correction of the deformity is therefore more challenging, and specialized techniques are often appropriate. Segmental fixation with Luque wires gained widespread acceptance in neuromuscular scoliosis before idiopathic scoliosis, and it is fair to say that radical destabilizing surgery, such as total spondylectomy and posterior vertebral column resection (PCVR), were adopted for neuromuscular curves before gaining widespread acceptance in idiopathic curves.

Pedicle screw fixation was adopted as the gold standard for fixation of neuromuscular curves long before it's almost universal prevalence in idiopathic scoliosis. Modi et al. [19] reviewed 52 patients with Cerebral Palsy (CP) scoliosis. They found good correction of scoliosis, but one patient had a temporary paresis secondary to a misplaced screw. There were also 2 haemothoraces – it is not clear if these were due to screw malposition The same author [20] found that the use of pedicle screws enabled a modest (25 %) correction of rotatory deformity. The mechanism of reduction of the deformity was not specified in his paper. However the reduction in rotation was independent of diagnosis.

Blood Loss

Blood loss is a particular issue in surgery for neuromuscular scoliosis. Patients with neuromuscular scoliosis have more extensive surgery than patients with idiopathic or congenital scoliosis, with more levels being fused. The curves are often worse; the surgery is technically difficult and takes longer. However, even when these factors are controlled for the blood loss in patients with neuromuscular scoliosis is considerably higher. Edler et al. [21]

found that even when the number of levels operated was controlled for patients having surgery for neuromuscular scoliosis had a seven times greater chance of having a blood loss of more than 50 % of their estimated blood volume.

Complications of Surgery

Complications are more common in patients with neuromuscular scoliosis. They have more co-morbidities and medical complications are more common. Wounds are more extensive and the patients are not well nourished and to a degree immuno-compromised. Children with neuromuscular scoliosis tend to have a higher length of stay and hospital mortality than those with other diagnoses [22].

Mohamad et al. [23] in a review of 175 patients, predominantly with cerebral palsy (129/175) found that complications were common. In his group there were 96 complications in 58 patients. Nine percent of the patients had respiratory complications and 8 % wound infections. 4 % had cardio-vascular complications – mainly coagulopathy secondary to bleeding. A higher rate of complications was associated with seizure disorder, longer operations, increased estimated blood loss and sacral pelvic fixation.

Sarwark and Sarwahi [24] looked at the determinants of survival in their population of patients with neuromuscular scoliosis. If their kyphosis was more than one standard deviation above the mean (the mean was 56°, one standard deviation above was 86°) there was an excess mortality of 122 %. Similarly those who spent more than 30 days on the Intensive Care Unit had a mortality of ten times those who did not.

Vitale et al. [25] found that the length of stay and complications were higher in patients whose treatment was funded by Medicaid than private insurers. Whether this was due to societal factors or factors in the delivery of care is not clear. They also found a relationship between the outcome and the volume of surgery undertaken at a given institution, but this effect had a very low floor, with no additional benefit being perceived for operating on more than five cases per annum.

Tsirikos et al. [26] examined life expectancy after surgery for cerebral palsy. They found that a number of surgical variables (as well as a number that correlated directly with disease severity) correlated with length of post-operative survival. These included spinal deformity, intra-operative blood loss, operative time, length of ICU stay and length of hospital stay. Whilst it could be argued that these variables are surrogates for disease severity, the importance of the avoidance of complications is highlighted. The mean survival time for globally affected children was 11 years 2 months.

Spinal Cord Monitoring

Spinal cord monitoring is possible in patients with neuromuscular scoliosis. In our own series using epidural electrodes we found that it was possible to monitor consistently except in patients with neurodegenerative diseases. [27]. The findings of Tucker et al. were similar [28]. Both of these authors reported series using epidural electrodes.

The situation with respect to cortical evoked potential monitoring is more difficult, and it may be harder to monitor in conditions affecting the cerebral pathways.

Considerations in Specific Diseases

Duchenne Muscular Dystrophy

Duchenne Muscular Dystrophy is the commonest muscular dystrophy, affecting about 1 in 3,500 – 6,000 male live births. It leads to progressive disability and although advances in treatment have seen life expectancy extended, boys with Duchenne Muscular Dystrophy usually die in their third decade [29].

Duchenne is inherited in an x-linked recessive manner but a third of cases are caused by new mutations. The locus of the genetic defect in Duchenne is Xp21. This is the dystrophin locus where dystrophin, a large but uncommon protein is encoded.

Dystrophin is active in the cell membrane of all muscles. It connects the sarcolemma to the muscle protein actin. Dystrophin is important in calcium transport and is thought to be essential for force transduction by linking the contractile mechanism to the extracellular matrix.

About two-thirds of boys with DMD have a gross rearrangement deletion, whereas the other third have duplications (10 %) or smaller point mutations (10 %). The smaller mutations may lead to a reduction rather than complete absence of dystrophin, leading to a milder phenotype (for example Becker Muscular Dystrophy) – rather than the more severe Duchenne. Boys with Duchenne generally have absence of dystrophin in skeletal and cardiac muscle. Some isoforms of dystrophin are also expressed in the brain and absence of these isoforms is responsible for the low intellect which complicates a proportion of cases of Duchenne.

Only one-third of cases are due to transmission from the mother. Advances in molecular genetics now allow precise evaluation of carrier status of females in the family of an affected individual. Determination of carrier status is important, because as well as for reasons of counselling and ante-natal diagnosis, carriers have a 10 % lifetime risk of developing cardiomyopathy and appropriate surveillance is clearly important [30].

Late diagnosis of Duchenne continues to be a problem [31–34], The reason for this delay may be that healthcare workers do not see children performing high demand activities such as running and rising from the floor which require well developed muscle power. Late motor development, frequent falls, waddling gait, persistent toe walking and difficulty running may be presenting features to the Orthopaedic surgeon.

The first investigation in such children should be a serum creatinine kinase (CK) which is always extremely elevated (10–100 x normal) in Duchenne. A high CK should instigate a referral to a specialist neuromuscular clinic for diagnosis. A normal CK at presentation excludes the diagnosis.

Scoliosis is common in boys with Duchenne, but only progresses once they become dependent upon a wheelchair [35].

There are a number of issues for the spinal surgeon which are unique to patients with Duchenne Muscular Dystrophy.

Natural History

Scoliosis is very common in boys with Duchenne Muscular Dystrophy once they are wheelchair-bound. Scoliosis in wheelchair-bound boys with Duchenne Muscular Dystrophy may be invariable if they are followed until death [36]. Galasko quotes the incidence to be over 90 %. [35, 37] Rideau [38] recognises different categories of severity of scoliosis in Duchenne Muscular Dystrophy, however all who were followed until death developed some degree of scoliosis. At the other end of the spectrum Brooke [39] found that almost 25 % of patients had "a relatively straight back". Factors which may modify the progression of scoliosis include prolongation of walking in long-leg callipers [35, 40] and prolongation of walking by the use of steroids [41].

A number of authors have reported the natural history of scoliosis in Duchenne Muscular Dystrophy. Although most boys with DMD develop a scoliosis, and it is progressive in most, some do not progress.

Kinali et al. [42] reported their experience in a large neuromuscular clinic. This unit had the policy of only offering surgery to those who developed curves of more than 50°. The authors question the need for spinal fusion in all who have a scoliosis, saying that perhaps 35 % do not need spinal surgery. However it is clear from their paper that a significant number of their patients with a larger scoliosis were not suitable for surgery because of lack of fitness. The current guideline [43] is that scoliosis surgery should be considered for patients whose curve reaches 20–40°.

The natural history of the Orthopaedic problems in Duchenne Muscular Dystrophy can be improved by the use of steroids. Houde et al. [44] found significant differences in patients treated with steroids when compared with those who were not. They found improved cardiac function, prolonged walking time and a decreased incidence of scoliosis. They hypothesise that the use of steroids may eliminate the need for spinal surgery. However vertebral crush fractures and stunted spinal growth were much more common in the steroid-treated group.

King et al. [45] in a study of a large number of patients found that the use of steroids delayed the age at which boys became wheelchair dependent by some 3.5 years. The prevalence of scoliosis was decreased from 91 % to 31 %, and when scoliosis occurred it was less severe (average Cobb angle of 11° against 32°). However 32 % of the treated group had concomitant vertebral fractures (none in the control group) and long bone fractures were 2.6 times more frequent. The boys treated with steroids were 13.9 kg heavier than those not treated with steroids. Overall they found that the risk of scoliosis surgery was reduced to one-third of the risk in the untreated group. However it would be clear to all surgeons that boys with Duchenne Muscular Dystrophy have a degree of osteoporosis, even without steroid treatment. The technical difficulty of spinal surgery in those who have had prolonged steroid treatment is greatly increased.

Blood Loss

Those familiar with spinal surgery in Duchenne Muscular Dystrophy will be aware of the technical difficulty of all aspects of the surgery. The dissection is difficult with the paraspinal muscles being replaced by a dense fibrotic mass, making dissection down to the posterior elements more difficult. Even with painstaking technique, the blood loss in boys with Duchenne Muscular Dystrophy is higher than for other forms of posterior spinal surgery. Noordeen et al. [46] compared the blood loss in patients with Duchenne Muscular Dystrophy with other neuromuscular groups and found a significantly higher blood loss in boys with Duchenne, even when other variables were corrected for. He hypothesised that this was due to a lack of dystrophin in the smooth muscle of the vessel walls, impairing the contractility and preventing haemostasis.

Turturro [47] found that boys with Duchenne Muscular Dystrophy had a higher peri-operative blood loss, independent of all other surgical variables. They found an increased bleeding time in Duchenne Muscular Dystrophy and examined the platelets of control patients who did not have DMD. No dystrophin was found in these non-Duchenne platelets and the suggestion that there may be a defect in platelet function was not supported. The authors suggested a primary defect of haemostasis possibly due to impaired vessel reactivity.

The measures which the surgeon can take to alleviate this effect, apart from meticulous attention to surgical detail and careful positioning, include the use of pharmacological anti-fibrinolytic agents. Aprotonin has been shown to be extremely efficacious in this regard. Its main use was in cardiac surgery and unfortunately because of problems in cardiac surgery its use has been discouraged. We no longer use aprotonin for patients with idiopathic scoliosis, but as it is still available on a named patient basis in the UK, we use it in patients with neuromuscular scoliosis However tranexamic acid has also been shown to reduce the blood loss significantly in patients with Duchenne Muscular Dystrophy [48].

Operative Technique and Fusion Levels

There remains debate as to the type of surgery to be performed in boys with Duchenne Muscular Dystrophy. All are agreed that a posterior spinal fusion is the operation of choice, with anterior surgery being precluded by the patient's respiratory function. Segmental fixation is universally accepted.

Gaine et al. [49] compared the use of Luque sublaminar wires with Isola hybrid instrumentation, with pedicle screws being used in the lumbar spine. They found that not only did the Isola instrumentation produce a better correction but there was less loss of correction post-operatively.

There is much debate about the caudal extent of spinal fusion in Duchenne Muscular Dystrophy. Some authorities maintain that it is not necessary to fuse past L5 whereas others argue that fusion to the sacro-pelvis produces better outcomes.

Mubarak et al. [50] examined 22 patients, of whom 12 were fixed to the pelvis and 10 to L5. All patients had small curves and pelvic obliquity was assessed clinically. No difference was seen between the two groups.

There are a number of papers which report good results in patients having long spinal fusions from the upper thoracic spine to the pelvis. However, Hahn et al. [51] were operating on

a relatively low risk population with an average 44° pre-operative Cobb angle and an average pre-operative forced vital capacity of 55 % of predicted. Notwithstanding this they had a 77 h intensive care length of stay and one intra-operative death. Similarly Mehta et al. [52] had a policy of pelvic fixation for pelvic obliquity of more than 15°. They also had one peri-operative death. Takaso et al. [53] examined 28 patients with large (75°) curves. All were fused to L5 with pedicle screws. All had a curve apex caudal to L2 though they found that an L5 tilt of less than 15° prognosticated for a good correction of pelvic obliquity. However if the L5 tilt was greater than 15° there was significant residual pelvic obliquity. The functional significance of this is not clear.

Alman & Kim [54] examined 48 patients treated by Luque Galveston surgery. 38 were fused to L5 and 10 with more pelvic obliquity were to the sacrum. They found that those whose curve apex was caudal to L1, if only fused to L5, had a much greater increase in pelvic obliquity when compared to those fused to S1. It can be argued that this paper examines historical surgical methodology which may not be directly applicable to the use of pedicle screw instrumentation.

Sengupta [55] compared two groups of patients, one group being operated early, the other late. The earlier operated group were treated by pedicle screws down to L5 whereas the later group were treated by Luque Galveston instrumentation down to the sacral pelvis. They found equally satisfactory results in terms of pelvic obliquity in those treated early and fused down to L5.

It is our experience that fusion to L5 with pedicle screw instrumentation leads to a satisfactory result in all but those with the most severe pelvic obliquity (Fig. 4).

Lung Function

A number of authors have examined the effects of spinal surgery on lung function in Duchenne Muscular Dystrophy. Untreated the respiratory function of boys with Duchenne progressively worsens as they age.

Galasko et al. [37] found that the performance of spinal stabilisation produced a 3 year plateau in the decline of forced vital capacity when

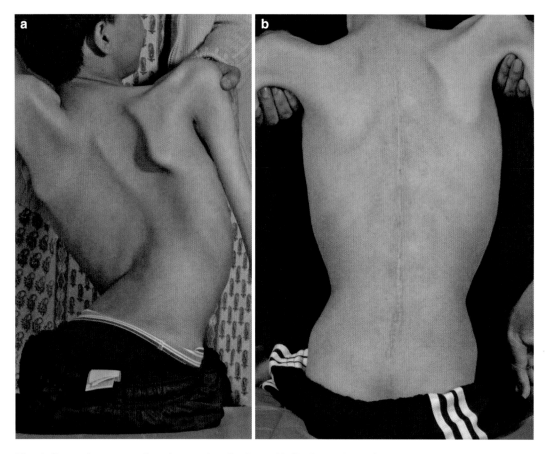

Fig. 4 Pre- and post-operative photographs of a boy with Duchenne Muscular Dystrophy showing satisfactory correction of pelvic obliquity with instrumentation to L5. (**a**) Pre-operative, (**b**) Post-operative

compared to an un-operated, and seemingly identical, cohort of patients who declined the offer of surgery. They also found that significantly more of the boys who accepted the offer of surgery were alive 5 years from the date of the offer.

Kennedy [56] examined 17 patients, some of whom had surgery and some of whom did not they found no difference in the rate of decline of respiratory function.

A number of other authors have found no difference in lung function between those operated and those not [57, 58] However Velasco [59] in a more recent paper concluded that posterior spinal fusion slowed the rate of respiratory decline in boys with Duchenne Muscular Dystrophy. Eagle et al. [60] found that the effects of spinal surgery and nocturnal home ventilation were additive. Patients having both ventilation

and surgery survived to 30 years, compared with 22.2 years for those who only had ventilation. Those who had neither lived to 17.2 years.

Galasko et al. [35] demonstrated that a standing regimen protected lung function and delayed the onset of progression of scoliosis. They reported a large series of patients who had no major complications from spinal surgery. Once again they reported that the forced vital capacity remained static for 36 months after spinal surgery. Significantly they found that 61 % of the cohort who accepted the offer of spinal surgery was alive at 5 years compared with 23 % of the matched cohort who declined the offer.

A number of papers have examined the effect of lung function on surgical prognosis. It is often quoted that spinal surgery should not be performed in boys with an FVC of less than 30 %.

Takaso et al. [61] examined 14 patients, all of whom had an FVC of less than 30 %. All had pedicle screw fixation with no complications. All of the patients and their parents thought that there was an appreciable quality of life gain. Marsh et al. [62] compared two groups of patients, one of whom had an FVC of greater than 30 % and one had an FVC of less than 30 % and found no difference in the surgical outcomes or rate of complications. Harper et al. [63] again compared those with an FVC of greater or less than 30 %. They found no difference but did suggest that in the group with the worst lung function weaning onto non-invasive ventilation may smooth the post-operative course. Bentley et al., in a seies of 64 patients with Duchenne Muscular Dystrophy with a range of 18–63 % forced vital capacity, found no influence on outcome [64].

In conclusion therefore spinal surgery in boys with Duchenne Muscular Dystrophy with scoliosis produces an appreciable quality-of-life gain and may well have a protective effect on respiratory function. It would seem to be advantageous to operate early, when the curve is 20–40° when respiratory and cardiac function are good. In this group, before significant pelvic obliquity has developed, fusion down to L5 with a pedicle screw system is probably adequate.

Boys with Duchenne Muscular Dystrophy have considerable co-morbidities and their safe management requires an experienced multi-disciplinary team. Such surgery should probably only be undertaken in centres which perform surgery for neuromuscular scoliosis regularly.

Spinal Muscular Atrophy

Spinal Muscular Atrophy (SMA) was first described independently in the early 1890s by Werdnig and Hoffman. It is a genetic disorder with a prevalence of 8 in 100,000 live births. It is the commonest fatal neuromuscular disease of infancy.

Spinal Muscular Atrophy has an autosomal recessive pattern inheritance with a slight male preponderance. Gilliam et al. [65] identified the gene locus in 1990 as 5q 11.2 – 13.3. The gene at

this site is the survival motor neurone gene (SMN1). This gene has deletions in greater than 98 % of patients with SMA [66] The function of the gene product encoded by the SMN1 gene is not clear.

SMA is characterised clinically by symmetrical muscle weakness affecting the legs more than the arms, proximal muscles more than distal ones and affecting the axial muscles and the intercostals selectively. The diaphragm is relatively spared, but bulbar involvement is common.

Byers and Banker [67, 68] based their classification on severity of disease and age of clinical onset. Type 1 is usually diagnosed in the first few months of life. The child has little useful motor function and death from respiratory failure is early. Type 2 is diagnosed later and children may sit without support. They rarely stand. Many patients now survive to the third or fourth decade. Type 3 is the mildest form and patients can often walk unassisted. They may lose the ability to walk as they grow older.

Many paediatric neurologists use a pragmatic classification [69] based on the onset of symptoms, with Type 1 patients seeing an onset before 6 months of age, and never sitting. Type 2 has an onset between 7 and 18 months of age and patients are able to sit. Type 3 has an onset older than 18 months, and these children can walk. Type 4 has an onset in adult life, usually the second or third decade.

Spinal Muscular Atrophy has a spectrum of severity. Survival depends on the degree of bulbar and respiratory involvement, which largely, but not completely mirrors the motor function on which the disease is classified.

There is no curative medical treatment for SMA but palliative methods such as nutritional and respiratory support have seen a significant improvement in quality of life and survival [70].

Scoliosis is the main functional problem of patients with SMA. Its prevalence and severity mirrors the severity of the disease [71, 72]. The onset of the scoliosis is earlier in patients with more severe disease, and once established the scoliosis is relentlessly progressive. A severe kyphoscoliosis with marked pelvic obliquity and painful costo-iliac impingement is very common.

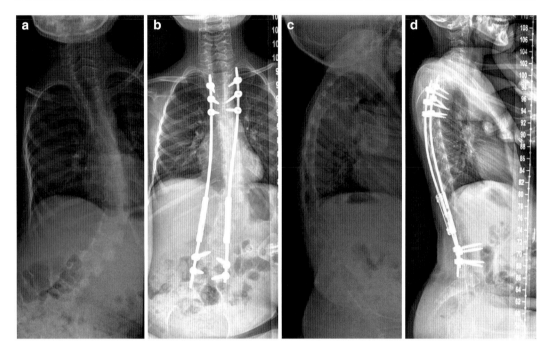

Fig. 5 Pre- and post-operative xrays of a child with Spinal Muscular Atrophy with growing rods (Case of Mr Rajat Verma). (**a**) A-P view, (**b**) lateral view, (**c**) A-P view, (**d**) lateral view

A number of authors have reported good surgical results in patients with SMA. Aprin et al. [73] operated on 15 patients. They concluded that short segment anterior fusion had a high respiratory complication rate and was accompanied by progressive deformity. Posterior spinal fusion seemed to reduce the rate of pulmonary deterioration but did not stop it. A number of other papers have reported good results of spinal surgery in patients with Spinal Muscular Atrophy. [74–79] All of the patients in these cohorts were relatively mature, being largely in their teens with an occasional patient in childhood. Bentley et al., in a study of 33 patients with Spinal Muscular atrophy, reported good outcomes over a 13-year period. They noted that it is necessary to avoid fusion below L.5 in ambulant patients because fixation of the pelvis could prevent the pelvic tilt required for walking [64].

A number of authors have examined lung function in Spinal Muscular Atrophy. Robinson et al. [80] found that the scoliosis in patients with SMA deteriorated in patients once they stopped standing. Even if they stood in orthoses scoliosis was prevented and lung function protected. They found an inverse relationship between the Cobb angle and percentage lung function. They reported good results in 16 patients operated. Chng et al. [81] studied 8 patients. They found a continuing decline in lung function even after spinal fusion, but the decline was slower than pre-surgery.

The dilemma now faced by contemporary surgeons is that medical advances have increased life expectancy of patients with what would have previously been a poor prognosis Spinal Muscular Atrophy. They are therefore presented with increasingly younger patients with severe scoliosis. Anterior surgery is precluded because of poor lung function whereas posterior only surgery invariably results in a recurrence of deformity, due to anterior spinal overgrowth ("crankshaft" effect).

These patients present a therapeutic dilemma. Conservative treatment in the form of corsetry or bracing is ineffective and has an inhibitory effect on lung function, whereas conventional surgical techniques will yield a poor result. In this cohort we have operated a number of patients by the use of growing rods (Fig. 5). This technique has been evaluated by other authors but no comprehensive follow-up is yet published [82, 83]. It is our experience that this is an efficacious means of controlling the curve in an otherwise difficult population. Clearly in commencing this treatment one is committed to a programme of treatment and in this population and multi-disciplinary approach is paramount. The decision to offer definitive spinal fusion is frequently made on the advice of the chest physician or neurologist because the child's lung function has declined sufficiently that the window for further surgery will soon close. Nonetheless we have found this to be a useful way out of a difficult situation.

Hereditary Sensory Motor Neuropathy (Charcot-Marie Tooth Disease)

Charcot-Marie Tooth Disease (CMT) is the most common inherited sensory neuropathy with an incidence rate of between 1 in 2,500 and 1 in 5,000 [1, 84]. The common orthopaedic manifestation is of cavovarus feet, but hip dysplasia is also more common. Scoliosis occurs in CMT with a higher prevalence than in the general population. The nature of the scoliosis is different from idiopathic scoliosis and the scoliosis is associated with some genotypes more than others. Walker et al. [85] reviewed 100 patients with electrophysiologically proven Charcot-Marie Tooth Disease. Of these, 89 had spinal x-rays with 37 having a spinal deformity. Of the 37, 17 had a kyphotic deformity with or without scoliosis.

Scoliosis seems to have been mild as only 2 patients underwent surgical treatment. Of those with x-rays at skeletal maturity 50 % had some degree of spinal deformity. Horacek [86] reviewed 175 patients with HSMN. They found that the incidence of scoliosis depended on the genotype. Those with deletional duplication at the PMP22 gene on chromosome 17 had a 56 % chance of spinal deformity. Those with a Cx32 gene mutation (typically CMTX) had an 18 % chance of scoliosis whilst those with the MPZ gene mutation, including those with Dejerine-Sottas syndrome, had a 13 % chance of scoliosis. Of those with spinal deformities 58 % had

scoliosis, 31 % kypho-scoliosis and 11 % an isolated hyper-kyphosis. Interestingly hyper-kyphosis was more common in patients with the MPZ mutation than PMP22 abnormalities. Karol & Ellison [87] examined 298 patients with Charcot-Marie Tooth Disease. 1 in 6 of these developed a scoliosis and of those followed two-thirds progressed. Progression was more common in those with a large curve at presentation and in those with hyper-kyphosis.

Of those treated surgically a long posterior spinal fusion with instrumentation was performed. It was not possible to get consistent SSEP monitoring and this latter coincides with our own findings [27].

Friedreich's Ataxia

Friedreich's Ataxia is a spinal cerebellar disease or hereditary ataxia. It is usually inherited as an autosomal recessive trait, due to mutations in the frataxin gene. Inheritance is variable. Patients with Friedreich's Ataxia usually present in early adolescence with an ataxic gait but may also present with scoliosis or foot deformity. The disease is generally progressive with increasing loss of mobility and eventual death from cardiomyopathy. The genetic defect has been identified on the locus 9q13. The absent gene product allows the accumulation of intramitochondrial iron and cell death [88, 89]. Cady and Bobechko [90] examined 42 patients. Of 34 for whom complete data were available 30 developed a scoliosis.

Daher et al. [91] examined 19 patients with a diagnosis of Friedreich's Ataxia and a scoliosis. Of these 8 had a degree of hyper-kyphosis and 12 came to surgery.

Labelle examined 56 patients with Friedreich's Ataxia [92]. All developed a scoliosis of more than 10° by the end of follow-up and of these two-thirds had some degree of hyper-kyphosis. Of those with long term follow-up [36] 20 proved to have progressive curves. The authors found no correlation of the risk of progression with disease severity but did find a correlation with the age of onset of scoliosis. They suggested that as the curve patterns resemble those of idiopathic scoliosis rather than neuromuscular scoliosis that scoliosis in Friedreich's Ataxia behaves more like idiopathic scoliosis than neuromuscular scoliosis.

Milbrandt et al. [93] found that 49 of the 77 patients whom they observed developed a scoliosis (63 %). Of these 49, 24 progressed and a third had come to surgery by the time the paper was written. Like Labelle these authors found that double major curve patterns predominated, but in contrast to Labelle's findings they found no relationship between the age at diagnosis of the scoliosis or curve magnitude and the risk of progression.

Furthermore, the authors illustrated their belief that these curves do not behave like idiopathic scoliosis using two examples. One had a selective thoracic fusion for a double major curve which was followed by severe progression of the lumbar curve and the other had severe proximal junctional kyphosis after a short fusion.

They found that somatosensory evoked potential monitoring was not possible.

Cerebral Palsy

Cerebral palsy (CP) is a neurological condition which results from a static lesion in the brain of a growing child. Cerebral palsy is the commonest cause of neuromuscular scoliosis.

It is hard to estimate the prevalence of scoliosis in cerebral palsy because cerebral palsy is a protean condition with manifestations ranging from the severely disabled child with whole body spastic cerebral palsy to those who are minimally affected whose problems can only be properly diagnosed by a skilled physician. Most estimates of the prevalence of cerebral palsy are based on severely affected individuals. For example, the incidence of scoliosis in the institutionalized population is some 60 % or 70 % [94]. Cerebral palsy has different manifestations. Spastic cerebral palsy is the most common but cerebral palsy may also cause movement disorders such as ataxia and athetosis. Madigan and Wallace [94] found a 69 % incidence of cerebral palsy in those with a spastic condition, 50 % in those with ataxia and 39 % of their "dyskinetic" group.

The incidence of scoliosis is greater in those with the greatest neurological affliction.

Like other neuromuscular scolioses cerebral palsy scoliosis has a propensity to deteriorate. Saito et al. [95] found that patients whose curves were 40° by the age of 15 years invariably progressed to more than 60°. Those with whole body cerebral palsy were more likely to deteriorate. These findings were confirmed by Majd et al. [96] who found that many relatively small (less than 50° curves) progressed after skeletal maturity, linking an increasing scoliosis to a decline in physical function. A number of the patients in their study went from being assisted sitters to being bed-bound as their scoliosis progressed.

The effect of scoliosis in cerebral palsy is functional. Loss of trunkal balance may deprive the ambulant patient of his ability to walk. The non-ambulant may lose their ability to sit, or need to use the arms to arrest declining sitting balance, rendering the patient a "functional quadriplegic." An increasing scoliosis and pelvic obliquity may make sitting impossible.

Pelvic obliquity leads to an increasing likelihood of development of pressure sores over the dependent ischial tuberosity, greater trochanter or sacrum. Once established it is very difficult to treat a decubitus ulcer without treating the underlying pelvic obliquity. Skin problems in the costo-iliac angle are also difficult to treat.

The scoliosis associated with cerebral palsy is sometimes painful. Pain is a frequent concern of the care givers but seems to be less prevalent than is sometimes imagined. Most children severely affected by cerebral palsy and scoliosis can communicate their discomfort to the care givers.

The aims of treatment in cerebral palsy are to maximize function, even in severe whole body CP. This is best done by minimizing trunkal imbalance. This can sometimes be achieved by the provision of a rigid polythene TLSO or by seating adaptations. The benefits which accrue to the patient from wearing a brace are immediate and functional. There is no convincing evidence that brace treatment in cerebral palsy affects the natural history of the condition.

Surgical treatment has the ultimate aim of restoring a balanced trunk over a level pelvis.

Scoliosis in cerebral palsy is often very severe before treatment and consideration is frequently given to destabilizing surgery to allow a better correction of the deformity.

This may take the form of an anterior release or more recently surgeons have used posterior vertebral column resection as a way of inducing flexibility in the spine [97]. With preliminary anterior surgery debate remains as to the pros. and cons. of sequential (that is to say under the same anaesthetic) anterior and posterior spinal surgery compared with staged (that is to say under two anaesthetics) surgery. This was examined by Tsirikos et al. [98]. They found that sequential procedures were associated with an increased intra-operative blood loss, prolonged operative time and an increased incidence of medical and surgical complications in a group of 45 patients. They concluded that staged surgery provided safer and more consistent results.

Outcome Measurement

The concept of measurement of outcome is essential to the science of surgery. In spinal deformity surgery the earliest outcomes measured were radiographic. However correction of Cobb angle has been shown to have a poor relationship with patient satisfaction and this has prompted the search for outcome measures which are more relevant to the patient. The Scoliosis Research Society (SRS) questionnaire is now accepted as a reliable and valid measurement of outcome for patients with adolescent idiopathic scoliosis.

In assessing outcome in neuromuscular scoliosis, function is of prime importance. Functional outcomes, or their surrogates have been used rather than cosmesis or deformity. As has been seen in this chapter respiratory function is frequently used as an outcome measure in neuromuscular scoliosis. Similarly, walking status may be used in the ambulant patient. A number of authors have made moves towards developing patient-related outcome measures. These may be condition specific (examples in low back surgery for example the Oswestry Disability Index

and the Low Back Outcome Score) or the general health-related quality-of-life questionnaire (e.g., SF36). The best assessment of outcome can be obtained by using a combination of a generic health-related outcome, condition-specific measures and a measurement of function.

A number of authors have developed questionnaires for use in patients with neuromuscular conditions. Bridwell et al. [99] evaluated 48 patients with SMA and DMD using a structured questionnaire of twenty questions covering the domains of function, satisfaction, quality of life and cosmesis. The questionnaire covered a range of issues specific for progressive flaccid neuromuscular scoliosis including questions from the SRS and American Academy of Orthopedic Surgeons questionnaires.

Wright et al. recently developed a muscular dystrophy spine questionnaire [100] In cerebral palsy. Narayanan et al. [101, 102] developed a questionnaire from interviews with health care providers and the care givers of children with cerebral palsy. The final questionnaire had 36 items in six domains, (personal care, position in transfer and mobility, communication and social interaction, comfort in motions and behaviour, health and quality-of-life). Reliability was established by a test/re-test performance with a very high correlation coefficient. A number of authors have used such outcome measures to assess the effects of scoliosis surgery. Watanabe et al. [103] examined 84 patients with cerebral palsy who underwent spinal fusion, Of 142 patients undergoing surgery 18 had re-located and a further 40 did not return the questionnaires (10 of this 40 did not return the questionnaire because the child had died).

The questionnaire used was a version of that developed by Bridwell et al. [99] addressing expectations, cosmesis, function, patient care, quality-of-life, pulmonary function, pain, comorbidity, self-image and satisfaction. Families of patients were given the questionnaires and asked to remember the child's pre-operative state. The authors results indicated that spinal deformity surgery was beneficial and that cosmesis improved dramatically after surgery. Interestingly, only 40 % of patients saw an improvement in function from surgery, whereas

72 % of the patients or carers reported an improved quality of life.

Larsson et al. [104] performed a functional assessment of 82 patients with neuromuscular scoliosis. The assessments comprised sitting, Cobb angle, lung function, reaching, pain and activities of daily living, care given and time used for resting. Post-operatively there were improvements in Cobb angle, lung function, seating, activities of daily living and resting time, allowing the authors to show that patients function was mostly improved.

References

1. Holmberg BH. Charcot-Marie-Tooth disease in northern Sweden: an epidemiological and clinical study. Acta Neurol Scand. 1993;87(5):416–22.
2. Gupta MC, et al. Reliability of radiographic parameters in neuromuscular scoliosis. Spine (Phila Pa 1976). 2007;32(6):691–5.
3. Yuan N, et al. The effect of scoliosis surgery on lung function in the immediate postoperative period. Spine (Phila Pa 1976). 2005;30(19):2182–5.
4. Ramappa M. Can 'sniff nasal inspiratory pressure' determine severity of scoliosis in paediatric population? Arch Orthop Trauma Surg. 2009;129(11):1461–4.
5. Almenrader N, Patel D. Spinal fusion in children with non-idiopathic scoliosis:is there a need for for routine postoperative ventilation? Br J Anaesth. 2006;97:851–7.
6. Bach JR, Sabharwal S. High pulmonary risk scoliosis surgery: role of noninvasive ventilation and related techniques. J Spinal Disord Tech. 2005;18(6):527–30.
7. Yuan N, et al. Preoperative predictors of prolonged postoperative mechanical ventilation in children following scoliosis repair. Pediatr Pulmonol. 2005;40(5):414–9.
8. Jesevar DS, Karlin LI. The relationship between preoperative nutritional status and complications after an operation for scoliosis in patients who have cerebral palsy. J Bone Joint Surg Am. 1993;75(6):880.
9. Allen BL, Ferguson R. The Galveston technique for L rod instrumentation of the scoliotic spine. Spine (Phila Pa 1976). 1982;7:276–84.
10. Peelle MW, et al. Comparison of pelvic fixation techniques in neuromuscular spinal deformity correction: Galveston rod versus iliac and lumbosacral screws. Spine (Phila Pa 1976). 2006;31(20):2392–8; discussion 2399.
11. Phillips JH, Gutheil JP, Knapp Jr DR. Iliac screw fixation in neuromuscular scoliosis. Spine (Phila Pa 1976). 2007;32(14):1566–70.
12. Takeshita K, et al. Analysis of patients with nonambulatory neuromuscular scoliosis surgically treated to the pelvis with intraoperative halo-femoral traction. Spine (Phila Pa 1976). 2006;31(20):2381–5.
13. Vialle R, Delecourt C, Morin C. Surgical treatment of scoliosis with pelvic obliquity in cerebral palsy: the influence of intraoperative traction. Spine (Phila Pa 1976). 2006;31(13):1461–6.
14. McCall RE, Hayes B. Long-term outcome in neuromuscular scoliosis fused only to lumbar 5. Spine (Phila Pa 1976). 2005;30(18):2056–60.
15. Emami A, et al. Outcome and complications of long fusions to the sacrum in adult spine deformity: luque-galveston, combined iliac and sacral screws, and sacral fixation. Spine (Phila Pa 1976). 2002;27(7):776–86.
16. Tsuchiya K, et al. Minimum 5-year analysis of L5-S1 fusion using sacropelvic fixation (bilateral S1 and iliac screws) for spinal deformity. Spine (Phila Pa 1976). 2006;31(3):303–8.
17. Edwards 2nd CC, et al. Long adult deformity fusions to L5 and the sacrum. A matched cohort analysis. Spine (Phila Pa 1976). 2004;29(18):1996–2005.
18. Modi HN, et al. Evaluation of pelvic fixation in neuromuscular scoliosis: retrospective study in 55 patients. Int Orthop. 2010;34(1):89–96.
19. Modi HN, et al. Surgical correction and fusion using posterior-only pedicle screw construct for neuropathic scoliosis in patients with cerebral palsy: a three-year follow-up study. Spine (Phila Pa 1976). 2009;34(11):1167–75.
20. Modi H, et al. Correction of apical axial rotation with pedicular screws in neuromuscular scoliosis. J Spinal Disord. 2008;21(8):606–13.
21. Edler A, Murray DJ, Forbes R. Blood loss during posterior spinal fusion in patients with neuromuscular disease: is there an increased risk? Paediatr Anaesth. 2004;13:818–22.
22. Barsdorf AI, Sproule DM, Kaufmann P. Scoliosis surgery in children with neuromuscular disease: findings from the US National Inpatient Sample, 1997 to 2003. Arch Neurol. 2010;67(2):231–5.
23. Mohamad F, et al. Perioperative complications after surgical correction in neuromuscular scoliosis. J Pediatr Orthop. 2007;27(4):392–7.
24. Sarwark J, Sarwahi V. New strategies and decision making in the management of neuromuscular scoliosis. Orthop Clin North Am. 2007;38(4):485–96, v.
25. Vitale MA, et al. The contribution of hospital volume, payer status, and other factors on the surgical outcomes of scoliosis patients: a review of 3,606 cases in the State of California. J Pediatr Orthop. 2005;25(3):393–9.
26. Tsirikos AI, et al. Life expectancy in pediatric patients with cerebral palsy and neuromuscular scoliosis who underwent spinal fusion. Dev Med Child Neurol. 2003;45(10):677–82.

27. Williamson JB, Galasko CS. Spinal cord monitoring in patients with neuromuscular scoliosis. J Bone Joint Surg Br. 1992;74B:870–2.

28. Tucker SK, Noordeen MHH, Pitt MC. Spinal cord monitoring in neuromuscular scoliosis. J Pediatr Orthop B. 2001;10:1–5.

29. Bushby K, et al. Diagnosis and management of Duchenne muscular dystrophy, part 1: diagnosis, and pharmacological and psychosocial management. Lancet Neurol. 2010;9(1):77–93.

30. Politano L, et al. Development of cardiomyopathy in female carriers of Duchenne and Becker muscular dystrophies. JAMA. 1996;275(17):1335–8.

31. Galasko CS. Incidence of orthopedic problems in children with muscle disease. Isr J Med Sci. 1977;13(2):165–76.

32. Mohamed K, Appleton R, Nicolaides P. Delayed diagnosis of Duchenne muscular dystrophy. Eur J Paediatr Neurol. 2000;4(5):219–23.

33. Read L, Galasko CS. Delay in diagnosing Duchenne muscular dystrophy in orthopaedic clinics. J Bone Joint Surg Br. 1986;68(3):481–2.

34. Marshall PD, Galasko CS. No improvement in delay in diagnosis of Duchenne muscular dystrophy. Lancet. 1995;345(8949):590–1.

35. Galasko CS, Williamson JB, Delaney CM. Lung function in Duchenne muscular dystrophy. Eur Spine J. 1995;4(5):263–7.

36. Smith AD, Koreska J, Moseley CF. Progression of scoliosis in Duchenne muscular dystrophy. J Bone Joint Surg Am. 1989;71(7):1066–74.

37. Galasko CS, Delaney C, Morris P. Spinal stabilisation in Duchenne muscular dystrophy. J Bone Joint Surg Br. 1992;74(2):210–4.

38. Rideau Y, et al. The treatment of scoliosis in Duchenne muscular dystrophy. Muscle Nerve. 1984;7(4):281–6.

39. Brooke MH, et al. Duchenne muscular dystrophy: patterns of clinical progression and effects of supportive therapy. Neurology. 1989;39(4):475–81.

40. Rodillo EB, et al. Prevention of rapidly progressive scoliosis in Duchenne muscular dystrophy by prolongation of walking with orthoses. J Child Neurol. 1988;3(4):269–74.

41. Alman BA, Raza SN, Biggar WD. Steroid treatment and the development of scoliosis in males with duchenne muscular dystrophy. J Bone Joint Surg Am. 2004;86-A(3):519–24.

42. Kinali M, et al. Management of scoliosis in Duchenne muscular dystrophy: a large 10-year retrospective study. Dev Med Child Neurol. 2006;48(6):513–8.

43. Muntoni F, Bushby K, Manzur AY. Muscular dystrophy campaign funded workshop on management of scoliosis in Duchenne muscular dystrophy 24 January 2005, London, UK. Neuromuscul Disord. 2006;16(3):210–9.

44. Houde S, et al. Deflazacort use in Duchenne muscular dystrophy: an 8-year follow-up. Pediatr Neurol. 2008;38(3):200–6.

45. King WM, et al. Orthopedic outcomes of long-term daily corticosteroid treatment in Duchenne muscular dystrophy. Neurology. 2007;68(19):1607–13.

46. Noordeen MH, et al. Blood loss in Duchenne muscular dystrophy: vascular smooth muscle dysfunction? J Pediatr Orthop B. 1999;8(3):212–5.

47. Turturro F, et al. Impaired primary hemostasis with normal platelet function in Duchenne muscular dystrophy during highly-invasive spinal surgery. Neuromuscul Disord. 2005;15(8):532–40.

48. Shapiro F, Zurakowski D, Sethna NF. Tranexamic acid diminishes intraoperative blood loss and transfusion in spinal fusions for duchenne muscular dystrophy scoliosis. Spine (Phila Pa 1976). 2007;32(20):2278–83.

49. Gaine WJ, et al. Progression of scoliosis after spinal fusion in Duchenne's muscular dystrophy. J Bone Joint Surg Br. 2004;86(4):550–5.

50. Mubarak SJ, Morin WD, Leach J. Spinal fusion in Duchenne muscular dystrophy–fixation and fusion to the sacropelvis? J Pediatr Orthop. 1993;13(6):752–7.

51. Hahn F, et al. Scoliosis correction with pedicle screws in Duchenne muscular dystrophy. Eur Spine J. 2008;17(2):255–61.

52. Mehta SS, et al. Pedicle screw-only constructs with lumbar or pelvic fixation for spinal stabilization in patients with Duchenne muscular dystrophy. J Spinal Disord Tech. 2009;22(6):428–33.

53. Takaso M, et al. Can the caudal extent of fusion in the surgical treatment of scoliosis in Duchenne muscular dystrophy be stopped at lumbar 5? Eur Spine J. 2010;19(5):787–96.

54. Alman BA, Kim HK. Pelvic obliquity after fusion of the spine in Duchenne muscular dystrophy. J Bone Joint Surg Br. 1999;81(5):821–4.

55. Sengupta DK, et al. Pelvic or lumbar fixation for the surgical management of scoliosis in duchenne muscular dystrophy. Spine (Phila Pa 1976). 2002;27(18):2072–9.

56. Kennedy JD, et al. Effect of spinal surgery on lung function in Duchenne muscular dystrophy. Thorax. 1995;50(11):1173–8.

57. Miller RG, et al. The effect of spine fusion on respiratory function in Duchenne muscular dystrophy. Neurology. 1991;41(1):38–40.

58. Granata C, et al. Long-term results of spine surgery in Duchenne muscular dystrophy. Neuromuscul Disord. 1996;6(1):61–8.

59. Velasco MV, et al. Posterior spinal fusion for scoliosis in duchenne muscular dystrophy diminishes the rate of respiratory decline. Spine (Phila Pa 1976). 2007;32(4):459–65.

60. Eagle M, et al. Managing Duchenne muscular dystrophy–the additive effect of spinal surgery and home nocturnal ventilation in improving survival. Neuromuscul Disord. 2007;17(6):470–5.

61. Takaso M, et al. Surgical management of severe scoliosis with high-risk pulmonary dysfunction in Duchenne muscular dystrophy. Int Orthop. 2010;34(3):401–6.

62. Marsh A, Edge G, Lehovsky J. Spinal fusion in patients with Duchenne's muscular dystrophy and a low forced vital capacity. Eur Spine J. 2003;12(5):507–12.

63. Harper CM, Ambler G, Edge G. The prognostic value of pre-operative predicted forced vital capacity in corrective spinal surgery for Duchenne's muscular dystrophy. Anaesthesia. 2004;59(12):1160–2.

64. Bentley G, Haddad F, Bull TM, Seingry D. The treatment of scoliosis in muscular dystrophy using modified Luque and Harrington-Luque instrumentation. J Bone Joint Surg Br. 2001;83-B(1):22–8.

65. Gilliam TC, et al. Genetic homogeneity between acute and chronic forms of spinal muscular atrophy. Nature. 1990;345(6278):823–5.

66. Rodrigues NR, et al. Deletions in the survival motor neuron gene on 5q13 in autosomalrecessive spinal muscular atrophy. Hum Mol Genet. 1995;4:631–4.

67. Byers RK, Banker BQ. Infantile muscular atrophy. Arch Neurol. 1961;5:140–64.

68. Byers RK, Banker BQ. Infantile muscular atrophy: an eleven year experience. Trans Am Neurol Assoc. 1960;85:10–4.

69. Munsat TL, Davies KE. International SMA consortium meeting. (26–28 June 1992, Bonn, Germany). Neuromuscul Disord. 1992;2(5–6):423–8.

70. Wang CH, et al. Consensus statement for standard of care in spinal muscular atrophy. J Child Neurol. 2007;22(8):1027–49.

71. Granata C, et al. Spinal muscular atrophy: natural history and orthopaedic treatment of scoliosis. Spine (Phila Pa 1976). 1989;14(7):760–2.

72. Merlini L, et al. Scoliosis in spinal muscular atrophy: natural history and management. Dev Med Child Neurol. 1989;31(4):501–8.

73. Aprin H, et al. Spine fusion in patients with spinal muscular atrophy. J Bone Joint Surg Am. 1982;64(8):1179–87.

74. Schwentker EP, Gibson DA. The orthopaedic aspects of spinal muscular atrophy. J Bone Joint Surg Am. 1976;58(1):32–8.

75. Riddick MF, Winter RB, Lutter LD. Spinal deformities in patients with spinal muscle atrophy: a review of 36 patients. Spine (Phila Pa 1976). 1982;7(5):476–83.

76. Evans GA, Drennan JC, Russman BS. Functional classification and orthopaedic management of spinal muscular atrophy. J Bone Joint Surg Br. 1981;63B(4):516–22.

77. Daher YH, et al. Spinal surgery in spinal muscular atrophy. J Pediatr Orthop. 1985;5(4):391–5.

78. Brown JC, et al. Surgical and functional results of spine fusion in spinal muscular atrophy. Spine (Phila Pa 1976). 1989;14(7):763–70.

79. Phillips DP, et al. Surgical treatment of scoliosis in a spinal muscular atrophy population. Spine (Phila Pa 1976). 1990;15(9):942–5.

80. Robinson D, et al. Scoliosis and lung function in spinal muscular atrophy. Eur Spine J. 1995;4(5):268–73.

81. Chng SY, et al. Pulmonary function and scoliosis in children with spinal muscular atrophy types II and III. J Paediatr Child Health. 2003;39(9):673–6.

82. Fujak A, et al. Treatment of scoliosis in intermediate spinal muscular atrophy (SMA type II) in childhood. Ortop Traumatol Rehabil. 2005;7(2):175–9.

83. Sponseller PD, et al. Pelvic fixation of growing rods: comparison of constructs. Spine (Phila Pa 1976). 2009;34(16):1706–10.

84. Skre H. Genetic and clinical aspects of Charcot-Marie-Tooth's disease. Clin Genet. 1974;6(2):98–118.

85. Walker JL, et al. Spinal deformity in Charcot-Marie-Tooth disease. Spine (Phila Pa 1976). 1994;19(9):1044–7.

86. Horacek O, et al. Spinal deformities in hereditary motor and sensory neuropathy: a retrospective qualitative, quantitative, genotypical, and familial analysis of 175 patients. Spine (Phila Pa 1976). 2007;32(22):2502–8.

87. Karol LA, Elerson E. Scoliosis in patients with Charcot-Marie-Tooth disease. J Bone Joint Surg Am. 2007;89(7):1504–10.

88. Alper G, Narayanan V. Friedreich's ataxia. Pediatr Neurol. 2003;28(5):335–41.

89. Campuzano V, et al. Friedreich's ataxia: autosomal recessive disease caused by an intronic GAA triplet repeat expansion. Science. 1996;271(5254):1423–7.

90. Cady RB, Bobechko WP. Incidence, natural history, and treatment of scoliosis in Friedreich's ataxia. J Pediatr Orthop. 1984;4(6):673–6.

91. Daher YH, et al. Spinal deformities in patients with Friedreich ataxia: a review of 19 patients. J Pediatr Orthop. 1985;5(5):553–7.

92. Labelle H, et al. Natural history of scoliosis in Friedreich's ataxia. J Bone Joint Surg Am. 1986;68(4):564–72.

93. Milbrandt TA, Kunes JR, Karol LA. Friedreich's ataxia and scoliosis: the experience at two institutions. J Pediatr Orthop. 2008;28(2):234–8.

94. Madigan RR, Wallace SL. Scoliosis in the institutionalized cerebral palsy population. Spine (Phila Pa 1976). 1981;6(6):583–90.

95. Saito N, et al. Natural history of scoliosis in spastic cerebral palsy. Lancet. 1998;351(9117):1687–92.

96. Majd ME, Muldowny DS, Holt RT. Natural history of scoliosis in the institutionalized adult cerebral palsy population. Spine (Phila Pa 1976). 1997;22(13):1461–6.

97. Suk SI, et al. Posterior vertebral column resection for severe spinal deformities. Spine (Phila Pa 1976). 2002;27(21):2374–82.

98. Tsirikos AI, et al. Comparison of one stage versus two stage antero-posterior spinal fusion in pediatric patients with cerebral palsy. Spine (Phila Pa 1976). 2003;28(12):1300–5.

99. Bridwell KH, et al. Process measures and patient/parent evaluation of surgical management of spinal deformities in patients with progressive flaccid neuromuscular scoliosis (Duchenne's muscular

dystrophy and spinal muscular atrophy). Spine (Phila Pa 1976). 1999;24(13):1300–9.

100. Wright JG, et al. Assessing functional outcomes of children with muscular dystrophy and scoliosis. J Pediatr Orthop. 2008;28:840–5.

101. Narayanan, U. G, et al. Care giver priorities in child health index of life with disabilities. Dev Med Child Neurol. 2004; 46 (Supplement 99): 6.

102. Narayanan UG, et al. Initial development and validation of the care giver priorities in child health index

of life with disabilities. Dev Med Child Neurol. 2006;48(10):804–12.

103. Watanabe K, et al. Is spine deformity surgery in patients with spastic cerebral palsy truly beneficial?: a patient/parent evaluation. Spine (Phila Pa 1976). 2009;34(20):2222–32.

104. Larsson EL, et al. Long-term follow-up of functioning after spinal surgery in patients with neuromuscular scoliosis. Spine (Phila Pa 1976). 2005;30(19): 2145–52.

Surgical Management of Adult Scoliosis

Norbert Passuti, G. A. Odri, and P. M. Longis

Contents

Keywords

Adult • Aetiology • Classification • Complications • Diagnosis • Pathomorphology • Pre-operative preparation • Scoliosis • Surgical techniques

Introduction

The natural course of idiopathic scoliosis during adult life is neither static nor benign. As the patient gets older, the deformed spinal column may show aggravation of the curves, increasing kyphosis, decompensation, and spondylotic changes. These pathologic changes may cause back pain, radiculopathy, cosmetic, and psychological problems, and cardiopulmonary compromise, possibly leading to increased mortality.

The prevalence of adult scoliosis in the general population has been reported as ranging from 1 % to 4 %. Physical deformity, significant pain and disability can develop. With the demographic shift involving an ageing population in the Western World and increased attention to quality of life issues, adult scoliosis is becoming a significant health-care concern. The progression of spinal deformities in the adult population, treatment approaches for adult scoliosis, and surgical techniques have consequently been reported frequently in the literature.

Adult scoliosis can be defined as a spinal deformity in a skeletally-mature patient with a Cobb angle greater than 10°. Although there are many known causes of spinal deformity in the adult, two

N. Passuti (✉) • G.A. Odri • P.M. Longis
Faculté de Médecine, Nantes, France
e-mail: norbert.passuti@chu-nantes.fr

G. Bentley (ed.), *European Surgical Orthopaedics and Traumatology*,
DOI 10.1007/978-3-642-34746-7_34, © EFORT 2014

categories embrace the largest number of scolioses. The first category includes patients with scoliosis during childhood and adolescence that may progress or become symptomatic as the patient ages. This type of scoliosis is often idiopathic and can be termed "adolescent scoliosis of the adult" (ASA).

The second category includes patients in whom a the spinal deformity developed after skeletal maturity. This type of scoliosis is often termed "DDS". Although the causes of ASA and DDS appear quite different, they may share a common pathway in symptomatic patients: gradual loss of intersegmental stability with ageing and consequent progressive deformity and pain. Certainly, some adult deformities may not fit clearly into the categories of ASA or DDS, such as traumatic, metabolic, osteoporotic, or iatrogenic deformities.

Progress in surgical techniques and technology has been significantly supported by progress in anaesthesia for spinal surgery and by more sophisticated and precise diagnostic imaging and differentiated application of invasive and functional diagnostic tests. Increased patient awareness, the patient's unwillingness to accept their limitations and pains, and the gradual shift in the demographics towards a "grey society", make adult scoliosis with all of its different forms and clinical presentations a much more frequent problem in a general spine practice than the scoliosis of children and adolescents. This trend is likely to continue when we consider the fact that in 25 years from now, a significant part (more than 10 %) of the population in the industrialized societies will be over 65 years old.

Aetiology, Classification and Pathomorphology

Aebi [1] described 3 types of adult scoliosis.

A scoliosis is diagnosed in adult patients when it occurs or becomes relevant after skeletal maturity with a Cobb angle of more than 10° in the frontal plain.

Type 1: Primary degenerative scoliosis ("de novo" form), mostly located in the thoracolumbar or lumbar spine.

Type 2: Progressive idiopathic scoliosis in adult life of the thoracic, thoracolumbar, and/or lumbar spine.

Type 3: Secondary degenerative scoliosis.

(a) Scoliosis following idiopathic or other forms of scoliosis or occurring in the context of a pelvic obliquity due to a leg-length discrepancy, hip pathology or a lumbosacral transitional anomaly, mostly located in the thoracolumbar, lumbar or lumbosacral spine.

(b) Scoliosis secondary to metabolic bone disease (mostly osteoporosis) combined with asymmetric arthritic disease and/or vertebral fractures.

Therefore, scoliosis can be present since childhood or adolescence and become progressive and/or symptomatic in adult life; or scoliosis may appear "de novo" in adult life without any precedence in earlier life.

Clinically, the most prominent groups are secondary (type 3) and primary (type 1) degenerative adult scoliosis. In elderly patients, both forms of scoliosis may be aggravated by osteoporosis, which also holds true for the type 2 scoliosis. All three types of scoliosis may appear at a certain stage as degenerative scoliosis, and degenerative scoliosis is therefore the main bulk of adult scoliosis. Beyond the above classification, the degenerative adult scoliosis can also be sub-divided into scoliosis which has its aetiology in the spine itself and scoliosis with an aetiology elsewhere. Schwab et al. proposed recently a radiographic classification including type I–III scoliosis, characterized by the a/p and lateral views in standing position. They correlated the classification I–III with increasing severity of self-reported pain and disability. Boachie-Adjei considered specifically the idiopathic adult scoliosis (our type 2 scoliosis) and uses the age as a classifying criterion combined with degenerative changes, that is, patients with idiopathic adult scoliosis below and above 40 years of age.

Degenerative adult scoliosis, specifically in the lumbar spine, is characterized by quite a uniform pathomorphology and pathomechanism. The asymmetric degeneration of the disc and/or the facet joints leads to an asymmetric loading of the spinal segment and consequently of a whole spinal area. This again leads to an asymmetric deformity, for example, scoliosis and/or kyphosis. Such a deformity again triggers asymmetric degeneration and induces asymmetric loading, creating a vicious circle and enhancing curve progression. On the one hand, the curve progression is caused by the pathomechanism of an adult degenerative curve, and on the other hand by the specific bone metabolism of the post-menopause female patients with a certain degree of osteoporosis, who are most frequently affected by the degenerative form of scoliosis. The potential of individual asymmetric deformation and collapse in the weak osteoporotic vertebra is clearly increased and contributes further to the curve progression.

The destruction of discs, facet joints and joints capsules usually ends in some form of uni-or multi-segmental sagittal and/or frontal latent or obvious instability. There may be not only a spondylolisthesis, meaning a slip in the sagittal plain, but also translational dislocation. The biological reaction to an unstable joint or, in the case of the spine, an unstable segment, with the formation of osteophytes at the facet joints (spondylosis), both contributing to the increasing narrowing of the spinal canal together with the hypertrophy and calcification of the ligamentum flavum and joint capsules, creating central and lateral recess spinal stenosis.

The osteophytes of the facet joints and the spondylotic osteophytes, however, may not sufficiently stabilize a diseased spinal segment; such a condition leads to a dynamic, mostly foraminal stenosis with radicular pain or claudication-type pain.

Diagnosis and Pre-Operative Preparation for Surgery

The adult scoliosis population is similar to most spinal disorder populations in that pain is the most common presentation, with reports of approximately 90 % of patients reporting pain as their primary complaint [3,8].

Pain that localizes over the convexity of the curve is often axial and diffuse in nature; it is believed to be the result of muscle fatigue and/or spasm of the paraspinal musculature. However, pain on the concavity of the curve may be localized to the back and nerve roots. This may be the result of disc rupture or facet hypertrophy narrowing nerve roots and a subsequent radiculopathy.

Pulmonary compromise with severe thoracic scoliosis (curve >80°) is well-recognized, due to loss of lung volume and inability to expand the thorax with inspiration. However, it is the exception for these patients to present to the spine surgeon because of respiratory issues and, in fact, they typically present before the scoliosis is this severe. As discussed earlier, some adolescent idiopathic scoliosis patients will experience progression of their curve even after skeletal maturity and present for evaluation.

In addition to a complete history and physical examination, there are additional areas that should be specifically reviewed when evaluating a patient with a spinal deformity. The aetiology of the patient's pain needs to be interpreted as caused by the progression of the deformity, neurological compromise, or de-conditioning. Details of the axial pain should include location, radiation, aggravating and alleviating factors, as well as the time course; specifically, nocturnal pain may suggest a neurogenic source (e.g., spinal cord tumour). It is important to rule out other sources of axial spinal pain, such as pathological fractures or infection. Family history and social history are relevant because patients with depression, nicotine use, and substance abuse have an increased risk for worse outcomes. In addition, physicians must be cautious in the patient with a rapidly-progressing curve because it may suggest an underlying neurological condition. Similarly, on physical examination, café au lait spots, naevi, skin dimpling, and hairy patches may all be hallmarks of an underlying neurogenic abnormality therefore necessitating a detailed imaging of the neuroaxis. If the patient has an abnormal neurological examination (e.g., radiculopathy, myelopathy), magnetic resonance imaging should be considered to determine any neurogenic cause of the scoliosis.

Perhaps the single most important principle in the surgical treatment of adult scoliosis is achieving and maintaining a proper sagittal and coronal balance such that the spine is oriented to have the cranium placed over the pelvis. Such a balanced spinal posture provides for decreased energy requirements with ambulation, limits pain and fatigue, improves cosmesis and patient satisfaction, and limits complications associated with unresolved (or new) deformities. The sagittal-vertical axis is determined and defined by a plumb line from the mid-C7 vertebral body on a lateral x-ray in the standing position. If this line falls anterior to the ventral S1 vertebra, it is referred to as positive (+) balance and if the line falls posterior it is called negative (−) balance. In a patient with a "normal" sagittal-balanced spine, the plumb line should pass 2–4cm posterior to the ventral S1 vertebra (negative 2–4 cm) or 1 cm posterior to the L5/S1 disc space. Any spine with a positive value is thought to be out of sagittal balance [4].

The centre sacral line is used to assess coronal balance. The centre sacral line is a line that bisects a line passing through both iliac crests and ascends perpendicularly. The vertebrae bisected most closely by this line are known as the "stable vertebrae".

The apical vertebra is the vertebra associated with the greatest segmental angulation at both its rostral and caudal disc interspaces, compared with all other disc interspaces in the curve. In general, it is located in the mid-portion or apex of the curve. Conversely, the neutral vertebra is the vertebra associated with little or no angulation at the rostral and caudal disc spaces of the curve. In general, an instrumentation construct should not terminate at or near an apical vertebra and should extend to a neutral vertebra to balance forces on the deformity.

Standing 36-in. x-rays (posteroanterior [PA], lateral and bending) can aid in determining the main or major curve, which is by definition a structural curve. Typically, a Cobb angle greater than 25° on lateral-bending x-rays defines a structural curve.

Additionally, structural curves are of greater magnitude and less flexible than compensatory curves. Curve magnitude, flexibility, and the apical vertebral translation of the thoracic and lumbar curves should be measured. Radiographic signs of degenerative disease are categorized, and listhesis (rotary and lateral) are noted. Degenerative segments often are associated with stenosis and this must be considered as well in the treatment algorithm.

One very important parameter is to precisely define the lumbo-pelvic parameters and particularly the pelvic incidence which is normally around 50°. The amount of sagittal correction will be correlated to the degree of the pelvic incidence which links to the sacral slope and the pelvic tilt (Figs. 1 and 2).

The importance of sagittal plane deformity has been well documented, particularly with reference to post-surgical flat back syndromes and post-traumatic kyphosis. Symptomatic deformity is often unresponsive to non-surgical treatment, and surgical treatment is complex. Several studies have shown that adequate restoration of sagittal plane alignment is necessary to improve significantly clinical outcome and avoid subsequent pseudarthrosis. Positive sagittal balance has also been identified as the radiographic parameter most highly correlated with adverse outcome measures in unoperated adult spinal deformity.

Despite this reported data, sagittal balance, like many radiographic measures, is still an inconsistent predictor of clinical symptoms. Studies in asymptomatic volunteers have shown that progressive positive sagittal balance is associated with normal ageing. In some instances, effective compensation mechanisms may develop in patients, which generate a more acceptable functional sagittal balance. Although some of these patients eventually decompensate, more sophisticated evaluation techniques, such as gait analysis, may be necessary to understand better the progression of these deformities [3,7].

These findings emphasize the importance of thoroughly accessing sagittal plane alignment in the treatment of spinal deformity. Although the response to non-operative treatment has not been systematically studied, the research suggest that methods directed at the improvement in standing balance might be beneficial. With surgical treatment, maintenance or restoration of lumbar

Fig. 1 Pelvic parameters

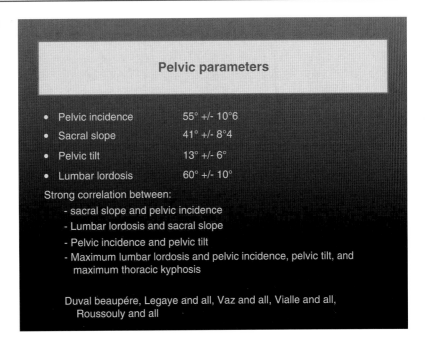

Fig. 2 Pelvic Incidence

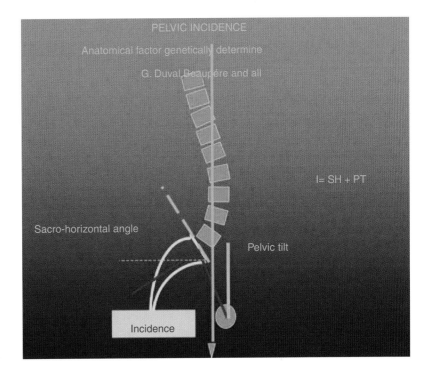

lordosis appears to be critical, particularly for patients with a positive sagittal balance before surgery. Most important, the literature emphasises the vital role of reproducible radiographic and clinical outcome measures such that our clinical experience can lead to more effective treatment paradigms for patients with adult deformity (Fig. 3).

Sagittal Balance

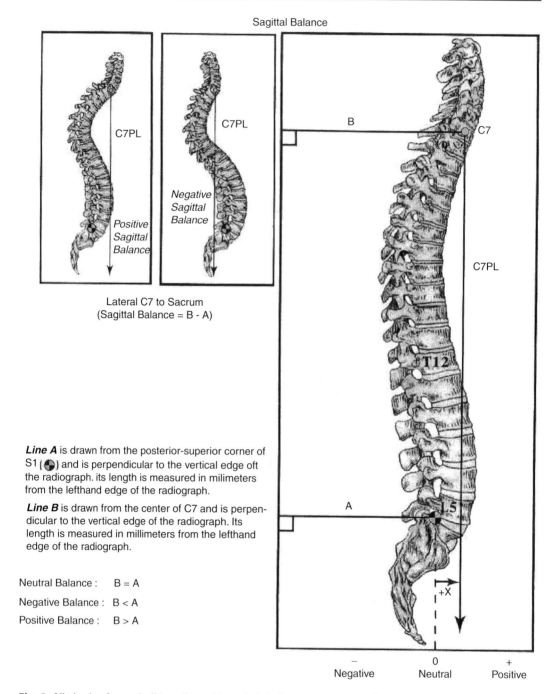

Lateral C7 to Sacrum
(Sagittal Balance = B - A)

Line A is drawn from the posterior-superior corner of
S1 (⬤) and is perpendicular to the vertical edge oft
the radiograph. its length is measured in milimeters
from the lefthand edge of the radiograph.

Line B is drawn from the center of C7 and is perpendicular to the vertical edge of the radiograph. Its
length is measured in millimeters from the lefthand
edge of the radiograph.

Neutral Balance :   B = A

Negative Balance :   B < A

Positive Balance :   B > A

Fig. 3 Vital role of reproducible radiographic and clinical outcome measures for efficient treatment paradigms for
patients with adult deformity (From S.D. Glassman [4])

Surgical Techniques

Once surgery is decided as the optimal treatment option, the correction of the deformity with incorporation of proper sagittal balance should be assessed because the loss of lumbar lordosis has been shown to be associated with poor outcomes. Glassman et al. also confirmed that restoration of proper sagittal balance is the most important factor associated with a good clinical outcome. The use of an operating table that produces extension of the hips and maximizes lumbar lordosis (e.g., Jackson) is biomechanically advantageous, particularly when fusing more than one lumbar segment. The ultimate choice of surgical approach for the treatment of lumbar adult scoliosis depends on the levels of the pain-generating segments, the flexibility of the curve, the tilt of the distal vertebrae, and the extent of the curve.

The aim of surgical treatment is correction and stabilization of the deformity and, therefore, an in-situ or on-lay fusion is an option for a minority of patients since this will not correct the deformity and lessens the chance of an arthrodesis. For example, it may become an option for an elderly patient with a small curve or deformity and poor bone quality. Therefore, an arthrodesis and correction of the deformity may be accomplished with a variety of methods, many of which require restoration of anterior column height. A lumbar interbody fusion (transforaminal lumbar interbody fusion or posterior lumbar interbody fusion) may achieve these goals through a posterior-only approach. To further assist in correction of the deformity, the cage may be biased to the concavity of the scoliosis deformity to address the coronal plane.

The "double major" curve describes a scoliosis in which there are two structural curves which are usually of equal size. Patients with double major adult scoliosis (most often a right thoracic curve in conjunction with a left lumbar curve of equal magnitude) may present with axial skeletal pain. However, the typical presentation is one of progression of the deformity manifested as changes in balance, ambulation, and cosmesis. The surgical treatment of a double major curve in adult scoliosis that is progressive in nature often requires anterior and posterior procedures. A long, relatively inflexible deformity may require anterior releases to accomplish effective reduction and fusion with posterior surgery. However, with the increased ability to manipulate a curve with modern instrumentation through a posterior approach, this may lessen the need for anterior releases. The curve stiffness is related to both patient age and curve magnitude. Flexibility decreases by 10 % with every 10° increase and by 5–10 % with each decade of life.

The primary structural goal is achieving a proper sagittal balance. Reduction of the coronal and rotational deformities follows in priority, with the goal of establishing coronal balance and reduction of rib asymmetry for enhanced cosmesis and patient satisfaction. Shoulder balance is particularly concerning for patient cosmesis and should be considered in deformity corrections.

The rostral construct should include the thoracic curve and should not stop caudal to any structural aspect of this portion. Adult thoracic deformity curves tend not to be flexible enough to correct significantly as opposed to the adolescent patient.

Therefore, all fixed deformities and subluxations should be included in the fusion. For relatively flexible rotational deformities, however, reduction can be achieved with effective improvement in trunk symmetry, which can significantly improve patient satisfaction. One technique is to use mono-axial or uni-axial screws, which are placed into the pedicles of the vertebra of the vertebrae that will be manipulated at the convexity.

After one pre-bent rod is placed and rotated in the usual manner to reduce the coronal deformity at the convexity and attain a proper sagittal relationship, it is secured and the contra-lateral rod is placed. The strength of the construct can be augmented with the use of rod cross-links since they can increase the stiffness of long constructs. Additional release manoeuvres may be necessary in stiff curves including thoracoplasty, concave rib osteotomies, and aggressive facetectomies.

The correction of a deformity is therefore achieved after an appropriate release either by step-wise correction though segmental instrumentation or by one or more segmental osteotomies for the frontal or sagittal re-alignment of the spine.

In case a lumbar curve is still flexible, which can be assessed by side-bending and flexion/extension views, and a certain compensation of the thoracic counter curve can be anticipated, a posterior correction, stabilization and fusion with or without decompression are sufficient. This is also done when a curve is clearly progressive.

If back pain is a leading symptom, with or without leg pain, a fusion is usually indicated. The levels to be included in the fusion can be difficult to determine.

Generally speaking, it is unfavourable to stop a fusion at L1 or even L2, i.e., below the thoracolumbar junction, because it may easily lead to decompensation above the fusion, with localized disc degeneration, segmental collapse, translational instability and secondary kyphosis [6].

The most critical segment to consider whether or not to include in a fusion is the lumbosacral junction. It takes all the movement from the lumbar spine and is the most difficult fusion to be achieved. A high percentage may remain with a non-union due to the unfavourable mechanical conditions of this junction between the two major lever arms of the fused spine and the rigid pelvis. The incidence of the non-union varies quite remarkably in the literature (5–30 %). Various types of instrumentation have been designed to enhance the fusion healing to the sacrum. They are mostly based on an increasingly more solid anchorage in the sacrum, or in the sacrum and iliac wings at the same time. None of these instrumentations have been clinically demonstrated to significantly overcome the problem of non-union in the complex pathology of degenerative scoliosis. The most certain approach to eliminate the problem of non-union is a 360° circumferential fusion at the lumbosacral junction. In order to avoid the anterior approach, unless needed for an extensive release, the refinement and standardization of

posterior lumbar interbody fusion (PLIF) technique using specifically-designed cages has become a well-controlled procedure [7].

Summary for Surgical Strategy

The complexity of the relationship between clinical signs, symptoms and pathophysiology of adult scoliosis remains a big challenge in spinal surgery. Radiographic correction is more effective in younger adults patients, pain improvement is a more reliable outcome in older patients, although younger patients rarely have severe pain symptoms, older patients may require extension of the fusion to lower segments because of a higher prevalence of degenerative changes but two problems could be encountered. First the risk of pseudarthrosis at level L5-S1 and the risk of proximal junctional kyphosis above the superior level of fixation. The strategy may be a more reliable technique for restoring sagittal balance which is the most significant parameter combined with functional outcomes but medical complications are a frequent occurrence with adult deformity spinal surgery. Pulmonary complications are among the most common life-threatening complications that occur. Awareness of the presentation, treatment and prevention of medical complications of deformity surgery may allow the spine surgeon to minimize their occurrence and optimize treatment.

Complications

The two most common mechanisms of failure are:

1. Fracture or late screw loosening of rostral instrumentation and
2. Late progressive kyphosis again at the rostral aspect of the construct. This risk of progressive post-operative kyphosis may be minimized by not ending the construct within a kyphotic or apical region of the spine. In addition, longer constructs over the thoracolumbar junction or apex of the kyphosis are preferred to avoid this phenomenon.

Fig. 4 A 56 year old female patient presented with a severe progressive adult scoliosis with frontal imbalance (6 cm right side) and sagittal imbalance (positive C7-plumb line +7 cm) and high pelvic incidence PI: 65

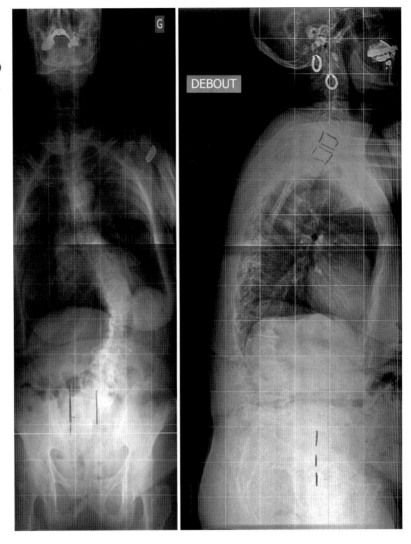

These longer constructs therefore, should not be presumed to be overly aggressive, particularly in the osteoporotic spine. However, each patient must be individually evaluated and the specific construct modified to meet the goals of the procedure. Many adult deformities are rigid and therefore require combined surgical approaches. "Same-day" or "combined" procedures may be preferable to "staged" procedures if they can be performed within a reasonable time period such as less than 12 h. If staged procedures are performed, care must be taken in proceeding with the second stage because the patient can become malnourished if the interval is too great. In a study by Dick et al., 7 of 11 staged procedure patients and 10 of 13 combined procedure patients developed postoperative malnutrition. However, the only infections occurred in the staged patients. Therefore, the combined group had 30 % less hospital costs and a shorter hospital stay; Furthermore, all patients reported that they would prefer to have both operations performed on the same day as opposed to staged operations [2].

Fig. 5 C7-plum line was achieved with an excellent clinical result at 3 years post-operatively

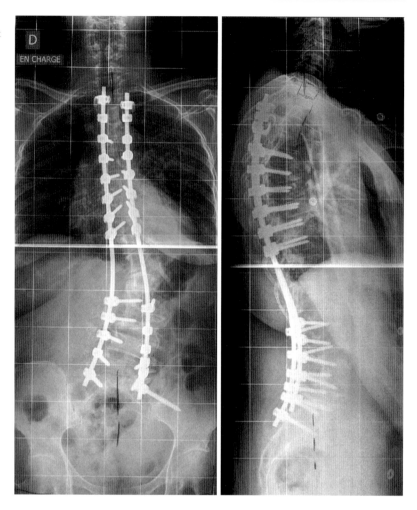

Lenke et al. prospectively demonstrated that it takes 6–12 weeks to return to baseline nutritional status and that as the number of fusion levels increase, the time to return to nutritional baseline increases. Therefore, if a surgical procedure needs to be staged, there should be supplemental nutrition between the stages to reduce the risk of malnutrition-related complications.

Infection rates depend on the approach and the age of the patient. Overall, infection rates in scoliosis surgery are reported at 3–5 %. Infection rates after anterior surgery alone is reported to be approximately 1 %. Despite a low rate of infection, a deep infection can have significant sequelae and may require multiple operations to eradicate the infection.

Pseudoarthrosis is another serious adverse consequence of an arthrodesis procedure that may require revision surgery if symptomatic. Weiss et al. reported a 38 % pseudoarthrosis rate at 37 months' follow-up that increased to 64 % if the sacrum was included in the fusion. Others have documented that posterior instrumentation and fusion alone to the sacrum carries a 15–20 % rate of pseudoarthrosis even with newer, stiffer instrumentation constructs.

Although major complications can occur, fortunately, neurological injury occurs in less than 1–5 % of cases. Significant risk factors for major intra-operative neurological deficits include hyperkyphosis and combined surgery.

Neurological deficits can manifest in a delayed manner. In fact, delayed paraplegia has been well-described and can occur several hours after spinal reconstruction surgery. Post-operative hypovolemia and mechanical tension on spinal vessels along the concavity of the curve have been implicated as the cause of spinal cord ischaemia which leads to delayed post-operative paraplegia. Therefore, it is important to maintain adequate volume and blood pressure in the patients during the post-operative period.

Case Report

A 56 year old female patient presented with a severe progressive adult scoliosis with frontal imbalance (6 cm right side) and sagittal imbalance (positive C7-plumb line +7 cm) and high pelvic incidence PI: 65° (Fig. 4)

There was severe lumbar pain in the standing position and radicular pain at the L4-L5 level on the right side.

Through a posterior approach:

Instrumentation from T3 to S1 was performed.

Segmental screw fixation and Smith Petersen osteotomies at levels L3-L4 and L5 were employed.

Good correction frontal balance and negative C7-plum line was achieved with an excellent clinical result at 3 years post-operatively (Fig. 5).

References

1. Aebi M. The adult scoliosis. Eur Spine J. 2005; 14:925–48.
2. Baron EM, Albert TJ. Medical complications of surgical treatment of adult spinal deformity and how to avoid them. Spine. 2006;31(19):S106–18.
3. Birknes JK, White AP, Albert TJ, et al. Adult degenerative scoliosis a review. Neurosurgery. 2008;63(3): A94–103.
4. Glassman SD, Bridwelle K, Dimar JR, et al. The impact of positive sagittal balance in adult spinal deformity. Spine. 2005;30(18):2024–9.
5. Kim YJ, Bridwell KH, Lenke L, et al. Sagittal thoracic decompensation following long adult lumbar spinal instrumentation and fusion to L5 or S1: causes, prevalence and risk factors analysis. Spine. 2006;31(20): 2359–66.
6. Kim YJ, Bridwelle KH, Lenke LG, et al. Proximal junctional kyphosis in adult spinal deformity after segmental posterior spinal instrumentation and fusion. Spine. 2008;33(30):2179–84.
7. Schwab FJ, Lafage V, Forcy J-P, et al. Predicting outcome and complications in the surgical treatment of adult scoliosis. Spine. 2008;33(20):2243–7.
8. Takahashi S, Delécrin J, Passuti N. Surgical treatment of idiopathic scoliosis in adults. Spine. 2002;27(16): 1742–8.

Spondylolysis With or Without Spondylolisthesis

Philippe Gillet

Contents

P. Gillet
Centre Hospitalier Universitaire, Liège, Belgium
e-mail: philippe.gillet@chu.ulg.ac.be

G. Bentley (ed.), *European Surgical Orthopaedics and Traumatology*,
DOI 10.1007/978-3-642-34746-7_28, © EFORT 2014

Abstract

Spondylolysis with or without spondylolisthesis is an often well-tolerated situation. However, growing or adult patients may experience severe back pain, referred pain or even neurological compromise that justifies surgical treatment. During growth, exceptionally in adult life, true instability with increase of the spondylolisthesis may also require stabilisation, in situ or after reduction of the deformity. Posterior, anterior and combined approaches intended to obtain correction and fusion have been described, the choice between available options remains difficult. The recent literature does not necessarily support procedures that seem more logical but are more invasive than others. While the importance of maintaining or restoring an adequate sagittal profile of the lumbar spine is universally well-accepted, the importance of slip correction is considered less important. This chapter intends to help the surgeon dealing with different situations encountered in spondylolysis and spondylolisthesis patients by first exposing the different techniques currently in use with their respective advantages and disadvantages and by considering the proper matching of the most logical procedure theoretically required by the anatomical situation and the functional expectations of the particular patient.

Keywords

Anterior interbody fusion • Diagnosis • Imaging-radiographs, C-T scanning, NMR • Natural history • Posterolateral fusion • Reduction of spondylolisthesis • Spondylolisthesis: aetiology and classification • Spondylosis • Surgical indications

Introduction

Spondylolisthesis is the anteroposterior displacement of a vertebra with regard to the lower vertebrae. It can be the result of a pars interarticularis defect called spondylolysis, degenerative disorders of the spine, dysplasia of posterior facet joints or severe trauma.

When spondylolisthesis is due to dysplasia of the lumbosacral facets or to degenerative conditions the whole vertebra including the posterior arch slips forward, causing central canal stenosis in addition to foraminal stenosis. Multiple root compromise can occur and may be severe. When a spondylolysis exists, associated or not with spondylolisthesis, back pain and referred leg pain, true sciatica or even neurological deficit and progressive deformity of the spine in the sagittal plane may occur. Multiple root compromise is exceptional but foraminal entrapment can occur. The condition is often well tolerated during lifetime and surgery is needed in a very restricted number of patients. In spondylolisthesis due to spondylolysis, many patients presenting with thigh or even leg pain do not really suffer from root entrapment but from referred pain. Even in the case of true radicular pain, it does not imply that a true decompression of the nerve root must necessarily be carried out. Root pain can be initiated by local inflammatory conditions due to excessive motion of the mobile segment. Fusion without decompression can lead to disappearance of radicular symptoms as well as back pain and muscle contracture. True entrapment of nerve roots may exist in severe slips and severe disk narrowing deforming the neural foramen or in the case of associated herniated discs.

Aetiology and Classification

A *spondylolysis* is a fatigue fracture thought to be the result of repetitive microtrauma. In some cases, the pars interarticularis can fracture and heal several times, leading to an elongated pars. Spondylolysis usually occurs in the youth. Male to female ratio is about 2:1. Spondylolysis is not accepted as a congenital disease, however genetic factors can influence the occurrence of isthmic spondylolisthesis but in a far lesser degree than in dysplastic types. A genetic influence is illustrated by a different prevalence of the disease in different races and greater prevalence in certain families. Repetitive stress on the pars, especially in extension, and hyperlordosis favour impingement on the affected pars by the distal aspect of the lower articular facet of the upper vertebrae. Adolescents practising sports involving hyperextension are at risk with up to 47 % of paediatric patients involved in comparison to a 5 % occurrence in the general adult population. The occurrence of spondylolysis is probably multi-factorial. Radiological peculiarities such as dysplasia of the vertebral body show that there can be a predisposition that weakens the pars, probably from genetic origin and further local repetitive microtrauma leads to the fracture.

A spondylolysis can lead to spondylolisthesis because of mechanical failure of the posterior arch and the overloaded disc and ligaments. Spondylolysis with or without spondylolisthesis occurs mostly at L5, followed by L4 and rarely more proximally.

A *degenerative spondylolisthesis* is the result of failure of the disc and ligaments, moreover, it produces severe alteration of the articular cartilage and deformation of the posterior facets leading to segmental hypermotion. Degenerative spondylolisthesis usually occurs at the L4-L5 level.

A *dysplastic spondylolisthesis* is the result of developmental malformation of the posterior facets, consisting of sagittal orientation of the articular processes with loss of their buttress effect or hypoplasia or aplasia of the facets. This condition occurs mostly at the lumbosacral junction.

A *traumatic spondylolisthesis* is the result of severe lesions of the posterior arch associated with disco-ligamentous injuries.

The *importance of spondylolisthesis* is described according to the Meyerding classification: grades 1, 2, 3, 4 correspond to more or less 25 %, 50 %, 75 % and, 100 % of anterior slip. When the slipped vertebra is anterior to the sacrum and usually tilted in kyphosis, the term spondyloptosis is used to describe the condition. A certain degree of kyphotic tilt can occur in grades 3 and 4 spondylolisthesis and must ideally be corrected more than the slip itself. A false L5-S1 spondylolisthesis is often described because of dysplasia of the L5 vertebral body: some patients show a trapezoidal-shaped vertebral body with a reduced anteroposterior diameter. This leads to the description of a spondylolisthesis because the posterior walls of L4, L5 and S1 are not aligned. However, the author has often noticed in such cases that the anterior borders of the vertebral bodies are

in a perfectly smooth sagittal alignment. The term spondylolisthesis should not be used in such cases since it can lead to misinterpretation of the local stability conditions of the lumbosacral junction. Such patients illustrate the role of genetic factors in the occurrence of isthmic spondylolysis since the vertebral body changes are not due to secondary remodelling as proved by the normal positioning of the vertebral body in regard to adjacent vertebrae.

The *kyphotic angle* can be measured in different ways, e.g. between a line drawn tangential to the posterior wall of S1 and the upper vertebral plate of L5 (slip angle).

It must be stressed that there is no relation between the importance of a slip and the mechanical or neurological symptoms in spondylolitic cases. Kyphotic spondylolitic spondylolisthesis is often more symptomatic. In degenerative cases and dysplasic cases, when the whole vertebra slips, neurologic compromise is often related to the severity of the stenosis.

Natural History of Spondylolysis

A spondylolysis can heal without sequelae or can persist until adulthood, with progressive pain presenting after decades of asymptomatic existence. Late onset symptoms can occur as the result of stress imposed on the various ligamentous structures because of the motion segment instability induced by the pars fracture. Potential intervertebral instability is theoretically greater for L4 or L3 spondylolysis than for L5 spondylolysis because of the absence of anatomical links such as the ilio-lumbar ligaments. Most of the slips are less than 30–50 %. Progressive slips are more often associated with local anatomical peculiarities such as a vertical sacrum, a dome-shaped sacrum, or a trapezoidal-shaped L5 with a short anteroposterior diameter of the vertebral body. A local kyphosis is more troublesome than the amount of slip. Progressive slip is unusual in adulthood but can be the result of degenerative disc disease with disc collapse leading to an added slight amount of spondylolisthesis. Important slips presenting in adult patients are generally present since adolescence. Early onset of pars fracture can increase the risk for progressive spondylolisthesis.

Progression of the slip usually occurs during the growth spurt. The more the slip is important during the growth period (more than grade 2), the more the patient is at risk for further displacement until skeletal maturity. A high slip angle is also associated with a risk of progression. Therefore, even in asymptomatic patients, there may be an occasional indication for fusion in severe spondylolisthesis. Spondylolisthesis occurs two times more often in males but the risk of increasing spondylolisthesis is four times greater in female than male patients.

If not the cause of spondylolysis, trauma can increase symptoms related to the anomaly and favour increase of the slip.

From a personal experience, spondylolysis with or without spondylolisthesis ultimately requiring surgical management is a problem of the young adult. In a series of 276 patients from 1986 to 2006, the mean age was 37 years with a range from 13 to 70 years; 75 % were between 20 and 50 years old.

Diagnosis

Clinical Findings

Spondylolysis and even spondylolisthesis are often diagnosed incidentally because they are asymptomatic. However, the patient, either child, adolescent or adult may present with common or acute back pain, thigh or leg pain – the latter can be mechanical pain radiating to the lower limb or true radicular pain- lumbar scoliosis, paravertebral muscle spasm, abnormal stance or gait. If symptoms are important, other pathological conditions of the spine should be ruled out since spondylolysis is often poorly symptomatic. Symptoms are not proportional to the importance of the pathological condition, spondylolysis without slip can be more painful than spondylolysis with obvious spondylolisthesis. Möller and co-workers found that symptoms were similar in adult patients with spondylolisthesis or with chronic non-specific low back pain probably related to degenerative conditions; however they found that the chronic low back pain group reported greater functional disability [17].

In degenerative spondylolisthesis and dysplastic spondylolisthesis, leg weakness can be observed on top of back pain and referred pain, true sciatica is also more common than with spondylolytic slips.

Imaging

Plain lateral, ap. and oblique radiographs are the first step in the evaluation of spondylolisthesis. Ideally, standing films should be obtained, centred on the lumbosacral area and not the lumbar spine. Spondylolysis can be missed on lateral views, oblique views centred on the pathological vertebra must be obtained when the abnormality is suspected. Even with perfect quality plain radiographs, spondylolysis, especially in the early stage, can be missed. **CT scan**, using particularly the reversed gantry technique, can be necessary to show the defect but is of low interest in the general set-up except in dysplastic and degenerative conditions. *Bone scans* are helpful to make the diagnosis of a pars defect at an early stage.

Dynamic lateral views can be helpful to evaluate the mobility of the abnormal vertebra. A *lateral full-length standing film* is recommended to judge the global sagittal alignment and balance of the spine, especially when a severe spondylolisthesis or lumbosacral kyphosis is present

The regular pre-operative imaging set-up for a spondylolysis with or without spondylolisthesis requires *NMR*. It will give the necessary information on the presence of and on the indication for removal of a intraforaminal herniated disc, on the possible choice between a reconstruction procedure of the pars if there is no degenerative disc disease at the level of the spondylolysis or some kind of intervertebral fusion if degenerative disc disease is present, and finally on the necessary length of such a fusion to stop it ideally at the level of an intact disc space (Fig. 1). If NMR gives doubtful results, a *provocative discography* can be performed, the procedure does however not

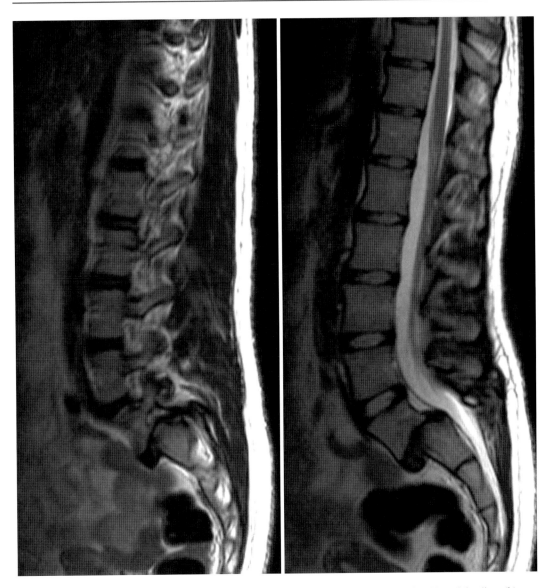

Fig. 1 Pre-operative NMR imaging is essential to evaluate the status of the neural foramina (**a**) and the discs (**b**)

seem innocuous [3]. NMR is the best procedure to evaluate central root compromise in degenerative and dysplastic spondylolisthesis but lacks dynamic information as does CT scanning.

Myelography has been and is still used by some teams to evaluate possible root compromise. In spondylolytic spondylolisthesis myelography is commonly normal: since the posterior arch remains in place, there is an increase in the anteroposterior diameter of the spinal canal, the possible root impingement is far lateral, in an area the contrast does not reach. Dynamic myelography is the sole dynamic procedure to date and may be useful in degenerative conditions when the importance of the slip can be underestimated by the supine position needed for CT and NMR. The association of NMR and dynamic plain films gives however the possibility to assess the possible neurological compromise occurring in dynamic conditions.

Radiological Peculiarities

In unilateral spondylolysis, a hypertrophy of the opposite pars or pedicle may occur due to by-pass of the loads through these structures. Differential diagnosis from osteoid osteoma must be made, especially if the patient has persistent pain. Unilateral pars defect with opposite pedicle lysis can be observed.

Indications for Surgery

General Principles for Treatment

Asymptomatic patients presenting with a spondylolysis and grade 0–2 spondylolisthesis should not be prevented from sports activities and strenuous work as long as such activities do not induce pain. In symptomatic patients without neurological compromise, adaptation of the lifestyle, which can mean change of work and refraining from sports, in association with conservative treatment, is the cornerstone of treatment [6, 19]. Fusion procedures should only be performed in the unusual cases where a great risk of increased spondylolisthesis is present, whether the patient is symptomatic or not, and in cases where conservative treatment has failed to relieve symptoms. There is a place for surgery in patients who are relieved by adaptation of their lifestyle but who want to regain normal work or sporting possibilities. If a reasonable surgical procedure can be proposed, surgical treatment, although invasive, may be considered in selected patients capable of making a well- understood decision with the surgeon.

Decompression procedures are usually associated with fusion, however, in a symptomatic stenosis due to degenerative spondylolisthesis, isolated fenestration may be contemplated if instability is low and will not be worsened by the decompression procedure.

Pre-Operative Preparation and Planning

Surgical options depend on the age of the patient, the existence or not of an associated degenerative disc disease and the presence of a true local instability. Where some kind of stabilization procedure is performed the possibilities include pars repair with no fusion of a motion segment, different posterior fusion procedures and interbody fusion by posterior or anterior approach. The number of motion segments to be fused must be estimated. The need for decompression of the nerve roots must be assessed but differential diagnosis between referred pain and true radicular symptoms is sometimes difficult. Reduction or not of an associated spondylolisthesis or lumbosacral kyphosis and the role of internal fixation must be discussed for each individual patient.

Author's Pre-Operative Imaging Strategy

The regular imaging set-up for spondylolysis with or without spondylolisthesis will require plain radiographs and NMR.

In dysplastic cases, an additional CT scan may be performed to perfectly assess the posterior arch anomalies.

In degenerative cases, plain radiographs with additional dynamic lateral views and NMR are performed.

Operative Techniques

The techniques are described for spondylolysis cases with or without spondylolisthesis; particularities for dysplastic and degenerative cases will be highlighted.

Patient Positioning and Approaches to the Spine

Approaches are described in another section of this treatise. While the posterior approach carries few risks, except when penetrating the spinal canal and performing the reduction, the anterior approach carries specific risks because of the anatomical structures that lie in front of the spine.

Patient positioning is important according to the specificity of the disease.

Patient Positioning for the Posterior Approach

The patient can be positioned on any operating table the surgeon is familiar with. However the sagittal alignment of the lumbosacral spine is important during a posterior approach. A decompression procedure and the access to the disc are easier with the patient in slight kyphosis. If a posterolateral fusion is performed without instrumentation, the sagittal alignment can correct itself in the post-operative brace to restore lordosis. If an instrumentation is performed or if interbody bone blocks or cages are inserted, a permanent sagittal mal-alignment of the lumbosacral spine may result from positioning the patient in a flexed position. When performing a procedure that fixes the spine in a definite position, one must ascertain that the patient's sagittal profile is adequate at the end of this procedure. Sagittal imbalance of the spine, especially in the lumbosacral area can be badly tolerated. The author uses a regular Hall frame with the hips slightly flexed at about 20°. This provides a slight amount of lordosis, usually not interfering with the decompression procedure if the latter is necessary while offering great ease to achieve adequate lordosis by simply fixing the spine in that position or by putting some compression between pedicle screws or by contouring the rods if more lordosis is desired. Another way to position the patients adequately is to put them in a kneeling position, taking care that the pelvis remains free to rotate around the hip joints. This position gives more freedom for reduction manoeuvres, allowing true anterior tilt of the pelvis and sacrum while pulling back the slipped vertebra. In any case abdominal pressure must be avoided to lessen epidural bleeding.

Patient Positioning for the Anterior Approach

The patient is positioned supine on the operating table. Traction and lordosis have been advocated to obtain partial slip correction if needed and to facilitate exposure of the spine [15]. However, too much lordosis can tighten the abdominal wall and pre-vertebral vascular structures, making retraction of these tissues more difficult. A neutral position of the spine may be preferred. A slight Trendelenbourg positioning is favourable to clear the bowels from the lumbosacral area.

Possible complications of the anterior approach to the lumbosacral spine include vascular, bowel and urogenital injury [1, 20, 26]. Anterior approaches should only be performed by properly trained Orthopaedic surgeons and with the assistance of a vascular surgeon if needed. The true frequency of urogenital complications (retrograde ejaculation and sterility) related to the anterior approach of the lumbosacral junction is difficult to evaluate; meticulous surgical technique and avoidance of monopolar electrocautery should keep this risk to a minimum [12, 15].

Decompression Procedures

If true neurological compromise is present, compression usually occurs at the level of the deformed foramina. Therefore, posterior decompression of the nerve roots, when necessary, is a more complete procedure than the usual laminectomy or fenestration for spinal degenerative stenosis. It includes the removal of the entire posterior arch and all bulky fibrocartilaginous tissue present at the level of the pars defect. It is indeed this fibrous tissue, in association with the slip, if present, that compresses the nerve roots. The procedure is known as the Gill procedure. Louis has described the most offending structure which is in fact the proximal pars remnant, it is called the "crochet isthmique" or isthmus hook, this particular structure may be responsible for stretching the nerve root when a spondylolisthesis is present. The decompression procedure must include thorough removal of this structure. It is preferable to remove it with a chisel than with Kerrisson rongeurs since the latter can compress the already compromised nerve root. Removal of all offending tissue is necessary flush with the inferior and internal border of the pedicle at the end of the procedure.

En bloc resection of the posterior arch is advised to obtain a bony structure from which cortico-cancellous bone blocs can be trimmed when interbody fusion is contemplated. If a posterolateral onlay graft or if cages are planned, the posterior arch may be removed piecemeal with rongeurs.

An isolated Gill procedure, without stabilisation, can increase the risk of progression and is not recommended, except in some elderly patients where degenerative disc space remodelling has re-established some local stability. If a herniated disk is present and is responsible for root compression, it should be removed; an isolated discectomy in a patient presenting with an otherwise asymptomatic spondylolysis may be considered.

Stabilisation Procedures

The various stabilisation procedures will be described here, their indications will be discussed at the end of this chapter.

Posterolateral Fusion With and Without Instrumentation

Posterolateral fusion is a common fusion procedure in the lumbosacral area, bone graft is packed against the lateral aspect of the articular processes, the posterior aspect of the transverse processes and the sacral ala. In spondylolysis and spondylolisthesis, it can be performed either in situ or after reduction of the slip.

General Principles for Posterolateral Fusion

The posterior aspect of the spine is exposed through a standard mid-line approach and subperiosteal muscle stripping. The exposure must extend to the tips of the transverse processes and to the ala of the sacrum. The small arterial branches close to the pars interarticularis are regularly sacrificed. The mid-line approach enables the surgeon to perform a decompression procedure if needed. If no decompression is contemplated, the Wiltse paraspinal approach is an option. The lateral extra-articular aspect of the articular processes and the posterior

aspect of the transverse processes or the ala of the sacrum are decorticated down to bleeding cancellous bone first with a rongeur and then with a large curette; care must be taken not to break the transverse processes which can be very thin (Fig. 2a–d). The strongest part of the transverse processes where most of the graft material should be laid is close to the articular processes (Fig. 2e). If an instrumentation is performed the bone chips can be inserted while the instrumentation is already in place, but it is strongly advised to make the decortication before putting the implants, as these can hinder adequate access to the bone and lead to inadequate preparation of the fusion bed, thus favouring non-union. It may be easier however to mark the insertion points for the implants before starting the decortication. During the decortication procedure as well as the introduction of pedicle screws, the articular capsules of the adjacent free motion segment must be preserved to lower the risk of secondary degenerative changes. Autologous bone graft can be harvested from the iliac crest, which is the "gold standard", either by a separate incision or through the mid-line approach. If a Gill procedure is performed, sufficient bone chips can often be trimmed from the posterior arch to perform a one level fusion. Bank bone or bone substitutes can be used as an adjunct to autologous bone.

In Situ Posterolateral Fusion

In situ posterolateral fusion, i.e. without any attempt to improve the sagittal alignment of the lumbosacral junction, has been described as a functionally successful treatment even in high grade spondylolisthesis in adolescents and even when mild nerve root irritation was present [11, 13, 21]. In situ fusion can be associated with posterior decompression. In the case of a narrow degenerative disc space, in situ posterolateral fusion can lead to secondary spontaneous fusion of the disc space (Fig. 3).

After-Treatment and Role of the Instrumentation

The use of a solid rod-screw type instrumentation spares the need for post-operative bracing in the author's experience. When no

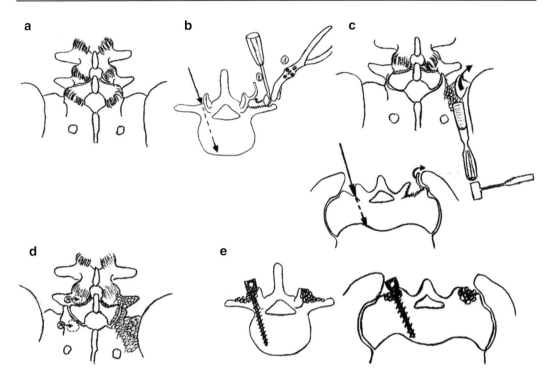

Fig. 2 Posterolateral L5-S1 fusion: the bone graft must be placed in a carefully decorticated area, using rongeurs, curettes and bone chisels (**a–d**). Pedicle screws must only be placed after proper bone grafting or at least decortication has been performed, pre-positioning the screws can hinder adequate fit of the bone graft; the direction of pedicle screws must follow the natural orientation of the pedicles (**e**)

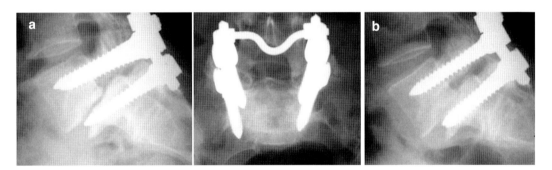

Fig. 3 Grade 2 spondylolisthesis in an adult patient. Severe back and buttock pain, no radicular pain though severe remodelling of the neural foramen. In the absence of no true instability at the L5-S1 level an in situ posterolateral L5-S1 fusion was performed associated with a Gill procedure. Radiographs at 1 month (**a**) and 2 years post-operative: (**b**) spontaneous fusion of the disc space

instrumentation is used, permanent rigid bracing, preferably including one thigh is recommended for 3 months. In any case, during the first 3 months after a posterolateral fusion, bending of the trunk is prohibited. Patients are encouraged to walk frequently but no specific rehabilitation is performed, it is even discouraged. Return to light work is allowed after 6–12 weeks, strenuous work is discouraged before 4–6 months [18].

Posterolateral Fusion with Reduction of the Spondylolisthesis

Reduction may be desirable if the slip is significant and especially if lumbosacral kyphosis is present. Techniques of reduction are described further in this chapter. Posterolateral fusion is performed after reduction in the same way as described above.

After-Treatment and Role of the Instrumentation

After reduction of the spondylolisthesis, the mechanical stress on the healing postero-lateral bone graft and the posterior instrumentation is much greater than with in situ fusion, this can augment the risk for non-union and lead to loss of correction. Post-operative immobilisation should be more rigorous. A semi-rigid or rigid brace may be considered; it has been the author's practice not to use bracing with the strong rod-screw instrumentations but to ensure strict respect for lumbosacral bolting by the trunk musculature during the first 3 months. Return to work follows the same rules as with in situ fusion. Though correction of the spondylolisthesis associated with posterolateral fusion is a classic procedure, the author favours interbody fusion when correction of the slip is performed to avoid excessive stress on the posterior graft and instrumentation.

Interbody Fusion

Posterolateral fusions are submitted to tension and bending stresses, reduction creates a new unstable condition until bone healing. Interbody fusions are more logical from a biomechanical point of view. They are submitted to a compression stress favourable to stability and fusion but some shear stress persist if the lumbosacral junction is very oblique. Compared to posterolateral fusion, the increased bony surface and superior vascularity of the interbody space provides a potentially superior biological environment for fusion [8, 14, 22, 25].

Posterior Lumbar Interbody Fusion (PLIF)

PLIF offers the opportunity to perform the whole surgical procedure through one single approach. The spine is exposed through a standard posterior approach. The posterior arch is removed -en bloc to provide bone graft- as well as the fibrous tissue and all other potentially offending structures at the level of the pars interarticularis and the neural foramen. The nerve roots must be free of any compression. The disc is excised completely, the dural sac being retracted alternatively to the left and right (Fig. 4a–d). Adequate decortication of the end-plates is carried out with rongeurs, curettes, side cutting spreaders in 1 or 2 mm increment sizes and rarely bone chisels in the case of dense cortical bone (Fig. 4e). Deep penetration down to cancellous bone must be avoided because it can lead to sinking of the bone grafts in the vertebra; subchondral end-plates should be respected while some bleeding of the end-plates must be obtained to ensure an ideal bed for the graft. Distraction between the end-plates must be maintained during the insertion of the grafts. This can be obtained by using the side-cutting intradiscal spreaders actually offered by most instrumentations. Distraction can also be obtained and maintained by pedicle screws and rods or plates. Since the distraction obtained with the posterior instrumentation can lead to segmental kyphosis, even with strong pedicle screws and rods, because the distraction force predominates at the posterior aspect of the spine (Fig. 5d), the author does recommend the use of incrementally-sized intradiscal speaders to obtain most of the distraction. The size of the last spreaders is slightly superior to the height of the future bone grafts, the distraction is then only maintained by the posterior instrumentation (Fig. 5a–c) and the corticocancellous bone blocs, or the cages filled with bone graft are alternatively placed at the left and right sides after the intradiscal speaders have been removed (Fig. 4f). Before placing the grafts, it is advised to take advantage of the distraction to improve if necessary the removal of all potential neurologically offending structures, especially in the foraminal area. When the bone grafts or cages have been placed in the intervertebral space, the locking nuts of the proximal of distal pedicle screws are released and compression is applied; finally all the locking nuts are tightened again.

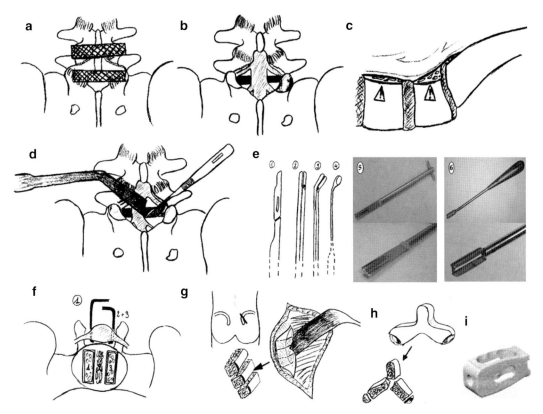

Fig. 4 Basic principles to perform posterior lumbar interbody fusion. The level of the disc spaces with regard to the posterior arch is showed (**a**). After removal of the posterior arch, the nerve roots are thoroughly decompressed and the disc exposed (**b**), bi-polar electrocautery is used to perform haemostasis at the level of the disc space; at the level of the vertebral body, especially at the area of the slip, epidural veins are difficult to control (**c**). The disc is removed and the end-plates are decorticated using specific instruments (**d**, **e**). Corticocancellous bone blocks from the iliac crest (**g**), from the posterior arch (**h**) or cages filled with autologous bone (**i**) are placed in the disc space; at least three bone blocks are put in place or two cages and one bone block in between (**f**)

This locks the grafts or cages in place and improves the lumbosacral lordosis (Fig. 5e, f). Adequate bending of the rods in the sagittal plane is mandatory. Corticocancellous bone grafts can be obtained from the posterior iliac crest or the removed posterior arch if the latter is large (Fig. 4g, h); cages filled with autologous bone graft are an option to diminish the removal from the donor sites (Fig. 4i). When using cages, it is recommended to pack bone also between the cages to augment the local bone stock and favour solid fusion (Fig. 4f). About a 1 cm height for the bone grafts seems necessary to avoid crushing and failure. When using cages, a greater height may lead to inadequate

revascularistion and healing at mid-height of the graft and to a locked non-union.

Drawbacks and Possible Complications

The anterior longitudinal ligament and anterior border of the disc should be respected to avoid great vessel injury [9, 19]. The dural sac and the nerve roots are at permanent risk throughout the procedure. The use of adequate retractors and cautious manipulation of the nerve roots while performing the discectomy and inserting the bone grafts or cages is mandatory to limit the risk for dural leaks. To facilitate haemostasis of the epidural plexus, it is advised to stay at the level of the disc space since profuse bleeding usually occurs

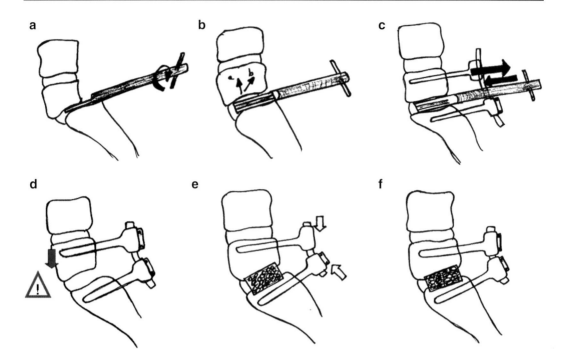

Fig. 5 Method to obtain distraction and perform interbody fusion by posterior approach. Using intradiscal spreaders, the disc space is restored, this also leads to partial reduction of the slip when present by tightening of the residual soft tissues surrounding the adjacent vertebrae (**a**, **b**), distraction using pedicle screws can also open the disc space but carry the risk of inducing kyphosis (**d**). With the spreaders and posterior instrumentation, the desired intervertebral space and reduction is obtained (**c**). After removal of the intradiscal instruments, the disc height is maintained by the posterior instrumentation (**d**), the bone grafts or cages are placed, compression is finally put on the pedicle screws to lock the grafts and improve the lumbosacral lordosis (**e**, **f**)

from veins at the level of the vertebral body (Fig. 4c). If bi-polar coagulation is insufficient, compression by gelfoam° or surgicel° is recommended. Controlled hypotension is a prerequisite to perform this procedure safely. Adequate decortication of the vertebral end-plates is difficult because the view is limited by the dural sac and any bleeding. Specific instruments such as lateral cutting shapers and broaches like those designed for the placement of cages help to perform the procedure safely, even if only corticocancellous bone blocks are used.

After-Treatment
In the author's experience, thanks to the stability of interbody bone grafts in combination with posterior instrumentation in compression, patients are allowed to ambulate immediately, according to post-operative pain, without a brace except if bone purchase of the pedicle screws is compromised by bad bone quality. With the exception of walking, exercises are however not recommended during the healing process of the graft for approximately 3 months. Return to physical work is allowed 3–6 months after surgery, according to the radiological appearances and the type of work and earlier in sedentary occupations. If PLIF is performed without posterior instrumentation, caution must be observed in mobilisation and rigid bracing is mandatory for 3 months. This procedure is not recommended by the author.

Anterior Lumbar Interbody Fusion (ALIF)
Anterior interbody fusion can be performed by transperitoneal or retroperitoneal approach. The disk space can be exposed with greater facility than through the spinal canal, allowing the placement of multiple corticocancellous bone grafts after discectomy and decortication of the endplates with rongeurs, curettes and bone chisels.

A technique using a fibular peg from the anterosuperior border of L5 down to the S1 vertebral body through the disc space has been described [15].

Drawbacks and Possible Complications

Isolated anterior interbody fusion plays a small role in the surgery for spondylolisthesis. It generally does not allow a safe reduction of the slip if no preliminary decompression of the nerve roots has been performed. If a nerve root entrapment is present, an isolated anterior interbody fusion may not be able to obtain decompression. However, if the entrapment is only present at the level of the foramina, the restoration of the normal disc height by the interbody graft may theoretically suffice to decompress the nerve root without a complementary posterior approach, but the risk of mobilising more disc in the foramen with increased root compression is present during reduction of the slip. Immediate intervertebral stabilisation is not obtained because of the vessels that almost precludes strong anterior internal fixation at the lumbosacral level which carries the risk of bone graft mobilisation. Anterior in situ fusion may be considered when the lumbosacral junction remains well balanced and no decompression or reduction is desired. Complications due to the anterior approach have been described earlier.

After-Treatment

Rigid bracing and avoidance of physical exercise during the healing period of an isolated anterior intervertebral fusion is mandatory.

Combined Anterior and Posterior Fusion

These procedures combine the techniques described above. Several authors [6, 11, 20, 26] have reported on combined or staged anterior and posterior approaches for spondylolysis with spondylolisthesis, usually for severe slips. The aim of this two or three-stage surgery is generally to obtain correction of the slip while improving the chances for solid fusion. The posterior approach permits adequate decompression of the nerve roots before any attempt at reduction, and a posterolateral fusion and pedicle screw instrumentation can help to obtain the reduction and promotes early stability of the operated mobile segment. The anterior approach is used to perform the interbody bone fusion, sometimes also the reduction with specific reduction instruments [20]. All these combined procedures can be performed in one operative setting or as staged operations, depending on the severity of the case, the surgical team and the general health status of the patient.

The author often uses the combined approach in one operative setting *in degenerative spondylolisthesis* when instability is significant. After completion of the posterior L4-L5 decompression and instrumentation, the patient is placed in right side decubitus and a small minimal invasive approach is performed anterolaterally by muscle splitting and retroperitoneal approach to put an interbody bone graft or cage in the disc space. Other authors favour a TLIF procedure in such cases which has the theoretical advantage of keeping the patient in a prone position. The combined approach is somewhat longer due to the two consecutive positionings of the patient but it gives a better view of the disc and favours a thorough debridment. Moreover, fluoroscopy is kept to a minimum.

Drawbacks and Possible Complications

The potential insufficiencies of an isolated posterior or anterior approach may be compensated for by the combination with other procedures. However, the possible complications linked to the specific techniques described earlier are cumulative.

After-Treatment

The immediate stability obtained with these techniques is usually excellent, the same post-operative rules as for instrumented PLIF are recommended.

Techniques of Reduction of the Spondylolisthesis

It seems logical that anatomical and biomechanical restoration of the lumbosacral sagittal balance should lead to better long-term results as far as back and thigh pain are concerned and that it should lessen the risk for a junctional-segment syndrome. Correction of the slip puts the posterolateral bone grafts in better mechanical conditions to ensure solid fusion. Restoration of normal or close to normal anatomical relationships also favours radicular decompression by opening the neural foramina. Lordosis is the aim, and correction of the kyphotic deformity, if present, is more important than the slip.

Reduction of the spondylolisthesis may be obtained pre-operatively or post-operatively using traction tables, halo-pelvic or halo-femoral traction. These procedures have the advantage of offering close neurological monitoring but are uncomfortable for the patient [5]. Correction of the deformity is generally obtained intra-operatively using some kind of instrumentation. The instrumentation has two aims: to obtain the desired reduction and to provide post-operative immobilization. In severe instability supplementary post-operative bracing must be considered. All techniques using distraction only favour loss of lumbosacral lordosis and must be abandoned. Pedicle screw fixation with plates or rods can be used to obtain and maintain correction while keeping the length of fusion to a minimum [2, 18].

A pre-requisite to obtain and maintain reduction is a firm fixation in the sacrum as well as in the slipped vertebra. Pedicle screws are the safest and strongest fixators. To improve the sacral fixation, another pair of pedicle screws can be put in the S2 pedicles, in the sacral ala and even in the iliac crest using special connectors. The different sacral fixation options are too numerous to be completely described in this chapter.

The sacrum is considered as the reference vertebra with regard to which the slipped vertebra must be reduced. The sacrum can be vertical in association with lumbosacral kyphosis in severe slips. Reduction of the slip must not re-align the posterior aspects of the vertebral bodies but above all correct the lumbosacral angle by tilting the sacrum forward and downwards under the lumbar vertebra while the latter is pulled backwards and in lordosis. Beforehand, a slight distraction may be necessary to de-co-apt the adjacent vertebrae and give the mobile segment the necessary freedom before correcting the slip and the kyphosis. Resection of the dome of the sacrum is sometimes required.

In low grade, i.e. grade 1 or 2 spondylolisthesis, the usefulness of reduction is questionable if there remains an adequate lumbosacral lordosis. If reduction is desired, it is easily obtained by putting pedicle screws in L5 and S1, fixing rods to the S1 screws and bringing the L5 pedicle screws and the L5 vertebra backward against the rods with the help of levers, rod pushers and rod introducers from the ancillary instrumentation. Partial re-alignment is often already obtained by the use of intra-discal spreaders: the spreaders not only restore the height of the disc space. Thanks to the remaining ligamentous structures and lateral and anterior parts of the annulus, there is a combined backwards movement of the upper vertebra while the disc space is distracted (Fig. 5a–b). Pulling the screws back against the rods or plates while pushing the sacrum under L5 to induce lordosis finalizes the reduction (Fig. 5c). The L5 rod screw fixations are tightened and a interbody or posterolateral bone fusion is performed. An interbody fusion is advised to minimise the risk of deformity recurrence if slip reduction has been obtained, even if a strong posterior instrumentation is used in combination with posterolateral fusion.

In severe slips, the correction is more difficult to obtain. In any case, a thorough decompression of the nerve roots must be obtained before any attempt of reduction. The disc space must be recognised, if necessary with the help of an image intensifier. Resection of the dome of the sacrum may be necessary to enter the disc space and perform the resection of the residual disc tissue. A spatula or the disc spreaders may be introduced in the disc space and used as a lever to disengage the slipped vertebra from its position (Fig. 5a). While doing this, some kind of the ancillary instruments such as rod introducers are used to try to pull the slipped vertebra backwards while tilting the sacrum forwards thanks to the screws and rods fixed to the vertebrae (Figs. 5c, 6). The correction may be stopped when an adequate lordosis of the lumbosacral area has been obtained. Complete reduction of the slip is not the aim and produces a greater risk of root tethering than angular correction. Posterolateral fusion, PLIF or ALIF is performed after the instrumentation has been tightened in place. If there is a contact between

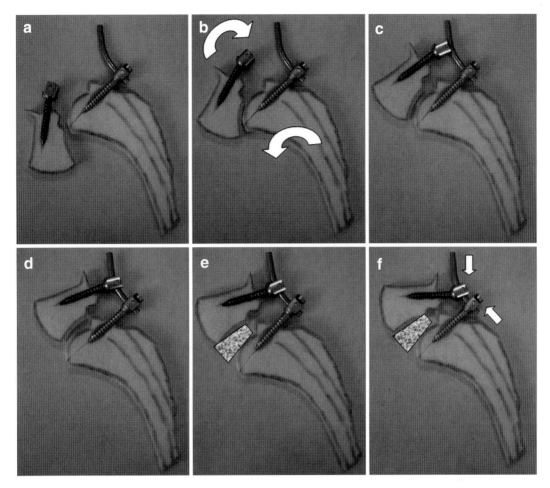

Fig. 6 Reduction of severe slips. A thorough posterior decompression is performed, pedicle screws are fixed in the sacrum and the slipped vertebra. The disc space is recognized with the help of an image intensifier and after resection of the dome of the sacrum if necessary (**a**, **b**). After removal of the disc, a lever is introduced in the disc space to de-coapt the adjacent vertebrae and induce correction of the lumbosacral deformity in combination with the posterior instrumentation and ancillary instruments such as rod introducers, trying to pull and tilt L5 and S1 in relationship to each other (**c**, **d**), the arrows show the resulting correcting forces that should be obtained. When correction of the slip is satisfactory, sagittal profile can be further increased by compression between the body of the screws, if adequate anterior bone support is present (**e**, **f**). The use of polyaxial screws at the lumbar level is necessary to obtain adequate fit and secure tightening between the screws and the rods

the decorticated adjacent end-plates after the reduction while there is no root compromise, a posterolateral fusion may be sufficient but if there is an anterior gap, it should be filled with an interbody fusion to avoid late recurrence of the deformity.

Because of the angular deformity, the use of regular monoaxial screws can be difficult because there will be a great sagittal angulation between the L5 screws and the rods fixed to the S1 screws before reduction is attempted.

When the desired reduction is obtained there can still be an great angulation between the screws and the rods making it impossible to assure solid tightening using the locking nuts. The use of polyaxial screws may help since the body of the screw may move to maintain adequate alignment with the rods during the whole phase of the correction. In the beginning, there will be a flexion tilt between the core of the screw and the body of the screw, while the reduction improves, this angle will lessen (Fig. 6b–d),

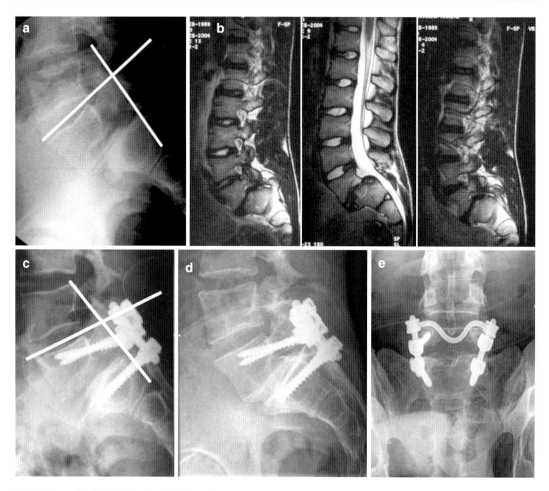

Fig. 7 Posterior lumbar interbody fusion with reduction in a patient with grade 2 L5-S1 spondylolisthesis in slight kyphosis, suffering from associated back and radicular pain, after return to full work (**a–d**). Slight residual slip remains but there is adequate sagittal profile

finally compression between the body of the screws to improve lordosis may even reverse the angle between the core and the body of the screw while maintaining adequate fit between the body of the screw and the rod (Fig. 6e, f). However, one must be aware that by using the mobility of polyaxial screws, there can be a risk of secondary loss of lordosis if there is no adequate anterior support or if the tightening of the screws against the rod is not perfect. Final compression between the screws should be performed after the interbody grafts or cages have been put in place, using the procedure with the spreaders in combination with the posterior instrumentation described above. The surgeon is encouraged to critically evaluate the

instrumentation he intends to use because its reliability can be highly manufacturer-related. When polyaxial screws are not really needed, the use of monoaxial screws remains recommended. When anterior interbody fusion is needed, it can be performed either by an anterior approach or by a posterior approach using the specific instruments described in the paragraph on posterior interbody fusion (Fig. 7).

In some cases, a supplementary L4 fixation can be useful to obtain reduction [23]. If the L4-L5 disc is intact, the rod may be cut between L4 and L5 and the L4 screws removed after L5-S1 fixation to regain the mobility of the L4-L5 segment. It may happen that the L5 pedicles are weak and in this case, temporary fixation without fusion to L4 can prevent screw pull-out at L5. The L4 fixation may be removed 6 months later. If the L4-L5 disc space remains very oblique or if L5-S1 sagittal alignment is unsatisfactory after L5-S1 fixation only, lengthening the fusion and instrumentation up to L4 may improve the global lumbar lordosis by adequately contouring the rods and compressing the posterior L4-L5 elements. A L4-S1 fusion may be preferable to a shorter L5-S1 fusion if the result is a better sagittal spine balance.

Drawbacks and Possible Complications
In severe slips, there can be a shortening of the L5 roots and these may be stretched during the reduction procedure, either closed or open, leading to severe deficit. Partial reduction of the deformity is often the safest procedure. Correction of the kyphosis, when present, is more important than reducing the translational slip.

One must be aware that when the reduction of a spondylolisthesis is obtained, this creates a new temporary unstable situation that is generally even worse than the one before the surgical procedure. The posterior instrumentation is submitted to a tremendous stress before bone fusion occurs. This carries the risk of slip recurrence depending of the type of bone graft, the strength of the internal fixation and the post-operative behaviour of the patient. Reduction by posterior instrumentation and posterolateral fusion only is at risk for secondary loss of correction because of the lack of an anterior weight-bearing bone graft. In situ fusion, even for high slips must be considered as a viable option [11, 13].

L5 Vertebrectomy and L4-S1 Fusion in High Grade Slips
Gaines has advocated a combined approach with removal of the L5 vertebral body and posterior arch and L4-S1 fusion in spondyloptosis [9]. The first stage is performed by an anterior retroperitoneal approach using a transverse skin and rectus abdominis muscle incision. Great care must be taken to control the vascular structures including exiting epidural veins at the level of the L4-L5 and L5-S1 foramina. The L5 pedicles define the posterior border of the anterior stage resection.

The L5 vertebral body is excised with the two adjacent disks and the lower L4 cartilage endplate is removed maintaining the subchondral bony end-plate. No attempt is made at that stage to reduce the deformation. The second, posterior stage consists in the removal of the L5 posterior arch, the positioning of pedicle screws in L4 and S1 and the progressive reduction of L4 on the sacral plateau which has been decorticated. Bone fragments obtained from the removed vertebral body are used to perform supplementary posterolateral fusion and to improve bone contact between the end-plates if necessary. Gaines observed no serious permanent root damage with this method but other authors reported complications [9].

Drawbacks and Possible Complications
The risks for complications are those of all combined procedures, with the increased difficulty to recognise anatomical elements such as the vessels and nerve roots due to the severe deformation of the lumbosacral area.

After-Treatment
A 4–6 weeks' bed rest in a crutch-type brace with leg extension is advised before the patient starts walking. Surgical inspection of the fusion mass and implant removal are usually performed at 4–6 months.

Pars Defect Reconstruction Procedures
A spondylolysis can induce pain even without associated degenerative disc disease, the hypermobility of the loose posterior arch stimulates the defect tissue which seems rich in nocioceptive nerve endings and the relative instability of the vertebral body induces excessive stress to the underlying disc. Removal of the soft tissue and bone grafting of the defect to restore the stabilising role of the posterior arch seems a logical form of treatment in this small group of patients, the theoretical advantage being the avoidance of any sacrifice of a motion segment. The procedure can be described as "isthmic reconstruction" or "direct repair" of the pars interarticularis. Most procedures include some sort of internal fixation in order to improve the fusion rate and favour more rapid return to active life without external support: a screw across the

pars, techniques using the passage of wires under the laminae and transverse processes, special screw-hook constructs or special plates. We described a technique using a V-shaped rod and pedicle screws, associated with direct bone grafting of the pars defect using a rod-screw instrumentation [10]. The optimal indication for pars defect reconstruction is isolated spondylolysis, pars reconstruction is not recommended if underlying disc degenerative disease is present. The following three methods have been used by the author.

V-Rod and Pedicle Screw Technique

By a posterior mid-line approach, the lumbosacral junction is exposed from the L4 to S1 spinous processes and laterally to the tips of the L5 transverse processes. To avoid stress being put on the isthmus of L5 by the overlying inferior L4 facets which could possibly lead to recurrence of the spondylolysis, [16], two or 3 mm of the distal aspect of these facets are removed with an osteotome, taking care to remove as little capsular structure as possible. The soft tissue situated in the pars defect is removed with rongeurs. If the pre-operative MRI has shown the absence of any root impingement, which is usually the case, a very thin layer of soft tissue is preserved at the bottom of the defect to avoid migration of the bone graft in the foramen. The sides of the defect, the upper half of the laminae and the lateral, extra-articular aspect of the upper zygapophyseal joint are exposed down to bleeding bone. Lumbar screws, about 35 mm. in length and 5 mm. in diameter, are inserted in the L5 pedicles, avoiding violation of the L4-L5 joint. Iliac bone graft is harvested and trimmed to be placed in the defect and on the posterior aspect of the laminae and lateral aspect of the zygapophyseal processes. A rod, usually 8–10 cm. in length, is bent in a V-shape and inserted under the L5 spinous process, after the L5-S1 interspinous ligament has been removed. The rod is firmly fixed against the spinous process and the laminae, offering the possibility of compressing the graft in the defect and to stabilise the posterior arch. A slight bending is made in the sagittal plane if necessary to achieve proper fit against the posterior arch of the vertebra and the grooves of the open pedicle screws; postero-anterior compression on the L5-S1 joints must be avoided. The pedicle screws are placed with their grooves oriented 30–45° to the longitudinal axis of the patient. Finally, the blocking elements are firmly tightened against the rod to fixed to the pedicle screws. Care is taken to avoid any impingement between the rod and the superior aspect of the S1 spinous process during extension of the spine (Fig. 8).

The same technique may be used at the L4 level.

After-Treatment

Patients are allowed to sit and walk 1 or 2 days after surgery and are usually discharged at day 4. No brace is recommended. Return to work is allowed between 6 and 12 weeks, sports after 3 months.

Limitations of the Technique

The presence of a spina bifida precludes the use of this technique.

Morscher Hook-Type Techniques

The spine is exposed and the pars defect is dissected as with the previous technique. After iliac bone blocks have been put in the defect, pedicle screws are fixed and the hooks are slid onto the rods and tightened against the inferior aspect of the laminae (Fig. 9).

After-Treatment

The original Morscher instrumentation is somewhat delicate and a brace is recommended for about 3–4 months. Stronger implants from most universal rod-screw-hook instrumentations may be used; the use of post-operative bracing is then optional [4].

Limitations of the Technique

The presence of a spina bifida precludes the use of this technique.

Butterfly-Plate Type Technique

The techniques described above carry the theoretical risk of shortening the posterior arch and creating mal-alignment of the L5-S1 articular facets. Louis recommended bone grafting of the pars defect followed by temporary fixation of the L5-S1 segment with a butterfly plate. This technique can be used in the case of associated spina bifida occulta and the mid-line defect is also grafted. Since the butterfly plate is not any more

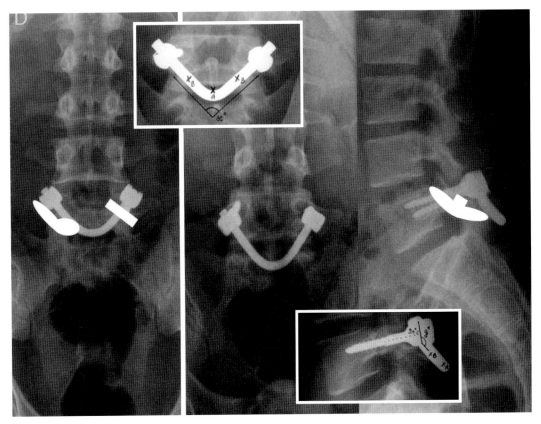

Fig. 8 Pars reconstruction with the V-rod technique which can be performed with any universal rod-screw instrumentation. Mono-axial screws must be used and adequate bending of the rod must be performed to obtain close fit on the posterior arch and immobilisation of the isthmic bone graft. Supplementary graft may be put on the lateral aspect of the facet down to the lamina. Care must be taken not to injure the nerve root in the foramen when fitting the bone graft in the decorticated defect

available, a temporary fixation of the L5-S1 segment may be performed with any instrumentation but taking care to stabilise the loose posterior arch, for instance, with supplementary wires [16].

After-Treatment

A light brace is recommended for 3 months. Secondary removal of the instrumentation is required, usually at 6 months, which is not an obligation with the other techniques.

Discussion

The usefulness and indication for surgical stabilisation in spondylolysis and spondylolisthesis have been questioned by many authors.

Indisputable data remain scarce; a recent study however showed that surgical treatment can improve pain status and allow for a more active lifestyle [19]. The role of instrumentation still remains a matter for debate, at least in posterolateral fusions [18]. On theoretical grounds its usefulness seems undisputable in severe unstable conditions, it also favours more comfortable postoperative conditions through the avoidance of cumbersome braces.

Length of Fusion

The length of the fusion is important to consider with regard to the activities the patient contemplates after the operation. It is reasonable to

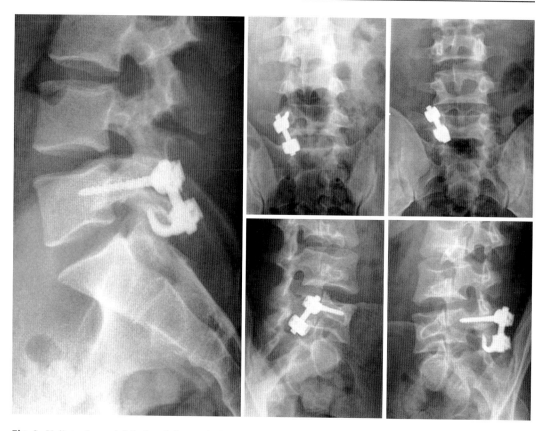

Fig. 9 Unilateral spondylolysis at L5 treated with a Morscher hook-type instrumentation using a custom made device constructed with a universal posterior instrumentation

assume that the longer the fusion, the more the residual free motion segments are at risk for junctional segment disease, a problem well-recognized in degenerative spine fusions [7]. Work and sport expectations of the patient must be considered to see if the length of fusion which appears necessary is compatible with such expectations. If the fusion involves only one motion segment (the lumbosacral or a floating lumbar segment), all types of work or sports may be allowed, as with a reconstruction procedure. A fusion length that does not exceed two levels is considered an acceptable procedure in most cases. However, strenuous work or sport should be discouraged. If more than two motion segments are involved with degenerative changes, decision- making becomes very difficult. Surgical treatment would not be advised except if unbearable pain is present and indisputably linked to the abnormalities. To evaluate the

respective role of spondylolysis, spondylolisthesis and degenerative disc disease, discograms of the different motion segments can be of help, not so much by the radiological image but more by the accompanying provocative pain test. In carefully selected cases and with a good understanding by the patient of a potentially less than optimal result, "compromise" reconstruction procedures or short fusions may be considered, as they may represent a more satisfactory surgical option than a fusion involving a great number of lumbar motion segments.

The Use of Interbody Fusion and Posterior Instrumentation

Posterior or anterior interbody fusion is recommended if anterior bone support is required: in heavy patients, when strenuous physical activity is anticipated, with normal or near-normal disc height, and after reduction of a spondylolisthesis since this creates an even greater, though temporary, unstable situation than pre-operatively.

Uninstrumented PLIF has been proposed but most authors have combined pedicle fixation and rods or plates with interbody fusion [8, 22, 25]. It is logical to perform posterior instrumentation in combination with posterior interbody fusion because facet joints must be largely resected to avoid root injury during the introduction of the bone blocks or cages; this leads to marked weakening of the posterior supportive structures. Since the posterior longitudinal ligament and the disc are also largely excised, the motion segment becomes highly unstable, and there is a real risk of secondary mobilisation of the grafts into the neural canal if the operated segment is not kept perfectly immobile until biological fusion is obtained. However the usefulness of internal fixation associated with interbody fusion to improve fusion rate and clinical results remains a matter for debate because few comparative studies have been reported. Though some authors have shown improved results using instrumentation, its use is mostly justified on theoretical grounds.

Summary: Suggested Choices

Spondylolysis Without Associated Disc Disease and Without Spondylolisthesis

A pars defect reconstruction is advised whenever possible to avoid loss of mobile segments and increased stress on adjacent structures. On occasions, when a L5 spondylolysis was present with an intact L5-S1 disc but with degenerative disc changes at L4-L5, isthmic reconstruction of L5 has been attempted to avoid L4-S1 fusion, hoping that in such cases, the L5 spondylolysis was the main cause of back pain. Results were satisfactory but inferior to those in the isolated spondylolysis cases. Such a therapeutic option should be considered with caution and only in carefully selected cases.

Spondylolysis With Associated Disc Disease and Grade 0 or 1 Spondylolisthesis

A posterolateral in situ fusion with or without posterior instrumentation is the classical procedure; reduction of a grade 1 slip is optional. If root entrapment is present, resection of the posterior arch should be performed and, if needed, removal of a herniated disc.

In heavy patients, if strenuous work is anticipated, if disc material has been removed or if the disc space is high, a PLIF with posterior instrumentation is a recommended option.

Spondylolysis With Associated Disc Disease and Grade 2 or 3 Spondylolisthesis

A PLIF with partial or total reduction of the slip and restoration of an adequate lumbosacral lordosis combined with posterior instrumentation is recommended. If the disc space is very narrow, if there is no significant loss of lumbosacral lordosis and if no neurological symptoms are present, a posterolateral in situ fusion with posterior instrumentation would be an option, especially in grade 2 slips.

Spondylolysis With Associated Disc Disease and Grade 4 Spondylolisthesis or Spondyloptosis

A posterior reduction with a PLIF, or a combined anterior and posterior approach with ALIF, posterolateral fusion and posterior instrumentation should be considered, remembering that correction of the lumbosacral kyphosis is more important than correction of the slip. If true spondyloptosis is present, the Gaines procedure may be an option. However, it must be stressed that in situ L4-L5-S1 posterior fusion remains a neurologically safe and valid option. It is recommended to obtain an adequate lordotic angle between the first upper free mobile segment and the sacrum at the end of the procedure to avoid junctional breakdown.

Lysis at the Level of the Pedicle

If a unilateral pedicle lysis associated with contralateral spondylolysis or if a bilateral pedicle lysis is present, the only option is an interbody fusion since a posterolateral bone graft will not stabilize the vertebral body and the motion segment; a PLIF would be our procedure of choice.

Dysplasic Spondylolisthesis

A thorough posterior mid-line and lateral decompression must be performed, keeping in mind that severe narrowing of the spinal canal may be present with severe compromise of the cauda equina. Further injury of the nerve roots must be avoided during the intra-canalicular use of surgical instruments. Reduction and fusion are performed according to the above-mentioned rules.

Degenerative Spondylolisthesis

In symptomatic degenerative spondylolisthesis, spinal stenosis is the rule and the main or the sole indication for surgical treatment is often the neurological deficit. In the event of primary severe instability or post-laminectomy instability, a posterolateral fusion, instrumented or not, a PLIF or a lateral retroperitoneal ALIF –since degenerative spondylolisthesis often occur at L4-L5- should be considered. The aim of the fusion in this specific indication is more often to avoid iatrogenic secondary increase of the spondylolisthesis than to treat back pain.

References

1. Berchuck M, Garfin S, Bauman T, Abitbol J. Complications of anterior intervertebral grafting. Clin Orthop. 1992;284:54–62.
2. Boos D, Marchesi D, Zuber K, Aebi M. Treatment of severe spondylolisthesis by reduction and pedicular fixation. Spine. 1993;18:1655–61.
3. Carragee EJ, Don AS, Hurwitz EL, Cuellar JM, Carrino JA, Hertzog R. Does discography cause accelerated progression of degenerative changes in the lumbar disc: a ten year matched cohort study. Spine. 2009;34:2338–45.
4. Debusscher F, Troussel S. Direct repair of defects in lumbar spondylolysis with a new pedicle screw hook fixation: clinical, functional and CT assessed study. Eur Spine J. 2007;16:1650–8.
5. Dubousset J. Treatment of spondylolysis and spondylolisthesis in children and adolescents. Clin Orthop. 1997;337:77–85.
6. Ekman P, Möller H, Hedlund R. The long term effect of posterolateral fusion in adult isthmic spondylolisthesis: a randomized controlled study. Spine J. 2005;5:36–44.
7. Ekman P, Möller H, Shalabi A, Yu YX, Hedlund R. A prospective randomised study on the long term effect of lumbar fusion on adjacent disc degeneration. Eur Spine J. 2009;18:1175–86.
8. Enker P, Steffee A. Interbody fusion and instrumentation. Clin Orthop. 1994;300:90–101.
9. Gaines RW. L5 vertebrectomy for the surgical treatment of spondyloptosis: thirty cases in 25 years. Spine. 2005;30:S66–70.
10. Gillet P, Petit M. Direct repair of spondylolysis without spondylolisthesis using a rod-screw construct and bone grafting of the pars defect. Spine. 1999;24:1252–6.
11. Grzegorzewski A, Kumar J. In situ posterolateral spine arthrodesis for grades III, IV and V spondylolisthesis in children and adolescents. J Ped Orthop. 2000;20:506–11.
12. Johnson R, McGuire E. Urogenital complications of anterior approaches to the lumbar spine. Clin Orthop. 1981;154:114–8.
13. Lamberg T, Remes V, Helenius I, Schlenzka D, Seitsalo S, Poussa M. Uninstrumented in situ fusion for high-grade childhood and adolescent isthmic spondylolisthesis: long-term outcome. J Bone Joint Surg Am. 2007;89:512–8.
14. Lin P. Posterior lumbar interbody fusion technique: complications and pitfalls. Clin Orthop. 1985;193:90–102.
15. Louis R. Fusion of the lumbar and sacral spine by internal fixation with screw plates. Clin Orthop. 1986;203:18–33.
16. Louis R. Reconstruction isthmique des spondylolyses par plaque vissée et greffes sans arthrodèse (Pars interarticularis reconstruction for spondylolysis by plate and screws with grafting without arthrodesis). Rev Chir Orthop. 1988;74:549–57.
17. Möller H, Sundin A, Hedlund R. Symptoms, signs and functional disability in adult spondylolisthesis. Spine. 2000;25:683–9.
18. Möller H, Hedlund R. Instrumented and noninstrumented posterolateral fusion in adult spondylolisthesis. Spine. 2000;25:1716–21.
19. Möller H, Hedlund R. Surgery versus conservative management in adult isthmic spondylolisthesis. Spine. 2000;25:1711–5.
20. Rajaraman V, Vingan R, Roth P, Keary R, Conclin L, Jacobs G. Visceral and vascular complications

resulting from anterior lumbar interbody fusion. J Neurosurg: Spine. 1999;91:60–4.

21. Remes V, Lamberg T, Tervahartiala P, Helenius I, Schlenzka D, Yrjönen T, Osterman K, Seitsalo S, Poussa M. Long-term outcome after posterolateral, anterior and circumferential fusion for high grade spondylolisthesis in children and adolescents: magnetic resonance imaging findings after average 17-year follow-up. Spine. 2006;31:2491–9.

22. Roca J, Ubierna M, Caceres E, Iborra M. One stage decompression and posterolateral and interbody fusion for severe spondylolisthesis. Spine. 1999;24:709–14.

23. Ruf M, Koch H, Melcher RP, Harms J. Anatomic reduction and monosegmental fusion in high-grade developmental spondylolisthesis. Spine. 2006;31:269–74.

24. Schlenzka D, Remes V, Helenius I, Lamberg T, Tervahartiala P, Yrjönen T, Tallroth K, Osterman K, Seitsalo S, Poussa M. Direct repair for treatment of symptomatic spondylolisis and low-grade isthmic spondylolisthesis in young patients: no benefit in comparison to segmental fusion after a mean follow-up of 14.8 years. Eur Spine J. 2006;15:1437–47.

25. Suk S, Lee C, Kim W, Lee J, Cho K, Kim H. Adding posterior lumbar interbody fusion to pedicle screw fixation and posterolateral fusion after decompression in spondylolytic spondylolisthesis. Spine. 1997;22:210–20.

26. Watkins R. Anterior lumbar interbody fusion, surgical complications. Clin Orthop. 1992;284:47–53.

Microdiscectomy

Trichy S. Rajagopal and Robert W. Marshall

Contents

Abstract

Microdiscectomy is the commonest spinal operation and the one that produces the most reliable outcomes from spinal surgery. The origins of the procedure are discussed from the time that disc herniations were mistaken for some form of chondral tumour to the proper identification of the pathology by Mixter and Barr in 1934. The natural history of disc herniations is outlined together with the clinical syndrome of back pain, sciatica and neurological dysfunction. As sciatica can resolve spontaneously with resorption of the herniated disc material a conservative approach to treatment is often possible with medications, perineural steroid injections and physiotherapy providing enough comfort to help the patient to manage the condition whilst buying time for the natural healing process to occur. There are absolute and relative indications for surgical intervention. Details of simple microdiscectomy techniques are shown, which are highly effective without the need for sophisticated instrumentation. Tips are given to improve level localisation and ensure that the procedure can be carried out safely through a small approach with minimal retaction. Complications and their avoidance are discussed.

T.S. Rajagopal • R.W. Marshall (✉)
Department of Orthopaedic Surgery, Royal Berkshire
Hospital, Reading, UK
e-mail: robmarshall100@hotmail.com

Keywords

Alternative treatment • Complications • Far lateral disc • History • Lumbar intervertebral

G. Bentley (ed.), *European Surgical Orthopaedics and Traumatology*,
DOI 10.1007/978-3-642-34746-7_89, © EFORT 2014

disc herniation • Microdiscectomy • Natural history • Post-discectomy back pain • Surgical technique

Historical Perspective

The surgical treatment of lumbar disc herniation has gradually evolved over the last century. Oppenheim and Krause were credited with the first report of surgery for lumbar disc herniation in 1909 [1]. The German surgeon, Fedor Krause, operated on a patient who had severe sciatic pain for many years, and presented with an acute cauda equina syndrome. The operation consisted of laminectomy from L2 to L4, a transdural approach to the intervertebral disc and removal of a small mass, which was erroneously believed to be a spinal tumour at that time. Similar reports were published by Steinke in 1918 [2], Adson in 1922 [3], Stookey in 1922 [4] and Dandy in 1929 [5]. In 1934 American Neurosurgeon, William Mixter and Orthopaedic Surgeon, Joseph Barr described 'the rupture of the intervertebral disc' in their historic paper where they reviewed the previous case reports and added 11 cases of their own. They described the pathophysiology of disc herniation and suggested surgical treatment by extensive laminectomy and removal of the ruptured disc by a transdural approach.

With the advent of the operating microscope, application of microsurgical techniques to the treatment of lumbar disc herniation became popular. In 1977, Yasargil from Switzerland and Caspar from Germany reported their experience in using the operating microscope for lumbar disc surgery [6, 7]. In the following year Williams who popularised microdiscectomy in the United States reported on a series of 532 patients [8]. Generally any new procedure is met with initial scepticism and microdiscectomy was no exception. However, the pioneering work of Caspar, Yasargil, Williams, Wilson and Goald confirmed the efficacy of microdiscectomy in reducing the incision size, soft-tissue disruption and morbidity. The vast majority of spinal surgeons now perform lumbar disc surgery with an operating microscope.

Natural History

The natural history of lumbar disc herniation is not well understood. However in the majority of patients this follows a favourable course. There are a few observational reports in the literature about the natural history of lumbar disc herniation especially in relation to surgical and non-surgical intervention. There are no conclusions about the duration or average course of the disease [9].

Usually the onset of sciatica correlates with the period of most intense pain. In the first 6 weeks the leg pain diminishes in about 70 % of the patients [10]. The residual pain remains more or less the same, or improves gradually for 1–3 months. Symptoms gradually subside after a few months and almost disappear in 70–90 % of the patients [11–13].

The natural course does not seem to be influenced by age or sex [14]. However co-existing spinal pathologies such as spinal canal stenosis or spondylolisthesis seem to influence it [13]. Smoking [15], psychosocial factors [14], repetitive heavy lifting [15], sedentary life style and obesity have been cited as important risk factors. The number of months required for spontaneous recovery from sciatica is variable and therefore uncertain.

There are a few randomised trials comparing surgical and non-surgical intervention for lumbar disc herniation [16–19]. These studies seem to indicate that the patients undergoing surgery achieve greater improvement than non-operatively treated patients in all primary and secondary outcome measures. However the relative benefit of surgery decreases over time.

Clinical Presentation

.... surgical treatment of spinal disorders produces the best results when clinical signs and symptoms are congruous and confirmed by carefully selected imaging studies, and when they have resulted in an unequivocal diagnosis amenable to surgical management...... (Frymoyer [81])

Most lumbar disc herniations occur between 30 and 50 years of age. Patients usually present with a history of low back pain which over a period of time radiates increasingly into one leg. Unilateral leg pain becomes the dominant complaint and radiates from buttock to calf (S1 nerve) or buttock to lateral aspect of the leg and ankle (L5 nerve) The cardinal symptoms of lumbar disc herniation include radicular leg pain, sensory loss and muscle weakness. These symptoms usually correspond to the sclerotome (dermatome and myotome) of the compressed nerve root [20]. It is important to ask specifically about symptoms of cauda equina syndrome which include severe or incapacitating back or leg pain, bilateral numbness or weakness, urinary retention or incontinence, faecal or flatulent incontinence and reduced perineal sensation. Other pertinent symptoms relating to lumbar disc herniation include radicular pain provoked by coughing and sneezing, paraesthesia in the affected dermatome and previous episodes of acute back pain. Children and adolescents with lumbar disc herniation usually present with back pain and hamstring tightness rather than characteristic sciatica.

Physical signs include alteration of the sagittal lumbar curve (flattening of the lordosis), a scoliotic list and painful restriction of spinal mobility especially forward flexion. A positive ipsilateral straight leg raising test with radiating pain below knee level seems to be associated with good sensitivity (72–97 %) but lower specificity (11–66 %) [20–22]. Restriction of the contralateral straight leg raise with cross-legged pain is more specific for a large disc herniation [23]. For the rarer syndromes of upper lumbar disc herniations affecting L2 to L4 nerve roots, the femoral nerve stretch test is often positive. Careful neurological examination including precise testing of dermatomal sensation and muscle power of the local extremities is of paramount importance. Neurological examination should also include testing of perianal sensation and the tone of the anal sphincter.

Investigations

Water-soluble contrast myelography and computerised axial tomography were of great value historically and are still used in cases where magnetic resonance imaging (M.R.I.) is contra-indicated, but the investigation of choice is undoubtedly M.R.I. However, M.R.I. is a very sensitive test and Boden et al. warned of the high incidence of lumbar disc abnormalities seen in asymptomatic individuals so the MRI will often reveal incidental pathology that has nothing to do with the patient's symptom complex [24].

Non-Surgical Treatment

The natural course of disc herniation involves a gradual process of spontaneous resolution, with respect to the symptoms and the volume of the disc herniation itself, justifying a conservative approach in the vast majority of patients. The goals of conservative management include [25]:

- Relief of pain
- Reduction of disability
- Restoration of pre-morbid level of spinal motion
- Regaining activities of daily living
- Return to work and leisure activities

Several factors have been associated with a favourable outcome in patients having non-operative treatment for lumbar disc herniation. These include [20]:

- Young age
- Small disc herniation
- Minor neurological compromise
- Mild disc degeneration
- Mild to moderate sciatica

The non-operative treatment options include

- A short period of bed rest – limited to under 3 days during the acutely painful phase
- Analgesia and anti-inflammatory medication
- Physiotherapy including exercise prescription, manual therapy and pain management
- Epidural and periradicular steroid injections

- Rehabilitation strategies including Cognitive Behavioural Therapy

During the acute period of sciatica, pain may be so severe that the patient cannot be mobilised. The primary goal at this stage is to control pain effectively and increase the physical activity. With regard to physiotherapy, specific supervised retraining of trunk stabilising muscles appears to be superior to general exercise programme in restoring spinal function [26, 27].

Epidural corticosteroid injections are still used in patients with radicular pain due to lumbar disc herniation but scientific evidence is lacking for the long-term effectiveness of this treatment [28]. Epidural corticosteroid injections were evaluated for the treatment of sciatica due to lumbar disc herniation in a randomised double-blind trial. The results showed that the epidural corticosteroid injections provided improvement in the leg pain and sensory deficit and reduced the need for analgesia in the first 6–12 weeks but after 3 months there was no difference between the patient groups. At 1 year there was no difference in the need for surgery [29]. Another prospective randomised study compared epidural corticosteroid injections and discectomy after 6 weeks of non-invasive treatment. Patients who underwent discectomy had better results (92–98 % effective) than patients in the epidural group (42–56 %).

Selective nerve root injections of corticosteroids have also been shown to be effective in the short term providing relief of symptoms [30]. A systematic review showed there is strong evidence that the selective nerve root block may relieve radicular nerve root pain in the short term [31]. The available literature is supportive of selective nerve root block as a diagnostic tool, especially in the presence of negative or inconclusive imaging studies.

Operative Treatment

The objectives of surgery in lumbar disc herniation include decompression of neural structures, removal of mechanical pressure and chemical irritation to the nerve root by excision of the disc material. Results of surgery for lumbar disc herniation are favourable when there is good correlation between clinical symptoms, physical signs and radiological evidence of disc herniation.

Even though there is controversy over the choice of treatment between non-operative and operative treatment, it is generally agreed that absolute indications for surgery include cauda equina syndrome and severe neurological deficit with weakness of MRC grade <3.

Relative indications include the presence of severe sciatica, persistent or progressive sensorimotor deficit, persistent radicular leg pain unresponsive to conservative treatment for 6–12 weeks and presence of concomitant spinal canal stenosis. The surgical techniques available in the treatment of lumbar disc herniation include:

- Microdiscectomy
- Open discectomy (laminotomy)
- Chemonucleolysis
- Minimally invasive techniques (Automated percutaneous discectomy and Endoscopic discectomy)

Microdiscectomy

Advantages of microdiscectomy include [32–34]:
- Smaller skin incision
- Reduced trauma to soft-tissues
- Improved illumination and magnification
- Provision of binocular vision
- Better haemostasis due to meticulous preparation of epidural veins
- Less post-operative pain
- Rapid mobilisation
- Reduced hospital stay
- Less scarring
  Disadvantages and potential pitfalls include:
- Limited exposure making it easier to operate at the wrong level
- Possibility of overlooking free fragments
- Inadequate decompression
- Learning curve involved in microsurgery
- Inadvertent neural or vascular injury

The indications for microdiscectomy are similar to those of open discectomy and both techniques are suitable for all forms of lumbar disc herniation.

Surgical Technique of Microdiscectomy

Check the Side and Level of the Disc Herniation and Correlate with MRI Findings

Pre-operatively the surgeon should check the scans and investigations, to confirm the level and side of the surgery (Fig. 1). It is also imperative to check the date of the MRI. Disc pathology evolves so if the scan is more than 6 months old the operative findings may be very different from those predicted by the scan. We recommend a new MRI if the original is greater than 6 months old. One should also make a careful assessment of segmentation anomalies of the vertebrae to avoid operating at the wrong level. Then the patient's signed consent to the procedure is checked.

Positioning of the Patient on the Operating Table

Microdiscectomy is usually performed under general anaesthesia. The procedure is most commonly performed in the prone position with flexion of the lumbar spine (Fig. 2).

Some prefer a lateral position with flexion of hips and knees to induce flexion of the lumbar spine (Fig. 3). Patient supports allow good flexion of the lumbar spine and do not interfere with the surgical approach (if placed over the upper lumbar spine and upper tibiae).

While most surgeons prefer the familiarity of the prone position, the lateral position allows optimal exposure of the interlaminar space and ligamentum flavum so that the fenestration into the canal can be made with minimal resection of the bony lamina. Another advantage is that the surgeon is seated upright, can see into the wound clearly with the microscope facing due laterally and can use instruments easily in this ergonomic posture (Fig. 4). The table can be tilted away from or towards the surgeon to improve the view as required.

Use of Fluoroscopy to Identify and Mark the Level of the Relevant Intervertebral Disc

Two of the uncommon but serious errors in disc surgery include operating at the wrong level and operating on the wrong side. When the wrong level is operated upon, it is usually the level above the intended one [34]. Therefore, it is imperative to have an on-table level check with an image intensifier. Besides ensuring that the correct level is treated, the x-ray guided marker will also allow optimal placement of the small skin incision (Figs. 5 and 6).

Skin Incision and Retraction of Soft Tissues

Once the disc level is identified radiologically the skin incision is made, bearing in mind that the disc space at L5-S1 is inter-laminar in location; at L4-5 the disc is partially covered by the L4 lamina and at proximal lumbar levels, the disc space is almost completely covered by the superior lamina [33]. The skin incision is carried down to the lumbar fascia, which is then incised close to the midline. When operating in the lateral position it is particularly important to ensure that no fascia or muscle is left medially, obscuring access to the medial portion of the interlaminar area. The fascial incision is usually longer than the skin incision to allow tension-free retraction of the paraspinal muscles. A Cobb elevator is used to reflect the muscle off the laminae and ligamentum flavum.

Once this soft tissue has been cleared a retractor is inserted. Retractors vary in design and sophistication. Some of the tubular systems are quite constraining and can interfere with access for instruments, so there are advantages to the simple but effective method of a curved Trethowan bone lever attached to a Charnley chain and weight (Fig. 7). The tip of the lever is inserted over the facet joint at the operated level and, once the weight and chain are attached, the soft tissues are tented laterally, giving the surgeon a triangular field of exposure that allows excellent

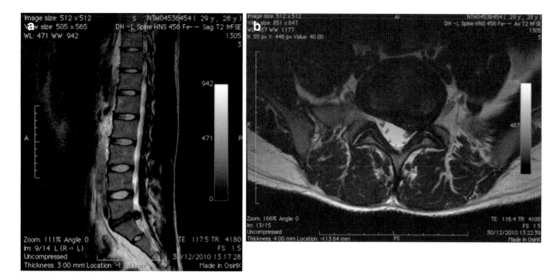

Fig. 1 Sagittal and axial T2 weighted images showing L5-S1 disc herniation

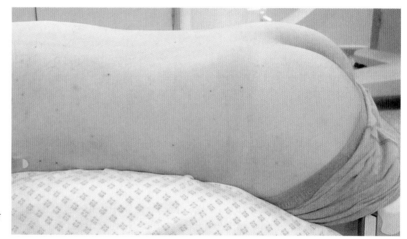

Fig. 2 Patient positioned prone on Wilson Frame with abdomen free of pressure. The frame is adjusted to allow flexion of the lumbar spine

visualisation of the anatomy with complete freedom to insert the operating instruments (Fig. 8).

Use of the Operating Microscope

The microscope is moved into position and focussed through the incision and onto the laminae and ligamentum flavum. If the patient is prone, the microscope is usually positioned on the far side and the surgeon stands on the near side (Fig. 9). If the lateral position is used, the

surgeon sits facing the exposed back and the microscope is placed on the opposite side and brought across the operating table.

Fenestration of the Ligamentum and Laminae

Any remaining muscle fibres are removed off the ligamentum flavum with pituitary rongeur forceps so that a clear view of the ligamentum and laminae is obtained (Fig. 10).

Fig. 3 Patient in the lateral position between hip supports to create flexion of hips, knees and lumbar spine

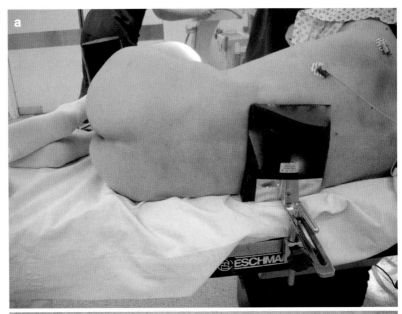

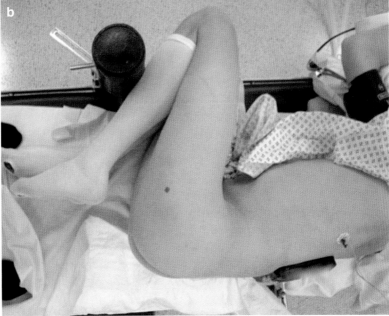

The ligamentum flavum is then incised quite medially and 2 or 3 mm inferior to the superior lamina. The medial entry point is chosen as there is more space here between the ligamentum and the nerve than out laterally where the nerve would be more vulnerable to injury (Fig. 11).

Once the entry point is made the ligamentum is cleared away, either by a flavectomy or by raising a medially based flaval flap, which has the theoretical benefit of less scarring and easier revision surgery if required. We prefer a flavectomy. Once an opening is made, this is carefully enlarged with Kerrison bone punches and a laminotomy is made to complete the fenestration. A cottonoid neuro-patty can be placed through the small fenestration to protect the nerves and dura while the opening is enlarged with Kerrison bone punches. It is important to

Fig. 4 With the patient in the lateral position the seated surgeon has a good ergonomic posture

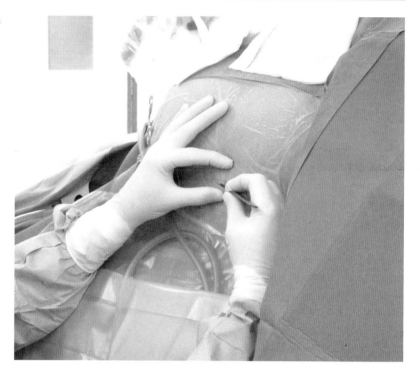

make a big enough window to see the nerve clearly and retract it. The window will be a square shape approximately 1 cm^2 but the opening may need to be larger in cases where the surgeon has to reach disc material that has become sequestrated higher or lower than the disc space itself (Figs. 12 and 13).

Location, Protection and Gentle Retraction of the Compressed Nerve Root

Lateral extension of the fenestration allows good exposure of the nerve root.

The nerve roots can be anomalous (conjoined) so there may be more than one nerve traversing the space. In order to avoid inadvertent damage to a second nerve, the Watson-Cheyne dissector is used as a probe to feel the pedicle and ensure that the lateral edge of the most lateral neural structure (usually the single traversing nerve) is visualized and carefully retracted. If the nerve cannot easily be retracted medially the fenestration is too small and more of the overhang should be removed inferolaterally, but also medially as

retained ligamentum can sometimes prevent medial retraction of the nerve.

Once the nerve root is adequately exposed the anterior epidural space is then prepared for discectomy. We recommend the use of two neuro-patties placed into the lateral recess, one packed superior to the nerve, and the other placed inferiorly to act as a gentle nerve retractor. These neuro-patties protect the nerve and dura mater, pack away the epidural veins and tamponade any bleeding (Fig. 14a).

Metal nerve root retractors can be used, but we prefer to avoid this unnecessary trauma to the nerve. In the case of large disc herniations, the nerve root is carefully mobilised over the protruding disc to ensure that the disc fragments are not removed through the axilla of the nerve root.

Intervertebral Disc Incision and Discectomy

The posterior annulus of the intervertebral disc may have been perforated by the herniating nucleus pulposus, extruding into the epidural

Fig. 5 Lateral imaging with a metal marker shown in the prone and lateral positions

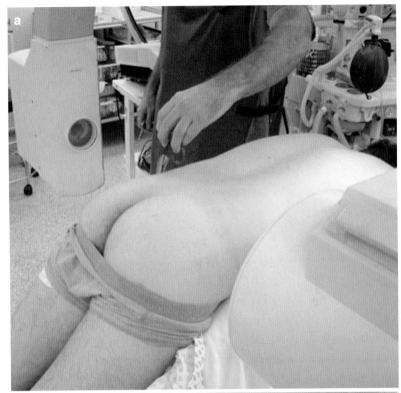

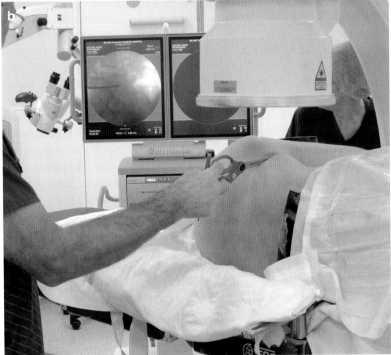

Fig. 6 The level of the
posterior edge of the disc
space is marked on the skin

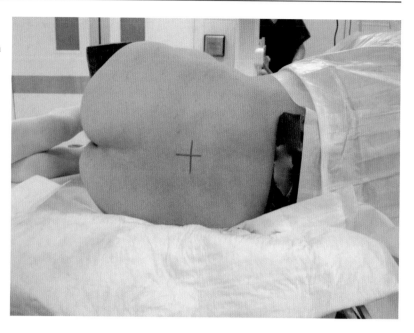

space, in which case the opening can be stretched with the jaws of the pituitary rongeur forceps and the space entered by removing degenerate disc material, but if the disc is bulging and not perforated it will be necessary to incise the annulus and then enter the disc space to remove the loose and degenerate nucleus pulposus (Fig. 14b).

Fine tipped, straight and angled pituitary forceps are used to remove loose fragments of nucleus pulposus from the disc space (Fig. 15).

How much to remove is the vexed question. Some favour minimal trauma to the disc, but evidence for worsening of disc function and back pain is lacking, so a careful but thorough disc clearance does not seem to have a worse long-term prognosis than the natural history of the disease. We favour removal of all loose fragments of nucleus pulposus, but do not advocate curettage of the end plates of the vertebrae. Once the disc space has been emptied with the pituitary rongeur forceps it can be washed out by flushing saline from a syringe with a blunt metal cannula placed through the opening in the annulus. This has the dual effect of flushing out any remaining small disc fragments and diluting the effects of the inflammatory chemicals that are contained within the nucleus pulposus.

It is important at this stage to ensure that the nerve root is adequately decompressed and that there are no free fragments of disc lying sequestrated in the spinal canal.

It must be remembered that the left common iliac artery runs across the anterior aspect of the L4-5 intervertebral disc and care should be taken while using the pituitary rongeurs to avoid a vascular injury, especially at this level. On occasions a pre-existing defect may be present in the anterior annulus and this provides a significant hazard [34]. Haemostasis of the epidural venous bleeding is achieved by bipolar diathermy or packing with neuro-patties. There is no convincing evidence in the literature regarding the efficacy of materials to reduce epidural fibrosis after disc surgery. Their routine use is not recommended.

We use intrathecal injection of morphine (300 μg) and 2 ml of 0.125 % bupivacaine for post-operative analgesia. This analgesic cocktail is injected into the cerebrospinal fluid through a very fine (25 gauge) spinal needle. A small piece of calcium alginate can be left overlying the fenestration to promote haemostasis, but beware – some haemostatic materials such as oxidised cellulose have been blamed for post-operative cauda equina syndrome.

Fig. 7 Curved Trethowan bone lever with its insertion and attachment to a Charnley weight (Prone position). The surgeon stands on the side of the disc pathology

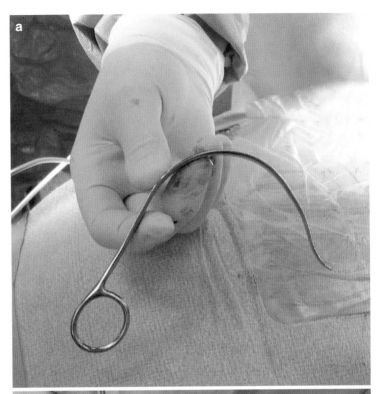

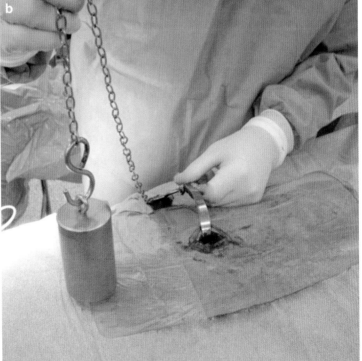

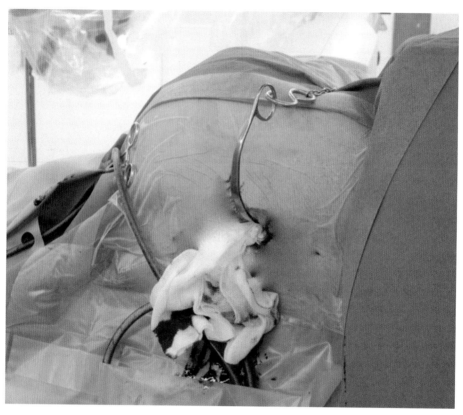

Fig. 8 In the lateral position the affected side is placed uppermost and the Trethowan bone lever is attached to the weight which is suspended over the far side of the operating table

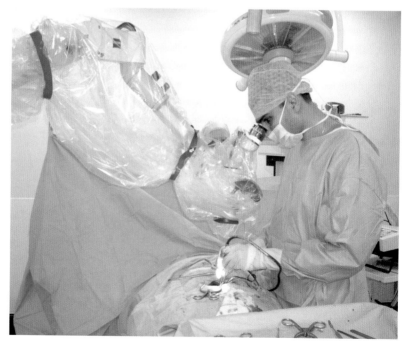

Fig. 9 Prone position – surgeon nearside and microscope across from the far side

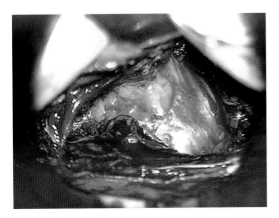

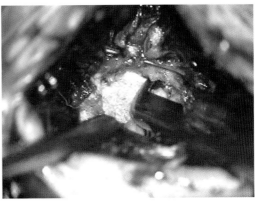

Fig. 10 Operating microscope view of ligamentum flavum. The white line shows the position of the lamina

Fig. 12 Kerrison bone punches are used to create a laminotomy. A neuro-patty has been placed through the small opening for safety

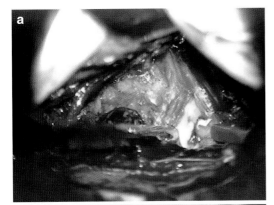

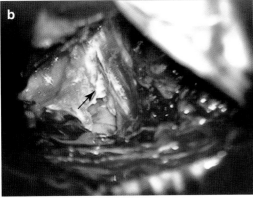

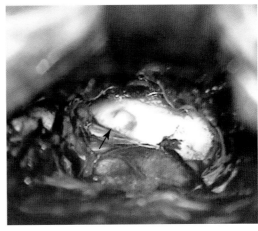

Fig. 13 Intervertebral disc is exposed as the nerve (*arrowed*) is retracted

The wound is closed in layers of absorbable suture material.

Post-Operative Care

Post-operatively the patients can be mobilised on recovery from anaesthesia and discharged home within 2 days. There are reports in the literature confirming the safety of day case microdiscectomy, but this is not widely practised.

Fig. 11 (**a**) Incision of ligamentum flavum close to midline and just beneath the upper lamina. (**b**) The epidural fat can be seen through the flaval opening (*arrowed*)

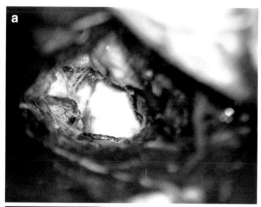

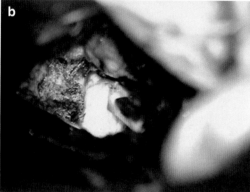

Fig. 14 (**a**) Disc pathology isolated by using neuro-patties as retractors. (**b**) Transverse incision of the bulging annulus of the disc

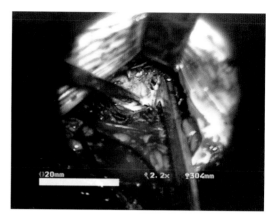

Fig. 15 Pituitary rongeur forceps teasing disc material through the annular opening

The patients are encouraged to make a graduated return to normal activities with return to sedentary work by 4 weeks and to manual work after 6 weeks. There is no rational basis for imposing or lifting restrictions after lumbar disc surgery [35].

Open Discectomy

Open discectomy is generally preferred in the following circumstances:

- Concomitant spinal stenosis
- Revision surgery
- Multi-segmental disease

Open discectomy involves unilateral laminotomy to create an inter-laminar window followed by flavectomy to expose the dura and the nerve root. While the procedure is similar to microdiscectomy, more lamina may be removed to improve the exposure; however this may not be always needed. A magnifying loupe and

headlight are used by some surgeons to improve the visibility. The ideal magnification would be 3–4 times and the optimal focal length (working distance) would be around 400 mm.

In cases of cauda equina syndrome, some surgeons employ a more extensive exposure with either a central approach removing the spinous process and laminae or a bilateral approach with a hemilaminectomy either side of the spinous process.

Review of early literature comparing open discectomy and microdiscectomy based on retrospective case series seems to indicate that microdiscectomy could provide a better outcome [36–38]. These reports also showed reduced blood loss, faster rehabilitation and improved functional results with microdiscectomy. In contrast, prospective clinical trials (some randomised) have failed to show any significant differences between the two surgical procedures including pre and post-operative pain scores, operative time, blood loss and functional outcome [39–42]. However one trial showed reduced hospital stay following microdiscectomy (mean – 2 days) compared to open discectomy (mean–7 days) [41].

Far Lateral Disc Herniation

The term 'far lateral' applies to a lumbar disc herniation which compresses the nerve root exiting at the same level, irrespective of its location. This is in contrast to classic posterolateral disc compression which affects the nerve root leaving at the level below. For example an L4-5 far lateral disc herniation would result in compression of the L4 nerve root as opposed to a posterolateral disc herniation which would result in L5 nerve root compression. The site of herniation is usually lateral to the pedicle in the region of the intervertebral foramen (Fig. 16). Failure to recognise its presence has often been responsible for a poor outcome and persistent sciatica after operation. Far lateral disc herniations account for between 6 % and 10 % of all lumbar disc herniations (Fig. 17) [43].

Foraminal steroid injections are often effective, but surgical treatment of a far lateral disc herniation involves a muscle splitting, inter-transverse approach through a paramedian incision. The alternative is an inter-laminar approach, but full exposure of the nerve root requires total resection of the facet joint and this may prejudice the subsequent stability of the spine. The advantages of the inter-transverse approach include direct access to the herniated disc, minimal soft tissue traumatisation and minimal resection of bone. The bony resection is usually limited to hypertrophied facets and to the L5-S1 level. The medial branch of the posterior primary ramus of the spinal nerve is a useful anatomical landmark in this approach, allowing early identification of the spinal nerve and dorsal root ganglion and safe dissection of the inter-transverse space. The use of an operating microscope helps to identify the posterior primary ramus of the spinal nerve where it passes through the medial aspect of the inter-transverse membrane, before distributing its branches to the dorsal musculature.

O'Hara and Marshall reported their results using the muscle splitting, inter-transverse approach, which were excellent in 60 %, good in 30 %, no improvement in 5 % and poor in 5 % [43]. Similar results have also been reported by other authors in the literature [44, 45].

Modern designs of retractors for minimally invasive surgery such as the "In-sight retractor" of Synthes or the "Quadrant retractors" of Medtronic allow very good access for microscopic far lateral discectomy as follows:

With the patient prone a guide wire is passed obliquely from a paramedian position 5 cm from the midline and is directed into the intertransverse area under fluoroscopy. A series of dilators are passed over the guide wire until the retractors can be inserted into the small incision (Fig. 18a, b) and expanded (Fig. 19).

The retractors expose the intertransverse space and allow the surgeon to work under the lateral aspect of the pars interarticularis and superior facet joint so that the intertranverse muscle and aponeurosis can be reflected. This reveals the much deeper position of the exiting nerve and its dorsal root ganglion. Venous bleeding is frequently encountered during this dissection and should be controlled by packing with neuropatties and bipolar diathermy. Gentle lateral retraction of the nerve exposes the intervertebral disc herniation. By working in the axilla of the nerve the disc space can be opened and emptied of the herniating disc material. Because one is starting very laterally, it is important to direct the pituitary rongeur forceps medially when clearing the disc (Fig. 20).

Chemonucleolysis

Chemonucleolysis involves intra-discal injection of a proteolytic enzyme, usually chymopapain to dissolve the nucleus pulposus of the intervertebral disc. Chymopapain is a sulfhydryl protease obtained from the purified extract of the papaya fruit [46]. Smith et al. in 1963 first reported the use of chymopapain injection into the intervertebral disc to treat intervertebral disc prolapse [47]. Since then it has been the subject of a number of randomised controlled trials.

In general the indications for chemonucleolysis are the same as those for discectomy for intervertebral disc prolapse. McCulloch published his criteria for selection of patients in 1977 [48]. These included unilateral leg pain, specific neurological symptoms involving a single nerve, limitation of straight leg raise with leg pain, neurological signs and a positive myelogram, which can be reasonably substituted by magnetic resonance imaging confirmation of disc prolapse. If the patient has three or more of these criteria then he or she should be considered

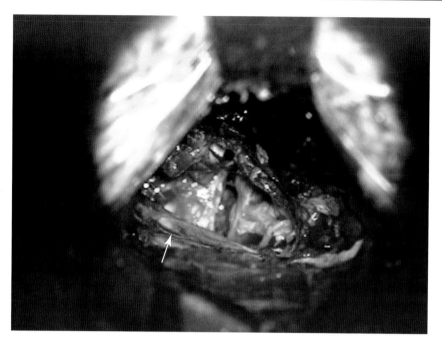

Fig. 16 Emptied disc space and decompressed nerve root (*white arrow*)

as a candidate for chemonucleolysis. The contraindications include sequestrated discs, hard discs, lateral recess or foraminal stenosis, fibrosis due to previous surgery, cauda equina syndrome and known chymopapain or papaya allergy.

A posterolateral approach is generally used under local anaesthesia with sedation or general anaesthesia. A transdural approach is strongly contraindicated. It is generally advisable to use discography to confirm the position of the needle before injecting the enzyme. The dosage has reduced from about 3,000–4,000 units down to 500–2,000 units. The disc height reduces by about one fourth after chymopapain injection. It may gradually recover over a period of 1 year.

Potentially serious complications are rare. Norby et al. examined the safety of chemonucleolysis reviewing the adverse effects reported in the United States between 1982 and 1991 [49]. There were seven reported cases of fatal anaphylaxis in 135,000 patients (0.0005 %); other complications included infection (24 patients), haemorrhage (32 patients), neurological complications (32 patients), the most serious

of which was transverse myelitis with paraplegia. Various other reports estimate that allergic reactions occur in 2–12 % of patients.

Chemonucleolysis is one of the most investigated interventions for the treatment of intervertebral disc prolapse. More than 20 randomised trials evaluated chemonucleolysis.

Gibson and Waddell published a Cochrane review, which included a systematic review of the chemonucleolysis [50]. Trials which compared chemonucleolysis and placebo injection consistently reported that chemonucleolysis was superior to placebo treatment [51–53]. Another trial found collagenase chemonucleolysis superior to placebo [54]. Trials comparing chemonucleolysis against either open surgery or microdiscectomy showed slightly less efficacy for chemonucleolysis compared to surgery in the short term, but fewer complications and long-term recurrences. The long-term results were comparable [55–57]. The results of surgery after failed chemonucleolysis are similar to those obtained after primary discectomy, indicating that failure to respond to chemonucleolysis does not compromise surgical discectomy. In spite of the favourable evidence for chemonucleolysis,

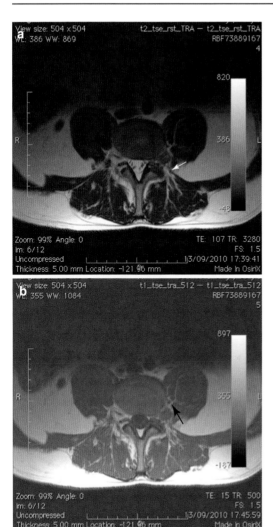

Fig. 17 M.R.I. T2 and T1 Axial images show a left sided, far lateral disc prolapse (*arrowed*) causing L4 nerve (*exiting*) compression

been investigated most include automated percutaneous lumbar discectomy and endoscopic discectomy.

Automated Percutaneous Lumbar Discectomy (APLD)

Automated Percutaneous Lumbar Discectomy is a procedure that involves percutaneous insertion of a cannula under fluoroscopic guidance using a posterolateral approach. A probe is then connected to an automated cutting and aspiration device, which is introduced through the cannula [58]. The disc is aspirated until no more nuclear material can be obtained. The procedure is performed under local anaesthesia with or without sedation. The indication for the procedure primarily involves patients with contained disc herniations or protrusions.

One randomised controlled trial compared automated percutaneous lumbar discectomy with microdiscectomy. This reported 29 % successful outcome with automated percutaneous lumbar discectomy compared with 80 % of patients with microdiscectomy, and the difference was statistically significant [59]. Another randomised controlled trial compared automated percutaneous lumbar discectomy with chemonucleolysis and found that significantly more patients had successful results after chemonucleolysis [60]. Grevitt et al. reported on 137 patients who had automated percutaneous lumbar discectomy. 52 % of patients had excellent or good outcome after a mean follow-up of 55 months [61]. However, with the advent of endoscopic procedures the popularity of automated percutaneous lumbar discectomy has declined.

Endoscopic Discectomy

Percutaneous endoscopic removal of the herniated lumbar disc can be performed through a midline posterior, posterolateral or transforaminal approach. Kambin is credited with the description of the first discoscopic view of a herniated disc, even though percutaneous techniques of disc removal have been described earlier. The development of appropriate surgical instrumentation and the description of a "triangular working zone" by Kambin were the basis for all further progress.

its use has been thwarted by worldwide shortage of the enzyme due to lack of production. There is a real opportunity for someone to resume manufacture and marketing of this useful agent.

Minimally Invasive Techniques

The perceived advantages of percutaneous techniques over those of open procedures include less damage to the soft tissues, shorter hospital stay and less scar formation. There are a number of techniques described but the ones that have

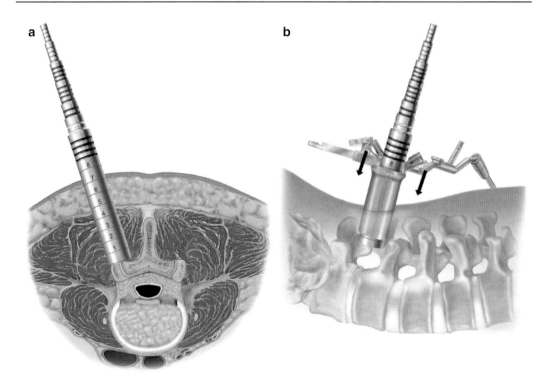

Fig. 18 (**a**) Serial dilators over a guide-wire. (**b**) Quadrant retractors inserted (Pictures with permission of Medtronic)

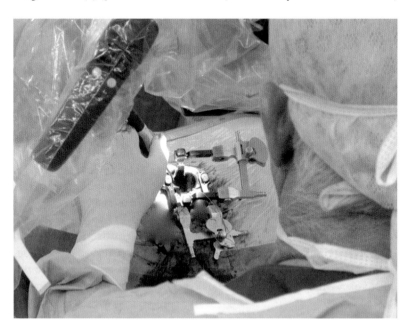

Fig. 19 Medtronic's "Quadrant" retractors in place (dilators removed)

He reported a favourable outcome in 87 % of the cases; a similar rate to open disc surgery [62]. Yeung reported on a series of 307 patients who underwent percutaneous endoscopic discectomy for lumbar disc herniation. 90.7 % of the patients were satisfied at the end of 1 year and he concluded that percutaneous endoscopic discectomy has comparable results to open microdiscectomy [63].

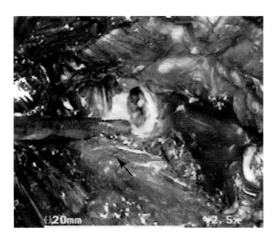

Fig. 20 Operating microscope view of emptied disc space in the axilla of the exiting nerve (*arrowed*) which is being retracted by the sucker tip. The broken white line indicates the overhanging bone of the pars interarticularis and superior facet joint

Ruetten et al. reported on a prospective series of 463 patients who underwent full endoscopic uniportal transforaminal approach using an extreme lateral access for lumbar disc herniation. They reported that 81 % of their patients had complete resolution of leg pain [64].

There has been a recent surge in the literature on endoscopic discectomy as a result of improvement in endoscopic techniques. The reported outcomes with endoscopic discectomy continue to improve and are equal to those of microdiscectomy. The advantages of endoscopic discectomy include outpatient surgery, less surgical trauma and early functional recovery. However, although the 2 year results were similar for the three groups in a prospective, randomized trial of 240 patients comparing endoscopic discectomy with microdiscectomy and conventional discectomy, the costs and complications were higher in the endoscopic group. Complications included dural tears, nerve injury and recurrent disc herniation [65].

Complications

Complications following microdiscectomy are generally rare but some can be serious and devastating. Complications can be classified as intra-operative, early or late complications. Intra-operative complications include those complications which are evident during the surgery or become apparent immediately afterwards. These include epidural bleeding, dural tears, nerve root injury and vascular injury.

Epidural Bleeding

Epidural venous bleeding may be minimised by positioning the patient prone with the abdomen hanging freely. Experienced surgeons feel that epidural venous bleeding usually stops when the disc fragment is removed and after the wound closure. Tamponading the epidural veins with neuro-patties is useful to reduce the bleeding; however the use of bipolar diathermy may be required to stop the bleeding. Excessive use of diathermy may be a cause of epidural fibrosis and post discectomy syndrome.

Dural Tears

Inadvertent injury to the dura with loss of cerebrospinal fluid can occur during any form of spinal surgery. When a dural tear is recognised it is important to localise and repair the defect. Usually it is necessary to enlarge the fenestration laminotomy to carry out a repair. Small punctures can be left alone. If dural repair is performed we prefer 6–0 Prolene sutures and a small fat graft from the subcutaneous tissue can be tied over the suture line to seal the leak. If light-headedness and headache result, the patient may need to be kept in bed for 24–48 h until the cerebrospinal fluid volume increases.

Various reports in the literature quote an incidence of 0.8–7.3 % of dural tears during discectomy. Consequences of dural tear include headache, cerebrospinal fluid fistula and post-operative pseudomeningocele which may require re-exploration and repair of the defect.

Nerve Root Injury

The incidence of nerve root injury during surgery has been estimated to be 0.2–1 %. Poor visibility, perineural adhesions, and congenital abnormalities of the nerve roots such as conjoined nerve roots are the most common causes of nerve root injury. Good lighting and visibility during microdiscectomy help to reduce the incidence of this complication.

Vascular Injury

Vascular injury is fortunately rare, but can be devastating. This happens when pituitary rongeurs penetrate the anterior annulus fibrosis inadvertently during removal of the disc. The most common vessel involved is the left common iliac artery during right-sided L4-5 microdiscectomy. The reported incidence of these injuries is in the order of 0.003 %. Some reports indicate that the mortality is about 50 %. Any dramatic unexplained fall in blood pressure and excessive haemorrhage from the disc should alert one to the possibility of unrecognised vascular injury. This should be treated with rapid wound closure, intravenous fluids and blood, and repositioning the patient for a trans-abdominal approach for a vascular repair. Some surgeons prefer to use rongeurs that have stops to prevent deeper insertion.

Wrong Level Surgery

Wrong level exploration is most likely to occur at L4-5 level or higher and is usually rare at L5-S1. It is therefore important to use x-ray confirmation pre-operatively and well as intra-operatively.

Infection

The reported rate of infection varies between 0.2 % and 1 %. Treatment of disc space infection involves aspiration of the disc to identify the organism and the use of appropriate antibiotics for a minimum of 6 weeks, or until the infection markers return to normal. In spite of successful treatment of infection, some patients end up with chronic back pain and require a surgical fusion later.

Persistent Leg Pain

Presence of persistent or residual leg pain after discectomy is uncommon; however if present one should look for a specific cause. Frequent causes of persistent sciatica after discectomy include:

- Wrong level surgery
- Residual disc fragment
- Nerve root injury
- Early recurrent disc herniation
- Unrecognised additional nerve root compression
- Inadequate decompression of concomitant spinal stenosis
- Extra-foraminal nerve compression
- Intrinsic neuropathy such as diabetes

If present, persistent sciatica should be investigated with further magnetic resonance imaging.

Cauda Equina Syndrome

Cauda equina syndrome can result from an epidural haematoma or from intra-operative nerve injury. If there is a concern about cauda equina injury, a thorough neurological examination should be carried out and immediate imaging performed. If a compressive lesion is identified immediate surgical decompression is indicated.

Recurrent Disc Herniation

The incidence of recurrent disc herniation after primary discectomy has been reported as 5–11 % [66–68]. Gaston and Marshall showed that survival analysis is a better method of estimating the recurrence [69]. In their series the rate continued to rise steadily with each year of follow-up; it was only 1.1 % at 1 year, 5.0 % at 5 years and 7.9 % at 8 years. No recurrences occurred after 8 years from the primary operation. The majority of recurrences occurred on the same side as previous discectomy with relatively few occurring on the contralateral side.

As in primary disc herniation, the extent of clinical symptoms is a critical determinant in deciding on surgical management. Persistent radicular pain in the distribution consistent with previously operated level, severely reduced walking ability, straight leg raising test positive at less than 30° and pain-free interval of at least a few months after prior discectomy increase the likelihood of true recurrent disc herniation [70].

Magnetic resonance imaging with intravenous gadolinium contrast is the imaging modality of choice to study recurrent disc herniation by comparing T_1-weighted images before and after injection of the contrast. Gadolinium enhances the vascularised soft tissue structures including epidural fibrosis and scar formation, which can be readily distinguished from a recurrent disc herniation that does not enhance. At the same time, conventional T_2 weighted sequences give information on disc herniation at another level, associated spinal stenosis or any other cause of sciatica.

The indications for surgery are similar to those for primary disc herniation. However it has been stated that a relatively smaller degree of disc herniation could cause severe symptoms in the presence of epidural fibrosis which might limit the mobility of the affected nerve root. The presence of epidural fibrosis on its own is not an indication for surgery, as the results of outcome for surgery on epidural fibrosis are not rewarding [71].

In terms of surgical technique, a wider surgical exposure is required compared to primary discectomy. A wider laminotomy or even a partial laminectomy may be required to enter the spinal canal through virgin territory and then work a way through the scar tissue. Using a high speed burr to thin the lateral aspect of the lamina can be a good way of approaching the lateral aspect of the nerve and then freeing the nerve in its bed of scar tissue and retracting it medially to expose the recurrent disc hernia. The use of an operating microscope assists this soft tissue dissection. Any lateral recess stenosis should be addressed by undercutting of the facet joint (partial medial facetectomy). The chance of a successful outcome is good after recurrent discectomy, provided that the patient has had a pain-free period of several months or years before recurrence. Review of literature suggests that the improvement of radicular leg pain, back pain and functional outcome is almost similar to that of primary discectomy [66, 71–73] The risk of yet another disc herniation at the same level is not clearly known [73, 74].

Post-Discectomy Back Pain: Spinal Fusion and Disc Replacement

Microdiscectomy and open discectomy are effective in relieving radicular leg pain, but a significant proportion of patients continue to have axial back pain. The term post-discectomy syndrome is loosely used, but this condition is not clearly defined. Review of the literature suggests that the incidence of recurrent or persistent back or leg pain varies from 7 % to 37 % depending on the criteria used [75]. Management of this group of patients is quite complex requiring a multidisciplinary approach including physiotherapists, psychologists and pain management services.

In considering surgical management, it is important to take into account a number of factors. It is also important to identify the pain generator, i.e. if the pain is arising from the degenerative disc or the facet joints, presence or absence of any neural compression and perineural or epidural fibrosis. The presence or absence of segmental instability also influences the choice of surgical treatment.

Non-operative treatment involves an aggressive regimen of physiotherapy and aerobic conditioning, involvement of pain specialists and cognitive behavioural therapy. Before considering any surgical intervention it is important to exclude infection by blood tests including full blood count, erythrocyte sedimentation rate and C-reactive protein. Standing flexion and extension lateral radiographs are taken to assess the presence or absence of segmental instability. The presence of any significant translation or angulation in the motion segment indicates instability.

The choice of surgical treatment is usually between fusion and disc replacement. There are very few reports in the literature that address the problem of post-discectomy back pain. The sparse literature indicates that successful functional outcome does not depend on the choice of surgical technique or the type of fusion [76, 77]. Various techniques such as anterior, posterior and trans-foraminal lumbar interbody fusion and posterolateral fusion have been successful in achieving a good outcome. Chitnavis et al. have reported on the use of posterior lumbar interbody fusion and were able to achieve 92 % improvement and 95 % radiological fusion rate [78]. Similar results have been reported with trans-foraminal [79] and anterior lumbar interbody fusion [80].

With regard to lumbar disc replacement, in one series 36 % of patients undergoing lumbar disc replacement had post-discectomy pain. The study confirmed satisfactory clinical results. However a slightly higher rate of complications was noted at L4-5 when compared to the L5-S1 level [76].

References

1. Oppenheim H, Krause F. Uber Einklemmung bzw. Strangulation der cauda equina. Dtsch Med Wochenschr. 1909;35:697–700.
2. Steinke CR. Spinal tumours: statistics on a series of 330 collected cases. J Nerv Ment Dis. 1918;47: 418–26.
3. Adson AW, Ott WO. Results of the removal of tumours of spinal cord. Arch Neurol Psychiatr (Chicago). 1922;8:520–38.
4. Stookey B. Compression of the spinal cord due to ventral extradural chordomas: diagnosis and surgical treatment. Arch Neurol Psychiatr (Chicago). 1928;20:275–91.
5. Dandy WE. Loose cartilage from intervertebral disk simulating tumour of spinal cord. Arch Surg (Chicago). 1929;19:660–72.
6. Yasargil MG. Microsurgical operation of herniated lumbar disc. In: Wullenweber R, Brock M, Hamer J, et al., editors. Advances in neurosurgery. Berlin/Heidelberg/New York: Springer; 1977. p. 81–2.
7. Caspar W. A new surgical procedure for lumbar disc herniation causing less tissue damage through a microsurgical approach. In: Wullenweber R, Brock M, Hamer J, et al., editors. Advances in neurosurgery. Berlin/Heidelberg/New York: Springer; 1977. p. 74–7.
8. Williams RW. Microlumbar discectomy: a conservative surgical approach to the virgin herniated lumbar disc. Spine (Phila Pa 1976). 1978;3(2):175–82.
9. Bendix T. Disc herniation: definition and types. In: Hea H, editor. The lumbar spine. Philadelphia: Lippincott Williams & Wilkins; 2004. p. 399–406.
10. Vroomen PC, de Krom MC, Knottnerus JA. Predicting the outcome of sciatica at short-term follow-up. Br J Gen Pract. 2002;52(475):119–23.
11. Weber H, Holme I, Amlie E. The natural course of acute sciatica with nerve root symptoms in a double-blind placebo-controlled trial evaluating the effect of piroxicam. Spine (Phila Pa 1976). 1993;18(11):1433–8.
12. Weber H. The natural course of disc herniation. Acta Orthop Scand Suppl. 1993;251:19–20.
13. Saal JA, Saal JS, Herzog RJ. The natural history of lumbar intervertebral disc extrusions treated nonoperatively. Spine (Phila Pa 1976). 1990;15(7): 683–6.
14. Rasmussen C. Lumbar disc herniation: social and demographic factors determining duration of disease. Eur Spine J. 1996;5(4):225–8.
15. Frymoyer JW, Pope MH, Clements JH, Wilder DG, MacPherson B, Ashikaga T. Risk factors in low-back pain. An epidemiological survey. J Bone Joint Surg Am. 1983;65(2):213–8.
16. Weber H. Lumbar disc herniation. A controlled, prospective study with ten years of observation. Spine (Phila Pa 1976). 1983;8(2):131–40.
17. Atlas SJ, Keller RB, Wu YA, Deyo RA, Singer DE. Long-term outcomes of surgical and nonsurgical management of sciatica secondary to a lumbar disc herniation: 10 year results from the maine lumbar spine study. Spine (Phila Pa 1976). 2005;30(8): 927–35.
18. Weinstein JN, Lurie JD, Tosteson TD, Tosteson AN, Blood EA, Abdu WA, et al. Surgical versus nonoperative treatment for lumbar disc herniation: four-year results for the Spine Patient Outcomes Research Trial (SPORT). Spine (Phila Pa 1976). 2008;33(25):2789–800.
19. Peul WC, van den Hout WB, Brand R, Thomeer RT, Koes BW. Prolonged conservative care versus early surgery in patients with sciatica caused by lumbar disc herniation: two year results of a randomised controlled trial. BMJ. 2008;336(7657):1355–8.
20. Leonardi M, Noos N. Disc herniation and radiculopathy. In: Boos N, Abei M, editors. Spinal disorders. Berlin/Heidelberg: Springer; 2008. p. 481–507.
21. Vroomen PC, de Krom MC, Knottnerus JA. Consistency of history taking and physical examination in patients with suspected lumbar nerve root involvement. Spine (Phila Pa 1976). 2000;25(1):91–6; discussion 97.
22. Hunt DG, Zuberbier OA, Kozlowski AJ, Robinson J, Berkowitz J, Schultz IZ, et al. Reliability of the lumbar flexion, lumbar extension, and passive straight leg raise test in normal populations embedded within a complete physical examination. Spine (Phila Pa 1976). 2001;26(24):2714–8.
23. Suk KS, Lee HM, Moon SH, Kim NH. Lumbosacral scoliotic list by lumbar disc herniation. Spine (Phila Pa 1976). 2001;26(6):667–71.
24. Boden SD, Davis DO, Dina TS, Patronas NJ, Wiesel SW. Abnormal magnetic-resonance scans of the lumbar spine in asymptomatic subjects. A prospectiive investigation. J Bone Joint Surg Am. 1990;72(3): 403–8.
25. Singer KP, Fazey PJ. Disc herniation: non-operative treatment. In: Hea H, editor. The lumbar spine. Philadelphia: Lippincott Williams & Wilkins; 2004. p. 427–36.
26. O'Sullivan PB, Phyty GD, Twomey LT, Allison GT. Evaluation of specific stabilizing exercise in the treatment of chronic low back pain with radiologic diagnosis of spondylolysis or spondylolisthesis. Spine (Phila Pa 1976). 1997;22(24):2959–67.

27. Danneels LA, Vanderstraeten GG, Cambier DC, Witvrouw EE, Bourgois J, Dankaerts W, et al. Effects of three different training modalities on the cross sectional area of the lumbar multifidus muscle in patients with chronic low back pain. Br J Sports Med. 2001;35(3):186–91.

28. Leonardi M, Pfirrmann CW, Boos N. Injection studies in spinal disorders. Clin Orthop Relat Res. 2006;443:168–82.

29. Carette S, Leclaire R, Marcoux S, Morin F, Blaise GA, St-Pierre A, et al. Epidural corticosteroid injections for sciatica due to herniated nucleus pulposus. N Engl J Med. 1997;336(23):1634–40.

30. Riew KD, Yin Y, Gilula L, Bridwell KH, Lenke LG, Lauryssen C, et al. The effect of nerve-root injections on the need for operative treatment of lumbar radicular pain. A prospective, randomized, controlled, double-blind study. J Bone Joint Surg Am. 2000;82-A(11): 1589–93.

31. Datta S, Everett CR, Trescot AM, Schultz DM, Adlaka R, Abdi S, et al. An updated systematic review of the diagnostic utility of selective nerve root blocks. Pain Physician. 2007;10(1):113–28.

32. Mayer HM. Principles of microsurgical discectomy in lumbar disc herniations. In: Mayer HM, editor. Minimally invasive spine surgery. 2nd ed. Berlin/Heidelberg/New York: Springer; 2006. p. 278–82.

33. Kraemer R, Wild A, Haak H, Herdmann J, Kraemer J. Microscopic lumbar discectomy. In: Hea H, editor. The lumbar spine. 3rd ed. Philadelphia: Lippincott Williams Wilkins; 2004. p. 453–63.

34. Greenough CG. Operative treatment of disc hernaition: laminotomy. In: Hea H, editor. The lumbar spine. 3rd ed. Philadelphia: Lippincott Williams Wilkins; 2004. p. 443–6.

35. Magnusson ML, Pope MH, Wilder DG, Szpalski M, Spratt K. Is there a rational basis for post-surgical lifting restrictions? 1. Current understanding. Eur Spine J. 1999;8(3):170–8.

36. Nystrom B. Experience of microsurgical compared with conventional technique in lumbar disc operations. Acta Neurol Scand. 1987;76(2):129–41.

37. Andrews DW, Lavyne MH. Retrospective analysis of microsurgical and standard lumbar discectomy. Spine (Phila Pa 1976). 1990;15(4):329–35.

38. Caspar W, Campbell B, Barbier DD, Kretschmmer R, Gotfried Y. The Caspar microsurgical discectomy and comparison with a conventional standard lumbar disc procedure. Neurosurgery. 1991;28(1):78–86; discussion 86-7.

39. Henriksen L, Schmidt K, Eskesen V, Jantzen E. A controlled study of microsurgical versus standard lumbar discectomy. Br J Neurosurg. 1996;10(3): 289–93.

40. Katayama Y, Matsuyama Y, Yoshihara H, Sakai Y, Nakamura H, Nakashima S, et al. Comparison of surgical outcomes between macro discectomy and micro discectomy for lumbar disc herniation: a prospective randomized study with surgery performed by the same spine surgeon. J Spinal Disord Tech. 2006;19(5): 344–7.

41. Lagarrigue J, Chaynes P. Comparative study of disk surgery with or without microscopy. A prospective study of 80 cases. Neurochirurgie. 1994;40(2): 116–20.

42. Kahanovitz N, Viola K, Muculloch J. Limited surgical discectomy and microdiscectomy. A clinical comparison. Spine (Phila Pa 1976). 1989;14(1): 79–81.

43. O'Hara LJ, Marshall RW. Far lateral lumbar disc herniation. The key to the intertransverse approach. J Bone Joint Surg Br. 1997;79(6):943–7.

44. Papavero L. The lateral, extraforaminal approach. In: Mayer HM, editor. Minimally invasive spinal surgery. 2nd ed. Berlin/Heidelberg/New York: Springer; 2006. p. 304–14.

45. Porchet F, Chollet-Bornand A, de Tribolet N. Long-term follow up of patients surgically treated by the far-lateral approach for foraminal and extraforaminal lumbar disc herniations. J Neurosurg. 1999;90(1 Suppl):59–66.

46. Fairbank J. Chymopapain and chemonucleolysis. In: Hea H, editor. The lumbar spine. 3rd ed. Philadelphia: Lippincott Williams Wilkins; 2004. p. 447–51.

47. Smith L, Garvin PJ, Gesler RM, Jennings RB. Enzyme dissolution of the nucleus pulposus. Nature. 1963;198:1311–2.

48. McCulloch JA. Chemonucleolysis. J Bone Joint Surg Br. 1977;59(1):45–52.

49. Nordby EJ, Wright PH, Schofield SR. Safety of chemonucleolysis. Adverse effects reported in the United States, 1982-1991. Clin Orthop Relat Res. 1993;293:122–34.

50. Gibson JN, Waddell G. Surgical interventions for lumbar disc prolapse: updated cochrane review. Spine (Phila Pa 1976). 2007;32(16):1735–47.

51. Dabezies EJ, Langford K, Morris J, Shields CB, Wilkinson HA. Safety and efficacy of chymopapain (discase) in the treatment of sciatica due to a herniated nucleus pulposus. Results of a randomized, double-blind study. Spine (Phila Pa 1976). 1988;13(5):561–5.

52. Fraser RD. Chymopapain for the treatment of intervertebral disc herniation. The final report of a double-blind study. Spine (Phila Pa 1976). 1984;9(8):815–8.

53. Javid MJ, Nordby EJ, Ford LT, Hejna WJ, Whisler WW, Burton C, et al. Safety and efficacy of chymopapain (chymodiactin) in herniated nucleus pulposus with sciatica. Results of a randomized, double-blind study. JAMA. 1983;249(18):2489–94.

54. Bromley JW, Varma AO, Santoro AJ, Cohen P, Jacobs R, Berger L. Double-blind evaluation of collagenase injections for herniated lumbar discs. Spine (Phila Pa 1976). 1984;9(5):486–8.

55. Muralikuttan KP, Hamilton A, Kernohan WG, Mollan RA, Adair IV. A prospective randomized trial of chemonucleolysis and conventional disc

surgery in single level lumbar disc herniation. Spine (Phila Pa 1976). 1992;17(4):381–7.

56. Ejeskar A, Nachemson A, Herberts P, Lysell E, Andersson G, Irstam L, et al. Surgery versus chemonucleolysis for herniated lumbar discs. A prospective study with random assignment. Clin Orthop Relat Res. 1983;174:236–42.

57. Crawshaw C, Frazer AM, Merriam WF, Mulholland RC, Webb JK. A comparison of surgery and chemonucleolysis in the treatment of sciatica. A prospective randomized trial. Spine (Phila Pa 1976). 1984;9(2):195–8.

58. National Institute of Clinical Excellence. Interventional procedures overview: automated percutaneous mechanical lumbar discectomy. London: National Institute of Clinical Excellence; 2004.

59. Chatterjee S, Foy PM, Findlay GF. Report of a controlled clinical trial comparing automated percutaneous lumbar discectomy and microdiscectomy in the treatment of contained lumbar disc herniation. Spine (Phila Pa 1976). 1995;20(6):734–8.

60. Revel M, Payan C, Vallee C, Laredo JD, Lassale B, Roux C, et al. Automated percutaneous lumbar discectomy versus chemonucleolysis in the treatment of sciatica. A randomized multicenter trial. Spine (Phila Pa 1976). 1993;18(1):1–7.

61. Grevitt MP, McLaren A, Shackleford IM, Mulholland RC. Automated percutaneous lumbar discectomy. An outcome study. J Bone Joint Surg Br. 1995;77(4):626–9.

62. Kambin P, Zhou L. History and current status of percutaneous arthroscopic disc surgery. Spine (Phila Pa 1976). 1996;21(24 Suppl):57S–61.

63. Yeung AT, Tsou PM. Posterolateral endoscopic excision for lumbar disc herniation: surgical technique, outcome, and complications in 307 consecutive cases. Spine (Phila Pa 1976). 2002;27(7): 722–31.

64. Ruetten S, Komp M, Godolias G. An extreme lateral access for the surgery of lumbar disc herniations inside the spinal canal using the full-endoscopic uniportal transforaminal approach-technique and prospective results of 463 patients. Spine (Phila Pa 1976). 2005;30(22):2570–8.

65. Teli M, Lovi A, Brayda-Bruno M, Zagra A, Corriero A, Giudici F, Minoia L. Higher risk of dural tears and recurrent herniation with lumbar micro-endoscopic discectomy. Eur Spine J. 2010;19(3):443–50.

66. Suk KS, Lee HM, Moon SH, Kim NH. Recurrent lumbar disc herniation: results of operative management. Spine (Phila Pa 1976). 2001;26(6):672–6.

67. Connolly ES. Surgery for recurrent lumbar disc herniation. Clin Neurosurg. 1992;39:211–6.

68. Fandino J, Botana C, Viladrich A, Gomez-Bueno J. Reoperation after lumbar disc surgery: results

in 130 cases. Acta Neurochir (Wien). 1993;122(1–2):102–4.

69. Gaston P, Marshall RW. Survival analysis is a better estimate of recurrent disc herniation. J Bone Joint Surg Br. 2003;85(4):535–7.

70. O'Sullivan MG, Connolly AE, Buckley TF. Recurrent lumbar disc protrusion. Br J Neurosurg. 1990;4(4): 319–25.

71. Jonsson B, Stromqvist B. Clinical characteristics of recurrent sciatica after lumbar discectomy. Spine (Phila Pa 1976). 1996;21(4):500–5.

72. Jonsson B, Stromqvist B. Repeat decompression of lumbar nerve roots. A prospective two-year evaluation. J Bone Joint Surg Br. 1993;75(6):894–7.

73. Cinotti G, Roysam GS, Eisenstein SM, Postacchini F. Ipsilateral recurrent lumbar disc herniation. A prospective, controlled study. J Bone Joint Surg Br. 1998;80(5):825–32.

74. Cinotti G, Gumina S, Giannicola G, Postacchini F. Contralateral recurrent lumbar disc herniation. Results of discectomy compared with those in primary herniation. Spine (Phila Pa 1976). 1999;24(8):800–6.

75. McGirt MJ, Ambrossi GL, Datoo G, Sciubba DM, Witham TF, Wolinsky JP, et al. Recurrent disc herniation and long-term back pain after primary lumbar discectomy: review of outcomes reported for limited versus aggressive disc removal. Neurosurgery. 2009;64(2):338–44; discussion 44–5.

76. Niemeyer T, Halm H, Hackenberg L, Liljenqvist U, Bovingloh AS. Post-discectomy syndrome treated with lumbar interbody fusion. Int Orthop. 2006; 30(3):163–6.

77. Sinigaglia R, Bundy A, Costantini S, Nena U, Finocchiaro F, Monterumici DA. Comparison of single-level L4-L5 versus L5-S1 lumbar disc replacement: results and prognostic factors. Eur Spine J. 2009;18 Suppl 1:52–63.

78. Chitnavis B, Barbagallo G, Selway R, Dardis R, Hussain A, Gullan R. Posterior lumbar interbody fusion for revision disc surgery: review of 50 cases in which carbon fiber cages were implanted. J Neurosurg. 2001;95(2 Suppl):190–5.

79. Chen Z, Zhao J, Liu A, Yuan J, Li Z. Surgical treatment of recurrent lumbar disc herniation by transforaminal lumbar interbody fusion. Int Orthop. 2009;33(1):197–201.

80. Choi JY, Choi YW, Sung KH. Anterior lumbar interbody fusion in patients with a previous discectomy: minimum 2-year follow-up. J Spinal Disord Tech. 2005;18(4):347–52.

81. Frymoyer JW. Radiculopathies: Lumbar disc herniation: Patient selection, predictors of success and failure and non-surgical treatment options. In: Frymoyer JW, editor. The Adult Spine. Philadelphia: Raven-Lippincott, 1997;1937–46.

Applications of Lumbar Spinal Fusion and Disc Replacement

Robert W. Marshall and Neta Raz

Contents

R.W. Marshall (✉)
Department of Orthopaedic Surgery, Royal Berkshire
Hospital, Reading, UK
e-mail: robmarshall100@hotmail.com

N. Raz
Department of Orthopaedic Surgery, Royal Berkshire
Hospital, Reading, UK

Bnai Zion Medical Center, Haifa, Israel

G. Bentley (ed.), *European Surgical Orthopaedics and Traumatology*,
DOI 10.1007/978-3-642-34746-7_214, © EFORT 2014

Abstract

Spinal fusion has been the operation of choice for degenerative back pain for almost a century. However, the desire to maintain movement and minimise the risk of biomechanical disturbance of adjacent levels has led to the development of intervertebral disc arthroplasty. Artificial disc replacement has increased in popularity, but the long term consequences are not yet known and the intended benefits are still to be proven. We trace the history of spinal fusion, including the many different ways to achieve arthrodesis of the diseased levels. The evidence for spinal fusion and disc arthroplasty together with the detailed results of existing clinical trials are considered. Surgical techniques are compared and contrasted.

Keywords

Adjacent segment degeneration • Anterior • Complications • Fusion-posterior • Lateral • Lumbar • Lumbar disc replacement-indications • Motion preservation • Outcomes • Spine • Surgical techniques • Spine • Cervical • Anterior fusion • Prosthetic disc replacement • History • Prosthetic design • Surgical indications • Fusion and disc replacement • Surgical management • Anterior decompression and fusion • Complications • Conclusions

Applications of Lumbar Spinal Fusion and Disc Replacement

In this section, the history of spinal fusion will be discussed, posterior un-instrumented fusions, the later addition of instrumentation, anterior and posterior lumbar interbody fusions, the more recent development of the transforaminal lumbar interbody technique and finally lumbar disc replacement. Indications, clinical results and complications of the different methods will be considered and the comparative studies of spinal fusion with lumbar disc arthroplasty will be analysed. Because of the strong similarity in surgical approach between anterior lumbar interbody fusion and lumbar disc replacement the operative anterior approach to the spine will be outlined in detail.

History of Fusion of the Lumbar Spine

The first published accounts of *posterior lumbar fusions* appeared in 1911 when Hibbs [1] devised a method of fusion for spinal deformity that involved excision of the facet joints and decortication of the laminae and spinous processes and later the same year Albee used tibial strut grafts placed between clefts created in the spinous processes, initially in the treatment of spinal tuberculosis [2] (Pott's disease).

Hibbs extended the indications to include treatment of back pain in 1914 and by 1929 he published his experience in 147 cases [3]. There were also publications on posterior fusion for poliomyelitis and scoliosis [4, 5], but tuberculosis remained the commonest indication [6].

The indications for posterior fusion in the absence of deformity or chronic infection were more controversial and usually included persistent back pain refractory to conservative treatment in the presence of radiographic changes of degeneration. The pain source was uncertain as were the number of levels that required to be fused. There was even a vogue for "trisacral fusion" from L4 to the sacrum with additional arthrodesis of the sacro-iliac joints [7]!

When Mixter and Barr published the evidence for herniation of lumbar intervertebral discs [8] posterior lumbar fusion operations were used even more freely, especially after their long follow-up study suggested that the outcome was slightly better after discectomy and fusion than after discectomy alone [9].

The various posterior methods of fusion, especially the Hibbs method were found to be associated with a pseudarthrosis rate of 20–40 % and 50 % in two level fusions [10–13].

In an attempt to improve the fusion rate alternative methods were developed – e.g. the intertransverse fusion of Watkins [14] and Adkins [15], posterior lumbar interbody fusion by Cloward 1953 [16], James and Nesbit 1953 [17], and Adkins 1955 [15] and anterior lumbar interbody fusion by Mercer 1936 [18], Harmon 1960 [19], and Freebody 1964 [20].

Internal fixation was introduced in an attempt to improve the fusion rate and also shorten the period of immobilisation. (King 1948 [21], Boucher 1959 [22]). Originally the internal fixation methods were not suitable for spondylolisthesis despite some attempts at stabilization involving support of the transverse processes of the displaced vertebra (Nelson [23]).

A large series of uninstrumented posterolateral fusions with iliac crest autografts and long follow-up was reported from the Mayo Clinic with a radiographic fusion rate of 80 % which correlated with a similar rate of clinical success [24].

Internal fixation devices for correction and fusion of scoliosis were developed [25–27] and whilst these could be used as supportive treatment for spinal fractures and after spinal tumour resections, they were not usually appropriate for back pain fusions for degenerative disc disease, which usually only involved one or two motion segments.

Adaptations were introduced to make the Luque wiring method more appropriate for lumbar fixation, resulting in the Hartshill Rectangle [28] with sublaminar wire fixation.

Cotrel and Dubousset designed special rods and hooks that allowed rotational control of the spine in the treatment of scoliosis [29].

Transpedicular screws and plate systems (later screws and rod fixation) revolutionised the internal fixation of the spine and allowed much stronger fixation than with any other fixation system [30–32]. These allowed stabilization, even when the spinous processes and laminae were missing. They allowed improved correction of spinal deformity, better reduction and stabilization of spinal fractures, spinal support after resection of primary tumours and spinal metastases, treatment of high grade spondylolisthesis, spinal instability and back pain due to degeneration – all these with

an acceptable complication rate and low incidence of neurological damage.

Although internal fixation became increasingly sophisticated and reliable there are a number of studies showing that the addition of internal fixation produced a higher rate of fusion, but this did not necessarily equate to an improved clinical outcome in patients treated for degenerative disc disease and chronic back pain. Internal fixation increased the cost of the procedure and the complication rate, but did not always produce improvement in outcome [33, 34]. However, instrumented fusion at the time of posterior decompression for stenosis and degenerative spondylolisthesis produced better fusion rates. It was originally thought that the results were no better than with uninstrumented posterolateral fusion [35], but later follow-up showed improved long term outcome [36] when fusion was achieved.

Besides posterolateral fusion, there was a vogue for *posterior lumbar interbody fusion*

The posterior lumbar interbody fusion (PLIF) procedure was first described in 1944 by Briggs and Milligan [37], who used laminectomy and bone chips in the disc space. In 1946, Jaslow modified the technique by positioning an excised portion of the spinous process within the intervertebral space [38].

Although Cloward used the technique of interbody fusion using iliac crest autograft blocks as early as 1940, it took him until 1953 to publish his experience [16]. His extensive use and expanded indications of the PLIF technique led to further publications of large series over the next 30 years [39, 40]. Although a better rate of spinal fusion was achieved, the increased complexity of the PLIF approach was associated with higher rates of dural and nerve injury. The higher complications discouraged many surgeons until the advent of interbody, moulded fusion cages, made either of carbon, stainless steel, titanium or polyether ether ketone (PEEK) and more sophisticated instrumentation to allow safer insertion of the interbody devices [41–43].

The cages were based upon a precursor used to fuse the cervical spine in horses with "wobbler syndrome" [44].

A modification of the lumbar interbody fusion technique- *transforaminal lumbar interbody fusion* was introduced by Harms and Jeszenszky in 1998 – 191 cases were treated in this way over a 4 year period with very satisfactory results in spondylolisthesis, post-discectomy syndrome, degenerative scoliosis and spinal stenosis [45]. The approach was unilateral with partial or total excision of the facet joint which allowed access to the foramen for the exiting nerve and a lateral entry point to the intervertebral disc for discectomy and preparation of the vertebral end-plates with insertion of a single cage packed with bone graft. The lateral approach increased the safety of the procedure and reduced the incidence of nerve damage and dural tears.

The transforaminal approach allows excellent decompression of the exiting nerve in the foramen and restoration of disc space height with concomitant enlargement of the foramen which makes it an ideal treatment for the lytic spondylolisthesis with nerve entrapment in the foramen. The unilateral approach carries the additional advantage of preserving the anatomy on the contralateral side.

Anterior Lumbar Interbody Fusion

The anterior approach to the lumbar spine was first used in the treatment of spondylolisthesis [18, 46, 47].

Case reports or small series of anterior interbody fusions prevailed until enthusiasts began to report much larger series with the extended indication of treating back pain due to degenerative disc disease [20, 48]. Improvement was reported in 90 % of cases and similar rates of sound fusion were found radiographically.

Despite these favourable reports the anterior lumbar fusion approach was discredited by review of a large series from the Mayo Clinic by Stauffer and Coventry [49]. They found improvement in only 36 % of patients and

a 44 % pseudarthrosis rate was reported. In addition to the unimpressive results, complications included thromboembolism, graft extrusion, paralytic ileus, cardiac arrest and infection.

Mayer re-kindled the interest in anterior lumbar interbody fusion by devising a less invasive "mini-ALIF" approach with excellent results and low morbidity [50]. This approach was often used in conjunction with posterior instrumentation in the form of pedicle screws or translaminar screw fixation, but there is evidence that stand-alone anterior lumbar fusions are just as good and there is probably no need for posterior fixation [51].

Some advocated revision surgery with anterior fusion in patients with persistent pain despite sound posterior fusions [52]. There was a perception that "discogenic pain" was not addressed fully by posterior surgery. This in turn increased the vogue for "360°" (Anterior, lateral and posterior) fusion surgery.

Lateral Transpsoas Interbody Fusion (Extreme Lateral Interbody Fusion – XLIF)

The trans-psoas approach to the lateral aspect of the spine employs sophisticated retraction and instrumentation systems that allow interbody fusions to be carried out through very small incisions with minimal soft tissue trauma [53]. The technique seems to be of particular value in the correction and fusion of adult degenerative scoliosis, but it is not without complications. Damage to the lumbar plexus can occur so that psoas weakness and thigh numbness are not uncommon. The precise place of this procedure is still uncertain.

Spinal Fusion for Degenerative Disc Disease

The surgical treatment of chronic back pain due to degenerative disease of the spine has become the commonest indication for spinal fusion surgery. Despite the enthusiasm for this treatment, favourable outcome is only achieved in around 60–70 % of cases and, in a multicenter randomised controlled trial, spinal fusion was no better than a structured functional restoration programme consisting of education, physiotherapy and the contribution of a clinical psychologist [54].

In analysis of outcome from the Swedish Spine Registry the results were equivalent for surgery undertaken posteriorly, posteriorly with instrumentation or through combined anterior and posterior surgery (circumferential or 360° fusion) [55].

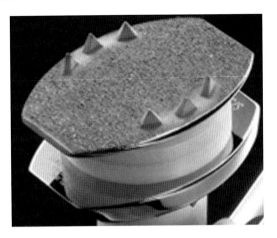

Fig. 1 The Charité III prosthesis. 'Reproduced with permission and copyright © of the British Editorial Society of Bone and Joint Surgery (Mayer HM. Total lumbar disc replacement. *J Bone Joint Surg [Br]* 2005;87-B: 1029-1037 – Fig. 4)

Lumbar Intervertebral Disc Replacement

Lumbar disc replacement or arthroplasty surgery developed for three reasons:

1. Dissatisfaction with the unpredictable results of spinal fusion for degenerative back pain.
2. The desire for preservation of motion in the diseased segment.
3. An attempt to reduce the potential for adverse biomechanical effects of fusion upon adjacent segments of the spine.

History of Lumbar Disc Replacement

There are currently large numbers of different lumbar disc replacement prostheses, but many only have very short follow-up and remain unproven. Therefore only three will be mentioned as they have had longer follow-up and have been subjected to greater scrutiny.

An excellent review of this topic was published by Mayer in 2005 [56].

The first attempt at disc replacement involved the use of stainless steel balls placed between the vertebral bodies. They were devised by Fernstrom and first implanted by Harmon [57, 58].

Although initial reports were favourable the technique never progressed, probably because of endplate penetration by the stainless steel spheres and inevitable subsidence [59].

At the Charité Hospital in East Germany a disc replacement was developed by Schellnack and Büttner-Janz in 1982 and modified to the type II in 1984 and Charité III version in 1987 [60, 61]. This is an unconstrained prosthesis consisting of metallic end-plates (Cobalt Chrome Molybdenum) lined by plasma sprayed Titanium and a coating of calcium phosphate to promote bone ingrowth. The core consists of biconvex ultra-high molecular weight polyethylene with freedom to move on the biconcave end-plates. Tooth-like projections allow primary stability whilst secondary stability results from bone ingrowth into the porous coating (Fig. 1).

The *Prodisc L prosthesis* (Synthes, Paoli, Pennsylvania) was developed in France in the 1980's and was reported by Marnay [62, 63]. This is a semi-constrained device consisting of two Cobalt Chrome Molybdenum alloy end-plates with an insert of UHMWPE inlay which clips into a fixed position during the procedure. The shape of the insert and the

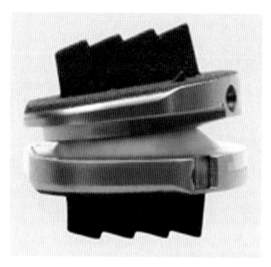

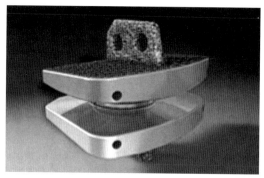

Fig. 3 The Maverick disc prosthesis (Reproduced with permission and copyright © of the British Editorial Society of Bone and Joint Surgery (Mayer HM. Total lumbar disc replacement. *J Bone Joint Surg [Br]* 2005;87-B:1029-1037 – Fig. 6))

Fig. 2 The Prodisc-L Prosthesis (Reproduced with permission and copyright © of the British Editorial Society of Bone and Joint Surgery (Mayer HM. Total lumbar disc replacement. *J Bone Joint Surg [Br]* 2005;87-B:1029-1037 – Fig. 5)

fact that it is not free to move mean that the axis of flexion and extension is fixed and the movements are semi-constrained. The device has central, sagittally-orientated keels which fit into slots created in the vertebrae by the specific instrumentation. This provides primary fixation and the plasma sprayed titanium coating allows for secondary fixation through bone ingrowth (Fig. 2).

The *Maverick disc prosthesis* (Medtronic Minneapolis Minnesota) is a metal-on-metal implant with a ball and socket design and a posteriorly situated, fixed axis of flexion and extension (semi-constrained). Good preliminary results were reported in 2004 [64] (Fig. 3).

Indications for Lumbar Disc Replacement

Whereas spinal fusions can be used to treat infection, spinal deformity, spondylolisthesis, tumour, fractures and degenerative back pain, the indications for disc replacement are much more restricted and are confined to degenerative disc disease, recurrent disc herniation and post-discectomy back pain.

Between 70 % and 85 % of the population suffer from low back pain at some time in their lives. The annual incidence of back pain in adults is 15 % and its point prevalence is approximately 30 %. Low back pain is the primary cause of disability in individuals younger than 50 years [65].

Potential sources of low back pain include the intervertebral discs, facet joints, vertebrae, neural structures, muscles, ligaments, and fascia.

Changes in disc volume and shape occur almost universally with aging. In as many as 90 % of individuals, the lumbar discs may develop degenerative changes by the age of 50 years.

Fissures and cracks usually develop between the lamellae and may establish channels of communication between the peripheral layers of the annulus and the nucleus. Disc tissue can herniate through these cracks.

The relationship between intervertebral disc degeneration and low back pain is not clearly understood. It appears that alteration in biomechanical properties of the disk structure, sensitization of nerve endings by neurovascular ingrowth into the degenerated disks all may contribute to the development of pain.

There is also a biochemical basis for discogenic pain with abnormal release of cytokines from degenerate discs These are pro-inflammatory mediators [66, 67].

Manifestation and Diagnosis of Discogenic Back Pain

Discogenic low back pain is non-radicular and occurs in the absence of spinal deformity, instability and signs of neural tension [68]. In the absence of evidence of disc pathology on radiological images, it may be impossible to localise a painful disc from the symptoms and the signs elicited on physical examination.

Although MRI may identify a degenerative disc (a "black disc"), it will not differentiate between a disc which is pathologically painful and one which is physiologically ageing.

Moreover, intervertebral disc degeneration is commonly seen on MRI in asymptomatic subjects [68].

Discography is used in diagnosing discogenic back pain, but its reliability is questionable. The key feature of discography is the reproduction of the pain felt by the patient on stimulation of the disc. Some claim high accuracy and specificity of discography [68], but Carragee assessed the outcome of fusion spinal surgery in patients with single level discogenic pain as confirmed by discography and concluded that discography failed to identify a single segment pain generator in 50 % of patients [69]. An association has been demonstrated between high intensity zones visible on MRI and the incidence of discogenic back pain [70].

Treatment Options for Discogenic Back Pain

Most of these individuals can be treated successfully without recourse to surgery, but some have persistent back pain which may be amenable to surgical treatment.

Traditionally, fusion has become the "gold standard" in the surgical treatment of degenerative disease in the lumbar spine, but in the light of unpredictable outcome after fusion, this accolade would seem unduly flattering.

Spinal fusion is an expensive procedure which can involve a long hospital stay. It has a significant rate of complications and considerable morbidity.

Recuperation is lengthy and return to work can be delayed.

The posterior approach to the spine inevitably causes damage to the paravertebral muscles which are so important in subsequent functional recovery. Failure of fusion remains a problem even with the use of sophisticated instrumentation.

The use of screws and cages tends to increase neurological and vascular risks. The reported incidence of these complications varies, but a meta-analysis of 47 publications found a 9 % risk of significant donor site pain and a pseudarthrosis rate of 14 % [71].

A particular concern with rigid fusion is the transfer of stress to adjacent segments.

This may cause symptomatic degenerative disease in the long term and may require further surgery in up to 20 % of patients in 5 years and perhaps even 37 % within a decade following 'successful' lumbar fusion.

This risk may lead to the exclusion of many very deserving patients from consideration for surgery if the adjacent segments show any existing sign of degeneration, even if this is asymptomatic [72–74].

An alternative surgical procedure, total disc replacement, has increased in popularity.

The purpose of this technique is to restore and maintain spinal segment motion, which is presumed to prevent adjacent level degeneration at the operated levels, while relieving pain [75].

The design of total disc prostheses needed to take into account the aims of total disc arthroplasty:
1. Restoration of physiological kinematics and mobility, whilst avoiding segmental instability;
2. Restoration of correct spinal alignment and sagittal balance;

3. Protection of the biological structures, such as the adjacent intervertebral discs, the facet joints and the ligaments, from increased loading which could lead to rapid degeneration;
4. Device stability and wear properties [76].

Significant facet joint osteoarthritis is a contra-indication to the procedure and yet, it is difficult to identify in its early stages. The use of total disc replacement may be limited to the treatment of early degenerative disc disease with preservation of disc height thereby eliminating its uses in the majority of patients [75]. The fate of facet joints following a total disc replacement is unknown and facet joint hypertrophy, which accelerates spinal stenosis, may be a potent long-term complication.

Anterior revision procedures are bound to be technically difficult with a significant risk of vascular injury, particularly at the L4/5 level.

A summary of the indications and contra-indications for disc replacement is as follows:

Young, active patients with chronic discogenic low back pain, reproduced by discography, little facet disease, and good bone stock, are the ideal candidates for arthroplasty.

Instability and deformity are strong contra-indications to lumbar arthroplasty, particularly with an unconstrained prosthesis design.

Although there are proponents of expanded indications for semi-constrained prostheses, evidence of safety and effectiveness in these patients has not been proven [77].

Motion Preservation

The whole concept of disc arthroplasty is based upon preservation of motion of the operated level so it is important to consider the evidence for motion preservation.

Many studies show results of relatively short follow-up with significant improvement and even restoration of a normal range of motion in the operated level.

In a prospective randomized trial FDA-supported multi-center study in the USA [78], 304 patients with DDD who failed conservative treatment were randomised for either lumbar total disc replacement with Charité disc or ALIF surgery using the BAK cage and iliac crest bone graft, and followed for 24 months. The range of motion in the operated level of the arthroplasty group gradually increased to a level of 113.6 % compared to pre-operative range of motion (final range of motion exceeded the pre-operative range by 13.6 %).

There was a mean range of motion of 7.5° at 24 months, including subjects with suboptimally-placed prostheses.

A prospective Canadian study that followed 57 patients with degenerative disc disease who underwent disc replacement with the Charité III prosthesis with average follow-up of 55 months (2–7 years) showed that motion was maintained at the replaced segment with a mean flexion-extension range of 6.5° that compares favourably with the sagittal rotation reported in the literature [79].

Cinotti et al. reported 46 patients undergoing artificial disc replacement with Charité SB III disc prosthesis with a mean follow-up of 3.2 years (range 2–5 years).

The vertebral motion averaged 9° (range 0–15) at the operated level with four patients developing spontaneous fusions [80].

Tropiano et al. reported on 53 patients who underwent Pro-Disc II lumbar disc replacement [63]. Forty patients had surgery at one level, 11 patients at two levels and two patients at three levels. The mean follow-up time was 1.4 years (range 1–2 years).

At L5–S1, the flexion/extension range of motion averaged 8° (range 2–12) at the operated level. At L4-5, the range of motion averaged 10° (8–18) at the operated level.

Bertagnoli and Kumar reported on 108 patients undergoing total disc replacement with the Pro-Disc II implant [81]. Ninety-four patients underwent surgery at one level, 12 at two levels and two at three levels.

Range of follow-up time varied from 3 months to 2 years, with 54 patients (50 %) having more than 1-year follow-up.

There were no implant failures and the average range of motion at L5–S1 was 9° (range 2–13) and at L4-5 was 10° (range 8–15).

The above studies had the limitation of a short follow-up. By contrast, Putzier's is the only long-term follow-up study and yielded much less favourable results with regard to motion preservation [82]. In this retrospective clinical and radiological analysis of 84 Charité discs (71 patients, operated between 1984–89) after an average follow up of 17.3 years (14.5–19.2 years) a segmental mobility of 3° or less was graded as "Ankylosed" whilst a segmental mobility of more than 3° was graded as "mobile".

The results of this study are not favourable and show that 60 % of the patients had definitive ankylosis at long term follow-up due to high grade anterior heterotopic ossification. One of the possible explanations for this high rate of heterotopic ossification is the surgical technique which included repair of the anterior longitudinal ligament, now known to trigger ossification.

There are two French studies with 10-year follow up where motion was preserved.

In Thierry's series of 106 patients, seven cases of ossification were found, four of them partial and asymptomatic. Mean range of motion at the operated level at the end of follow up was 10.1° of flexion-extension and 4.4° of lateral bending [77].

Lemaire et al, retrospectively reported on 107 patients (147 implants) following Charité disc replacement between 1989 and 1993 and followed for an average of 11.3 years [83]. Three cases of heterotopic ossification were noted, 2 of them affecting the implant mobility. Mean range of motion was 10.4° of flexion-extension and 5.4° of lateral bending.

The differences in these series raise questions about prosthetic design and the influence of surgical technique upon the rate of heterotopic ossification.

Adjacent Segment Degeneration

The second main theoretical benefit behind disc replacement is preservation of the "adjacent segment".

Maintaining motion at the operated segment can theoretically reduce the over-loading and subsequent rapid degeneration of the adjacent motion segments.

One should remember that it is difficult to differentiate between "true surgery-related adjacent segment degeneration" and the natural process of spinal degeneration.

There is considerable debate in the available literature regarding the definition and prevalence of adjacent segment degeneration (ASD) following spinal fusion and disc arthroplasty and the actual clinical significance of the changes.

General Definitions

After lumbar spinal surgical intervention such as arthrodesis or arthroplasty, the *radiographic* presence of disc deterioration adjacent to the surgically-treated disc is referred to as: "Adjacent Segment Degeneration" (ASDeg).

This must be differentiated from Adjacent Segment Disease (ASDis) which is the development of clinically symptomatic junctional degeneration [84]. ASDis may lead to additional surgery and thus impact negatively on functional outcome, as opposed to ASDeg which is purely a radiographic finding without associated symptoms.

ASDeg and ASDis Following Lumbar Fusion

There is wide variation in the reports regarding the incidence of lumbar ASDeg (5.2–100 %) and ASDis (5.2–18.5 %) following lumbar arthrodesis [84].

Ghiselli *et al* reported the largest single series of patients managed with a posterior lumbar arthrodesis in which junctional degeneration was assessed. 215 patients were assessed at an average follow up of 6.7 years. They found an incidence of ASDis of 16.5 % at 5 years and 36.1 % at 10 years. Perhaps surprisingly, there was no correlation between the number of levels of fused, i.e. the length of the lever-arm and the degree of degeneration at adjacent levels [74]. In Brantigan's study adjacent segment degeneration occurred in 61 % of patients, but was clinically significant only in 20 % at 10 years after lumbar fusion [85].

The systematic literature review by Harrop et al calculated the incidence of ASDeg to be around 34 % and the incidence of ASDis to be approximately 14 % following a lumbar arthrodesis [84].

In an attempt to evaluate the rate of "natural ageing process" of the non-operated spine, Hassett et al assessed the incidence of degenerative spinal disease in a population of women over a 9 year period and found it to progress at an incidence of 3–4 % per year. This seems similar to the spinal fusion population and suggests that ASDeg following spinal fusion is not significantly different from the natural ageing process of the non-operated spine [86].

Adjacent segment degeneration and adjacent segment disease following lumbar disc replacement.

Most studies involve short follow-up and cannot address the long term process of ASD.

The available data are products of the few long-term studies. The systematic literature review by Harrop et al. found that 9 % of arthroplasty patients were noted to have ASDeg and only 1 % clinically symptomatic ASDis.

This low level of symptomatic disease was also reported by David -100 single level (L4–L5 or L5–S1) arthroplasty patients with a 13.2 year average follow-up and 2.8 % incidence of ASDis [87].

Huang et al, using graphic motion analysis found 24 % of patients developed radiographic evidence of ASDeg [87]. The authors noted that disc degeneration correlated with a decreased overall lumbar range of motion. Patients with motion of 5° or greater had a 0 % prevalence of ASD degeneration, whereas patients with less than 5° motion had a 34 % prevalence of ASD degeneration. However, despite these radiographic changes there was no significant correlation with clinical outcome.

Putzier reported on 53 patients that underwent a Charité I to III disc arthroplasty procedure with a follow up over 17 years and found a 17 % (9/53) incidence of ASDeg changes [82]. However, in keeping with Huang's findings, the degenerative changes only occurred in arthroplasty cases which had ankylosed and had limited motion.

The arthroplasty patients that maintained their motion (40 %) did not develop any evidence of adjacent segment degeneration.

Whilst lumbar disc replacement reduces the load on adjacent segments of the spine, it is known to increase the load on the facet joints at the operated level (which are off-loaded following successful fusion surgery), and that is why "facet arthrosis" is considered to be a contra-indication to disc replacement. A 2.5-fold increase in facet joint loading was measured following lumbar total disc replacement [88, 89].

Complications of Lumbar Disc Arthroplasty

Complications can be divided into:
1. Those related to surgical approach;
2. Those related to implant survival and function.

The complications of the surgical approach should be the same for lumbar disc replacement and anterior lumbar fusion as the surgical technique is virtually identical. They include the risk of bleeding from the iliac vessels (the bifurcation of the aorta and vena cava is located just anterior to the vertebral column at L4-5 level), injury to the superior hypogastric plexus of nerves which in males can lead to retrograde ejaculation.

Poor positioning of the implants or over-distraction of the disc space can endanger the nerve roots.

Post-operatively, the circumstances are different as fusion involves a "static implant" and the main anticipated complication is failure of fusion (pseudarthrosis) that could lead to pain and even implant failure.

When solid fusion is achieved the implant is "off loaded", leaving mainly the adjacent segment degeneration as a continuing concern.

Lumbar disc replacement employs a "dynamic implant", and with time there is an increased likelihood of implant failure or even unintended ankylosis of the treated motion segment.

The relative impact of the two treatments upon adjacent segment degeneration has been discussed above and is more favourable for the motion-preserving arthroplasty.

In a meta-analysis of 47 papers on lumbar fusions the most common problems following spinal fusions were: Pseudo-arthrosis (14 %) and chronic pain at the iliac crest bone graft donor site. Less frequent complications were venous thrombo-embolism (3.7 %) and neurological injury (2.8 %) [71, 90].

Implant failure:

In the 17-year follow up study after disc arthroplasty 23 % needed fusion surgery for implant failure or pain [81].

There were two reports of cohorts of patients referred to a tertiary center in the Netherlands following an unsuccessful lumbar disc replacement [59, 92].

In the first series of 27 patients [59], early complications included 2 cases of early prosthesis dislocation, 2 cases of erectile dysfunction and retrograde ejaculation and 4 cases of abdominal wall or retro peritoneal hematomas. Late complications included: degeneration of facet joints at the same level, degeneration of facet joints and discs at neighboring levels, as well as subsidence and migration of the prosthesis. In one patient, signs of polyethylene breakdown were seen.

In the second series (75 patients) [91] the causes of persisting pain were thought to be related to the following late-complications: subsidence (39 cases), adjacent degeneration in various combinations (36 cases), facet joint degeneration according to CT scan (25 cases), prosthesis migration(6 cases) and wear of the disc prosthesis (5 cases).

Van Ooij et al pointed out that whilst degenerative disc disease is supposed to be the main cause of the symptoms, it is possible that the facet joints play a role in the pain syndrome of most of these patients [60]. Obviously, replacing only the intervertebral disc would not address this pain source. A normal intervertebral disc has a shock-absorbing function. The current prostheses, made from metal and polyethylene or from metal alone, have little shock-absorbing capacity, and this should be a matter of concern.

The fixation of a disc prosthesis onto the vertebral end-plates is questionable and some suggest that press-fit fixation components with spikes, pegs, and posts are inadequate after tensile loading and may be effective only for the relatively short term [92]. Subsidence of prostheses is encountered and it is known that the central end-plate is relatively weak and that only the outer rim of the end-plates contains stronger bone. This implies that the metal plates must be large enough to rest on the periphery of the end-plates. A disadvantage of larger plates is that they carry more risk for compression of the exiting nerve roots posterolaterally and on the great vessels ventrally.

In males, temporary or permanent retrograde ejaculation can result from damage to the superior hypogastric plexus of nerves on the anterior aspect of the lumbosacral spine. This risk has been reported in from 2–7 % [93]. Sasso et al found that the risk was substantially greater with transperitoneal compared to retroperitoneal approaches [94].

The problems of polyethylene and metal debris caused by wear have been investigated extensively in hip and knee replacements, but little evidence exists regarding these issues following lumbar disc arthroplasty.

Although the clinical significance is not yet known, a recent study on metal-on-metal disc replacements showed cobalt and chromium levels that were elevated at all post-operative time points, and similar in magnitude to those seen in well-functioning metal-on-metal surface replacements of the hip and in metal-on-metal total hip replacements [95].

Reports of osteolysis after disc arthroplasty exist [60, 96], but Lemaire et al in a prospective report of 100 followed for a mean of 11.3 years after implantation of Charité disc replacements noted no patients with signs of osteolysis [83].

Relative Safety of Spinal Fusion and Lumbar Disc Replacement

Comparative studies show a similar rate of complications for lumbar fusion and arthroplasty at 2 and 5 years

A prospective, randomized, multicenter FDA study of 304 patients who underwent either lumbar total disc replacement with the CHARITÉ™ artificial disc or ALIF surgery, with 2 year follow-up, showed the following results:

1. Neurological complications were the same in the two groups.
2. Pain at the bone graft donor site occurred in 18 (18.2 %) of the ALIF patients.
3. Device failures necessitating re-operation, revision, or removal occurred in 11 (5.4 %) patients in the disc replacement group and 9 (9.1 %) patients in the ALIF group.
4. There were no catastrophic device failures resulting in death or injury in either group.
5. Approach-related complications occurred in 20 (9.8 %) of the disc arthroplasty patients and 10 (10.1 %) of the ALIF patients.
6. The overall complication rate was similar.
7. The short follow up did not permit assessment of the impact of the procedures upon the adjacent segments of the spine [97].

Clinical Outcomes After Lumbar Disc Replacement and Lumbar Fusion

In the randomised controlled trial that compared the 2 year results of 304 patients with degenerative disc disease randomised for either Charité lumbar disc replacement or anterior lumbar interbody fusion using the BAK cage packed with iliac crest bone graft both patient groups demonstrated significant improvement in the Oswestry Disability Index (ODI, functional self assessment) and the pain levels determined by the visual analogue scale [97].

The disc replacement group demonstrated better results at all stages of follow-up. Patient satisfaction was also higher in the LTDR group (73 % vs. 59 %) and when asked whether they would have the same treatment again the answer at the end of follow-up was positive in 69.9 % of the patients in the disc replacement group but only in 50 % of the ALIF group ($p = 0.006$) [97].

The need for narcotics for pain control was lower in the disc replacement group compared to the ALIF group at all stages of follow-up (at 24 months: 64 % vs. 80 %, $p = 0.004$) [97].

Assessment of the work status before and after surgery showed no significant difference between the groups.

At the end of follow-up the clinical success rate at the lumbar disc arthroplasty group was 63.9 % compared to 56.8 % in the ALIF group ($p = 0.0004$) [97].

In a prospective study of 57 patients who underwent disc replacement (Charité III) and followed for an average of 55 month (2–7 years) an improvement of 50 % in ODI, VAS and SF-36 was achieved compared to pre-operative scores [79].

In Lemaire's prospective report of 100 patients followed for a mean of 11.3 years excellent clinical outcome was achieved in 62 % of the patients, good in 28 % and 10 % of patients experienced a poor outcome [83].

In four published randomised studies comparing disc prosthesis with fusion, the clinical

Fig. 4 Supine, Trendelenburg position with pillow to flex knees and hips. A urinary catheter and intermittent calf compression are in place

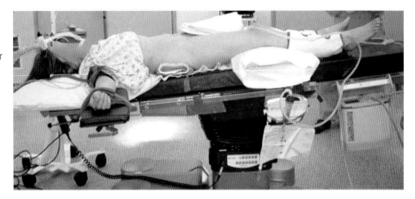

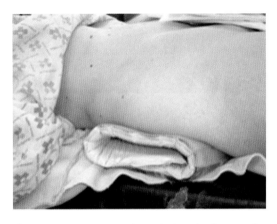

Fig. 5 A gel pad is placed beneath the spine for posterior support

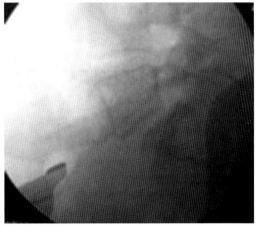

Fig. 7 A metal marker is used with fluoroscopy to mark the ideal skin incision for access to the correct level of the spine – in this case L5-S1 with lytic spondylolisthesis

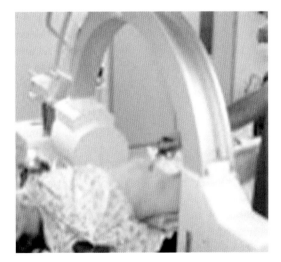

Fig. 6 A metal marker is used with fluoroscopy to mark the ideal skin incision for access to the correct level of the spine – in this case L5-S1 with lytic spondylolisthesis

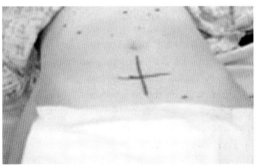

Fig. 8 A metal marker is used with fluoroscopy to mark the ideal skin incision for access to the correct level of the spine – in this case L5-S1 with lytic spondylolisthesis

Fig. 9 The surgeons attach
the synframe and make sure
that there is no pressure
upon the patient

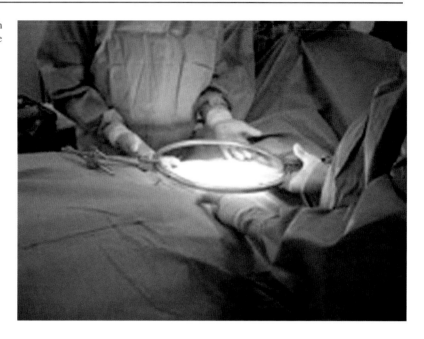

outcome of disc prosthesis was at least equivalent
to that of fusion [97–100].

A recent Norwegian study has shown
better improvement of function (measured
by the Oswestry Disabiity Index) after disc
replacement in comparison to a rehabilitation
programme involving a multidisciplinary team
using cognitive therapy and physiotherapy [101].

Operative techniques for lumbar disc replacement and spinal fusion

We will concentrate upon the similarities of
the anterior approach for the two operations.
The surgical approach is usually retroperitoneal
for the L4-5 and higher lumbar levels, but the
L5-S1 level can be approached retroperitoneally
or transperitoneally. For the purposes of illustration only, we shall describe the transperitoneal
access to L5-S1 for an anterior lumbar
interbody fusion using a Synfix cage (Synthes)
and graft and the retroperitoneal approach to the
L4-5 level for a Prodisc II (Synthes) lumbar disc
replacement.

For both procedures a general anaesthetic is
administered via a cuffed endotracheal tube.

Prophylactic antibiotics are administered with
the induction of anaesthesia and currently we use
the combination of Teicoplanin and Gentamicin.

Abdominal surgery should be accompanied by
effective thromboprophylaxis using the combination of intra-operative and post-operative intermittent calf compression boots and low molecular
weight heparin administered 6 h after completion
of the operation and continued until the patient is
discharged from hospital.

The position on the operating table is
supine with a pillow beneath the lower limbs to
keep the hips and knees slightly flexed (Fig. 4).
This takes the tension off the iliac vessels
and lumbosacral plexus, thus making retraction
safer [102]. The Trendelenburg position is
helpful in keeping the small bowel retracted
during a transperitoneal approach.

In order to provide posterior support
and prevent sagging of the vertebral column,
a gel pad can be placed beneath the patient.
(Fig. 5)

By placing a metal marker on the anterior
abdominal wall and using fluoroscopy the ideal
location of the skin incision can be marked.
(Figs. 6–8).

The synframe retractor (Synthes) is attached
to its table mountings and placed carefully in
order to avoid pressure upon the patient's
abdomen (Fig. 9).

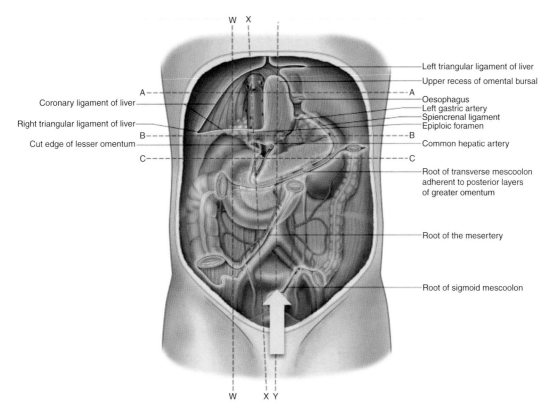

W X

Left triangular ligament of liver
Upper recess of omental bursal

A - A
Coronary ligament of liver
Oesophagus
Left gastric artery
Spiencrenal ligament
Right triangular ligament of liver
Epiploic foramen
B - B
Cut edge of lesser omentum
Common hepatic artery
C - C

Root of transverse mescoolon
adherent to posterior layers
of greater omentum

Root of the mesertery

Root of sigmoid mescoolon

W   X Y

Fig. 10 Transperitoneal approach – directly between iliac vessels. (reproduced from Gray's Anatomy with kind permission from Elsevier)

Transperitoneal Approach to L5-S1

The spine at L5-S1 can be approached retroperitoneally or transperitoneally. As the procedure is carried out in the mid-line between the iliac vessels, the transperitoneal approach gives rapid, direct access to the anterior aspect of the lumbosacral junction (Fig. 10).

Through a vertical mid-line skin incision below the umbilicus, the rectus sheath is exposed and the linea alba incised in the midline. This allows access to the peritoneal sac which is elevated on a clip and incised (Figs. 11–13).

Moist packs are used to keep the small bowel retracted and expose the posterior peritoneum overlying the spine (Fig. 14). After incising the posterior peritoneum, it and the autonomic nerves of the superior hypogastric plexus are carefully peeled away from the spine and retracted gently (Fig. 15).

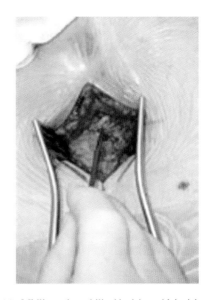

Fig. 11 Midline sub-umbilical incision with incision along the linea alba to part the rectus abdominis muscles. The peritoneum is picked up and opened with dissecting scissors

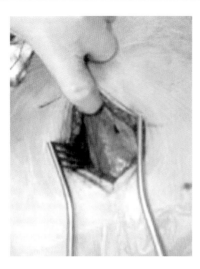

Fig. 12 Midline sub-umbilical incision with incision along the linea alba to part the rectus abdominis muscles. The peritoneum is picked up and opened with dissecting scissors

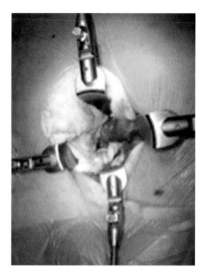

Fig. 14 Moist swabs pack the loops of small bowel away and the posterior peritoneum is exposed overlying the disc

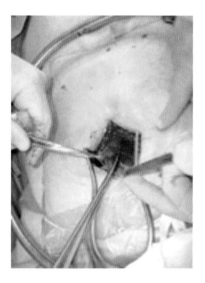

Fig. 13 Midline sub-umbilical incision with incision along the linea alba to part the rectus abdominis muscles. The peritoneum is picked up and opened with dissecting scissors

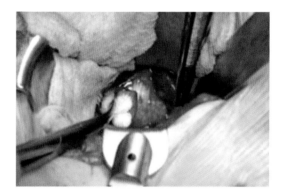

Fig. 15 The posterior peritoneum is incised and carefully cleared using a Lahey swab to expose the anterior longitudinal ligament and intervertebral disc

Once the vertebral column is well visualized the synframe bone levers can be placed either side of it and attached to the synframe. Because they have sharp points that can find their way into the spinal foramina, it is neccessary to wrap some Surgicel around the tips of the levers to prevent damage to the exiting spinal nerves.

With the bone levers placed laterally, the Synframe retractors are inserted superiorly and inferiorly to allow good access to the disc space (Fig. 16).

When safe access is established, the intervertebral disc can be excised and removed (Figs. 17 and 18).

The vertebrae are distracted by insertion of a spreader and this allows thorough curettage of the end-plates to remove all disc remnants and the end-plate cartilage (Figs. 19 and 20).

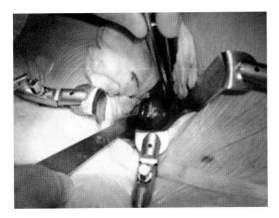

Fig. 16 A Synframe bone lever is placed on either side of the intervertebral disc and synframe retractor blades placed superiorly and inferiorly

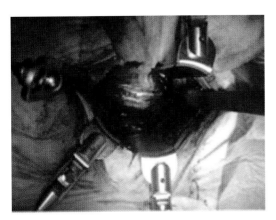

Fig. 17 The intervertebral disc is incised and removed with rongeurs

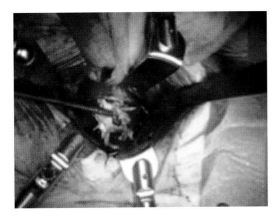

Fig. 18 The intervertebral disc is incised and removed with rongeurs

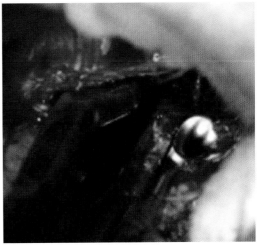

Fig. 19 Using an intervertebral spreader and curettes, the cartilaginous end-plates are removed to expose bleeding bone

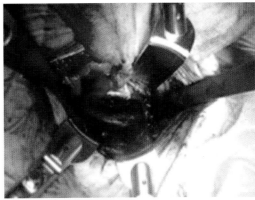

Fig. 20 Using an intervertebral spreader and curettes, the cartilaginous end-plates are removed to expose bleeding bone

When the disc space has been cleared the Synfix trial can be used to judge the optimal size of cage to be used. As large a footprint as possible should be used and at L5-S1 angled end-plates are necessary – usually requiring a 12° cage. Fluoroscopy is used to help judge the choice of cage (Figs. 21 and 22).

The Synfix cage is filled with bone graft. This can be autogenous or allograft bone, but we prefer synthetic bone in the form of tricalcium phosphate granules in a conformable

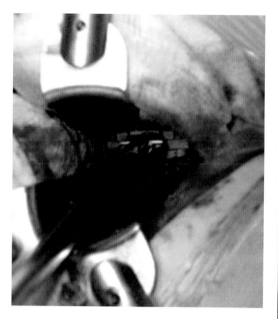

Fig. 21 Trial Synfix cage introduced with fluoroscopy to check ideal size and placement

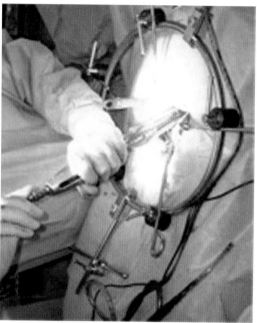

Fig. 23 "The squid" is used to introduce the Synfix cage containing bone graft

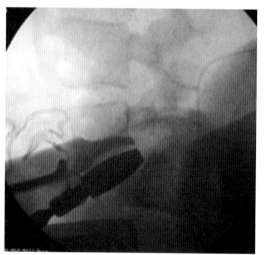

Fig. 22 Trial Synfix cage introduced with fluoroscopy to check ideal size and placement

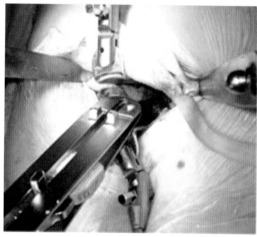

Fig. 24 "The squid" is used to introduce the Synfix cage containing bone graft

gel (Actifuse ABX). The specially designed "squid introducer" allows ready insertion of the device into the disc space (Figs. 23 and 24).

The well-seated cage is fixed into place using four cancellous screws which anchor the cage securely and also have a thread which engages firmly into the threaded holes in the cage (Fig. 25). Radiographic confirmation of position and fixation is important (Figs. 26 and 27).

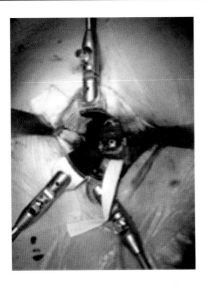

Fig. 25 Synfix cage fixed in place with 4 cancellous screws

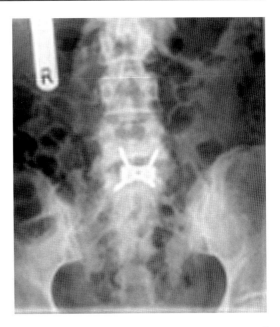

Fig. 27 Show radiographic appearances – lateral and anteroposterior views

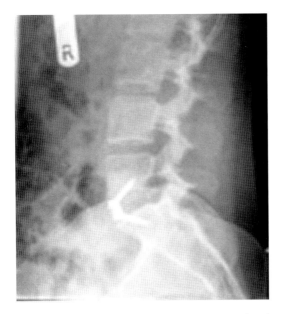

Fig. 26 Show radiographic appearances – lateral and anteroposterior views

Retroperitoneal Approach to L4-5

The anaesthetic and positioning are identical to the transperitoneal approach described above. However, for the retroperitoneal approach to the higher levels, a transverse skin incision is favoured. This is done on the left side to allow the peritoneum and peritoneal contents to be retracted to the right (Fig. 28).

Through the transverse skin incision, placed optimally after fluoroscopic marking, the rectus sheath is exposed in the mid-line and to the left side. Then the left anterior rectus sheath is exposed vertically (Figs. 29 and 30).

The left rectus is freed from the anterior sheath and retracted medially. (Figs. 31 and 32). The posterior rectus sheath is thus exposed.

By going below the arcuate line of the posterior rectus sheath, the peritoneum can be separated off the sheath. Then the arcuate line and posterior sheath itself are incised to allow better access (Fig. 32).

The peritoneal sac and its contents can be reflected medially until the vertebral column is exposed (Figs. 33 and 34). It is important to retract the left common iliac vessels carefully to avoid damage to them and particular to the iliolumbar veins which have variable anatomy and, if torn, can lead to brisk haemorrhage. In dealing with these veins it is also possible for them to pull off the iliac vein resulting in

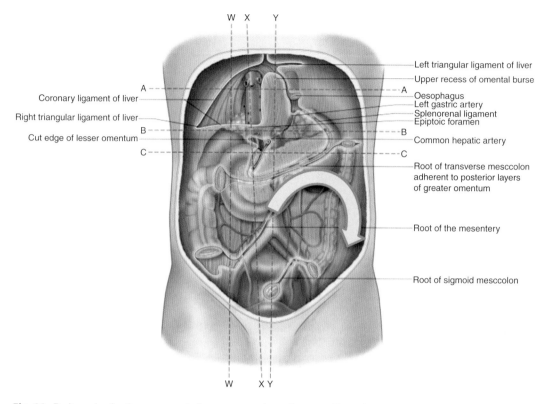

Fig. 28 Peritoneal reflections – arrow indicates retroperitoneal access. (Reproduced from Gray's Anatomy with kind permission from Elsevier)

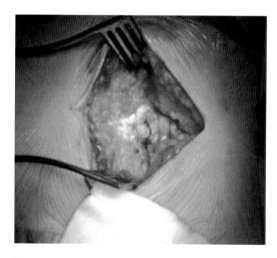

Fig. 29 A transverse skin incision is followed by a vertical splitting of the left anterior rectus sheath

an even more major bleed from the common iliac vein itself. A cadaveric study has highlighted the hazards of variable anatomy and the proximity of the lumbosacral plexus to these veins [103].

Once the spine is exposed, fluoroscopy in the anteroposterior plane is used to locate the midline with an injection needle. Then, an osteotome is used to mark the mid-line across the adjacent vertebrae (Figs. 35–37).

Then the intervertebral disc is totally excised (Fig. 38).

Once the disc has been excised and the endplates cleared of all disc and cartilage it is important to release the posterior longitudinal ligament all the way across using fine Kerrison rongeur punches (Fig. 39). Without this step the prosthesis will be under posterior tension, cannot articulate properly and tends to be extruded.

Trial implants are used to determine the ideal size for the patient (Fig. 40). Then the trial is placed with a stop to prevent it extending too far posteriorly while the chisel is passed through the slot in the trial. This cuts the slots in the vertebral end-plates for the keels on the prosthesis (Figs. 41 and 42).

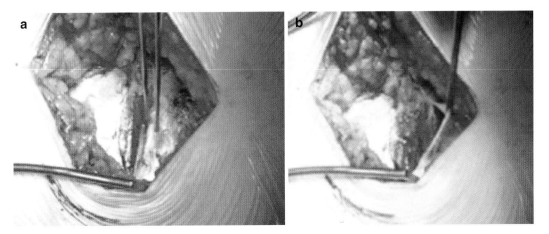

Fig. 30 Transverse skin incision is followed by a vertical splitting of the left anterior rectus sheath

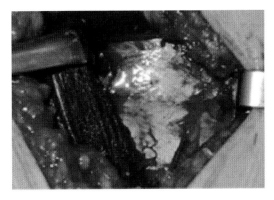

Fig. 31 After opening the left rectus sheath the left rectus abdominis muscle is retracted medially to expose the posterior rectus sheath

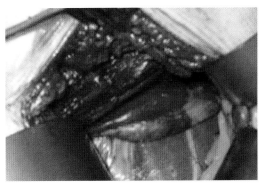

Fig. 33 The peritoneal sac and contents are reflected off the posterior abdominal wall revealing the psoas muscle

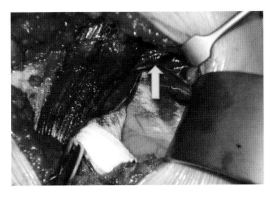

Fig. 32 Arrow shows arcuate line of posterior rectus sheath incised after separating it from the peritoneum

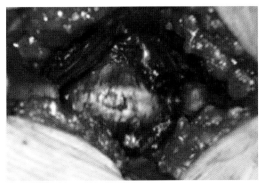

Fig. 34 Retraction medially allows exposure of the intervertebral disc

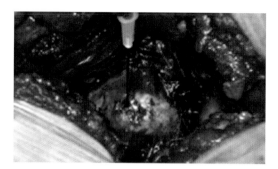

Fig. 35 The mid-line is determined with an injection needle and fluoroscopy

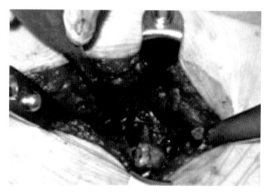

Fig. 36 The mid-line is marked on the adjacent vertebral bodies using an osteotome

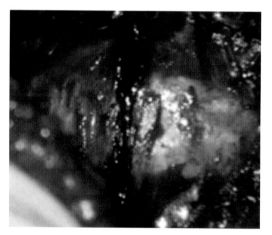

Fig. 37 Shows mid-line marking

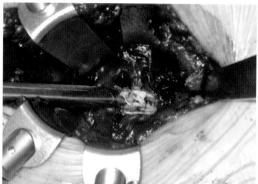

Fig. 38 Shows excision of the intervertebral disc

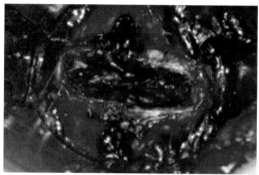

Fig. 39 Disc clearance and division of the posterior longitudinal ligament

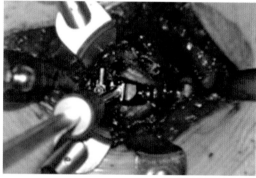

Fig. 40 Shows insertion of trial implant with adjustable stop

The end plates of the Prodisc C prosthesis are fitted onto the introducer and locked in place. After engaging the keels in the vertebral end-plate slots the prosthesis is tapped into place with a mallet. This process must be done with fluoroscopic control. Once the end-plates of the prosthesis are securely fixed within the vertebral bodies, the polyethylene insert is passed along

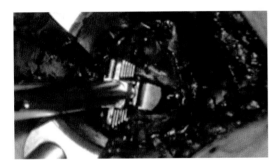

Fig. 41 Chisel inserted to cut the slots for the keel

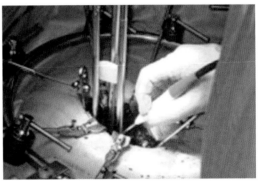

Fig. 44 Polyethylene insert sliding down introducer

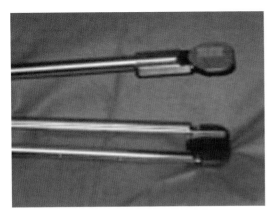

Fig. 42 End-plates of the prosthesis on inserter

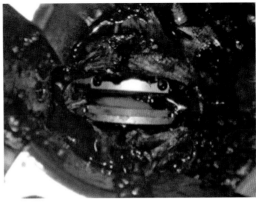

Fig. 45 Prodisc C prosthesis and insert in place

Wound Closure

The wound is closed in layers with synthetic, absorbable sutures (Polyglycolic acid), taking care to close any inadvertent openings in the peritoneum and both layers of the rectus sheath are repaired. After the mid-line approach a strong loop PDS suture is used for a mass closure of the anterior abdominal wall. The skin is approximated with a subcuticular stitch and steristrips.

No drains are necessary.

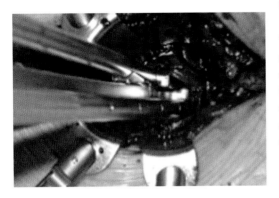

Fig. 43 Prosthesis inserted

Post-Operative Care

grooves in the introducer and clicked into place (Figs. 43–45).

Satisfactory seating of the device is confirmed on fluoroscopy (Figs. 46 and 47).

The patient receives opiate analgesia which can be in the form of patient controlled analgesia via an intravenous line and infusion pump, but we

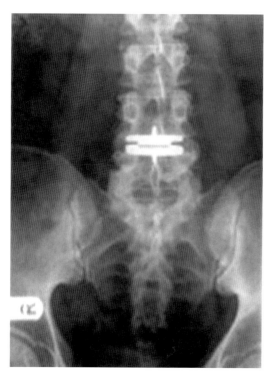

Fig. 46 A-P and lateral radiographs post-operatively

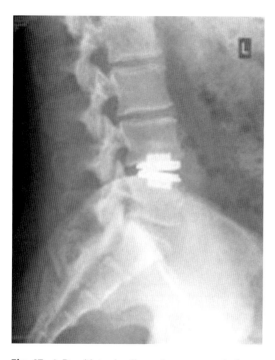

Fig. 47 A-P and lateral radiographs post-operatively

favour the use of a small dose of morphine and Bupivicaine injected into the CSF via a a 25 Guage spinal needle. This is given at the end of the operation and provides excellent analgesia for the first 12–24 h.

Sometimes a paralytic ileus occurs post-operatively, but is usually of short duration so we do not restrict fluids or food intake for more than a few hours after surgery.

The patient sits out and walks on the first post-operative day and when they can manage to visit the bathroom the urinary catheter is removed.

The low molecular weight heparin injections and mechanical DVT prophylaxis (calf compression) continue until the patient is fully mobile and ready for discharge from hospital. They are usually ready for discharge after 3–4 days.

For fusion or disc replacement we use a lumbar support for the first 4 weeks after which physiotherapy exercises commence. Activities are increased according to comfort.

Post-operative radiographic and clinical checks are at 6 weeks, 3 months and 6 months.

Times to return to work and to active sport vary according to the patient and their perceived progress. We impose as few restrictions as possible and encourage resumption of all activities in a graduated way.

Summary and Conclusions

1. Spinal fusions have been carried out in various forms for over 100 years and have a proven record in dealing with a whole range of spinal pathology.
2. Lumbar disc arthroplasty is a more recent development with restricted indications including degenerative disc disease, post-discectomy back pain and recurrent disc herniation.
3. Comparative randomised controlled trials have shown that lumbar disc arthroplasty is at least equivalent to spinal fusion after follow-up for 5 years.
4. Both procedures can be carried out anteriorly through a retroperitoneal approach so the complications are similar and mainly approach-related.

5. The long term effects of polyethylene and metal wear debris remain uncertain, but may produce late complications of disc arthroplasty.

6. The benefits to the neighbouring spinal motion segments of maintaining movement are still being evaluated and there is no definite proof of reduction of degenerative disc disease in adjacent segments.

References

1. Hibbs RA. An operation for progressive spinal defor-mities. NY Med Jour. 1911;93:1013.

2. Albee FH. Transplantation of a portion of the tibia into the spine for Pott's disease. JAMA. 1911;57:885.

3. Hibbs RA, Swift WE. Developmental abnormalities of the lumbosacral juncture. Surg Gynec Obst. 1929;68:604.

4. Hibbs RA. Treatment of deformities of the spine caused by poliomyelitis. JAMA. 1917;69:787.

5. Hibbs RA. A report of 59 cases of scoliosis treated by the fusion operation. J Bone Joint Surg. 1924;6:3.

6. Hibbs RA. Treatment of vertebral tuberculosis by the fusion operation: report of 210 cases. JAMA. 1918;71:1372.

7. Chandler FA. Trisacral fusion. Surg Gynec Obst. 1929;48:501.

8. Mixter WJ, Barr JS. Rupture of the inter-vertebral disc with involvement of the spinal canal. New Eng J Med. 1934;211:210–5.

9. Barr JS, Mixter WJ. Posterior protrusion of the lum-bar intervertebral discs. J Bone Joint Surg. 1941;23:444–56.

10. Thompson WAL, Ralston EL. Pseudarthrosis follow-ing spine fusion. J Bone Joint Surg. 1949;31A:400.

11. Newman PH. Symposium on lumbosacral fusion and low back pain. J Bone Joint Surg. 1955;37B:164.

12. Shaw EG, Taylor JG. The results of lumbosacral fusion for low back pain. J Bone Joint Surg. 1956;38B:485–97.

13. Eriksen B. Lumbosacral fusion. J Bone Joint Surg. 1960;42B:660.

14. Watkins MB. Posterolateral fusion of the lumbar and lumbosacral spine. J Bone Joint Surg. 1953;35A:1014.

15. Adkins EW. Lumbosacral arthrodesis after laminectomy. J Bone Joint Surg. 1955;37B:208.

16. Cloward RB. The treatment of ruptured lumbar intervertebral discs by ven- tral fusion: indications, operative technique, after care. J Neurosurg. 1953;10:154.

17. James A, Nesbit NW. Posterior intervertebral fusion of the lumbar spine: preliminary report of a New operation. J Bone Joint Surg. 1953;35B:181.

18. Mercer W. Spondylolisthesis. Edinburgh Med J NS. 1936;43:545.

19. Harmon PH. Anterior extraperitoneal lumbar disk excision and vertebral body fusion. ClinOrthop. 1961;18:169.

20. Freebody D, Bendall R, Taylor RD. Anterior transperitoneal lumbar fusion. J Bone Joint Surg Br. 1971;53(4):617–27.

21. King D. Internal fixation for lumbosacral fusion. J Bone Joint Surg. 1948;30A:560.

22. Boucher HH. A method of spinal fusion. J Bone Joint Surg. 1959;41B:248–59.

23. Nelson MA. A long-term review of posterior fusion of the lumbar spine. Proc Roy Soc Med. 1968; 61:558–9.

24. Stauffer RN, Coventry MB. Posterolateral lumbar-spine fusion. Analysis of mayo clinic series. J Bone Joint Surg Am. 1972;54(6):1195–204.

25. Harrington PR. Treatment of scoliosis. Correction and internal fixation by spine instrumentation. J Bone Joint Surg Am. 1962;44-A:591–610.

26. Luque ER. Segmental spinal instrumentation for cor-rection of scoliosis. Clin Orthop Relat Res. 1982;163:192–8.

27. Luque ER. The anatomic basis and development of segmental spinal instrumentation. Spine. 1982;7(3): 256–9.

28. Dove J. Internal fixation of the lumbar spine. The hartshill rectangle. Clin Orthop Relat Res. 1986;203:135–40.

29. Cotrel Y, Dubousset J. Nouvelle technique d'ostheosynthèse rachidienne sègmentaire par voie postèrieure. Rev Chir Orthop. 1984;70:489–95.

30. Roy-Camille R, Saillant G, Mazel C. Plating of tho-racic, thoracolumbar, and lumbar injuries with pedi-cle screw plates. Orthop Clin North Am. 1986;17(1):147–59.

31. Roy-Camille R, Saillant G, Mazel C. Internal fixation of the lumbar spine with pedicle screw plating. Clin Orthop Relat Res. 1986;203:7–17.

32. Steffee AD, Sitkowski DJ, Topham LS. Total vertebral body and pedicle arthroplasty. Clin Orthop Relat Res. 1986;203:203–8 instrumentation for scoliosis deformities. Clin Orthop Relat Res 264:103–110.

33. Sidhu KS, Herkowitz HN. Spinal instrumentation in the management of degenerative disorders of the lum-bar spine. Clin Orthop Relat Res. 1997;335:39–53.

34. Brox JI, Sørensen R, Friis A, Nygaard Ø, Indahl A, Keller A, Ingebrigtsen T, Eriksen HR, Holm I, Koller AK, Riise R, Reikerås O. Randomized clinical trial of lumbar instrumented fusion and cognitive intervention and exercises in patients with chronic low back pain and disc degeneration. Spine. 2003;28(17):1913–21.

35. Fischgrund JS, Mackay M, Herkowitz HN, Brower R, Montgomery DM, Kurz LT. Volvo award winner in clinical studies. Degenerative lumbar spondylo-listhesis with spinal stenosis: a prospective,

randomized study comparing decompressive laminectomy and arthrodesis with and without spinal instrumentation. Spine. 1997;22(24):2807–12.

36. Kornblum MB, Fischgrund JS, Herkowitz HN, Abraham DA, Berkower DL, Ditkoff JS. Degenerative lumbar spondylolisthesis with spinal stenosis: a prospective long-term study comparing fusion and pseudarthrosis. Spine. 2004;29(7):726–33 (Phila Pa 1976).

37. Briggs H, Milligan P. Chip fusion of the low back following exploration of the spinal canal. J Bone Joint Surg. 1944;26:125–30.

38. Jaslow I. Intracorporeal bone graft in spinal fusion after disc removal. Surg Gynecol Obstet. 1946;82:215–22.

39. Cloward RB. Spondylolisthesis: treatment by laminectomy and posterior interbody fusion: review of 100 cases. Clin Orthop. 1981;154:74–82.

40. Cloward RB. Posterior lumbar interbody fusion updated. Clin Orthop Relat Res. 1985;193:16–9.

41. Brantigan JW, Steffee AD, Geiger JM. A carbon fiber implant to aid interbody lumbar fusion. Mechanical testing. Spine. 1991;16:S277–82.

42. Ray CD. Threaded titanium cages for lumbar interbody fusions. Spine. 1997;22:667–79.

43. Bagby G. The bagby and kuslich (BAK) method of lumbar interbody fusion. Spine. 1999;24:1857.

44. Wagner P, Grant B, Bagby G. Evaluation of cervical spinal fusion as a treatment in the equine "wobbler" syndrome. Vet Surg. 1979;8:84–9.

45. Harms JG, Jeszenszky D. Die posteriore, lumbale, interkorporelle fusion in unilateraler transforaminaler technik. Oper Orthop Traumatol. 1998;10:90–102. (German).

46. Capener N. Spondylolisthesis. Br J Surg. 1932;19:374.

47. Burns BH. An operation for spondylolisthesis. Lancet. 1933;1:1233.

48. Sacks S. Anterior interbody fusion of the lumbar spine. J Bone Joint Surg. 1965;47:2ll–23.

49. Stauffer RN, Coventry MB. Anterior interbody lumbar spine fusion: analysis of mayo clinic series. J Bone Joint Surg Am. 1972;54:756–68.

50. Mayer HM. A new microsurgical technique for minimally invasive anterior lumbar interbody fusion. Spine. 1997;22(6):691–9 (Phila Pa 1976), ; discussion 700.

51. Strube P, Hoff E, Hartwig T, Perka CF, Gross C, Putzier M. Stand-alone anterior versus anteroposterior lumbar interbody single-level fusion after a mean follow-up of 41 months. J Spinal Disord Tech. 2012;25(7):362–9.

52. Weatherley CR, Prickett CF, O'Brien JP. Discogenic pain persisting despite posterior fusion. JBJS. 1986;68-B(1):142–3.

53. Ozgur BM, Aryan HE, Pimenta L, Taylor WR. Extreme lateral interbody fusion (XLIF): a novel surgical technique for anterior lumbar interbody fusion. Spine J. 2006;6(4):435–43.

54. Fairbank J, Frost H, Wilson-MacDonald J, Ly-Mee Y, Barker K, Collins R. Randomised controlled trial to compare surgical stabilisation of the lumbar spine with an intensive rehabilitation programme for patients with chronic low back pain: the MRC spine stabilisation trial. BMJ. 2005;330(7502):1233.

55. Fritzell P, Hägg O, Wessberg P, Nordwall A. Chronic low back pain and fusion: a comparison of three surgical techniques: a prospective multicenter randomized study from the Swedish lumbar spine study group. Spine. 2002;27:1131–41.

56. Mayer HM. Total lumbar disc replacement. J Bone Joint Surg Br. 2005;87-B:1029–37.

57. Harmon P. Anterior excision and vertebral body fusion operation for intervertebral disk syndromes of the lower lumbar spine: three-to five-year results in 244 cases. Clin Orthop Relat Res. 1963;26:107–27.

58. Fernstrom U. Arthroplasty with intercorporal endoprosthesis in herniated disc and in painful disc. Acta Chir Scand. 1966;357:154–9.

59. Siemionow KB, Hu X, Lieberman IH. The fernstrom ball revisited. Eur Spine J. 2012;21(3):443–8.

60. Van Ooij A, Oner FC, Verbout AJ. Complications of artificial disc replacement: a report of 27 patients with the SB Charité disc. J Spinal Disord Tech. 2003;16:369–83.

61. Büttner-Janz K. The development of the artificial disc: SB charité. Dallas: Huntley & Associates; 1992.

62. Marnay T. The ProDisc: clinical analysis of an intervertebral disc implant. In: Kaech DL, Jinkins JR, editors. Spinal restabilization procedures. Amsterdam: Elsevier Science BV; 2002. p. 317–31.

63. Tropiano P, Huang RC, Girardi FP, Marnay T. Lumbar disc replacement: preliminary results with ProDisc II after a minimum follow-up period of 1 year. J Spinal Disord Tech. 2003;16:362–8.

64. Le Huec JC, Aunoble S, Friesem T, Mathews H, Zdeblick T. Maverick total lum- bar disk prosthesis: biomechanics and preliminary clinical results. In: Gunzburg R, Mayer HM, Szpalski M, Aebi M, editors. Arthroplasty of the spine. Berlin: Springer-Verlag; 2004. p. 53–8.

65. Biyani A, Andersson GB. Low back pain: pathophysiology and management. J Am Acad Orthop Surg. 2004;12:106–15.

66. Burke JG, Watson RWG, McCormack D, et al. Intervertebral discs which cause low back pain secrete high levels of proinflammatory mediators. J Bone Joint Surg Br. 2002;84-B:196–201.

67. Hadjipavlou AG, Tzermiadianos MN, Bogduk N, Zindrick MR. The pathophysiology of disc degeneration. A critical review. J Bone Joint Surg Br. 2008;90-B:1261–70.

68. Peng B, Wu W, Hou S, Li P, Zhang C, Yang Y. The pathogenesis of discogenic low back pain. J Bone Joint Surg Br. 2005;87-B:62–7.

69. Carragee E, Alamin T, Carragee J, Van der Haak E. Clinical outcomes after solid ALIF for presumed lumbar 'discogenic' pain in highly selected patients: an indirect indication of diagnostic failure.

Annual meeting of the International Society for the Study of the Lumbar Spine. Porto: Portugal, 2004.

70. Aprill C, Bogduk N. High intensity zone: a diagnostic sign of painful lumbar disc on magnetic resonance imaging. Br J Radiol. 1992;65:361–9.

71. Turner JA, Ersek M, Herron L. Patient outcomes after lumbar spinal fusions. JAMA. 1992;268:907–11.

72. Gillet P. The fate of the adjacent motion segments after lumbar fusion. J Spinal Disord Tech. 2003;16:338–45.

73. Etebar S, Cahill DW. Risk factors for adjacent segment failure following lumbar fixation with rigid instrumentation for degenerative instability. J Neurosurg. 1999;90:163–9.

74. Ghiselli G, Wang JC, Bhatia NN, Wellington KH, Dawson EG. Adjacent segment degeneration in the lumbar spine. J Bone Joint Surg Am. 2004;86: 1497–503.

75. van den Eerenbeemt KD, Ostelo RW, van Royen BJ, Peul WC, van Tulder MW. Total disc replacement surgery for symptomatic degenerative lumbar disc disease: a systematic review of the literature. Eur Spine J. 2010;19:1262–80.

76. Galbusera F, Bellini CM, Zweig T, Ferguson S, Raimondi MT, Lamartina C, Brayda-Bruno M, Fornari M. Design concepts in lumbar total disc arthroplasty. Eur Spine J. 2008;17:1635–50.

77. David T. Long-term results of One-level lumbar arthroplasty minimum 10-year follow-up of the charite'artificial disc in 106 patients. Spine. 2007;32(6):661–6.

78. McAfee P, Cunningham B, Holsapple G, Adams K, Blumenthal S, Guyer RD, Dmietriev A, Maxwell Regan JJ, Isaza J. A prospective, randomized, multicenter food and drug administration investigational device exemption study of lumbar total disc replacement with the CHARITÉ™ artificial disc *versus* lumbar fusion part II: evaluation of radiographic outcomes and correlation of surgical technique accuracy with clinical outcomes. Spine. 2005;30(14):1576–83.

79. Katsimihas M, Bailey CB, Issa K, Fleming J, Rosas-Arellano P, Bailey SI. Prospective clinical and radiographic results of CHARITÉ III artificial total disc arthroplasty at 2- to 7-year follow-up: a Canadian experience. J Can Chir. 2010;53(6): 408–4145.

80. Cinotti G, David T, Postacchini F. Results of disc prosthesis after a minimum follow-up period of two years. Spine. 1996;21:995–1000.

81. Bertagnoli R, Kumar S. Indications for full prosthetic disc arthroplasty: a correlation of clinical outcome against a variety of indications. Eur Spine J. 2002;11: S130–6.

82. Putzier M, Funk JF, Schneider SV, Gross C, Tohtz SW, Khodadadyan-Klostermann C. Charité total disc replacement—clinical and radiographical results after an average follow-up of 17 years. Eur Spine J. 2006;15:183–95.

83. Lemaire J, Carrier H, Ali E, Skalli W, Lavaste F. Clinical and radiological outcomes with the Charité TM artificial disc 10-year minimum follow-Up. J Spinal Disord Tech. 2005;18(4):353–9.

84. Harrop JS, Youssef JA, Maltenfort M, Vorwald P, Jabbour P, Bono CM, Goldfarb N, Vaccaro AR, Hilibrand AS. Lumbar adjacent segment degeneration and disease after arthrodesis and total disc arthroplasty. Spine. 2008;33(15):1701–7.

85. Brantigan JW, Neidre A, Toohey JS. The lumbar I/F cage for posterior lumbar interbody fusion with the variable screw placement system: 10-year results of a food and drug administration clinical trial. Spine J. 2004;4:681–8.

86. Hassett G, Hart DJ, Manek NJ, et al. Risk factors for progression of lumbar spine disc degeneration: the Chingford study. Arthritis Rheum. 2003;48: 3112–7.

87. Huang RC, Girardi FP, Cammisa FP, et al. Correlation between range of motion and outcome after lumbar total disc replacement: 8.6-Year follow-up. Spine. 2005;30:1407–11.

88. Dooris AP, Goel VK, Grosland NM, Gilbertson LG, Wilder DG. Load-sharing between anterior and posterior elements in a lumbar motion segment implanted with an artificial disc. Spine. 2001;26(6): E122–9.

89. Lemaire JP, Skalli W, Lavaste F, Templier A, Mendes F, Diop A, Sauty V, Laloux E. Intervertebral disc prosthesis. Results and prospects for the year 2000. Clin Orthop. 1997;337:64–76.

90. Turner JA, Herron L, Deyo RA. Meta-analysis of the results of lumbar spine fusion. Acta Orthop Scand. 1993;64 Suppl 251:120–2.

91. Punt IM, Visser VM, van Rhijn LW, Kurtz SM, Antonis J, Schurink GW, van Ooij A. Complications and reoperations of the SB Charité lumbar disc prosthesis: experience in 75 patients. Eur Spine J. 2008;17:36–43.

92. Hedman TP, Kostuik JP, Fernie GR, Hellier WG. Design of an intervertebral disc prosthesis. Spine. 1991;16(6 Suppl):S256–60 (Phila Pa 1976).

93. Penta M, Fraser RD. Anterior lumbar interbody fusion. A minimum 10-year follow-up. Spine. 1997;22(20):2429–34 (Phila Pa 1976).

94. Sasso RC, Kenneth Burkus J, LeHuec JC. Retrograde ejaculation after anterior lumbar interbody fusion: transperitoneal versus retroperitoneal exposure. Spine. 2003;28(10):1023–6.

95. Gornet MF, Burkus JK, Harper ML, Chan FW, Skipor AK, Jacobs JJ. Prospective study on serum metal levels in patients with metal-on-metal lumbar disc arthroplasty. Eur Spine J. 2012;22:741–6.

96. van Ooij A, Kurtz SM, Stessels F, Noten H, van Rhijn L. Polyethylene wear debris and long-term clinical failure of the charite' disc prosthesis a study of 4 patients. Spine. 2007;32(2):223–9.

97. Blumenthal S, McAfee PC, Guyer RD, Hochschuler SH, Geisler FH, Holt RT, Garcia R,

Regan JJ, Ohnmeiss DD. A prospective, randomized, multicenter food and drug administration investigational device exemptions study of lumbar total disc replacement with the CHARITÉ™ artificial disc *versus* lumbar fusion part I: evaluation of clinical outcomes. Spine. 2005;30(14): 1565–75.

98. Zigler J, Delamarter R, Spivak JM, Linovitz RJ, Danielson 3rd GO, Haider TT, Cammisa F, Zuchermann J, Balderston R, Kitchel S, Foley K, Watkins R, Bradford D, Yue J, Yuan H, Herkowitz H, Geiger D, Bendo J, Peppers T, Sachs B, Girardi F, Kropf M, Goldstein J. Results of the prospective, randomized, multicenter food and drug administration investigational device exemption study of the ProDisc-L total disc replacement versus circumferential fusion for the treatment of 1-level degenerative disc disease. Spine. 2007;32(11):1155–62.

99. Guyer RD, McAfee PC, Banco RJ, Bitan FD, Cappuccino A, Geisler FH, et al. Prospective, randomized, multicenter food and drug administration investigational device exemption study of lumbar total disc replacement with the Charité artificial disc versus lumbar fusion: five-year follow-up. Spine J. 2009;9:374–86.

100. Berg S, Tullberg T, Branth B, Olerud C, Tropp H. Total disc replacement compared to lumbar fusion: a randomised controlled trial with 2-year follow-up. Eur Spine J. 2009;18:1512–9.

101. Hellum C, Johnsen LG, Storheim K, Nygaard OP, Brox JI, Rossvol I, Rø M, Sandvik L, Grundnes O. Surgery with disc prosthesis versus rehabilitation in patients with low back pain and degenerative disc: two year follow-up of randomised study. BMJ. 2011;342:2786.

102. Pastefanou SL, Stevens K, Mulholland RC. Femoral nerve palsy. An unusual complication of anterior lumbar interbody fusion. Spine. 1994;19(24): 2842–4.

103. Jasani V, Jaffray D. The anatomy of the iliolumbar vein. A cadaver study. J Bone Joint Surg. 2002; 84-B(7):1046–9.

Spinal Osteotomy – Indications and Techniques

Enric Cáceres Palou

Contents

Abstract

Corrective osteotomies are used to treat sagittal and coronal imbalance of the spine in patients with a variety of spinal deformities. It is important to be able to recognize the type and underlying cause of the deformity so that the most appropriate osteotomy can be chosen.

The *Smith-Petersen osteotomy* is relatively simple compared with the other osteotomies and can typically be used to treat type-1 deformities. Also, curves that have a relatively smooth kyphosis instead of a sharp angular kyphosis can be treated with a Smith-Petersen osteotomy. Multiple Smith-Petersen osteotomies can be used to achieve the necessary amount of correction.

Pedicle subtraction osteotomy is typically used in patients with greater imbalances in the sagittal plane of the spine and when a minimum of 30° of correction is needed.

Vertebral column resection is reserved for deformities, such as those in both the sagittal and the coronal plane, that are not amenable to treatment with either a Smith-Petersen osteotomy or a pedicle subtraction osteotomy, or a combination of the two.

Recent results have shown high patient satisfaction rates and good functional outcomes after spinal osteotomies done to treat a variety of disorders. As the level of complexity of the osteotomy increases, so does the potential for complications.

E.C. Palou
Department Hospital Vall d'Hebron, Autonomous
University of Barcelona, Barcelona, Spain
e-mail: ecaceres@vhebron.net

G. Bentley (ed.), *European Surgical Orthopaedics and Traumatology*,
DOI 10.1007/978-3-642-34746-7_223, © EFORT 2014

Keywords

Complications • Indications • Osteotomy-Smith-Peterson, pedicle subtraction, vertebral column resection • Spine • Techniques

Introduction

Most patients with spinal sagittal imbalance have a fusion mass that is either kyphotic or hypolordotic, with segments above or below the fusion that have subsequently degenerated. The four most common presentations include a patient who had a long fusion for adolescent idiopathic scoliosis with subsequent degeneration distally; a patient with degenerative sagittal imbalance in whom fusions have initially been performed in the distal lumbar spine in a somewhat hypolordotic or kyphotic position with subsequent degeneration of segments above the fusion; a patient with post-traumatic kyphosis; and a patient with an ankylosing spondylitis.

The surgical solutions usually involve a combination of osteotomies through the fusion mass and extension of the fusion to include degenerated segments.

The usual goal is to normalize the regional segmental spinal alignment as much as possible and to achieve global balance. Global balance is confirmed when the C7 plumb line falls over the lumbosacral discon a standing long lateral radiograph.

Most patients should have at least 10–20° more lumbar lordosis than thoracic kyphosis. Usually a Smith-Petersen osteotomy will achieve 10° of correction and a pedicle subtraction osteotomy will produce 30–35° of lordosis of the spine.

Sagittal Imbalance

Sagittal balance is most frequently defined by the position of the C7 plumb line on a standing lateral radiograph (Fig. 1). When a C7 plumb line is dropped, neutral balance is suggested if the plumb line falls through the lumbosacral disc. If the C7 plumb line falls behind the lumbosacral disc; sagittal balance is defined as negative, whereas if it falls in front of the lumbosacral disc it is positive. The most commonly used specific reference point for the C7 plumb line is the posterior aspect of the L5-S 1 disc. Most investigators consider normal sagittal balance as the C7 plumb line falling through disc or 2 on in front 01' behind it. It is known that the C7 plumb line and the centres of gravity are not identical. In most circumstances the centre of gravity falls in front of the C7 plumb line and slightly behind the hip joints. There is a range of sagittal imbalance (Fig. 1). Booth and associates [1] refer to a type 1 imbalance as a segmental kyphosis, with global balance in which the C7 plumb line (on a long cassette standing radiograph) falls over the lumbosacral disc. Patients with this type of imbalance frequently have to hyperextend segments above or below the kyphosis to maintain balance. It is believed that this compensatory mechanism predisposes the patient to accelerated disc degeneration. In a type II sagittal imbalance, the C7 plumb is so far anterior to the lumbosacral disc that the patient is not able to compensate to maintain global balance. In this situation, there is usually substantial disc degeneration above or below an area of prior fusion or pathology that makes it impossible for the patient to hyperextend segments enough to maintain balance. Sagittal imbalance is the most poorly tolerated and debilitating form of adult deformity. The intersection between this line and a line that is perpendicular to the L5-S 1 endplate determines the pelvic incidence.

Initial Work-Up

When a patient has a substantial deformity, the initial work-up always includes an assessment of flexibility of the spine. This can be determined both clinically and radiographically. At times, if a patient stands with a sagittal imbalance, the surgeon may find that if the patient

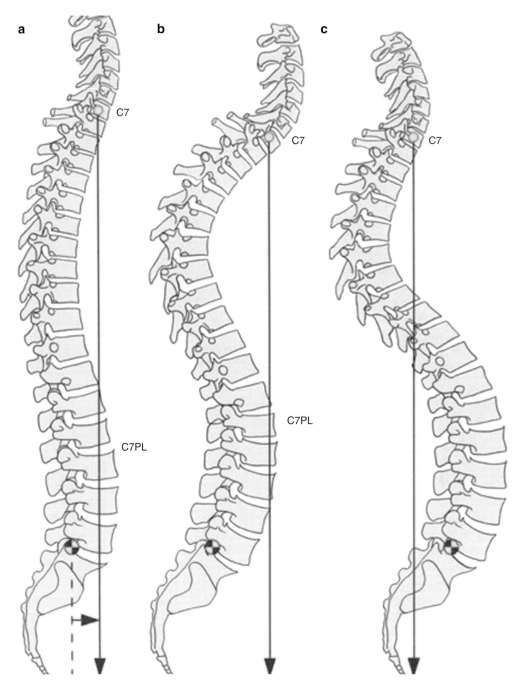

a

C7

C7PL

b

C7

C7PL

c

C7

Fig. 1 (**a**) The spine is sagittally balanced when the plumb line from C7 touches the posterior edge of S1. (**b**) Spinal imbalance is positive when the line falls in front of this point. (**c**) It is negative when the plumb line falls behind this point

lies supine or prone, this imbalance corrects to some extent through mobile segments. Therein, part of the assessment is to compare standing long-cassette anteroposterior and lateral radiographs to either long-cassette anteroposterior and lateral supine or prone radiographs. The patient's spine will fall into one of three categories:

1. Totally flexible, meaning that the spinal deformity corrects simply by being in a supine or prone unweight position;
2. A deformity that partially corrects through mobile segments, but not entirely.
3. A totally inflexible deformity with no correction in the recumbent position, meaning that the spine is entirely fused throughout the thoracic and lumbar spine.

Fixed sagittal imbalance (a syndrome in which the patient is only able to stand with the weight-bearing line in front of the sacrum) has many aetiologies. The most commonly reported technique for correction is the Smith-Petersen osteotomy. Few reports on pedicle subtraction procedures (resection of the posterior elements, pedicles, and vertebral body through a posterior approach) are available in the peer-reviewed literature. We are aware of no report involving a substantial number of patients with co-existent scoliosis who underwent pedicle/vertebral body subtraction for the treatment of fixed sagittal imbalance.

Treatment of fixed sagittal imbalance involves performing osteotomies to shorten the spine. One option is to perform multiple Smith-Petersen procedures, which do not directly address the anterior column of the spine.

Many factors contribute to fixed sagittal imbalance. A hypolordotic or hyperkyphotic fusion mass with subsequent disk degeneration above or below the fusion is common. Subsequent disc degeneration leads to loss of anterior column height and increased kyphosis. In most patients, both ageing and iatrogenic factors contribute to fixed sagittal imbalance.

Assessment of Correction

Pelvic incidence
• Duval-Beaupère and associates defined the term "pelvic incidence" (Fig. 2). Pelvic incidence measures a combination of pelvic tilt and sacral slope. The higher the pelvic incidence the more lumbar lordosis a patient needs to maintain balance. A higher pelvic incidence is

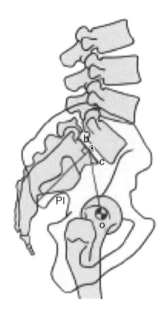

Fig. 2 Pelvic incidence (PI) is defined as the angle subtended by a line that is drawn from the centre of the femoral head to the mid-point of the sacral end-plate and a line perpendicular to the centre of the sacral end-plate

associated with a more horizontal sacrum: the hip joints are situated more anterior to the L5-S1 disc. The measurement of pelvic incidence is made by drawing a line between the mid-point of the L5-S1 disc connecting the mid-point of the femoral heads.

Thoracic kyphosis relative to lumbar lordosis
• There is a wide variation in the normal range of the measurements of thoracic kyphosis and lumbar lordosis. The middle of the bell-shaped curve is 30–35° of thoracic kyphosis measured from T5 to T12 and 55–60° of lumbar lordosis measured from T12 to the sacrum. Lumbar lordosis usually begins at T12-L1. Between two-thirds and three-fourths of lumbar lordosis is located in the distal two discs. However, there is substantial individual variation. If a patient has only 10° of thoracic lordosis, then less lumbar lordosis is required to maintain balance. One guideline is that the measurement of lumbar lordosis from T12 to S1

should exceed the measurement of thoracic kyphosis from T5 to T12 by at least 10–20°.

The C7 plumb line
• The C7 plumb line will be affected by the patient's positioning. When a long cassette lateral radiograph is taken, the patient is usually asked to extend the shoulders and arms out in front of the trunk to allow the spine to be seen on the radiograph. This positioning may have a tendency to posteriorly displace the C7 plumb line. The effect of arm position on the C7 plumb line was studied and it was concluded that a position in which the shoulders are flexed approximately 30° and the fists are placed in the supraclavicular fossa was the most desirable position to allow for visualization of the anatomical landmarks. The C7 plumb line is the best assessment for sagittal balance, but it is not perfect because it does not always directly correlate with the centre of gravity, which is the element that is actually being assessed. A patient's centre of gravity should always fall either through the hip joints or somewhat behind it.

Deformity Correction

Most spinal osteotomies are based on a combination of two traditional osteotomies: the Smith-Peterson and the pedicle subtraction osteotomies. Both techniques were originally described for the management of flexion deformities that occurred in rheumatoid and ankylosing spondylitis patients and have since been extensively modified. Frequently, as in patients with unsegment bars; an asymmetric osteotomy aimed at addressing the specific vertebral anomaly should be designed as necessary. A thin-slice or spiral CT scan is essential for preoperative surgical planning, which can be performed through either a single posterior approach or a combined approach. The inherent neurologic risks of such techniques must be well understood before undertaking such a procedure. Placement of segmental instrumentation for

provisional stabilization prior to completing the osteotomy can help to reduce the risk of uncontrolled translation of the spine with corresponding neurologic injury.

Smith-Petersen Osteotomy (Posterior Element Wedge Resection)

Smith-Petersen et al. first described this osteotomy as an operative technique for the treatment of kyphotic deformity caused by ankylosing spondylitis [4] (Fig. 3). Smith-Petersen et al. recommended a single-stage posterior wedge resection of the mid-lumbar spine in a chevron arrangement with controlled fracturing of the ossified anterior longitudinal ligament.

Surgical Technique
Like all osteotomies, the Smith-Petersen osteotomy can be performed on an open-frame spine table and should take advantage of any flexibility in the deformity. The hips of the patient may need to be flexed initially and then extended to help close the osteotomy site. Once the appropriate level for the Smith-Petersen osteotomy is identified, the lamina, ligamentum flavum, and superior and inferior articular processes are removed bilaterally. Typically, the width of the osteotomy is 7–10 mm. A rough guideline to follow is that every 1 mm. of resection results in 1° of correction, resulting in approximately 10° of correction at each level at which the Smith-Petersen osteotomy is performed. An open disc space is a prerequisite for closure of the Smith-Petersen osteotomy site. If the disc is collapsed, then it may limit the amount of correction that can be obtained. Additionally, a Smith-Petersen osteotomy cannot be done at a level at which a spinal arthrodesis has been previously performed, since the disc is no longer mobile. Once the osteotomy site has been closed with the aid of rods and pedicle screws, through gradual compression, it is important to ensure that the neural elements are free and not compressed in the osteotomy site.

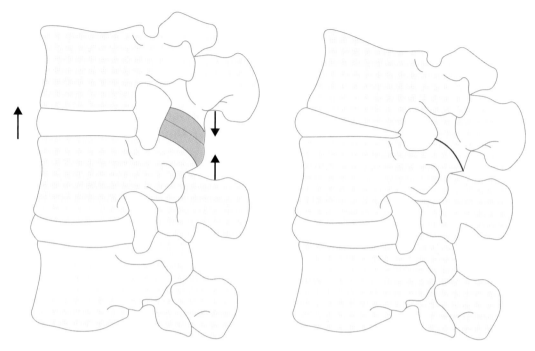

Fig. 3 Smith-Petersen osteotomy

The lumbar region is more favourable than the thoracic, since the latter commonly presents ankylosedcostovertebral joints rendering correction difficult, if notimpossible. Selection of the lumbar level or levels at which the osteotomy is to be performed depends on the roentgenographic findings; the less marked the ossification, the better the chanceof correction.

Pedicle Subtraction Osteotomy

Another option is to perform a pedicle subtraction osteotomy, which usually achieves about 30° of lordosis (Fig. 4). Performance of that procedure amounts to performing two Smith-Petersen osteotomies as well as resection of the pedicles and vertebral body bilaterally from a posterior approach. This accomplishes approximately as much correction as can be achieved with three Smith-Petersen osteotomies, but it is technically much more demanding. The advantage of the pedicle subtraction osteotomy is that, when

the osteotomy is completed, there is bone-on-bone contact throughout all three columns of the spine.

Surgical Technique

Step 1: Prior to the initiation of the osteotomy, the fixation points should be placed (Fig. 5). Next, a laminectomy is performed and the necessary posterior elements are resected. If there is no coronal plane deformity, the wedge should be made symmetrically on both sides. When resecting the posterior elements, the surgeon should start off using hand instruments such as Leksell rongeurs, osteotomes, and curettes to try to retain as much bone graft as possible. Then, if needed, a high-speed air-drill is used to thin the posterior elements. Finally, a Kerrison rongeur is used to surround the pedicles. The first step of surrounding the pedicles is to resect bone centrally and then to perform, in essence, a Smith-Petersen osteotomy both cephalad to and caudad to the pedicles on both sides. This involves

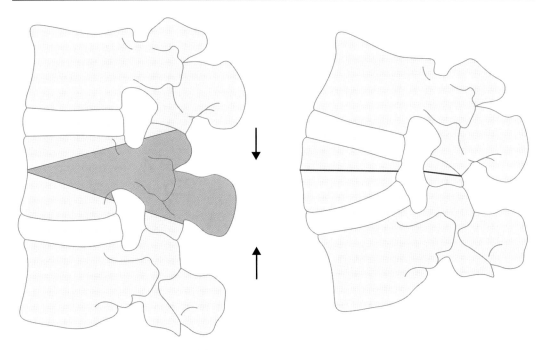

Fig. 4 Pedicle Substraction Ostetomy (PSO)

exposing the nerve root caudad to the pedicle, which, in the case illustrated, is the L3 nerve root. As the pedicles are circumferentially surrounded, they are detached from the transverse processes.

Step 2: The next step is to "decancellate" the pedicles and vertebral body (Fig. 2). The medial wall of the pedicle is identified, and the thecal sac and the nerve root are retracted with a Penfield retractor to identify the posterior wall of the vertebral body. It is helpful to move straight and curved curettes and Woodson elevators back and forth from one side to the other until the resection of the vertebral body connects one side to the other. If there is bleeding from epidural vessels cephalad and caudad to the pedicles, it is best controlled with a surface haemostatic agent and packing with "cottonoids". At this point of the procedure, one should try to preserve the medial wall of the pedicle.

Step 3: Next, the pedicle stump is resected on both sides flush with the vertebral body.

This is done with a combination of a Kerrison rongeur from within the pedicle and a thin Leksell rongeur from without. Care should be taken to retract the neural elements so that the exiting nerve root is not injured during the process.

Step 4: The next step is to finish the resection of the posterior wall of the vertebral body. Working underneath the posterior vertebral cortex, the surgeon thins the cortex as much as possible with curettes and Woodson elevators. Once the posterior wall of the vertebral body is thin enough, a Woodson elevator or a substantial reverse-angled curette is placed between the anterior dura and the posterior vertebral cortex and pushed anteriorly to create a greenstick fracture of the posterior vertebral cortex. The fractured posterior cortex is then removed. At this point, the osteotomy is still stable because the lateral vertebral body walls remain intact. The amount of the posterior wall that is removed should be asymmetrical.

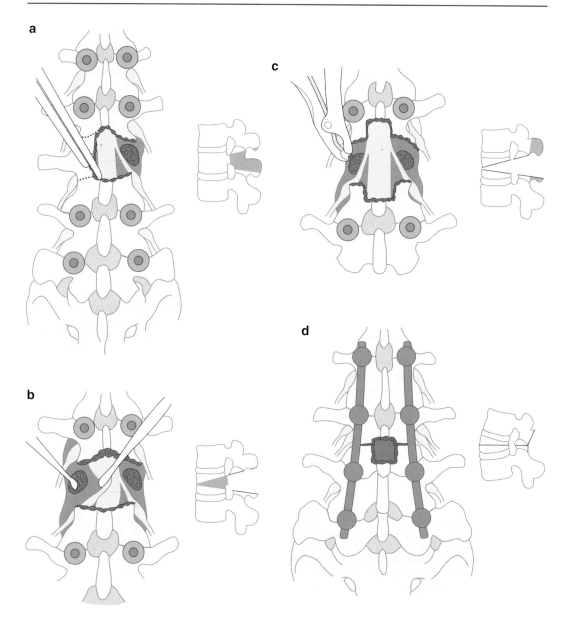

Fig. 5 (**a**) The initial resection of the posterior elements and surrounding of the pedicles. The amount of bone resected is demonstrated in the lateral view in this figure (**b**) Decancellation of the pedicles and the vertebral body.

(**c**) Resection of the lateral walls and central canal enlargement (**d**) Closure of the osteotomy and final instrumentation

Step 5: Next, the spinal canal is enlarged centrally somewhat more with use of Kerrison rongeurs, but the surgeon must be sure that the lateral masses remain symmetrical. In preparation for resection of the lateral vertebral body walls, the surgeon first dissects them with a small Cobb or Penfield elevator.

The lateral vertebral cortex should be hugged during the dissection so that the segmental vessel is not injured. Then, a rongeur is used to resect the lateral vertebral body walls down to, but not through, the anterior cortex. Once this is accomplished on both sides, the osteotomy is complete.

Step 6: The final step is to close the osteotomy. Depending on the circumstances, this can be accomplished by either applying compression or cantilevering the spine. Also, hyperextending the patient's chest and lower extremities may accomplish closure. Sometimes, when this step is performed, subluxation occurs, most commonly with the proximal elements subluxating dorsally on the distal elements. If this does occur, the subluxation needs to be reduced anatomically as the final implants are placed. When the construct is complete and the osteotomy is closed on both sides, the spinal canal is dissected, first with a nerve hook and then with a Woodson elevator to confirm that there is no dorsal compression of the dural sac. The lateral masses should be squeezed together very tightly to promote stability and osteogenesis.

Vertebral Column Resection

Vertebral column resection has been described for the treatment of spinal column tumours (Fig. 6), spondyloptosis, and congenital kyphosis as well as for hemivertebrae excision. It is defined as a resection of one or more vertebral segments, including the posterior elements (spinous process and lamina), pedicles, vertebral body, and discs cephalad and caudad to the vertebral body. Vertebral column resection has been suggested for use in deformity-correcting operations when the deformity is not amenable to other osteotomy techniques such as the Smith-Petersen osteotomy or the pedicle subtraction osteotomy. The vertebral column resection is performed either through a combined anterior and posterior approach or through a posterior approach only.

Surgical Technique

First, the posterior elements (spinous process and lamina), including the pedicles, are removed. A wide lateral dissection to the transverse processes is done to facilitate the vertebral body resection. This wide lateral resection will avoid violation of the thecal sac when it is performed more cephalad than L2 and prevent excessive retraction on the thecal sac when it is performed caudad to L2. In the thoracic spine, costotransversectomies are performed to facilitate removal of the vertebral body. Unlike the previously discussed osteotomies, bone-on-bone contact is not achieved, as the vertebral body is completely removed. Therefore, reconstruction of the spinal column is needed after the deformity is corrected. A metal cage, structural autograft, or allograft may be used to reconstruct the vertebral column after correction of the deformity. This reconstruction of the vertebral column is supplemented with pedicle screws and rods. The instrumentation also helps to achieve the desired deformity correction once the vertebral column resection is done. Finally, an arthrodesis of the spine that is equal to the length of the instrumentation is done to further stabilize the spine.

In the Fig. 7 we can observe a PSO for a severe cervico-thoracic post-traumatic spine deformity.

Selection of the Appropriate Osteotomy and Spinal Level

Selecting the appropriate osteotomy and level at which to perform it is critical to the success of the procedure. The osteotomies are typically performed in the region of the relative kyphosis and maximal deformity, which can be in the cervical, thoracic, or lumbar spine [15]. The amount of correction needed can be estimated from the pre-operative radiographic measurements indicating the degree of curvature in the sagittal plane [6]. A Smith-Petersen osteotomy can be used if $<30°$ of correction is needed. A sagittal deformity that is combined with coronal imbalance is better treated with an asymmetric pedicle subtraction osteotomy or even a vertebral column resection so that the coronal deformity is corrected rather than exacerbated. The Smith-Petersen osteotomy or a symmetric pedicle subtraction osteotomy will correct the sagittal deformity and allow the coronal deformity to decompensate as these osteotomies

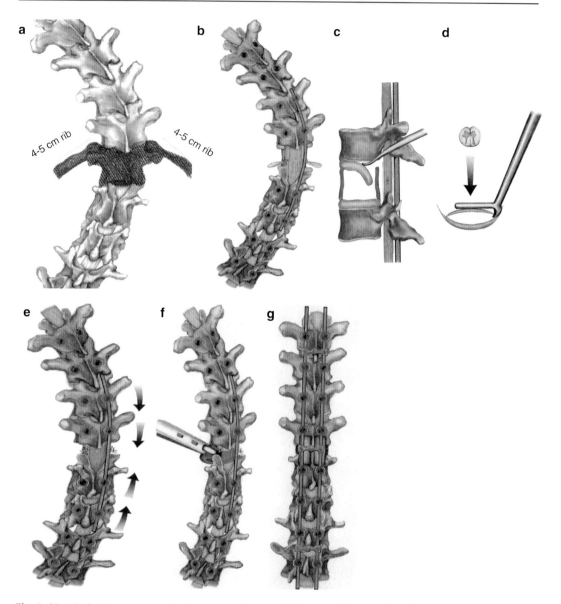

Fig. 6 Vertebral column resection. (**a**) In order to address the vertebral body above we resect about 3–5 cm. bilateral rib (**b**) Image of vertebral body resection by posterior approach (**c**) Discectomy above and below the osteotomy

(**d**) Image of impactation of vertebral body after bone resection (**e**) Concavity rod compression (**f**) Placement of an interbody cage (**g**) Final correction

cannot correct a coronal deformity. The level of the osteotomy is also important in that the more caudad the osteotomy, the fewer vertebrae there are for fixation, placing greater stress on the instrumentation and potentially leading to hardware failure prior to osseous union.

Once the selected osteotomy is done, an adequate number of vertebrae need to be included in the instrumentation and arthrodesis. Instrumentation that is too short (encompassing two or three vertebrae) may result in junctional kyphosis cephalad or caudad to the

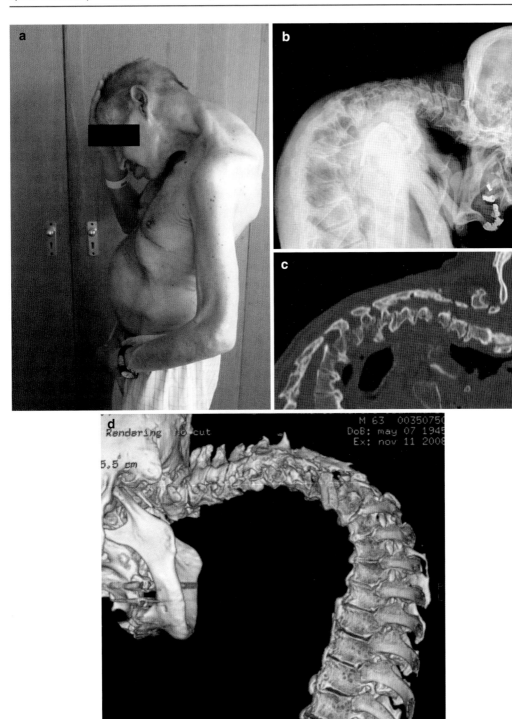

Fig. 7 (continued)

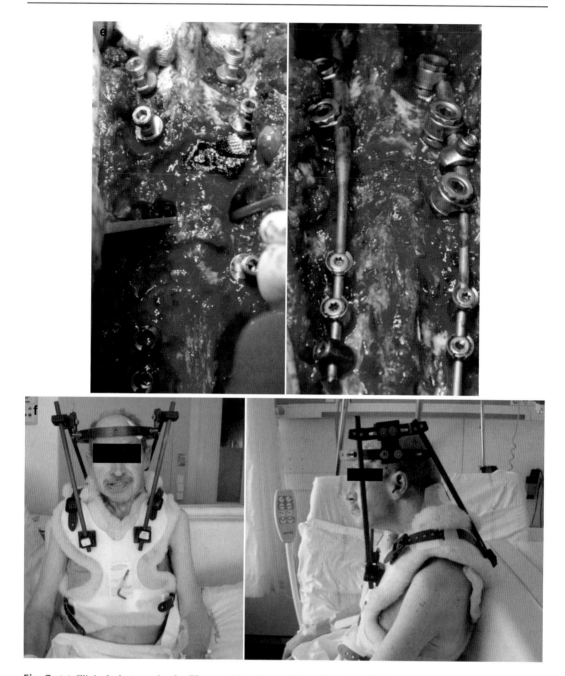

Fig. 7 (a) Clinical photograph of a 72 year old patient with severe cervico-thoracic coronal and sagittal deformity after polytrauma injury (b) Radiological image of the cervico-thoracic deformity (c) CT scan sagittal view (d) Three-dimensional CT reconstruction of the cervico-thoracic deformity (e) Intra-operative image of the pedicle subtraction osteotomy at T2 (f) Post-operative appearance after osteotomy

operative construct. Additionally, the operative construct should not end at the apex of the curve as this may exacerbate the curve or lead to loss of fixation. The caudad end of the construct should end, if possible, cephalad to the L5 vertebra, with the L4-L5 and L5-S1 disc spaces left open. A construct that ends at L5 may accelerate degeneration of the L5-S1 disc.

Indications for Specific Osteotomies

Smith-Petersen osteotomy
- Indications for the Smith-Petersen osteotomy depend on the extent of the deformity, the degree of functional impairment of the patient, the age and condition of the patient, and the feasibility of correction. The Smith-Petersen osteotomy is typically performed in the thoracic spine. In addition, multiple Smith-Petersen osteotomies can be done throughout the thoracic spine, and even the lumbar spine, to achieve the desired correction.
- Multiple Smith-Petersen osteotomies are very useful for treating a fixed imbalance in the sagittal plane of the spine caused by a loss of lumbar lordosis following operative treatment of spinal deformities, particularly idiopathic scoliosis. These patients were typically treated with a posterior distraction instrumentation system such as the Harrington rods [25]. Smith-Petersen osteotomies are also beneficial for patients with a degenerative imbalance in the sagittal plane of the spine. This condition typically occurs in the lumbar spine in older individuals (more than 50 years of age). These patients typically have substantial intervertebral disc collapse, facet arthropathy, and vertebral end-plate osteophytes causing the deformity.

Pedicle subtraction osteotomy
- The pedicle subtraction osteotomy is useful for treating patients with ankylosing spondylitis and an imbalance in the sagittal plane of the spine. Unlike the Smith-Petersen osteotomy, the pedicle subtraction osteotomy is mainly useful for deformities with an apex in the lumbar spine. The pedicle subtraction osteotomy is historically performed at L2 or L3, and an ideal candidate for the procedure typically has a positive sagittal imbalance of >12 cm. The pedicle subtraction osteotomy is also indicated for patients who have had a circumferential fusion along multiple vertebrae, which pre- vents the performance of a Smith-Petersen osteotomy since osteoclasis cannot be done through a fused intervertebral disc.

Vertebral column resection
- Patients with a severe and rigid imbalance in the sagittal plane of the spine that is not amenable to treatment with a Smith-Petersen osteotomy or a pedicle subtraction osteotomy are candidates for a vertebral column resection. A type-II sagittal deformity with coronal imbalance of the spine requires a vertebral column resection, as an asymmetric pedicle subtraction osteotomy would not fully correct the coronal deformity. Additional indications for a vertebral column resection include congenital kyphosis, a hemi- vertebra, L5 spondyloptosis, and resection of a spinal tumour.

Complications with Osteotomies

Spinal osteotomies are extensive and complex procedures. As the level of complexity increases, so does the risk of complications. As in any spinal procedure, major neurologic problems can occur, especially when there is manipulation of the foraminal space, retraction of the thecal sac and nerve roots, and shortening of the spinal column and segments. Therefore, it is important to perform proper spinal cord monitoring. A wake-up test after the osteotomy site has been closed may be the most accurate way to assess spinal cord and nerve root function.

A Smith-Petersen osteotomy shortens the posterior column while lengthening the anterior column. There is a concern that this could result in injury of the major vessels, particularly the abdominal aorta, although we are not aware of any reported case of an aortic injury. Specific to the Smith-Petersen osteotomy are complications such as intraspinal haematoma and intestinal obstruction or superior mesenteric artery syndrome. Cho et al. found that the most frequent complications after a Smith-Petersen osteotomy were superficial wound infections and substantial coronal imbalance of >4 cm.

when three or more Smith-Petersen osteotomies had been done.

Pedicle subtraction osteotomies are technically demanding and involve substantial mobilization of the dura, and the blood loss is greater than that associated with the Smith-Petersen osteotomy. A retrospective analysis of data obtained prospectively in a study of 46 patients who were 60 years of age or older showed that patients who underwent a pedicle subtraction osteotomy were seven times more likely to have at least one major complication compared with patients who underwent a different spinal procedure (odds ratio, 6.96; 95 % confidence interval, 1.10–79). Major complications included neurologic deficits; deep wound infection, pulmonary embolus, pneumonia, and myocardial infarction. Increasing age was a significant predictor of a complication ($p < 0.05$). The investigators concluded that the age at which patients are able to tolerate a major procedure such as a pedicle subtraction osteotomy might be lower than the age at which they can tolerate other common spinal procedures. Buchowski et al. reported the prevalence of intra-operative and post-operative neurological deficits to be 11.1 % and the prevalence of permanent deficits to be 2.8 % in a study of 108 patients who had undergone a pedicle subtraction osteotomy [3]. In a study by Bridwell et al., five (15 %) of 33 patients who had undergone a pedicle subtraction osteotomy for the treatment of an imbalance in the sagittal plane experienced a transient neurological deficit. In a recent retrospective study, Yang et al. found the prevalence of intra-operative or post-operative neurological deficits to be 4 % (1 of 28 patients) after lumbar or thoracic pedicle subtraction osteotomy for the treatment of an imbalance in the sagittal plane [42]. This single deficit was thought to be most likely due to nerve root compression.

In a cervical extension osteotomy, neurologic complications can arise from a variety of causes. When the osteotomy site is closed, neural elements including the spinal cord and nerve roots may be compressed if enough bone was not removed from the posterior elements (spinous process and lamina). Also, the C8 nerve roots may be compressed in their intervertebral foramen if not enough bone was removed from the pedicles cephalad and caudad to the osteotomy. In addition, instability and subluxation at the osteotomy site may lead to neurologic complications. If subluxation occurs, there is a high probability that it will lead to non-union at the osteotomy site, which may require an anterior spine arthrodesis [1].

Suk et al. retrospectively evaluated the complication rate following a vertebral column resection in 16 patients with rigid scoliosis [30]. Complications, including one complete paralysis, one haematoma, one haemopneumothorax, and one proximal junctional kyphosis, developed in four of these patients. In another retrospective study, a complication developed in 20 % (five) of 25 patients who had had a vertebral column resection to treat a fixed lumbosacral deformity.

The complications included two cases of radicular pain that resolved in 6 months, two compression fractures, and one pseudarthrosis. The investigators reported a mean blood loss of 2,810 mL (range, 320–5,460 mL), indicating that a substantial amount of blood loss can occur in association with this procedure.

Conclusions

Spinal deformities can result in increasing thoracic kyphosis or loss of lumbar lordosis, leading to imbalance in the sagittal plane. Such deformities can be functionally and psychologically debilitating. The Smith-Petersen osteotomy can achieve approximately 10° of correction in the sagittal plane at each spinal level at which it is performed. This osteotomy is beneficial for patients who have a degenerative imbalance in the sagittal plane. The pedicle subtraction osteotomy can achieve approximately 30–40° of correction in the sagittal plane at each spinal level at which it is performed. It is the preferred osteotomy for patients with ankylosing spondylitis who have an imbalance of the spine in the sagittal plane. The cervical extension osteotomy is performed in the cervical spine, at the cervico-thoracic junction, in patients who have a cervical flexion deformity that impedes their ability to look straight ahead while walking or who have difficulty swallowing. The vertebral column resection is used when the imbalance is severe enough that the other osteotomies cannot correct the deformity, especially in patients who have a combined sagittal and coronal spinal imbalance. Neurologic problems, whether transient or permanent, are the most commonly encountered complications following these procedures. Recent results have shown a high patient satisfaction rate and good functional outcomes after spinal osteotomies performed to treat a variety of disorders.

References

1. Booth KC, Bridwell KH, Lenke LG, Baldus CR, Blanke KM. Complications and predictive factors for the successful treatment of flatback deformity *fixed sagittal imbalance. Spine. 1999;24:1712–20.
2. Glassman SD, Berven S, Bridwell K, Horton W, Dimar JR. Correlation of radiographic parameters and clinical symptoms in adult scoliosis. Spine. 2005;30:682–8.
3. Duval-Beaupère G, Schimdt C, Cosson P. A barycentemetric study of sagittal shape of spine and pelvis: the conditions required for an economic standing position. Ann Biomed Eng. 1992;20:451–62.
4. Mac-Thiong J, Berthonnaud E, Dimar Jr II, Betz RR, Labelle H. Sagittal alignment of the spine and pelvis during growth. Spine. 2004;29:1642–7.
5. Legaye J, Duval-Beaupère G, Hecquet J, Marty C. Pelvic incidence: a fundamental pelvic parameter for three-dimensional regulation of sagittal curves. Eur Spine J. 1998;7:99–103.
6. Wambolt A, Spencer DL. A segmental analysis of the distribution of lumbar lordosis in the normal spine. Orthop Trans. 1987;11:92–3.
7. Hehne HJ, Zielke K, Bohm H. Polysegmental lumbar osteotomies and transpedicular fixation for correction of long-curved kyphotic defoprmities in ankylosing spondylitis: report of 177 cases. Clin Orthop. 1990;258:49–55.
8. Bernhard M, Bridwell KH. Segmental analysis of the sagittal plane alignment of the normal thoracic and lumbar spines and thoracolumbar junction. Spine. 1989;14:717–21.
9. Cho K, Bridwell KH, Reitenbach AK. Preoperative gait comparisons between adults undergoing long spinal deformity fusion surgery and controls. Spine. 2001;26:2020–8.
10. McMaster MJ. Osteotomy of the cervical spine in ankylosing spondylitis. J Bone Joint Surg Br. 1997;79:197–203.
11. Booth KC, Bridwell KH, Lenke LG, Baldus CR, Blanke KM. Complications and predictive factors for the successful treatment of flatback deformity (fixed sagital imbalance). Spine. 1999;24:1712–20.
12. Buchowski JM, Bridwell KH, Lenke LG, Kuhns CA, Lehman Jr RA, Kim YJ, Stewart D, Baldus C. Neurologic complications of lumbar pedicle subtraction osteotomy: a 10-year assessment. Spine. 2007;32:2245–52.
13. Smith-Petersen MN, Larson CB, Aufranc OE. Osteotomy of the spine for correction of flexion deformity in rheumatoid arthritis. J Bone Joint Surg Am. 1945;27:1–11.
14. Thomasen E. Vertebral osteotomy for correction of kyphosis in ankylosing spondylitis. Clin Orthop Relat Res. 1985;194:142–52.
15. Wang MY, Berven SH. Lumbar pedicle subtraction osteotomy. Neurosurgery. 2007;60(2 Suppl 1):ONS140–6.
16. Bridwell KH, Lewis SJ, Lenke LG, Baldus C, Blanke K. Pedicle subtraction osteotomy for the treatment of fixed sagittal imbalance. J Bone Joint Surg Am. 2003;85:454–63.
17. Bridwell KH, Lewis SJ, Rinella A, Lenke LG, Baldus C, Blanke K. Pedicle subtraction osteotomy for the treatment of fixed sagittal imbalance. Surgical technique. J Bone Joint Surg Am. 2004;86 Suppl 1:44–50.
18. Urist MR. Osteotomy of the cervical spine; report of a case of ankylosing rheumatoid spondylitis. J Bone Joint Surg Am. 1958;40:833–43.
19. Van Royen BJ, Slot GH. Closing-wedge posterior osteotomy for ankylosingspondylitis. Partial corporectomy and transpedicular fixation in 22 cases. J Bone Joint Surg Br. 1995;77:117–21.
20. Lazennec JY, Saillant G, Saidi K, Arafati N, Barabas D, Benazet JP, Laville C, Roy-Camille R, Ramaré S. Surgery of the deformities in ankylosing spondylitis: our experience of lumbar osteotomies in 31 patients. Eur Spine J. 1997;6:222–32.
21. Bridwell KH. Decision making regarding Smith-Petersen vs. pedicle subtraction osteotomy vs. vertebral column resection for spinal deformity. Spine. 2006;31(19 Suppl):S171–8.
22. Sansur CA, Fu KM, Oskouian Jr RJ, Jagannathan J, Kuntz 4th C, Shaffrey CI. Surgical management of global sagittal deformity in ankylosing spondylitis. Neurosurg Focus. 2008;24:E8.
23. Cho KJ, Bridwell KH, Lenke LG, Berra A, Baldus C. Comparison of Smith-Petersen versus pedicle subtraction osteotomy for the correction of fixed sagital imbalance. Spine. 2005;30:2030–8.
24. Kuklo TR, Bridwell KH, Lewis SJ, Baldus C, Blanke K, Iffrig TM, Lenke LG. Minimum 2-year analysis of sacropelvic fixation and L5-S1 fusion using S1 and iliac screws. Spine. 2001;26:1976–83.

25. Kornblatt MD, Casey MP, Jacobs RR. Internal fixation in lumbosacral spine fusion. A biomechanical and clinical study. Clin Orthop Relat Res. 1986;203:141–50.

26. Macagno AE, O'Brien MF. Thoracic and thoracolumbar kyphosis in adults. Spine. 2006;31(19 Suppl):S161–70.

27. Lebwohl NH, Cunningham BW, Dmitriev A, Shimamoto N, Gooch L, Devlin V, Boachie-Adjei O, Wagner TA. Biomechanical comparison of lumbosacral fixation techniques in a calf spine model. Spine. 2002;27:2312–20.

28. McCord DH, Cunningham BW, Shono Y, Myers JJ, McAfee PC. Biomechanical analysis of lumbosacral fixation. Spine. 1992;17(8 Suppl):S235–43.

29. Edwards 2nd CC, Bridwell KH, Patel A, Rinella AS, Jung Kim Y, Berra AB, Della Rocca GJ, Lenke LG. Thoracolumbar deformity arthrodesis to L5 in adults: the fate of the L5-S1 disc. Spine. 2003;28:2122–31.

30. Polly Jr DW, Hamill CL, Bridwell KH. Debate: to fuse or not to fuse to the sacrum, the fate of the L5-S1 disc. Spine. 2006;31(19 Suppl):S179–84.

31. Kuhns CA, Bridwell KH, Lenke LG, Amor C, Lehman RA, Buchowski JM, Edwards 2nd C, Christine B. Thoracolumbar deformity arthrodesis stopping at L5: fate of the L5-S1 disc, minimum 5-year follow-up. Spine. 2007;32:2771–6.

32. Lagrone MO, Bradford DS, Moe JH, Lonstein JE, Winter RB, Ogilvie JW. Treatment of symptomatic flatback after spinal fusion. J Bone Joint Surg Am. 1988;70:569–80.

33. Bridwell KH, Lewis SJ, Edwards C, Lenke LG, Iffrig TM, Berra A, Baldus C, Blanke K. Complications and outcomes of pedicle subtraction osteotomies for fixed sagittal imbalance. Spine. 2003;28:2093–101.

34. Berven SH, Deviren V, Smith JA, Emami A, Hu SS, Bradford DS. Management of fixed sagittal plane deformity: results of the transpedicular wedge resection osteotomy. Spine. 2001;26:2036–43.

35. Hoh DJ, Khoueir P, Wang MY. Management of cervical deformity in ankylosing spondylitis. Neurosurg Focus. 2008;24:E9.

36. Bradford DS, Tribus CB. Vertebral column resection for the treatment of rigid coronal decompensation. Spine. 1997;22:1590–9.

37. Suk SI, Chung ER, Kim JH, Kim SS, Lee JS, Choi WK. Posterior vertebral column resection for severe rigid scoliosis. Spine. 2005;30:1682–7.

38. Suk SI, Kim JH, Kim WJ, Lee SM, Chung ER, Nah KH. Posterior vertebral column resection for severe spinal deformities. Spine. 2002;27:2374–82.

39. Bradford DS, Boachie-Adjei O. One-stage anterior and posterior hemivertebral resection and arthrodesis for congenital scoliosis. J Bone Joint Surg Am. 1990;72:536–40.

40. Ponte A. Posterior column shortening for Scheuermann's kyphosis: an innovative one-stage technique. In: Haher TR, Merola AA, editors. Surgical techniques for the spine. New York: Thieme Medical; 2003. p. 107–13.

41. Geck MJ, Macagno A, Ponte A, Shufflebarger HL. The Ponte procedure: posterior only treatment of Scheuermann's kyphosis using segmental posterior shortening and pedicle screw instrumentation. J Spinal Disord Tech. 2007;20:586–93.

42. Kim YJ, Bridwell KH, Lenke LG, Cheh G, Baldus C. Results of lumbar pedicle subtraction osteotomies for fixed sagittal imbalance: a minimum 5-year follow-up study. Spine. 2007;32:2189–97.

43. Suk SI, Kim JH, Lee SM, Chung ER, Lee JH. Anterior-posterior surgery versus posterior closing wedge osteotomy in posttraumatic kyphosis with neurologic compromised osteoporotic fracture. Spine. 2003;28:2170–5.

44. Belanger TA, Milam 4th RA, Roh JS, Bohlman HH. Cervicothoracic extensión osteotomy for chin-on-chest deformity in ankylosing spondylitis. J Bone Joint Surg Am. 2005;87:1732–8.

45. Suk SI, Chung ER, Lee SM, Lee JH, Kim SS, Kim JH. Posterior vertebral column resection in fixed lumbosacral deformity. Spine. 2005;30:E703–10.

46. Adams JC. Technique, dangers and safeguards in osteotomy of the spine. J Bone Joint Surg Br. 1952;34:226–32.

47. McMaster MJ. A technique for lumbar spinal osteotomy in ankylosing spondylitis. J Bone Joint Surg Br. 1985;67:204–10.

48. Daubs MD, Lenke LG, Cheh G, Stobbs G, Bridwell KH. Adult spinal deformity surgery: complications and outcomes in patients over age 60. Spine. 2007;32:2238–44.

49. Yang BP, Ondra SL, Chen LA, Jung HS, Koski TR, Salehi SA. Clinical and radiographic outcomes of thoracic and lumbar pedicle subtraction osteotomy for fixed sagittal imbalance. J Neurosurg Spine. 2006;5:9–17.

Posterior Decompression for Lumbar Spinal Stenosis

Franco Postacchini and Roberto Postacchini

Contents

Keywords

Definition and classification • Microsurgery • Posterior decompression • Spinal stenosis • Surgical indications • Surgical treatment-decompression, laminectomy, laminotomy, spinal fusion

Definition of Lumbar Stenosis

Lumbar spinal stenosis can be defined as *an abnormal narrowing of the osteoligamentous vertebral canal and/or the intervertebral foramina, which is responsible for compression of the thecal sac and/or the caudal nerve roots; narrowing of the vertebral canal may involve one or more levels and, at a single level, may affect the entire canal or a part of it* [1]. Thus, abnormal narrowing of the spinal canal may be considered as stenosis if two criteria are fulfilled: the narrowing involves the osteoligamentous spinal canal and causes compression of the neural structures.

If the concept of stenosis is not limited to the osteoligamentous canal, even disc herniation in a normally-sized spinal canal might be considered a stenotic condition because it causes a pathological narrowing of the canal.

The second criterion emphasizes the concept of compression of the thecal sac and nerve roots. The term stenosis indicates a disproportion between the calibre of the container and the volume of the content. If the content is solid or semi-fluid, as in the vertebral canal, the dimensional disproportion results in compression of the content by the walls of

F. Postacchini (✉)
Department of Orthopaedic Surgery, University "Sapienza", Rome, Italy
e-mail: franco.postacchini@hotmail.com

R. Postacchini
Department Orthopaedic Surgery Israelitic Hospital, IUSM, Rome, Italy
e-mail: robby1478@hotmail.com

G. Bentley (ed.), *European Surgical Orthopaedics and Traumatology*,
DOI 10.1007/978-3-642-34746-7_37, © EFORT 2014

the container. If the narrowing is not severe enough to cause compression of the neural structures, the spinal canal should be considered narrow but not stenotic. Therefore, the diagnosis of stenosis cannot be based on measurements of the size of the vertebral canal or the area of the thecal sac in the axial sections. Diagnosis can be based only on the evidence of compression of the neural structures (symptomatic or asymptomatic) by an abnormally narrow osteoligamentous spinal canal (Fig. 1).

Classifications of Lumbar Stenosis

Site of Constriction

Lumbar stenosis can be distinguished as stenosis of the spinal canal, isolated stenosis of the nerve root canal, and stenosis of the intervertebral foramen [2].

In stenosis of the spinal canal, both the central portion of the canal and the lateral parts occupied by the emerging nerve roots, are usually constricted. Therefore, the expression stenosis of the spinal canal is more correct than that of central stenosis, which would indicate constriction only of the central area. However, the expression *central stenosis* will be used because it has become the one generally adopted. As a rule, central stenosis is located at the level of the intervertebral space, where there are the anatomical structures, such as the intervertebral disc, the apophyseal joints and the ligamenta flava, which can change with ageing or disease.

In isolated stenosis of the nerve root canal, or radicular canal, only this part of the spinal canal is constricted (Fig. 2). This canal (more an anatomical concept than a true canal) is the semi-tubular structure in which the nerve root exiting from the thecal sac runs before entering the intervertebral foramen Similarly to the central form the term *lateral stenosis* has become the most widely used for this type of stenosis.

The intervertebral foramen, which begins and ends at the level of the medial and the lateral border of the pedicle, respectively, should be considered as a distinct anatomical entity compared to the spinal canal. Therefore, stenosis of

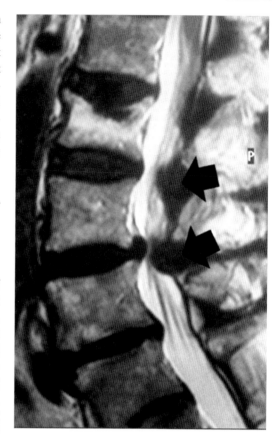

Fig. 1 T-2 weighted MR midsagittal scan showing spinal stenosis at L4-L5 and L3-L4. The thecal sac is compressed by the posterior elements of the spinal canal, namely the posterior joints and the ligamentum flavum (*arrows*)

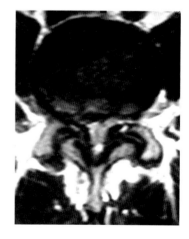

Fig. 2 Axial MR scan of isolated stenosis of the nerve root canal at L4-L5. The articular processes encroach only on the lateral portions of the spinal canal

the foramen should be differentiated from the other two forms of stenosis, although it can be associated with them.

Types of Stenosis

Three aetiological forms of stenosis can be identified: primary, secondary and combined [2].

Primary Forms
Central Stenosis
This form includes congenital and developmental stenosis. *Congenital stenosis*, which is exceedingly rare, is due to congenital malformations of the spine.

Developmental stenosis, a term introduced by Verbiest [3], includes achondroplastic and constitutional forms [4]. In achondroplasia, stenosis is due to abnormal shortness of the pedicles. In constitutional stenosis, in which the cause of the defective vertebral development is unknown, two types of anatomical abnormality may be identified:
(a) A short mid-sagittal diameter of the spinal canal.
(b) An exceedingly sagittal orientation of the laminae and/or shortness of the pedicles. In the latter type, the spinal canal is abnormally narrow, mainly or only, in the interarticular diameter.

Lateral Stenosis
This may result from abnormal shortness of the pedicles, even more so if associated with a trefoil configuration of the spinal canal or anomalous orientation and/or shape of the superior articular process. In this form, a primary role may be played by the intervertebral disc because even a mild bulging of the annulus fibrosus may be enough to cause symptoms.

Stenosis of the Intervertebral Foramen
Primary forms are found almost exclusively in the presence of abnormally short pedicles associated with decrease in height of the intervertebral disc [5].

Secondary Forms
Central Stenosis
If the dimensions of the spinal canal are primarily normal, or at the lower limits, compression of the caudal nerve roots is the result of one or more acquired conditions, such as spondylotic changes of the facet joints, abnormal thickening of the ligamenta flava and bulging of the intervertebral discs. We define this form as *simple degenerative stenosis* (Fig. 1).

Very often, however, degenerative spondylolisthesis of the cranial vertebra of the motion segment is also present, at one or, occasionally, two or more levels. Degenerative spondylolisthesis is mostly responsible for spinal stenosis (Fig. 3). However it may cause narrowing of the spinal canal with no neural compression. This is because the presence, type and severity of stenosis is related to several factors, such as the constitutional dimensions of the spinal canal, the orientation (more or less sagittal) and the severity of degenerative changes of the facet joints, and the amount of vertebral slipping, which however may play no or a minor role. The type of stenosis, central or lateral, depends on the orientation of the articular processes, and the length of the pedicles. Usually stenosis is lateral initially, and central in later stages. Whatever the type, we call this form of stenosis *degenerative stenosis associated with degenerative spondylolisthesis.*

Instability, that is hypermobility on flexion-extension radiographs, is one of the main characteristics of degenerative spondylolisthesis; in these case, we define instability as "actual". When there is no appreciable hypermobility of the slipped vertebra, we consider the condition as a "potential" instability of the slipped vertebra, which can become unstable as a result of surgery with removal of a large part of the facet joints or disc excision. In degenerative spondylolisthesis, the intervertebral disc often bulges into the intervertebral foramen causing constriction of the foramen. However, true stenosis is rarely present as the foramen becomes larger in the sagittal dimensions in the presence of slipping of the cranial vertebra [5].

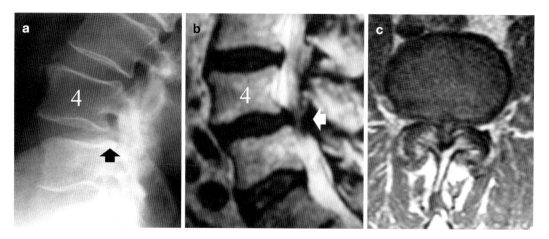

Fig. 3 Degenerative spondylolisthesis of L4. (**a**) Lateral radiograph of the lumbar spine showing slipping of the L4 vertebra (*arrow*). (**b**) Midsagittal MR scan showing compression of the neural structures (*arrow*). (**c**) Axial MR scan shows severe central spinal stenosis

A particular form of degenerative stenosis is that associated with degenerative scoliosis, in which a role may be played by the scoliotic curve as well as the degenerative changes of the facet joints, particularly on the concave side.

Other forms of secondary stenosis include late sequelae of fractures or infectious diseases of the spine, and Paget's disease.

Lateral Stenosis

Most often, this form of stenosis is degenerative in nature. Usually degenerative stenosis involves the lateral portions of the spinal canal in the initial stages and becomes central in more advanced stages. A particular form of lateral stenosis is that due to a cyst of the facet joint, compressing the emerging root in the nerve root canal.

Stenosis of the Intervertebral Foramen

This is rare especially as an isolated condition. In most cases, foraminal stenosis is associated with central or lateral stenosis. At times, root compression occurs when there is a lateral disc herniation or disc bulge in the presence of advanced degenerative changes of the articular processes.

Combined Forms

These forms occur when primary narrowing of the spinal canal, the nerve root canal or the intervertebral foramen, is associated, at the same vertebral level, with secondary narrowing due to spondylotic changes.

Indications for Surgery

Decompressive surgery is contra-indicated for a narrow spinal canal, not causing any compression of the neural structures. In these cases, in the presence of a herniated disc, only discectomy should be performed. Generally, decompressive surgery is not indicated in patients who complain only of back pain, in the absence of deformities, such as degenerative spondylolisthesis or scoliosis. In patients with an unstable motion segment who have only back pain it is usually sufficient to perform a fusion alone if stenosis is mild, because it is unlikely that neural compression will significantly increase and become symptomatic over time after fusion. Neural decompression may instead be performed if stenosis is severe, because it can be responsible for the onset of radicular symptoms in the months or years following surgery.

In patients with leg symptoms, surgery is indicated when conservative management carried out for 4–6 months has led to no significant improvement. The exception is the patient with severe motor and/or sensory deficit in the lower limbs or a cauda equina syndrome,wich requires emergent neural decompression.

In the presence of fixed motor deficits only (with no radicular pain), surgery is usually indicated when stenosis is marked, the deficits are severe and their duration is less than few months. In the presence of severe paresis or paralysis lasting more than 6–8 months there can be no indication for decompression because there are few or no chances of improvement of muscle function.

The best candidates for surgery are those patients who have no co-morbid diseases, a severe or very severe stenosis, long-standing leg symptoms and severe intermittent claudication, moderate or no motor deficits, and mild or no back pain. This is in contrast to patients who have mild stenosis, mild or inconstant leg symptoms with no precise radicular distribution, a history of claudication after many hundreds metres, no motor deficit and back pain of similar severity to, or more severe than, leg symptoms. A less predictable outcome is associated with surgery in this group.

In patients with no degenerative spondylolisthesis or other forms of "actual" or "potential" instability before surgery, there is usually no need for spinal fusion. However, arthrodesis should be planned when, prior to surgery, wide surgical decompression risking the development of post-operative instability, is previewed. Spine fusion, or some form of stabilization, may be indicated for patients with chronic back pain and severe degeneration of the disc(s) or facet joints in the area of decompression.

Age

Lumbar stenosis is usually diagnosaed and treated surgically betwen 50 and 70 years. However, surgical decompression may offer significant relief of symptoms also to patients older than 70 years, provided the patient's general health is satisfactory [6, 7]. There is no significant difference in the results of surgery between patients in early senile age and those aged 80 years or even more.

Co-Morbidity

A high rate of co-morbid illnesses was found to be inversely related to the rate of satisfactory results following surgery [8] In one study, comparing the long-term results of surgery in 24 diabetic and 22 non-diabetic patients, the rate of satisfactory outcomes was 41 % in the diabetic, compared to 90 % in the non-diabetic, group [9] However, different results were observed in a similar study [10], in which the outcome was satisfactory in 72 % of the diabetic and 80 % of the non-diabetic patients. Neither the duration of the diabetes before surgery nor its type correlated with the outcome. A mistaken pre-operative diagnosis was the main cause of failure in diabetic patients, in whom diabetic neuropathy or angiopathy may mimic the symptoms of stenosis. It is thus mandatory to carry out electrophysiological studies in diabetic or non-diabetic patients who have symptoms in the lower limbs not typical of lumbar stenosis to exclude a peripheral neuropathy.

Type and Level of Stenosis

There is no significant difference in the outcomes between the various types of central stenoses. However, patients with degenerative or combined stenosis at a single level are the best candidates for surgery because they tend to have better results than those with stenosis at multiple levels. In patients with constitutional stenosis, the intervertebral disc may play a significant role in the compression of the neural structures. When the disc bulges considerably in the spinal canal, but it is not truly herniated, it may be difficult to eliminate the anterior compression of the neural structures and this may lead to less satisfactory results than in the cases in which the neural

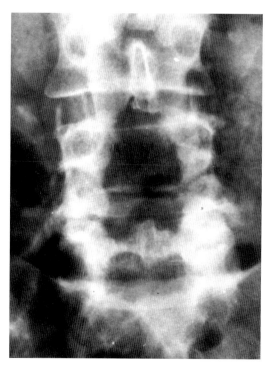

Fig. 4 Anteroposterior radiograph showing total laminectomy from the caudal border of L3 to the cranial part of L5 for severe central stenosis at L4-L5

compression is caused exclusively by the posterior vertebral arch. Nevertheless, discectomy should not usually be performed in these cases because the intervertebral disc is an important stabilizing structure and removal of a not herniated nucleus pulposus exposes more to the risk of recurrent herniation.

Patients with lateral stenosis, particularly at a single level, tend to have better results than those with central stenosis, provided the nerve-root compression is severe and the leg symptoms have a precise dermatomal distribution.

Surgical Management

Definition of Terms

Decompression of the lumbar spinal canal can be carried out by bilateral laminectomy, also defined as total laminectomy (Fig. 4). More focal decompression can be accomplished

with a laminotomy, also called keyhole laminotomy or hemilaminectomy or partial hemilaminectomy. Laminotomy consists in the removal of the caudal portion of the proximal lamina, the cranial portion of the distal lamina and a varying portion of the articular processes, which should not usually exceed the medial half, and ligamentum flavum on the side of surgery. Laminotomy can be performed at a single level on one side or both sides (Fig. 5). When necessary, it is performed at multiple levels. An alternative to bilateral laminectomy or bilateral laminotomy is bilateral decompression by a unilateral approach, performed with the use of the operating microscope (Fig. 10).

The term foraminotomy indicates removal of a part of the posterior wall of the intervertebral foramen, while the term foraminectomy refers to complete excision of the wall of the foramen.

Operative Planning

General Concepts

Surgical treatment is aimed at decompressing the neural structures by means of a bilateral laminectomy or laminotomy at one or more vertebral levels.

It is crucial to plan accurately the extent of decompression before surgery because during the operation it may be difficult to determine whether, at a given level, the central or lateral canal is stenotic, particularly if stenosis is mild. Lack of sufficient care in planning the operation may give rise to inadequate decompression, which can leave areas of stenosis, or a too wide decompression, which may cause iatrogenic instability.

Types of Stenosis
Stenosis with no Degenerative Spondylolisthesis or Scoliosis
Central Stenosis

Number of levels to decompress. The stenotic levels should be distinguished accurately as levels at which the need for decompression is absolute and levels where the need is relative.

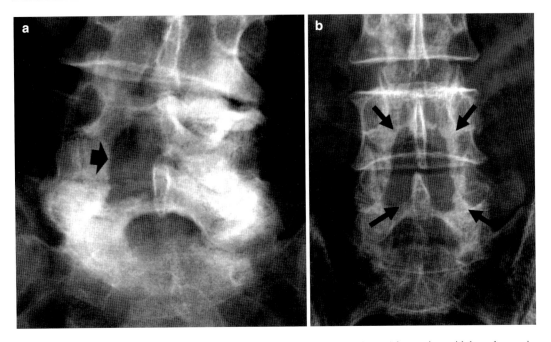

Fig. 5 (**a**) Anteroposterior radiograph showing L4-L5 unilateral laminotomy (*arrow*) in a patient with lateral stenosis. (**b**) Bilateral laminotomy at the same level (*arrows*) for central stenosis at L4-L5

In the former case, compression of the neural structures is marked or, regardless of the severity, is responsible for clinical symptoms and signs. In the latter case, neural compression is mild and asymptomatic. In many instances, there are one or two levels contiguous to the area of symptomatic stenosis.

The usefulness of prophylactic surgery at the levels at which there is a relative need for decompression stems from the evaluation of several factors, such as the patient's age, the amount of constriction, the site of stenosis (central or lateral), the presence of disc abnormalities and the vertebral stability.

In patients aged over 75 years the need for a prophylactic decompression is less than in middle-aged patients. Posterior compression of the thecal sac due to mild central stenosis is less likely to become symptomatic than constriction of the lateral spinal canal where the nerve roots run close to the facet joints. Marked bulging of the annulus fibrosus, which may become symptomatic over time, may represent an indication for prophylactic decompression. The presence of intersomatic osteophytes producing spontaneous vertebral

fusion represents a guarantee against post-surgical instability, which may be worrying when decompression has to be carried out at high lumbar levels. At these levels, in fact, a larger removal of the articular processes in the transverse plane is needed to decompress the lateral part of the spinal canal since the facets are orientated more sagittally than at the lower lumbar levels.

Unilateral or bilateral decompression. For the intervertebral levels at which the need for decompression is absolute and stenosis is bilateral, the decompression should be performed bilaterally either in patients with bilateral leg symptoms and/or signs, and in those with unilateral symptoms. When, at a given level, stenosis is severe and symptomatic on one side and milder and asymptomatic on the other, unilateral decompression may be considered, particularly when operative time should be limited due to the old age or co-morbidities of the patient, or discectomy has to be performed.

For levels with relative stenosis, the choice between unilateral or bilateral decompression should be made taking into consideration the severity of stenosis on the two sides, and the factors considered in determining the number of levels to decompress.

Extent of decompression. The long-term results of surgery may deteriorate with time because of re-growth of the resected portion of the posterior vertebral arch [12]. This is more likely to occur when a narrow decompression is performed. We believe that decompression should be as wide as possible in the lateral portion of the spinal canal, while preserving at the same time vertebral stability. The optimal facetectomy is that in which the medial two-thirds of the superior and inferior articular processes are removed. An important concept is that in lumbar stenosis radicular symptoms usually originate from compression of the nerve root after it has emerged from the thecal sac, that is in the radicular canal, rather than within the thecal sac.

Compression of the thecal sac and nerve roots usually occurs at intervertebral level. To be adequate, decompression should involve the whole area facing the intervertebral disc. That is, decompression should extend as far as half of the height of the vertebrae above and below the stenotic area.

Methods of Decompression

Surgery for lumbar stenosis is aimed at adequately decompressing the neural structures, particularly the nerve roots in the extrathecal course, with no significant compromise of vertebral stability, whilst not causing or worsening back pain after surgery.

In the last two decades, the technique of multiple laminotomy has become widely used in the treatment of central spinal stenosis because it preserves vertebral stability better than central laminectomy [11, 12]. More recently, bilateral decompression with unilateral approach has gained popularity because it allows even better preservation of the facet joints contralateral to the side of direct approach. However, a major role is still played by total laminectomy, which may allow a more effective decompression of the neural structures and often implies a shorter operative time compared to the other decompressive methods. It should be taken in to account, however, that re-growth of posterior vertebral arch, which tends to occur over time, may "re-stabilze" partially destabilized motion segments [13] (Fig. 6).

Multiple laminotomy is the treatment of choice for constitutional stenosis because the patients are usually middle-aged, the stenosis is rarely severe, and disc excision may be necessary [12]. Multiple laminotomy is also preferred for degenerative or combined stenosis when narrowing of the spinal canal is mild or moderate, particularly if disc excision has been planned. The same is true for bilateral decompression with unilateral approach, which is also indicated for simple degenerative stenosis of moderate severity, particularly in those patients in whom leg symptoms prevail on one side, or in the presence of mild degenerative spondylolisthesis when the surgeon decides against a concomitant spine fusion because the slipped vertebra shows no or very mild hypermobility on pre-operative flexion-extension radiographs. Total laminectomy is usually indicated for very severe stenosis in patients with bilateral leg symptoms, providing that the involved segments are stable pre-operatively, or when a fusion has been planned due to a clear-cut vertebral instability.

Spine Fusion

In addition to degenerative spondylolisthesis with moderate or severe instability of the slipped vertebra and to degenerative scoliosis, spinal fusion should be planned if the area to be decompressed is unstable or when total laminectomy and bilateral discectomy are to be performed. Spine fusion should also be planned when there are high chances that, at surgery, the articular processes will be completely removed on both sides or they will be excised on one side and discectomy performed bilaterally, and in patients complaining of severe chronic back pain determined to originate from the motion segment needing decompression.

Fig. 6 (**a**) Anteroposterior radiograph taken a few weeks afte total laminectomy performed from L2 to L5 for central stenosis at L2-L3, L3-L4 and L4-L5, with generous resection of the facet joints. (**b**) Radiograph obtained after 4 years of the operation. The posterior verbral arch has undergone partial regrowth, thus "restabilizing" the operated vertbral segments

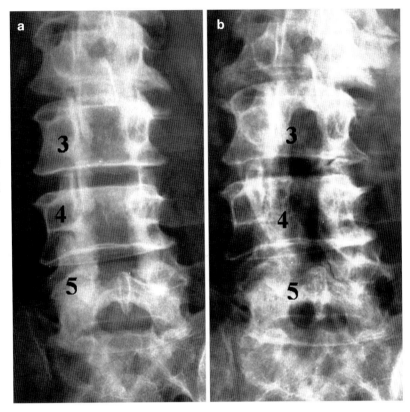

Except for these situations there is no need for spinal fusion in stenotic patients [2, 14].

Isolated Lateral Stenosis

Usually a single vertebral level is involved.

In patients with radicular symptoms on both sides, bilateral decompression should be carried out, even if on one side leg symptoms are mild and no neurological abnormalities are present.

When stenosis is bilateral and the patient complains of radicular symptoms on only one side, bilateral decompression is usually indicated particularly in middle-age patients or in those with electrophysiological evidence of nerve-root deficit on the asymptomatic side. However, in the elderly patient, a unilateral decompression may be indicated if the surgical procedure should preferably be rapid due to co-morbid diseases.

If pre-operative MRI shows a bulging disc at the stenotic level, a possible discectomy has to be planned. However, the final decision should be taken intra-operatively based on the severity of bulging and the degree of softness of the disc on pressure by a blunt probe. A hard disc should not generally be excised unless there is a clear evidence that it contributes to compression of the neural structures.

Generally there is no indication for spinal fusion, unless bilateral decompression is performed at a pre-operatively unstable level, particularly when disc excision is carried out, or the patient complains of chronic low back pain due to disc degeneration.

Stenosis of the Intervertebral Foramen

MRI or CT often show narrowing of the neuroforamen. However, in the vast majority of these cases the nerve running in the foramen is not compressed. Decompression of the neuroforamen is rarely needed unless the narrowing is associated to a severe annular bulging or a herniated disc.

Stenosis with Degenerative Spondylolisthesis

In this type of stenosis, like that with no degenerative olisthesis, decompression of the neural strucures may be carried out by unilateral or bilateral laminotomy, bilateral decompression by unilateral approach or total laminectomy. Furthermore, the presence of degenerative spondyolisthesis does not necessarily require a spinal fusion.

The indications for unilateral laminotomy with no fusion are: moderate central stenosis in elderly patients with unilateral symptoms; lateral stenosis only on one side; an additional condition, such as a synovial cyst, on the side of the radicular symptoms; and no chronic back pain. Bilateral laminotomy may be carried out with no concomitant fusion in the presence of mild olisthesis, no vertebral hypermobility on functional radiographs, moderate central stenosis or any degree of isolated lateral stenosis, and mild or no back pain. In these cases, bilateral decompression by a unilateral approach, rather than bilateral laminotomy, has the advantage of preserving better vertebral stability.

Patients with severe central stenosis and severe leg symptoms usually need total laminectomy which allows the neural structures to be decompressed as widely as necessary. In these cases a pedicle screw instrumentation and a vertebral fusion is usually needed, particularly if the olisthetic vertebra is hypermobile on functional radiographs and/or in the presence of a history of chronic low back pain (Fig. 7). However, in elderly patients with co-morbid diseases, fusion may be avoided especially when the olisthetic vertebra shows no hypermobility on functional radiographs (Fig. 8). An alternative, in these cases, is to perform a unilateral instrumentation with unilateral intertransverse fusion.

Stenosis and Degenerative Scoliosis

When lumbar degenerative scoliosis is associated with spinal stenosis, decompression of the nerural structures may lead to aggravation of the curve or an increase of lateral vertebral slipping where this is present. This may occur if total laminectomy is performed, but also when bilateral, or even unilateral, laminotomy is carried out. The increase in amount of the curve is responsible for worsening of the back pain, which usually is a prominent component of the patient's symptoms.

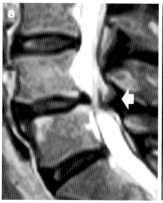 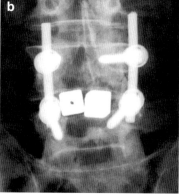 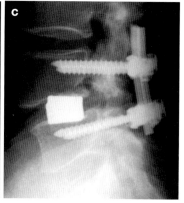

Fig. 7 Spine fusion at L4-L5 carried out by pedicle screw instrumentation and PLIF with blocks of trabecular metal in a patient with degenerative spondylolisthesis, central stenosis and chronic low back pain. (**a**) Preoperative MR scan, the arrow pointing to constriction of the neural structures. (**b**) and (**c**) Postoperative radiographs

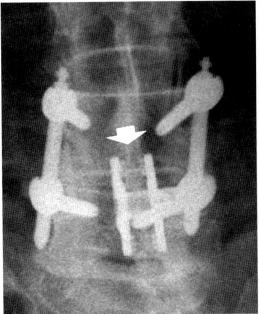 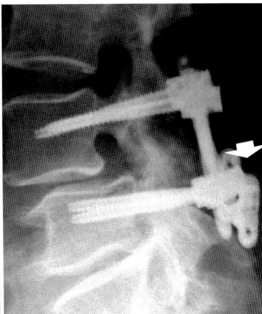

Fig. 8 Postoperative anteroposterior and lateral radiographs of a 76-year-old man with spinal stenosis and degenerative spondylolisthesis of L4 whose functional radiographs showed no hypermobility of the slipped vertebra. After bilateral laminotomy, pedicle screw instrumentation was applied and interspinous stabilization was performed with a system of two interconnected plates (Aspen) fixed to the spinous processes of L4 and L5 (*arrows*)

In the presence of mild scoliosis and bilateral symptoms, there may be an indication for bilateral decompression by unilateral approach and no fusion. On the other hand, when scoliosis is severe, total laminectomy performed at the stenotic levels should be associated with spinal fusion after correction of the curve using pedicle screw instrumentation. The latter should often be extended to the lower thoracic spine when scoliosis involves the entire lumbar spine.

Surgical Technique

Total Laminectomy

Skin Incision and Superficial Haemostasis

The skin incision extends from the cranial edge of the spinous process above to the caudal edge of the spinous process below that of the vertebra, or the group of vertebrae, needing decompression.

Dermal and subdermal vessels may be cauterized or clamped, together with a small portion of superficial subcutaneous tissue; clamps are turned outwards of the wound and held together with an elastic band for 15–20 min. This method makes haemostasis of the superficial vessels very rapid.

Dis-Insertion of Paraspinal Muscles

The thoracolumbar fascia is incised, starting on the side of the surgeon, immediately adjacent and parallel to the spinous processes using an electric cautery knife.

Dis-insertion of the paraspinal muscles starts from the most caudal of the exposed vertebrae [2]. A periosteal elevator is introduced deep to the muscle mass and allowed to slip along the outer surface of the spinous process and lamina to detach the paraspinal muscles from the bone surface until the lateral border of the facet joints. Dry sponges are packed beneath the muscle mass to arrest bleeding. The sponge packed at one extremity of the motion segment is then removed and, while retracting the muscle mass, the residual musculo-tendinous attachments to the base of the spinous processes and interspinous ligaments are sectioned. The other sponge is then removed and haemostasis is completed. When decompression is needed at more than one motion segment, dry sponges are again packed into the depth of the wound and the vertebrae and intervertebral spaces are exposed. The manoeuvres described above are then performed on the opposite side.

One or two self-retaining retractors are applied and remnants of muscle and fat tissue still adherent to the laminae, facet joints and ligamentum flavum are removed using a large curette or a bone rongeur.

Opening of the Spinal Canal

After exposure of the ligamenta flava and interspinous ligaments, the vertebrae included in the operative field are identified by locating the lumbosacral interspace, when exposed. In the doubt, the level or levels to be decompressed should be identified using fluoroscopic imaging after inserting a spinal needle into one, or two contiguous, interspinous spaces.

When a single intervertebral level has to be decompressed, the cranial half of the spinous process of the distal vertebra and the caudal half or two-thirds of the spinous processes of the proximal vertebra together with the interspinous ligament are resected as far as their base.

For decompression of a motion segment, the ligamentum flavum is detached from the deep surface of the proximal laminae using a small curette. Laminectomy is started in the central portion of the laminar arch, that is, at the level of the posterior angle of the spinal canal, not occupied by the thecal sac. The lamina on each side can be removed using a bone rongeur or small or medium-bite Kerrison rongeurs. Laminectomy is then continued, alternately on one side and the other, after further detachment of the ligamenta flava from the ventral aspect of the laminae. The ligaments are then detached from the proximal border of the laminae of the distal vertebra. The cut edge of the ligament is picked up with a forceps, sectioned longitudinally using a thin scalpel, and removed as

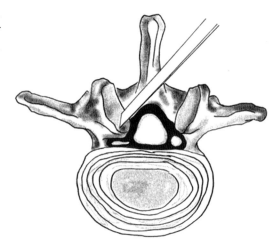

Fig. 9 Drawing showing how the chisel should be oriented to carry out the undercutting facetectomy

extensively as possible. The lateral portion of the laminae and the inferior articular processes are removed using a bone rongeur or Kerrison punches.

An alternative technique, that we prefer, is to perform lamino-arthrectomy using chisels. After removal of the spinous processes and detachment of the ligamentum flavum from the laminae of the proximal vertebra, a chisel is used, on each side, to remove the caudal half of the lamina of the proximal vertebra and the medial half of the inferior articular process of the same vertebra. The proximal portion of the lamina of the distal vertebra can be removed partly by a chisel and partly using Kerrison rongeurs. After removal of the ligamentum flavum and exposure of the thecal sac, the residual lateral portions of the articular processes are removed using either chisels or punch rongeurs. When using chisels, undercutting facetectomy can be performed by orienting the instrument at 45° in a medio-lateral and postero-anterior direction to undermine the articular processes, that is to remove only the ventral portion of the bone in order to preserve vertebral stability (Fig. 9) [15].

If total laminectomy has to be performed at multiple contiguous levels the spinous processes located between the most proximal and distal vertebra is excised completely. Since stenosis occurs at the intervertebral level, when performing decompression at multiple levels, laminectomy is extended, proximally and distally, beyond the intervertebral discs located at the extremities of the stenotic area.

Exploration of Intervertebral Discs and Spinal Nerve Roots

The spinal canal is opened laterally until the nerve root emerging from the thecal sac is visualized. The emerging root and the thecal sac are then retracted medially and the disc is exposed at each of the intervertebral levels included in the area of laminectomy. Consistency of the annulus fibrosus is tested with a blunt probe. If the annulus is hard in consistency, the disc should not be excised.

A right-angled blunt probe is used to evaluate the width of the intervertebral foramen. If this is constricted, foraminotomy is continued until complete decompression of the root is obtained. However, foraminectomy is very rarely necessary. If bilateral foraminectomy is performed, spine fusion may be necessary, especially when the disc has been excised.

Wound Closure

At the site of laminectomy, the paraspinal muscles of the two sides are sutured by interrupted sutures. The thoracolumbar fascia is closed with a continuous suture. Where the spinous processes have not been resected, the fascia is anchored to the supraspinous ligament.

Post-operative haematoma between the subcutaneous tissue and thoracolumbar fascia is avoided by passing a few sutures both in the deep subcutaneous layer and the fascia.

Laminotomy

Single Level

Skin incision extends from the cranial border of the spinous process of the proximal vertebra to the caudal border of the spinous process of the distal vertebra.

When performing unilateral laminotomy, the thoracolumbar fascia is incised only on the symptomatic side just laterally to the spinous processes. The paraspinal muscles are detached from the spinous processes, the laminae and the facet joint. Bleeding can be controlled using small dry sponges packed in the osteo-muscular space. After a few seconds, one of the sponges is removed and bleeding vessels are coagulated by bi-polar cautery. The same is done for the other sponges.

For retraction of the paraspinal muscles, we use a Taylor retractor of appropriate width, installed against the lateral aspect of the articular processes and held by a metal weight of two kilograms or less. A large curette is used to clean up the proximal and distal lamina and the ligamentum flavum. The ligament is detached from the deep surface of the proximal lamina using a small curette, and the distal one-third to half of the lamina is excised using a Kerrison rongeur. The ligamentum flavum is dis-inserted from the proximal border of the distal lamina to allow removal of the proximal one-third of that lamina with a Kerrison rongeur. The medial one-third to half of the facets are excided together with the ligamentum flavum using Kerrison rongeurs.

When the interlaminar space is very narrow, the inferior articular process of the proximal vertebra can be intially removed with a chisel, until the superior articular process of the vertebra below is exposed. The chisel can be replaced by a high speed microdrill. The ligamentum flavum is then detached from the border of the distal lamina to allow a small-bite Kerrison to be inserted under the lamina to initiate removal of the proximal part of it. The remaining ligament is then removed in a caudo-cranial direction using Kerrison rongeurs. Alternatively, a thin dissector is carefully introduced between the layers of the central part of the ligament to progressively dissect them until the thecal sac is exposed. A Kerrison rongeurs is then inserted between the sac and the ligament and the latter is gradually and carefully removed. Afterwards, the remaining lateral part of the ligament is excised together with the medial part of the articular processes by inserting Kerrison rongeurs beneath the facets.

Facetectomy should be extended laterally to expose the emerging nerve root. By retracting the sac and the root medially, the intervertebral disc is exposed and the degree of its prominence and consistency is evaluated. Disc excision should be done only when the disc is prominent and soft in consistency, and appears to contribute significantly to compression of the neural structures.

Lamino-arthrectomy of the cranial vertebra should be continued proximally as far as a few millimetres cranially to the disc. Laminotomy of the distal vertebra should proceed until the caudal part of the pedicle. A blunt probe can then be used to assess the width of the neuroforamen. Generally the latter is not constricted. In the rare cases in which it appears stenotic, formaninotomy is performed until complete decompression of the nerve root is achieved.

For bilateral laminotomy at a single level, the procedure described above is then performed on the opposite side.

Multiple Levels

Unilateral or bilateral laminotomy can be performed at two or more adjacent intervertebral levels. The surgical technique is similar to that described for single level laminotomy. However, when performing laminotomy at two adjacent levels on the same side, care should be taken to leave intact, for at least five millimeters, the lamina between the two motion segments.

Laminotomy at multiple levels may be indicated for any type of stenosis, but particularly for:
(a) Constitutional stenosis in which constriction of the spinal canal is usually moderately severe and disc excision is often necessary,
(b) Isolated lateral stenosis at multiple levels,
(c) Simple degenerative central stenosis when constriction of the spinal canal is not particularly severe,
(d) Degenerative spondylolisthesis when spinal fusion has not been planned.

Microsurgery

One of the main difficulties in performing laminotomy, particularly at a single level, is related to poor lighting of the deep operative field when using a short skin incision. These difficulties may be overcome with the use of the operating microscope.

The microscope provides excellent lighting, regardless of the extent of surgical exposure, which is 2–3 or 4–6 cm long for one or two levels, respectively. Furthermore, by slanting the objective, any part of the operative field can be illuminated. Thus, surgical manoeuvres can be performed with greater precision, the causes of compression of the neural structures can be more easily identified and fewer risks are run of causing undue trauma to the emerging nerve root or thecal sac. Moreover, only occasionally is an excessively large portion of the articular processes excised or a complete facetectomy inadvertently performed.

Laminotomy using the microscope is performed with the same instruments used for the naked eye procedure. The exception is the paraspinal muscle retractor, which should be as narrow as possible, at least for one level laminotomy. Many surgeons use the Caspar retractor. We use a Taylor retractor about one-third in width of the standard instrument. Even the chisel or a bone rongeur can be used for removal of the inferior articular process of the proximal vertebra. However, many surgeons use high speed microdrill to a large extent to perform the lamino-arthrectomy.

The operating microscope is indispensable to carry out bilateral decompression with a unilateral approach (Fig. 10). After laminotomy has been performed on one side (usually the one in which the radicular symptoms are more severe) with the operating table placed parallel to the floor, decompression is continued towards the opposite side after inclining the table and slanting the microscope towards that side by some 10°. The base of the spinous processess and the most medial part of the laminae is removed with a Kerrison rongeur or a high speed microdrill. This allows the surgeon to see the top of the thecal sac. The table is further inclined by some 25° with respect to the floor and the microscope is slanted enough to see the medial part of the articular processes which are removed until the contra-lateral border of the the thecal sac is clearly visible and the emerging nerve root is at least glimpsed. The articular processes of the contra-lateral side are removed using a kerrinson punches, a microdrill or a thin chisel (Fig. 9).

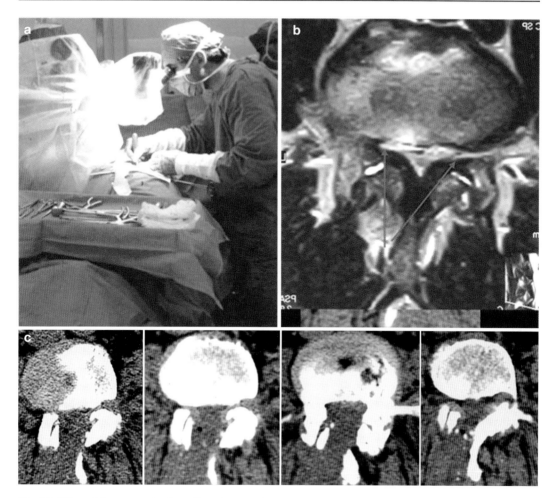

Fig. 10 Bilateral decompression by unilateral approach. (**a**) Photograph of the use of the operating microscope to perform the procedure. (**b**) Scheme of the surgical procedure: on the right side a laminotomy is performed and then the decompression is carried out obliquely on the opposite side. (**c**) Postoperative CT scans showing the decompression performed for a central stenosis; the lamina and articular processes are partially resected also on the left side, thus decompressing the central area of the spinal canal and the lateral canal

Interspinous Distraction Devices

In the last few years several interspinous devices have been developed to obtain indirect decompression of neural structures by posterior segmental distraction. The implant most often used has been the X-Stop, which is inserted by open surgery, through an approach centred on the interspinous space to be treated. Successively, other devices haved been introduced that can be applied percutaneously, i. e. through a 2–3 cm. skin incision carried out 8–10 cm. from the spinous processes (Fig. 11).

Recently there has been a widespread use of interspinous distraction devises in patients with central or lateral lumbar stenosis of any severity. However, the clinical results of these devices, evaluated in all studies by the Zurich Claudication Questionnaire (ZCQ), are contrroversial. In a multi-centre study on patients followed-up for 2 years, a clinically significant improvement in

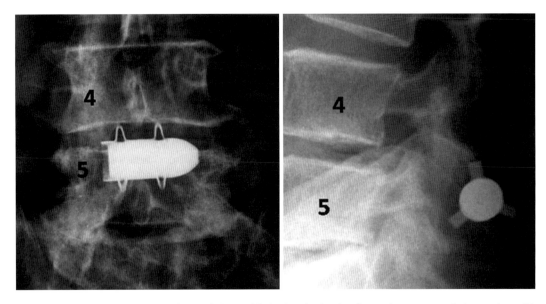

Fig. 11 Posterior segmental distraction carried out with the Aperius implant inserted percutaneously in a patient with moderate central stenosis at L4-L5 level

the Symptoms Severity and the Physical Function domains of the ZCQ was found in 60 % and 57 % of patients, respectively, while 73 % were at least somewhat satisfied in the Patient Satisfaction domain [16]. By contrast, in another study [17] a good outcome, when considering all three domains of the ZCQ, was obtained only by 31 % of patients 1 year on average after operation.

Only one study compared the result of operation after a mean of 2 years in a group of patients who had a distraction device inserted percutaneously and a group submitted to open surgical decompression (laminotomy or total laminectomy) [18]. In the former group, a good outcome was found in 60 % of patients with moderate stenosis and only in 31 % of those with very severe stenosis, while in the open decompression group the outcomes were satisfactory in 69 % of moderate stenoses and 89 % of severe stenosss. These findings suggest that, at present, interspinous distraction devices are poorly indicated in patients with severe stenosis.

However, they may represent an alternative to open decompression as a preventive measure in patients with relative stenosis (mild and asymptomatic) located above or below levels undergoing laminotomy or laminectomy for symptomatic stenosis.

References

1. Postacchini F. Lumbar spinal stenosis and pseudostenosis. Definition and classification of of pathology. Ital J Orthop Traumatol. 1983;9:339–51.
2. Postacchini F. Lumbar spinal stenosis. Wien/ NewYork: Springer Verlag; 1989.
3. Verbiest H. A radicular syndrome from developmental narrowing of the lumbar vertebral canal. J Bone Joint Surg Br. 1954;36-B:230–7.
4. Postacchini F. Management of lumbar spinal stenosis. J Bone Joint Surg Br. 1996;75-B:154–64.
5. Cinotti G, De Santis P, Nofroni I, Postacchini F. Stenosis of the intervertebral foramen. Anatomic study on predisposing factors. Spine. 2002;27:223–9.
6. Herron LD, Mangelsdorf C. Lumbar spinal stenosis: results of surgical treatment. J Spinal Disord. 1991;4:26–33.
7. Sanderson PL, Wood PLR. Surgery for lumbar spinal stenosis in old people. J Bone Joint Surg Br. 1993;75B:393–7.
8. Katz IN, Lipson SJ, Larson MG, et al. The outcome of decompressive laminectomy for degenerative

lumbar stenosis. J Bone Joint Surg Am. 1991;73A:809–11.

9. Simpson JM, Silveri CP, Balderstone RA, et al. The results of operations on the lumbar spine in patients who have diabetes mellitus. J Bone Joint Surg Am. 1993;75A:1823–9.

10. Cinotti G, Postacchini F, Weinstein JN. Lumbar spinal stenosis and diabetes. Outcome of surgical decompression. J Bone Joint Surg Br. 1994;76B:215–9.

11. Aryanpur J. Ducker T: multilevel lumbar laminotomies: an alternative to laminectomy in the treatment of lumbar stenosis. Neurosurgery. 1990;26:429–33.

12. Postacchini F, Cinotti G, Perugia D, Gumina S. The surgical treatment of central lumbar stenosis. Multiple laminotomy compared with total laminectomy. J Bone Joint Surg Br. 1993;75B:386–92.

13. Postacchini F, Cinotti G. Bone regrowth after surgical decompression for lumbar spinal stenosis. J Bone Joint Surg Br. 1992;74-B:862–9.

14. Grob D, Humke T, Dvorak J. Degenerative lumbar spinal stenosis. decompression with and without arthrodesis. J Bone Joint Surg Am. 1995;77A:1036–41.

15. Getty CJM. Lumbar spinal stenosis. The Clinical spectrum and the results of operation. J Bone Joint Surg Br. 1980;62B:481–5.

16. Zucherman JF, Hsu KY, Hartjen CA, Mehalic TF, Implicito DA, Martin MJ, Johnson 2nd DR, Skidmore GA, Vessa PP, Dwyer JW, Puccio ST, Cauthen JC, Ozuna RM, Zucherman JE, Hsu KY, Charles A. A multicenter, prospective, randomized trial evaluting the X STOP Interspinous process decompression system for the treatment of neurogenic intermittent claudication: two-year follow-p results. Spine. 2005;30:351–1358.

17. Brussee P, Hauth J, Donk RD, Verbeek AL, Bartels RH. Self-rated evaluation of outcome of the implantation of interspinous process distraction (X-Stop) for neurogenic claudication. Eur Spine J. 2008;17:200–3.

18. ostacchini F, Ferrari E, Faraglia S, Menchetti PPM, Postacchini R. Aperius interspinous implant versus open surgical decompression in lumbar spinal stenosis. Spine J. 2011;11:933–9.

Minimally-Invasive Anterior Lumbar Spinal Fusion

H. Michael Mayer

Contents

Abstract

Less invasive anterior approaches to the lumbar spine have been developed and become popular within the last 20 years. Although the influence of mid-term and long-term outcomes is yet unclear, they have significantly reduced peri-operative morbidity such as tissue trauma, blood loss, hospitalisation time and post-operative pain. This chapter describes the retroperitoneal lateral approaches as well as anterior retroperitoneal midline approaches to the lumbar levels L2-S1. These approaches can be used for various type of interbody fusion as well as for total disc replacement. They require a detailed knowledge of the individual topographic anatomy of and around the lumbar spine. With this information, individualized approaches can be planned and performed, which employ the most convenient access with the least risk potential in each individual case.

Keywords

Anatomy • Anterior fusion • Complications • Critical evaluation • Indications • Lumbar spine • Minimally-invasive • Operative techniques-L4-5 disc, L5-S1 disc • Principles

General Introduction

The term 'minimally invasive' has been used in the surgical scientific literature since the introduction of microsurgical and endoscopic surgical approaches. It has been applied in various fields

H.M. Mayer
Spine Centre Munich, Schön Klinik München Harlaching,
München, Germany
e-mail: MMayer@schoen-kliniken.de

G. Bentley (ed.), *European Surgical Orthopaedics and Traumatology*,
DOI 10.1007/978-3-642-34746-7_33, © EFORT 2014

mainly in abdominal surgery, gynaecological or thoracic surgery [9, 18, 21]. Although arthroscopic techniques in the peripheral joints or microsurgical techniques for discectomy or decompression have been used for many years in Orthopaedic surgery, the term 'minimally-invasive' was very rarely used or associated with these procedures. In fact, it has only come to our perception in the last years, when it was increasingly used to describe or characterize procedures or surgical approaches for the treatment of degenerative disc disorders of the lumbar spine.

For the surgical treatment of degenerative disorders of the lumbar spine a variety of minimally-invasive techniques have been developed in the last 15 years. All these techniques have in common to represent surgical **approaches** which are less invasive than the standard approaches which have been used hitherto [12].

This leads us to a very fundamental but important statement to avoid misunderstandings and misinterpretations: whenever we talk about minimally-invasive surgery for the curative treatment of segmental lumbar disc degeneration we talk about *minimally-invasive approaches* to perform 'target surgery' such as disc excision, fusion or disc replacement which in all cases is still as (maximal) invasive as it ever was.

Wrong indications for surgery, undesired side – effects, complications and bad results are strongly determined or influenced by the surgical approach to the target area [2, 13]. Less invasive techniques in general decrease the degree of 'iatrogenic' surgical trauma. They ameliorate early post-operative morbidity and enable early and aggressive rehabilitation of the patient without an increase in complications. The following chapter describes the rationales and goals of fusion surgery for degenerative lumbar spine disorders, and the implementation of minimally-invasive techniques into the surgical standard strategies.

General Principles

Disc degeneration is a key pathomechanism which, per se, can lead to clinical symptoms ('discogenic' low back pain). However, low back pain due to disc degeneration is in most cases 'multifactorial'. Whereas pure discogenic back pain is mainly found in a younger patient population, the majority of patients presents with a mixture of discogenic, arthrogenic and musculo-ligamentous symptoms. Surgical procedures to deal with these symptoms have different goals in common: the excision or elimination of pain source(s), the elimination of pain-generating biomechanical mechanisms, the restoration and retention of the physiological segmental curvature as well as the restoration of disc – and foraminal – height especially in cases with lateral recess and/or foraminal stenosis. There is no doubt, that all these goals can best be achieved by 360° or 270° fusion of one or several lumbar segments. Using this technique, the pain sources (disc, end-plates, facet joints, facet joint capsules) are excised. Pathologic load patterns due to loss in disc height as well as macro-instabilities (e.g., degenerative spondylolisthesis) are eliminated by the fusion. Disturbances of lumbar curvature in the sagittal (kyphosis, hyperlordosis) as well as frontal (degenerative lumbar scoliosis, segmental tilt) planes can be reduced and retained by posterior instrumentation. Disc height as well as foraminal height can be restored in cases with root symptoms associated with low back pain. Thus spinal fusion is the only 'curative' salvage procedure to treat degenerative low back pain.

Indications and Patient Selection

There is consensus that spinal fusion in degenerative conditions of the lumbar spine should be the last therapeutic step when non-invasive or semi-invasive conservative measures have failed or in cases where total disc arthroplasty or other motion-preserving techniques are contra-indicated. However, there is no international consensus on the type of fusion which should preferably be used in different pathologies [3, 4, 6, 8, 11]. The most often-used techniques are listed in Tables 1 and 2.

Table 1 Minimally invasive access surgery for fusion and disc reconstruction

Laparoscopic anterior interbody fusion [18, 19]
Percutaneous posterolateral interbody fusion [8]
Mini-open microsurgical posterolateral fusion [15]
Mini-ALIF [10]
Mini-open total disc replacement [14]

Table 2 Spinal fusion techniques

Posterolateral (intertransverse)	180° post
TLIF/PLIF	270° post
Percutaneous PLIF	180° ant
ALIF	180° ant
Post/ALIF	270° post/ant

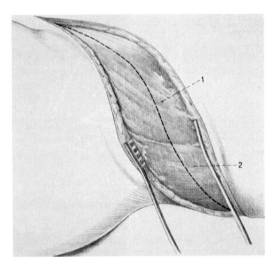

Fig. 1 'Tradtional' anterior approach for lumbar interbody fusion [7] (*1* external oblique muscle, *2* quadratus lumborum muscle)

Minimally-Invasive Anterior Approaches for Interbody Fusion

In 1990 Obenchain first described a laparoscopic approach to the L5/S1 disc [16]. This 'key' publication triggered the development of a variety of less invasive anterior accesses to the lumbar spine, which dominated the 90s of the last century. Laparoscopic surgery soon turned out to be associated with a variety of technical pitfalls and hazards and has never reached the status of a 'routine-procedure' in spine centres around the world [17, 19, 20]. However, the need for less invasive anterior approaches was obvious since 360° or 270° fusion seemed to achieve the highest fusion rates of all fusion techniques used hitherto [5, 11, 14]. In 1997, the author described two 'mini-open' access-techniques to the lumbar levels for anterior interbody fusion [10]. They were based on the application of microsurgical philosophy to the well-known standard anterior approaches.

Operative Techniques

Lateral Retroperitoneal Approaches (L2-L5)

Mono- as well as multi-segmental anterior fusion is performed through a standard anterior approach to the lumbar levels L2-L5. With this technique,

the abdominal muscle layers were cut irrespective of their orientation and the lumbar segment(s) were approached anterior to the psoas – muscle [7] (Fig. 1).

The Microsurgical (Mini-Open) Access
Pre-Operative Planning and Preparation of the Patient

The surgical approach is performed from the left side. Thus, topographical anatomy of the anterior-lateral circumference of the target segment must be studied carefully before the operation. In addition to information about the underlying pathology, MRI of the lumbar spine and its surrounding structures gives all the anatomical information which is needed to perform meticulous pre-operative planning (Fig. 2).

It facilitates the operation if the surgeon is well informed and aware of the size, shape, and localization of the psoas muscle in relation to the anterior – lateral border of the lumbar spine, and the size and course of the retroperitoneal vessels. For the approach to L4/5, MRI examination should be focused, in particular, on the size and shape of the common iliac vein as well as on the presence and size of an ascending lumbar vein on the left side.

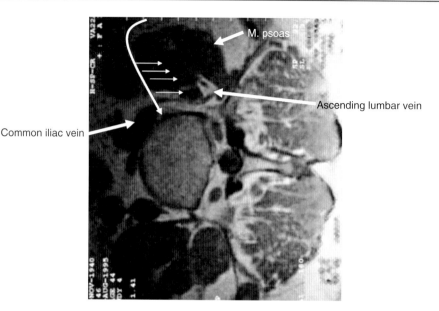

Fig. 2 MRI T2-axial view of the disc space level L4-5. Watch the surrounding anatomic structures retroperitoneal vessels, Psoas

Pre-operative conventional X-rays of the lumbar spine in two planes are mandatory in order to gain enough information on the spine curvature as well as the height of the intervertebral space to be approached. Additional information on the shape of the inferior borders of the rib cage, which is important for the approach to L2/3, can also be obtained. It is important to notice that there might be huge lateral osteophytes of the vertebral bodies adjacent to the segment which is to be fused.

Starting 24 h prior to surgery, the patients are treated with routine mechanical large bowel preparations to empty the colon.

Anatomical Considerations

The disc spaces L2/3, L3/4, and L4/5 are reached through a left-sided retroperitoneal approach. The disc space is reached through an antero-lateral route along the medial border of the psoas muscle. A trans-psoas approach, has a significantly higher risk for damaging of lumbar plexus nerves within the psoas muscle. Especially in young athletic patients the psoas muscle reaches a thickness of more than 5–7 cm, which makes it difficult to cross it (Fig. 3). The other advantage of this antero-lateral dissection is that no nerve monitoring is necessary.

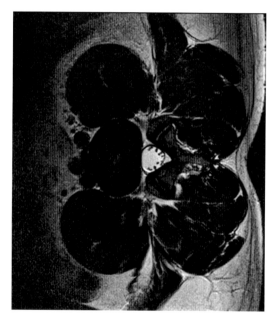

Fig. 3 Psoas thickness in a young athlete. High risk of muscular damage or lumbar plexus damage if a transpsoas approach would be used

To facilitate the surgical preparation (especially in obese patients), the patient is placed in a right lateral decubitus position. In contrast to the conventional macro-surgical approach, the

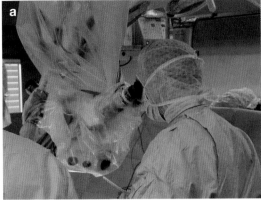
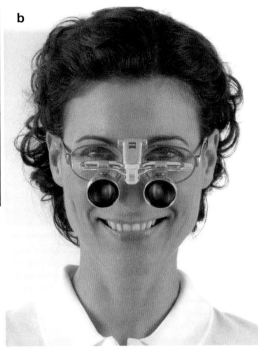

Fig. 4 (**a**) and (**b**) A surgical microscope or loupes should be used in difficult anatomic situations

segmental lumbar arteries and veins are not routinely exposed nor do they need to be dissected in the majority of cases. However, one has to be aware of the segmental vessels since they are at risk for indirect tension due to retraction of their "mother vessels" (vena cava, aorta, common iliac vein).

Optical Aids

The use of a bright head lamp (Xenon Light source) and optical aids (surgical microscope; loupes) is recommended especially in difficult anatomic situations (obese patients, re-operations, difficult vascular situation in the retroperitoneal space) (Fig. 4).

Positioning

The operation is performed with the patient in a right lateral decubitus position on an adjustable surgical table. The table is slightly tilted (legs down) to increase the distance between the iliac crest and the inferior border of the rib cage. Due to this positioning, the surgical approach is facilitated especially in obese patients since

all the abdominal contents "fall away" from the surgical field making way for the approach corridor (Fig. 5).

According to the level to be approached, the table is then tilted backward 20° in the axial plane for (L4/5), 30° (L3/4), or 40° (L2/3). The orientation of the lumbar motion segment is then checked with lateral fluoroscopy. If necessary, the tilt of the table is adjusted in order to achieve a parallel projection of the vertebral end-plates of the level to be approached. The orientation of the disc level ("orientation line"), as well as the centre of the disc space ("centre line"), are marked on the skin. The line of the skin incision is centred over the target point (intersection of the orientation and centre lines) in an oblique direction (parallel to the fibre orientation of the external oblique abdominal muscle) (Fig. 6).

Surgical Steps
Skin to Retroperitoneal Space

A 4-cm skin incision is sufficient for the exposure of one segment. The retroperitoneal space is exposed through a blunt, muscle-splitting approach.

Fig. 5 Positioning of the patient (right lateral decubitus for left lateral approach)

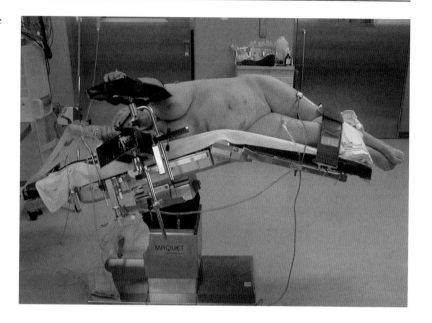

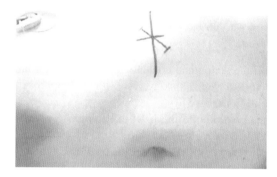

Fig. 6 Localization of target segment

Each muscular layer (external oblique, internal oblique, transverse abdominal muscle) is dissected in the direction of their fibre orientation (Fig. 7).

The branches of the intercostal nerves 10–12 as well as the iliohypogastric/ilioinguinal nerves, which occasionally cross the surgical field at the level of L4/5 between the layers of the internal oblique and transverse abdominal muscles, are the only structures at risk during muscle splitting. They must be preserved in order to maintain innervations of the rectus abdominis muscle. Blunt splitting of the transverse abdominal muscle should be performed as far lateral as possible to avoid accidental opening of the peritoneum. Even in very slim patients, there is usually enough retroperitoneal fat tissue beneath the lateral part of the transversus muscle and the peritoneum, which is more adherent to the inner fascia of the medial part of this muscle.

Retroperitoneal Space to Intervertebral Region

Blunt dissection is continued in the retroperitoneal space using peanut swabs and modified Langenbeck hooks for preparation. Small bridging veins between the fat tissue and the inner wall of the lateral abdomen are closed with bipolar coagulation and dissected. The anterior and medial circumference of the psoas muscle is identified. The peritoneal sack as well as the ureter and the common iliac artery at L4/5 are gently retracted toward the midline using the blunt hooks. Anteromedial attachments of the psoas muscle to the lumbar spine can be identified and incised and sharply dissected from the anterolateral circumference of the disc space and adjacent vertebral body borders after bipolar coagulation. Dissection should not be extended posterior to the pedicle entrance in order to avoid irritation of the lumbar nerve roots. Very rarely the segmental vessels of the inferior vertebral body need to be ligated with clips, cut, and dissected from the vertebral surface.

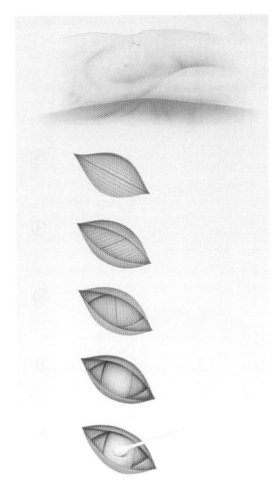

Fig. 7 Blunt, muscle-splitting access to retroperitoneal cavity

At L4/5, the common iliac vein may cover the mediolateral aspect of the intervertebral space. The vein can be gently retracted after mobilization in most of the cases. However, this may be a very difficult task in patients with spondylitis/spondylodiscitis since there are often adhesions between the vessel and the infectious granulation tissue. The use of the surgical microscope is helpful in such situations. The main branch of the sympathetic chain can now be identified. It can occasionally be mobilized and preserved; however, in the majority of cases cauterization and dissection is necessary.

The lateral border of the anterior longitudinal ligament is now visible and blunt dissection is completed when 5–10 mm of the adjacent vertebral bodies are exposed.

Retractor blades are attached to a self-retaining frame-type retractor (Synframe; SynthesOberdorf, Switzerland). The retractor ring is fixed to the surgical table, and the retractor blades can be adjusted according to the individual anatomical situation (Fig. 8).

Interbody Fusion
Discectomy and Preparation of Graft Bed
The annulus fibrosis is incised from the middle of the anterior longitudinal ligament to the medial border of the incised psoas muscle. The anterolateral annulus as well as the nucleus pulposus are removed with curettes and rongeurs. In patients with inferior bone quality due to osteoporosis, care must be taken not to injure the subchondral bone. The cartilaginous end-plates are removed carefully with curettes. The subchondral bone is then smoothed with a high-speed drill. The height and depth of the graft or cage needed is measured with a sliding caliper after completion of graft bed preparation.

The type of anterior fusion is optional once the target area is exposed. All types of fusion techniques are possible (autologous bone graft; cages (PEEK, Titanium) combined with bank bone, autologous bone; femoral ring grafts or BMP, "stand alone" ALIF cages etc.) (Figs. 9 and 10).

Wound Closure
At the end of the operation, the interbody space is covered with surgicell. A drain usually is not necessary. The muscle layers are re-co-apted with resorbable sutures. The skin is closed with resorbable sub- and intra-cutaneous sutures.

Since all patients are treated either with additional posterior fixation or with stand-alone anterior constructs, they are allowed to mobilize 8–12 h after surgery. A brace is recommended for 12 weeks post-operatively (Fig. 11).

Mid-Line Approaches to the Levels L2/3, L3/4, L4/5, L5/S1

There are no general contra-indications for mini-open anterior mid-line accesses, however for the levels L4-5 and higher, they are only used as an

Fig. 8 Synframe (Synthes, Oberdorf, Switzerland) ring-retractor

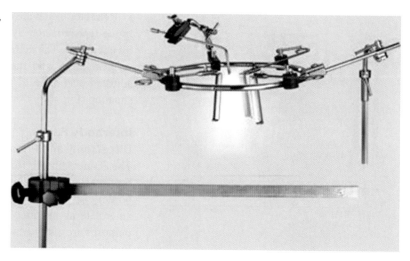

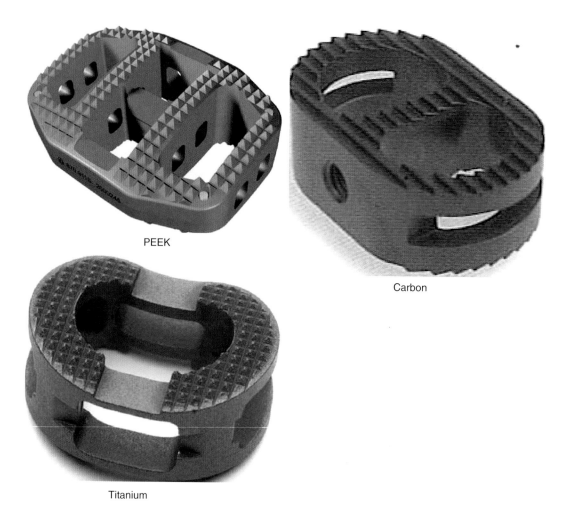

PEEK

Carbon

Titanium

Fig. 9 Different types of anterior interbody cages

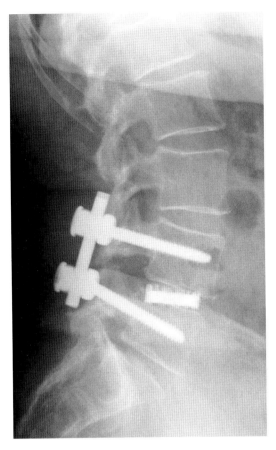

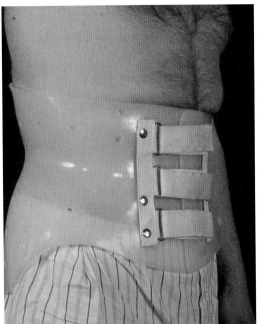

Fig. 11 Typical post-operative lumbar brace

Fig. 10 Anterior lumbar interbody fusion L4-5. X-ray lateral projection post-operatively

alternative to the lateral approach in case stand-alone cages or total disc replacement is performed which, for technical reasons, usually requires a mid-line approach (Fig. 12). For the level L5-S1 we use this approach as a standard.

This type of mini-open access may be modified in patients with difficult vascular situations or severe intra-abdominal scarring following previous abdominal operations.

Pre-Operative Work-Up
Meticulous pre-operative planning is necessary to avoid vascular complications.

Imaging
Plain x-rays of the lumbar spine including flexion-extension views are standard. They give information about the curvature, disc space height as well as about the anterior bony circumference of the disc space to be approached.

The pre-operative planning should also include MRI investigation of the lumbar spine to show the target pathology, the surrounding structures in the spinal canal, the degree of disc degeneration as well as the type of degenerative changes in the adjacent vertebral bodies.

The knowledge of the vascular topography of the retroperitoneal blood vessels allows the planning of individualized approaches. We thus routinely include a 3-D-CT– angiography to evaluate the size, shape and the topography of the retroperitoneal blood vessels (Fig. 13). Venous and arterial bifurcation can be clearly visualized as well as the entrance and topography of the ascending lumbar vein and the segmental arteries and veins. The topographical relationship between the arterial and venous branches and the underlying lumbar spine can be shown. The knowledge of the individual vascular situation of the patient influences the surgical technique and, in rare cases, might lead to a contra-indication for disc replacement (e.g., venous bifurcation

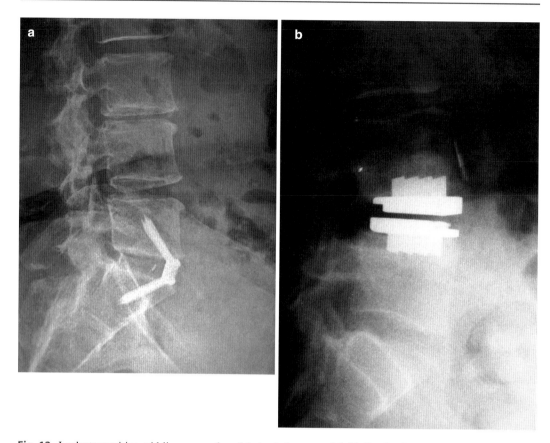

Fig. 12 Implants requiring mid-line approaches: (**a**) stand-alone cage L5-S1 (Synfix, Synthes, Siwtzerland) (**b**) total disc replacement L4-5 (prodisc L, Synthes Switzerland)

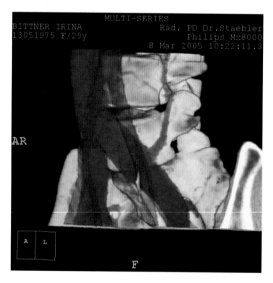

Fig. 13 3-D-colour-coded CT angiography. Note the ascending lumbar vein

covering completely the anterior circumference of the target disc space). It also helps to decide, whether the help or the availability of a vascular surgeon is necessary during the operation to avoid medico-legal problems in case of complications.

Patient Positioning

The patients are placed in a 'Da-Vinci–position' (supine, arms abducted 90°, legs abducted 25° each) (Fig. 14). The supine-position should be neutral, hyperextension of the lumbar spine should be avoided. A surgical table, which allows intra-operative tilting of the legs, is recommended. The orientation of the disc space can then be adjusted to fit the visual axis of the surgeon.

Localization

The target level is localized under a.p. and lateral fluoroscopic control and marked on the skin.

In slim patients, the abdominal wall is slightly indented with a metal marker to show the position of the marker on the skin surface in relation to the anterior border of the target disc space (Fig. 15). All implantations are performed through small 4–5 cm. transverse skin incisions Because of anatomical and topographical details each level has very specific technical demands.

L5/S1

There are three options to approach the L5-S1 disc space (Fig. 16):

1. The first choice of access to the L5-S1 disc is retroperitoneal from the right side. The right side is chosen to decrease the risk of injury to the superior hypogastric plexus in men and women and to leave the left approach-side untouched for a potential future approach to the level L4-5 (e.g., in adjacent level degeneration requiring an anterior approach).

2. The second choice is retroperitoneal from the left side. This approach is alternatively chosen in cases with previous abdominal surgery in the lower right quadrant (e.g., appendectomy, gynaecological operations, operation for abdominal hernia).

3. The third choice is transperitoneal, which we prefer in extremely obese patients (see below).

The skin incision is either placed in the midline in slim patients or slightly asymmetric to the approach side in obese patients or in patients with a very wide stature (Fig. 17).

This is the easiest segment to approach. After exposure of the anterior rectus fascia, the linea alba is split in the mid-line. The rectus abdominis is then visible on both sides. Sometimes there are adhesions between the ligamentum urachi and the pre-peritoneal fat pad, which have to be dissected sharply. A soft tissue spreader with blunt blades is then inserted to retract both rectus muscles from the midline. This leads to exposure of the peritoneum.

Retroperitoneal access from the right side: The peritoneum is bluntly detached from the inner abdominal wall on the right side. The transverse fascia has to be incised to mobilize the abdominal contents adequately. The psoas muscle, as well as the common iliac artery with the ureter, are identified. Preparation is continued

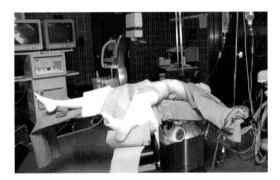

Fig. 14 'Da-Vinci-position'

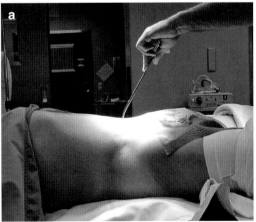
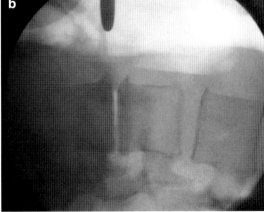

Fig. 15 (**a** and **b**) Localization of disc space with lateral fluoroscopic control

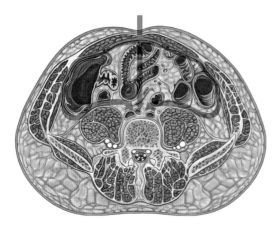

Fig. 16 Three approaches to L5-S1

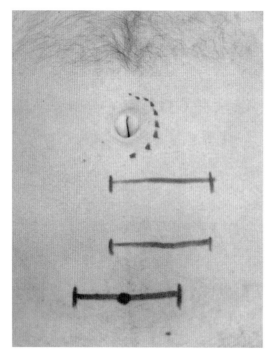

Fig. 17 Skin incisions for different levels L2-3 to L5-S1

fat tissue including the plexus exposes the medial sacral artery and vein, which can then be clipped or coagulated and dissected. Thus L5/S1 can be exposed easily. The left common iliac vein can be retracted carefully to the left. This is the safest and easiest 3.2.4 Approach to L5/S1 Disc.

Retroperitoneal access from the left side: Dissection process is the same as on the right side. Dissection is performed across the common iliac vein to the disc space L5/S1. This can be difficult especially if the vein has a large diameter and covers part of the disc space. The superior hypogastric plexus has to be pushed medially with care avoiding any coagulation. These two factors make this approach the 'second-choice-approach'; however, exposure of L5/S1 can be achieved as properly as from the right side.

Transperitoneal access: The fat pad in front of the peritoneum is mobilized from lateral to medial in order to expose the peritoneum and to facilitate laparotomy. The peritoneum is then opened and armed with four sutures placed at the cranial and caudal edges. The mesentery with the ileum is carefully pushed into the upper left abdominal cavity using the Langenbeck hooks for blunt dissection and small abdominal towels to hold the abdominal contents in place. The same is done to the sigmoid colon, which is carefully retracted to the left. A soft tissue retractor with blunt blades is inserted in order to retract the bowel to the right and to the left after identification of the common iliac artery and the retroperitoneal course of the ureter on the right side. Thus, the promontory is exposed. The retractor is then completed with two other blades. Once these are positioned between the bifurcation in front of the lower anterior part of the L5 – vertebral body, the other one is centred in the pre-sacral space. Now, the corridor to the anterior circumference of L5/S1 is free.

The peritoneum in front of the promontory is incised with micro-scissors. The incision is made about 2 cm. lateral to the mid-line on the right side and completed in a semi-circular manner. The reason for this is the fact, that the main branches of the superior hypogastric plexus usually are located in the medial and left aspect of the pre-vertebral space at L5/S1. On the right lateral

towards the mid-line between the ureter (displaced medially) and the artery. Medial to the common iliac artery, the lateral circumference of L5/S1 can be exposed. In this area, the superior hypogastric plexus is very thin with rare and small branches, which decreases the risk of damaging this plexus. Blunt dissection of the pre-vertebral side, you can only find very small fibres of the plexus, which can be identified easily under the surgical microscope. Dissection is performed bluntly and the pre-vertebral fat tissue including the superior hypogastric plexus is gently pushed away from the anterior disc circumference from the right to the left using cotton wool pads. Only bi-polar coagulation is allowed. Thus, the anterior circumference of L5/S1 as well as the median sacral vessels are exposed. The vessels are closed with vascular clips, dissected and retracted from the disc surface.

The retractor blades can now be re-adjusted underneath the peritoneum in order to retract the peritoneum and the pre-vertebral tissues from the surgical field.

In very obese patients, in patients who have had conventional abdominal surgery and in revision cases, the transperitoneal minimally-invasive approach is the adequate technique. It is the most direct way to L5/S1 and can be performed easily even in obese and previously-operated patients.

Approach to L4/5 Disc

The anterior access to L4-5 is from the right side. A retroperitoneal approach is the first choice. This is the most difficult level to access because of the vascular anatomy. The disc space is, in most cases, covered by vascular structures. Vascular anatomy thus determines the approach to L4/5. Due to the venous anatomy, the retroperitoneal approach from the left side has been preferred in conventional anterior approaches. However, vascular mobilization across the mid-line has its limitations using a minimally-invasive approach. Mobilization of the abdominal contents is more difficult through a 4–5 cm. skin incision. The same is true for preparation and retraction of the blood vessels. Since vascular injury or arterial occlusion can result in a life-threatening situation, all efforts should be directed to avoid such type of complication. An individualized access, which considers the individual vascular topography is recommended to access the L4-5 disc space. Pre-operative 3-D-CT angiography determines the individual mobilisation of the blood vessels. Intra-operative monitoring includes the continuous measurement

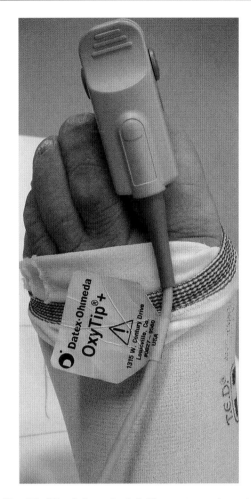

Fig. 18 "Oxytip" on the left big toe to continuously measure the oxygen-saturation in the left leg

of oxygen saturation in the left big toe to avoid prolonged ischaemia of the leg due to retractor pressure on the arteries (Fig. 18).

After localization of the level of the skin incision it is placed slightly paramedially to the left side (Fig. 17). The rectus fascia is exposed from the linea alba to its lateral border. It is then incised transversely to allow mobilization of the rectus muscle (Fig. 19).

The muscle belly is then mobilized medially to expose the posterior rectus sheath and the linea arcuata. The posterior rectus sheath is the incised longitudinally and the peritoneum is exposed (Fig. 20). Care has to be taken not to open the peritoneum. The retroperitoneal space is entered

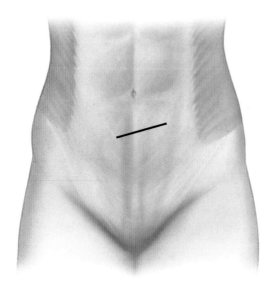

Fig. 19 Incision of the anterior rectus sheath

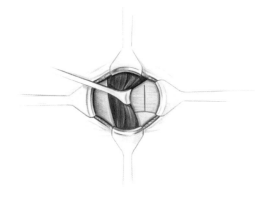

Fig. 20 Incision of the arcuate line (posterior rectus sheath)

lateral to the rectus muscle, to facilitates vascular preparation and dissection in the lower left quadrant with only low retraction pressure on the rectus muscle. The peritoneum is then mobilized from the lateral abdominal wall and the psoas muscle is identified. Medial to the psoas muscle, the common iliac vein and artery are exposed. The ureter is dissected from the common iliac artery and mobilized medially together with the peritoneum. The lateral border of the disc space

L4-5 is then identified. The next surgical target is the lateral border of the common iliac vein and the entry of the iliolumbar – and ascending lumbar venous branches. It is essential to first identify these venous branches. They have to be occluded with sutures or vascular clips and dissected. This surgical step is paramount since in the majority of the cases, the common iliac vein cannot be mobilized without the risk of a tear injury to the iliolumbar and ascending lumbar branches. The mobilization of the common iliac artery is simple, since there are no exiting branches in this region.

Once this step is completed, the retroperitoneal space lateral to the rectus muscle is left and is entered again medial to the muscle belly.

Further mobilization of the vascular structures should follow the individual vascular anatomy. Although, 3D-CT angiography shows a great variety of vascular situations in front of the L4-5 disc space, there are three variations of vascular mobilization which are recommended.

Variation 1

If venous and arterial bifurcation are located cranial to the superior border of the L4-5 disc space, the access can be between the bifurcations. In this situation, mobilization and dissection of the ascending lumbar veins is not necessary. The median sacral vessel however should be ligated and dissected. This is a rare situation at the level L4-5 (Fig. 21a).

Variation 2

If the arterial bifurcation is located on the level of the disc space, it should be mobilized together with the venous structures across the mid-line. However, it is recommended to carefully monitor the oxygen saturation in the left big toe and, if necessary, to relieve the pressure of the retractor blades on the artery every 30–40 min. With this type of mobilization, ligature of the left segmental artery and vein L4 is mandatory (Fig. 21b).

Variation 3

If the arterial bifurcation alone is well above the disc space L4-5, a dissection between the arteries is recommended. Only the common iliac vein

Fig. 21 Low-risk vascular mobilization in minimally-invasive mid-line approaches (**a**) left-to-right: if aorta is close to the mid-line and vena cava right to the mid-line (**b**) between aorta and vena cava: if aorta far left and vena cava close to the mid-line (**c**) below bifurcation: if arterial and venous bifurcation are above L4-5 disc space level

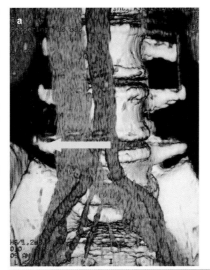

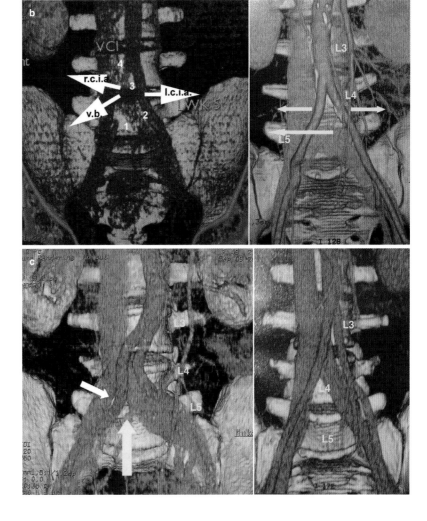

or the inferior cava vein is mobilized across the mid-line, whereas the common iliac arteries are slightly pushed to both sides of the disc space. Ligature of the segmental vein L4 on the left side is necessary (Fig. 21c).

A direct, transperitoneal approach would be the second-choice approach. The superior hypogastric plexus and the perivascular tissues have to be dissected carefully. The mobilization of the blood vessels will be the same as described above.

Approach to L 2/3/4 Disc

The approach to L3/4 and L2/3 needs modifications on the skin-to-spine-route. The skin incision is usually at the level or above the umbilicus (Fig. 17). If it is at the umbilical level, a small, longitudinal paramedian incision on the left side is preferred. Retroperitoneal exposure is much more difficult at these levels, since the peritoneum is adherent to the posterior rectus sheet. Innervation of the rectus muscle must be preserved and the integrity of the fascial indentations at these levels must be respected. It is thus recommended to expose the retroperitoneal space in two steps: Longitudinal midline incision of the anterior rectus sheet 5 mm lateral to the linea alba and exposure of the left rectus muscle. Then, dissection from anterior to the muscle to its lateral border and opening of the retroperitoneal space is performed.

Thus, the peritoneum can be detached from the posterior rectus sheet from left- lateral to the mid-line. The exposure is then continued by opening of the posterior rectus sheath close to the mid-line and retroperitoneal dissection from the left to the right. In obese patients again, a transperitoneal route is recommended.

At the level L2-3, care should be taken for the renal vessels to avoid tethering or indirect rupture.

Exposure of the Disc Space

Once the peritoneum and the vascular structures are shifted away from the anterior circumference of the spine, the disc space can be exposed (Fig. 22). The approach corridor is then secured by the insertion of a frame-type retractor.

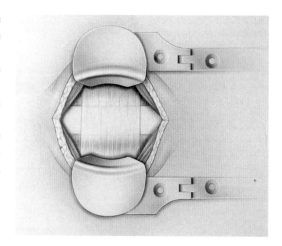

Fig. 22 Exposure of the disc space (L4-5). Synframe retractor in place

Hazards and Complications

Lateral Approach L2-L5

There are a variety of potential complications, pitfalls, and hazards which can arise at various steps of the operation:

Wrong positioning of the patient: It is common to all microsurgical procedures that positioning of the patients significantly contributes to the success of the operation. The patient should be positioned as described above. Special attention must be made to the parallel orientation of the disc space borders as well as to the tilt of the surgical table. This is emphasized because all anatomical landmarks (iliac crest, psoas muscle, anterior longitudinal ligament) are helpful and valid only when they are oriented the right way. Take care that the end-plates are in a parallel projection. If there is a tilt which cannot be corrected it is necessary to modify the insertion of the anchoring screws in a way that perforation of the tip of the anchoring screw into the intervertebral space is avoided.

Skin incision too close to iliac crest: This can happen in patients with "high" iliac crests. If this situation occurs during localization of the skin incision (usually at L4/5), I recommend to tilt the table slightly more backward which will shift the incision line more anteriorly. The same is valid for patients with hypertrophy of the psoas muscle.

High muscle tension due to insufficient relaxation of the patient: Note that the patient has to be completely relaxed otherwise high forces are needed to retract the abdominal muscles.

Ureter: The ureter is rarely seen during exposure of the target area. It usually courses in the retroperitoneal fat, which is mobilized anteriorly.

Common iliac artery: The left common iliac artery can only be exposed at L4/5. In patients with severe arteriosclerosis, the vessels might kink laterally and thus reach into the approach corridor. It is not a problem to retract the vessel. However, if there are calcifications the retraction should be very gentle in order to avoid lesions to the calcified wall of the vessel.

Genitofemoral nerve: This nerve courses on the medial surface of the psoas muscle. It is exposed to damage by pressure of the retractor blade or by bipolar coagulation. The nerve should be preserved since irritation causes post-operative paresthesias, pain, and discomfort projecting into the groin and medial thigh.

Donor site complications: The most common post-operative complications at the iliac crest are pain, irritation of the lateral femoral cutaneous nerve, haematoma, and fatigue fracture of the anterior superior iliac spine. Most of these complications can be avoided if the graft is taken at least 4 cm. lateral to the anterior superior iliac spine. This helps to preserve the lateral femoral cutaneous nerve, decreases the risk of fatigue fracture as well as post-operative pain. Haematomata can be avoided by meticulous haemostasis, including the use of bone wax, as well as by sufficient wound drainage.

Transperitoneal Approach to L5-S1

Approach: Pitfalls might be wrong positioning of the patient and inadequate localization of the corridor line. If the patient does not have a Trendelenburg positioning the angle between the L5/S1 interspace and the surgeon's visual axis increases and might make it impossible to have a good insight into the disc space.

Exact localization of the corridor line is paramount since mobility of the skin of the patient is limited once the surgical approach is too far cranial or caudal.

Retraction of the abdominal contents gets extremely difficult if the bowel is not empty and relaxed. So pre-operative bowel preparation is one of the keys to a successful operation.

Microsurgical dissection in front of the peritoneum is safe. However it should be performed bluntly with small swabs, the use of bipolar coagulation must be restricted to a minimum.

Dissection in the retroperitoneal space in front of the promontory must start from the right side in order to decrease the risk of injury to the superior hypogastric plexus.

The opening of the retractor in the retroperitoneal space must be performed very gently in order to avoid over-distraction of the venous bifurcation. If there is an overlap of the medial aspect of the left common iliac vein with the L5/S1 disc space, the vein should be retracted gently by the assistant.

There is sometimes bleeding from intraosseous veins of the sacrum, which might occur after resection of the end-plate. This can be controlled with bone-wax, which is distributed on the bony surfaces with the high-speed diamond burr.

The peri-operative complication rate is less than 10 %.

Critical Evaluation

Results

Results of Mini-open anterior fusion have already been described [10, 11, 14]. The combination of mini-open anterior fusion with pedicle instrumentation leads to excellent and good results in 75–85 % of the patients. The pseudoarthrosis rate is 3 % and the rate of complications due to the anterior approach is 5.2 %. Decrease in peri-operative morbidity however seems to be the most striking advantage of this technique and the clinical results seem to be comparable to conventional fusion techniques [1].

Minimally-invasive approaches for spinal fusion or reconstruction in degenerative diseases have replaced the standard anterior approaches in the last 10 years. Pre-operative planning, modification of surgical strategies and innovative instruments and implants are the key factors for a safe and successful performance. It is mandatory for the spine surgeon to face the challenges of these surgical techniques and, if necessary for medico-legal reasons, to involve vascular or general surgeons in planning and performing the access to the surgical target area. The main advantages are the reduction of peri-operative morbidity as well as the possibility of early and aggressive mobilization and rehabilitation of the patient.

The use of these approaches for total lumbar disc replacement has opened a new era for a wider application spectrum for less-invasive surgical approaches [12].

References

1. Brau SA. Mini-open approach to the spine for anterior lumbar interbody fusion: description of the procedure, results and complications. Spine J. 2002;2:216–23.
2. Faciszewski T, Winter RB, Lonstein JE, Denis F, Johnson L. The surgical and medical perioperative complications of anterior spinal fusion surgery in the thoracic and lumbar spine in adults. Spine. 1995;20:1592–9.
3. Greenough CG, Taylor LJ, Fraser RD. Anterior lumbar fusion. A comparison of noncompensation patients with compensation patients. Clin Orthop. 1994;300:30–7.
4. Greenough CG, Taylor LJ, Fraser RD. Anterior lumbar fusion: results, assessment techniques and prognostic factors. Eur Spine J. 1994;3:225–30.
5. Grob D, Scheier HJG, Dvorak J, Siegrist H, Rubeli M, Joller R. Circumferential fusion of the lumbar and lumbosacral spine. Arch Orthop Trauma Surg. 1991;111:20–5.
6. Herkovitz HN, Kurz LT. Degnerative lumbar spondylolisthesis with spinal stenosis: a prospective study comparing decompression with decompression

and intertransverse process arthrodesis. J Bone Joint Surg Am. 1991;73A:802–8.
7. Hodgson AR, Wong AK. A description of a technique and evaluation of results in anterior fusion for deranged intervetebral disk and spondylolisthesis. Clin Orthop. 1968;56:133–61.
8. Kambin P. Arthroscopic lumbar interbody fusion. In: White AH, editor. Spine care. St. Louis: C.V. Mosby; 1996. p. 1055–66.
9. Mack MJ, Aronoff RJ, Acuff TE, Douthit MB, Bowman RT, Ryan WH. Present role of thoracoscopy in the diagnosis and treatment of diseases of the chest. Ann Thorac Surg. 1992;54:403–9.
10. Mayer HM. A new microsurgical technique for minimally invasive anterior lumbar interbody fusion. Spine. 1997;22:691–700.
11. Mayer HM. Microsurgical approaches for anteriorinterbody fusion of the lumbar spine. In: McCulloch JA, Young PA, editors. Essentials of spinal microsurgery. Philadelphia: Lippincott-raven; 1998. p. 633–49.
12. Mayer HM, editor. Minimally invasive spine surgery. Berlin/Heidelberg/New York: Springer; 2000.
13. Mayer HM, Korge A. Non-fusion technology in degenerative lumbar spinal disorders: facts, questions, challenges. Eur Spine J. 2002;11 Suppl 2: 85–91.
14. Mayer HM, Wiechert K, Korge A, Qose I. Minimally invasive total disc replacement: surgical technique and preliminary clinical results. Eur Spine J. 2002;11 Suppl 2:124–30.
15. McCulloch JA. Posterolateraluninstrumented lumbar fusion. In: Mcculloch JA, Young PA, editors. Essentials of spinal microsurgery. Philadelphia: Lippincott-Raven; 1998. p. 531–52.
16. Obenchain TG. Laparoscopic lumbar discectomy. J Laparoendoc Surg. 1991;3:145–9.
17. Pellissé F, Puig O, Rivas A, Bagó J, Villanueva C. Low fusion rate after L5-S1- laparoscopic anterior lumbar interbody fusion using twin stand-alone carbon fibre cages. Spine. 2002;27:1665–9.
18. Reddick EJ, Olson DO. Laparoscopic laser cholecystectomy: a comparison with mini-lap cholecystectomy. Surg Endosc. 1989;3:131–3.
19. Regan JJ. Endoscopic applications of the BAK system. In: Regan JJ, McAfee PC, Mack MJ, editors. Atlas of endoscopic spine surgery. St. Louis: Quality Medical Publishing; 1995. p. 321–31.
20. Sachs B, Schweitzberg SD. Lumbosacral discectomy and interbody fusion technique. In: Regan JJ, McAfee PC, Mack MJ, editors. Atlas of endoscopic spine surgery. St. Louis: Quality Medical Publishing; 1995. p. 275–91.
21. Steptoe PC, editor. Laparoscopy in gynaecology. Edinburgh: E&S Livingstone; 1967.

Sub-Total and Total Vertebrectomy for Tumours

Stefano Boriani, Joseph Schwab, Stefano Bandiera, Simone Colangeli, Riccardo Ghermandi, and Alessandro Gasbarrini

Contents

S. Boriani (✉) • S. Bandiera • S. Colangeli •
R. Ghermandi • A. Gasbarrini
Department of Oncologic and Degenerative Spine
Surgery, Istituto Rizzoli, Bologna, Italy
e-mail: stefanoboriani@gmail.com

J. Schwab
Department of Orthopedic Surgery, Massachusetts
General Hospital, Boston, MA, USA

Abstract

En bloc resections in the spine involve sub-total and total vertebral body excision depending on the location of the tumour. The goal of these procedures is to obtain tumour-free margins and conform surgical planning to the oncological indications proposed by Enneking and validated later in the treatment of primary tumours. The spine imposes significant anatomical constraints which make wide margins more difficult to achieve when compared to extremity surgery.

There are three techniques one can use:

- The first is a combination of anterior and posterior approaches to perform the en bloc resection of the vertebral body/ies In selected cases -when the tumour is not expanding anteriorly- this procedure can be performed by posterior-only approach.
- The second is an anterior and posterior approach (or posterior approach alone if feasible) to perform a sagittal resection of the vertebrae.
- The third is the resection of posterior elements by posterior approach alone. All three are technically challenging and complications should be anticipated.

The Weinstein, Boriani, Biagini staging system can be used to help assess spine tumours as well as to plan the resection.

The epidural extension of a tumour may prevent the obtaining of negative margins. A very morbid choice like dura resection and

G. Bentley (ed.), *European Surgical Orthopaedics and Traumatology*,
DOI 10.1007/978-3-642-34746-7_38, © EFORT 2014

inclusion in the specimen can be considered and weighed against the risks.

The risks of surgery must always be balanced against the risks of avoiding surgery. When non-oncologically appropriate treatment is performed most of these patients will experience local recurrences and undergo further surgery and possibly die of the disease.

Keywords

Aetiology and classification • Anatomy and pathology • Complications • Diagnosis • Indications for surgery • Operative techniques-vertebrectomy-posterior approach, sagittal resection, combined approach • Spine • Subtotal and total vertebrectomy • WBB Staging

General Introduction

Primary tumours of the spine are exceedingly rare. Owing to their rarity, few surgeons had gained enough experience and insight into their management until the 1970s when B. Stener first applied oncological criteria to the resection of spinal tumours. Spinal tumours had been treated with intra-lesional curettage prior to this period. It is important to acknowledge that Stener was the first to plan and perform en bloc tumour resections in the spine using oncological principles previously outlined in tumours of the gastro-intestinal tract. His works are still an unsurpassed example of adapting surgery to tumour size and anatomical constraints to achieve an en bloc resection with negative margins.

Later on R. Roy Camille popularized a technique to standardize en bloc resection in the thoracic spine using a posterior approach and in the lumbar spine by combined posterior and anterior approach. Some years later K. Tomita proposed a similar technique that entailed removing the posterior arch en bloc followed by removing the vertebral body en bloc using a saw finer than the Gigli saw. However what is missing in those excellent contributions, which represent the foundations upon which other surgeons have further advanced, is any consideration to the margins to be achieved. The oncological value of such procedures must be considered in terms of the margin they provide.

An oncologically appropriate surgery in primary bone tumours of the spine should be accomplished by planning surgery based on oncological and surgical staging. Following appropriate guidelines allows one to achieve a margin that is oncologically sound for each tumour as dictated by its aggressiveness [1]. Many examples are reported in the most recent literature of highly technically-demanding surgical procedures performed either in tumours of the cervical or cervico-thoracic spine [2–6] or including the dural sac and neurological structures in order to obtain an appropriate oncological margin [7, 8].

Several different techniques are therefore described and detailed in this chapter together with the basic principles of surgical staging and planning. Using these principles one can adapt the techniques described to each individual case as the tumour demands. Furthermore, we have also included tips that can be used to avoid problems and thereby reducing morbidity.

Aetiology and Classification

Fewer than 5 % of the 2,500 primary malignant bone tumours that present each year in the United States occur in the spine [9–11]. For that reason, there are few centres that gained a critical level of experience in the management of these tumours. Furthermore, the terminology utilized to describe these tumours had tended to vary considerably from one region to the next. In addition, there were no staging systems that helped one decide which type of surgery to perform. All of these reasons entered into our decision to help develop the Weinstein, Boriani, Biagini (WBB) surgical staging system. This system is designed to unify the ways by which tumours are described in order to facilitate communication between physicians. In addition, once a common descriptive language is accepted it helps to facilitate research efforts. Finally, the WBB system helps guide the surgeon with regard to what type of resection is possible.

The WBB divides the axial presentation of the vertebrae involved with tumour into 12 zones

Fig. 1 WBB Staging System. The transverse extension of the tumour is described with reference to 12 radiating zones (numbered *1–12* in anti-clockwise direction starting from the left half of the spinous process) and to five concentric layers (*A–E*)

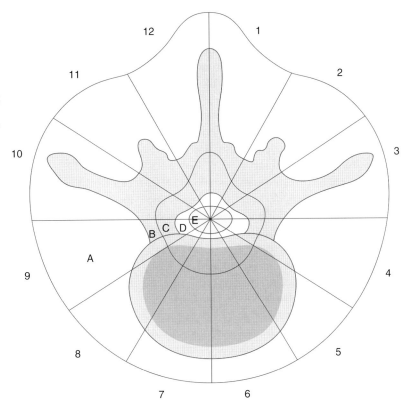

similar to a clock face (Fig. 1). Position number 1 begins at the left half of the spinous process and position 12 ends at the right half of the spinous process. Zones 4 and 9 are particularly important to know because they define respectively the left and the right pedicle. Vertebrectomy with adequate surgical margins depends upon one of these two zones to be free of tumour. The vertebra is further divided into radial zones. The radial zones define the depth of tumour invasion. For instance, zone A represents a soft tissue mass extending beyond the confines of the bony cortex. Zone B describes tumour within the superficial bony vertebrae, whereas zone C defines tumour within the deep bony vertebrae. Zone D describes epidural tumour involvement and zone E is intradural. It is also important to describe the longitudinal extent of the tumour.

As an example, a tumour of a lumbar vertebra involving the left pedicle and the vertebral body, extending into the psoas and the epidural space can be described based on the distribution within the WBB staging system as involving zones 4 through 8 with extension into zones A and D.

Relevant Applied Anatomy, Pathology and/or Basic Science, e.g., Biomechanics

Fundamental knowledge of the relevant anatomy for each region of the spine is imperative when planning en bloc excision of tumours. The tumour leads the surgeon into areas of the spine that are not often encountered in the average practice of degenerative spine surgery. Each vertebrae receives segmental arterial contributions from two vessels. These are matched by two veins leading to the azygos or hemi-azygos in the chest and the vena cava in the abdomen. While the artery is often considered, avulsion of a vein is more likely and more difficult to manage. The vessels travel from the aorta towards the neural foramina along the osseous portion of the vertebral leaving the disc spaces relatively free of major vessel attachment. The blood supply to the spinal cord enters through the neural foramina, inside the nerve roots (radicular artery) and reaches the terminal territory by the so called artery of Adamkiewicz (radiculare magna a.) Some segmental contributions are more vigorous than others, and the major supply to the lower thoracic/lumbar spine is classically described as arising from one segmental artery. This view is not confirmed by dynamic angiographic and MRI studies. There are animal data that suggest that ligation of fewer than four segmental vessels inclusive of the arteria radicularis magna does not result in spinal cord dysfunction [12–14]. Furthermore, Kawahara et al. reported the ligation of the arteria radicularis magna in 14 patients without neurologic compromise [15]. However, it is commonly accepted that there is an increasing risk of spinal cord injury when the arteria radicularis magna – as discovered on angiography- is injured or ligated. This must be discussed with the patient prior to surgery.

The specific type of tumour also has an impact on surgical preparation. For instance, Ewing's sarcoma and osteosarcoma are often treated with neoadjuvant chemotherapy. These patients are often mal-nourished and immuno-compromised which makes their ability to heal and recover from surgery sub-optimal. It is imperative to consider nutritional optimization of these patients prior to surgery. In addition to chemotherapy, it is important to determine whether the patient has received radiation therapy previously. Radiation therapy given pre-operatively has been shown to increase the rate of wound complications in extremity sarcoma [16]. Furthermore, a remote history of radiation should signal to the surgeon that a significant amount of scar tissue may be encountered making dissection much more dangerous, with risk of injury to the vessels, the dura, and the ureters.

Diagnosis

A differential diagnosis for primary malignant bone tumours of the spine can be made based on the patient's history and plain radiographs. Axial

imaging is imperative for surgical staging and planning. A tissue sample is also crucial. CT-guided biopsies have become more accurate and are the procedure of choice for obtaining a tissue diagnosis [17]. However, they carry a non-diagnostic rate of nearly 10 % and they are inaccurate in about 2 % of cases [17]. In cases where the diagnosis is in question, an open biopsy is warranted. In general, a transpedicular approach is best. The entry site can be filled with methylmethacrylate to help mitigate tumour spillage. An open biopsy can also be performed at the time of surgical resection by frozen section. However, the surgeon should exchange the instruments used for biopsy with new ones. In addition, the surgeons should change their gown, gloves and re-drape prior to proceeding with resection.

Indications for Surgery

Surgery is indicated when one is attempting to cure a patient for their primary sarcoma. Surgery may also be indicated for palliative treatment due to the ability to allow a long time for local control of the disease, but, in general, en bloc surgery should be reserved for those patients who have a meaningful chance of long-term survival. The morbidity associated with en bloc resection is not in keeping with the goals of palliation.

A frank discussion must occur with the patient prior to proceeding with surgery. The goal of surgery is to remove the tumour with an oncologically-acceptable margin. For malignant tumours this means removal of tumour with a layer of normal tissue surrounding it. In cases where nerve root resection will lead to significant motor deficit, the patient must be made aware. Furthermore, there may arise a situation where a meaningful surgical margin is not possible without transaction of the spinal cord. This option must be discussed with the patient. For some patients, the idea of paralysis is not worth considering, however there are others who may wish to accept paralysis in exchange for possible cure. This is clearly a decision that only a patient should make in conjunction with the counsel of their surgeon.

Pre-Operative Preparation and Planning

As mentioned above, the WBB system is helpful in planning for surgery. A pre-operative MRI is an important part of the WBB system as it provides the necessary image quality used in the WBB staging system. The goal of surgery should be to obtain a negative margin. This is possible when the tumour spares at least one pedicle (zones 4 or 9). Extension into zone D may preclude the obtaining of a negative margin unless a layer of healthy tissue (pseudocapsule) exists between the tumour and the dura. It is not always possible to know this until the time of surgery. Close attention should be paid to zone A extension. The anterior approach should be directed towards the side with maximum zone A involvement to allow for best visualization. In addition, one must pay close attention to the cephalo-caudal extent of the tumour. This will help determine whether the transverse cuts should occur through a disc or vertebrae. If a foramen is involved, then the nerve root in that foramen will need to be taken with the tumour in order to obtain a tumour-free margin. Furthermore, it may be necessary to remove a nerve root to facilitate tumour exposure even on the non-tumour side of the vertebrae. This is generally done in the thoracic spine.

It is imperative to plan ahead when en bloc resection is entertained. A team must be assembled in order to perform this procedure. This team may include a thoracic surgeon, vascular surgeon and/or general surgeon among others. Skilled anaesthesia is critical and post-operative intensive care should be anticipated. Blood products must be at the ready in case rapid infusion is necessary to counteract hypovolaemia.

There are four general types of en bloc resection in the thoracic and lumbar spine. There is the posterior-only approach for anterior vertebral tumours, a staged approach for anterior vertebral tumours, a staged sagittal resection and a posterior-only resection for posteriorly based tumours.

While en bloc excision from a posterior only approach is possible, it provides an adequate oncological margin only for tumours without extension into zone A. For all tumours that extend into zone A we recommend a staged posterior followed by anterior procedure, or an anterior release as first step It is our opinion that the staged approaches are safer and allow for best oncological margins. For this reason we generally stage our anteriorly and sagittally-based tumours. We will describe our technique for removing these tumours as well as our technique for removing a sagittally-based tumour and tumours of the posterior elements. It is important to remember that these techniques were first described by Stener and Roy Camille [18, 19].

Operative Technique

Vertebrectomy

Posterior Approach for a Vertebrectomy

The patient is placed in the prone position with both the hips and the knees flexed. Care is taken to avoid compression of the abdominal compartment. The shoulders and iliac crests must be protected to avoid skin breakdown.

A standard mid-line incision is utilized to elevate the paraspinal muscles for at least two levels above and below the site of the tumour (Fig. 2). For low lumbar tumours this includes exposing the sacrum.

Prior to addressing the tumour, spinal instrumentation is inserted (Fig. 3). In general we insert pedicle screws two levels above and two below the affected vertebra. However, hooks can also be used. One of the advantages of pedicle screws, aside from providing more rigid fixation to bone, is that the pedicle screws can be inserted into the anterior construct. This is particularly true when carbon fibre cages are used.

We usually instrument two levels above and two below, but there are exceptions to this rule. We avoid ending our instrumentation at the apex of a curve. The apex must be assessed on pre-operative standing radiographs. If a hook construct is utilized in the thoracic spine, we may extend the fixation upwards by a level or two.

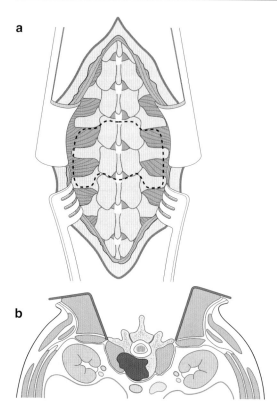

Fig. 2 Lumbar vertebrectomy (L3). Posterior approach. Patient prone. Midline posterior skin incision extending 3 levels above and below the affected vertebra. (**a**) Posterior view. Exposure of the posterior elements and removal of all the posterior elements not affected by the tumour. (**b**) Transverse view. A dissection of muscle connections from the vertebral body opposite to the tumour expansion is then performed and haemostatic sponges are left (see also Fig. 7). Avoid any digital or instrumental manoeuvres in the area occupied by the tumour growth to avoid entering the mass and producing tumour contamination of the surrounding tissue

Once the instrumentation is inserted, then one can begin excision of the posterior elements. All the posterior elements not involved with tumour are removed. This is necessary to allow visualization of the structures anterior to the spinal cord (Fig. 3b). Obviously, if tumour involves a portion of the posterior elements such as a pedicle, then it is left untouched to be removed during the anterior approach. If both pedicles are involved with tumour, it is still possible to remove the tumour en bloc, but it is less likely that an appropriate margin will be obtainable. The uninvolved pedicle is removed with a rongeur or high speed burr.

In the thoracic spine we remove ribs from a level above and below the tumour. The ribs are also removed from the level of the tumour if they do not have tumour involvement. We generally remove about 10–15 cm. of the rib from the rib head distally. The pleura is carefully dissected and pushed anteriorly.

Once the posterior elements are removed, then the lateral aspects of the vertebral bodies must be bluntly dissected. Again, if one side of the vertebral body has a soft tissue extension, then the opposite side should be approached from posteriorly. The side with the soft tissue mass will be approached anteriorly. Blunt dissection of the lateral aspect of the vertebral body necessarily involved identification and ligation of the segmental blood vessels. Remember that they course along the sides of the vertebral body towards the neural foramina. It is important to ligate the vessels on the uninvolved side of the vertebrae. This will be the "blind side" when the anterior approach is carried out. Once this dissection has taken place, then sponges can be packed into the dead space created. These will be removed on the anterior approach.

Prior to beginning the osteotomy, it is wise to place a rod on the side opposite to that on which the bone is being cut. When one moves to the other side for the osteotomy, then the rod can be placed on the opposite side again. This is to prevent any sudden movement if the spine were to fracture through the osteotomy. Now the osteotomy can begin. Abundant bleeding should be anticipated during osteotomy. One should communicate with the anaesthesiologists that blood loss is expected. The decision whether to make the cut through the discs or through the vertebral body will have been made based on the pre-operative imaging. If the discs are the site of the cut, then the discs are removed in their entirety. It is particularly important to remove the annulus fibrosis form the "blind side". This is the side opposite where the anterior approach will occur. If an osteotomy is chosen, then the cuts should be made most aggressively on the "blind side".

The posterior longitudinal ligament (PLL) must be transected at the level of the osteotomy. In addition, the potential space between the dura

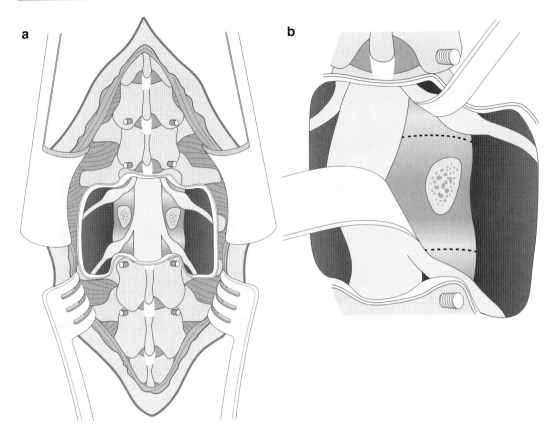

Fig. 3 Lumbar vertebrectomy (L3). Posterior approach. (**a**) The posterior elements have been removed and the pedicular screws introduced. (**b**) The dural sac is separated from the tumour, if growing in the epidural space. Section of the annulus and longitudinal ligament. If the pre-operative plan requires section of the vertebral body, the selected area for performing the osteotomy will be isolated. The nerve roots will be sacrificed if included in the tumour mass or if preventing a complete separation of the dura from the tumour

and the PLL should be developed in order to allow a sheath to be placed. This sheath will be helpful during the anterior approach as it will help to identify the dura. It will be removed during the anterior approach.

At this point the rods are place into the screws and the screw caps are positioned and hand-tightened (Fig. 4). They are not tightened with the torque wrench as the rods will be removed during the anterior approach. The wound is closed loosely.

Anterior Approach for a Vertebrectomy

The patient is placed on the side in a secure position (Figs. 5, 6). A posterolateral skin incision is performed. Depending on the level, a thoracotomy, throracolumbar or retroperitoneal approach (Fig. 7) is used. The soft tissues are identified and retracted away from the tumour. Segmental vessels are identified and ligated. A malleable retractor is placed between the large vessels and the vertebral body (Fig. 8). Now the posterior incision is re-opened. Nearly two-thirds of the vertebral body/tumour can now be visualized. The "blind side" is not visualized, but the dissection from the posterior approach has addressed this. The sheath between the dura and vertebral body is identified and removed. The spinal cord is protected.

The remaining disc or bone can now be cut or removed. The osteotomy is finished with an osteotome, burr or gigli saw. Copious bleeding should be anticipated during osteotomy. The tumour is now delivered en bloc (Figs. 9, 10, 11).

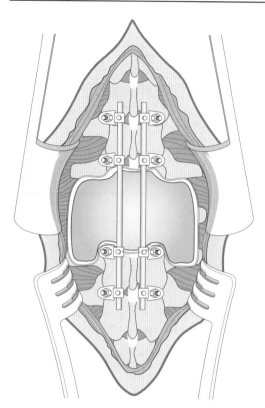

Fig. 4 Lumbar vertebrectomy (L3). End of the posterior stage. A posterior stabilisation system has been implanted. Haemostatic sponges are positioned to fill the defect and around the dura

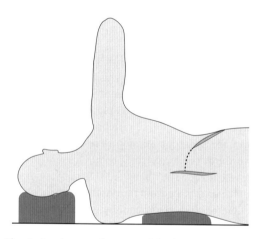

Fig. 5 Lumbar vertebrectomy (L3). Stage 2. Patient in a lateral position. An anterolateral retroperitoneal approach is performed which, in selected cases, can arrive at the midline approach forming a T shaped incision. The T incision should be limited to those cases in which the tumour is growing in the spinal muscles, to resect such structures en bloc. The posterior approach is opened again

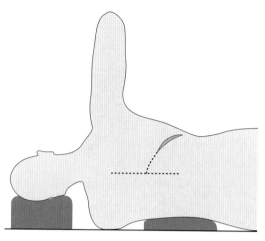

Fig. 6 Thoracic vertebrectomy. Stage 2. Patient in a lateral position. Skin incisions: the posterior midline approach is opened again after the change of position. The thoracotomy is classically performed one level above the lesion. A T shaped incision is advised whenever the tumour grows posteriorly, to include a muscle shell around the tumour mass

Reconstruction of the defect can now ensue. The size of the defect can be measured, and appropriately-sized cage can be inserted. The cage is filled with local bone obtained during the previous exposure. Note, if iliac crest bone is to be used, then a separate set of instruments and drapes should be used. We often use a carbon fibre cage, because we like to connect the screws from the posterior construct into the cage (Fig. 12). Once the cage is secure and the rods are again in place posteriorly, then the screw caps are tightened with a torque wrench.

Sagittal Resection

Posterior Approach for a Sagittal Resection

One of the key differences between the sagittal resection and the vertebrectomy is that the neural foramina are usually involved with tumour and the corresponding nerve root will need to be sacrificed in order to obtain a tumour-free margin. The positioning is similar to that for the posterior portion of the vertebrectomy. The posterior dissection is also performed in a manner similar to the posterior portion of the

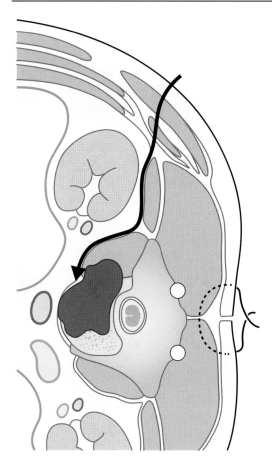

Fig. 7 Lumbar vertebrectomy (L3). Stage 2. Anterior retroperitoneal approach. Note the haemostatic sponges positioned around the dura and between the vertebral body and the muscle insertion on the contralateral side to the approach

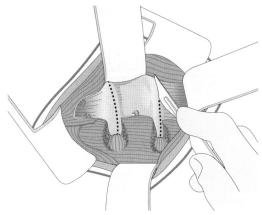

Fig. 8 Lumbar vertebrectomy (L3). Stage 2. Anterior retroperitoneal approach. Segmental vessels sectioned between ligatures. Malleable retractors positioned around the vertebral body. The psoas is left over the tumour mass and the level of osteotomy is decided according to pre-operative planning. Section of the discs above and below the tumour, when located inside the vertebral body

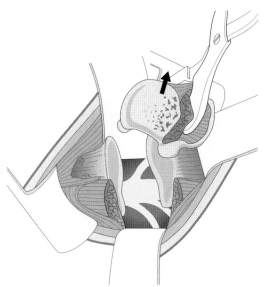

Fig. 9 En bloc removal of L3 vertebral body

vertebrectomy with one exception. The tumour often involves a portion of the posterior elements on one side and so the posterior dissection must respect this area and leave it untouched in order to obtain a margin. This may require that a cuff of muscle be left on the transverse process or ribs if there is a soft tissue mass extending posteriorly. The uninvolved posterior elements are removed. The dura needs to be exposed on the side opposite the tumour as well as the entire dura above and below the level of the tumour. A plane must be developed between the tumour and the muscles of the lumbar spine on the side of the spine with the tumour. At least one nerve root will be taken with the specimen and it should be identified as it leaves the mass so that it can be ligated. In the

thoracic spine the rib above and below must be prepared for excision. The ribs should be cut distal to the extent of the tumour on the involved side (Fig. 13).

Pedicle screws should be placed into two levels above and below the site of resection. The osteotomes will often be placed between the tumour and the dura on the side of the spine

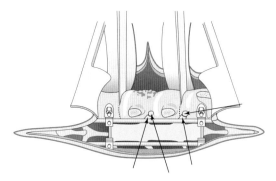

Fig. 10 Thoracic vertebrectomy. Stage 2. Patient in a lateral position. Combined posterior and anterior approach through the T shaped incision (horizontal incision over the midline, transverse incision over the 9th rib). A couple of malleable retractors (*arrows*) displace and protect the mediastinum structures and the lung. A couple of chisels (*arrow head*) are used to complete the resection

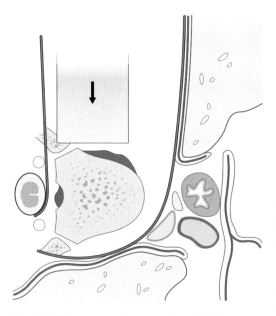

Fig. 11 Thoracic vertebrectomy. Stage 2. Transverse section of Fig. 10. A malleable retractor not illustrated in Fig. 10 is introduced between the posterior wall and the dura to protect from the chisels (*arrow*). Note the circumferential protection obtained by the malleable retractor displacing the viscerae (*arrow*, see Fig. 10)

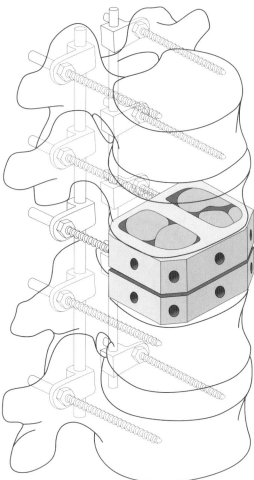

Fig. 12 Carbon fibre cages are stacked together according to the required length and filled with autogenous cortico-cancellous bone. A circumferential reconstruction of the spine by connecting the prosthesis with the posterior stabilisation system is performed

involved. Haemostasis is critical and bi-polar cautery is often very helpful. Gelfoam mixed with thrombin and/or fibrin glue can also be helpful. The dural sac will necessarily be moved slightly to place the osteotome. It is critical to remove the contralateral pedicle so that the dura is not retracted into it's hard surface. Rods are placed into position, but the screw caps are only tightened manually without the use of the torque wrench. The wound is closed loosely in preparation for it to be re-opened.

Anterior Approach for a Sagittal Resection

The positioning is similar to that for the anterior approach. The incision is made and planes of dissection chosen based on the location of the tumour. The same "T" incision is made to

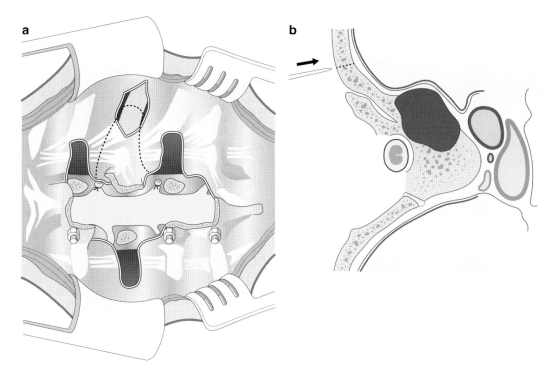

Fig. 13 Sagittal resection of a thoracic vertebra. Stage 1. Posterior approach. Removal of the healthy elements of the posterior arch, to visualise the epidural space and dissect the dura from the tumour pseudocapsule, if required. (**a**) Posterior view. (**b**) Transverse section

connect with the posterior incision. The lung is collapsed and the pleura is incised around the tumour mass to be used as a margin. The ribs will be cut at this time if they have not already been cut on the posterior approach. In the lumbar spine the soft tissues around the tumour are sectioned including the psoas or portions of the diaphragm. The segmental vessels are ligated which will allow for a malleable retractor to be placed between the large vessels and the spine.

The posterior incision should be re-opened. An osteotome can now be placed between the dura and the tumour. The direction of the osteotome will be determined based on the extent of vertebral body involvement with tumour. The malleable retractor should serve as a barrier between the osteotome as it comes out the cortex and the vessels (Fig. 14). Once the vertical cut has been made, then two horizontal cuts are made at each end of the vertical cut to complete the osteotomy. The tumour is removed in one piece.

Reconstruction of the spine can be as simple as removing remaining discs and placing intebody cages filled with bone, or a reconstructive cage can be used if more than 1/3 of the vertebral body has been taken. When we use a cage that is not connected to the posterior hardware, we will use a plate along the sides of the vertebrae for extra support. The rod is now replaced back into the posterior screw heads and the screw caps are tightened with a torque wrench.

Posterior Resection

The posterior resection requires that both pedicles are free of tumour in order to obtain a margin. The patient is placed prone as described above. A cuff of normal tissue is left over the tumour in the posterior elements (Fig. 15). The spine is exposed subperiosteally above and below this level. The spine must be exposed lateral to the end of the transverse processes in the lumbar

a

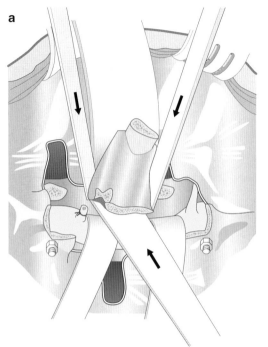

b

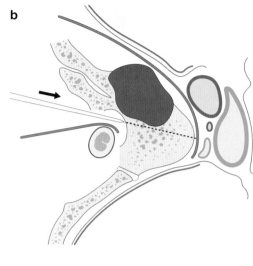

Fig. 14 Sagittal resection. Stage 2. Combined posterior and anterior approach through a T shaped incision which is always required for leaving an appropriate shell of healthy tissue around the tumour. (**a**) Posterior view. The dural sac is carefully retracted. The section of at least two nerve roots prevents excessive traction on the cord.

A couple of chisels cut the spine above and below the tumour. A chisel directed posterior to anterior according to the pre-operative planning completes the resection. (**b**) Transverse section. A malleable retractor protects the mediastinum structures from the chisel (*arrow*) directed posterior to anterior

spine and lateral to the angle of the ribs in the thoracic spine. The dura must be exposed above and below the level of the tumour. Both pedicles must be exposed without contaminating the field. The pedicles must be transected (Fig. 16). There are several ways to do this. One way is to use the "T" saw. The saw must be passed around the pedicle with the use of a guide. Once the saw is in place, the bone is cut by using a back and forth motion with the saw. This technique was described by Tomita [20]. Alternatively, a high speed burr can be used. We prefer a diamond burr as it is less likely to injure the dura as long as it is kept cool with irrigation. Curved rongeurs can also be used to cut the pedicles. The tumour can be lifted away and any further soft tissue attachments can be removed bluntly or sharply as required (Fig. 17). The spine is reconstructed with posterior instrumentation as described above.

Post-Operative Care and Rehabilitation

The vertebrectomies and sagittal resections require a stay in the intensive care unit post-operatively. This is usually not the case for posterior-only resections. Once the patient is out of the intensive care unit, we allow them to bear weight. In many cases we use a 3-point orthosis. This is discontinued at about 2 months.

Complications

Complications are very common after en bloc surgery in the spine. We have a team dedicated to the management of spine tumours, and 1 out 3 patients in our series sustained a complication [21].

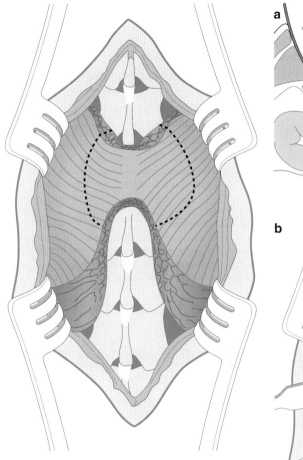

Fig. 15 Posterior resection. Patient prone. Midline approach. A muscle shell is left over the tumour

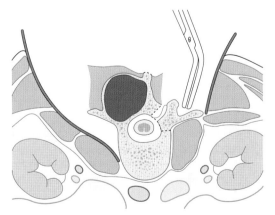

Fig. 16 Posterior resection. Circumferential dissection around the tumour in the lumbar spine (sectors 10 to 12)

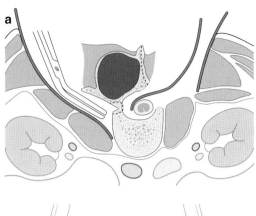

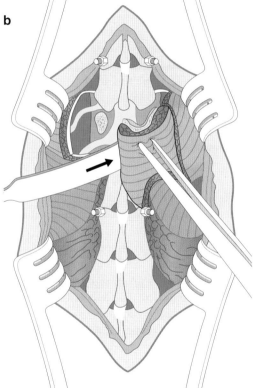

Fig. 17 Posterior resection. Final stage of resection in the lumbar spine (sectors 10 to 12). (**a**) Transverse view. (**b**) Posterior view

The rate of complication goes up with when surgery is for a recurrence or if more than one level is involved. Staged procedures had a higher rate of complication when compared to single-stage approaches [21]. This reflects the more technically-challenging cases since they are most likely to require staged approaches.

The technical challenges of these procedures cannot be emphasized enough. Some of these tumours are quite adherent to the dura making dural tear more likely. Previously irradiated tissues have a higher rate of complications. In this setting, a dural tear may not heal even with primary closure of the durotomy. A lumbar drain is sometimes necessary to help with closure. A blood patch can also be utilized. Dural tears can lead to C.S.F. leak and depletion with possible subdural hematoma. Infectious meningitis is another possible sequel.

Damage to the large vessels in the abdomen or chest can lead to rapid blood loss and death. It is wise to consider having a vascular surgeon available to help with large vessel management.

Infections are a problem in part due to the long operative times as well as to the tissue that is necessarily removed leading to a potential dead space. This is made worse in patients who have been treated with chemotherapy or who are malnourished.

Non-union and hardware failure are also problems. Again, large portions of bone are removed making fusion more difficult. It is important to have very stable anterior and posterior stabilization to help mitigate the loss of bone.

Our mortality rate from these surgeries is 2 % [21]. Unfortunately, these tumours will eventually cause the demise of most of these patients if they are not removed. This is a critical point to remember. Local recurrence, metastases and death are all the enemies of these patients. The surgeon carries a large burden when he attempts to remove a spine tumour en bloc. The surgery is extensive and death is a possibility from the surgery itself. The patient, and the surgeon, must understand this before engaging in these cases.

Conclusions

Subtotal and total vertebrectomies are technically challenging procedures. They require careful planning. Current staging systems are available to help organize the surgical plan. Staged procedures are often necessary and the specific type of resection is dictated by the location of the tumour. We have described the details of three major types of en bloc resections in the thoracic and lumbar spine. The purpose of removing tumours en bloc is to obtain an oncologically-sound margin. While complications remain high for these resections, one must remember that the tumour itself will cause it's own set of complications if untreated.

Acknowledgments We are deeply indebted to Prof. M. Campanacci, who spent a long time teaching us how to understand the biological behaviour of bone tumours and how to establish the treatment strategy on the complete analysis of each single case. To his memory this work is dedicated.

A special thank to Carlo Piovani for his assistance in preparing the preliminary drawings and for the daily work of imaging elaboration and archive.

References

1. Talac R, Yaszemski MJ, Currier BL, et al. Relationship between surgical margins and local recurrence in sarcomas of the spine. Clin Orthop Relat Res. 2002;397:127–32.
2. Fujita T, Kawahara N, Matsumoto T, Tomita K. Chordoma in the cervical spine managed with en bloc excision. Spine. 1999;24(17):1848–51.
3. Rhines LD, Fourney DR, Siadati A, Suk I, Gokaslan ZL. En bloc resection of multilevel cervical chordoma with C-2 involvement. Case report and description of operative technique. J Neurosurg Spine. 2005;2(2):199–205.
4. Bailey CS, Fisher CG, Boyd MC, Dvorak MF. En bloc marginal excision of a multilevel cervical chordoma. Case report. J Neurosurg Spine. 2006;4(5):409–14.
5. Currier BL, Papagelopoulos PJ, Krauss WE, Unni KK, Yaszemski MJ. Total en bloc spondylectomy of C5 vertebra for chordoma. Spine. 2007;32(9):E294–9.
6. Leitner Y, Shabat S, Boriani L, Boriani S. En bloc resection of a C4 chordoma: surgical technique. Eur Spine J. 2007;16(12):2238–42.
7. Biagini R, Casadei R, Boriani S, et al. En bloc vertebrectomy and dural resection for chordoma: a case report. Spine. 2003;28(18):E368–72.
8. Keynan O, Fisher CG, Boyd MC, O'Connell JX, Dvorak MF. Ligation and partial excision of the cauda equina as part of a wide resection of vertebral osteosarcoma: a case report and description of surgical technique. Spine. 2005;30(4):E97–102.
9. American Cancer Society. Facts and figures 2008. http://www.americancancersociety.org. Accessed 2008.
10. Dahlin DC, Unni KK. In Bone tumors. General aspects and data on 8,542 cases. 4th ed. Springfield: Charles C Thomas; 1986.

11. Campanacci M. Bone and soft tissue tumors. 2nd ed. New York: Springer; 1999.
12. Woodard JS, Freeman LW. Ischemia of the spinal cord; an experimental study. J Neurosurg. 1956;13(1):63–72.
13. Fujimaki Y, Kawahara N, Tomita K, Murakami H, Ueda Y. How many ligations of bilateral segmental arteries cause ischemic spinal cord dysfunction? An experimental study using a dog model. Spine. 2006;31(21):E781–9.
14. Kato S, Kawahara N, Tomita K, Murakami H, Demura S, Fujimaki Y. Effects on spinal cord blood flow and neurologic function secondary to interruption of bilateral segmental arteries which supply the artery of Adamkiewicz: an experimental study using a dog model. Spine. 2008;33(14):1533–41.
15. Kawahara N, Tomita K, Murakami H, Demura S. Total en bloc spondylectomy for spinal tumors: surgical techniques and related basic background. Orthopedic Clin N Am. 2009;40(1):47–63, vi.
16. O'Sullivan B, Davis AM, Turcotte R, et al. Preoperative versus postoperative radiotherapy in soft-tissue sarcoma of the limbs: a randomised trial. Lancet. 2002;359(9325):2235–41.
17. Yang J, Frassica FJ, Fayad L, Clark DP, Weber KL. Analysis of nondiagnostic results after image-guided needle biopsies of musculoskeletal lesions. Clin Orthop Relat Res. 2010;468(11):3103–11.
18. Roy Camille R, Mazel CH, Saillant G, Lapresle Ph. Treatment of malignant tumours of the spine with posterior instrumentation. In: Sundaresan N, Schmidek HH, Schiller AL, Rosenthal DI, editors. Tumours of the spine. Philadelphia: WB Saunders; 1990.
19. Stener B, Johnsen OE. Complete removal of three vertebrae for giant-cell tumour. J Bone Joint Surg Br. 1971;53(2):278–87.
20. Tomita K, Kawahara N, Baba H, Tsuchiya H, Fujita T, Toribatake Y. Total en bloc spondylectomy. A new surgical technique for primary malignant vertebral tumors. Spine. 1997;22(3):324–33.
21. Boriani S, Bandiera S, Donthineni R, et al. Morbidity of en bloc resections in the spine. Eur Spine J;19(2):231–41.

Computer-Aided Spine Surgery

Teija Lund, Timo Laine, Heikki Österman, Timo Yrjönen, and Dietrich Schlenzka

Contents

Abstract

Recent literature has shown that computer-aided techniques increase the accuracy of pedicle screw insertion. In the past 10–15 years, various navigation systems have been introduced to clinical practice. Each computer-aided technique has its advantages and disadvantages, but the theoretical principles remain the same. Thorough understanding of and adherence to these principles is mandatory for successful application of computer-aided technology in the operating theatre. The present chapter outlines the theoretical basis of computer-aided spine surgery, as well as the principles of applying this technology in the clinical setting to avoid any possible pitfalls. The specific features of different navigation techniques are discussed, and the justification of computer-aided spine surgery is addressed based on available evidence.

Keywords

Computer-aided • Computer-assisted • Navigation • Pedicle screw • Spine • Surgery-indications, techniques and rehabilitation

Introduction

The basic principles of computer-aided surgery (image guidance, navigation) date back to early 1900's, when Clarke and Horsley introduced an apparatus for precise location of intracranial

T. Lund • T. Laine • H. Österman • T. Yrjönen •
D. Schlenzka (✉)
ORTON Orthopaedic Hospital, Helsinki, Finland
e-mail: dietrich.schlenzka@invalidisaatio.fi

G. Bentley (ed.), *European Surgical Orthopaedics and Traumatology*,
DOI 10.1007/978-3-642-34746-7_25, © EFORT 2014

lesions during surgery [1]. The three components of their device were similar to any modern computer-aided surgery system: the surgical object (herein a brain tumour), the virtual object (a brain atlas), and a navigator (an outer frame attached to the patient's head). While these frame-based techniques are still used in neurosurgical procedures, it was not until frameless techniques became possible, that computer-aided surgery was introduced to orthopaedics, and specifically to spine surgery. Pedicle screw insertion, a technically demanding procedure with the risk of significant neurologic, vascular or visceral injury, was chosen as the first clinical application. In the mid-1990s several research groups independently published their first laboratory and clinical results using computer-aided techniques for pedicle screw insertion [2–5].

While several additional applications for computer-aided techniques have been introduced in spine surgery, pedicle screw insertion remains the most widely used. Hence, this chapter concentrates on computer-aided pedicle screw insertion. First, the basic principles of computer-aided surgery will be discussed. Second, the clinical application of computer-aided pedicle screw insertion is described, along with the possible pitfalls of the technique. Finally, a discussion on the justification of computer-aided spine surgery, based on existing literature, will be conducted.

Basic Principles of Computer-Aided Spine Surgery

The navigation apparatus of Clarke and Horsley was based on the principle of stereotaxis, a method of localizing surgical objects within the body without direct access to its interior. The stereotactic concept consists of the three above-mentioned basic components: the surgical object (e.g. the vertebra to be instrumented), the virtual object (e.g. the CT image of that vertebra), and a navigator to link these two objects. In addition, conventional surgical tools slightly modified to fulfill the requirements of computer-aided surgery are needed for execution of surgical procedures. In stereotactic surgery, all surgical objects (e.g. the vertebrae)

and tools are assumed to be rigid bodies, i.e. they should not deform during the procedure. Despite apparent differences between various navigational systems available to date, they are all based on these fundamental principles.

Although the vertebra with its distinctive anatomical features is an ideal object for stereotactic surgery, the concept was introduced to spine surgery only after a functional alternative for a frame of reference, and modern motion analysis systems were available for clinical use. The navigator of the stereotactic apparatus is basically a position-tracking device with an ability to determine the three-dimensional co-ordinates of the surgical object (the vertebra) and the surgical tools in the space. From various available methods, opto-electronic tracking based on a camera system registering the position data of the surgical object and tools remains the most widely used. For the cameras to be able to track the location and orientation of the tools used in surgery, the tools need to be equipped with either infra-red light emitting diodes (LEDs) in systems using active markers, or passive light- reflecting spheres. In the latter, LEDs emitting infra-red light are positioned around the camera; this light is then reflected by the spheres, and further registered by the opto-electronic camera. For reasons of simplicity, this chapter will concentrate on active navigation systems, but the same principles apply for passive systems as well. For the opto-electronic camera to be able to register the position of the vertebra to be instrumented, the vertebra needs to be equipped with a frame of reference. Therefore, a bone clamp mounted with LEDs (dynamic reference base, DRB) needs to be attached to the spinous process of the vertebra in question. Rigid fixation of the DRB to the surgical object compensates for the motion of both the patient (e.g. due to ventilation) and the opto-electronic camera during the subsequent procedure. Finally, the central control unit (CCU) of the navigational system is used for storage and reconstruction of image data to create the virtual object, as well as real-time visualization of the surgical tools based on position data provided by the opto-electronic camera. The basic components of a navigation system are illustrated in Fig. 1.

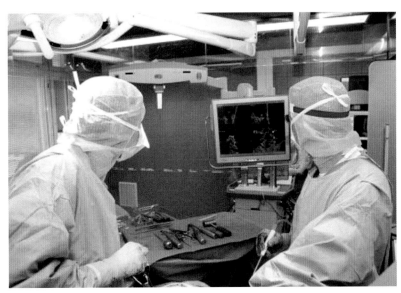

Fig. 1 Navigation set-up in the operation theatre. The opto-electronic camera (**a**) positioned to the foot end of the operation table such that direct line of sight between the camera and the navigational tools is maintained throughout the navigation, and the computer screen of the central control unit (**b**) with real-time display of the navigational instruments superimposed on the virtual image of the vertebra are the basic hardware components of all currently available systems

Skeletal registration (matching) is the process linking the real surgical object (the vertebra) to its virtual representation (e.g. a CT image of that particular vertebra) by means of the navigator´s co-ordinate system. This is the most crucial phase of any computer- aided surgery, and allows for the determination of the location of the various surgical instruments in reference to the patient's anatomy. The most frequently used options for skeletal registration in spine surgery are discussed in the next chapter on the technique of computer-aided pedicle screw insertion.

Technique of Computer-Aided Pedicle Screw Insertion

The ultimate aim of computer-aided surgery is to give the surgeon the possibility to follow his/her actions in real time on a computer screen. The navigation systems used in spine surgery are based on imaging of the area to be operated on, either pre-operatively or intra-operatively. The first clinical applications of computer-aided spine surgery relied upon pre-operative imaging of the relevant anatomy, usually with computed tomography (CT) for a so called CT-based navigation. Later, intra-operative fluoroscopy

enabling navigation with 2D and/or 3D reconstructions of the vertebrae was introduced.

For CT-based computer-aided pedicle screw insertion, pre-operative CT images of the area to be operated on are acquired using a specific imaging protocol, and transferred to the central control unit of the navigation system. The software of the system then reconstructs and displays 3D images of the surgical object, as well as multiple 2D views, usually in frontal, sagittal and axial planes. These reconstructions are used for the pre-operative planning of the computer-aided pedicle screw insertion. For skeletal registration, three to six distinctive anatomical landmarks are identified from each vertebra to be instrumented. These landmarks need to be easily identifiable from the patient's anatomy during the surgery; the authors recommend one to two points from the tip of the spinous process, the most dorsal points of the superior articular processes, and the tips of the transverse processes. The pre-operative planning also allows for definition of ideal pedicle screw trajectories, as well as careful analysis of the patient's surgical anatomy.

All available computer-aided navigation systems aim to interfere with the surgical procedure as little as possible. For CT-based navigation, it is important to preserve the bony surfaces during exposure for subsequent skeletal registration.

The dynamic reference base (DRB) is fixed to the spinous process of the vertebra to be instrumented. Stable fixation of the DRB is essential, as its position in space is the only means for the navigation system to "see" the vertebra of interest. The required connection between the patient's "real" anatomy and the virtual images stored in the CCU is established through a specific registration process (matching). For the *paired-point matching*, all the anatomical landmarks selected from the pre-operative CT are identified from the actual vertebra, and digitized with a pointer. The navigation system then finds the best fit for these two sets of points, the selected points on the virtual image, and the "real" points from the patient's anatomy for a mean registration error (MRE). It is important to realize that this is a mathematically calculated figure, and does not necessarily correlate to the clinical accuracy of the navigation system in that particular case. To ensure the clinical accuracy of the navigation system, the surgeon selects random points from the vertebra with the pointer to confirm that the computer screen display corresponds to the anatomy of the patient (confirmation or verification of the matching). Based on this crucial phase of any navigation procedure the surgeon decides either to continue with screw tract preparation or to further improve the matching with *a surface matching* for better clinical accuracy. The *surface matching* implies digitizing a minimum of 20–30 random points from the bony surfaces of the vertebra of interest. For this purpose, the posterior surfaces of the laminae and both sides of the spinous process usually provide sufficient data [6]. The surface matching algorithm of the navigation system then fits this acquired cloud of points to the virtual representation of the vertebra. The time required to register one vertebra using both paired-point and surface matching techniques averages close to 2 min [7]. After a repeated confirmation to exclude any translational or rotational inaccuracies, the surgeon can proceed to the actual screw tract preparation. The location of the tip and the orientation of the surgical tools in reference to the patient's anatomy are now displayed in multiple planes on the computer screen. Figure 2 (a) through (e) illustrate the different stages of computer-aided pedicle screw insertion using the CT-based technique.

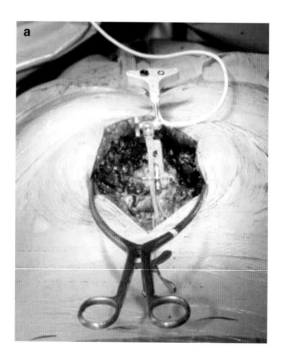

Fig. 2 (continued)

In 2000, Nolte et al. published the first report on computer-aided spine surgery based on conventional 2D fluoroscopy, also called virtual fluoroscopy [8]. For fluoroscopy- based surgical navigation, calibration of the C-arm is required to track its position and orientation during the image acquisition, and to eliminate the problem of distorsion associated with standard fluoroscopic images. Hence, a calibration ring equipped with LEDs needs to be fixed to the C-arm. Like CT-based navigation, virtual fluoroscopy begins with securing the DRB to a vertebra. Fluoroscopic images are then acquired and automatically registered by simultaneous tracking of the DRB and the calibration ring attached to the C-arm. Adherence to a strict imaging protocol

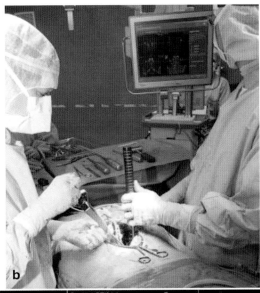

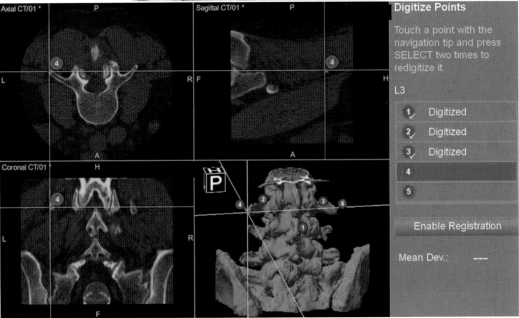

Fig. 2 (continued)

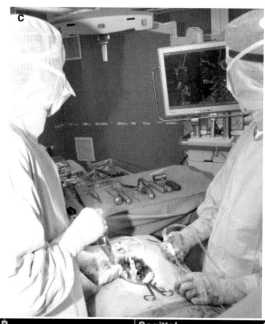

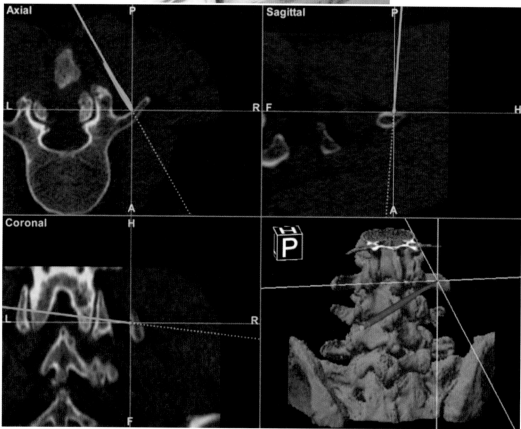

Fig. 2 (continued)

is of highest importance for successful navigation. True antero-posterior (spinous process centered between the pedicles) and lateral (parallel end-plates and pedicles) images are a minimum requirement, additional oblique views are optional. After image acquisition the C-arm can be removed to provide the surgeon with an unrestricted access to the operative field. The need for intra-operative anatomic registration is eliminated, as the registration process is entirely automatic. The acquired images can be used for screw tract preparation in a way comparable to continuous fluoroscopy. Figure 3 illustrates the display and the principle of 2D fluoroscopy-based pedicle screw insertion.

Intra-operative 3D fluoroscopy provides us with another technique of computer- aided pedicle screw insertion with automatic registration. Again, a DRB rigidly fixed to a vertebra will provide the information needed for the location of the surgical object; likewise, the iso-centric C-arm needs to be fitted with a calibration ring. For image acquisition and registration purposes the C-arm rotates continuously around the patient, at the same time keeping the relevant area (the vertebral levels of interest) in the centre of the rotating motion. By definition, multiple vertebral levels can be registered simultaneously, averaging three lumbar and six cervical levels per spin of the C-arm [9]. The image acquisition, automatic registration, and reconstruction of the images take on average 8.5 min [9]. The continuous iso-centric rotation of the C-arm creates a set of 2D projections of the anatomy, out of which the software reconstructs a 3D image dataset with additional axial, frontal and sagittal planes. The actual surgical procedure is then similar to that of CT-based navigation described earlier.

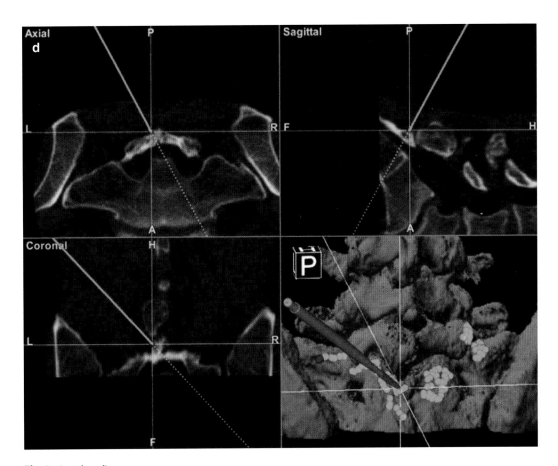

Fig. 2 (continued)

Figure 4 (a) and (b) illustrate some specific features of the 3D-fluoroscopy navigation.

Direct comparison of the different navigation techniques is difficult. A recent systematic review and meta-analysis found more data on virtual fluoroscopy and CT-based navigation than on 3D-fluoroscopic navigation [10]. The clinical accuracy of the navigation techniques available to date will be discussed in the chapter on the justification of computer-aided pedicle

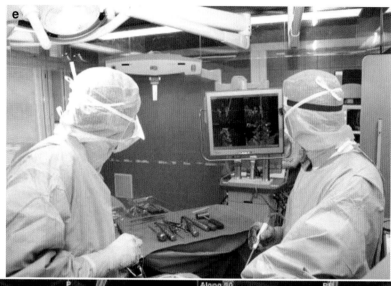

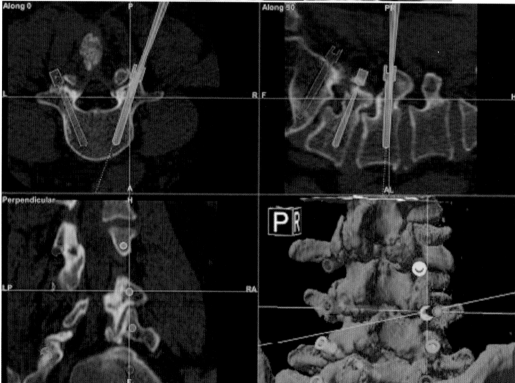

Fig. 2 (continued)

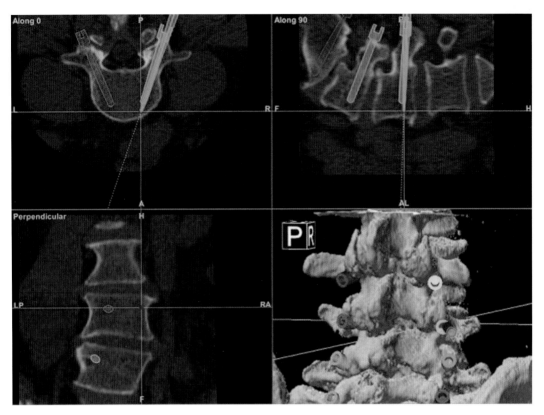

Fig. 2 (**a**) The dynamic reference base (DRB) rigidly attached to the vertebra to be instrumented. The DRB consists of a clamp equipped with a probe mounted with at least three non-collinear light emitting diodes (LEDs). (**b**) In CT-based navigation, the anatomical landmarks selected from the pre-operative CT-images (here the tip of the left transverse process) are identified from the patient's real anatomy and digitized. Based on these digitized points the system performs the so called paired-point matching. (**c**) Confirmation of the registration includes selection of several random points from the patient's anatomy to verify that the computer display corresponds to the real anatomical situation. The *green line* represents the axis of the instrument. On the computer screen display, the tip of the surgical instrument is on the bony surface of the right transverse process. (**d**) In the so called surface matching, 20–30 random points from the bony surface of the vertebra are selected to create a cloud of points which is then matched to the virtual images from the same vertebra. The example herein shows verification after surface matching for the S1 vertebra. The *green dots* on the display represent the points selected randomly by the surgeon. (**e**) After registration and verification the system is ready for screw tract preparation, here for the right-sided L4 pedicle screw. The *light blue* graphic screw corresponds to the planned screw trajectory, and the *green bar* represents the orientation and location of the surgical tool superimposed on the virtual image

screw insertion. As far as CT-based navigation is concerned, experimental studies have evaluated the accuracy of the different registration (matching) methods. Holly et al. found that although paired-point matching combined with surface matching significantly improved the calculated accuracy compared to paired-point matching alone, the clinical accuracy of the two techniques was equivalent [11]. In another comparison on artificial models of the lumbar spine, paired-point matching proved to be more precise than a modified surface matching technique [12]. In vitro studies comparing the three navigation techniques suggest that CT-based navigation provides better accuracy than virtual fluoroscopy [13, 14], but no significant difference exists between CT-based and 3D-fluoroscopy-based navigation [15].

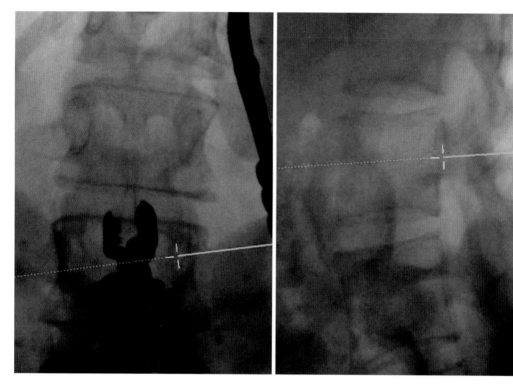

Fig. 3 Example of a computer screen display from 2D fluoroscopy based navigation for upper lumbar spine pedicle screw insertion. True lateral and antero-posterior fluoroscopy images are paramount for this technique. The *light blue line* represents the position and orientation of the surgical instrument. By definition, no axial views are available, but medial perforation of the pedicle cortex is unlikely if the tip of the instrument on the antero-posterior view does not cross the medial limit of the pedicle when the tip of the instrument on the lateral view is just entering the vertebral body. This situation is illustrated herein

The advantages and disadvantages of the different navigational techniques are summarized in Table 1.

Pitfalls of Computer-Aided Spine Surgery

As with any new surgical technique, the introduction of computer assistance to the operation theatre involves a certain learning curve, even for experienced spine surgeons [16]. In one clinical series on the introduction of 3D fluoroscopic navigation into the clinical practice, a sharp decrease in the mean operative time and pedicle screw misplacement rate was noticed after 6 months of experience [17]. Thorough understanding of the underlying theoretical principles, and in vitro practice with e.g. artificial lumbar spine models and animal models are pre-requisites for a successful introduction of computer-aided spine surgery into the clinical setting. The following paragraphs discuss the additional pitfalls of computer- aided spine surgery concentrating on the clinical aspects of navigation. It is important to bear in mind that any inaccuracies of navigation are always a combination of technical and human (surgeon dependent) factors, out of which the latter are usually more relevant.

Any image-based navigation technique relies upon good-quality medical imaging of the surgical area. No surgery should be conducted based on less than optimal imaging. The quality of the fluoroscopically-generated 2D imaging may vary significantly from one fluoroscope to another. Moreover, in both 2D and 3D fluoroscopy, the acquired images in especially obese or

Fig. 4 (**a**) An iso-centric 3D image intensifier. When the C-arm is used for computer aided surgery, it needs to be equipped with an additional calibration ring. For image acquisition, the C-arm rotates iso-centrically around the patient, after which the acquired images are reconstructed and automatically registered such that computer aided pedicle screw tract preparation is possible in axial, sagittal and frontal views (**b**) (Pictures courtesy of Dr. X. Ma, Shanghai, China)

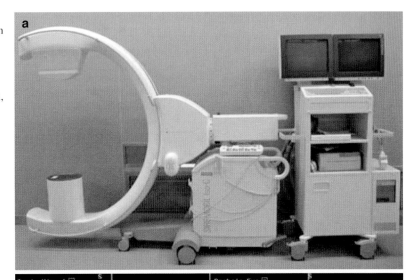

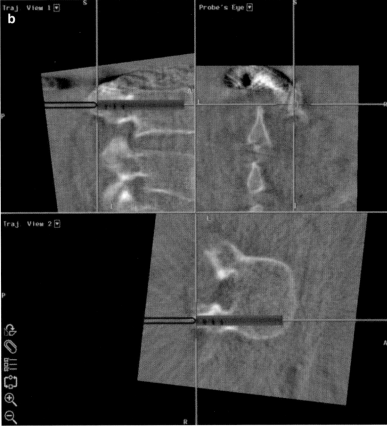

osteoporotic patients may not be sufficient for navigation purposes.

Navigation technology based on opto-electronic tracking requires direct line of sight at all times from the DRB and the surgical tools to the camera. This may cause some changes to the traditional layout of the operation theatre, which are to be taken into account when positioning the camera. In case of a passive navigation system based on reflective spheres, any

Table 1 Advantages and disadvantages of the different computer-aided techniques

Computer-aided technique	Advantages	Disadvantages
2D fluoroscopy-based ("Virtual fluoroscopy")	No pre-operative preparation needed	No possibility for precise pre-operative planning
	Virtual images obtained intra-operatively with the patient in the prone position	Inferior image quality in obese and osteoporotic patients
	Suitable for minimally- invasive procedures	Accuracy sufficient for lower thoracic and lumbar spine only
	Automatic registration	No axial images available
	Reduced radiation exposure	
3D fluoroscopy-based	No pre-operative preparation needed	No possibility for precise pre-operative planning
	Virtual images obtained intra-operatively with the patient in the prone position	Inferior image quality in obese and osteoporotic patients
	Automatic registration	Expensive equipment
	Multiple levels registered simultaneously	
	Suitable for minimally- invasive procedures	
	Possibility for post-procedure imaging before wound closure	
	Reduced occupational radiation exposure	
CT- based	Possibility for precise pre-operative planning	Requires pre-operative CT imaging with a specific protocol
	Strict adherence to the principles of navigation possible	Surgeon-dependent registration process (learning curve)
	Optimal quality of imaging	Separate registration usually needed for every level
		Not ideal for minimally- invasive applications

contamination of the spheres with blood or irrigation fluid may change their reflective qualities, and thus induce inaccuracies into the procedure.

Computer-aided techniques in general cannot ensure that the surgery is performed at the right levels. If the posterior anatomy from vertebra to vertebra is almost identical, it is possible to obtain satisfactory accuracy by chance with anatomical landmarks from the adjacent vertebra. Thus, the surgeon needs to use other measures to verify the correct levels before starting with navigation.

In CT-based computer-aided surgery, meticulous attention has to be paid to the registration (matching) process to avoid any inaccuracies in the actual navigation procedure. Fixation of the DRB to the vertebra in question needs to be stable such that there is no relative motion between the vertebra and the DRB. Further, any undetected change in the relative position of the DRB after the registration is completed leads to inaccuracies

in navigation [18]. The former of course applies as well to fluoroscopy-based navigation. Thus, selecting a position for the DRB such that it will not interfere with the surgical instruments, as well as protecting this position throughout the navigation phase, is mandatory. Frequent accuracy checks during the surgery, especially if movement of the DRB is suspected, are strongly recommended.

CT-based navigation technique, by definition, is based on pre-operative CT images acquired with the patient lying supine. Relative motion between the vertebrae from this position to the prone position during the operation may lead to navigational errors if it is not accounted for. For this reason adherence to the rigid body principle, i.e. registration of each vertebral level separately *and* fixation of the DRB to the level in question, is strongly recommended for improved accuracy [19]. Sometimes it is not possible to fully follow the rigid body principle, e.g. if the posterior elements of the vertebrae are missing due to previous surgery. In such cases the DRB needs to be fixed to the nearest possible vertebra, and the deviation from the principles reckoned. If no relative intervertebral motion has occurred from the pre-operative to the intra-operative situation, it is possible – after verification of the matching accuracy – to operate on adjacent vertebrae with one single registration. However, in one clinical series, adequate navigation accuracy was confirmed in only 13 % of the adjacent vertebral levels [7]. The surgeon-dependent registration procedure shows a considerable learning curve over time [5].

In either 2D- or 3D-fluoroscopy-based navigation, the DRB often is attached to a vertebra other than that to be instrumented, or e.g. to the posterior iliac crest for minimal invasive surgery. In 2D-fluoroscopic navigation this has proven highly inaccurate. In a cadaveric study with thoracic spine specimens, significantly better accuracy was achieved by adhering to the rigid body principle, i.e. acquiring several sets of fluoroscopic images for navigation with the DRB attached to the index level [20]. Furthermore, fixation of the DRB to the vertebra in question excludes inaccuracies due to intra-operative motion between the vertebrae. If the DRB is attached to a remote vertebra, and excessive manipulation of the vertebra is unavoidable due to sclerotic bone, significant differences between the reality and display on the computer screen may exist, even though the images have been acquired intra-operatively using 2D or 3D fluoroscopy.

In the stereotactic concept, all navigated surgical tools are treated as rigid bodies, i.e. the navigation system assumes the instruments do not bend. However, tension from paraspinal muscles or space constraints by retractors may cause bending of the tools. In these instances, the information displayed on the computer screen does not correspond to reality, and care must be taken to evaluate the situation based on those views only where the instrument is not manipulated.

Inept use of navigation in the operation theatre is associated with significant risks and less than ideal results. Thorough understanding and strict adherence to the underlying principles is the only means to avoid these mistakes. Furthermore, to assure adequate skill level in handling the navigation system by all members of the operation team, the technique should be used on a regular basis, and not reserved only for the more difficult operations [21].

Is Computer-Aided Pedicle Screw Insertion Justified?

Although computer-aided spine surgery has been a clinical reality for more than 15 years, its routine use has not gained widespread acceptance amongst spine surgeons [14, 20, 22]. When inserting pedicle screws, spine surgeons have traditionally relied upon anatomical landmarks, the tactile feedback of probing the prepared screw channel, and confirmation by conventional fluoroscopy. Especially in the lumbar spine the routine use of computer-aided surgery is deemed unnecessary because of the relatively consistent anatomy of that region [14]. On the other hand, wide variance in the three-dimensional anatomy of the vertebrae has been shown [23–25], making pedicle screw insertion based on anatomical landmarks unreliable.

Pedicle screw misplacement rates with the conventional insertion technique and adequate post-operative CT examination have ranged from 5 % to 29 % of the screws in the cervical spine [26–32], from 3 % to 58 % in the thoracic spine [33–45], and from 6 % to 41 % in the lumbosacral region [46–58]. Despite these relatively high pedicle perforation rates, the incidence of screw-related complications in the above mentioned studies has remained low. Interestingly, the highest rates of neurovascular injuries have been reported from the lumbosacral spine in up to 17 % of the patients [48].

In their clinical study on accuracy of pedicle screw insertion, Gertzbein and Robbins introduced a hypothetical 4-mm "safe zone" in the thoracolumbar spine for medial encroachment, consisting of 2-mm of epidural and 2-mm of subarachnoid space [49]. Later, several authors have found the safety margins to be significantly smaller [59–62], suggesting that the "safe zone" thresholds of Gertzbein and Robbins do not apply to the thoracic spine, and seem to be too high even for the lumbar spine [20]. The mid-thoracic and mid-cervical spine, as well as the thoracolumbar junction set the highest demands for accuracy in pedicle screw insertion, with e.g. no room for either translational or rotational error at T5 [63].

Although the reported incidence of pedicle screw-related complications remains low, every pedicle screw violating especially the inferior or medial pedicle cortex increases the risk of neurologic injury. Moreover, it only takes one cortical breach per individual patient for a potentially catastrophic complication to occur. Studies on the proportion of patients having misplaced pedicle screws have reported alarming results: up to 72 %, 54 %, and 80 % of patients with cervical, thoracic and lumbosacral pedicle screws, respectively, have at least one misplaced pedicle screw, and thus are at risk of neuro-vascular complications [28, 44, 51, 56].

Clinical studies on the accuracy of computer-aided pedicle screw insertion have reported misplacement rates ranging from 0 % to 34 % of the screws in the cervical spine [64–72], from 2 % to 19 % in the thoracic spine [73–79], and from 0 % to 23 % in the lumbosacral spine [80–95]. Comparing the results from these studies is, however, difficult, as different criteria for accurate and "acceptable" screw position have been used. With CT-based and 3D fluoroscopy based navigation some of the lateral pedicle perforations are likely intentional, e.g. in an effort to protect the upper facet joint. Moreover, in the thoracic spine, the "in-out-in" technique of pedicle screw insertion is clinically acceptable, although it results in lateral perforation of the pedicle cortex reported in some of the above-mentioned studies. Very few screw-related neurovascular injuries have been published: none in the cervical or thoracic spine, and in up to 1.4 % of patients in the lumbosacral spine [89, 94], even if one clinical series on percutaneous placement of lumbosacral pedicle screws with 2D virtual fluoroscopy reports a significantly higher pedicle perforation rate of 23 % and a 10 % incidence of screw-related neurological injury [91]. Two randomized

controlled trials have compared the accuracy of computer-aided pedicle screw insertion to the conventional technique [76, 86]. Rajasekaran et al. inserted 236 thoracic pedicle screws under fluoroscopic control, and 242 screws using a 3D fluoroscopy-based navigation system for deformity correction [76]. Post-operative CT examination showed a misplacement rate of 23 % in the conventional group and 2 % in the navigation group. In the study of Laine et al., 277 pedicle screws were inserted using the conventional technique with anatomical landmarks, and 219 pedicle screws with navigation based on pre-operative CT imaging [86]. Post-operative CT control showed a significant reduction of screw misplacement rate in the navigation group: 4.6 % of the navigated pedicle screws violated the pedicle cortex, as opposed to 13.4 % of the screws in the conventional group. In addition to a quantitative difference, these two studies demonstrated a qualitative difference in the placement of pedicle screws. Laine et al. reported a medial or inferior misplacement of pedicle screws in 10.1 % and 0.4 % of their patients in the conventional and navigation group, respectively. This corresponded to 40 % of the patients in the conventional group, and 2.4 % of the patients in the navigation group having a pedicle screw perforation into these more hazardous directions. A significant reduction in inferior, medial and/or anterior misplacement was reported by Rajasekaran et al. as well. Finally, several meta-analyses from the existing literature have demonstrated a higher accuracy of pedicle screw insertion with computer-aided techniques compared to conventional methods [10, 96–98].

Some specific circumstances exist for computer-aided surgery in the different regions of the spine. Irrespective of the technique used, highest precision in pedicle screw insertion is needed when the screw diameter approximates the dimensions of the pedicle. Thus, cervical pedicles can be regarded as objects of marginal size for any computer-aided system available to date [99]. In one experimental study on human cadaveric cervical spines, greater risk of injuring a critical structure with either conventional technique or CT-based navigation was demonstrated if the pedicle screw was placed in a pedicle less than 4,5-mm in diameter [100]. The C3 to C5 pedicles have the smallest diameter and largest transverse angle in the cervical spine, and the importance of precise registration and extreme caution in applying computer-aided techniques in this region cannot be overemphasized [23]. At the mid-thoracic spine (T3-T7) extremely small translational and rotational error margins for the placement of pedicle screws have been demonstrated [63]. The accuracy requirements at these levels may well be beyond the clinical accuracy of current computer-aided systems. Thus, expecting the navigation systems to perform with absolute accuracy is not realistic or feasible.

Some studies have specifically compared the different available computer-aided techniques for pedicle screw insertion accuracy. In the cervical spine, pedicle screw misplacement rates seem to be significantly higher with virtual fluoroscopy (based on 2D fluoroscopy) than with either 3D fluoroscopy or CT-based navigation; between the latter two no significant difference was noticed [69]. No significant difference between 2D and 3D fluoroscopy navigation could be shown in pedicle screw insertion accuracy in the thoracic spine [75]. A recent meta-analysis, however, concluded that CT-based computer-aided technology is associated with a reduced risk of pedicle screw misplacement compared to the 2D fluoroscopy- based technique at the thoracic level [97]. At the lumbar level no significant differences between the different computer-aided techniques were noticed. Not surprisingly, the accuracy of 2D fluoroscopy-based navigation is better in the sagittal than in the axial plane [82]. Thus, the use of this navigation technique should probably be limited to the lower thoracic and lumbar spine in patients with no anatomic abnormalities.

Added operative time is one of the concerns associated with computer-aided pedicle screw insertion. In the randomized controlled trial of Laine et al., the average time needed to insert one pedicle screw was significantly longer in the navigation group than in the conventional group, but this did not reflect to the total operative time [86]. Rajasekaran et al., on the other hand, could demonstrate in a randomized setting that the time required to insert pedicle screws in deformity patients was significantly shorter in the navigation group than in the conventional group [76]. Our clinical experience further confirms that especially in those patients with significant deformities or altered posterior anatomy e.g. due to previous fusion, computer-aided technology reduces the operative time. Moreover, with experience the time needed for computer-aided pedicle screw insertion decreases significantly [17].

Introduction of computer-aided techniques into clinical practice have decreased the radiation exposure for both the patient and the surgical team. Significantly lower radiation doses and fluoroscopy times have been shown with fluoroscopy-based computer- aided pedicle screw insertion techniques compared with the conventional technique using repetitive fluoroscopic imaging [101–104]. In the CT-based computer-aided techniques, however, higher organ and effective doses for the patient have been reported compared to the fluoroscopy-based computer-aided technology [105]. Although the radiation dose from CT imaging for computer-aided surgery is well below that of the diagnostic examinations, close attention to the imaging protocol is recommended with modifications to reduce the radiation dose to the patient [106].

Computer-aided spine surgery involves expensive equipment. In an era of continuously increasing health-care costs and funding problems, it may be difficult to justify acquisition of such costly technology. No evidence exists to suggest better functional outcomes after computer-aided spine surgery compared to conventional techniques [98]. But evidence does show computer-aided pedicle screw insertion to be more accurate than the conventional technique. The low incidence of clinical complications with the latter, however, may give a false sense of security with no need for added effort to ensure better performance. Safer surgeries with computer-aided technology may well be worth the financial investment.

Summary

Computer-aided technology increases the accuracy of pedicle screw insertion. Although the reported rates of serious complications related to pedicle screw misplacement with the conventional technique remain low, reliance on the "safe zone" concept is not based on hard evidence. Consequently, surgeons should welcome every technical innovation that makes spine surgery safer for the patient. Various navigational systems are available for image-guided spine surgery, with no significant difference between the different commercial systems. Each navigation technique has its advantages and disadvantages, and the choice between them should be determined by the individual surgeon based on his/her preferences and clinical needs. Thorough understanding of and strict adherence to the principles of computer-aided spine surgery is mandatory when using this technology. Finally, computer-aided techniques can never substitute for knowledge of the complex three-dimensional anatomy of the spine, accurate clinical judgement, and meticulous surgical technique. Appropriate skill level in conventional pedicle screw insertion is mandatory for any spine surgeon using computer-aided technologies.

References

1. Clarke RH, Horsley V. On a method of investigating the deep ganglia and tracts of the central nervous system (cerebellum). Br Med J. 1906;2:1799–800.
2. Amiot LP, Labelle H, DeGuise JA, et al. Computer-assisted pedicle screw fixation: a feasibility study. Spine. 1995;20:1208–12.
3. Kalfas IH, Kormos DW, Murphy MA, et al. Application of frameless stereotaxy to pedicle fixation of the spine. J Neurosurg. 1995;83:641–7.
4. Nolte L-P, Zamorano L, Jiang Z, et al. Image-guided insertion of transpedicular screws: a laboratory set-up. Spine. 1995;20:497–500.
5. Nolte L-P, Zamorano L, Visarius H, et al. Clinical evaluation of a system for precision enhancement in spine surgery. Clin Biomech. 1995;10:293–303.
6. Tamura Y, Sugano N, Sasama T, et al. Surface-based registration accuracy of CT-based image-guided spine surgery. Eur Spine J. 2005;14:291–7.
7. Nottmeier EW, Crosby TL. Timing of paired points and surface matching registration in three-dimensional (3D) image-guided spinal surgery. J Spinal Disord Tech. 2007;20:268–70.
8. Nolte L-P, Slomczykowski MA, Berlemann U, et al. A new approach to computer-aided spine surgery: fluoroscopy-based surgical navigation. Eur Spine J. 2000;9(Suppl 1):S78–88.
9. Nottmeier EW, Crosby TL. Timing of vertebral registration in three-dimensional, fluoroscopy-based, image-guided spinal surgery. J Spinal Disord Tech. 2009;22:358–60.
10. Tian N-F, Huang Q-S, Zhou P, et al. Pedicle screw insertion accuracy with different assisted methods: a systematic review and meta-analysis of comparative studies. Eur Spine J 2010, ePub ahead of print
11. Holly LT, Bloch O, Johnson JP. Evaluation of registration techniques for spinal image guidance. J Neurosurg Spine. 2006;4:323–8.
12. Schäffler A, König B, Haas NP, et al. Best matching. Experimental comparison of different matching procedures for use in computer navigation. Unfallchirurg. 2009;112:809–14.
13. Arand M, Schempf M, Fleiter T, et al. Qualitative and quantitative accuracy of CAOS in a standardized in vitro spine model. Clin Orthop Relat Res. 2006;450:118–28.
14. Austin MS, Vaccaro AR, Brislin B, et al. Image-guided spine surgery. A cadaver study comparing conventional open laminoforaminotomy and two image-guided techniques for pedicle screw placement in posterolateral fusion and nonfusion models. Spine. 2002;27:2503–8.
15. Geerling J, Gosling T, Gosling A, et al. Navigated pedicle screw placement: experimental comparison between CT- and 3D-fluoroscopy based techniques. Comput Aided Surg. 2008;13:157–66.
16. Richards PJ, Kurta IC, Jasani V, et al. Assessment of CAOS as a training model in spinal surgery: a randomised study. Eur Spine J. 2007;16:239–44.
17. Bai Y, Zhang Y, Chen Z, et al. Learning curve of computer-assisted navigation system in spine surgery. Chin Med J. 2010;123:2989–95.
18. Citak M, Board TN, Sun Y, et al. Reference marker stability in computer aided orthopaedic surgery: a biomechanical study in artificial bone and cadavers. Technol Health Care. 2007;15:407–14.
19. Lee T-C, Yang L-C, Liliang P-C, et al. Single versus separate registration for computer-assisted lumbar pedicle screw placement. Spine. 2004;29:1585–9.
20. Mirza SK, Wiggins GC, Kuntz C, et al. Accuracy of thoracic vertebral body screw placement using standard fluoroscopy, fluoroscopic image guidance, and computed tomographic image guidance. A cadaver study. Spine. 2003;28:402–13.
21. Tjardes T, Shafizadeh S, Rixen D, et al. Image-guided spine surgery: state of art and future directions. Eur Spine J. 2010;19:25–45.

22. Assaker R, Reyns N, Vinchon M, et al. Transpedicular screw placement. Image-guided versus lateral-view fluoroscopy: in vitro simulation. Spine. 2001;26:2160–4.

23. Ludwig SC, Kramer DL, Balderston RA, et al. Placement of pedicle screws in the human cadaveric cervical spine. Comparative accuracy of three techniques. Spine. 2000;25:1655–67.

24. Robertson PA, Novotny JE, Grobler L, et al. Reliability of axial landmarks for pedicle screw placement in the lower lumbar spine. Spine. 1998;23:60–6.

25. Zindrick MR, Wiltse LL, Doornik A, et al. Analysis of the morphometric characteristics of the thoracic and lumbar pedicle. Spine. 1987;12:160–6.

26. Abumi K, Shono Y, Ito M, et al. Complications of pedicle screw fixation in reconstructive surgery of the cervical spine. Spine. 2000;25:962–9.

27. Kotil K, Bilge T. Accuracy of pedicle and mass screw placement in the spine using fluoroscopy: a prospective clinical study. Spine J. 2008;8:591–6.

28. Neo M, Sakamoto T, Fujubayashi S, et al. The clinical risk of vertebral artery injury from cervical pedicle screws inserted in degenerative vertebrae. Spine. 2005;30:2800–5.

29. Yoshimoto H, Sato S, Hyakumachi T, et al. Spinal reconstruction using a cervical pedicle screw system. Clin Orthop Relat Res. 2005;431:111–9.

30. Yoshimoto H, Sato S, Hyakumachi T, et al. Clinical accuracy of cervical pedicle screw insertion using lateral fluoroscopy: a radiographic analysis of the learning curve. Eur Spine J. 2009;18:1326–34.

31. Yukawa Y, Kato F, Yoshihara H, et al. Cervical pedicle screw fixation in 100 cases of unstable cervical injuries: pedicle axis views obtained using fluoroscopy. J Neurosurg Spine. 2006;5:488–93.

32. Yukawa Y, Kato F, Ito K, et al. Placement and complications of cervical pedicle screws in 144 cervical trauma patients using pedicle axis view techniques by fluoroscope. Eur Spine J. 2009;18:1293–9.

33. Belmont PJ, Klemme WR, Dhawan A, et al. In vivo accuracy of thoracic pedicle screws. Spine. 2001;26:2340–6.

34. Belmont PJ, Klemme WR, Robinson M, et al. Accuracy of thoracic pedicle screws in patients with and without coronal plane spinal deformities. Spine. 2002;27:1558–66.

35. Boachie-Adjei O, Girardi FP, Bansal M, et al. Safety and efficacy of pedicle screw placement for adult spinal deformity with a pedicle–probing conventional anatomic technique. J Spinal Disord. 2000;13:496–500.

36. Carbone JJ, Tortolani PJ, Quartararo LG. Fluoroscopically assisted pedicle screw fixation for thoracic and thoracolumbar injuries. Technique and short-term complications. Spine. 2003;28:91–7.

37. Guzey FK, Emel E, Seyithanoglu MH, et al. Accuracy of pedicle screw placement for upper and middle thoracic pathologies without coronal plane spinal deformity using conventional methods. J Spinal Disord Tech. 2006;19:436–41.

38. Karapinar L, Erel N, Ozturk H, et al. Pedicle screw placement with a free hand technique in thoracolumbar spine: is it safe? J Spinal Disord Tech. 2008;21:63–7.

39. Kim YJ, Lenke LG, Cheh G, et al. Evaluation of pedicle screw placement in the deformed spine using intraoperative plain radiographs: a comparison with computerized tomography. Spine. 2005;30:2084–8.

40. Lehman RA, Lenke LG, Keeler KA, et al. Computed tomography evaluation of pedicle screws placed in pediatric deformed spine over a 8-year period. Spine. 2007;32:2679–84.

41. Liljenqvist UR, Halm HFH, Link TM. Pedicle screw instrumentation of the thoracic spine in idiopathic scoliosis. Spine. 1997;22:2239–45.

42. Modi HN, Suh SW, Fernandez H, et al. Accuracy and safety of pedicle screw placement in neuromuscular scoliosis with free-hand technique. Eur Spine J. 2008;17:1686–96.

43. Samdani AF, Ranade A, Saldanha V, et al. Learning curve for placement of thoracic pedicle screws in the deformed spine. Neurosurgery. 2010;66:290–4.

44. Schizas C, Theumann N, Kosmopoulos V. Inserting pedicle screws in the upper thoracic spine without the use of fluoroscopy or image guidance. Is it safe? Eur Spine J. 2007;16:625–9.

45. Wang VY, Chin CT, Lu DC, et al. Free-hand thoracic pedicle screws placed by neurosurgery residents: a CT analysis. Eur Spine J. 2010;19:821–7.

46. Amato V, Giannachi L, Irace C, et al. Accuracy of pedicle screw placement in the lumbosacral spine using conventional technique: computed tomography postoperative assessment in 102 consecutive patients. J Neurosurg Spine. 2010;12:306–13.

47. Brooks D, Eskander M, Balsis S, et al. Imaging assessment of lumbar pedicle screw placement. Sensitivity and specificity of plain radiographs and computer axial tomography. Spine. 2007;32:1450–3.

48. Castro WHM, Halm H, Jerosch J, et al. Accuracy of pedicle screw placement in lumbar vertebrae. Spine. 1996;21:1320–4.

49. Gertzbein SD, Robbins SE. Accuracy of pedicle screw placement in vivo. Spine. 1990;15:11–5.

50. Haaker RG, Eickhoff U, Schopphoff E, et al. Verification of the position of pedicle screws in lumbar spinal fusion. Eur Spine J. 1997;6:125–8.

51. Laine T, Mäkitalo K, Schlenzka D, et al. Accuracy of pedicle screw insertion: a prospective CT study in 30 low back patients. Eur Spine J. 1997;6:402–5.

52. Mavrogenis AF, Papagelopoulos PJ, Korres DS, et al. Accuracy of pedicle screw placement using intraoperative neurophysiologic monitoring and

computed tomography. J Long Term Eff Med Implants. 2009;19:41–8.

53. Odjers CJ, Vaccaro AR, Pollack ME, et al. Accuracy of pedicle screw placement with the assistance of lateral plain radiography. J Spinal Disord. 2006;9:334–8.

54. Ringel F, Stoffel M, Stuer C, et al. Minimally invasive transmuscular pedicle screw fixation of the thoracic and lumbar spine. Neurosurgery. 2006;59(Suppl 2):361–7.

55. Sapkas GS, Papadakis SA, Stathakopoulos P, et al. Evaluation of pedicle screw position in thoracic and lumbar spine fixation using plain radiographs and computed tomography. A prospective study of 35 patients. Spine. 1999;24:1926–9.

56. Schizas C, Michel J, Kosmopoulos V, et al. Computer tomography assessment of pedicle screw insertion in percutaneous posterior transpedicular stabilization. Eur Spine J. 2007;16:613–7.

57. Schulze CJ, Munzinger E, Weber U. Clinical relevance of accuracy of pedicle screw placement: a computed tomographic-supported analysis. Spine. 1998;23:2215–20.

58. Wiesner L, Kothe R, Schulitz K-P, et al. Clinical evaluation and computed tomography scan analysis of screw tracts after percutaneous insertion of pedicle screws in the lumbar spine. Spine. 2000;25:615–21.

59. Ebraheim NA, Jabaly G, Xu R, et al. Anatomic relations of the thoracic pedicle to the adjacent neural structures. Spine. 1997;22:1553–6.

60. Ebraheim NA, Xu R, Darwich M, et al. Anatomic relations between the lumbar pedicles and the adjacent neural structures. Spine. 1997;22:2338–41.

61. Soyuncu Y, Yildirim FB, Sekban H, et al. Anatomic evaluation and relationship between the lumbar pedicle and adjacent neural structures: an anatomic study. J Spinal Disord. 2005;18:243–6.

62. Lien SB, Liou NH, Wu SS. Analysis of anatomic morphometry of the pedicles and the safe zone for through-pedicle procedures in the thoracic and lumbar spine. Eur Spine J. 2007;16:1215–22.

63. Rampersaud YR, Simon DA, Foley KT. Accuracy requirements for image-guided spinal pedicle screw placement. Spine. 2001;26:352–9.

64. Hott JS, Papadopoulos SM, Theodore N, et al. Intraoperative Iso-C C-arm navigation in cervical spinal surgery. Review of the first 52 cases. Spine. 2004;29:2856–60.

65. Ishikawa Y, Kanemura T, Yoshida G, et al. Clinical accuracy of three-dimensional fluoroscopy-based computer-assisted cervical pedicle screw placement: a retrospective comparative study of conventional versus computer-assisted cervical pedicle screw placement. J Neurosurg Spine. 2010;13:606–11.

66. Ito Y, Sugimoto Y, Tomioka M, et al. Clinical accuracy of 3D fluoroscopy-assisted cervical pedicle screw insertion. J Neurosurg Spine. 2008;9:450–3.

67. Kamimura M, Ebara S, Itoh H, et al. Cervical pedicle screw insertion: assessment of safety and accuracy with computer-assisted image guidance. J Spinal Disord. 2000;13:218–24.

68. Kotani Y, Abumi K, Ito K, et al. Improved accuracy of computer-assisted cervical pedicle screw insertion. J Neurosurg. 2003;99(3 Suppl):257–63.

69. Liu Y, Tian W, Liu B, et al. Comparison of the clinical accuracy of cervical (C2-C7) pedicle screw insertion assisted by fluoroscopy, computed tomogarphy-based navigation, and intraoperative three-dimensional C-arm navigation. Chin Med J. 2010;123:2995–8.

70. Rajan VV, Kamath V, Shetty AP, et al. IsoC-3D navigation assisted pedicle screw placement in deformities of the cervical and thoracic spine. Indian J Orthop. 2010;44:163–8.

71. Rajasekaran S, Kanna PRM, Shetty TAP. Intraoperative computer navigation guided cervical pedicle screw insertion in thirty-three complex cervical spine deformities. J Cranio-vertebr Junction Spine. 2010;1:38–43.

72. Richter M, Mattes T, Cakir B. Computer-assisted posterior instrumentation of the cervical and cervico-thoracic spine. Eur Spine J. 2004;13:50–9.

73. Bledsoe JM, Fenton D, Fogelson JL, et al. Accuracy of upper thoracic pedicle screw placement using three-dimensional image guidance. Spine J. 2009;9:817–21.

74. Kotani Y, Abumi K, Ito M, et al. Accuracy analysis of pedicle screw placement in posterior scoliosis surgery. Comparison between conventional fluoroscopic and computer-assisted technique. Spine. 2007;32:1543–50.

75. Lekovic GP, Potts EA, Karahalios DG, et al. A comparison of two techniques in image-guided thoracic pedicle screw placement: a retrospective study of 37 patients and 277 pedicle screws. J Neurosurg Spine. 2007;7:393–8.

76. Rajasekaran S, Vidyadhara S, Ramesh P, et al. Randomized clinical study to compare the accuracy of navigated and non-navigated thoracic pedicle screws in deformity correction surgeries. Spine. 2007;32:E56–64.

77. Sugimoto Y, Ito Y, Tomioka M, et al. Clinical accuracy of three-dimensional fluoroscopy (IsoC-3D)-assisted upper thoracic pedicle screw insertion. Acta Med Okayama. 2010;64:209–12.

78. Takahashi J, Hirabayashi H, Hashidate H, et al. Accuracy of multilevel registration in image-guided pedicle screw insertion for adolescent idiopathic scoliosis. Spine. 2010;35:347–52.

79. Youkilis AS, Quint DJ, McGillicuddy JE, et al. Stereotactic navigation for placement of pedicle screws in the thoracic spine. Neurosurgery. 2001;48:771–8.

80. Amiot L-P, Lang K, Putzier M, et al. Comparative results between conventional and computer-assisted pedicle screw installation in the thoracic, lumbar, and sacral spine. Spine. 2000;25:606–14.

81. Carl AL, Khanuja HS, Gatto CA, et al. In vivo pedicle screw placement: image-guided virtual vision. J Spinal Disord. 2000;13:225–9.
82. Fu TS, Chen LH, Wong CB, et al. Computer-assisted fluoroscopic navigation of pedicle screw insertion: an in vivo feasibility study. Acta Orthop Scand. 2004;75:730–5.
83. Girardi FP, Cammisa FP, Sandhu HS, et al. The placement of lumbar pedicle screws using computerised stereotactic guidance. J Bone Joint Surg Br. 1999;81-B:825–9.
84. Idler C, Rolfe KW, Gorek JE. Accuracy of percutaneous lumbar pedicle screw placement using the oblique or "owl's-eye" view and novel guidance technology. J Neurosurg Spine. 2010;13:509–15.
85. Laine T, Schlenzka D, Mäkitalo K, et al. Improved accuracy of pedicle screw insertion with computer-assisted surgery: a prospective clinical trial of 30 patients. Spine. 1997;22:1254–8.
86. Laine T, Lund T, Ylikoski M, et al. Accuracy of pedicle screw insertion with and without computer assistance: a randomized controlled clinical study in 100 consecutive patients. Eur Spine J. 2000;9:235–40.
87. Merloz P, Troccaz J, Vouaillat H, et al. Fluoroscopy-based navigation system in spine surgery. Proc Inst Mech Eng H. 2007;221:813–20.
88. Nakashima H, Sato K, Ando T, et al. Comparison of the percutaneous screw placement precision of isocentric C-arm 3-dimensional fluoroscopy-navigated pedicle screw implantation and conventional fluoroscopy method with minimally invasive surgery. J Spinal Disord Tech. 2009;22:468–72.
89. Nottmeier EW, Seemer W, Young PM. Placement of thoracolumbar pedicle screws using three-dimensional image guidance: experience in a large patient cohort. J Neurosurg Spine. 2009;10:33–9.
90. Rampersaud YR, Pik JHT, Salonen D, et al. Clinical accuracy of fluoroscopic computer-assisted pedicle screw fixation: a CT analysis. Spine. 2005;30:E183–90.
91. Ravi B, Zahrai A, Rampersaud R. Clinical accuracy of computer-assisted two-dimensional fluoroscopy for the percutaneous placement of lumbosacral pedicle screws. Spine. 2010;36:84–91.
92. Schwarzenbach O, Berlemann U, Jost B, et al. Accuracy of computer-assisted pedicle screw placement: an in vivo computer tomography analysis. Spine. 1997;22:452–8.
93. Sugimoto Y, Ito Y, Tomioka M, et al. Upper lumbar pedicle screw insertion using three-dimensional fluoroscopy navigation: assessment of clinical accuracy. Acta Med Okayama. 2010;64:293–7.
94. Villavicencio AT, Burneikiene S, Bulsara KR, et al. Utility of computerized isocentric fluoroscopy for minimally invasive spinal surgical techniques. J Spinal Disord Tech. 2005;18:369–75.
95. Wood M, Mannion R. A comparison of CT-based navigation techniques for minimally invasive lumbar pedicle screw placement. J Spinal Disord Tech 2010, ePub ahead of print
96. Kosmopoulos V, Schizas C. Pedicle screw placement accuracy. A meta-analysis. Spine. 2007;32:E111–20.
97. Tian N-F, Xu H-Z. Image-guided pedicle screw insertion accuracy: a meta-analysis. Int Orthop. 2009;33:895–903.
98. Verma R, Krishan S, Haendlmayer K, et al. Functional outcome of computer-assisted spinal pedicle screw placement: a systematic review and meta-analysis of 23 studies including 5992 pedicle screws. Eur Spine J. 2010;19:370–5.
99. Reinhold M, Bach C, Audige L, et al. Comparison of two novel fluoroscopy-based stereotactic methods for cervical pedicle screw placement and review of the literature. Eur Spine J. 2008;17:564–75.
100. Ludwig SC, Kowalski JM, Edwards CC, et al. Cervical pedicle screws. Comparative accuracy of two insertion techniques. Spine. 2000;25:2675–81.
101. Kim CW, Lee YP, Taylor W, et al. Use of navigation-assisted fluoroscopy to decrease radiation exposure during minimally invasive spine surgery. Spine J. 2008;8:584–90.
102. Kraus MD, Krischak G, Keppler P, et al. Can computer-assisted surgery reduce the effective dose for spinal fusion and sacroiliac screw insertion? Clin Orthop Relat Res. 2010;468:2419–29.
103. Linhardt O, Perlick L, Luring C, et al. Extracorporeal single dose and radiographic dosage in image-controlled and fluoroscopic navigated pedicle screw implantation. Z Orthop Ihre Grenzgeb. 2005;143:175–9.
104. Smith HE, Welsch MD, Sasso RC, et al. Comparison of radiation exposure in lumbar pedicle screw placement with fluoroscopy vs computer-assisted image guidance with intraoperative three-dimensional imaging. J Spinal Cord Med. 2008;31:532–7.
105. Schaeren S, Roth J, Dick W. Effective in vivo radiation dose with image reconstruction controlled pedicle instrumentation vs. CT-based navigation. Orthopade. 2002;31:392–6.
106. Slomczykowski M, Roberto M, Schneeberger P, et al. Radiation dose for pedicle screw insertion. Fluoroscopic method versus computer-assisted surgery. Spine. 1999;24:975–83.

General Management of Spinal Injuries

César Vincent and Charles Court

Contents

Abstract

Spinal trauma is a serious issue with a tremendous impact in western countries. Patients are usually very young, involved in high energy trauma but spinal trauma is more and more frequent in the elderly. Sequelae can be devastating and irreversible. The social impact of spinal trauma is considerable. Efforts are being made in prevention and in managing patients with spinal injuries. Many studies tried to evaluate neuro-protective agents to enhance recovery. Although the AO classification is being widely used in Europe, new classifications have been published to help physicians in understanding mechanisms and treatment rationales. Conservative treatment can give good results mainly with low energy trauma and no neurological impairment. Surgery is being indicated to ensure good fracture reduction and neural decompression. Surgical techniques are based on fusion by posterior or anterior approaches. No approach has proven to give better long-term results and no consensus has been found with respect to posterior fusion or fixation extent. New minimally-invasive techniques have recently emerged in an effort to decrease surgical morbidity especially in elderly and polytrauma patients. These techniques need to be confirmed by large prospective randomized studies with long-term follow-up.

C. Vincent • C. Court (✉)
Spine Unit, Orthopaedic Department, Bicetre University
Hospital, AP-HP Paris, Université Paris-Sud ORSAY,
Le Kremlin Bicêtre, France
e-mail: cesar.vincent@bct.aphp.fr;
charles.court@bct.aphp.fr

G. Bentley (ed.), *European Surgical Orthopaedics and Traumatology*,
DOI 10.1007/978-3-642-34746-7_30, © EFORT 2014

Keywords

Biomechanics and Classifications • Clinical
assessment • General Management • Imaging-
radiographs, CT Scanning, MR Scanning •
Injuries • Neurological assessment • Neuro-
protection • Spine • Treatment-non-operative,
operative

Introduction

Spinal trauma can lead to dramatic functional
sequelae when neurological lesions are present.
In treating such lesions, the surgeon must
conduct a general examination to look for
associated lesions, as well as a precise
neurological examination. Imaging studies are
warranted and are oriented by the physical
findings. CT scan is the "gold standard" in
assessing the entire spine, fractures lines and
spinal canal compromise. Magnetic resonance
imaging is of value to look for ligamentous
injuries and medullar lesions. Classifications
are derived from imaging studies. Numerous
classifications exist based on the anatomical
lesion, mechanism lesion or the clinical and
mechanical lesion. Their use is necessary to
determine spine stability and decide treatment.
The choice between Orthopaedic conservative
or surgical treatment is not straightforward as
guidelines are lacking.

General Considerations

Injuries of the thoracic and lumbar spine occur in
two categories of patients. In the first one,
patients are mainly young and active people
and injuries are caused by high-energy trauma,
while in the others, spine injuries are related to
low-energy trauma in patients with altered bone
density and involve older patients especially
post-menopausal women.

High energy trauma is caused mainly by motor
vehicle accidents (drivers, passengers and pedes-
trian) [1–3], falls [4], gunshots [5] and sports
[6–11]. Efforts have been made to diminish the

risk of injury to drivers and passengers. Not only
have restraints and airbags diminished the severity of injuries, but also they changed the pattern
of thoraco-lumbar fractures in patients involved
in car accidents [12–15].

In a multi-centre study of the Scoliosis
Research Society including 1,019 patients, 16 %
of injuries occurred between T1 and T10, 52 %
between T11 and L1, and 32 % between L1
and L5 [16]. Multi-level fractures occur in up to
25 % of patients [17, 18]. Any spine fracture can
be associated with another non-contiguous spine
fracture in up to 15 % of cases [17], so these
fractures can be overlooked if not systematically
looked for, and consequently thoraco-lumbar
fractures are missed more frequently in
polytrauma patients [14].

Clinical Assessment

In high-energy trauma patients, life-threatening
lesions should be suspected and actively looked
for. These include abdominal, thoracic, head and
vascular lesions. Polytrauma patients with severe
lesions are usually admitted to resuscitation areas
which have been developed in an effort to minimize the adverse effects of major trauma [19, 20].
Management is usually conducted by a multi-
disciplinary trauma team where the spine surgeon
plays a key role.

On admission, the patient is usually placed
on a hard spinal board and the cervical
spine is immediately immobilized with a rigid
Philadelphia collar if it has not been done earlier.
It is important to limit the time on the rigid
backboard to avoid the development of skin
breakdown [21].

The ABC rules (ensuring airway, breathing
and circulation) should be applied. Airway
clearance should be assured by removing any
mechanical obstruction (teeth, tongue, clots...),
and performing intubation if necessary. The team
should have a good experience with intubation
techniques [22] which can be more challenging
with an immobilized spine.

Breathing can be jeopardized in thoracic
trauma (lung contusion and alveolar bleeding,

haemothorax, tension pneumothorax, flail chest). Haemothorax and tension pneumothorax, interfering with ventilation, should be drained urgently. To ensure normal breathing, mechanical ventilation may be necessary especially in thoracic trauma and comatose patients. Intubation and sedation could be also indicated secondarily for pain management. In case of sternal fracture and great vessels injury should be ruled out.

Circulation is monitored by heart rate and arterial blood pressure. In 2003, French experts [23] recommended the correction of any systolic pressure below 90 mmHg and the maintenance of a mean blood pressure greater than 80 mmHg. They also pointed to the fact that a mean blood pressure greater than 110 mmHg should be controlled to avoid spinal cord oedema.

A femoral catheter is usually used for precise pressure monitoring and drug administration. Shock in polytrauma patients is usually hypovolaemic due to bleeding but may be of cardiogenic or neurogenic origin. Shock may lead to prolonged severe hypotension which can worsen traumatic spinal cord damage.

Haemorragic shock should be treated initially by colloid perfusion. If necessary, blood should be transfused as soon as possible to minimize hypoxaemia especially in spinal cord trauma [21]. Arterial embolization may be indicated in case of continuous arterial bleeding especially for pelvic or spine lesions. Cardiogenic shock should be suspected in association with thoracic trauma. Tamponade should be ruled out and immediately addressed by aspiration. Shock could be also caused by cardiac contusion with myocardial function. Neurogenic shock usually responds to perfusion and vasopressive drugs.

Once the patient is haemodynamically stable, secondary assessment is made.

In case of head or facial trauma, cervical fracture is found in up to 10 % of cases [24, 25].

The anterior wall of the abdomen and chest are inspected. The spine surgeon should look for abdominal wall contusion, bruising over the iliac crest and "seat-belt" sign for their association with spinal injuries. Chapman et al. found that "seat-belt" sign has a positive predictive value of 0.59 and a negative predictive value of 0.93 for intra-abdominal lesions and is present in around half of flexion-distraction injuries [26, 27]. Abdominal injuries including solid organs (liver, kidney, spleen...) or hollow viscus (bowel, stomach and mesentery) are associated with lumbar flexion-distraction in up to 55 % of patients [26]. The thoracic wall should be examined for deformity, bruising or signs of flail chest. A special search should be made to look for sternal fracture (swelling, deformity or pain) and anterior shoulder bruising since it can be associated with unstable upper thoracic spine fractures. Many authors have highlighted the need to have a high index of suspicion not to overlook these fractures [28, 29].

Patients with normal neurological examination are carefully log- rolled into the lateral position with the cervical spine protected by a rigid collar [30–32]. In cases of neurological impairment, log-rolling of the patient may be postponed after obtaining X-rays to evaluate spine stability.

The posterior chest wall should be inspected for bruising, wounds or skin lacerations, cerebrospinal fluid leakage, haematomata, contusions and subcutaneous degloving (Morel Lavallee syndrome, in which the skin is separated from fascia), especially in falls, since it can interfere with surgical approach. The spinous processes should be palpated systematically to detect any abnormal spacing or palpable step. In the case of an alert patient, the surgeon should look for pain over the midline. Pain can be spontaneous or caused by palpation over mid-line. Hsu et al. [33] assessed the value of clinical examination in detecting spine fracture. They found pain to be the most sensitive sign (sensitivity of 62 %) and palpable mid-line step being the most specific sign (specificity of 100 %). The spine surgeon should keep in mind that cervico-thoracic lesion causes pain in the interscapular region. Unsurprisingly, clinical examination is less reliable in the case of patients with altered Glascow score, drug or alcohol intoxication, and a major painful distraction lesion. In these cases, the surgeon should have a high index of suspicion and get radiographic examinations to clear the spine.

Neurological Assessment

Neurological examination is conducted and may be difficult depending on the patient's level of consciousness.

In patients with head trauma or multiple injuries or in those who are sedated for any reason, the motor function cannot be assessed reliably. Sometimes, curare action can be reversed to test motor function but examination is less reliable. In confused unresponsive patients, the spine surgeon should observe the patient's spontaneous movements and detect any reluctance in moving a limb. This raise the possibility of neurologic impairment, but bearing in mind that this can also be due to associated limb skeletal trauma. The tone of the anal sphincter should be assessed in all cases as it can be the only indication of spinal damage.

In alert patients, neurologic examination should include sensory, motor, reflex and pelvic examination according to the ASIA score (Fig. 1).

Sensory examination tests both dorsal columns (*light touch,*) and spinothalamic tract (*pain*). Sensory examination should proceed by dermatomes (key dermatomes are T4: nipples, T6: xyphoid, T10: umbilicus, T12: groin).

Motor function is assessed in the upper and lower limbs by testing key muscles [34]. Muscles are tested bilaterally against resistance and gravity. Force is quoted using the Medical Research Council grading system as follows [35–37]:
0: Absent Total paralysis
1: Trace of palpable or visible contraction
2: Poor Active movement through a range of motion with gravity eliminated
3: Fair Active movement through a range of motion against gravity
4: Good Active movement through a range of motion against resistance
5: Normal power

In all patients, assessment of sacral roots is performed by testing the anal tone. In alert patients, anal contractility should be tested for intensity and symmetry. Sensory loss of the perineum is assessed and urinary retention is looked for in alert patients. Reflexes should be obtained-

the "anal wink" (S2-S4) and bulbocavernosus reflex (S3-S4). The bulbocavernous reflex is the most distal reflex. Spinal shock is a kind of spinal cord impairment after trauma which can last up to 48 h in most cases. The neurological examination in this period is not reliable. The bulbocavernous reflex being the most distal, is the first to be active after spinal shock but this concept has been recently questioned [38]. Reflexes of the abdominal wall and limbs are tested systematically.

Several grading systems for neurological status have been described. Frankel [39] described a system in 5 grades which has been widely used in the evaluation of neurological recovery [40, 41]. In the early 1990s, the American Spine Injury Association (ASIA) along with the International Medical Society of Paraplegia (IMSOP) published the "International Standards for Neurological and Functional Classification of Spinal Cord Injury" which clarified the incomplete lesions described in the Frankel grading system in an effort to improve reliability [34, 42]. With the new ASIA/IMSOP International Standards for Neurological and Functional Classification of Spinal Cord Injury (ISCSCI), Grade A is a complete injury with no motor or sensory function preserved below the level of injury including most caudal sacral segments. Grades B, C, and D are incomplete injuries. In grade B, sensory but not motor function is preserved below the neurologic level. In grade C, motor function in the majority of key muscles below the neurological level has a muscle grade less than 3 (this is replacing "useless function" in the Frankel system) while in grade D motor function is greater than 3 (replacing "useful function" in the Frankel system). In grade E, the neurologic examination is normal.

Moreover, incomplete injuries may be distinguished in clinical spinal cord syndromes: central cord syndrome (CCS), anterior cord syndrome (ACS), posterior cord syndrome and Brown-Sequard syndrome. Moreover, two syndromes (not purely spinal cord) are well-known in spine trauma: conus medullaris syndrome and cauda equina syndrome [43].

Central Cord Syndrome, first described by Schneider in 1954 [44], is the most common incomplete spinal cord injury syndrome.

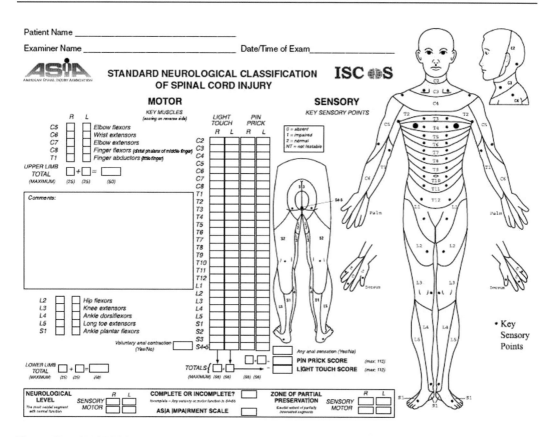

Fig. 1 The ASIA/ISCOS classification

It is characterized by more severe motor impairment of upper limbs, bladder dysfunction and variable sensory impairment. This syndrome is seen after cervical trauma with hyperextension mechanism in older patients. It can be seen also in immature patients (known as SCIWORA spinal cervical injury without radiological anomalies) with a congenital or acquired narrow cervical spine canal. It is very rare in thoracic spine trauma in mature patients and vascular injury should be ruled out [45].

In ACS, the lesion affects the two anterior thirds of the spinal cord, with paralysis, loss of temperature and pain sensation. Dorsal column function is preserved (light touch, 2-point discrimination, vibration) [43]. It's mostly seen in flexion injuries of thoracic spine or vascular injuries. The prognosis is usually poor.

Brown-Sequard syndrome is defined as a hemi-section of spinal cord and is usually associated with penetrating trauma (gunshots or stab wounds) [46] or rotational injury. It's characterized by ipsilateral proprioceptive and motor loss and contralateral loss of sensitivity to pain and temperature below lesion's level. Brown-Sequard syndrome carries the best prognosis of the SCI clinical syndromes (up to 90 %).

Posterior cord syndrome is a selective lesion to the posterior neurologic columns (light touch, 2-point discrimination, vibration) and is the least common of the SCI syndromes [43].

Conus Medullaris Syndrome is an injury of the ending of the spinal cord at thoraco lumbar junction (T10-L1). It's characterized by a combination of lesions in the spinal cord and nerves roots. Clinical manifestations include saddle anaesthesia, bladder and bowel dysfunction, lower limbs paralysis or paresis [40, 43, 47].

Cauda equina syndrome is not a spinal cord syndrome since it's an injury of the lumbar and sacral nerve roots (lower motor neurons). It presents like Conus Medullaris Syndrome (saddle anaesthesia, bladder and bowel dysfunction, variable lower extremity involvement) but with no upper motor neuron signs. It may have a better prognosis for neurological regeneration than spine cord injuries [43, 48, 49].

Neuro-Protective Therapy

Secondary neurological damage is thought to be caused by ischaemic and inflammatory mechanisms and may cause secondary deterioration of neurological status [50]. Many drugs have been investigated in an effort to limit secondary damage and to enhance recovery.

Corticosteroids have been largely used in acute spinal damage. Three prospective randomized studies have been conducted to attempt to prove their efficiency (*National Acute Spinal Cord Injury Study NASCIS*) and patients have been followed for 1 year. In the first NASCIS [51], 100 mg daily for 10 days was compared to 1,000 mg. daily for 10 days in 330 patients. No difference in neurological recovery between both groups was noted.

The second NASCIS [52, 53] was a randomized, double-blind, placebo-controlled trial including 487 patients in three groups: the first had been given methylpredinsolone (30 mg/kg in 1 h then 5.4 mg/kg/h for 23 h), the second received naloxone (5.4 mg/kg iv in 1 h then 4 mg/kg/h for 23 h) and the third group received placebo. Only patients treated by methylprednisolone in the first 8 h after trauma showed improved neurologic recovery. The three groups showed equal mortality and the steroid treatment was considered safe by authors [54]. Authors recommended the usage of high dosage of methylprednisolone only if it could be started in the first 8 h after trauma. While this study aroused enthusiasm among physicians and surgeons dealing with spinal cord trauma, its methodology was largely debated [55–57] and concerns were aroused about infectious complications [58]. Other studies failed to show improvement

under massive dosage of methylprednisolone in closed injury [59, 60] while showing deterioration of neurologic function or increased infectious complications in penetrating trauma [61–63]. The third NASCIS III [64, 65] compared methylprednisolone for 24 h to methylprednisolone for 48 h at the same dosage of 30 mg/kg in 1 h then 5.4 mg/kg/h and to tirilazad mesylate. Authors concluded that methylprednisolone should be maintained for 24 h if begun in the first 3 h after trauma and for 48 h if begun between 3 and 8 h. The statistical methods of these studies were criticized and there were concerns about randomization and clinical end-points, to a such point that many authors rejected or questioned methylprednisolone protocols as standard of care [66–72]. In Europe, the use of methylprednisolone is still controversial and not accepted as standard of care [73]. In France, experts' report have not recommended the use of methylprednisolone until it is proven safe and efficient [23].

Imaging

Several imaging methods are available for use to depict thoraco-lumbar traumatic injuries. Plain radiographs, computed tomography scan, magnetic resonance imaging and sonography have been used in the emergency setting.

Plains Radiographs

They have been the mainstay of the radiographic assessment of trauma patients in the emergency department. In a review of literature in 2005, France et al. [74] stated that "surgeons agreed that the mainstay of initial radiographic evaluation of the spine after acute trauma remains plain radiographs".

In 1994, Frankel et al. [75] defined their indications for obtaining thoracic and lumbar spine radiographs: back pain, fall of more than 3 ft, ejection from motorcycle or motor vehicle crash of more than 50 mph, Glascow score ≤ 8, and neurologic deficit. They stated as well that the absence of back pain does not exclude significant thoraco-lumbar fracture. In cases of spine trauma, plain radiographs are sometimes difficult to obtain, especially in polytrauma patients and are often of poor quality. One of the most difficult areas to assess with plain radiographs is the cervico-thoracic junction and the upper thoracic spine down to T5. In this region, the shoulders' projection makes the vertebral bony contours less visible [28, 76, 77]. Fractures in this region should suspected especially in case of associated sternal fracture [76].

In a review of the literature and according to the opinion of an experienced group of spine surgeons, Keynan et al. [78] listed the parameters to use for vertebral assessment:
1. The Cobb angle, to assess sagittal alignment;
2. Vertebral body translation percentage, to express traumatic anterolisthesis;
3. Anterior vertebral body compression percentage, to assess vertebral body compression;
4. The sagittal-to-transverse canal diameter ratio, and canal total cross-sectional area (measured or calculated);
5. The percentage canal occlusion, to assess canal dimensions.

Daffner [79] identified many signs of instability:
1. Displacement implies injury to major ligamentous and articular structures;
2. A wide interlaminar space implies injury to the posterior ligamentous structures and the facet joints;
3. Wide facet joints imply injury to the posterior ligamentous structures;
4. A disrupted posterior vertebral body line implies burst injury with disruption of anterior bony and posterior ligamentous structures;
5. A wide vertebral canal implies injury to the entire vertebra in the sagittal plane.

Many trauma centres have protocol imaging for polytraumatized patients including an AP view of pelvis and a lateral view of cervical spine. The first will detect displaced fractures of the pelvis which could be a possible cause of major bleeding. The second will help in managing the immobilization of the cervical spine and the attention that should be paid to intubation.

CT Scan

More recently, trauma teams use helical CT Scanning as a tool for injury screening in high energy trauma. Helical CT Scans reduce the time needed to get a total body examination including mainly head, thorax, abdomen, cervical and thoraco-lumbar spine and pelvis. Many investigators reported the usefulness of such screening tools: Sampson et al. [80] reported on over a 7-year period 296 multi-trauma CT scans with positive findings in 86.2 % of cases. They also found 19 cervical spine fractures and 26 pneumothoraces not detected on plain radiographs. Antevil et al. [81] compared spiral CT scan with plain radiographs to evaluate spine trauma. They concluded that spiral CT Scan is a more rapid and sensitive modality than plain radiographs. It delivers less radiation than plain radiography in thoraco- lumbar spine evaluation but with a higher cost. Based on these facts, they concluded that spiral CT scan may replace plain radiography as the standard of care for evaluation of the spine in trauma patients. Campoginis et al. [82] reported on motorcycle accident victims and found that more than half with significant CT scan findings had normal physical examination, thus recommending lower thresholds for CT scan use in blunt trauma. Other authors [83] reported on usage of spiral CT scan in initial evaluation of spine trauma. Brown et al. [84] identified 99.3 % of spine fractures using spiral CT Scan and they stated that plain radiographs are no longer necessary for blunt trauma. Brandt et al. [85] found that using CT Scan images of chest, abdomen and pelvis obtained to evaluate visceral injuries are sufficient to rule out spine injuries.

The fine analysis of fracture line and the existence of spinal canal narrowing are important in choosing the treatment modality. The ability of plain radiograph to differentiate compression fracture from burst fracture was questioned. In 1992, Ballock et al. [86] studied the sensitivity of plain radiographs in detecting burst fracture comparing with CT Scans and found that a quarter of burst fractures would have been mis-diagnosed relying solely on plain radiographs. In an effort to increase the sensitivity of plain radiographs in detecting burst fractures, McGrory et al. [87] used the posterior vertebral body angle and found a sensitivity of 75 %. Bernstein et al. [27], in their review of 53 patients with Chance-type fractures, found that the fracture line in posterior elements may be very subtle on plain radiographs and that there was an associated burst fracture in nearly half of the cases.

Dai et al. [88] evaluated the role of CT Scans in treatment planning of thoraco-lumbar fractures. They found that treatment planning with plain radiographs remained unchanged in only 56 % of cases when using CT Scans for same cases. In fact, plain radiographs were less reliable for the evaluation of vertebral body comminution and thus for assessment of vertebral stability.

Fontijne et al. [89] studied the usefulness of CT Scan in predicting neurological impairment in burst fracture. They found that high level of fracture and increased amount of spinal canal narrowing were correlated with the presence of neurological abnormalities but not with the severity of neurological impairment.

The CT Scan is the "gold standard" for measuring spinal cord narrowing, to find and to study fractures lines. Reconstructed slices are especially useful to measure spinal canal dimensions in different plane inclinations. CT scan can study the entire spine looking for multi-level injuries.

Magnetic Resonance Imaging

MRI is known for its high sensitivity in soft tissue imaging. In spine trauma, MRI is the best tool to evaluate discs, ligaments and neural elements, but it is not routinely used because of the time necessary to complete examination, examination availability and cost considerations. In their review on management of spine trauma with associated injuries, Harris et al. [21] stated that "MRI is most useful in patients whose plain radiographs or CT results fall short of explaining their full clinical picture". This result is most common in the neurologically-impaired victim with "normal" appearing plain films. Schoenwaelder et al. [90] evaluated the

usefulness of complementary MRI for ligamentous injuries to the cervical spine and found that all unstable lesions were correctly detected by CT Scan and that 18 % of disc and ligamentous lesions were missed by CT Scan comparing to MRI. Other authors recommended the association of CT scan and MRI for cervical spine clearance [91], but such recommendations were not formulated for thoraco-lumbar trauma.

Dai et al. [92] found that MRI was reliable in detecting posterior ligamentous injuries in burst fractures but that these injuries were not correlated with the fracture severity nor with the neurological status thus making MRI unnecessary in treatment planning. Lee et al. [93] suggested that signal modification of fat-suppressed sequences correlated with ligament disruption. Thereafter, many authors pointed to the fact that relying solely on MRI to define stability of fractures may lead to unnecessary surgery [94]. In fact, it seems that many false positive results are associated with MRI evaluation of ligamentous injury, perhaps due to ligament elongation and not rupture. In a survey of the members of the Spine Trauma Group, surgeons considered signs on plain radiographs to be the most useful for diagnosing PLC injury, ranking them higher than other radiological modalities and physical signs [95]. The same group considered MRI more useful than CT Scan in detecting PLC lesion [96]. More recently, Vaccaro et al. [97] found little correlation between MRI findings and intra-operative findings, concluding that MRI should not be used in isolation to diagnose the PLC injury, contradicting the former findings of Haba et al. [98].

Ultrasonography

Ultrasonography is a tool used regularly in soft tissue investigation. It has been used in spine as well [99] to look for posterior ligamentous complex lesions in thoraco-lumbar trauma. Although it is less reliable than MRI, it is a useful tool in cases when MRI is contra-indicated [100, 101].

Biomechanics and Classification

Several authors have described classifications for thoraco-lumbar fractures in an effort to simplify the understanding of these complex lesions. Classifications aim to make reporting on these fractures easier and treatment decisions more straightforward.

In the third decade of last century, Böhler classified thoraco-lumbar injuries into five injury types taking into consideration anatomic definition and mechanisms of injury: compression fractures, flexion-distraction injuries, extension fractures, shear fractures and rotational injuries.

In the 1960s, Holdsworth [102, 103] introduced the concept of spine columns describing the spine as including two columns: an anterior column formed by vertebral bodies and discs acting in compression and a posterior column formed by pedicles, pars interarticularis, facet joints, laminae, spinous processes and ligaments, acting in tension. For Holdsworth, the posterior column is sufficient to maintain stability, thus he described burst fractures as stable fractures.

In the 1970s, Louis [104] described the concept of three columns: one anterior column composed of vertebral bodies and discs, and two posterior columns each composed of pars interarticularis and intervertebral articulations. Pedicles and laminae are described as structures linking these columns (the anterior with each posterior and the posterior with each other).

With the development of imaging technologies, CT Scan gave surgeons a "new look" for spine fractures by allowing fine analysis of fracture patterns.

In 1983, Denis [105] published his now worldwide-used classification based on a new concept of the three-column model: the anterior column is composed of the anterior longitudinal ligament and the anterior half of the intervertebral discs and vertebral bodies, the middle column is composed of the posterior half of the intervertebral discs and bodies and the posterior longitudinal ligament, the posterior column includes the neural arc, posterior ligaments (ligamentum flavum, articular complexes, posterior spinous ligamentous complex).

This concept highlighted the importance of the middle column for mechanical stability. The fracture severity was correlated to the number of injured columns. A long time before, in 1958, Decoulx and Rieunau [106] had pointed out this middle column, which they called the posterior wall, as a key factor for stability. Denis defined four distinct fractures types: I- compression fractures (anterior column), II- burst fractures (anterior and middle columns), III- seatbelt injuries and fracture-dislocations (all columns) with 16 total groups after subclassification.

Several authors criticized this classification. Lee et al. pointed out the inaccuracy of oversimplifying the concept of stability of the lesion of more than one column, which could lead to indicate surgical treatment for all burst fractures. In fact, many authors reported good results for burst fracture treated solely with bracing. Guigui et al. [107] underlined the fact that this classification is confusing with respect to the mechanism of injury. For these authors, a same fracture (e.g. a burst fracture of the vertebral body (type IIB)) could be the consequence of different mechanisms thus having very different progression prognosis depending on associated posterior lesions.

In 1984, Ferguson et al. [108] described a mechanistic classification of spinal fractures with seven categories based on the mechanical mode of failure of vertebral bodies.

In 1994, Magerl et al. [109] published what is now known as the AO (Association for Orthopaedics) classification. This classification appeared as the most inclusive of all classifications yet published with a total of 218 lesion types. The AO classification is based on mechanism of injury with three main groups: A- Compression fractures, B- Flexion-Distraction fractures, C- Translation/rotation fractures (Fig. 2). Each group is then sub-divided in sub-groups with sub-divisions (Fig. 3). The AO classification has the advantage of serving as a guide for treatment indications since the grading system is correlated with lesion severity. Indeed, the higher a fracture is graded, the higher is the risk for neurological injury or for instability. This classification was widely accepted especially in Europe [110].

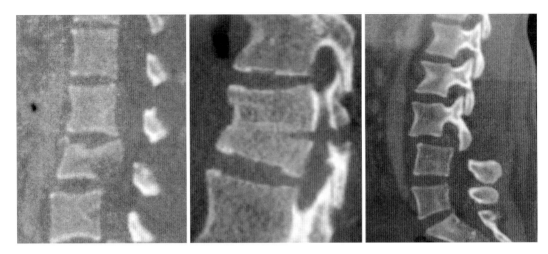

Fig. 2 The Magerl classification (AO classification): A-type compression fracture; B-type flexion-distraction fracture; C-type rotational component fracture

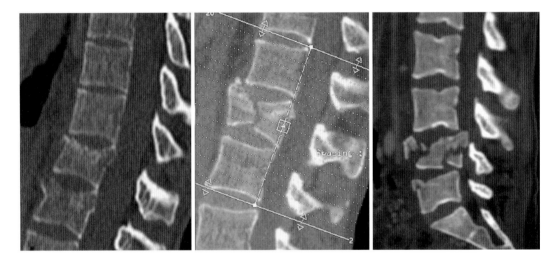

Fig. 3 AO classification A-type sub-groups: A1, A2, A3

In daily practice and for treatment decision, it is sufficient to use the three main groups and only few sub-groups (especially for burst fractures).

In classifying fractures using the AO classification, it is essential that surgeon treating spine trauma be familiar with the algorithm used in this classification. When analyzing the images the, surgeon should look first for signs of rotation or translation (type C fractures): spinous process step-off, unilateral facet joint fracture with contralateral facet joint dislocation, multiple transverse process fractures (lumbar level fractures) or multiple rib fractures or dislocations (thoracic level) in levels adjacent to the fracture level, rotational displacement of vertebral bodies on CT scan transverse view, asymmetrical vertebral body fracture with lateral bony fracture detached from the vertebral plateau and neural arc asymmetrical fracture[107]. If such radiological signs are lacking a type C fracture is ruled out. Then the surgeon should search for signs of anterior compression and posterior distraction corresponding to a type B fracture. Distraction signs are found on reconstructed sagittal CT Scan views: increased interspinous space, facet joint incongruity, horizontal fracture lines of laminae or pars interarticularis or facets joint. Anteriorly the vertebral body is compressed. Depending on the posterior lesion, the fracture is further classified as type B1 if the posterior lesion is predominantly ligamentous or B2 if this lesion is mainly osseous (the so-called Chance fracture is a typical B2 fracture). Inversely Type B3 corresponds to anterior distraction, identified by anterior disk space widening, and posterior compression. If no sign of distraction is found then fracture is classified as a compression fracture (type A). With new imaging techniques the posterior lesions are detected more frequently.

At the same time, in 1994, McCormack et al. [111] reviewed retrospectively 28 patients with failure of short segment fixation and described a new classification to assess the anterior column integrity. This classification, based on post operative CT Scan, is known now as the "Load Sharing Score" and is based on granting points to
1: Amount of damaged vertebral body,
2: The spread of fragments in the fracture site,
3: The amount of corrected trauma. This classification appears to be reliable with good reproducibility [112] and useful in assessing the acute instability of thoraco-lumbar fractures [113] and the need for anterior column graft or augmentation after posterior stabilization and reduction.

More recently, Vaccaro et al. [114] described a new classification system, the thoraco- lumbar injury classification system (TLICS) (Table 1). The aim of the author is to describe an easy-to-use system oriented toward clinical decision. The system is based on three determinants: fracture morphology, neurological status and posterior ligament complex integrity [115]. Each determinant is given points and a score is computed. The higher points are given according to severity of injury and/or emergency character of treatment. With respect to morphology of the lesion, distraction is given 4 points while rotation or translation are given three points, with respect to neurological status, the higher points are given to incomplete cord syndromes or cauda equina syndromes. A score less than or equal to 3 suggests that patient may treated non-operatively, while a score greater or equal to five suggests operative treatment and in between both

Table 1 Thoracolumbar Injury Classification and Severity Score (TLICS) [114]

Injury Morphology	
Compression	1
Burst	2
Rotation/translation	3
Distraction	4
Integrity of Posterior Ligamentous Complex	
Intact	0
Suspected/Intermediate	2
Injured	3
Neurological Status	
Intact	0
Root injury	2
Complete cord/conus medullaris injury	2
Incomplete cord/conus medullaris injury	3
Cauda equina	3
	10

Scoring ≤3 non-operative treatment should be considered
Scoring ≥5 operative treatment should be considered
Scoring ranging from 3 to 5 both treatments can be considered

treatments can be applied [116]. This system has the advantage over other systems of taking into consideration clinical findings and the neurological status. Including PCL in point-granting has the advantage of underlining its importance in stability. Rotation or distraction highly suggests that PCL is injured, so giving PCL points in this case may be questionable. In case of burst fracture, PCL status is of high importance and would influence the indication for surgery. But it is in this case that PCL assessment is the most difficult [92, 95, 97, 98, 101, 117].

Many investigators assessed the reliability of TLICS. Many authors found the TLICS user-friendly, reliable and useful [116], with good intra-observer and inter-observer reliability both in US and non-US surgeons [118–120]. The ability of TLICS to predict surgery was found good in a retrospective study and was correlated to the AO classification [121]. TLICS showed limitations in predicting surgery in cases of multiple contiguous fractures or fractures in the ankylosed spine [122]. In a review of the literature, Oner et al. [123] considered TLICS to be the most useful system for therapeutic decision-making in thoraco-lumbar spine injuries. In comparing three classification systems, TLICS showed good reliability when compared to AO or Denis classifications [124].

Treatment

Several treatment modalities have been described in the literature: functional treatment with early ambulation, Orthopaedic treatment with bracing or casting (Fig. 4), surgical treatment with posterior or anterior or combined approaches and more recently less invasive anterior or posterior fixation techniques are all being investigated.

Several authors compared non-operative to operative treatment trying to define clearly the indications for surgery.

In 1975, Bedbrook et al. [125] stated that ninety percent of thoracic and lumbar spine fractures with paraplegia or paraparesis could be treated and reduced by closed methods. Harris [126] stated that "the natural course of thoraco-lumbar fracutes is usually benign and the non-surgical methods should be the standard treatment with few exceptions".

Many regimens for non-operative treatment exist but most of them include an initial period of bed rest (which can be as long as 3 months in some cases) with special attention to lordotic posture to reduce or limit kyphosis, followed by ambulation with a cast or plaster. No study has compared different regimens so treatment protocol is chosen according to the surgeon's estimation of fracture stability, the patient's characteristics and his/her ability to comply with the treatment plan. The need for an orthosis is not very well proven [127, 128] and some authors did not find any difference in stable burst fractures treated with or without orthosis [129]. Cantor et al. [130] reported on a series of fractures without posterior column disruption with good functional results from early ambulation with total contact orthosis. They attributed their good results to the fact that the posterior column was intact. Chow et al. [131] disagreed with this conclusion and reported on a series of burst fractures treated by hyperextension cast

with good results. They stated that posterior column disruption was not a contra-indication to non-operative treatment. Mumford et al. [132] reported good results in burst fractures treated non-surgically. McEvoy et al. [133] reported on a series of burst fractures and concluded that non-operative treatment was a sound choice for neurologically-intact patients, but in cases of neurological impairment, improvement is unlikely with non-operative treatment and that deterioration could occur. Tezer et al. [134] recommended conservative treatment in cases with no neurologic involvement and no posterior column disruption (MRI to define in cases with kyphosis greater than 30°). Moller et al. [135] retrospectively evaluated 27 patients at a mean follow-up of 27 years and found that results are stable in time but with reduction of height of adjacent discs. Agus et al. [136] treated successfully two- and three-columns fractures non-surgically. Shen et al. [137] reported a case of a three columns ankylosed spine fracture treated successfully by non surgical treatment, introducing the concept of a fourth column consisting of sternum and ribs. Tropiano et al. [138] reported on a series of thoraco-lumbar fractures treated by reduction and casting (Böhler technique) with good functional results. Kyphosis recurred at fourth months but lesser than the amount before reduction. In a survey for Canadian spine surgeons in 1994, Findlay et al. reported that the treatment of choice for burst fractures in Canada was essentially surgical [139]. Post et al. [140] reported good functional results of non-surgical treatment for compression fractures (AO classification's type A) at 4 and 10 years follow-up.

Many authors compared conservative and surgical treatment. Knight et al. [141] found no difference in functional results between non-operative and operative treatment for two- or three-column burst fractures. Buttler et al. [142] compared retrospectively two groups of L1 burst fractures and found that burst fractures managed conservatively had better functional results than those treated surgically, and that clinical outcome was not correlated with vertebral collapse, kyphosis or canal narrowing. In a prospective randomized study

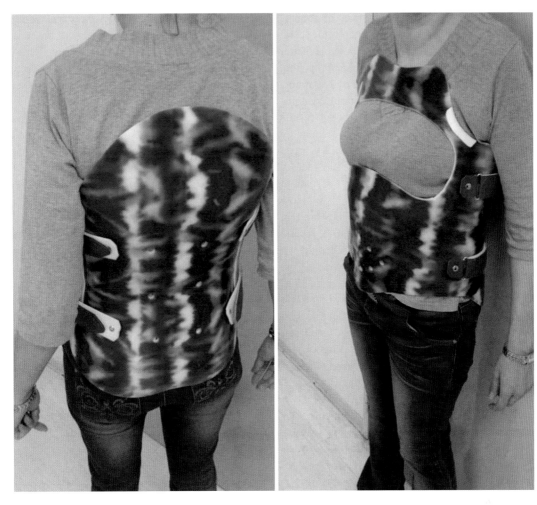

Fig. 4 Orthopedic treatment with brace

comparing operative and non-operative treatment for stable burst fractures, Wood et al. [143] found no long term advantage for operative treatment. In a systematic review of the literature, Thomas et al. [144] concluded that there is no evidence proving superiority of one treatment for burst fractures without neurological deficit. More studies are still needed to establish treatment guidelines.

Timing of Surgery

Urgent surgery was proposed to enhance neurologic recovery or to limit morbidity in polytrauma patients. Questions concerning the risks of urgent operation or whether its advantages outweigh the risks have been largely debated. Krengel et al. [145] found that early decompression and fixation for thoracic fracture with incomplete neurologic impairment was safe and improved neurologic recovery. In a review of literature conducted in 1999, Fehlings [146] concluded that animal studies suggested a benefit of early decompression for neurologic recovery but that solid proof in human studies was lacking. Many authors [147] found no correlation between initial spinal canal narrowing and neurological recovery and that remodelling of the canal diameter was seen in patients many years after trauma [148], thus questioning the utility of surgical decompression [149].

Zelle et al. [150] in a small series of patients suffering neurological impairment from sacral fracture, found that decompression gave better neurological recovery and better physical function.

Rath et al. [151] reported a series of 42 patients treated by open fixation and fusion and decompression. They found significantly better results in neurological outcome in patients treated by very early decompression (less than 24 h).

Muchaty et al. [152] reported satisfactory results with a specific protocol for patient selection: ASIA B, C, D, and ASIA A below T10 patients were operated within 8 h as surgical emergencies, and ASIA A from T1 to T 10 and ASIA E were operated on a regular schedule.

In 2006, Rutgers et al. [153] reviewed the available data on timing of surgery for spinal cord injury in thoraco-lumbar fractures. They found that the studies' results with respect to neurological outcome are contradictory so no conclusion can be drawn. On the other hand, early surgery was shown to be beneficial for respiratory complications and hospital stay in trauma patients.

Cengiz et al. [154] prospectively followed two groups of thoraco-lumbar fracture patients with neurological impairment: 12 patients were operated within 8 h and 15 patients between 3 and 15 days. They found better neurologic recovery in the group with early surgery.

More recently, in a prospective survey of 971 spine surgeons investigating timing of surgery in spinal cord injury, Fehlings et al. [65, 155] found that the majority of spine surgeons prefer to decompress the injured spinal cord within 24 h.

Early surgical fixation, with or without decompression, was also advocated to limit morbidity [156, 157] and respiratory complications (more prevalent in upper thoracic injuries in comparison to lower injuries [158]).

Kerwin et al. [159] reviewed retrospectively the records of 16,812 patients who underwent surgical fixation for thoraco-lumbar fractures (National Tauma Data Bank). They found that patients operated within 3 days from trauma had less complications than those operated later. Schinkel et al. [160] reviewed the German National Trauma Database and concluded that patients operated in the first 3 days had better outcome that those operated later on and reduced mortality. In a recent review of English literature, Bellabarba et al. [161] drew the same conclusions, recommending that patients with unstable thoraco-lumbar fractures be operated within 3 days from trauma to decrease respiratory complications, ICU and hospital stay for thoracic fractures and hospital stay for lumbar fractures. The effect of early stabilization on mortality was less clear. Kerwin et al. [162] reported better results for early surgery (before 3 days) in majority of patients but some of them operated on early had poorer outcome. These authors do not recommend rigid protocol for polytrauma patients but a protocol that can be tailored for every specific patient.

In conclusion, it appears that polytrauma patients with or without neurologic involvement benefit from early stabilization in the first 3 days after trauma to facilitate nursing and patient mobilization. Even though there is no strong proof, most spine surgeons recommend operating on patients with incomplete neurologic impairment within 24 h and some of them within 8 h.

Summary

Injuries to the thoracic and lumbar spine are frequent and can be devastating. It happens mainly in young patients due to falls, sport or traffic accidents. They can be associated with other vital system injuries. Their management often needs a multidisciplinary team. The initial medical management is described in this chapter. The main classifications are discussed and the treatment orientation is described. Physicians taking care of trauma emergencies, and especially orthopedic surgeons, need to have good knowledge of clinical examination, radiologic assessment and the main treatment options. When surgery is indicated and the timing is discussed in this chapter. The different surgical options and techniques are discussed in detail in an another chapter.

References

1. Richards D, et al. Incidence of thoracic and lumbar spine injuries for restrained occupants in frontal collisions. Annu Proc Assoc Adv Automot Med. 2006;50:125–39.

2. Robertson A, et al. Spinal injuries in motorcycle crashes: patterns and outcomes. J Trauma. 2002;53(1):5–8.

3. Robertson A, et al. Spinal injury patterns resulting from car and motorcycle accidents. Spine (Phila Pa 1976). 2002;27(24):2825–30.

4. Hahn MP, et al. Injury pattern after fall from great height. An analysis of 101 cases. Unfallchirurg. 1995;98(12):609–13.

5. Farmer JC, et al. The changing nature of admissions to a spinal cord injury center: violence on the rise. J Spinal Disord. 1998;11(5):400–3.

6. Etminan M, et al. Revision strategies for lumbar pseudarthrosis. Orthop Clin North Am. 2002;33(2):381–92.

7. Wolf BR, et al. Injury patterns in division I collegiate swimming. Am J Sports Med. 2009;37(10):2037–42.

8. Tator CH, Carson JD, Edmonds VE. New spinal injuries in hockey. Clin J Sport Med. 1997;7(1):17–21.

9. Press JM, et al. The national jockey injury study: an analysis of injuries to professional horse-racing jockeys. Clin J Sport Med. 1995;5(4):236–40.

10. Kruse D, Lemmen B. Spine injuries in the sport of gymnastics. Curr Sports Med Rep. 2009;8(1):20–8.

11. Franz T, et al. Severe spinal injuries in alpine skiing and snowboarding: a 6-year review of a tertiary trauma centre for the Bernese Alps ski resorts, Switzerland. Br J Sports Med. 2008;42(1):55–8.

12. Blacksin MF. Patterns of fracture after air bag deployment. J Trauma. 1993;35(6):840–3.

13. Kuner EH, Schlickewei W, Oltmanns D. Protective air bags in traffic accidents. Change in the injury pattern and reduction in the severity of injuries. Unfallchirurgie. 1995;21(2):92–9.

14. Anderson S, Biros MH, Reardon RF. Delayed diagnosis of thoracolumbar fractures in multiple-trauma patients. Acad Emerg Med. 1996;3(9):832–9.

15. Inamasu J, Guiot BH. Thoracolumbar junction injuries after motor vehicle collision: are there differences in restrained and nonrestrained front seat occupants? J Neurosurg Spine. 2007;7(3):311–4.

16. Gertzbein SD. Scoliosis research society. Multicenter spine fracture study. Spine (Phila Pa 1976). 1992;17(5):528–40.

17. Henderson RL, Reid DC, Saboe LA. Multiple noncontiguous spine fractures. Spine (Phila Pa 1976). 1991;16(2):128–31.

18. Arthornthurasook A, Thongmag P. Thoracolumbar burst fracture with another spinal fracture. J Med Assoc Thai. 1990;73(5):279–82.

19. Kossmann T, et al. Damage control surgery for spine trauma. Injury. 2004;35(7):661–70.

20. Nirula R, Brasel K. Do trauma centers improve functional outcomes: a national trauma databank analysis? J Trauma. 2006;61(2):268–71.

21. Harris MB, Sethi RK. The initial assessment and management of the multiple-trauma patient with an associated spine injury. Spine (Phila Pa 1976). 2006;31 Suppl 11:S9–15; discussion S36.

22. Langeron O, Birenbaum A, Amour J. Airway management in trauma. Minerva Anestesiol. 2009;75(5):307–11.

23. Groupe Experts. Prise en charge d'un blessé adulte présentant un traumatisme vertébro-médullaire. SFCR, Editor; 2003.

24. Mithani SK, et al. Predictable patterns of intracranial and cervical spine injury in craniomaxillofacial trauma: analysis of 4786 patients. Plast Reconstr Surg. 2009;123(4):1293–301.

25. Mulligan R, Mahabir R. The prevalence of C-spine injury and/or head injury with isolated and multiple craniomaxillofacial fractures. Plast Reconstr Surg. 2010;126:1647–51.

26. Chapman JR, et al. Thoracolumbar flexion-distraction injuries: associated morbidity and neurological outcomes. Spine (Phila Pa 1976). 2008;33(6):648–57.

27. Bernstein MP, Mirvis SE, Shanmuganathan K. Chance-type fractures of the thoracolumbar spine: imaging analysis in 53 patients. AJR Am J Roentgenol. 2006;187(4):859–68.

28. van Beek EJ, et al. Upper thoracic spinal fractures in trauma patients – a diagnostic pitfall. Injury. 2000;31(4):219–23.

29. Nork SE, et al. Percutaneous stabilization of U-shaped sacral fractures using iliosacral screws: technique and early results. J Orthop Trauma. 2001;15(4):238–46.

30. Del Rossi G, et al. Spine-board transfer techniques and the unstable cervical spine. Spine (Phila Pa 1976). 2004;29(7):E134–8.

31. Del Rossi G, et al. The 6-plus-person lift transfer technique compared with other methods of spine boarding. J Athl Train. 2008;43(1):6–13.

32. Horodyski M, et al. Motion generated in the unstable lumbar spine during hospital bed transfers. J Spinal Disord Tech. 2009;22(1):45–8.

33. Hsu JM, Joseph T, Ellis AM. Thoracolumbar fracture in blunt trauma patients: guidelines for diagnosis and imaging. Injury. 2003;34(6):426–33.

34. Cohen ME, et al. A test of the 1992 international standards for neurological and functional classification of spinal cord injury. Spinal Cord. 1998;36(8):554–60.

35. Lucas JT, Ducker TB. Motor classification of spinal cord injuries with mobility, morbidity and recovery indices. Am Surg. 1979;45(3):151–8.

36. Bondurant FJ, et al. Acute spinal cord injury. A study using physical examination and magnetic resonance imaging. Spine (Phila Pa 1976). 1990;15(3):161–8.

37. Bhardwaj P, Bhardwaj N. Motor grading of elbow flexion – is Medical Research Council grading good enough? J Brachial Plex Peripher Nerve Inj. 2009;4:3.

38. Ko HY, et al. The pattern of reflex recovery during spinal shock. Spinal Cord. 1999;37(6):402–9.

39. Frankel HL, et al. The value of postural reduction in the initial management of closed injuries of the spine with paraplegia and tetraplegia I. Paraplegia. 1969;7(3):179–92.

40. Toh E, et al. Functional evaluation using motor scores after cervical spinal cord injuries. Spinal Cord. 1998;36(7):491–6.

41. Wells JD, Nicosia S. Scoring acute spinal cord injury: a study of the utility and limitations of five different grading systems. J Spinal Cord Med. 1995;18(1):33–41.

42. El Masry WS, et al. Validation of the American Spinal Injury Association (ASIA) motor score and the National Acute Spinal Cord Injury Study (NASCIS) motor score. Spine (Phila Pa 1976). 1996;21(5):614–9.

43. McKinley W, et al. Incidence and outcomes of spinal cord injury clinical syndromes. J Spinal Cord Med. 2007;30(3):215–24.

44. Schneider RC, Cherry G, Pantek H. The syndrome of acute central cervical spinal cord injury; with special reference to the mechanisms involved in hyperextension injuries of cervical spine. J Neurosurg. 1954;11(6):546–77.

45. Zipfel B, et al. Traumatic transection of the aorta and thoracic spinal cord injury without radiographic abnormality in an adult patient. J Endovasc Ther. 2010;17(1):131–6.

46. Reinke M, et al. Brown-Sequard syndrome caused by a high velocity gunshot injury: a case report. Spinal Cord. 2007;45(8):579–82.

47. van der Linden E, Kroft LJ, Dijkstra PD. Treatment of vertebral tumor with posterior wall defect using image-guided radiofrequency ablation combined with vertebroplasty: preliminary results in 12 patients. J Vasc Interv Radiol. 2007;18(6):741–7.

48. Harrop JS, Hunt Jr GE, Vaccaro AR. Conus medullaris and cauda equina syndrome as a result of traumatic injuries: management principles. Neurosurg Focus. 2004;16(6):e4.

49. Kingwell SP, Curt A, Dvorak MF. Factors affecting neurological outcome in traumatic conus medullaris and cauda equina injuries. Neurosurg Focus. 2008;25(5):E7.

50. Marshall LF, et al. Deterioration following spinal cord injury. A multicenter study. J Neurosurg. 1987;66(3):400–4.

51. Bracken MB, et al. Methylprednisolone and neurological function 1 year after spinal cord injury. Results of the national acute spinal cord injury study. J Neurosurg. 1985;63(5):704–13.

52. Bracken MB, et al. A randomized, controlled trial of methylprednisolone or naloxone in the treatment of acute spinal-cord injury. Results of the second national acute spinal cord injury study. N Engl J Med. 1990;322(20):1405–11.

53. Bracken MB, et al. Methylprednisolone or naloxone treatment after acute spinal cord injury: 1-year follow-up data. Results of the second national acute spinal cord injury study. J Neurosurg. 1992;76(1):23–31.

54. Shepard MJ, Bracken MB. The effect of methylprednisolone, naloxone, and spinal cord trauma on four liver enzymes: observations from NASCIS 2. National acute spinal cord injury study. Paraplegia. 1994;32(4):236–45.

55. Hanigan WC, Anderson RJ. Commentary on NASCIS-2. J Spinal Disord. 1992;5(1):125–31; discussion 132–3.

56. Young W, Bracken MB. The second national acute spinal cord injury study. J Neurotrauma. 1992;9 Suppl 1:S397–405.

57. Young W. Secondary injury mechanisms in acute spinal cord injury. J Emerg Med. 1993;11 Suppl 1:13–22.

58. Gerndt SJ, et al. Consequences of high-dose steroid therapy for acute spinal cord injury. J Trauma. 1997;42(2):279–84.

59. Gerhart KA, et al. Utilization and effectiveness of methylprednisolone in a population-based sample of spinal cord injured persons. Paraplegia. 1995;33(6):316–21.

60. Ito Y, et al. Does high dose methylprednisolone sodium succinate really improve neurological status in patient with acute cervical cord injury?: a prospective study about neurological recovery and early complications. Spine (Phila Pa 1976). 2009;34(20):2121–4.

61. Prendergast MR, et al. Massive steroids do not reduce the zone of injury after penetrating spinal cord injury. J Trauma. 1994;37(4):576–9; discussion 579–80.

62. Levy ML, et al. Use of methylprednisolone as an adjunct in the management of patients with penetrating spinal cord injury: outcome analysis. Neurosurgery. 1996;39(6):1141–8; discussion 1148–9.

63. Heary RF, et al. Steroids and gunshot wounds to the spine. Neurosurgery. 1997;41(3):576–83; discussion 583–4.

64. Bracken MB, et al. Administration of methylprednisolone for 24 or 48 hours or tirilazad mesylate for 48 hours in the treatment of acute spinal cord injury. Results of the third national acute spinal cord injury randomized controlled trial. National acute spinal cord injury study. JAMA. 1997;277(20):1597–604.

65. Bracken MB, et al. Methylprednisolone or tirilazad mesylate administration after acute spinal cord injury: 1-year follow up. Results of the third national acute spinal cord injury randomized controlled trial. J Neurosurg. 1998;89(5):699–706.

66. Molloy S, Middleton F, Casey AT. Failure to administer methylprednisolone for acute traumatic spinal cord injury-a prospective audit of 100 patients from a regional spinal injuries unit. Injury. 2002;33(7):575–8.

67. Coleman WP, et al. A critical appraisal of the reporting of the National Acute Spinal Cord Injury Studies (II and III) of methylprednisolone in acute spinal cord injury. J Spinal Disord. 2000;13(3):185–99.

68. Nesathurai S. Steroids and spinal cord injury: revisiting the NASCIS 2 and NASCIS 3 trials. J Trauma. 1998;45(6):1088–93.

69. Bracken MB, et al. Clinical measurement, statistical analysis, and risk-benefit: controversies from trials of spinal injury. J Trauma. 2000;48(3):558–61.

70. Short D. Is the role of steroids in acute spinal cord injury now resolved? Curr Opin Neurol. 2001;14(6):759–63.

71. Sayer FT, Kronvall E, Nilsson OG. Methylprednisolone treatment in acute spinal cord injury: the myth challenged through a structured analysis of published literature. Spine J. 2006;6(3):335–43.

72. O'Connor PA, et al. Methylprednisolone in acute spinal cord injuries. Ir J Med Sci. 2003;172(1):24–6.

73. Molloy S, Price M, Casey AT. Questionnaire survey of the views of the delegates at the European Cervical Spine Research Society meeting on the administration of methylprednisolone for acute traumatic spinal cord injury. Spine (Phila Pa 1976). 2001;26(24):E562–4.

74. France JC, Bono CM, Vaccaro AR. Initial radiographic evaluation of the spine after trauma: when, what, where, and how to image the acutely traumatized spine. J Orthop Trauma. 2005;19(9):640–9.

75. Frankel HL, et al. Indications for obtaining surveillance thoracic and lumbar spine radiographs. J Trauma. 1994;37(4):673–6.

76. Hills MW, Delprado AM, Deane SA. Sternal fractures: associated injuries and management. J Trauma. 1993;35(1):55–60.

77. el-Khoury GY, Whitten CG. Trauma to the upper thoracic spine: anatomy, biomechanics, and unique imaging features. AJR Am J Roentgenol. 1993;160(1):95–102.

78. Keynan O, et al. Radiographic measurement parameters in thoracolumbar fractures: a systematic review and consensus statement of the spine trauma study group. Spine (Phila Pa 1976). 2006;31(5):E156–65.

79. Daffner RH, et al. The radiologic assessment of post-traumatic vertebral stability. Skeletal Radiol. 1990;19(2):103–8.

80. Sampson MA, Colquhoun KB, Hennessy NL. Computed tomography whole body imaging in multitrauma: 7 years experience. Clin Radiol. 2006;61(4):365–9.

81. Antevil JL, et al. Spiral computed tomography for the initial evaluation of spine trauma: a new standard of care? J Trauma. 2006;61(2):382–7.

82. Compoginis JM, Akopian G. CT imaging in motorcycle collision victims: routine or selective? Am Surg. 2009;75(10):892–6.

83. Griffey RT, Ledbetter S, Khorasani R. Changes in thoracolumbar computed tomography and radiography utilization among trauma patients after deployment of multidetector computed tomography in the emergency department. J Trauma. 2007;62(5):1153–6.

84. Brown CV, et al. Spiral computed tomography for the diagnosis of cervical, thoracic, and lumbar spine fractures: its time has come. J Trauma. 2005;58(5):890–5; discussion 895–6.

85. Brandt MM, et al. Computed tomographic scanning reduces cost and time of complete spine evaluation. J Trauma. 2004;56(5):1022–6; discussion 1026–8.

86. Ballock RT, et al. Can burst fractures be predicted from plain radiographs? J Bone Joint Surg Br. 1992;74(1):147–50.

87. McGrory BJ, et al. Diagnosis of subtle thoracolumbar burst fractures. A new radiographic sign. Spine (Phila Pa 1976). 1993;18(15):2282–5.

88. Dai LY, et al. Plain radiography versus computed tomography scans in the diagnosis and management of thoracolumbar burst fractures. Spine (Phila Pa 1976). 2008;33(16):E548–52.

89. Fontijne WP, et al. CT scan prediction of neurological deficit in thoracolumbar burst fractures. J Bone Joint Surg Br. 1992;74(5):683–5.

90. Schoenwaelder M, Maclaurin W, Varma D. Assessing potential spinal injury in the intubated multitrauma patient: does MRI add value? Emerg Radiol. 2009;16(2):129–32.

91. Sekula Jr RF, et al. Exclusion of cervical spine instability in patients with blunt trauma with normal multidetector CT (MDCT) and radiography. Br J Neurosurg. 2008;22(5):669–74.

92. Dai LY, et al. Assessment of ligamentous injury in patients with thoracolumbar burst fractures using MRI. J Trauma. 2009;66(6):1610–5.

93. Lee HM, et al. Reliability of magnetic resonance imaging in detecting posterior ligament complex injury in thoracolumbar spinal fractures. Spine (Phila Pa 1976). 2000;25(16):2079–84.

94. Rihn JA, et al. Using magnetic resonance imaging to accurately assess injury to the posterior ligamentous complex of the spine: a prospective comparison of the surgeon and radiologist. J Neurosurg Spine. 2010;12(4):391–6.

95. Vaccaro AR, et al. Assessment of injury to the posterior ligamentous complex in thoracolumbar spine trauma. Spine J. 2006;6(5):524–8.

96. Lee JY, et al. Assessment of injury to the thoracolumbar posterior ligamentous complex in the setting of normal-appearing plain radiography. Spine J. 2007;7(4):422–7.

97. Vaccaro AR, et al. Injury of the posterior ligamentous complex of the thoracolumbar spine: a prospective evaluation of the diagnostic accuracy of magnetic resonance imaging. Spine (Phila Pa 1976). 2009;34(23):E841–7.

98. Haba H, et al. Diagnostic accuracy of magnetic resonance imaging for detecting posterior ligamentous complex injury associated with thoracic and lumbar fractures. J Neurosurg. 2003;99 Suppl 1:20–6.

99. Gillis C. Spinal ligament pathology. Vet Clin North Am Equine Pract. 1999;15(1):97–101.

100. Moon SH, et al. Feasibility of ultrasound examination in posterior ligament complex injury of thoracolumbar spine fracture. Spine (Phila Pa 1976). 2002;27(19):2154–8.

101. Vordemvenne T, et al. Is there a way to diagnose spinal instability in acute burst fractures by performing ultrasound? Eur Spine J. 2009;18(7):964–71.

102. Holdsworth FW. Diagnosis and treatment of fractures of the spine. Manit Med Rev. 1968;48(1):13–5.

103. Holdsworth FW. Fractures and dislocations of the lower thoracic and lumbar spines, with and without neurological involvement. Curr Pract Orthop Surg. 1964;23:61–83.

104. Louis R. Unstable fractures of the spine. III. Instability. A. Theories concerning instability. Rev Chir Orthop Reparatrice Appar Mot. 1977;63(5):423–5.

105. Denis F. The three column spine and its significance in the classification of acute thoracolumbar spinal injuries. Spine (Phila Pa 1976). 1983;8(8):817–31.

106. Decoulx P, Rieunau G. [Fractures of the dorsolumbar spine without neurological disorders]. Rev Chir Orthop Reparatrice Appar Mot. 1958;44(3–4):254–322.

107. Guigui PLB, Deburge A. Fractures et luxations récentes du rachis thoracique et lombaire de l'adulte. Encyclopédie Médico-Chirurgical; 1998.

108. Ferguson RL, Allen Jr BL. A mechanistic classification of thoracolumbar spine fractures. Clin Orthop Relat Res. 1984;189:77–88.

109. Magerl F, et al. A comprehensive classification of thoracic and lumbar injuries. Eur Spine J. 1994;3(4):184–201.

110. Aebi M. Classification of thoracolumbar fractures and dislocations. Eur Spine J. 2010;19 Suppl 1: S2–7.

111. McCormack T, Karaikovic E, Gaines RW. The load sharing classification of spine fractures. Spine (Phila Pa 1976). 1994;19(15):1741–4.

112. Dai LY, Jin WJ. Interobserver and intraobserver reliability in the load sharing classification of the assessment of thoracolumbar burst fractures. Spine (Phila Pa 1976). 2005;30(3):354–8.

113. Wang XY, et al. The load-sharing classification of thoracolumbar fractures: an in vitro biomechanical validation. Spine (Phila Pa 1976). 2007;32(11):1214–9.

114. Vaccaro AR, et al. A new classification of thoracolumbar injuries: the importance of injury morphology, the integrity of the posterior ligamentous complex, and neurologic status. Spine (Phila Pa 1976). 2005;30(20):2325–33.

115. Buchowski JM, et al. Surgical management of posttraumatic thoracolumbar kyphosis. Spine J. 2008;8(4):666–77.

116. Rihn JA, et al. A review of the TLICS system: a novel, user-friendly thoracolumbar trauma classification system. Acta Orthop. 2008;79(4):461–6.

117. Terk MR, et al. Injury of the posterior ligament complex in patients with acute spinal trauma: evaluation by MR imaging. AJR Am J Roentgenol. 1997;168(6):1481–6.

118. Ratliff J, et al. Regional variability in use of a novel assessment of thoracolumbar spine fractures: United States versus international surgeons. World J Emerg Surg. 2007;2:24.

119. Patel AA, et al. The adoption of a new classification system: time-dependent variation in interobserver reliability of the thoracolumbar injury severity score classification system. Spine (Phila Pa 1976). 2007;32(3):E105–10.

120. Harrop JS, et al. Intrarater and interrater reliability and validity in the assessment of the mechanism of injury and integrity of the posterior ligamentous complex: a novel injury severity scoring system for thoracolumbar injuries. Invited submission from the Joint Section Meeting On Disorders of the Spine and Peripheral Nerves, March 2005. J Neurosurg Spine. 2006;4(2):118–22.

121. Joaquim AF, et al. Evaluation of the thoracolumbar injury classification system in thoracic and lumbar spinal trauma. Spine (Phila Pa 1976). 2011;36(1):33–6.

122. Lenarz CJ, Place HM. Evaluation of a new spine classification system, does it accurately predict treatment? J Spinal Disord Tech. 2010;23(3):192–6.

123. Oner FC, et al. Therapeutic decision making in thoracolumbar spine trauma. Spine (Phila Pa 1976). 2010;35 Suppl 21:S235–44.

124. Lenarz CJ, et al. Comparative reliability of 3 thoracolumbar fracture classification systems. J Spinal Disord Tech. 2009;22(6):422–7.

125. Bedbrook GM. Treatment of thoracolumbar dislocation and fractures with paraplegia. Clin Orthop Relat Res. 1975;112:27–43.

126. Zdeblick TA, et al. Surgical treatment of thoracolumbar fractures. Instr Course Lect. 2009;58:639–44.

127. Giele BM, et al. No evidence for the effectiveness of bracing in patients with thoracolumbar fractures. Acta Orthop. 2009;80(2):226–32.

128. Rohlmann A, et al. Braces do not reduce loads on internal spinal fixation devices. Clin Biomech (Bristol, Avon). 1999;14(2):97–102.

129. Bailey CS, et al. Comparison of thoracolumbosacral orthosis and no orthosis for the treatment of thoracolumbar burst fractures: interim analysis of a multicenter randomized clinical equivalence trial. J Neurosurg Spine. 2009;11(3):295–303.

130. Cantor JB, et al. Nonoperative management of stable thoracolumbar burst fractures with early ambulation and bracing. Spine (Phila Pa 1976). 1993;18(8):971–6.

131. Chow GH, et al. Functional outcome of thoracolumbar burst fractures managed with hyperextension casting or bracing and early mobilization. Spine (Phila Pa 1976). 1996;21(18):2170–5.

132. Mumford J, et al. Thoracolumbar burst fractures. The clinical efficacy and outcome of nonoperative management. Spine (Phila Pa 1976). 1993;18(8):955–70.

133. McEvoy RD, Bradford DS. The management of burst fractures of the thoracic and lumbar spine. Experience in 53 patients. Spine (Phila Pa 1976). 1985;10(7):631–7.

134. Tezer M, et al. Conservative treatment of fractures of the thoracolumbar spine. Int Orthop. 2005;29(2):78–82.

135. Moller A, et al. Nonoperatively treated burst fractures of the thoracic and lumbar spine in adults: a 23- to 41-year follow-up. Spine J. 2007;7(6):701–7.

136. Agus H, Kayali C, Arslantas M. Nonoperative treatment of burst-type thoracolumbar vertebra fractures: clinical and radiological results of 29 patients. Eur Spine J. 2005;14(6):536–40.

137. Shen FH, Samartzis D. Successful nonoperative treatment of a three-column thoracic fracture in a patient with ankylosing spondylitis: existence and clinical significance of the fourth column of the spine. Spine (Phila Pa 1976). 2007;32(15):E423–7.

138. Tropiano P, et al. Functional and radiographic outcome of thoracolumbar and lumbar burst fractures managed by closed orthopaedic reduction and casting. Spine (Phila Pa 1976). 2003;28(21):2459–65.

139. Findlay JM, et al. A survey of vertebral burst-fracture management in Canada. Can J Surg. 1992;35(4):407–13.

140. Post RB, et al. Nonoperatively treated type A spinal fractures: mid-term versus long-term functional outcome. Int Orthop. 2009;33(4):1055–60.

141. Knight RQ, et al. Comparison of operative versus nonoperative treatment of lumbar burst fractures. Clin Orthop Relat Res. 1993;293:112–21.

142. Butler JS, Walsh A, O'Byrne J. Functional outcome of burst fractures of the first lumbar vertebra managed surgically and conservatively. Int Orthop. 2005;29(1):51–4.

143. Wood K, et al. Operative compared with nonoperative treatment of a thoracolumbar burst fracture without neurological deficit. A prospective, randomized study. J Bone Joint Surg Am. 2003;85-A(5):773–81.

144. Thomas KC, et al. Comparison of operative and nonoperative treatment for thoracolumbar burst fractures in patients without neurological deficit: a systematic review. J Neurosurg Spine. 2006;4(5):351–8.

145. Krengel 3rd WF, Anderson PA, Henley MB. Early stabilization and decompression for incomplete paraplegia due to a thoracic-level spinal cord injury. Spine (Phila Pa 1976). 1993;18(14):2080–7.

146. Fehlings MG, Tator CH. An evidence-based review of decompressive surgery in acute spinal cord injury: rationale, indications, and timing based on experimental and clinical studies. J Neurosurg. 1999;91 Suppl 1:1–11.

147. Shuman WP, et al. Thoracolumbar burst fractures: CT dimensions of the spinal canal relative to postsurgical improvement. AJR Am J Roentgenol. 1985;145(2):337–41.

148. Dai LY. Remodeling of the spinal canal after thoracolumbar burst fractures. Clin Orthop Relat Res. 2001;382:119–23.

149. Duh MS, et al. The effectiveness of surgery on the treatment of acute spinal cord injury and its relation to pharmacological treatment. Neurosurgery. 1994;35(2):240–8; discussion 248–9.

150. Zelle BA, et al. Sacral fractures with neurological injury: is early decompression beneficial? Int Orthop. 2004;28(4):244–51.

151. Rath SA, et al. Neurological recovery and its influencing factors in thoracic and lumbar spine fractures after surgical decompression and stabilization. Neurosurg Rev. 2005;28(1):44–52.

152. Mouchaty H, et al. Assessment of three year experience of a strategy for patient selection and timing of operation in the management of acute thoracic and lumbar spine fractures: a prospective study. Acta Neurochir (Wien). 2006;148(11):1181–7; discussion 1187.

153. Rutges JP, Oner FC, Leenen LP. Timing of thoracic and lumbar fracture fixation in spinal injuries: a systematic review of neurological and clinical outcome. Eur Spine J. 2007;16(5):579–87.

154. Cengiz SL, et al. Timing of thoracolomber spine stabilization in trauma patients; impact on neurological outcome and clinical course. A real prospective (rct) randomized controlled study. Arch Orthop Trauma Surg. 2008;128(9):959–66.

155. Fehlings MG, et al. Current practice in the timing of surgical intervention in spinal cord injury. Spine (Phila Pa 1976). 2010;35 Suppl 21:S166–73.

156. Frangen TM, et al. The beneficial effects of early stabilization of thoracic spine fractures depend on trauma severity. J Trauma. 2010;68(5):1208–12.

157. McLain RF, Benson DR. Urgent surgical stabilization of spinal fractures in polytrauma patients. Spine (Phila Pa 1976). 1999;24(16):1646–54.

158. Cotton BA, et al. Respiratory complications and mortality risk associated with thoracic spine injury. J Trauma. 2005;59(6):1400–7; discussion 1407–9.

159. Kerwin AJ, et al. Best practice determination of timing of spinal fracture fixation as defined by analysis of the National Trauma Data Bank. J Trauma. 2008;65(4):824–30; discussion 830–1.

160. Schinkel C, et al. Timing of thoracic spine stabilization in trauma patients: impact on clinical course and outcome. J Trauma. 2006;61(1):156–60; discussion 160.

161. Bellabarba C, et al. Does early fracture fixation of thoracolumbar spine fractures decrease morbidity or mortality? Spine (Phila Pa 1976). 2010;35 Suppl 9: S138–45.

162. Kerwin AJ, et al. The effect of early spine fixation on non-neurologic outcome. J Trauma. 2005;58(1):15–21.

Injuries of the Cervical Spine

Spiros G. Pneumaticos, Georgios K. Triantafyllopoulos, and Peter V. Giannoudis

Contents

S.G. Pneumaticos • G.K. Triantafyllopoulos
3rd Department of Orthopaedic Surgery, School of Medicine, University of Athens, Athens, Greece

P.V. Giannoudis (✉)
Academic Department of Trauma and Orthopaedics, School of Medicine, University of Leeds, Leeds, UK
e-mail: pgiannoudi@aol.com

Abstract

The incidence of cervical spine injuries ranges from 2 %–4.2 % among polytrauma patients. They may be accompanied with significant neurological impairment due to spinal cord involvement. High-energy trauma is the main cause of cervical spine injuries in younger populations, while falls are recognized as the main cause in older patients. The cervical spine is divided into two functional units, the upper or axial and the lower or sub-axial cervical spine. In the following chapter, the general approach for a patient with cervical spine trauma is discussed and specific injury types of both the upper and lower cervical spine are overviewed, with regards to clinical presentation, classification and treatment.

Keywords

Anatomy and Epidemiology • Cervical spine injuries • Classification • Conservative treatment • Neurological and imaging assessment • Operative techniques for 11 specific injuries • Operative treatment-goals

Epidemiology

Cervical spine trauma represents only a small percentage of all skeletal injuries, with an incidence ranging from 2 %–4.2 % among patients with blunt trauma [1, 2]. However, it poses a significant socio-economic problem, due to complications and sequelae related to spinal cord

G. Bentley (ed.), *European Surgical Orthopaedics and Traumatology*,
DOI 10.1007/978-3-642-34746-7_39, © EFORT 2014

involvement. Injuries of the cervical spine affect predominantly men, with the age distribution curve showing a double-peak pattern, in the third and sixth decades of life. High-energy trauma, including motor vehicle accidents, sports injuries, diving injuries, falls from heights and gunshot injuries are the most common causes of cervical spine trauma in young populations [1, 3–5]. On the other hand, falls, even from the standing or sitting position, are implicated as the major cause of cervical spine trauma in the elderly [1, 3–5]. Hence, in younger patients, injuries of the cervical spine are more likely to be related with concomitant injuries [4]. Among patients with spinal cord injury, trauma to the cervical spine is identified as the cause in approximately 53 % of cases, with the majority involving the C5 level [6]. In these patients, pulmonary complications are an important factor in morbidity [5].

Anatomy

The cervical spine is made up of seven vertebrae (C1-C7) and can be divided into two functional units, the upper and lower, or sub-axial, cervical spine. The upper cervical spine consists of the C1 vertebra, or atlas, and the C2 vertebra, or axis, and includes the complex occcipito-cervical junction, by which the cervical spine articulates with the occipital condyles of the cranium. The atlas and the axis exhibit unique anatomic characteristics when compared to the vertebrae of the sub-axial cervical spine. The atlas lacks a vertebral body, is ring-shaped and consists of the anterior and posterior arch and two lateral masses, surrounding the spinal foramen. The lateral masses have superior and inferior articular surfaces, which articulate with the oval occipital condyles and the superior facets of the axis, respectively. The axis is the thickest and strongest of the cervical vertebrae. Its main characteristic is the odontoid process or "dens", a cylindrical cephalad projection of the anterior aspect of the body, 12–16 mm in length. The anterior surface of the dens articulates with the anterior arch of the atlas, while posteriorly lies the transverse ligament. The atlas also exhibits a vertebral body, two lateral masses with superior and inferior facets, and a pedicle and lamina bilaterally. The laminae converge posteriorly in the midline to the spinous process, forming the spinal foramen.

The C3–C7 vertebrae have similar anatomic features, consisting of a vertebral body, two lateral masses and one pedicle and lamina on each side, which form the neural arch and surround the spinal foramen. The spinal foramina of all cervical vertebrae form the cervical spinal canal, within which lies the cervical spinal cord. Each lateral mass exhibits superior and inferior facets, with a 45° inclination from the horizontal plane. The transverse processes project laterally from the pedicle on each side, while posteriorly, the spinous process is formed in the mid-line by the convergence of the laminae. The inferior pedicle surface of the overlying vertebra and the superior pedicle surface of the underlying vertebra form the intervertebral foramen, one on either side, through which the corresponding nerve root exits the spinal canal.

In the upper cervical spine there are six joints, two atlanto-occipital (one on each side) and four atlanto-axial. Each atlanto-occipital joint is formed by the concave superior facet of the atlas and the corresponding occipital condyle, an anterior and posterior capsule and the tectorial membrane. The atlanto-axial articulations include the two facet joints laterally, between the inferior facets of the atlas and the superior facets of the axis, and the median atlanto-axial joints, one between the anterior surface of the dens and the posterior surface of the anterior arch of the atlas, and another between the posterior surface of the dens and the transverse ligament. The apical and alar ligaments provide further stability through their attachment to the apex of the dens. There is no intervertebral disc between the atlas and the axis. The atlanto-axial articulation is responsible for 50 % of total rotation of the cervical spine. In the sub-axial cervical spine, intervertebral discs are interposed between the vertebral bodies, which also articulate with the uncovertebral joints (joints of Luschka), on the posterolateral aspect. The facet, or zygoapophyseal, joints are formed on each side by the inferior facet of the overlying vertebra and the superior facet of the underlying vertebra. Even though these joints allow little movement between two consecutive vertebrae, the cervical spine as a functional whole is the most mobile part of the spine.

The anterior longitudinal ligament (ALL) and the posterior longitudinal ligament (PLL) attach on the anterior and posterior surface of the vertebral bodies and resist hyperextension and hyperflexion, respectively. The proximal extension of the PLL is the tectorial membrane. The facet joints are surrounded by a capsule and ligaments. The ligamentum flavum connects the laminae, while between the spinous processes lie the interspinous ligaments. The ligamentum nuchae extends from the occiput and dorsal to the spinous processes, and below C7 continues as the supraspinous ligament.

The spinal cord is constituted by H-shaped grey matter, with anterior and posterior horns, surrounded by white matter. Grey matter mainly includes neuronal bodies, while white matter is made up of axons. Within the white matter, the axons are organized in distinct tracts, both ascending and descending. These include the ventral and lateral spinothalamic tracts, which transmit pain and temperature sensation, the lateral corticospinal tracts, which transmit motor signals from the brain, and the posterior columns (fasciculus cuneatus and fasciculus gracillis), responsible for deep sensation, vibration and sensation of the body position in space (proprioception). There are eight pairs of spinal nerve roots, exiting the spinal canal from the corresponding intervertebral foramina. The C1 root exits above the C1 vertebra, the C2 exits below the C1 vertebra and the C8 exits below the C7 vertebra. The C5-T1 roots form the brachial plexi bilaterally, which innervate the upper extremities.

Initial Evaluation and Management

The correct and timely treatment of the patient with cervical spine trauma is very important, as it can diminish complications and sequelae related with these injuries. Every patient suffering from trauma must be considered as having a cervical spine injury, until proven otherwise. Thus, immobilization of the cervical spine with a rigid collar, a spine board and tapes, sandbags or rolled-up pieces of clothing must be performed at the site of injury and discontinued only when, after complete evaluation, an injury of the cervical spine is excluded. Flexion, extension or rotation of an unstable cervical spine can cause secondary damage to the spinal cord, resulting in quadriplegia or even death. The National Emergency X-ray Utilization Study (NEXUS) [7] has provided low-risk criteria for the diagnosis of cervical spine trauma. A patient without posterior mid-line cervical spine tenderness, without evidence of intoxication, with a normal level of alertness, without focal neurological deficit and painful, distracting injuries can be safely cleared from cervical spine trauma, without imaging studies. However, this tool cannot determine the best imaging modality for diagnosis, in a patient not fulfilling these criteria.

In a patient with blunt trauma, a hierarchical evaluation of the airway, breathing and circulation is performed. Hypoxia and hypotension should be avoided, especially in patients with suspected spinal cord injury, as they can both further impair spinal cord function [8]. High level spinal cord injuries (higher than C5) can cause respiratory failure, due to paralysis of the intercostal muscles and diaphragm. These patients should be closely monitored, as they may require early intubation. Concomitant injuries of the head and chest may further compromise the airway and respiratory function, and must be appropriately evaluated and treated. Generally, intubation and mechanical ventilation can secure both the airway and respiration. Major abdominal or chest trauma may cause hypovolaemic shock, which must be addressed. However, one should keep in mind that, in case of spinal cord injury, hypotension may occur even with normal blood volume. This is called neurogenic shock, it is caused by sympathetic impairment, and is further distinguished from hypovolaemic shock by the accompanying bradycardia. It has been suggested that, in patients with spinal cord injury, the mean arterial pressure should be kept >90 mmHg [8]. This can be accomplished by administration of crystalloid and colloid solutions, as well as blood, while in case of neurogenic shock, vasoconstricting agents

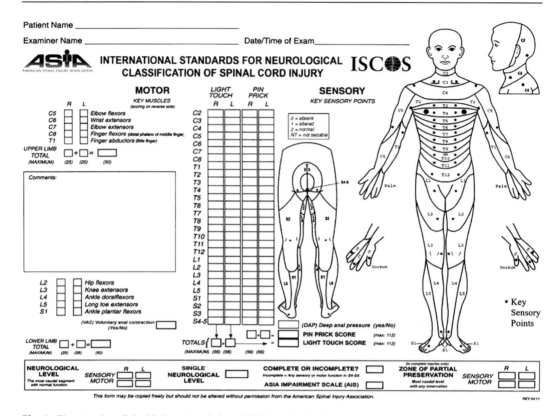

Fig. 1 The American Spinal Injury Association (ASIA) evaluation sheet

may also help. Examination of the spine takes place during secondary survey, with inspection and palpation. In up to 11 % of polytrauma patients, cervical injury may be associated with concomitant thoraco-lumbar injuries [9].

A thorough neurological examination is also necessary. Light touch and pin-prick sensation are tested in each dermatome and the result is graded as 2 (normal), 1 (impaired) or 0 (complete loss). The last normal dermatome is noted on each side. Examination of the sacral dermatomes and determination of peri-anal sensation should not be missed. Sensory examination can provide a quick overview of the patient's neurological status and the level of injury, but on the other hand it is highly subjective, as it depends greatly on the patient's perception of stimuli.

Motor function is evaluated by testing strength of certain key muscles that are predominantly innervated by the corresponding nerve roots. Each muscle receives a grade from a six-grade system, with 5 being normal muscle strength;

4, active movement with full range of motion against moderate resistance; 3, full range of motion against gravity; 2, full range of motion with gravity neutralized; 1, palpable or visible contractions; and 0, total paralysis. Voluntary contraction of the anal sphincter should always be included in the examination. Neurological examination should also include superficial and deep reflexes, as well as search for pathological reflexes (e.g. Babinski's sign). The American Spinal Injury Association (ASIA) evaluation sheet aids in obtaining a rapid, yet thorough assessment of a spinal cord injury (Fig. 1).

Spinal shock is a transient state of complete loss of neurological function, characterized by areflexia below the level of injury, along with flaccid paralysis and loss of sensation. The duration of spinal shock ranges from hours to days and its end is marked by the re-emergence of the reflex arcs below the level of injury, classically including the bulbocavernosus reflex. After spinal shock has resolved, the degree of the patient's

Table 1 The Frankel's grading system and the ASIA impairment scale are used to determine the neurologic status of a patient with a spinal cord injury

	Grade				
	A	B	C	D	E
Frankel's grading system	Complete paralysis	Preserved sensory but not motor function below the level of injury	Preserved sensory function, non-useful motor function (grade 2/5-3/5) below the level of injury	Preserved sensory function, useful motor function (grade 4/5) below the level of injury	Normal sensorimotor function
ASIA Impairment Scale	No sensory or motor function preserved in the S4–S5 segments	Sensory function preserved below the level of injury (including the S4–S5 segments). Absence of motor function more than three levels below the motor level on either side of the body	Preservation of motor function below the neurological level, with >50 % of key muscles with a grade less than 3/5	Preservation of motor function below the neurological level, with at least 50 % of key muscles with a grade ≥3/5	Normal sensorimotor function

neurological impairment can be determined, using either the Frankel's grading system, or the ASIA Impairment Scale (Table 1). Frequent serial neurological evaluations should be performed, in order to document any improvement of patient's neurologic status over time.

The topography of spinal cord injury determines clinical presentation, according to the affected spinal tracts. At the level of the cervical spinal cord, four distinct syndromes may be encountered, including the anterior, the posterior and the central cord syndrome, as well as the Brown-Séquard syndrome.

The anterior cord syndrome is caused by injuries of the anterior two-thirds of the spinal cord, commonly by a combination of flexion and compression forces. It is characterized by loss of motor function and pain and temperature sensation, but preservation of position and vibratory sensation. In case of a posterior spinal cord syndrome, the damage involves the posterior columns, with subsequent loss of deep sensation. A central cord syndrome, most frequently caused by hyperextension injury of a spondylotic cervical spine, involves the central portion of the cord and presents with paresis, which is more severe in the upper extremities, as the efferent and afferent

tracts responsible for upper extremity function lie more centrally in the spinal cord, than those designated to more distal parts of the body. Finally, the Brown-Séquard syndrome is caused by unilateral injuries (typically penetrating trauma) and is characterized by ipsilateral paresis, ipsilateral loss of position and vibratory sensation and contralateral loss of pain and temperature sensation, three dermatomes below the affected level. This clinical presentation is due to the different decussation patterns of the sensory and motor tracts, as the spinothalamic tracts decussate three levels after entering the spinal cord, while the corticospinal tracts decussate at the medulla oblongata (pyramidal decussation).

The National Acute Spinal Cord Injury Study (NASCIS) II and III trials showed improved prognosis in patients with incomplete spinal cord injury, after administration of high doses of methylprednisolone [10]. If the patient is admitted within 3 h after injury, an initial bolus dose of 30 mg/kg of methylprednisolone is administered within 15 min, followed by a 45-min pause, and a 23-h continuous infusion of 5.4 mg/kg/h. If the patient is admitted between 3 and 8 h after injury, infusion is continued for 48 h. Recently, however, the efficacy of this therapeutic scheme has been questioned [11]. Gangliosides(GM-1) have been also suggested as a potential treatment to improve recovery, but clinical trials failed to prove their effectiveness [12]. The effectiveness of other proposed agents, including naloxone, thyrotropin-releasing hormone and erythropoietin has not been confirmed in clinical trials [8].

Imaging Studies

It has already been stated that the NEXUS criteria do not determine the ideal imaging method for the diagnosis of cervical spine trauma. Plain radiography is the most widely available modality and, in most circumstances, is the first imaging study a patient with blunt trauma will undergo, if cervical spine injury is suspected. The lateral view, either in the erect or the supine (cross-table) position, can identify most fractures and dislocations of the cervical spine. In the upper cervical spine, the relationships between the skull, the atlas and the axis can be evaluated, whereas the atlas and the axis can be fully visualized. In the lower cervical spine, the vertebral bodies, the intervertebral disc spaces, the facet joints, and the spinous processes can be identified. Furthermore, the four contour lines of the cervical spine can be evaluated (Fig. 2).

A lateral view without depiction of the C7 vertebra must not be accepted, as injuries at this level can frequently be missed. In the anteroposterior view, the vertebral bodies of C3 to C7 can be visualized, as well as the Luschka joints, the disc spaces and the spinous processes. The open-mouth view is an anteroposterior view

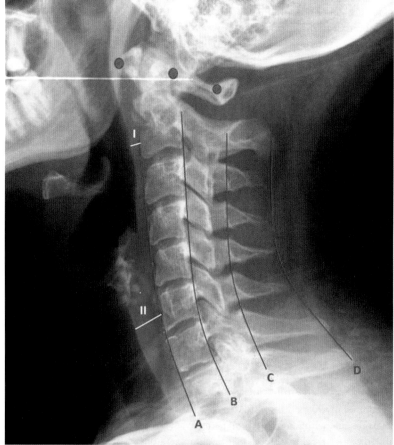

Fig. 2 Lateral radiograph of the cervical spine in a 23 year-old female with a fracture of the C2 odontoid process. The four contour lines include *A*: the anterior vertebral line along the anterior margins of the vertebral bodies, *B*: the posterior vertebral line along the posterior margins of the vertebral bodies, *C*: the spinolaminar line which outlines the posterior border of the spinal canal and *D*: the posterior spinous line along the tips of the spinous processes through C2–C7. The retropharyngeal space (*I*) should be ≤7 mm, while the retrotracheal space (*II*) should be <22 mm in adults and <14 mm in children. In this case, disruption of the *A*, *B* and *C* lines can be noted

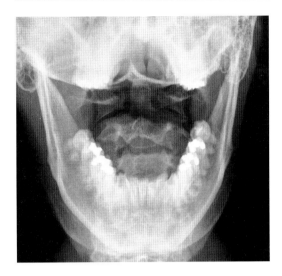

Fig. 3 Open-mouth view of the upper cervical spine

of the cervical spine, centred over the first two vertebrae. It provides full visualization of the dens, the body of the axis, the lateral masses of both the atlas and the axis and the lateral atlanto-axial joints (Fig. 3). The lateral, anteroposterior and open-mouth views are included in the standard radiographic imaging of the patient with suspected cervical spine injury. If they are negative and there is still high suspicion of injury, several other projections may be used, including the pillar view, the oblique view and the swimmer's view (Fig. 4). Dynamic radiographs in flexion and extension may reveal instability that cannot be identified in standard views. They are indicated in conscious, co-operative patients, who can actively flex and extend their neck. The presence of more than 3.5 mm of intervertebral translation or 11° of angulation is indicative of instability. Passive flexion-extension radiographs in the unconscious patient should generally be avoided, as they may result in secondary neurological sequelae [13]. Despite its simple nature and widespread availability, plain radiography may be time-consuming [14] and inadequate in detecting all cervical spine injuries [15], while repeated imaging is frequently required, because of poor visualization.

CT scanning is commonly used in the evaluation of cervical spine trauma, as it can more accurately detect fractures of the C1 arches, the dens and the occipital condyles. Moreover, it can provide valuable information about soft-tissue injuries, clinically insignificant injuries that require only symptomatic treatment, as well as the involvement of the spinal canal. CT is more sensitive than plain radiography in detecting cervical spine fractures, with a sensitivity of up to 98 %, versus 52 % for plain X-rays [16]. However, this does not justify the routine use of CT scanning for the screening of all patients with suspected cervical spine injury, as it is related to higher doses of ionizing radiation, with special consideration of the thyroid gland, and is a more expensive procedure. Hence, efforts have been made to establish clinical criteria for selecting those patients who would benefit from CT scanning of the cervical spine [17, 18]. Nevertheless, the development of newer and faster, multi-detector scanners has led many authors to reconsider these limitations [16].

Magnetic resonance imaging (MRI) is a valuable adjunct to cervical spine trauma evaluation, as it can accurately depict soft-tissue and spinal cord injuries. MRI can provide multiplanar images, revealing even minimal trauma of the spinal cord and the ligamentous structures (Fig. 5). It is also useful in cases of Spinal Cord Injuries Without Obvious Radiological Abnormalities (SCIWORA), as all other imaging modalities are negative [19]. It is interesting that, in patients with neurological deficit, MRI findings are well correlated with long-term outcomes [6, 20]. On the other hand, MRI requires time, which may not be available in the case of a yet unstable patient. Furthermore, patients are quite often immobilized with metallic traction devices, which are not compatible with a strong magnetic field. Finally, it is an expensive method and, as plain X-rays and CT can better visualize bony structures, it is usually used in cases of neurologic impairment, in order to define the extent of spinal cord injury.

Myelography is another modality widely used in the past. However, as novel techniques were developed, including CT and MRI, myelography is now rarely used in acute cervical trauma and mostly serves as an adjunct to CT scanning, if the patient is unable to undergo MRI.

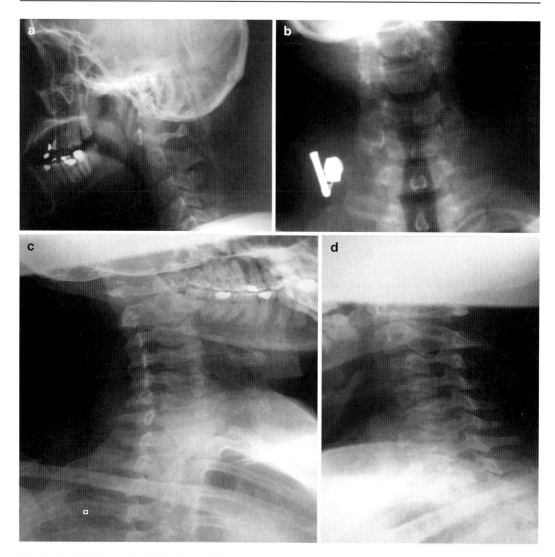

Fig. 4 (**a** and **b**) Lateral and AP views of the cervical spine of a 26 year-old male involved in a motor vehicle accident, who presented with complete C5 quadriplegia. The lateral view failed to demonstrate the vertebrae below C5, while in the AP view, only the decreased height of the C6 vertebral body raises suspicion of a fracture. Subsequently, *left* (**c**) and *right* (**d**) oblique views were obtained, demonstrating a burst fracture of the C6 vertebra with spinal canal compromise

General Considerations Regarding Treatment

Treatment of cervical spine fractures can be either non-operative or operative, depending on the type of injury, the degree of instability and the presence of neurological deficit.

Non-Operative Treatment

Non-operative measures include immobilization with skeletal skull traction, semi-rigid and rigid collars, cervico-thoracicorthoses and the Halo vest.

Skeletal skull traction involves applying weight traction to the skull, via tongs (Crutchfield or Gardner-Wells) placed 1 cm above the pinna,

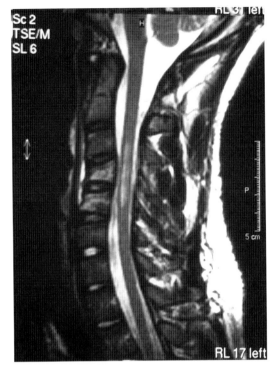

Fig. 5 Sagittal T2-weighted MRI of a patient with fractures of the C4 and C5 vertebrae and quadriplegia. Abnormal signal is noted within the substance of the spinal cord. The presence of haematoma between the anterior longitudinal ligament and the anterior margins of the vertebrae is demonstrated, while significant edema and injury of the posterior ligamentous structures can also be identified

standard for the total weight that may be applied. After reduction, however, it is limited to 10–20 lb. Moreover, distraction of a disc level for more than 1 cm precludes further weight application. If the patient is unconscious, closed reduction with skull traction should not be attempted without previous MRI. This is to exclude a protruding herniated disc at the level of the dislocation, which could result in post-reduction cord compression and quadriplegia. A CT scan or an MRI is done after successful reduction.

Semi-rigid and rigid collars are usually the first measure for cervical spine immobilization at the site of injury. When combined with sandbags and tapes, they provide optimal immobilization for patients' transfer. They include the Philadelphia collar, the Miami collar, the Aspen collar etc., and may be used in the treatment of stable cervical spine fractures. However, stand-alone semi-rigid collars still allow significant motion of the cervical spine, especially lateral bending and rotation. By incorporating the thorax, cervico-thoracic orthroses (e.g. the sterno-occipito-mandibular immobilizer – SOMI and the Minerva brace) provide better immobilization than collars, especially to the lower cervical spine and cervico-thoracicjunction. They are usually used in the treatment of stable fractures of the lower cervical spine. Collars and cervico-thoracic orthoses are mainly associated with skin complications, including ulcerations and allergic reactions, but they may also be related with muscle atrophy and pain.

The Halo vest represents the stiffest means of external immobilization and can be used either as a stand-alone treatment, or as an adjunct to cervical spine surgery. It consists of a ring, secured to the skull with pins and connected with rods to an upper torso vest. The ring is selected to the appropriate size and connected with four pins, two anterior and two posterior. The patient is supine, with the cervical spine provisionally immobilized with a collar. Under local anaesthesia, the pins are inserted into pre-defined sites of the skull and below its equator, with the use of a torque screwdriver in order to perforate only the outer cortex of the skull. The anterior pins are placed within a safe zone >1 cm above the orbital rim and along its

below the skull equator. A Halo ring may be used as well, especially if the Halo vest is planned to be the definitive treatment. Skeletal skull traction is used for reduction of acute dislocations and subluxations, as well as for immobilization of the cervical spine in critical care patients with upper or lower C-spine fractures. It is contra-indicated in patients with skull fractures. The patient is placed in a reverse Trendelenburg position and should ideally be conscious, in order to immediately recognize any acute deterioration in the neurological status during the procedure. Initially, a weight of 10 lb is placed, which is increased by 5 lb per level in 20–30 min intervals, in order to allow for muscle spasm subsidence. After each increase, a lateral radiograph is taken and a full neurological examination is carried out. Generally, there is no

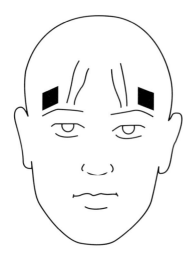 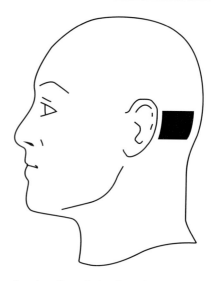

Fig. 6 Application of the "Halo". The safe zones for pin insertion are shaded. Anteriorly, an area 10 mm above the lateral third of the eyebrow will avoid the cutaneous nerves and frontal sinuses medially, and will be over the relatively thick plate of bone at the fronto-temporal junction. Posteriorly, the safe zone lies over the thick bone of the external occipital protruberance, avoiding branches of the occipital nerve posteriorly, and branches of the auricular nerves more anteriorly

lateral two thirds, where important structures, including the frontal sinus, the supra-orbital and supra-trochlear nerves, and the temporal artery are avoided (Fig. 6). During anterior pin placement, the patient should keep his/her eyelids closed, to avoid skin tethering. The posterior pins are placed opposite to the anterior pins. A vest of the appropriate size is applied and connected symmetrically to the ring with rods (Fig. 7). Before securing the rods to the vest, the alignment of the cervical spine to the head and chest is checked, in order to confirm proper fracture reduction. Moreover, malalignment could result in swallowing and eating problems, as well as ambulation difficulties, as the patient cannot see his/her feet. Pins and screws are re-tightened 24 h and 1 week after Halo vest placement, and weekly thereafter, while pin insertion sites are cleaned with hydrogen peroxide twice a day and observed for signs of infection. In paediatric patients, up to ten pins may be required to obtain stable fixation of the ring to the skull. Pin site infection, pin loosening, ring migration and pin discomfort are the most frequent complications of this method [21].

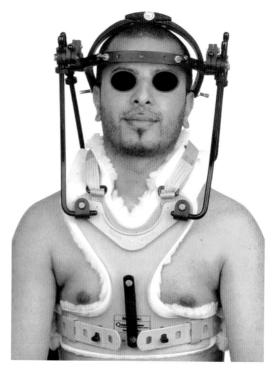

Fig. 7 Application of an appropriate size Halo-vest is illustrated

Operative Treatment

The goals of operative treatment include restoration of alignment, stabilization of the C-spine, and decompression of neural elements. It includes anterior and posterior procedures. Anterior procedures are indicated in cases of anterior column insufficiency or anterior spinal cord compression (e.g. burst fractures). On the other hand, in the presence of facet dislocations or trauma with significant posterior element compromise, posterior surgery is usually preferred. The detailed description of each surgical technique is beyond the scope of this chapter, however general points are discussed in the corresponding sections for specific C-spine injuries. The timing of surgery depends on the type of injury and the presence and progression of neurologic deficit. For example, a progressive neurological deficit in a patient with a fracture causing compression to the spinal cord requires surgical intervention. On the contrary, surgery could be delayed in patients without neurological impairment. However, early surgery permits patient mobilization and decreases morbidity related to prolonged recumbency.

A suggested treatment algorithm for cervical spine injuries is provided in Fig. 8.

Specific Injuries of the Cervical Spine

Upper Cervical Spine

Occipital Condyle Fractures

Occipital condyle fractures are classically described together with other injuries of the cervical spine. Typically, they result from axial compression or lateral bending forces to the head. They may be accompanied by head injuries, as well as fractures of the upper and lower cervical spine, which can make clinical diagnosis difficult. Clinical presentation is non-specific and may include pain and tenderness at the occipito-cervical region and torticollis [22]. The presence of neurologic deficit is variable and mostly involves the lower cranial

nerves IX, X, XI and XII (Collet-Sicard syndrome) [23]. Late neurologic deficit may be observed, due to fragment displacement, fibrosis or nerve edema. Plain X-rays are usually insufficient for diagnosis and, in case of a patient with a suspected occipital condyle fracture, CT scanning should be performed. Anderson and Montesano proposed a classification for occipital condyle fractures based on CT scan findings, recognizing three different types:

Type I includes comminuted fractures, with minimal or no displacement into the foramen magnum. The contra-lateral alar ligament and the tectorial membrane are intact, thus these fractures are considered stable.

Type II fractures are typically an extension of a basilar skull fracture to the base of the condyle. Stability is maintained by the intact ligamentous structures.

Type III fractures are avulsion fractures of the occipital condyles, and are considered potentially unstable. Treatment is in the majority of cases non-operative and includes immobilization with the use of a semi-rigid or rigid collar. If the fracture is considered unstable, then a Halo vest may provide a more rigid immobilization (Table 2).

Occipito-Atlantal Dislocation

Occipito-atlantal dislocation is recognized as the cause of 6–8 % of deaths among motor vehicle accident victims and accounts for 20–30 % of deaths from cervical spine injuries [24, 25]. In the past, these injuries were infrequently reported, but with the improvement of pre-hospital care, diagnostic modalities and management over the years, an increasing number of patients with such injuries subsequently survived and were diagnosed. Clinically, patients usually have concomitant injuries to other organs, as occipito-atlantal dislocation results from high-energy trauma. The vertebral arteries, cranial nerves, brainstem and spinal cord are also in danger. However, the absence of neurological deficit is also possible [26]. Occipito-atlantal dislocations

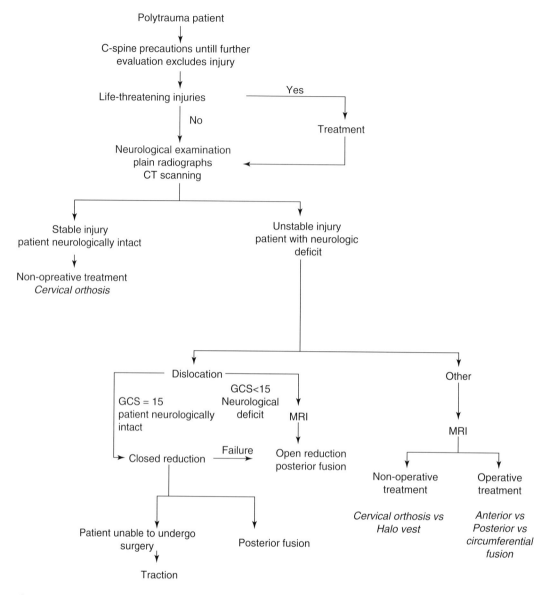

Fig. 8 Treatment algorithm for cervical spine injuries

are classified according to Traynelis into three types:

Type I involves anterior translation of the occiput in relation to the atlas.

Type II result from vertical distraction forces.

Type III are characterized by posterior dislocation of the occiput over the atlas. Nevertheless, the relationship of the occiput to the atlas is highly dependable on the position of the patient, limiting the accuracy of the Traynelis classification, as small changes in neck position may result in a totally different occipito-atlantal pattern.

In plain X-rays, several measurements have been proposed for determination of occipito-cervical dissociation. The distance from the basion to the posterior arch of the atlas, divided by the distance between the opisthion to the anterior arch of the atlas is called Power's ratio, with normal values less or equal than 1.0 (Fig. 9a).

The basion-dens interval can also be measured, with a distance of more than 10 mm in adults or 12 mm in children being abnormal (Fig. 9b). A condyle-C1 interval of more than 2 mm in adults or more than 5 mm in children is also indicative of occipito-atlantal dislocation (Fig. 9c). The X-line method involves drawing two lines, one from the basion to the C2 spinolaminar junction, and another from the opisthion to the postero-inferior corner of the C2 body. Normally, the first line intersects C2 and the second intersects C1 (Fig. 9d). CT imaging can be further used to evaluate occipito-atlantal

Table 2 Summary of treatment options for specific cervical spine injuries

Type of Injury		Treatment Modality		Operative
		Non-Operative		
Upper cervical spine				
Occipital condyle fractures		Semi-rigid or rigid collar immobilization		
		Halo vest immobilization may be considered in certain Type III fractures		
Occipitoatlantal dislocation				Occipitocervical fusion with wiring, rod and wire fixation and rod and screws (posterior approach), after initial skeletal skull traction
Fractures of the atlas	*Transverse ligament intact*	Semi-rigid or rigid collar immobilization		
	Transverse ligament disrupted	*Bony avulsion*	Halo vest immobilization	
		Non bony avulsion		Occipitocervical fusion (posterior approach)
Rotatory atlantoaxial dislocation		Closed reduction with skeletal skull traction + Halo vest immobilization		Open reduction and posterior C1–C2 fusion with wiring techniques or transarticular screws
Fractures of the axis	*Odontoid process (dens) fractures*	*Type I*	Semi-rigid or rigid collar immobilization	
		Type II	Halo vest immobilization (high rates of non-union)	Odontoid screw fixation (transoral approach)
				C1–C2 fusion (posterior approach) with the use of wires or cables, interlaminar clamps, transarticular screw fixation, crossed C2 intralaminar screws and rod and screw fixation
		Type III	Halo vest immobilization	
Traumatic spondylolisthesis of the axis	*Type I*	Rigid collar immobilization		
	Type II	Halo vest immobilization		
	Type III			Open reduction – C2-C3 fusion (posterior approach)
Lower cervical spine				
Burst fractures				Anterior decompression and fusion vs. combined procedures (in case of posterior elements' injury)
Flexion teardrop fractures				Anterior decompression and fusion vs. posterior fusion vs. combined procedures

(continued)

Table 2 (continued)

Type of Injury		Treatment Modality	
		Non-Operative	Operative
Facet fractures and dislocations	*Undisplaced unilateral facet fractures*	Semi-rigid or rigid collar immobilization	
	Bilateral facet fractures	Semi-rigid or rigid collar immobilization	Anterior vs. posterior fusion in case of translation >3.5 mm
	Lateral mass fracture separations		Anterior vs. posterior fusion
	Unilateral facet dislocations	Immobilization with a cervical orthosis may be considered in case of stable injuries, without neurologic deficit	Open reduction and posterior fusion with screws and rods
	Bilateral facet dislocations		Closed vs. open reduction and posterior fusion with screws and rods

dislocation in multiple planes. MRI is very useful for evaluation of ligamentous and neural tissue injuries, and can reveal abnormalities indicative of instability, even in the setting of normal radiographic or CT findings.

Treatment of these injuries includes initial immobilization by skeletal skull traction or a Halo vest. Skull traction is however contraindicated in type II injuries. The Halo vest may also be the definitive treatment in patients with normal CT findings and a borderline MRI [27]. However, in the vast majority of cases, instability is addressed with occipito-cervical fusion (Table 2). This can be achieved with different techniques, including wiring, rod and wire fixation and rod and screws fixation. Wiring techniques require post-operative use of a Halo vest for additional immobilization. Screws to the occiput are placed in the midline and have preferably bi-cortical purchase, while trans-articular screws are used for C1-C2 fixation and lateral mass screws for sub-axial vertebrae, if fusion must extend below C2.

Fractures of the Atlas

Fractures of the atlas represent 3–13 % of injuries to the cervical spine in adults and 3.5 % in children [28]. Motor vehicle accidents and falls are the main causes of atlas fractures, with a combination of axial loading, flexion, extension and lateral bending forces resulting in compression of the atlas between the occiput and the axis. Atlas fractures are therefore frequently accompanied with head injuries and other fractures of the cervical spine. The areas of transition between the lateral masses and the anterior and posterior arches represent the weakest points of the vertebra and it is at these sites that fractures occur during axial compression. If axial compression is combined with lateral bending, the result is usually a fracture of the lateral mass. Clinically, an atlas fracture presents with pain, tenderness and muscle spasm. Symptoms from injury of the C2 nerve root and the vertebral artery may also be encountered. As fractures of the atlas usually cause the spinal canal to expand, neurological deficit is unusual in cases of isolated atlas fractures. Jefferson's classification includes five types of fractures:

Type I and type II are isolated fractures of the posterior and anterior arch respectively.

Type III fractures are the classic Jefferson burst fractures of the atlas, involving bilateral posterior arch fractures and unilateral or bilateral fractures of the anterior arch.

Type IV fractures involve the lateral mass.

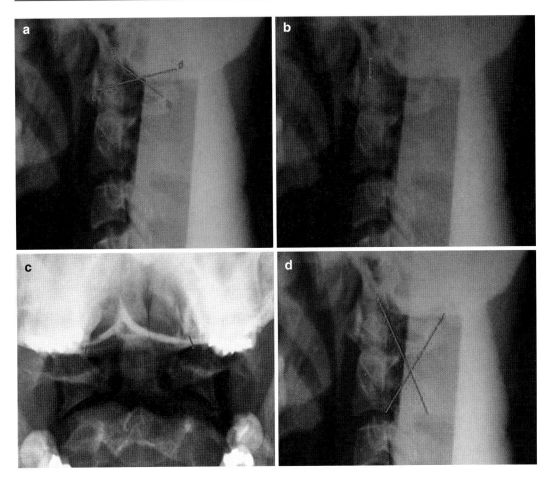

Fig. 9 (**a**) Power's ratio = ab/dc. Normal values ≤1. (**b**) Basion-dens interval. Normal values <10 mm in adults, <12 mm in children. (**c**) Condyle-C1 interval. Normal values <2 mm in adults, <5 mm in children. (**d**) The X line method

Type V include transverse fractures of the anterior arch.

Plain X-rays may demonstrate fractures of the posterior and anterior arch, while in the open-mouth view, fractures and displacement of the lateral masses may be noted. A sum of lateral mass diastasis of more than 6.9 mm is suggestive of transverse ligament insufficiency [29]. Flexion and extension X-rays can rule out instability. CT scanning provides a more detailed evaluation of the bony injuries (Fig. 10), while MRI may be used in order to evaluate the transverse ligament.

Treatment of atlas fractures consists of external immobilization with a Halo vest for 12 weeks (Table 2). Isolated posterior arch fractures may be treated with a cervical collar. After removal of the Halo vest, stability is confirmed with flexion and extension X-rays. Operative treatment is indicated in cases of non-bony avulsion of the transverse ligament or if residual instability is present after immobilization and includes posterior Occ-C1 and C1-C2 fusion.

Rotatory Atlanto-Axial Dislocation

Traumatic rotatory atlanto-axial dislocation, although common in children, is rarely described in adults. The main cause is motor vehicle accidents. Pain and restriction of neck's range of motion are the main clinical findings. Neurologic deficit may also be present, even though injury to

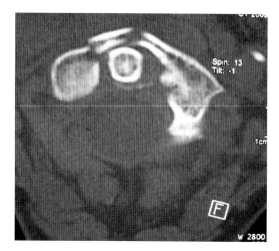

Fig. 10 Axial CT image of the C1 vertebra in a 74 years-old female who sustained a fall from a height. A fracture of the anterior arch of the C1 is demonstrated

the spinal cord at this level is frequently lethal. Rotatory atlanto-axial dislocation may be accompanied by rupture of the transverse ligament. The latter is classified into two types according to Dickman et al. [30]: type I includes rupture at the mid-portion of the transverse ligament or at its insertion point, while type II injuries represent bony avulsions of the ligament. Fielding's classification describes four patterns of rotatory atlanto-axial dislocation: type 1 includes rotatory displacement without shift, with the transverse ligament intact; type 2 involves 3–5 mm anterior displacement of the anterior arch in relation to the dens, with a lateral mass pivot; in type 3 injuries, displacement is more than 5 mm; finally, type 4 dislocations include posterior translation of the atlas in relation to the axis. Type 2 and 3 injuries are characterized by insufficient transverse and alar ligaments, while type 4 is associated with odontoid process fractures.

In plain X-rays, the atlanto-dens interval can be measured, with values >5 mm being indicative of instability. CT scanning is the diagnostic method of choice, as axial images can accurately depict C1–C2 rotatory translation. Again, MRI is useful in evaluation of ligamentous injuries.

Non-operative treatment includes skeletal skull traction for up to 3 weeks, in order to achieve reduction, followed by Halo vest immobilization for 12 weeks. If closed reduction is not possible, open reduction and C1–C2 fusion is indicated, with the use of wiring techniques or C1–C2 trans-articular screws (Table 2).

Fractures of the Axis
Odontoid Process (Dens) Fractures

Dens fractures are the most common fractures of the axis and result from flexion or extension forces, due to falls or motor vehicle accidents. Their sole clinical manifestation may be pain, making their diagnosis difficult. In the setting of an emergency department, these injuries are quite often missed. Anderson and D'Alonzo proposed the most widely-used classification of dens fractures, which includes three types:

Type I represents avulsion fractures of the tip of the dens, where the alar ligaments are attached.

Type II fractures occur at the junction of the dens to the C2 body (Fig. 11).

Type III fractures include injuries where the fracture line extends to the body of the axis (Figs. 2 and 12).

Diagnosis can be made with plain X-rays, but CT scanning provides multi-planar images and a more thorough evaluation of the fracture.

Treatment depends on the type of fracture (Table 2).

Type I fractures are treated non-operatively, with external immobilization in a cervical collar. However, in some cases, type I fractures may be associated with occipito-atlantal instability, which should always be evaluated. Non-operative treatment of type II fractures is related with high rates of non-union [31]. This is mainly due to the relatively poor blood supply of the dens base. Other factors include the lack of periosteal blood supply to the dens and the distractional forces applied by the intact alar ligaments. External immobilization in a Halo vest is a reasonable option, with total non-union rates ranging from 26 % to 29.7 % [32–35].

A displacement of 6 mm or more and an age ≥50 years are related with higher rates of non-union with Halo vest immobilization [35, 36]. In these patients, surgical management is the treatment of choice. Operative treatment includes odontoid process osteosynthesis and C1–C2

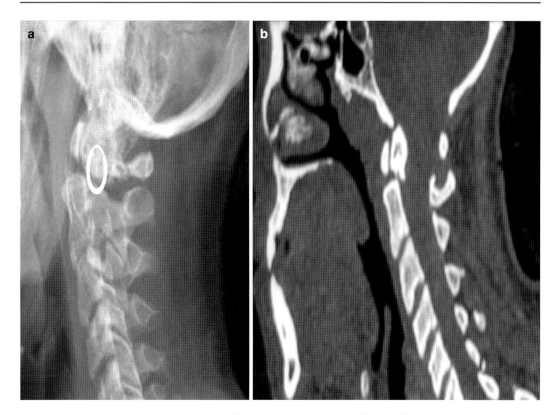

Fig. 11 (a) Lateral radiograph and (b) sagittal CT reconstruction image of a 19 year-old male with a type II fracture of the odontoid process, after a motor vehicle accident

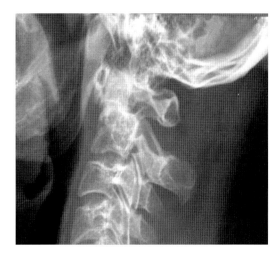

Fig. 12 Type III fracture of the odontoid process in a 34 year-old male who sustained a motor vehicle accident. The patient was neurologically intact and was treated non-operatively, with Halo-vest immobilization

fusion. Odontoid screw fixation has the theoretical advantage of preserving rotation between the atlas and the axis. Reported fusion rates are up to 88 % [37]. Contra-indications to this technique include disruption of the transverse ligament (absolute contra-indication), osteopenia, fractures older than 6 months, fractures with a direction from antero-inferiorly to postero-superiorly and poor general health. Moreover, the transoral approach is associated with high rates of complications. C1–C2 fusion may be achieved with several techniques, including use of wires or cables (Gallie fusion, Brooks and Jenkins fusion), interlaminar clamps, trans-articular screw fixation, crossed C2 intra-laminar screws [38] and rod fixation with C1 lateral mass screws and C2 pedicle screws (Harms and Melcher fixation [39]). Fusion rates up to 100 %

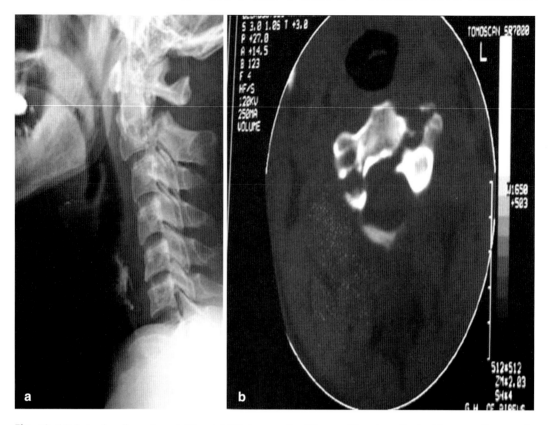

Fig. 13 (**a**) Lateral radiograph and (**b**) axial CT image of a 28 year-old male patient with a type I traumatic spondylolisthesis of the axis

have been reported [39], however C1-C2 fusion sacrifices 50 % of cervical spine rotation.

Type III injuries are typically treated with Halo vest immobilization, with bony union rates ranging from 84 % to 100 % [32, 33]. Failure of non-operative treatment, defined as mal-union or non-union, requires surgical intervention.

Traumatic Spondylolisthesis of the Axis (Hangman's Fracture)

The incidence of traumatic spondylolisthesis of the axis varies and has been reported up to 38 % [40]. This pattern of axis fracture was first described in death-sentenced convicts, who were executed by hanging. Today, motor vehicle accidents and falls from height are the primary causes (Fig. 13). Levine and Edwards [41] modified the Effendi [42] classification and described three types of fractures:

Type I fractures show displacement less than 3 mm without angulation, caused by a combination of hyperextension and axial loading.

Type II refers to fractures with displacement more than 3 mm and angulation more than 10°, caused by a sequence of hyperextension-axial loading and flexion.

Type IIa is a sub-group of type II fractures caused by flexion and distraction and characterized by widening of the posterior intervertebral space between C2 and C3. Type III fractures are additionally accompanied by unilateral or bilateral facet dislocation.

Treatment of type I fractures consists of rigid cervical collar immobilization for 12 weeks. Halo vest immobilization is the treatment of choice for type II fractures. On the other hand, type IIa and type III fractures are best treated surgically, with open reduction of the dislocation (type III) and posterior C2-C3 fusion (Table 2).

Lower Cervical Spine

The Allen-Ferguson classification [43] divides injuries of the lower (sub-axial) cervical spine into six categories, according to the mechanism of injury: extension-distraction, extension-compression, compression, flexion-compression, flexion-distraction injuries and lateral flexion injuries. Each of these categories is further subdivided in stages of increasing severity. Recently, the Cervical Spine Injury Severity Score (CSISS) [44] and the Sub-axial Cervical Injury Classification System (SLIC) [45] have been proposed, in order to guide therapeutic decision-making. The CSISS is obtained by the sum of analog scale points representing the degree of osseous and ligamentous injury of each of the four cervical spine columns (anterior, posterior, left and right pillar). A total of points ≥7 is suggestive for surgical management. The SLIC takes into account the injury morphology, the extent of disco-ligamentous complex involvement and the neurological status of the patient. If the score is ≥5, then operative treatment is recommended.

Burst Fractures
Burst fractures of the cervical spine result from vertical compression loads applied to the head, with the cervical spine in the neutral position. This leads to comminution and loss of height of the vertebral body. Retropulsion of bone fragments into the spinal canal may provoke spinal cord injury, with varying degrees of neurologic deficit, usually presenting as an anterior cord syndrome. Plain X-rays and CT scanning are the initial diagnostic modalities, with MRI being of vital importance in case of neurologic deficit (Fig. 14).

Cervical burst fractures are treated operatively, with anterior decompression and fusion being the procedure of choice. However, in certain circumstances, a burst fracture can be accompanied by significant posterior element injury, and circumferential fusion may be indicated (Table 2).

Flexion "Teardrop" Fractures
Flexion teardrop fractures are the result of flexion and compression forces to the cervical spine and are characterized by marked instability. They most often involve C4, C5 and C6 vertebrae. Typically, the vertebral body presents with a coronal fracture line, leading to a smaller, anterior fragment and a larger posterior fragment. The typical "teardrop" appearance of the fracture in the lateral radiograph is attributed to the anterior fragment. Frequently, the posterior fragment splits sagittally and protrudes into the spinal canal, compromising the spinal cord [46]. In addition to the vertebral body fracture, the posterior elements are disrupted, resulting in spinous process diastasis or even facet dislocation. Plain radiographs show the typical signs of a flexion teardrop fracture, including the triangular anterior fragment, the posterior translation of the cervical spine cephalad to the fracture and facet joint and interspinous space widening. Axial CT images can accurately depict the characteristic pattern of vertebral body fracture, as well as spinal canal narrowing. MRI can demonstrate the extent of spinal cord and ligamentous injury (Fig. 15).

The treatment of these significantly unstable injuries is mainly operative, especially in cases of complete or incomplete neurologic deficit (Table 2). Nevertheless, non-operative treatment with Halo vest immobilization has also been proposed [47], but its results are less predictable. Surgical treatment includes anterior decompression and fusion, posterior fusion or combined techniques.

Facet Fractures and Dislocations
Facet injuries range from unilateral undisplaced fractures to complete bilateral dislocations. Unilateral facet injuries account for approximately 6 % of all cervical spine injuries [48]. Facet fractures usually involve the superior facet, but the inferior facet may be affected as well. Although unilateral facet fractures are generally considered as stable injuries, they may be accompanied by ligamentous injury of the contralateral facet joint capsule, as well as injury of the posterior portion of the annulus fibrosus. This is a result of the mechanism of injury, which involves lateral bending or extension and rotation of the cervical spine. Bilateral facet fractures represent a more unstable

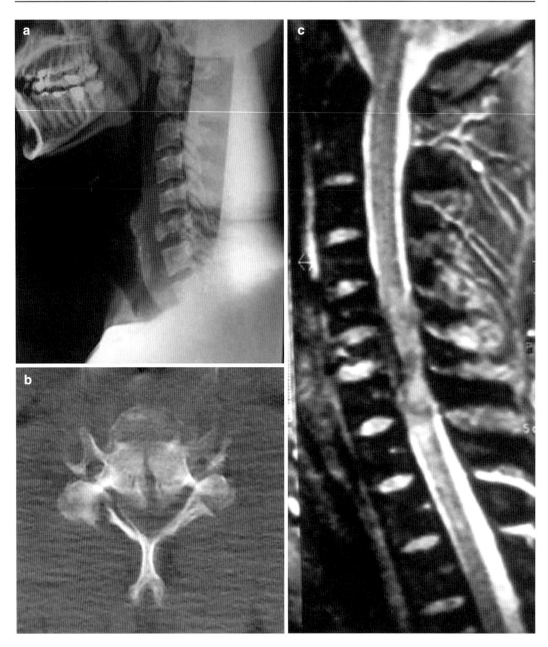

Fig. 14 (**a**) Lateral radiograph of a 27 year-old male with a burst fracture of the C6 vertebra and complete quadriplegia, after a motor vehicle accident. (**b**) CT scanning demonstrates in detail the vertebral body comminution and spinal canal compromise. (**c**) T2-weighted sagittal image showing extended spinal cord injury at the levels from C5 to C7

entity and are associated with a higher incidence of intervertebral disc injury. Fracture separations of the lateral mass (floating lateral mass) result from a concurrent fracture of the pedicle and the ipsilateral lamina, usually due to extension and rotation. Plain radiographs may not be conclusive. On the other hand, CT-scan can demonstrate the fracture pattern in detail. Undisplaced unilateral facet fractures are usually treated conservatively, with the use of a semi-rigid or rigid collar.

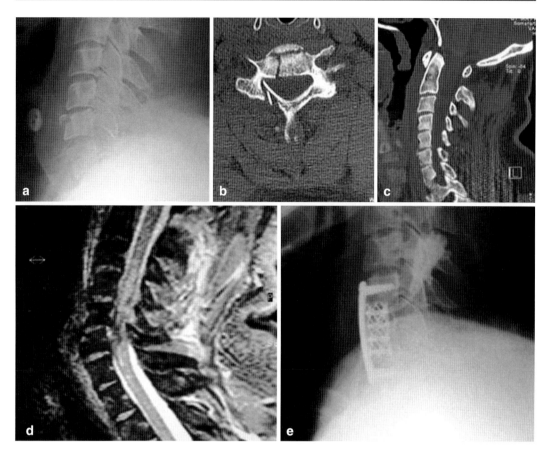

Fig. 15 A 36 year-old male, victim of a motor vehicle accident, was admitted with complete quadriplegia. (a) Lateral radiograph showing fracture of the C6 vertebra. (b) Axial and (c) sagittal CT images, demonstrating the typical appearance of a flexion teardrop fracture, with a fracture line in the coronal plane and another fracture line in the sagittal plane. (d) The MRI shows extended injury and oedema to the spinal cord. (e) The patient underwent anterior C6 corpectomy and C5–C7 fusion

However, when significant rotational instability is present, operative management with anterior or posterior fusion is indicated. Bilateral facet fractures may also be treated with conservative measures, except for those exhibiting translation greater than 3.5 mm. Fracture separations of the lateral mass create instability over two vertebral levels and thus are best treated surgically, with anterior or posterior fusion (Table 2).

Unilateral facet subluxations and dislocations result from concurrent flexion-distraction and rotation of the cervical spine. The axis of rotation is centred over a facet joint, thus provoking injury of the capsule and ligaments of the contra-lateral facet joint and subluxation or dislocation. The anterior and posterior longitudinal ligaments remain intact. On the other hand, bilateral facet dislocations are caused from flexion and distraction injuries, without a rotational component, and are characterized by initial disruption of the posterior ligamentous structures, followed by injury of the middle and anterior ligaments in more severe cases. The anterior translation of the cephalad vertebra may reach or even exceed 50 % of the superior end-plate of the caudal vertebra. The neurological status of patients with facet subluxations or dislocations ranges from normal to complete quadriplegia. Radicular symptoms are usually related with unilateral dislocations.

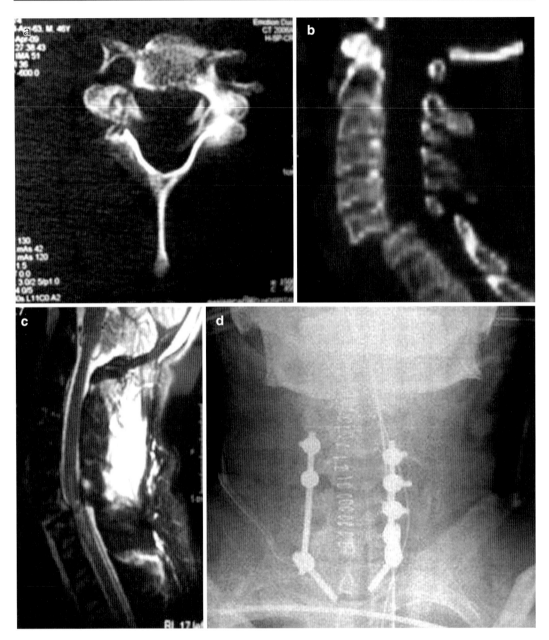

Fig. 16 A 46 year-old male was involved in a car accident and presented with a complete quadriplegia. (**a**) Axial and (**b**) sagittal CT images, demonstrating a C6–C7 bilateral facet dislocation. (**c**) The MRI revealed injury of the spinal cord, consistent with the patient's clinical presentation. (**d**) The patient underwent open reduction and posterior C4-T1 fusion

Radiographic evaluation consists of lateral, anteroposterior and oblique views, where perching or locking of the facets may be identified, with concomitant anterior translation of the overlying vertebra and kyphosis. Imaging also includes CT scanning, with a high sensitivity in detecting facet subluxations or dislocations, and MRI, particularly in cases with neurological deficit (Figs. 16 and 17). Reduction and surgical stabilization are the treatment principles of

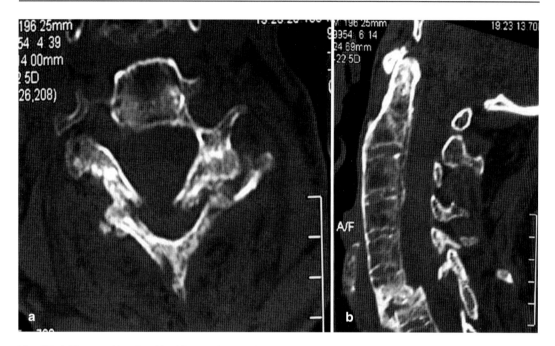

Fig. 17 A 71 year-old male with a history of ankylosing spondylitis sustained a C6–C7 fracture-dislocation without neurologic deficit, after falling from height. He was treated with a Halo- vest for 12 weeks. (**a**) Axial and (**b**) sagittal CT images of the patient's C-spine at 12 weeks, demonstrating C6-C7 spontaneous fusion

bilateral facet dislocations (Table 2). Stable unilateral injuries without neurologic deficit may be treated with external immobilization [49]. However, conservative treatment has been associated with poor outcomes [50, 51]. The closed reduction technique with skeletal traction has been described previously in this chapter. The necessity of obtaining a pre-reduction MRI to demonstrate a herniated disc at the level of dislocation remains a topic of controversy [52]. Generally, in the conscious, co-operative patient, closed reduction may be performed safely without previous MRI imaging [52–54], provided that an accurate and detailed neurologic evaluation is done after each increase of the weight applied. Open reduction is indicated in concussed patients, as well as in patients with failed attempts of closed reduction [52]. Surgical stabilization is done through a posterior approach, with instrumented fusion and/or decompression. However, anterior fusion has also been reported in cases of unilateral dislocations without neurologic deficit [55].

Paediatric Cervical Spine Injuries: SCIWORA

The paediatric cervical spine exhibits distinct anatomic features. The presence of synchondroses and ossification centres may confuse the radiographic evaluation of a child with cervical spine injury. Moreover, the increased elasticity of the spinal ligaments and overall cervical spine mobility lead to unique injury patterns [56]. Spinal Cord Injury Without Obvious Radiologic Abnormalities (SCIWORA) represents up to 38 % of cervical spine injuries in children [56]. Clinically, a paediatric patient with SCIWORA presents with neurologic deficit of variable severity, but plain radiography fails to demonstrate any pathology. The extent of spinal cord injury and soft-tissue trauma can be evaluated with the use of MRI. Treatment of SCIWORA consists of supportive measures and external immobilization, with prognosis depending on initial neurologic presentation [57].

References

1. Richards PJ. Cervical spine clearance: a review. Injury. 2005;36(2):248–69; discussion 270.
2. Milby AH, Halpern CH, Guo W, Stein SC. Prevalence of cervical spinal injury in trauma. Neurosurg Focus. 2008;25(5):E10.
3. Watanabe M, Sakai D, Yamamoto Y, Sato M, Mochida J. Upper cervical spine injuries: age-specific clinical features. J Orthop Sci. 2010;15(4):485–92.
4. Leucht P, Fischer K, Muhr G, Mueller EJ. Epidemiology of traumatic spine fractures. Injury. 2009;40(2):166–72.
5. Martin ND, Marks JA, Donohue J, Giordano C, Cohen MJ, Weinstein MS. The mortality inflection point for age and acute cervical spinal cord injury. J Trauma. 2011;71(2):380–5; discussion 385–6.
6. National Spinal Cord Injury Statistical Center. Annual report for the spinal cord injury model systems. 2010. https://www.nscisc.uab.edu/public_content/annual_stat_report.aspx
7. Hoffman JR, Mower WR, Wolfson AB, Todd KH, Zucker MI. Validity of a set of clinical criteria to rule out injury to the cervical spine in patients with blunt trauma. National Emergency X-Radiography Utilization Study Group. N Engl J Med. 2000;343(2):94–9.
8. Gupta R, Bathen ME, Smith JS, Levi AD, Bhatia NN, Steward O. Advances in the management of spinal cord injury. J Am Acad Orthop Surg. 2010; 18(4):210–22.
9. Terregino CA, Ross SE, Lipinski MF, Foreman J, Hughes R. Selective indications for thoracic and lumbar radiography in blunt trauma. Ann Emerg Med. 1995;26(2):126–9.
10. Bracken MB. Steroids for acute spinal cord injury. Cochrane Database Syst Rev. 2002;(3):CD001046.
11. Ito Y, Sugimoto Y, Tomioka M, Kai N, Tanaka M. Does high dose methylprednisolone sodium succinate really improve neurological status in patient with acute cervical cord injury?: a prospective study about neurological recovery and early complications. Spine (Phila Pa 1976). 2009;34(20):2121–4.
12. Chinnock P, Roberts I. Gangliosides for acute spinal cord injury. Cochrane Database Syst Rev. 2005;(2): CD004444.
13. Davis JW, Parks SN, Detlefs CL, Williams GG, Williams JL, Smith RW. Clearing the cervical spine in obtunded patients: the use of dynamic fluoroscopy. J Trauma. 1995;39(3):435–8.
14. Daffner RH. Cervical radiography for trauma patients: a time-effective technique? AJR Am J Roentgenol. 2000;175(5):1309–11.
15. Tins BJ, Cassar-Pullicino VN. Imaging of acute cervical spine injuries: review and outlook. Clin Radiol. 2004;59(10):865–80.
16. Holmes JF, Akkinepalli R. Computed tomography versus plain radiography to screen for cervical spine injury: a meta-analysis. J Trauma. 2005; 58(5):902–5.
17. Hanson JA, Blackmore CC, Mann FA, Wilson AJ. Cervical spine injury: a clinical decision rule to identify high-risk patients for helical CT screening. AJR Am J Roentgenol. 2000;174(3):713–17.
18. Goergen SK, Fong C, Dalziel K, Fennessy G. Can an evidence-based guideline reduce unnecessary imaging of road trauma patients with cervical spine injury in the emergency department? Australas Radiol. 2006;50(6):563–9.
19. Kothari P, Freeman B, Grevitt M, Kerslake R. Injury to the spinal cord without radiological abnormality (SCIWORA) in adults. J Bone Joint Surg Br. 2000;82(7):1034–7.
20. Machino M, Yukawa Y, Ito K, et al. Can magnetic resonance imaging reflect the prognosis in patients of cervical spinal cord injury without radiographic abnormality? Spine (Phila Pa 1976). 2011;36(24): E1568–72.
21. Botte MJ, Byrne TP, Abrams RA, Garfin SR. Halo skeletal fixation: techniques of application and prevention of complications. J Am Acad Orthop Surg. 1996;4(1):44–53.
22. Karam YR, Traynelis VC. Occipital condyle fractures. Neurosurgery. 2010;66 Suppl 3:56–9.
23. Sharma BS, Mahajan RK, Bhatia S, Khosla VK. Collet-Sicard syndrome after closed head injury. Clin Neurol Neurosurg. 1994;96(2):197–8.
24. Alker Jr GJ, Oh YS, Leslie EV. High cervical spine and craniocervical junction injuries in fatal traffic accidents: a radiological study. Orthop Clin North Am. 1978;9(4):1003–10.
25. Adams VI. Neck injuries: III. Ligamentous injuries of the craniocervical articulation without occipito-atlantal or atlanto-axial facet dislocation. A pathologic study of 21 traffic fatalities. J Forensic Sci. 1993;38(5):1097–104.
26. Horn EM, Feiz-Erfan I, Lekovic GP, Dickman CA, Sonntag VK, Theodore N. Survivors of occipitoatlantal dislocation injuries: imaging and clinical correlates. J Neurosurg Spine. 2007;6(2):113–20.
27. Bellabarba C, Mirza SK, West GA, et al. Diagnosis and treatment of craniocervical dislocation in a series of 17 consecutive survivors during an 8-year period. J Neurosurg Spine. 2006;4(6):429–40.
28. Kakarla UK, Chang SW, Theodore N, Sonntag VK. Atlas fractures. Neurosurgery. 2010;66 Suppl 3:60–7.
29. Spence Jr KF, Decker S, Sell KW. Bursting atlantal fracture associated with rupture of the transverse ligament. J Bone Joint Surg Am. 1970;52(3): 543–9.
30. Dickman CA, Greene KA, Sonntag VK. Injuries involving the transverse atlantal ligament: classification and treatment guidelines based upon experience with 39 injuries. Neurosurgery. 1996;38(1):44–50.

31. Wang GJ, Mabie KN, Whitehill R, Stamp WG. The nonsurgical management of odontoid fractures in adults. Spine (Phila Pa 1976). 1984;9(3):229–30.

32. Greene KA, Dickman CA, Marciano FF, Drabier JB, Hadley MN, Sonntag VK. Acute axis fractures. Analysis of management and outcome in 340 consecutive cases. Spine (Phila Pa 1976). 1997;22(16):1843–52.

33. Julien TD, Frankel B, Traynelis VC, Ryken TC. Evidence-based analysis of odontoid fracture management. Neurosurg Focus. 2000;8(6):e1.

34. Polin RS, Szabo T, Bogaev CA, Replogle RE, Jane JA. Nonoperative management of Types II and III odontoid fractures: the Philadelphia collar versus the halo vest. Neurosurgery. 1996;38(3):450–6; discussion 456–7.

35. Hadley MN, Browner C, Sonntag VK. Axis fractures: a comprehensive review of management and treatment in 107 cases. Neurosurgery. 1985;17(2):281–90.

36. Lennarson PJ, Mostafavi H, Traynelis VC, Walters BC. Management of type II dens fractures: a case–control study. Spine (Phila Pa 1976). 2000;25(10):1234–7.

37. Apfelbaum RI, Lonser RR, Veres R, Casey A. Direct anterior screw fixation for recent and remote odontoid fractures. J Neurosurg. 2000;93 Suppl 2:227–36.

38. Wright NM. Posterior C2 fixation using bilateral, crossing C2 laminar screws: case series and technical note. J Spinal Disord Tech. 2004;17(2):158–62.

39. Harms J, Melcher RP. Posterior C1-C2 fusion with polyaxial screw and rod fixation. Spine (Phila Pa 1976). 2001;26(22):2467–71.

40. Burke JT, Harris Jr JH. Acute injuries of the axis vertebra. Skeletal Radiol. 1989;18(5):335–46.

41. Levine AM, Edwards CC. The management of traumatic spondylolisthesis of the axis. J Bone Joint Surg Am. 1985;67(2):217–26.

42. Effendi B, Roy D, Cornish B, Dussault RG, Laurin CA. Fractures of the ring of the axis. A classification based on the analysis of 131 cases. J Bone Joint Surg Br. 1981;63-B(3):319–27.

43. Allen Jr BL, Ferguson RL, Lehmann TR, O'Brien RP. A mechanistic classification of closed, indirect fractures and dislocations of the lower cervical spine. Spine (Phila Pa 1976). 1982;7(1):1–27.

44. Anderson PA, Moore TA, Davis KW, et al. Cervical spine injury severity score. Assessment of reliability. J Bone Joint Surg Am. 2007;89(5):1057–65.

45. Patel AA, Hurlbert RJ, Bono CM, Bessey JT, Yang N, Vaccaro AR. Classification and surgical decision making in acute subaxial cervical spine trauma. Spine (Phila Pa 1976). 2010;35 Suppl 21:S228–34.

46. Kim KS, Chen HH, Russell EJ, Rogers LF. Flexion teardrop fracture of the cervical spine: radiographic characteristics. AJR Am J Roentgenol. 1989;152(2):319–26.

47. Rockswold GL, Bergman TA, Ford SE. Halo immobilization and surgical fusion: relative indications and effectiveness in the treatment of 140 cervical spine injuries. J Trauma. 1990;30(7):893–8.

48. Dvorak MF, Fisher CG, Aarabi B, et al. Clinical outcomes of 90 isolated unilateral facet fractures, subluxations, and dislocations treated surgically and nonoperatively. Spine (Phila Pa 1976). 2007;32(26):3007–13.

49. Spector LR, Kim DH, Affonso J, Albert TJ, Hilibrand AS, Vaccaro AR. Use of computed tomography to predict failure of nonoperative treatment of unilateral facet fractures of the cervical spine. Spine (Phila Pa 1976). 2006;31(24):2827–35.

50. Lee SH, Sung JK. Unilateral lateral mass-facet fractures with rotational instability: new classification and a review of 39 cases treated conservatively and with single segment anterior fusion. J Trauma. 2009;66(3):758–67.

51. Rorabeck CH, Rock MG, Hawkins RJ, Bourne RB. Unilateral facet dislocation of the cervical spine. An analysis of the results of treatment in 26 patients. Spine (Phila Pa 1976). 1987;12(1):23–7.

52. Lee JY, Nassr A, Eck JC, Vaccaro AR. Controversies in the treatment of cervical spine dislocations. Spine J. 2009;9(5):418–23.

53. Vaccaro AR, Falatyn SP, Flanders AE, Balderston RA, Northrup BE, Cotler JM. Magnetic resonance evaluation of the intervertebral disc, spinal ligaments, and spinal cord before and after closed traction reduction of cervical spine dislocations. Spine (Phila Pa 1976). 1999;24(12):1210–17.

54. Cotler JM, Herbison GJ, Nasuti JF, Ditunno Jr JF, An H, Wolff BE. Closed reduction of traumatic cervical spine dislocation using traction weights up to 140 pounds. Spine (Phila Pa 1976). 1993;18(3):386–90.

55. Nassr A, Lee JY, Dvorak MF, et al. Variations in surgical treatment of cervical facet dislocations. Spine (Phila Pa 1976). 2008;33(7):E188–93.

56. Jones TM, Anderson PA, Noonan KJ. Pediatric cervical spine trauma. J Am Acad Orthop Surg. 2011;19(10):600–11.

57. Pang D, Wilberger Jr JE. Spinal cord injury without radiographic abnormalities in children. J Neurosurg. 1982;57(1):114–29.

Treatment of Thoraco-Lumbar Spinal Injuries

Antonio A. Faundez

Contents

A.A. Faundez
Department of Surgery, Service de Chirurgie
Orthopédique et Traumatologie de l'Appareil Moteur,
University of Geneva Hospitals and Faculty of Medicine,
Geneva, Switzerland
e-mail: antonio.faundez@hcuge.ch

G. Bentley (ed.), *European Surgical Orthopaedics and Traumatology*,
DOI 10.1007/978-3-642-34746-7_9, © EFORT 2014

Abstract

Non-osteoporotic thoraco-lumbar fractures result from high energy trauma and affect mainly young people. Whereas the treatment management of fractures with neurologic deficit does not usually pose decisional issues, much more controversy surrounds fractures without neurologic deficit. It should be recalled that non-surgical treatment can still be applied to most of the thoraco-lumbar fractures diagnosed. On the other hand, marked improvements have been made in the development of less invasive surgical techniques in an effort to provide the best possible care to a usually young active population that requires to resume normal activity as soon as possible. There also is a trend in the literature to define more accurately the optimal treatment of fractures without neurologic deficit in light of sagittal spino-pelvic balance parameters, as well as from an economic point of view. An overview of current treatment options available is presented in this article.

Keywords

Classification types • Epidemiology • Fractures • Imaging • Minimally -invasive techniques • Recent advances • Surgical treatment • Thoraco-Lumbar Spinal injuries • Spine • Epidemiology • Initial management • Imaging • Classification • Non-operative treatment • Surgical treatment • Recent techniques

Introduction

Thoraco-lumbar fractures (Th10-L2) in young adults are common and often associated with profound socio-economic consequences [1]. Most of these result from motor vehicle accidents and falls from heights, which involve high kinetic energy and affect mainly males. Very often, patients are polytraumatized and present with associated thoracic and/or abdominal injuries. Initial in-hospital management is carried out following the Advanced Trauma Life Support (ATLS) guidelines, where priority is given to stabilization of vital functions and

only then to neurologic functions. The traumatized spine is assessed using standard radiologic imaging, as well as CT scan. MRI can provide valuable information about neural tissue and disco-ligamentous injuries. Specific treatment decisions will then rely on both intrinsic (e.g., fracture morphology, neurologic status, mechanical instability) and extrinsic factors (e.g., age, occupation, level of physical activity). The main goal of surgical treatment is to protect the neural tissue by mechanically stabilizing the spine and additionally decompressing the spinal canal if necessary. We present here an overview of current treatment options available to surgeons for the treatment of thoraco-lumbar fractures.

Epidemiology of Spinal Injuries

Thoraco-lumbar fractures affect mostly males between 20 and 30 years old and are due to high energy trauma, mostly motor vehicle accidents (40–50 %) and falls (around 20 %) [2]. It is difficult to present exact numbers for the incidence of spine fractures because of inconsistent data collection amongst Trauma centres. In a recent epidemiological review, it was estimated that the incidence of adult thoraco-lumbar fractures in the United Kingdom is around $117/10^5$ inhabitants/year [3]. The incidence of spinal cord injuries is better documented and is reported to range between 27 and 47 per million population in North America, with an acute mortality rate that has dramatically decreased from 38 % to 15.8 % over the past 30 years [1]. Major improvements have been made in pre- and in-hospital spinal cord injury management, as well as in surgical implants and techniques, thus allowing provision of better trauma care today.

Initial Management of Polytrauma Patients with an Associated Spine Injury

Patients with spine injuries are often polytraumatized. Strict adherence to ATLS guidelines is required before and upon arrival to the trauma centre [4]. Taking pictures of the scene of the accident can be very useful to determine the mechanism of trauma and is a current practice now in several paramedic teams. The patient should be adequately ventilated and oxygenated and the cervical spine immediately immobilized in a rigid collar. In the emergency room, after vital functions have been stabilized, a detailed physical examination and a thorough neurologic clinical assessment is performed in the conscious patient. As polytrauma patients frequently present with altered consciousness, they are usually immediately screened with a total body CT scan that also allows detection of occult fractures of the spine, which are frequently overlooked in this category of patient [5]. If a spinal cord injury is diagnosed, neurologic impairment is evaluated according to the American Spinal Injury Association (ASIA) classification (Fig. 1). Mean blood pressure should be maintained above 90 mmHg to protect the cord from secondary ischaemic injury [2]. Until relatively recently, the administration of steroids was also considered as a standard of care [6]. However, various methodological flaws of the clinical trials conducted by the National Acute Spinal Cord Injury (NASCIS) Study Group have seriously questioned the validity of their conclusions, and because of possible serious adverse effects, steroids should no longer be administered without further clinical research [7, 8]. A more detailed description of the medical management of spinal cord injury is provided in the article by Bernhard and colleagues published in 2005 [2]. Once urgent care has been delivered, treatment strategy decisions for the spinal injury need to be developed, also including possible fractures of the appendicular skeleton.

Thoraco-Lumbar Trauma Imaging

Polytraumatized patients are often immediately taken to the radiology departement for a total body CT scan once vital functions have been stabilized. However, standard radiologic imaging must still be part of the initial assessment as it provides an aerial view of the osseous lesions of the spine that cannot be completely replaced yet by the CT scan. Several basic pathomorphologic signs can already be identified on plain radiographs, such as the amount of height loss of the vertebral body, the interpedicular distance on antero-posterior views, interspinous distance and interruption of the posterior wall on lateral views, and the amount of kyphotic deformity. CT scan is useful to precisely analyze the bony contour of the spinal canal, but also the amount of vertebral body destruction, comminution and spread of fragments.

MRI is another important tool for the analysis of spinal cord and ligamentous injuries that cannot readily be detected on plain radiographs or CT scan, and often shows the real extent of vertebral injury by detecting changes of bone marrow signal intensity. It has been evaluated for the characterization of spine injuries since 1989 [9] and proposed for inclusion in future spine trauma classification schemes as early as 1995 [10]. Only more recent studies have investigated its clinical validity in the management of thoraco-lumbar fractures [11–13]. However, in an article by Dai and colleagues published in 2009, the practical role of MRI in clinical decision-making was questioned, in particular for burst fractures [11]. The authors argued that although it may be a reliable instrument for the assessment of ligamentous injuries, it did not correlate with neurologic status or fracture severity, and as such should not be used routinely. Further studies are awaited to better define indications for MRI investigation of non-osteoporotic spinal fractures.

Classification Systems

A variety of thoraco-lumbar fracture classifications have been described in the literature, but none has reached a consensus amongst Spine and Trauma surgeons. The most frequently cited classifications systems are the Denis classification (three-column theory), the load-sharing classification, and the AO classification (named after the founding Swiss group "Arbeitsgemeinschaft für Osteosynthesefragen").

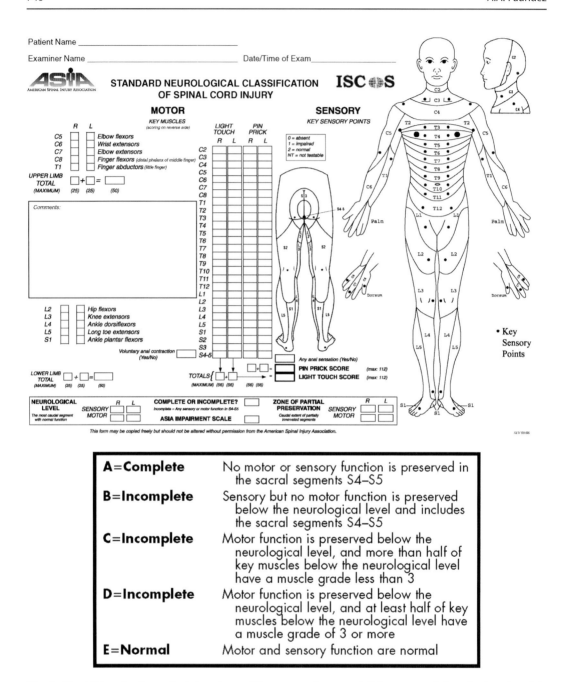

Fig. 1 *The ASIA scale of neurologic impairment.* The motor and sensory deficits are recorded on the data sheet *left.* The scale of impairment (*A, B, C, D, E*) is detailed on the *right*

Evolution of Classification Systems

Lorenz Boehler (1885–1973) was one of the first Trauma surgeons in Europe, and head of the first hospital for labourers, based in Vienna. His seminal work on the treatment of fractures was first published in 1929 [14]. Despite difficulties to achieve publication, the book encountered an important success and was soon translated into English and later into other languages.

Boehler's book is richly illustrated with drawings and pictures of various thoracic and lumbar fracture types and their long-term deformity if not treated appropriately. He described five categories of thoracolumbar injuries which served later as a basis for the Watson-Jones' classification in 1938 [15]. Holdsworth was the first to use the term "burst fracture" [16]. He also introduced the concept of "column", dividing the spine into an anterior (vertebral body and disc) and a posterior column (posterior facet joints and posterior ligamentous complex [PLC]) Some of the aspects of Holdsworth's classification were later redefined by Kelly and Whitesides [17] and served as the basis of the more recent AO classification published in 1994 by Magerl and colleagues [18].

Denis Classification (1983)

A major stage was reached in the management of spine trauma with the advent of CT scan imaging in the eighties. Using this new radiologic tool, Denis reviewed 412 patients with thoraco-lumbar fractures and published in 1983 one of the most frequently-cited thoraco-lumbar fracture classification systems today [19]. The results of this study and the concept of "middle column" originated from the observation that during scoliosis surgery, where he would release both anterior and posterior columns, he did not observe any major mechanical instability as defined in Holdsworth's classification. Denis concluded that the middle column had to be disrupted to result in a clinically significant instability. Four major types were defined: compression fracture, burst fracture, seat belt fracture and fracture-dislocation (flexion injury). It is often claimed that Denis' classification is incomplete, and does not describe other pathomorphologic fracture types, e.g., the "lumberjack" fracture type, which was however described by himself later in 1992 [20, 21].

The Load-Sharing Classification (1994)

In 1994, McCormack and Gaines described their load-sharing classification in an attempt to help

the surgeon to predict the risk of implant failure in short-posterior segment constructs, such as the ones obtained using the AO internal fixation device [22] (Fig. 2). They proposed a decisional algorithm to decide whether an additional reconstruction of the anterior column was necessary in burst fractures based on three criteria: comminution of the vertebral body; apposition of fragments of the vertebral body; and reducibility of sagittal deformation. Although a few studies have reported its validity in clinical decision-making [24–26], the disadvantage of this algorithm is that it does not take into account the neurologic status of the patient, which is a major drawback in clinical care.

The AO Classification (1994)

In 1994, Magerl and colleagues proposed the AO classification of thoraco-lumbar fractures following a review of 1445 cases [18]. Fractures are classified according to three pathomorphologic types: type A (flexion-compression fractures); type B (distraction); and type C (rotational-shearing) (Fig. 3). In an attempt to design a system describing every possible fracture, the authors further divided each type into sub-groups, sub-types and sub-divisions, resulting in a total of 53 patterns.

The Thoraco-Lumbar Injury Classification and Severity System (TLICS, 2005)

At present, none of these classifications has been adopted as a universal reference, mainly because of their poor intra- and inter-observer reliability [28]. The latest classification system described in the literature is the Thoraco-lumbar Injury Classification and Severity System (TLICS) [29, 30] that results from another classification system initially called the Thoraco-lumbar Injury Severity Score (TLISS). TLICS is a spine trauma evaluation score that considers three parameters: (1) the fracture morphology, based on the main mechanisms described in the AO classification;

Comminution/Involvement (A1-3)

1 Little = <30% comminution on sagittal
          section CT
2 More = 30%-60% comminution
3 Gross ≥ 60% comminution

Apposition of fragments (B1-3)

1 Minimal displacement on axial CT scan
2 Spread = At least 2mm displacement of
         <50% cross section of body
3 Wide = At least 2mm displacement of
       >50% cross section of body

Deformity correction

1 Little = Kyphotic correction ≤3° on
         lateral plain films
2 More = Kyphotic correction 4°-9°
3 Most = Kyphotic correction ≥10°

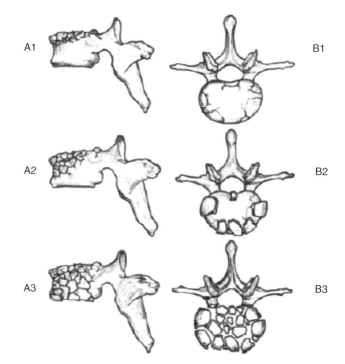

Fig. 2 *The load-sharing classification of Burst fractures* (Adapted from [22, 23]). The classification was proposed in an attempt to predict the risk of implant failure in short-posterior segment constructs. Three items are considered: (1) comminution; (2) apposition of fragments; (3) reducibility of the deformity. Each item is given a numerical value. Originally, the authors concluded that a score equal or greater than seven represented a high risk of failure of short segment fixations

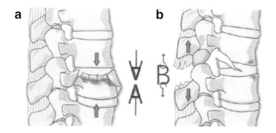
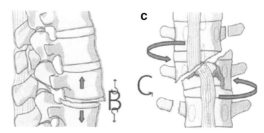

Fig. 3 *The AO classification of fractures* (with permission from Aebi et al. [27]). Three major traumatic mechanisms were described: *A.* flexion-compression fractures; *B.* distraction injuries, either in hyperflexion or hyperextension; *C.* rotational-shear fractures. There is a progressive scale of severity of the injury from type A to type C with a reported frequency of neurologic deficit of 14 % in type A, 32 % in type B and 55 % in type C

(2) the neurologic status; (3) the integrity of the PLC, inferred by clinical and radiologic examination, including MRI (Fig. 4). A numerical value is assigned for each injury subcategory, depending on the severity of injury. The sum of each numerical values is used to guide the treatment decision: a score of 5 or more suggests a surgical treatment; a score of 3 or less, a conservative treatment. For a score of 4, either surgical or conservative treatment can be recommended, also based on other confounding factors, such as the age of the patient, amount of kyphosis, quality of bone, etc. [29]. TLICS has shown improved intra- and

Fig. 4 *The Thoraco-Lumbar Injury Classification and Severity System* (TLICS adapted from [29]). The classification is based on three items: (1) Injury morphology; (2) Neurological status; (3) Integrity of PLC. A numerical value is attributed to each item and a total score is calculated: if ≤3, non-surgical treatment is advocated; if ≥5, surgical treatment is recommended; for a score of 4, either non-surgical or surgical treatment can be decided based on other confounding factors

Category	Points
injury morphology	
compression	1
burst	+1
translational/rotational	3
distraction	4
neurological status	
intact	0
nerve root	2
cord, conus medullaris	
incomplete	3
complete	2
cauda equina	3
PLC	
intact	0
injury suspected/indeterminate	2
injured	3

interrater reliability in recent studies, but only within the group of physicians who developed the system [30, 31], and further studies are needed to more widely validate this promising classification system.

Non-Surgical Treatment of Thoraco-Lumbar Fractures

AO Types A1 and A2

With the advent of less-invasive surgical techniques, there will probably be a future shift towards surgical treatment for lesions that would have been classically treated conservatively. Nevertheless, conservative treatment of thoraco-lumbar fractures still has a role to play at present. It can be divided into functional treatment or bracing with or without external reduction manoeuvres. In our institution, functional treatment (isometric muscular exercises) is applied for AO fractures of type A1 (impaction and wedge fractures, 5° vertebral kyphotic angulation). For most of type A2 (split fractures), we recommend bracing, usually a three-point thoraco-lumbar orthosis, for 6–12 weeks, depending on the radiologic follow-up. As already pointed out by Boehler at the beginning of the twentieth century, intensive and immediate physical therapy with the brace in place should be an integral part of the treatment plan [14]. In the particular case of the pincer-type fracture (A2.3), surgical treatment is recommended because of a high risk of non-union [18].

Burst Fractures (AO Type A3)

There is no consensus in the literature on the treatment of burst fractures [23, 32]. In our institution, mainly complete burst fractures (AO A3.3) are treated surgically. Incomplete burst fractures with acceptable sagittal deformity, up to 15° in the thoraco-lumbar junction, can be handled with a custom-made brace. However, despite an ongoing debate for years over the amount of tolerable kyphotic deformity of the thoraco-lumbar junction, it is interesting to note that only recent studies have started to focus on global sagittal balance and thoraco-lumbar fractures. Koller and colleagues published a retrospective study analyzing the long-term radiologic and clinical outcome for regional post-traumatic kyphosis of conservatively-treated thoraco-lumbar and lumbar burst fractures according to the global spino-pelvic alignment of each patient [33]. They concluded that the patient's global spine compensates for the post-traumatic regional kyphosis within the limits dictated by their pelvic geometry, in particular the pelvic incidence. They also found that clinical outcome correlated with regional kyphosis. Finally, the authors recommended that fractures with a load-sharing classification score of more than 6 should be treated by aggressive surgical reconstruction.

AO Fractures Type B and C

Except for type B2.1, also known as "Chance fracture" [34], which can be successfully treated by bracing, surgical treatment is recommended for most type B as well as type C injuries. Type B and C fractures result from very high energy trauma and usually include ligamentous disruptions that have a very poor healing potential. These fracture types are also associated wtih neuro-logic symptoms in 32 % and 55 % of patients, respectively [18]. As for the strategy of stabilization and reconstruction, the same principles of amount of kyphosis and vertebral body destruction apply (see chapter ▶ "Fractures with Arterial Injury"). It is important to recall, however, that not all neurologic symptoms imply surgical treatment. In a well-done Instructional Lecture course, Rechtine lists other similar myths around treatment indications for thoraco-lumbar fractures [35, 36].

Surgical Treatment

Surgical Treatment for Fractures with Neurological Deficit

As mentioned above, type B and C injuries usu-ally require surgical treatment and are character-ized by serious biomechanical instability and deformity, frequently accompanied by neural tis-sue damage. A treatment strategy is quite simple to define for patients with immediate and com-plete spinal cord damage. If any intervention is to be planned, it should be carried out only once vital functions have been stabilized, keeping in mind that the primary goal of surgery is to enhance nursing care and rehabilitation [37, 38]. For incomplete or progressive lesions, it is accepted that surgical decompression and stabili-zation should be performed within 6 to a maximum of 24 h from injury [39]. Posterior decompression and stabilization can be recommended as a first emergency procedure. However, it is not mandatory that any residual anterior compression be relieved as an emer-gency. Even if it is now suggested that the amount of canal narrowing is strongly associated with severity of the neurologic deficit [40, 41], it does not correlate with the prognosis of func-tional recovery. In other words, the removal of a large intra-canalar bone fragment will not nec-essarily improve the chances of neurologic recovery.

Surgical Treatment for AO Type A and B Fractures Without Neurologic Deficit

The treatment decision for thoraco-lumbar frac-tures of AO types A and B (predominantly osse-ous injury) without neurologic deficit remains very controversial and it must recalled that there is a very real risk to end up with irreversible iatrogenic nerve tissue damage. However, as described by Boehler and others [14, 23, 33], there is a rationale to treat these patients surgi-cally given the risk of mid- to late onset deformity

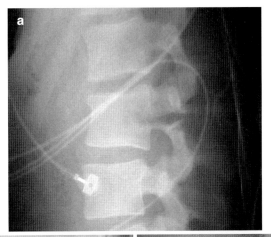

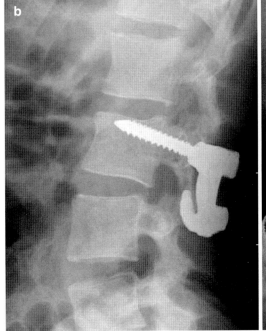

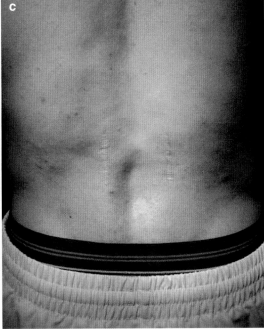

Fig. 5 Chance fracture of L2 (AO type B2.1) in a young male patient involved in a car accident, without neurologic deficit. Decision was taken with the patient to surgically treat the fracture using a minimally-invasive technique to avoid external reduction and bracing. At 2 year follow-up, the patient was symptom-free and the fracture radiologically healed. (**a**) Pre-operative Xray. (**b**) Post-operative Xray. (**c**) Skin incisions at 2 years follow-up

and its possible progressive cord compression and/or chronic disabling pain. Indications for surgical treatment of fractures without neurologic deficit should be based on the amount of deformity and weighed against its anatomical location, and on the amount of mechanical instability inferred by the analysis of radiologic documentation, including MRI (fracture classification). As an example, for burst fractures (AO type A3) of

the thoraco-lumbar junction, a maximum of 15° of regional kyphosis (measured between the upper end-plate of the vertebra above and the lower end-plate of the vertebra below) is usually tolerated for non-surgical treatment. However, it will also depend on the amount of destruction of the vertebral body. An incomplete burst fracture (AO 3.1) with 10–15° of regional kyphosis will be treated by external reduction

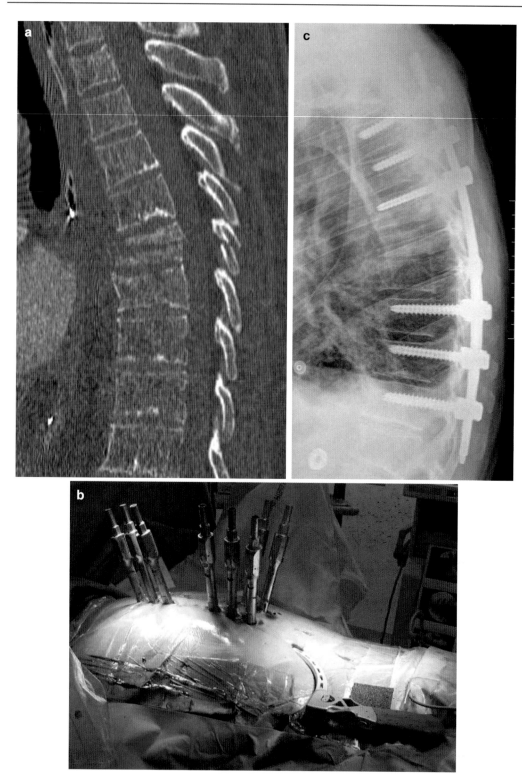

Fig. 6 (continued)

and bracing in our institution. But if the burst is complete (AO 3.3), reaching a high level of instability in compression, we will treat it surgically [23, 33].

A further decision, even more controversial, has to be made for complete burst fractures, i.e., whether a short posterior fusion will be enough or if an anterior approach and vertebral body reconstruction is needed, according to the load-sharing classification [22]. We continue to use the AO "fixateur interne" as a posterior stabilization implant. The technique is based on the principles of posterior short segment stabilization and ligamentotaxis: the indirect reduction of sagittal deformity and intra-canalar bone fragments of the posterior wall through posterior longitudinal ligament (PLL) retensioning [42, 43]. The success of the technique obviously relies on the integrity of the PLL. The "reverse cortical sign" is a radiologic sign corresponding to a 180° flip of the postero-superior wall fragment and a consequent rupture of the PLL [44]. If present, this sign normally precludes any efficiency of ligamentotaxis alone for reduction of the fragment and an additional anterior approach for direct decompression should then be considered. Of note, despite previous recommendations to remove intra-canalar bone fragments [45], the compromise of the spinal canal is not in itself an indication for surgical treatment in the absence of neurologic symptoms [35]. In a mimimum 5-year follow-up study, Wessberg and colleagues have confirmed that intra-canalar fragments stemming from the posterior wall are subject to remodelling

and that the cross-sectional area of the spinal canal recovers up to 87 % of its normal value without surgery [46]. If an anterior vertebral reconstruction is deemed necessary, it can be done by a classic open approach, for example the extra-pleural approach of the thoraco-lumbar junction, or by a video-assisted, less invasive approach [47]. More recently, vertebral body augmentation with calcium-phosphate cement has gained popularity and might be an alternative to more aggressive surgery in fractures without neurologic injury, but the risk of intra-canalar cement extravasation has to be assessed. In addition, improvements in cement resistance are required before it can be recommended as a routine procedure.

Some AO type B fractures can also be treated either surgically or non-surgically. Figure 5 presents a typical case of a young male patient who suffered a bi-column fracture (AO type B2.1 or Chance type). The accident occurred in an old car with only two- point seat belts and he suffered from splenic and hepatic contusions, in addition to a hyperflexion fracture. It is known that these types of fractures with a predominant osseous instability respond very well to external reduction and bracing [18]. For various reasons, bracing can be very impractical (hot weather, very active patient, overweight patient, etc.) and surgery can reasonably be proposed. However, it is of the utmost importance that the decision is taken together with the patient, and not by the surgeon alone. As for any other treatment, risks and benefits have to be discussed and weighed against each other.

Fig. 6 A two-level fracture (Chance type of Th7 with also some amount of height loss and compression fracture of Th8) in a 57-year-old male patient involved in a motorcycle accident. He also sustained multiple rib fractures and a haemo-pneumothorax precluding any bracing technique. To stabilize the fractures while easing nursing care, we performed a multiple-level percutaneous pedicle screw fixation. Blood loss was minimal and the patient recovered from surgery uneventfully. Initially, we had planned to also provide a cement augmentation to the vertebral bodies, but for technical reasons it could not be done simultaneously. Once discharged from the intensive care unit, the patient eventually declined to undergo the cementoplasty and at 3-month follow-up we did not observe further vertebral collapse on radiographs; the patient was also symptom-free. (**a**) Pre-operative CT scan re-formatting showing the hyperflexion type of injury with fracture of posterior elements. (**b**) Intra-operative picture of percutaneous pedicle screw and rod insertion. The fracture was stabilized in situ. No additional fusion was necessary as the lesion was predominantly osseous. (**c**) Post-operative lateral X-Ray at 3 months. The patient was symptom-free

Less-Invasive and Recent Surgical Techniques

Major improvements have been made during the past decade in spine surgical techniques and new instruments have been developed to insert implants through small incisions. For instance, surgeons have acquired an expertise in endoscopic treatment of vertebral fractures and extensive exposure of the thoraco-lumbar junction is no longer necessary to perform corpectomies and vertebral reconstructions with structural allografts or cages [47]. Pedicle screws can also be inserted percutaneously, with the consequence of lowering blood loss and operative time. An example of a fracture treated by percutaneous pedicle screws and rod placement is shown in Fig. 6. A technique that has recently gained popularity is cement augmentation of the vertebral body. It has been used for treatment of osteoporotic fractures for a long time, but only more recently for high energy spine fractures [48]. A few prospective non-randomized and non-controlled studies have been published and suggest that stand-alone vertebral body augmentation with calcium phosphate cements might become an alternative to bracing in non-osteoporotic AO type A1 up to A3.1 fractures [49, 50]. Bone resorption around the calcium phosphate cement has been reported in type A3.2 and A3.3 fractures and, for this reason, it probably should not be recommended in these types as a "stand-alone" technique. An additional posterior short segment construct could be added percutaneously to increase stability and avoid possible complications from cement resorption [51]. Other cement compositions are being currently tested, for instance, calcium phosphate cements with various Amounts of poly-methyl-methacrylate (PMMA) as well as ceramic cements. However, at present, there are not sufficiently clear data in the literature to recommend cement augmentation as a routine procedure for non-osteoporotic thoraco-lumbar fractures.

Recent Developments in Computer-Assisted Surgery

Development of less invasive surgical treatment techniques for thoraco-lumbar fractures is appraisable for polytraumatized patients, to decrease further tissue trauma and bleeding for instance. Less invasive techniques have also broadened the spectrum of treatment possibilities for fractures without neurological deficit, which were usually treated conservatively. But procedure safety becomes a major concern with narrowing of the surgical field and use of indirect techniques.

Thus additional intra-operative imagery becomes mandatory. It has to be accurate, reliable, but not expose the patient to increased radiation doses.

Improved computer-assisted surgery (CAS) tools have emerged in recent years meeting these goals. In our institution, acquisition of an O-ARM (Medtronic, Memphis, USA), which allows us to perform an intra-operative CT-scan and traditional scopic images, profoundly changed our surgical practice in spinal trauma. Surgical navigation with modern infra-red cameras, to insert pedicle screws has become much easier. Immediate verification of screw position and fracture fragments reduction also represents a major breakthrough.

In addition, these new navigation tools allow us to better plan and perform tumoural resections, whether primary, like osteoid osteomata, or metastases.

Navigation for Percutaneous Pedicle Screw Placement

Percutaneous pedicle screw stabilization of a thoracolumbar fracture follows the principle of internal splinting. This means, that fusion is usually not the goal, otherwise either a larger classic incision is to be done, or an additional mini- invasive technique has to be performed to fuse the posterior facet joints. pedicle screw insertion should be limited to fractures without posterior ligament complex (PLC) injury.

Because fusion is not possible, indications for percutaneous, MRI is thus mandatory to exclude complete rupture of especially the supraspinous ligament and if the images are equivocal, we would not recommend stabilization without fusion.

Typical indications for percutaneous pedicle screw stabilization would be thoraco-lumbar fractures AO type A3.2 and A3.3, in combination with cement vertebral body augmentation [51].

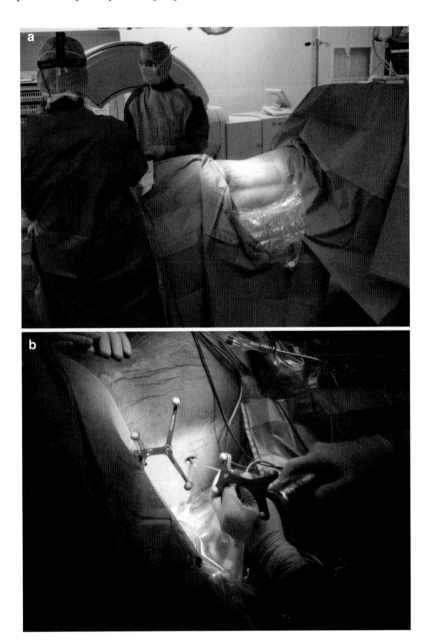

Fig. 7 (continued)

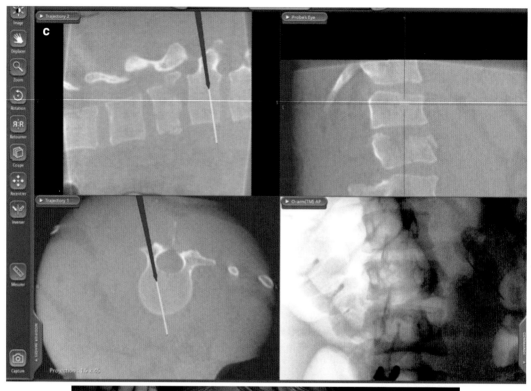

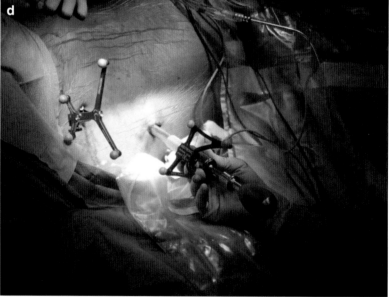

Fig. 7 (continued)

Navigation for Combined Approaches in Thoraco-Lumbar Fractures

Surgical navigation and intra-operative imaging are extremely helpful tools to optimize surgical technique safety. For some time now, we have been using surgical navigation to perform simultaneous posterior and anterior approaches for AO type A3.3 thoracolumbar fractures with indications for a corpectomy. With a dynamic reference base attached to a spinous process of the patient, as close as possible to the fracture, navigation can first be used to insert pedicle screws, percutaneously or by an open technique.

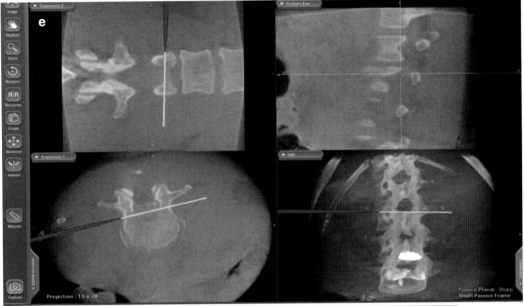

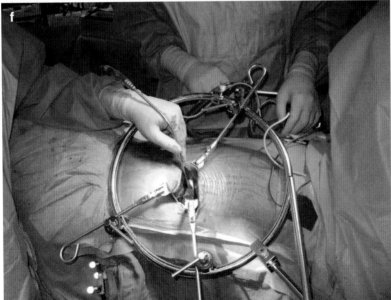

Fig. 7 (continued)

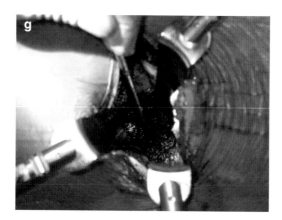

Fig. 7 (**a–d**): patient is placed in right lateral position. The reference frame is attached to the spinous process of L3, the fracture is at the level L2 (Burst fracture, patient had some left leg paresthesia). Pedicle screws are inserted percutaneously. (**e–g**): exposure of the anterior approach is planned with the help of navigation. Intra-operatively, navigation is also used to locate the intra-canicular fragments and ease removal

At the same time, after having planned the position,a second surgeon can start the anterior approach and length of the incision using the projection of a navigated pointer on the intra-operative CT scan images (Fig. 7).

The most efficient way to reduce a kyphotic deformity is by blocking the sliding of the pedicle screws on the rod and sagittaly diverging them, which is usually referred to as "ligamentotaxis". Different sets of tools to achieve this goal are available, according to the rod and screw system used by the surgeon. If an significant reduction has been obtained, it would be recommended to repeat the intra-operative CT scan before carrying on with the anterior approach and corpectomy, as the accuracy of navigation could be challenged.

Surgical Technique for Combined Anterior-Posterior Approach of Thoraco-Lumbar Fractures

We start with pedicle screw insertion. The patient is placed in a right lateral position on a Jackson table. We use pubic and sacral pads to stabilize the patient and an inflatable cushion under the right axilla. The dynamic reference frame is attached to the spinous process immediately distal to the fractured vertebra. For fractures below L4, the sacral pad and the lumbar lordosis could hide the the reference frame from the infrared camera, impeding accurate navigation. The frame can be placed on the posterior iliac crest, but this could decrease accuracy because of the distance from the fracture. Navigated instruments are calibrated, the CT scan is done and the OARM is pulled out during the surgery. Pedicle screws are inserted percutaneously, any kyphosis reduced by shaping the rod adequately or by ligamentotaxis when possible. The reference frame is left in place and the anterior surgical incision drawn by using the navigated pointer to aim at the fracture and thus planning the adequate surgical incision and exposure. In the example shown, the fracture was at the level L2 in a male patient with a very large psoas muscle. After placing retractors, navigation was very helpful to dissect the muscle while taking care of the lumbar nerve plexus. Navigation was again efficient in helping to perform the corpectomy in a narrow surgical field.

For fractures at the level L1 or T12, we approach the fracture through an extrapleural phrenectomy. There's thus no need for a chest tube.

The surgical technique for this combined approach shown here is for treating fractures from T5 to L3 (Fig. 7).

Conclusions

Spine injuries in polytrauma patients with cord injury do not usually pose decisional problems for their management strategy. Priority should be given to cardiopulmonary resuscitation with adequate oxygenation and mechanical protection of the cervical spine to avoid additional injury. The treatment decision, non-surgical versus surgical, is made after vital functions have been stabilized. There is still some controversy as to the optimal timing of surgery, but it is generally accepted that emergency surgical decompression and stabilization should be performed within 6–24 h after injury. Additional specific therapy, in particular the use of steroids, is not to be recommended given the current status of scientific evidence.

Non-surgical (conservative) treatment remains the treatment of choice for the majority of thoraco-lumbar fractures without neurological deficit and can be applied even in some cases of incomplete and complete neurological injuries. Surgical treatment of thoraco-lumbar fractures without neurologic deficit remains a controversial issue and care should be taken not to overtreat patients, an upcoming trend to be faced given the recent advent of less invasive and less time-consuming surgical procedures. Precise data are still lacking in the literature, but it has to be recalled that surgical treatment still induces today probably more pain and higher direct medical costs than non-surgical treatment [32, 52]. In non-osteoporotic spine fractures, cement augmentation techniques seems to be a promising alternative to bracing or as an additional technique to a posterior stabilization, but further research is needed.

References

1. Fisher CG, Noonan VK, et al. Changing face of spine trauma care in North America. Spine (Phila Pa 1976). 2006;31(11 Suppl):S2–8; discussion S36.
2. Bernhard M, Gries A, et al. Spinal cord injury (SCI) – prehospital management. Resuscitation. 2005;66(2):127–39.
3. Court-Brown CM, Caesar B. Epidemiology of adult fractures: a review. Injury. 2006;37(8):691–7.
4. Driscoll P, Wardrope J. ATLS: past, present, and future. Emerg Med J. 2005;22(1):2–3.
5. Anderson S, Biros MH, et al. Delayed diagnosis of thoracolumbar fractures in multiple-trauma patients. Acad Emerg Med. 1996;3(9):832–9.
6. Bracken MB, Shepard MJ, et al. Methylprednisolone or tirilazad mesylate administration after acute spinal cord injury: 1-year follow up. Results of the third National Acute Spinal Cord Injury randomized controlled trial. J Neurosurg. 1998;89(5):699–706.
7. Fehlings MG. Summary statement: the use of methylprednisolone in acute spinal cord injury. Spine. 2001;26(24 Suppl):S55.
8. Miller SM. Methylprednisolone in acute spinal cord injury: a tarnished standard. J Neurosurg Anesthesiol. 2008;20(2):140–2.
9. Emery SE, Pathria MN, et al. Magnetic resonance imaging of posttraumatic spinal ligament injury. J Spinal Disord. 1989;2(4):229–33.
10. Petersilge CA, Pathria MN, et al. Thoracolumbar burst fractures: evaluation with MR imaging. Radiology. 1995;194(1):49–54.
11. Dai LY, Ding WG, et al. Assessment of ligamentous injury in patients with thoracolumbar burst fractures using MRI. J Trauma. 2009;66(6):1610–5.
12. Lee HM, Kim HS, et al. Reliability of magnetic resonance imaging in detecting posterior ligament complex injury in thoracolumbar spinal fractures. Spine. 2000;25(16):2079–84.
13. Lee JY, Vaccaro AR, et al. Assessment of injury to the thoracolumbar posterior ligamentous complex in the setting of normal-appearing plain radiography. Spine J. 2007;7(4):422–7.
14. Böhler L. Die Technik der Knochenbruchbehandlung. Wien: Maudrich; 1929.
15. Watson-Jones R. The results of postural reduction of fractures of the spine. J Bone Joint Surg Am. 1938;20(3):567–86.
16. Holdsworth F. Fractures, dislocations, and fracture-dislocations of the spine. J Bone Joint Surg Am. 1970;52(8):1534–51.
17. Kelly RP, Whitesides Jr TE. Treatment of lumbodorsal fracture-dislocations. Ann Surg. 1968;167(5):705–17.
18. Magerl F, Aebi M, et al. A comprehensive classification of thoracic and lumbar injuries. Eur Spine J. 1994;3(4):184–201.
19. Denis F. The three column spine and its significance in the classification of acute thoracolumbar spinal injuries. Spine (Phila Pa 1976). 1983;8(8):817–31.
20. Burkus JK, Denis F. Hyperextension injuries of the thoracic spine in diffuse idiopathic skeletal hyperostosis. Report of four cases. J Bone Joint Surg Am. 1994;76(2):237–43.
21. Denis F, Burkus JK. Shear fracture-dislocations of the thoracic and lumbar spine associated with forceful hyperextension (lumberjack paraplegia). Spine (Phila Pa 1976). 1992;17(2):156–61.

22. McCormack T, Karaikovic E, et al. The load sharing classification of spine fractures. Spine. 1994;19(15): 1741–4.

23. Siebenga J, Leferink VJ, et al. Treatment of traumatic thoracolumbar spine fractures: a multicenter prospective randomized study of operative versus nonsurgical treatment. Spine (Phila Pa 1976). 2006;31(25):2881–90.

24. Dai LY, Jiang LS, et al. Conservative treatment of thoracolumbar burst fractures: a long-term follow-up results with special reference to the load sharing classification. Spine (Phila Pa 1976). 2008;33(23):2536–44.

25. Liu S, Li H, et al. Monosegmental transpedicular fixation for selected patients with thoracolumbar burst fractures. J Spinal Disord Tech. 2009;22(1):38–44.

26. Parker JW, Lane JR, et al. Successful short-segment instrumentation and fusion for thoracolumbar spine fractures: a consecutive 41/2-year series. Spine (Phila Pa 1976). 2000;25(9):1157–70.

27. Aebi M, Arlet V et al. (2007). AOSpine Manual, Thieme.

28. Wood KB, Khanna G, et al. Assessment of two thoracolumbar fracture classification systems as used by multiple surgeons. J Bone Joint Surg Am. 2005; 87(7):1423–9.

29. Patel AA, Dailey A, et al. Thoracolumbar spine trauma classification: the thoracolumbar injury classification and severity score system and case examples. J Neurosurg Spine. 2009;10(3):201–6.

30. Vaccaro AR, Lehman Jr RA, et al. A new classification of thoracolumbar injuries: the importance of injury morphology, the integrity of the posterior ligamentous complex, and neurologic status. Spine. 2005;30(20): 2325–33.

31. Patel AA, Vaccaro AR, et al. The adoption of a new classification system: time-dependent variation in interobserver reliability of the thoracolumbar injury severity score classification system. Spine (Phila Pa 1976). 2007;32(3):E105–10.

32. Wood K, Buttermann G, et al. Operative compared with nonoperative treatment of a thoracolumbar burst fracture without neurological deficit. A prospective, randomized study. J Bone Joint Surg Am. 2003;85-A (5):773–81.

33. Koller H, Acosta F, et al. Long-term investigation of nonsurgical treatment for thoracolumbar and lumbar burst fractures: an outcome analysis in sight of spinopelvic balance. Eur Spine J. 2008;17(8):1073–95.

34. Chance GQ. Note on a type of flexion fracture of the spine. Br J Radiol. 1948;21(249):452.

35. Rechtine GR. Nonsurgical treatment of thoracic and lumbar fractures. Instr Course Lect. 1999;48:413–6.

36. Rechtine 2nd GR. Nonoperative management and treatment of spinal injuries. Spine (Phila Pa 1976). 2006;31(11 Suppl):S22–7; discussion S36.

37. Capen DA. Classification of thoracolumbar fractures and posterior instrumentation for treatment of thoracolumbar fractures. Instr Course Lect. 1999;48:437–41.

38. Harris MB, Sethi RK. The initial assessment and management of the multiple-trauma patient with an associated spine injury. Spine (Phila Pa 1976). 2006;31(11 Suppl):S9–15; discussion S36.

39. Fehlings MG, Perrin RG. The timing of surgical intervention in the treatment of spinal cord injury: a systematic review of recent clinical evidence. Spine (Phila Pa 1976). 2006;31(11 Suppl):S28–35; discussion S36.

40. Meves R, Avanzi O. Correlation among canal compromise, neurologic deficit, and injury severity in thoracolumbar burst fractures. Spine (Phila Pa 1976). 2006;31(18):2137–41.

41. Mohanty SP, Venkatram N. Does neurological recovery in thoracolumbar and lumbar burst fractures depend on the extent of canal compromise? Spinal Cord. 2002;40(6):295–9.

42. Dick W, Kluger P, et al. A new device for internal fixation of thoracolumbar and lumbar spine fractures: the 'fixateur interne'. Paraplegia. 1985;23(4):225–32.

43. Lindsey RW, Dick W. The fixateur interne in the reduction and stabilization of thoracolumbar spine fractures in patients with neurologic deficit. Spine (Phila Pa 1976). 1991;16(3 Suppl):S140–5.

44. Arlet V, Orndorff DG, et al. Reverse and pseudoreverse cortical sign in thoracolumbar burst fracture: radiologic description and distinction – a propos of three cases. Eur Spine J. 2009;18(2):282–7.

45. Wannamaker GT. Spinal cord injuries; a review of the early treatment in 300 consecutive cases during the Korean Conflict. J Neurosurg. 1954;11(6):517–24.

46. Wessberg P, Wang Y, et al. The effect of surgery and remodelling on spinal canal measurements after thoracolumbar burst fractures. Eur Spine J. 2001;10(1):55–63.

47. Verheyden AP, Hoelzl A, et al. The endoscopically assisted simultaneous posteroanterior reconstruction of the thoracolumbar spine in prone position. Spine J. 2004;4(5):540–9.

48. Voormolen MH, Mali WP, et al. Percutaneous vertebroplasty compared with optimal pain medication treatment: short-term clinical outcome of patients with subacute or chronic painful osteoporotic vertebral compression fractures. The VERTOS study. AJNR Am J Neuroradiol. 2007;28(3):555–60.

49. Maestretti G, Cremer C, et al. Prospective study of standalone balloon kyphoplasty with calcium phosphate cement augmentation in traumatic fractures. Eur Spine J. 2007;16(5):601–10.

50. Schmelzer-Schmied N, Cartens C, et al. Comparison of kyphoplasty with use of a calcium phosphate cement and non-operative therapy in patients with traumatic non-osteoporotic vertebral fractures. Eur Spine J. 2009;18(5):624–9.

51. Verlaan JJ, Dhert WJ, et al. Balloon vertebroplasty in combination with pedicle screw instrumentation: a novel technique to treat thoracic and lumbar burst fractures. Spine (Phila Pa 1976). 2005;30(3):E73–9.

52. van der Roer N, de Bruyne MC, et al. Direct medical costs of traumatic thoracolumbar spine fractures. Acta Orthop. 2005;76(5):662–6.

Kyphoplasty - the Current Treatment for Osteoporotic Vertebral Fractures

Guillem Saló

Contents

Abstract

Vertebral osteoporotic fractures are the most frequent fractures in older patients with low mineral bone density. Kyphoplasty is a technique that tries to recover the height of the fractured vertebral body and support this fracture with the injection of cement into the vertebral body. This procedure is usually performed percutaneously and requires appropriate training so as to avoid potential complications. This chapter reviews the indications, pre-operative preparation and planning, operative technique guidelines, post-operative care and rehabilitation and the complications that might appear during and after this procedure.

Keywords

Complications • Indications for surgery • Kyphoplasty • Minimally-invasive surgery • Osteoporotic vertebral fractures • Operative technique-inflatable bone tamps • Rehabilitaion • Vertebral augmentation

General Introduction

Osteoporosis is the most common metabolic bone disorder. It affects two hundred million individuals worldwide [1]. Vertebral compression fractures are a frequently encountered clinical problem in these patients and are becoming increasingly more important as the median age of the population continues to rise. Patients with

G. Saló
Orthopaedic Department, Spine Unit, Universitat Autònoma de Barcelona, Barcelona, Spain
e-mail: Gsalo@hospitaldelmar.cat

painful vertebral compression fractures may have severe pain for prolonged periods of time. When such a fracture does cause pain, it can usually be successfully managed with a combination of medications, activity modification, and occasionally bracing [2]. In a patient who does not respond to this initial treatment, an internal splinting of the vertebral body with percutaneously injected methylmethacrylate may provide adequate pain relief that allows the patient to return to his or her previous level of functioning. In this way, the key principles of the percutaneous cement augmentation techniques are the immediate stabilization of vertebral body fractures to decrease pain or prevent further collapse of the vertebral body.

Percutaneous kyphoplasty is the placement of balloons in the vertebral body with a one-off inflation/deflation sequence that creates a cavity before the cement (generally polymethylmethacrylate) is injected. This procedure is most often performed percutaneously on an outpatient (or short-stay) basis. Kyphoplasty was developed in an attempt to reduce the deformity of the vertebral body and subsequent kyphosis while providing pain relief similar to that provided by vertebroplasty [2–12]. This should decrease the associated risks related to the deformity, increase filling control, stabilize the vertebra and, thereby safely decrease pain and improve mobility [12].

The exact mechanism of the analgesic effect of vertebral augmentation remains unclear. Some investigators attribute the reduction of pain to the toxic and/or thermal effect of the polymethylmethacrylate (PMMA) cement by the destruction of nerve fibres [13, 14]. A more mechanical viewpoint attributes the effect to the fixation of fragments and reduction of micro-motion and the associated irritation of periosteal nerve fibres [15].

Indications for Kyphoplasty

Percutaneous vertebral augmentation (vertebroplasty or kyphoplasty) is indicated for painful osteoporotic vertebral compression fractures

Table 1 Summary of guidelines for percutaneous vertebroplasty and percutaneous kyphoplasty according to the Society of Interventional Radiology and Cardiovascular and Interventional Radiological Society of Europe

Indications
Painful osteoporotic VCF refractory to 3 weeks of analgesic therapy
Painful vertebrae due to benign or malignant primary or secondary bone tumours
Painful VCF with osteonecrosis (Kummell's disease)
Re-inforcement of vertebral body before surgical procedure
Chronic traumatic VCF with non-union
Absolute contra-indications
Asymptomatic VCF
Patient improving on medical therapy
Active infection
Prophylaxis in osteoporotic patient
Uncorrectable coagulopathy
Myelopathy secondary to retropulsion of bone/canal compromise
Allergy to PMMA or opacification agent
Relative contra-indications
Radicular pain
VCF > 70 % height loss
Severe spinal stenosis, asymptomatic retropulsion
Tumour extension into canal/epidural space
Lack of surgical backup

[16–21] or lytic tumours, such as plasmocytoma or multiple myeloma [22], metastasis [23] and painful hemangiomata [24]. Evidence favours the use of this procedure for the pain associated with these disorders. The indications and contra-indications of this procedure are summarized in Table 1. Indications for kyphoplasty in osteoporotic fractures extend to vertebral fractures of less than 8 weeks with an increasing deformity of the vertebra. This is so even in cases of significant posterior wall disruption as well as in fractures with non-union with an intravertebral vacuum phenomenon [25, 26]. In the classification by Magerl, the fractures thereby suitable for augmentation are the A1.1 (end-plate impression), the A1.2 (wedge fracture), the A1.3 (vertebral collapse) and the A3.1 (incomplete burst fracture) types. A new indication for kyphoplasty in combination with posterior short-segment instrumentation has recently been described for the treatment of patients with traumatic burst fractures (non-osteoporotic). This combination has proven to provide good results [27–32].

The exclusion criteria for balloon kyphoplasty include vertebral fractures that are not painful or that are not the primary source of pain, the presence of local or systemic infection, arterio-venous malformations, bone fragments retropulsed into the vertebral canal or an epidural extension of a tumour [26]. Balloon inflation for the kyphoplasty procedure might force material into the spinal canal and thus cause cord compression. There are also relative contra-indications to kyphoplasty.

First, there must be sufficient residual height for the instruments used with kyphoplasty to be inserted in the compressed vertebral body.

Second, small pedicles may also be a limiting technical factor. When the pedicles appear to be too small to accommodate the instruments, a parapedicular approach can be utilized. Kyphoplasty can be performed safely from L5 to T7 in most patients [33].

Third, this technique is not recommended in high-energy injuries with concomitant ligamentous or posterior element injury. In this case, posterior instrumentation should be added.

Controversy exists concerning the specific indications for kyphoplasty as opposed to vertebroplasty [34]. As a review of the literature shows, the pain relief and biomechanical stability resulting from both procedures are comparable [35] although other factors need to be taken into account in choosing one of these techniques over the other. Fracture reduction and restoration of vertebral body height may be achieved through kyphoplasty. However, severe loss of height and an older fracture age may limit the aforementioned effects to a minimum [35]. The most valuable effect achievable through kyphoplasty is the markedly reduced rate of cement leakage [36] through the injection of high-viscosity bone cement into the cavity that is created.

Pre-Operative Preparation and Planning

Patients with a symptomatic vertebral fracture typically present with severe back pain following a minor injury [37]. The pain is made worse by standing erect and occasionally even by lying flat. The spine shows exaggerated thoracic kyphosis and the pain is typically reproduced by deep pressure over the spinous process at the involved level. Neurological deficits are rarely associated with these fractures, but they must always be ruled out [37, 38].

Pre-operative planning includes obtaining a detailed history and performing a thorough physical examination [39]. The proper identification of the painful vertebrae can sometimes be difficult and the patient's symptoms need to be linked to the vertebral compression fracture. Diagnostic studies usually include anteroposterior and lateral plain X-rays of the spine and magnetic resonance imaging (MRI) [39].

Radiographs show the osteopenia characteristic of these patients [40]. The vertebral body shows a fracture with loss of height and wedging and occasionally retropulsion of osseous fragments into the spinal canal. Fractures commonly occur in the thoracolumbar region, but they may be present anywhere in the spine [40]. If nonunion of a fracture is suspected, flexion and extension lateral X-rays can be helpful in assessing the degree of fracture healing and mobility. Magnetic resonance imaging of the spine is probably the single most useful test for determining fracture age, the ruling out of a malignant tumour and selection of the appropriate treatment [41]. MRI has the advantage of revealing additional spinal conditions that may contribute to the pain syndrome; in particular degenerative spinal disease, infections, injury of the disk or ligaments. In the acute period following a vertebral fracture, magnetic resonance imaging shows a geographic pattern of low-intensity-signal changes on T1-weighted images and high-intensity-signal changes on T2-weighted images [41]. In addition to that,

Fig. 1 T1-weighted, T2-weighted and Short Tau Inversion Recovery (*STIR*) magnetic resonance image showing increased signal through the L2 vertebrae, suggesting a recent fracture

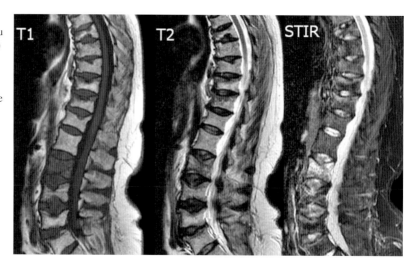

fat-signal suppressing STIR (short tau inversion recovery) of the MRI is particularly helpful in differentiating between fresh and healed fractures [41] (Fig. 1).

Scintigraphy in combination with CT can also be used as an alternative to locate the affected vertebrae in patients with a contra-indication to MRI, such as brain aneurysm clips or cardiac pacemakers [42]. Scintigraphy provides useful information about bone turnover and thereby identifies any vertebral fracture that has an on-going healing process. Bone scans are sensitive enough for the detection of fractures, but they have low specificity for the diagnosis of another underlying disease. An additional limitation of bone-scanning is that increased bone turnover can be detected as long as 2 years following a vertebral fracture [42]. The long term bone turnover period shown on scintigraphy limits the ability of a bone scan to demonstrate the acuity of an osteoporotic vertebral fracture and is not helpful in determining the source of the pain or the predictability of the response to treatment.

Computed tomography (CT) scan provides excellent detail of the bony structures and is the best imaging procedure for assessing the vertebral body deformity and the posterior wall and end-plate involvement. Furthermore, it is necessary to precisely classify the fracture type. It is also important to distinguish between a compression fracture with a collapse of the anterior vertebral cortex and a burst fracture in that the posterior wall is fractured as well [43].

The character of the fracture and bone quality must be assessed during the pre-operative evaluation [21]. In the osteoporotic vertebrae with a rarefied trabecular structure, fractures tend to result in varying degrees of vertebral body collapse with possible retropulsion of the posterior wall into the spinal canal. In contrast to fractures in non-osteoporotic vertebrae, splitting or severe fragmentation occur less frequently. A secondary indicator of posterior wall compromise is the presence of an epidural haematoma. This suggests that the fracture communicates directly with the epidural space and thus may be a conduit for cement leakage. Percutaneous kyphoplasty should only be pursued with great caution. The likelihood of restoring vertebral body height depends largely on the density of the bone and the acuteness of the fracture [18]. Fractures treated within 1–3 weeks of the event are much less likely to have experienced substantial healing and provide the best opportunity for height restoration.

Vertebral compression fractures can be caused by pathological conditions. Unless the diagnosis of osteoporosis is well-established, a biopsy is recommended. In patients who have a dual-energy x-ray absorptiometry (DEXA) study consistent with osteoporosis, no history of malignancy, and a previously known osteoporotic vertebral compression fracture, a biopsy is not necessary.

Operative Technique

The patient should be placed in a prone position on a radiolucent surgical table. Gentle lordotic positioning allows some postural reduction in certain fractures. The procedure can be performed with local anaesthetic in many patients, but the patient should be able to lie prone for at least 1 h without significant pain or respiratory difficulties [44]. The anaesthetic injection under the periosteum at the entry point decreases pain during trocar insertion and is recommended even in patients under general anaesthesia for peri-operative and post-operative pain control. A gentle intravenous sedation can be added to decrease pain during the procedure. If general anaesthesia is utilized, the patient must be handled gently. Rib fractures may occur as a result of undue pressure in the course of patient positioning and during impacting manoeuvres to insert the trocar into the thoracic vertebral body [45]. During multi-level injections, the cement load is greater. Toxic monomeric constituents have the potential to cause cardio-respiratory collapse. The anaesthetist must be alert at the time of each injection procedure. Vasoactive substances to treat sudden hypotension must be readily available [14, 44–46].

The use of bi-planar fluoroscopy greatly aids cannula insertion and cement injection [44, 47, 48]. Bi-planar fluoroscopy is readily obtained by using two separate C-arms (Fig. 2). The lateral image is bought over the top and the arc, leaning away toward the patient's head. The anteroposterior image is brought in diagonally with the image intensifier directly over the target site. It is most convenient to obtain a true anteroposterior image first because the diagonal entry makes this process challenging. Meticulous attention should be paid to obtaining true anteroposterior and lateral images of the target vertebrae. On the AP plane, the pedicles should be symmetrical in shape. The lateral edge of the

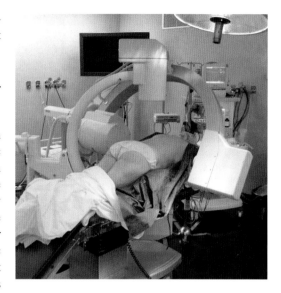

Fig. 2 Operative set-up for the percutaneous Kyphoplasty under bi-planar fluoroscopic guidance, with positioning of the patient and typical arrangement of the both C-arms

vertebral body should be equidistant from both pedicles and the spinous process should be centred between the pedicles (Fig. 3). Caution should be exercised when using the spinous process to obtain a true AP image because there is a significant anatomical variation in the shape of the spinous process [49]. Intra-operative fluoroscopic imaging of the mid-thoracic spine can be challenging in the severe osteoporotic patient. The image can be improved by halting respiration and bringing the x-ray tube closer to the patient. This magnifies the image and decreases beam scatter.

The entry point to the pedicle is marked using high-quality bi-planar images. It is necessary to obtain a true AP view of the pedicle with an oval shape in order to avoid lesions of the surrounding neural structures (Fig. 4). A trocar needle is inserted into the vertebral body either with a transpedicular or extrapedicular approach (Fig. 5). The transpedicular approach is best suited for large pedicles such as those in the lumbar and lower thoracic spine. Localization of the pedicles is performed in a manner similar to that used for vertebroplasty. A posterior approach with a slight ipsilateral obliquity of 10–25° is preferred [49–51]. The medial wall

Fig. 3 Intra-operative
fluoroscopy. The AP view
is adjusted with the spinous
process of the targeted
vertebral body in the exact
mid-line, end-plates
parallel and pedicles placed
symmetrically in the upper
lateral quadrant of the
projection of the vertebral
body. The lateral view is
adjusted with pedicles
superimposed, end-plates
parallel and the posterior
wall aligned with a single
contour

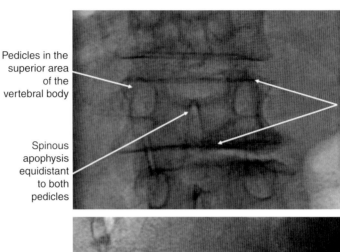

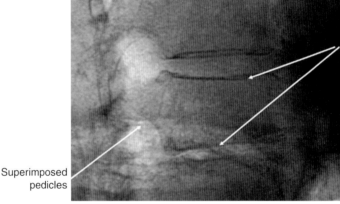

of the pedicle must be well visualized. The extrapedicular approach is best suited for the mid-thoracic spine. The entry point for the extrapedicular approach lies between the lateral edge of the pedicle and the costovertebral joint [44, 45, 48]. The rib head helps direct the needle into the vertebral body. The extrapedicular approach allows a trajectory more latero-medial, thereby accessing the central portion of the vertebral body. The approach is usually bilateral. However, adequate cement distribution into the vertebral body can be accomplished through a unilateral injection site with this technique.

The kyphoplasty procedure requires an 11- or 13-gauge bone entry needle, a scalpel, a kyphoplasty kit, inflatable balloon tamps, sterile barium sulphate or another opacifier, and bone cement. The surgical steps involved in transpedicular placement of a kyphoplasty balloon are shown in Fig. 6.

First, is necessary to place the needle (usually an 11-G Jamshidi needle) at the pedicle entry site at the angle between the upper articular process and the transverse process [44]. The needle targets a starting point just superior and lateral to the pedicle. One must be cautious to avoid injuring the exiting nerve roots and the beginning point must not be so far lateral as to puncture the bowel or kidney [45]. Oblique views should also be used to confirm proper positioning. The needle should pass through the pedicle centre without perforating the medial pediclar cortex, and go on to enter the vertebral body. Only now does the tip of the needle cross the projection of the medial pediclar cortex, as viewed from the rear. The optimal final placement of the needle should be in the anterior third of the vertebral body [47].

After needle insertion, the trocar is removed. A Kirschner wire is then directed through the needle and into the bone to act as a guide-wire. The cannula is inserted over the guide-wire and

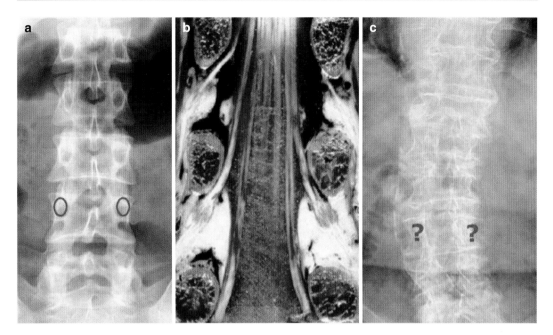

Fig. 4 (**a**) X-ray of a patient with a good visualization of the cross-section of the pedicles in the AP view. (**b**) Anatomical coronal cut across the pedicles, showing the neural structures around the pedicles that we must avoid during the procedure. (**c**) X-Ray of a patient with a bad visualization of the cross section of the pedicles in the AP view. In this case, is not possible to perform a safe technique and we recommend that the procedure be aborted because there is a high risk of neurological injury

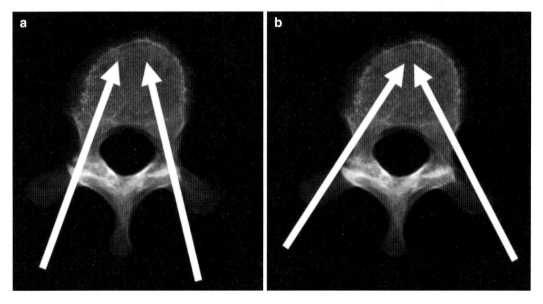

Fig. 5 Axial view demonstrating the trajectory of the needle in a transpedicular approach (**a**) and in a parapedicular approach (**b**). In the parapedicular approach, the needle follows the junction of the rib and transverse process of the vertebra and enters the vertebral body along the lateral margin of the pedicle

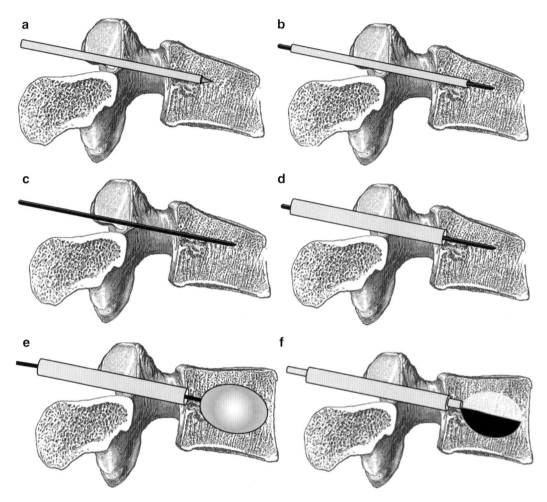

Fig. 6 Schematic diagram of a transpedicular kyphoplasty of a lumbar vertebral body. The surgical steps involved are: (**a**) placing the biopsy needle at the pedicle entry site at the angle between the upper articular process and the transverse process. (**b**) Kirschner wire fed through the biopsy needle and acting as a guide. (**c**) The biopsy needle is removed. (**d**) Introduction of the cannulated trocar via guide-wire. (**e**) Positioning the kyphoplasty balloon in the drilled channel in the fracture zone. Pressure-controlled inflation of the kyphoplasty balloon and the simultaneous gain in height of the vertebral body. (**f**) The cavity that remains after the kyphoplasty balloon has been removed is filled with high-viscosity augmentation material through the cannula

into the vertebral body. The operating surgeon should always have control of the proximal end of the Kirschner wire because the sharp tip could easily and inadvertently penetrate soft bone and breach the anterior vertebral cortex [44]. A skin incision is then made to accommodate the working cannula, which is advanced through the soft tissues and through the pedicle to rest at the posterior aspect of the vertebral body. A plastic handle can be placed on the hub of the cannula to advance it manually into the vertebral body, or a mallet can be used to tap the plastic handle, driving the cannula into the vertebral body [47]. The cannula is inserted approximately 2–3 mm. past the posterior vertebral body wall. If there is considerable resistance to placing the working cannula, the cannula handle can be rotated in an alternating clockwise-counter clockwise motion to help breach the cortex and facilitate advancement [46, 49]. The guide-wire is removed and a drill is used to create a path for the inflatable balloon tamp. If a biopsy is needed, a biopsy trocar is used to sample the vertebral bone prior to drilling the vertebral body. A 3 mm. drill is advanced through the cannula and multi-planar fluoroscopy is used to re-check the orientation of the working cannula. The drill is then ideally directed along a slightly posterolateral to anteromedial trajectory into the vertebra until the tip of the drill is 3 mm. posterior to the anterior margin of the vertebral body [47]. Extreme caution should be used to avoid breaching the anterior cortex of the vertebral body with the drill. For bilateral transpedicular or extrapedicular approaches, the sequence of events is repeated on the contralateral side [47].

After this, the kyphoplasty balloon is positioned in the drilled channel in the fracture zone. If the clinician feels resistance in the passageway of the drilled hole, perhaps secondary to small shards of bone, the drill or bone filler device can be inserted and withdrawn once or twice along the path to clear it of debris. Thereupon, the balloon tamp can be inserted without difficulty. The inflatable balloon tamp is available in different sizes. Each balloon has markers to delineate its distal and proximal extents. Once both balloons are in the vertebral body, they are pressure-controlled inflated with a radio contrast medium (for visualization) simultaneously under bi-planar fluoroscopy so as to gain height of the vertebral body. The inflatable bone tamp compacts the cancellous bone and re-expands the body. Before inflation, air is purged from the balloons, and the reservoir of an angioplasty injection device (incorporating a pressure monitor) is filled with 10 ml. of diluted iodine contrast material. Inflation via the injection device is begun under continuous fluoroscopy, increasing balloon pressure to approximately 50 psi. to secure the balloon in position. Balloon inflation should be performed slowly and progressively by half-millilitre increments. There should be frequent pauses to check for pressure decay, which occurs as the adjacent cancellous bone yields and compacts [49, 50]. If the bone is osteoporotic, pressure decay may be immediate. If the bone is quite dense, there may be little or no pressure decay, even at pressures up to 180 psi. The balloon system is raised to 180 psi., with

Table 2 End-points of balloon inflation during kyphoplasty

1. Restoration of the vertebral body height to normal position
2. Flattening of the balloon against an end-plate without accompanying height restoration
3. Appearance of a small outward bleb in the balloon
4. Contact with a lateral cortical margin
5. Inflation without further pressure decay
6. Reaching the maximum volume of the balloon
7. Reaching the maximum pressure of the balloon

a practical maximum of 220 psi. The possible end-points of inflation are shown in Table 2. The operating surgeon must maintain both visual and manual control throughout the entire inflation process and should record the amount of fluid used to inflate the balloon when the end-point has been achieved [47]. This volume indicates the size of the cavity that has been created and it will serve as an estimate of the amount of cement to be delivered. In some cases, reduction of the vertebral body can be accomplished. If substantial height restoration has not been achieved, careful repositioning of the bone tamps and re-inflation can be helpful [45]. The reduction manoeuvre is best accomplished when the balloon pushes up against the end-late and shows a flattened appearance on fluoroscopic image. When positioned properly, this technique elevates the end-plates without expanding the fractured vertebral body laterally or posteriorly. Two balloons are generally used to provide a greater reduction. Rupture of the balloon (who rarely occurs) is not a hazard, other than that of exposure to small volumes of radio contrast medium. If a balloon ruptures, it is simply withdrawn through the working cannula and replaced. The inflation of the balloon should be stopped before causing a cortical fracture, which is revealed by the appearance of a small outward bleb in the balloon [44].

The cavity that remains after the kyphoplasty balloon has been removed is filled with high-viscosity augmentation material through the cannula and the cement can be deposited under low pressure. Once adequate inflation has been achieved, the cement is mixed in a manner similar to that for vertebroplasty. The cement mixture is transferred to a bone filler device [14]. Once the bone cement has undergone transition from a liquid to a cohesive, doughy consistency (about 5 min after mixing, depending on the cement), the bone filler devices are passed through the working cannula and into the anterior aspect of the vertebral cavities. Small volumes of cement (about 0.5 cm [3]) are injected in a step-wise fashion with fluoroscopic visualization. The volume of cement for injection is approximately 1 ml. more than the volume of the cavity created by each inflatable balloon tamp [52]. In addition to filling the void created by the ballon tamp, additional cement is needed to allow integration of the cement into the surrounding trabecular bone. This serves to "lock in" the cement. If a quantity of cement is equal to or less than the volume of the cavity, the vertebra will not be re-inforced and may lead to further re-collapse of the surrounding bone due to excessive motion at the bone-cement interface. The cement should be injected into the anterior two-thirds of the vertebral body and the cavity should be filled from the anterior to the posterior aspect of the vertebra. By avoiding the posterior one third, the risk of cement leakage into the spinal canal is minimized [46]. Continuous fluoroscopic monitoring is maintained to identify leakage of cement into the spinal canal, paraspinous veins, inferior vena cava, or disc space [49]. When cement leakage is observed, injection should be halted immediately. The cannula is re-positioned to another location and another attempt at injection may be pursued after adequate time has passed to allow the first injection to polymerize. In most cases, cement leakage is clinically inconsequential. If a significant leak is suspected, a "wake-up" test is performed prior to departing the operation room. If there are clinical signs and symptoms of neurologic compromise, emergency decompression should be considered.

Treatment of multiple levels can be performed using a single batch of cement. The cement is stored in a sterile ice-water bath to slow the polymerization process. The guide-wires are inserted into all the target vertebral bodies. The first site in then drilled, the balloon tamp deployed, and the cement injected. The next level is then drilled, treated with the balloon tamp, and subsequently injected. A third site can be treated thereafter in the same sequence. This step-wise sequence allows use a single pair of balloon tamps for the treatment multiple levels. The limitation of the number of levels is dictated by the cement load. The risk of cement toxicity increases with the number of levels treated. As a general rule, no more than three levels should be treated during a single procedure [44].

Maintenance of reduction can be difficult in certain fractures, particularly in fractures with an intravertebral vacuum phenomenon. Once a balloon is deflated, the fracture may collapse again. The reduction can be maintained by the "eggshell technique" [44]. A small amount of cement ($0.5-1$ cm^3) is injected into the cavity. The balloon tamp is re-inserted and gently re-elevated. The small cement bolus is then spread around the balloon to create a thin eggshell of cement. When the balloon is removed, the eggshell mantle holds the reduction until the remainder of the cement is injected. This technique can also be utilized to control cement leakage [44].

When cement filling of the cavity has been confirmed fluoroscopically from both the lateral and anteroposterior views, the bone filler devices are partially withdrawn to allow complete filling of the cavity. They are then used to tamp the bone cement in place before being completely withdrawn. The patient remains prone on the table and is not moved until the remaining cement in the mixing bowl has hardened completely [15].

Post-Operative Care and Rehabilitation

The patients can be mobilized immediately after surgery without restrictions and without external support. When calcium phosphate has been used, we prescribe 12-h bed-rest as the process of hardening takes longer [44].

Pain relief occurs within 1 or 2 days in most cases and it has been correlated with fracture reduction. The patient is dismissed with routine pain medications and a graduated resumption of activity.

Discharge instructions for the patient should include: a call to the physician for the onset of new back pain, chest pain, lower extremity weakness or fever. The first follow-up after the procedure is at 1 week [47] and after this the patient should come back to the office at 1 month and at 3 months after the procedure. Six months after the procedure the patient can be definitively discharged.

As vertebral augmentation techniques cannot be shown to reduce the rate of further vertebral fractures, additional medical treatment for osteoporosis and physiotherapy are required [49].

Complications

The overall risks of the procedure are low, but serious complications (including spinal cord compression) can occur. With good patient selection and careful technique, these complications are avoidable and make the risk-to-benefit ratio highly favourable [53, 54].

Early complications of kyphoplasty are divided in three groups:
(a) systemic complications
(b) local complications related to the technique or to the placement of hardware in an incorrect location
(c) local complications due to extrusion of cement outside of the vertebra.

Delayed complications include a re-fracture or an insufficiency fracture of the cemented vertebrae, fractures of the adjacent level and delayed dislocation of the cement [14, 55–57].

Early systemic complications include cardiovascular changes, fat embolism and fever that are usually resolved in 2–4 days. It may occur as a result of inflammation or infection at the site of injection or as a result of exothermic effects of the cement [58, 59]. Unreacted monomer from the cement can have systemic cardiopulmonary effects resulting in hypoxia and embolism.

Infectious complications, although rare, have been reported. There are several reports of osteomyelitis requiring corpectomy [53]. Meticulous attention to sterile technique is warranted, including pre-operative intravenous antibiotic administration.

Complications related to the technique include, post-operative epidural bleeding, injury to the neural elements, temporary radicular pain, vascular injuries, dural tears and rib, pedicle or sternum fractures. Rib fractures are also known to happen as a result of pressure on the back and chest occurring during needle placement while the patient is prone [58]. New osteoporotic rib fractures are thought to occur when the patient is placed in prone position on the table for and during the procedure. However, they might significantly bias the clinical outcome relative to pain relief and should be treated with analgesic medications for an appropriate period. Pedicle fractures may be a primary finding of the vertebral compression or might be induced by the passage of the cannula during the procedure. Complications resulting from improper needle placement or inattention to fluoroscopic patterns of cement distribution during injection are dependent on operator training and experience.

Complications secondary to extrusion of cement include pulmonary embolism and nerve or spinal cord compression by cement. The most frequent problem is a transient radicular pain due to cement leakage into the radicular veins in proximity to the vertebral foramina. Cement leakage into peridural veins can, in the worst case, lead to para- or tetraplegia by compression of the thecal sac and its contents. In a group of thirty patients who underwent kyphoplasty, Lieberman et al. reported cement leakage into the epidural space in one patient, into a disc space on two occasions, and into the paraspinal tissues in three patients [33]. Cement leakage can occur less often in kyphopasty than vertebroplasty. The incidence of cement extrusion outside of bone occurring during kyphoplasty has been reported to be 8.6–33 %. In contrast to this, cement extrusion with vertebroplasty has been reported to occur in 3–70 % of cases [59].

Cement leakage into the paravertebral soft tissues or veins is generally asymptomatic. Cement leakage into the disc space is controversial because some studies have shown an increased risk for subsequent fractures of adjacent vertebral bodies [60–62], whereas others have claimed that cement leakage into the disc space is of no clinical significance [54, 57]. The incidence of cement leakage following either procedure can be higher than that seen on radiographs. Yeom et al. found that computerized tomography revealed cement leakage 1.5 times more frequently than did radiographs [63]. Garfin et al. reported on two patients with spinal cord injury following kyphoplasty [17]. Phillips et al. evaluated whether the creation of a bone void during kyphoplasty reduced the risk of cement leakage [36]. Under fluoroscopic control, they injected radiopaque contrast material into the vertebral body prior to and following the creation of a void within the vertebra. There was less extra-vertebral leakage of the contrast material into the epidural vessels, inferior vena cava and transcortically following the creation of the cavity, suggesting that cement leakage may be less likely following kyphoplasty [64]. Because cement extrusion outside of the vertebral body is usually asymptomatic with either vertebroplasty or kyphoplasty, it makes more sense to monitor and compare symptomatic complications rather than the incidence of cement extrusion.

Cement propagation via paravertebral veins into the inferior vena cava and pulmonary embolism has been described in several case reports as a possible cause for hypotension, arrhythmia, and hypocapnia [65, 66]. In a retrospective analysis, pulmonary cement embolism has been described in 4.6–8.1 % of the cases of vertebropasty, with 1.1 % of patients being symptomatic [67]. Experimental data have demonstrated that high-viscosity cements might probably reduce the leakage rate to avoid those complications completely in future. A decrease in the potential for cement extrusion with kyphoplasty has been suggested because of the cavity formed and a more viscous cement that results in the need for less injection pressure [67]. Highly vascular lesions and a liquid consistency of cement may also cause leakage of methylmethacrylate into perivertebral veins. In such cases, injection should immediately be discontinued so as to avoid pulmonary embolism from the cement.

In addition to the short-term peri-procedural risk of kyphoplasty, there can be an additional risk of new fracture development subsequent to the treatment. New vertebral fractures are reported in numerous patients subsequent to kyphoplasty. They usually occurred within the first year after treatment [68]. The hypothesis is that the restored stiffness of the augmented vertebra itself might propagate secondary fractures in adjacent non-augmented vertebrae. Because new vertebral fractures can occur in osteoporotic patients simply secondary to disease progression rather than as a result of vertebroplasty or kyphoplasty [69, 70], it is difficult to determine the added risk of fracture resulting from these procedures.

In general, kyphoplasty is a relatively safe procedure when performed by skilled operators. The overall symptomatic complication rate reported for kyphoplasty as a treatment for osteoporotic compression fractures is less than 1–6 %. They mostly consist of minor complications such as rib fractures and temporary radicular pain [19, 45, 47]. Major complications, such as permanent neurological injury or serious pulmonary embolism are rare. They occur in less than 1 % of cases [45].

A prospective, randomized trial directly comparing outcomes of kyphoplasty and vertebroplasty would be necessary to accurately compare the relative safety of both procedures.

Summary

In conclusion, kyphoplasty is a good technique for the treatment of osteoporotic vertebral fractures in order to relieve pain and restore vertebral body height. On the other hand, this procedure has serious potential complications that can lead to irreversible consequences for the patient, even to death. Following the guidelines set out above along with proper training allows for the carrying out of this technique with a low complication rate and with good results.

References

1. Lin JT, Lane JM. Osteoporosis: a review. Clin Orthop Relat Res. 2004;425:126–34.
2. Rao RJ, Manoj MD. Current concepts review. Painful osteoporotic vertebral fracture pathogenesis, evaluation and roles of vertebroplasty and kiphoplasty in its management. J Bone Joint Surg Am. 2003;85-A:10.
3. Hiwatashi A, Moritani T, Numaguchi Y, et al. Increase in vertebral body height after vertebroplasty. AJNR Am J Neuroradiol. 2003;24:185–9.
4. Teng MM, Wei CJ, Wei LC, et al. Kyphosis correction and height restoration effects of percutaneous vertebroplasty. AJNR Am J Neuroradiol. 2003;24:1893–900.
5. Carlier RY, Gordji H, Mompoint DM, et al. Osteorotic vertebral collapse: percutaneous vertebroplasty and local kyphosis correction. Radiology. 2004;233:891–8.
6. Dublin AB, Hartman J, Latchaw RE, et al. The vertebral body fracture in osteoporosis: restoration of height using percutaneous vertebroplasty. AJNR Am J Neuroradiol. 2005;26:489–92.
7. Rhyne 3rd A, Banit D, Laxer E, et al. Kyphoplasty: report of eighty-two thoracolumbar osteoporotic vertebral fractures. J Orthop Trauma. 2004;18:294–9.
8. Majd ME, Farley S, Holt RT. Preliminary outcomes and efficacy of the first 360 consecutive kyphoplasties for the treatment of painful osteoporotic vertebral compression fractures. Spine J. 2005;5:244–55.
9. Voggenreiter G. Balloon kyphoplasty is effective in deformity correction of osteoporotic vertebral compression fractures. Spine. 2005;30:2806–12.
10. Pradhan BB, Bae HW, Kropf MA, et al. Kyphoplasty reduction of osteoporotic vertebral compression fractures: correction of local kyphosis versus overall sagittal alignment. Spine. 2006;31:435–41.
11. Shindle MK, Gardner MJ, Koob J, et al. Vertebral height restoration in osteoporotic compression fractures: kyphoplasty balloon tamp is superior to postural correction alone. Osteoporos Int. 2006;17:1815–9.
12. Grohs JG, Matzner M, Trieb K, et al. Minimal invasive stabilization of osteoporotic vertebral fractures: a prospective nonrandomized comparison of vertebroplasty and balloon kyphoplasty. J Spinal Disord Tech. 2005;18:238–42.
13. Belkoff SM, Maroney M, Fenton DC, et al. An in vitro biomechanical evaluation of bone cements used in percutaneous vertebroplasty. Bone. 1999;25(2 Suppl):23S–6.
14. Jensen ME, Evans AJ, Mathis JM, et al. Percutaneous polymethylmethacrylate vertebroplasty in the treatment of osteoporotic vertebral body compression fractures: technical aspects. AJNR Am J Neuroradiol. 1997;18:1897–904.
15. Armsen N, Boszczyk B. Vertebro-/kyphoplasty: history, development, results. Eur J Trauma. 2005;31:433–41.
16. Berlemann U, Franz T, Orler R, Heini PF. Kyphoplasty for treatment of osteoporotic vertebral fractures: a prospective non-randomized study. Eur Spine J. 2004;13:496–501.
17. Garfin SR, Yuan HA, Reiley MA. New technologies in spine: kyphoplasty and vertebroplasty for the treatment of painful osteoporotic compression fractures. Spine. 2001;26:1511–5.
18. Cortet B, Cotten A, Boutry N, et al. Percutaneous vertebroplasty in the treatment of osteoporotic vertebral compression fractures: an open prospective study. J Rheumatol. 1999;26:2222–8.
19. Heini PF, Wälchli B, Berlemann U. Percutaneous transpedicular vertebroplasty with PMMA – a prospective study for the treatment of osteoporotic compression fractures. Eur Spine J. 2000;9:445–50.
20. Heini PF, Orler R. Kyphoplasty for treatment of osteoporotic vertebral fractures. Eur Spine J. 2004;13:184–92.
21. Lieberman I, Reinhardt MK. Vertebroplasty and kyphoplasty for osteolytic vertebral collapse. Clin Orthop Relat Res. 2003;415S:S176–86.
22. Lane JM, Hong R, Koob J, et al. Kyphoplasty enhances function and structural alignment in multiple myeloma. Clin Orthop. 2004;426:49–53.
23. Pflugmacher R, Taylor R, Agarwal A, et al. Balloon kyphoplasty in the treatment of metastatic disease of the spine: a 2-year prospective evaluation. Eur Spine J. 2008;17:1042–8.
24. Hadjipavlou A, Tosounidis T, Gaitanis I, et al. Balloon kyphoplasty as a single or as an adjunct procedure for the management of symptomatic vertebral haemangiomas. J Bone Joint Surg Br. 2007;89(4):495–502.
25. Jang JS, Kim DY, Lee SO. Efficacy of percutaneous vertebroplasty in the treatment of intravertebral pseudarthrosis associated with noninfected avascular necrosis of the vertebral body. Spine. 2003;28(14):1588–92.
26. McGraw JK, Cardella J, Barr JD, et al. Society of interventional radiology quality improvement guidelines for percutaneous vertebroplasty. J Vasc Interv Radiol. 2003;14:S311–5.
27. Hauck S, Beisse R, Bühren V. Vertebroplasty and kyphoplasty in spinal trauma. Eur J Trauma. 2005;31:453–63.
28. Oner FC, Verlaan JJ, Verbout AJ, Dhert WJ. Cement augmentation techniques in traumatic thoracolumbar spine fractures. Spine. 2006;31(11):S89–95.
29. Verlaan JJ, Dhert WJ, Verbout AJ, et al. Balloon vertebroplasty in combination with pedicle screw instrumentation: a novel technique to treat thoracic and lumbar burst fractures. Spine. 2005;30:E73–9.

30. Verlaan JJ, van de Kraats EB, Oner FC, et al. The reduction of endplate fractures during balloon vertebroplasty. A detailed radiological analysis of the treatment of burst fractures using pedicle screws, balloon vertebroplasty, and calcium phosphate cement. Spine. 2005;30(16):1840–5.

31. Pflugmacher R, Agarwal A, Kandziora F, Klostermann C. Balloon kyphoplasty combined with posterior instrumentation for the treatment of burst fractures of the spine – 1-year results. J Orthop Trauma. 2009;23(2):126–31.

32. Korovessis P, Repantis T, Petsinis G, et al. Direct reduction of thoracolumbar burst fractures by means of balloon kyphoplasty with calcium phosphate and stabilization with pedicle-screw instrumentation and fusion. Spine. 2008;33(4):E100–8.

33. Lieberman IH, Dudeney S, Reinhardt MK, et al. Initial outcome and efficacy of "kyphoplasty" in the treatment of painful osteoporotic vertebral compression fractures. Spine. 2001;26:1631–8.

34. Mathis JM. Percutaneous vertebroplasty or kyphoplasty: which one do I choose? Skeletal Radiol. 2006;35:629–31.

35. Boszczyk BM, Bierschneider M, Schmid K, et al. Microsurgical interlaminary vertebroplasty and kyphoplasty for severe osteoporotic fractures. J Neurosurg Spine. 2004;100(1 Suppl):32–7.

36. Phillips FM, Wetzel FT, Lieberman I, et al. An in vivo comparison of the potential extravertebral cement leak after vertebroplasty and kyphoplasty. Spine. 2002;27:2173–9.

37. Lee YL, Yip KM. The osteoporotic spine. Clin Orthop. 1996;323:91–7.

38. Peh WC, Gilula LA, Peck DD. Percutaneous vertebroplasty for severe osteoporotic vertebral body compression fractures. Radiology. 2002;223:121–6.

39. McKiernan F, Jensen R, Faciszewski T, et al. The dynamic mobility of vertebral compression fractures. J Bone Miner Res. 2003;18:24–9.

40. Yamato M, Nishimura G, Kuramochi E, Saiki N, Fujioka M. MR appearance at different ages of osteoporotic compression fractures of the vertebrae. Radiat Med. 1998;16:329–34.

41. Oner FC. MRI findings of thoracolumbar spine fractures: a categorization based on MRI examinations of 100 fractures. Skeletal Radiol. 1999;28:433–43.

42. Maynard AS, Jensen ME, Schweickert PA, Marx WF, Short JG, Kallmes DF. Value of bone scan imaging in predicting pain relief from percutaneous vertebroplasty in osteoporotic vertebral fractures. AJNR Am J Neuroradiol. 2000;21:1807–12.

43. Spivak JM, Johnson MG. Percutaneous treatment of vertebral body pathology. J Am Acad Orthop Surg. 2005;13:6–17.

44. Kim CW, Garfin SR. Percutaneous cement augmentation techniques (vertebroplasty, kyphoplasty). Spine surgery. Tricks of the trade (Chap. 66). 2nd ed. New York: Thieme; 2009.

45. Bierschneider M, Boszczyk BM, Schmid K, et al. Minimally invasive vertebral augmentation techniques in osteoporotic fractures. Eur J Trauma. 2005;31:442–52.

46. Hillmeier J, Meeder PJ, Nöldge G, et al. Minimally invasive reduction and internal stabilization of osteoporotic vertebral body fractures (balloon kyphoplasty). Eur J Trauma. 2005;31:280–90.

47. Mathis JM, Deramond H, Belkoff S, editors. Percutaneous vertebroplasty and kyphoplasty. 2nd ed. New York: Springer; 2006.

48. Cloft HJ, Jensen ME. Kyphoplasty: an assessment of a new technology. AJNR Am J Neuroradiol. 2007;28:200–3.

49. Franck H, Boszczyk BM, Bierschneider M, Jaksche H. Interdisciplinary approach to balloon kyphoplasty in the treatment of osteoporotic vertebral compression fractures. Eur Spine J. 2003;12 Suppl 2:S163–7.

50. Manson NA, Phillips FM. Minimally invasive techniques for the treatment of osteoporotic vertebral fractures. J Bone Joint Surg Am. 2006;88-A (8):1862–72.

51. Phillips FM. Minimally invasive treatments of osteoporotic vertebral compression fractures. Spine. 2003;28(15S):S45–53.

52. Belkoff SM, Mathis JM, Deramond H, Jasper LE. An ex vivo biomechanical evaluation of a hydroxyapatite cement for use with kyphoplasty. AJNR Am J Neuroradiol. 2001;22:1212–6.

53. Layton KF, Thielen KR, Koch CA, et al. Vertebroplasty, first 1000 levels of a single center: evaluation of the outcomes and complications. AJNR Am J Neuroradiol. 2007;28:683–9.

54. Mathis JM. Percutaneous vertebroplasty: complication avoidance and technique optimization. AJNR Am J Neuroradiol. 2003;24:1697–706.

55. Laredo JD, Hamze B. Complications of percutaneous vertebroplasty and their prevention. Skeletal Radiol. 2004;33:493–505.

56. Hulme PA, Krebs J, Ferguson SJ, et al. Vertebroplasty and kyphoplasty: a systematic review of 69 clinical studies. Spine. 2006;31:1983–2001.

57. Wong W, Mathis JM. Vertebroplasty and kyphoplasty: techniques for avoiding complications and pitfalls. Neurosurg Focus. 2005;18:e2.

58. Taylor RS, Taylor RJ, Fritzell P. Balloon kyphoplasty and vertebroplasty for vertebral compression fractures: a comparative systematic review of efficacy and safety. Spine. 2006;31:2747–55.

59. Eck JC, Nachtigall D, Humphreys SC, et al. Comparison of vertebroplasty and balloon kyphoplasty for treatment of vertebral compression fractures: a meta-analysis of the literature. Spine J. 2008;8:488–97.

60. Syed MI, Patel NA, Jan S, et al. Intradiskal extravasation with low-volume cement filling in percutaneous vertebroplasty. AJNR Am J Neuroradiol. 2005;26:2397–401.

61. Lin EP, Ekholm S, Hiwatashi A, et al. Vertebroplasty: cement leakage into the disc increases the risk of new fracture of adjacent vertebral body. AJNR Am J Neuroradiol. 2004;25:175–80.

62. Komemushi A, Tanigawa N, Kariya S, et al. Percutaneous vertebroplasty for osteoporotic compression fracture: multivariate study of predictors of new vertebral body fracture. Cardiovasc Intervent Radiol. 2006;29:580–5.

63. Yeom JS, Kim WJ, Choy WS, Lee CK, Chang BS, Kang JW. Leakage of cement in percutaneous transpedicular vertebroplasty for painful osteoporotic compression fractures. J Bone Joint Surg Br. 2003;85:83–9.

64. Ryu KS, Park CK, Kim MC, et al. Dose-dependent epidural leakage of polymethylmethacrylate after percutaneous vertebroplasty in patients with osteoporotic vertebral compression fractures. J Neurosurg. 2002;96:S56–61.

65. Padovani B, Kasriel O, Brunner P, et al. Pulmonary embolism caused by acrylic cement: a rare complication of percutaneous vertebroplasty. AJNR Am J Neuroradiol. 1999;20:375–7.

66. Choe DH, Marom EM, Ahrar K, et al. Pulmonary embolism of polymethylmethacrylate during percutaneous vertebroplasty and kyphoplasty. AJR Am J Roentgenol. 2004;183:1097–102.

67. Pitton MB, Herber S, Koch U, Oberholzer K, Drees P, Düber C. CT-guided vertebroplasty: analysis of technical results, extraosseous cement leakages, and complications in 500 procedures. Eur Radiol. 2008;18:2568–78.

68. Bouza C, Lopez T, Magro A, et al. Efficacy and safety of balloon kyphoplasty in the treatment of vertebral compression fractures: a systemic review. Eur Spine J. 2006;21:1–18.

69. Syed MI, Patel NA, Jan S, et al. New symptomatic vertebral compression fractures within fractures within a year following vertebroplasty in osteoporotic women. AJNR Am J Neuroradiol. 2005;26:1601–4.

70. Grafe IA, Da Fonseca K, Hillmeier J, et al. Reduction of pain and fracture incidence after kyphoplasty: 1-year outcomes of a prospective controlled trial of patients with primary osteoporosis. Osteoporos Int. 2005;16:2005–12.

Strategies for Low Back Pain

Richard Eyb and G. Grabmeier

Contents

Keywords

Clinical assessment • Diagnostic strategies • Imaging • Low back pain • Natural history • Risk factors • Therapy-activity and physiotherapy, surgery

Strategies and Management

Non-specific low back pain is second to upper respiratory problems as a reason to visit general physicians and the first to visit an Orthopaedic Surgeon's office. The reported prevalence is as high as 73 % [1]. For active adults not seeking medical attention, the annual incidence of significant low back pain (visual analogue scale VAS 4 on a ten-point scale) with functional impairment ranges between 10 and 15 % [2]. These numbers are for low back pain without sciatica, stenosis, instability or deformity. If low back pain occurs acutely (3–6 weeks previously), it usually resolves after several weeks [3]. The problem is the persistent or chronic disabling back pain.

Diagnostic Strategies

History

Before starting an exhaustive diagnostic procedure it is useful to address three questions
1. Is a systemic disease causing the pain?
2. Are there social or psychological disorders?
3. Is there neurological compromise? [4]

R. Eyb (✉) • G. Grabmeier
Orthopädische Abteilung, Sozialmedizinisches Zentrum
Ost Donauspital, Wien, Austria
e-mail: richard.eyb@wienkav.at

G. Bentley (ed.), *European Surgical Orthopaedics and Traumatology*,
DOI 10.1007/978-3-642-34746-7_35, © EFORT 2014

Table 1 Differential diagnosis of low back pain [4]

Mechanical (97 %)	Non mechanical (1 %)	Visceral disease (2 %)
Unspecific LBP **80 %**	**Neoplasia 0.7 %**	**Disease of pelvic organ**
Degenerative Discs and facets **10 %**	Multiple myeloma	Prostatitis
Disc herniation **4 %**	Metastasis	Endometriosis
Spinal stenosis **3 %**	Retroperitoneal tumours	**Renal diseases**
Osteoporotic fracture **4 %**	Primary vertebral tumours	Nephrolithiasasis
Olisthesis **2 %**	**Infection 0.01 %**	Pyelonephritis
Traumatic fracture <**1 %**	Osteomyelitis	**Aortic aneurysm**
Congenital deformity <**1 %**	Discitis	**Gastro-intestinal diseases**
Kyphosis, scoliosis	Epidural abscess	Pancreatitis
	Rheumatoid arthritis 0.3 %	Cholecystitis
	Ankylosing spondylitis	Gastric ulcer
	Psoriatric arthritis	
	Reiter syndrome	
	Scheuermann disease	
	Paget's disease	

With these questions the medical history can be briefly elicited:

Systemic diseases include the history of cancer, chronic infection or chronic polyarthritis.

Neurological involvement includes usually sciatica or spinal claudication combined with paraesthesia and numbness of one or both legs. Disc herniation with neurological impairment usually increases with sneezing, coughing or abdominal pressure. A massive mid-line herniation can lead to a cauda syndrome with bladder or bowel dysfunction and sensory loss in a "saddle" distribution and bilateral gait weakness.

Psychosocial reasons maybe found in depression, job or family problems, somatisation, litigation involvement and/or disability compensation issues.

If dealing with low back pain in adolescence the following risk factors have been pointed out [5]:
1. Rapid growth
2. Smoking
3. Tight quadriceps femoris
4. Tight hamstrings
5. Working during the school year
6. Poor mental health (but no correlation to Schober sign).

If dealing with older adults the diagnosis probabilities change: cancer, compression fractures, spinal stenosis and aortic aneurysm become more common. Osteoporotic fractures may even occur in the absence of a recognised trauma.

An overview of differential diagnosis of low back pain is shown in Table 1.

Clinical Examination

1. Muscle tenderness is almost always found but without specificity and is not reproducible.
2. Spinal stiffness is not strongly associated with any diagnosis, but may help in monitoring physical therapy [6].
3. Lasgues' test can be an indicator of nerve root irritation (straight-leg rising with symptoms of sciatica if elevation is less than 60°). Crossed Lasegues' test is sensitive but highly specific [7].
4. Further examination should include hip motion and tests of the sacro-iliac joint (Menell and Patrick's test), to exclude possible L3 symptoms.
5. Motor weakness of L5 and S1 nerve root (great toe dorsiflexion and plantar flexion).

Table 2 Red flags [8]

"Red flags" indicate possible underlying spinal pathology [8]
1. Onset age <20 or >55
2. Non-mechanical pain
3. Previous history of carcinoma, steroids, HIV
4. Thoracic pain
5. Feeling unwell
6. Weight loss
7. Neural symptoms
8. Structural deformity

6. Dermatomal sensory loss indicative of L5 or S1 nerve root lesions, which are approximately 95 % of lumbar disc herniations [4].
7. Reflexes of the patellar tendon (L4) and Achilles tendon (S1) conclude the neurologic "overview" to exclude serious neurological pathology (Table 2).

Imaging

Plain radiography should be limited to patients with:
1. Suggestion of systemic disease
2. History of trauma
3. Weight loss
4. Fever
5. History of cancer
6. Age over 50
7. Alcohol, drug abuse, HIV
8. Neural deficit
9. Pain duration >6 weeks [9].

CT and MRI should be reserved for patients with strong clinical suggestion of infection, cancer and neurological pathology. Both CT and MRI are equivalent for detecting spinal stenosis and disc herniation, but MRI is more sensitive for cancer, infection, neural tumours and fracture (bone marrow oedema) [10].

On the other hand these techniques show often "false positive" results: herniated discs are frequently seen especially in older patients who are asymptomatic [11]. In symptomatic individuals with low back pain this may lead to over-diagnosis, dependence on medical care and unnecessary treatment, and even to surgery.

Only in cases with "red flags" are these imaging tests are indicated, but the prevalence of these specific pathologies is low.

Natural History

Prognosis of unspecific low back pain is that about one-third of patients substantially recover within 1 week, two-thirds at 7 weeks [12]. Forty percent suffer recurrences within 6 months. Most of these recurrences are not disabling, but the result is frequently that of a chronic problem with intermittent acute phases. Low back pain is rarely permanently disabling [13].

Nevertheless there is a certain risk of chronicity and on-going research is looking for the identification of patients with acute low back pain who are individuals with high likelihood to become chronic low back pain patients. Certain risk factors can be worked out (Table 3).

Therapy

Non-steroidal anti-inflammatory drugs are effective for symptom relief, the evidence compared to placebo is strong. The same is true for muscle relaxants but with side effects which are drowsiness and sedation. Medication should be taken regularly rather than on an "as needed" basis [14].

Spinal manipulation and physical therapy have limited effects [15], strong evidence shows that bed rest and specific back exercises (strengthening, flexibility, stretching, flexion and extension exercises) are not effective in the acute phase. For most patients the best recommendation is rapid return to their daily activities with neither exercises nor bed rest in the acute phase, but heavy lifting, trunk twisting and vibrating work should be avoided. Back exercises are useful for later preventing recurrences and for treating chronic low back pain [16] (Table 4).

If low back pain becomes chronic, exercise and intensive multi-disciplinary pain

Table 3 Risk factors for LBP (van Tulder 1997)

Risk factors	Occurrence	Chronicity
Individual	Age, physical fitness	Obesity
		Low educational level
		High level of pain and disability
Psychosocial		Distress
	Negative emotions	Depressive mood
	Poor cognitive function	Somatisation
	Pain behaviour	
Occupational	Manual material handling	Job dissatisfaction
	Bending and twisting	Unavailability of light duty on return to work
	Whole body vibration	Heavy lifting work
	Job dissatisfaction	
	Monotonous tasks	
	Poor work relationship	

Table 4 Recommendations for acute LBP [8]

Recommendations – clinical guidelines for acute LBP
1. Re-assure patients
2. Advise patients to stay active
3. Prescribe medication (preferably) at fixed time intervals:
Paracetamol
NSAIDs
Muscle relaxants or weak opioids
4. Discourage bed rest
5. Consider spinal manipulation
6. Do not advise back-specific exercises

treatment have been shown to be effective. Some evidence supports the effectiveness of behaviour therapy, analgesics, antidepressive medication, NSAIDs, "back school" and manipulations.

No evidence was found for steroid injections, traction and lumbar support.

But many commonly used therapies lack sufficient evidence of clinically relevant long-term effects [17].

Acupuncture, spinal manipulation and massage are popular alternative therapies. Systemic reviews have found little positive effect from acupuncture [18], but some support for massage and spinal manipulation [15].

Available data suggests that a combination of medical care with physical therapy may be moderately more effective in reducing pain and disability than is a single method of treatment.

For patients with chronic low back pain intensive exercises improve function and reduce pain [19, 20]. It is however difficult to maintain these exercise regimes for a long period of time.

Antidepressant drug therapy is useful for one-third of patients with low back pain and depression. Conflicting evidence is found for patients without depression [21].

Opioids are also proposed and may have a greater effect on pain and mood than NSAIDs, but they seem not to raise the activity level and cause side-effects such as headache, nausea and constipation.

Referral to multi-disciplinary pain centre may be appropriate for patients with chronic low back pain. These centres combine cognitive behaviour therapy patient education, supervised exercise, selective nerve blocks and other strategies to relieve pain and improve function. Complete relief is unrealistic and therapeutic goals are necessary to be re-focussed to keep the level of function obtained in these centres [4].

Even for effective treatment, the effects are usually small and short term. Many commonly-used therapies lack sufficient evidence for clinically relevant long term effects [17] (Table 5).

Table 5 Recommendations for Chronic LBP [8]

European clinical guidelines for chronic LBP
Recommended:
Cognitive behaviour treatment
Supervised exercise therapy
Brief educational interventions
Multi-disciplinary (biopsychosocial) treatment
Short-term use of NSAID and weak opioids
Consider:
Short courses of manipulation and mobilisation
Antidepressants
Muscle relaxants
Not recommended:
Passive treatment (ultrasound, short wave)
Gabapentin
Invasive treatment

Invasive treatments for chronic low back pain reveal a wide variability of techniques such as facet joint, epidural, trigger point and sclerosant injections.

In randomized trials however they have not clearly improved outcomes, if the patient had no radiculopathy. Radio-frequency ablation of the small nerves of facet joints showed at best a moderate effect which lasted only for 4 weeks [22]. It may have possible benefit in patients with low back pain who respond to placebo-controlled anaesthetic blocks [23].

Other techniques advocated include percutaneous heat or radiofrequency application directly at the disc altering the internal mechanics or innervation. Data supporting their use are lacking Randomized trials showed no effect [24] or a benefit in only a small proportion of highly selected patients [25].

The role of surgery for chronic low back pain is under debate. The most common surgical treatment for persistent low back pain with degenerative changes is spinal fusion. One randomized trial comparing spinal fusion versus a rehabilitation programme showed no difference at 1 year in back pain, function, use of medication, working status and general satisfaction [26].

Another randomized study revealed better results in the level of back pain and improvement of function after 2 years in the group of patients who had been managed with spinal fusion [27]. The study showed no clear benefit of fusion surgery 5 years post-operatively.

The outcome of spinal fusion surgery can be improved for patients with isolated one- or two-level degenerative disc diseases, if patients are carefully selected and only individuals without co-existing psychosocial disorders, distress or other chronic pain are identified [27].

The expectations of the patient about the benefit of surgery should be discussed in advance. In a study of patients scheduled for fusion surgery due to degenerative disc diseases, 90 % indicated as an acceptable outcome: return to some gainful work, no more use of analgesics and a high level of physical function [28]. These expectations are not realistic and patients should be informed that pain reduction will be at about 50 %, recurrent back pain will be common and further activity will be necessary to keep their function level acceptable.

Conclusions and Future Perspectives

Treatment should mainly be distinguished between acute and chronic back pain patients. For both, natural history is favourable and patients need this reassurance. In the case of acute low back pain pharmacologic treatment should be recommended. The patient should know that there is no danger of serious neurological injury, bed rest will not help, and return to daily activity as soon as possible will be the best course.

In cases of chronicity again pharmacological treatment in combination with intensive multidisciplinary exercise and cognitive behaviour therapy is the best choice. The patient should understand that the primary goal of treatment is to maximize function and that some on-going or recurrent back pain is likely but not dangerous.

Imaging like plain radiography should only be performed if there is suspicion of an underlying systemic disease. Advanced imaging can be reserved for potential candidates for surgery. Generally, imaging is of little help due to the poor association between symptoms and morphologic findings. In the absence of severe spinal disease or radiculopathy, surgery should generally be avoided.

On-going research focuses mainly on possible prevention of chronicity of low back pain and identifying sub-groups of patients, for whom specific treatment modalities are helpful. There are numbers of randomized trials and systemic reviews (and epidemiologic studies) regarding the value of specific therapeutic interventions for low back pain treatment, few of which are conclusive.

References

1. Cassidy JD, Carroll LJ, Côté P. The Saskatchewan health and back pain survey. The prevalence of low back pain and related disability in Saskatchewan adults. Spine. 1998;23(17):1860–6.
2. Carragee E, Cohen S. Reliability of LBP history in asymptomatic subjects? The prevalence and incidence of reported back pain correlates with surveillance frequency [abstract]. Proceedings of the 14th Annual Meeting of the North American Spine Society; 2004 Oct 26–30: 216; Chicago. p. 216.
3. Pengel LH, Herbert RD, Maher CG, Refshauge KM. Acute low back pain: systematic review of its prognosis. BMJ. 2003;327(7410):323.
4. Deyo RA, Weinstein JN. Low back pain. N Engl J Med. 2001;344(5):363–70.
5. Feldman DE, Shrier I, Rossignol M, Abenhaim L. Risk factors for the development of low back pain in adolescence. Am J Epidemiol. 2001;154(1):30–6.
6. Deyo RA, Rainville J, Kent DL. What can the history and physical examination tell us about low back pain? JAMA. 1992;268(6):760–5.
7. Vroomen PC, de Krom MC, Knottnerus JA. Diagnostic value of history and physical examination in patients suspected of sciatica due to disc herniation: a systematic review. J Neurol. 1999;246(10):899–906.
8. Koes BW, van Tulder MW, Thomas S. Diagnosis and treatment of low back pain. BMJ. 2006; 332(7555):1430–4.
9. Bigos S, bowyer O, Braen G et al. Acute low back pain problems in adults. Clinical practice guidelines no.14 Rockville, MD.: Adency for Health Care Policy and Research. December 19CPR publication no. 95–0642.
10. Thornbury JR, Fryback DG, Turski PA, Javid MJ, McDonald JV, et al. Disk-caused nerve compression in patients with acute low-back pain: diagnosis with MR, CT myelography, and plain CT. Radiology. 1993;186(3):731–8.
11. Bochen SD, Davos DO, Dina TS, Patronas NJ, Wiesel SW. Abnormal magnetic resonance scans of the lumbar spine in asymptomatic subjects: a prospective investigation. J Bone Joint Surg Am. 1990;72:403–8.
12. Cherkin DC, Deyo RA, Street JH, Barlow W. Predicting poor outcomes for back pain seen in primary care using patients' own criteria. Spine. 1996;21(24):2900–7.
13. Carey TS, Garrett JM, Jackman A, Hadler N. Recurrence and care seeking after acute back pain: results of a long-term follow-up study. North Carolina Back Pain Project. Med Care. 1999;37(2):157–64.
14. Fordyce WE, Brockway JA, Bergman JA, Spengler D. Acute back pain: a control-group comparison of behavioral vs traditional management methods. J Behav Med. 1986;9(2):127–40.
15. Andersson GB, Lucente T, Davis AM, Kappler RE, Lipton JA, Leurgans S. A comparison of osteopathic spinal manipulation with standard care for patients with low back pain. N Engl J Med. 1999; 341(19):1426–31.
16. Lahad A, Malter AD, Berg AO, Deyo RA. The effectiveness of four interventions for the prevention of low back pain. JAMA. 1994;272(16):1286–91.
17. Van Tulder MW, Koes BW. Low back pain: chronic, clinical evidence. London: BMJ; 2006.
18. Van Tulder MW, Ostelo R, Vlaeyen JW, et al. Behavioral treatment for chronic low back pain: a systematic review within the framework of the Cochrane Back Review Group. Spine. 2001;26:270–81.
19. Manniche C, Hesselsøe G, Bentzen L, Christensen I, Lundberg E. Clinical trial of intensive muscle training for chronic low back pain. Lancet. 1988; 2(8626–8627):1473–6.
20. Frost H, Lamb SE, Klaber Moffett JA, Fairbank JC, Moser JS. A fitness programme for patients with chronic low back pain: 2-year follow-up of a randomised controlled trial. Pain. 1998;75(2–3):273–9.
21. Turner JA, Denny MC. Do antidepressant medication relieve chronic low back pain? J Fam Pract. 1993;37:545–50.
22. Van Kleef M, Barendse GA, Kessels A, Voets HM, et al. Randomized trial of radiofrequency lumbar facet denervation for chronic low back pain. Spine. 1999;24:1937–42.
23. Dreyfuss P, Halbrook B, Pauza K, Joshi A, et al. Efficacy and validity of radiofrequency neurotomy for chronic lumbar zygapophysial joint pain. Spine. 2000;25:1270–7.
24. Barendse GA, van Den Berg SG, Kessels AH, Weber WE, van Kleef M. Randomized controlled trial of percutaneous intradiscal radiofrequency thermocoagulation for chronic discogenic back pain: lack of effect from a 90 s 70° lesion. Spine. 2001;26:287–92.
25. Pauza KJ, Howell S, Dreyfuss P, Peloza JH, Dawson K, Bogduk N. A randomized, placebo-controlled trial of intradiscal electrothermal therapy for the treatment of discogenic low back pain. Spine J. 2004; 4(1):27–35.

26. Ivar Brok J, Sorenson R, Friis A, et al. Randomized clinical trial for lumbar instrumented fusion and cognitive intervention and exercises in patients with chronic low back pain and discs degeneration. Spine. 2003;28:1913–21.

27. Fritzell P, Hägg O, Wessberg P, Nordwall A, Swedish Lumbar Spine Study Group. 2001 Volvo Award Winner in Clinical Studies: lumbar fusion versus nonsurgical treatment for chronic low back pain: a multicenter randomized controlled trial from the Swedish lumbar spine study group. Spine. 2001;26:2521–32.

28. Carragee E, Alamin T. A prospective assessment of patient expectations and statisfaction in spinal fusion surgery [abstract]. Proceedings of the 30th Annual meeting of the International Society for the study of the lumbar spine; 2003 May 13–17; Vancouver.

Treatment of the Aging Spine

Max Aebi

Contents

Previously published in G. Bentley (ed.), European Instructional Lectures, European Instructional Lectures 13, DOI 10.1007/978-3-642-36149-4_11, © EFORT 2013

M. Aebi
MEM Research Center, University of Bern and Orthopaedic Department, Hirslanden-Salem Hospital, Bern, Switzerland
e-mail: max.aebi@MEMcenter.unibe.ch

Keywords
Aging • Osteoporosis • Spine • Spine and I.V. disc degeneration

Introduction

The aging of the population in the industrialised countries appears to be a non-reversible phenomenon. Increasing life expectancy, due in a great part to the improvement of healthcare, combined with a drastic decrease in birth rate, has led to this situation [41]. The world demographic situation has shifted from a pattern of high birth rates and high mortality rates to one of low birth rates and delayed mortality [23, 41]. In Europe, the proportion of subjects over 65 was 10.8 % in 1950, 14 % in 1970, 19.1 % in 1995 and is projected by some sources at 30.1 % in 2025 and 42.2 % in 2050 [20]. The proportion of subjects over 75 has grown from 2.7 % in 1950 to 5.2 % in 1995 and is projected at 9.1 % in 2025 and 14.6 % in 2050 [20]. However, this trend is not limited to industrialised countries: The developing countries' share of the world's population above 65 is projected to increase from 59 % to 71 %. The global consequences of this distortion of the age pyramid on healthcare development, access and costs are huge [29]. For instance approximately 59 % of US residents over 65 are affected by osteoarthritis, which is the main cause of disability. Back and neck pain are amongst the most frequently encountered complaints of all people and the nature of the spine renders those problems highly complex to investigate and to treat.

Ostoporosis

Furthermore, osteoporotic compression fractures of vertebral bodies is another increasing problem due to aging of the Western population as well as the Japanese and Chinese population, with an increasing number of severely osteoporotic subjects, mostly women. Recent studies have shown that osteoporotic vertebral fractures are associated with an increased risk of mortality and a decreased quality of life. The prevalence in those fractures is around 39 % in subjects over 65 years (National Center for chronic disease prevention, [31]).

Spinal and I.V. Disc Degeneration

Degeneration of the spinal structures induces interactive alterations at many levels: bones, discs, facet joints, ligaments. Some of these degenerative lesions can be responsible for compressive damage to the neural elements as in the case of disc herniations or spinal stenosis.

Disc degeneration begins when the balance between synthesis and degradation of the matrix is disrupted; i. e., at the microscopic level, disc degeneration includes a net loss of water as a consequence of a breakdown of proteoglycans in so-called short chains, which are unable to bind water [30, 35]. Furthermore, there is disruption of collagen fibre organisation, specifically in the annulus, and increased levels of proteolytic enzymes. Disc degeneration can be seen in 20 year-old people in about 16 %, whereas this phenomenon is found in 98 % in 70 year-old people and older [8, 9] (Fig. 1).

Women reach the same level of degeneration about 10 years later than men (Fig. 1). In the aging of the spine there is a predetermined cell viability (endogenous = genetic) and/or decreasing cellular activity in the disc over the years due to exposure of the disc to repetitive mechanical loads [2, 35]. This leads to a loss of extracellular matrix with proteoglycans degrading and decreased capability to bind water. The collagen organisation is dissociated which leads to a loss of the height of the disc. This is always combined with a secondary deterioration of the facet joints, ligaments and muscles. Through this process, the boundaries between the annulus and nucleus are less distinct and the collagen is increasing in the nucleus and replacing the proteoglycans. With that we see concentric fissuring at radial tears which weakens the disc, starting in the third and fourth decade of life. However, there are substantial differences in this whole cascade of events. These changes have clearly biomechanical consequences for the motion segment [2].

The role of vascularisation in the aging spine is most crucial: The nutritional supply of the cells in the disc diminishes because the adjacent vertebral end-plate permeability is decreasing, leading to a blood supply decrease with a secondary tissue breakdown, which starts in the nucleus, and a mechanical impact on the cells (sensitive to mechanical sickness) which leads to a qualitative and quantitative modulation of the matrix proteins [10, 19, 43]. The variation of the proteoglycan content as well as the water content is age-dependent and runs in parallel: more degradation of the proteoglycans, less water content and higher probability of disintegration of the disc (Fig. 2).

The aging of the spine is characterised by two major parallel, however (at least at the beginning), independent processes, which lead to different clinical pictures:

1. The reduction of bone mineral density, hence bone mass.
2. The development of degenerative changes of the discoligamentous complex (discs, ligaments, facet joint capsules and facet joints) with consequences of instability, deformity and narrowing of the spinal canal and the exit of the nerve roots (spinal and foraminal stenosis) with secondary neurological problems such as

Fig. 1 The prevalence of macroscopic disc degeneration based on autopsies by age for men and women. The women reach the same level of degeneration about a decade later than the men. (based on data from the study of Heine (8a), cited from Battié MC et al. Spine 2004; 29, Nr. 23 (8)

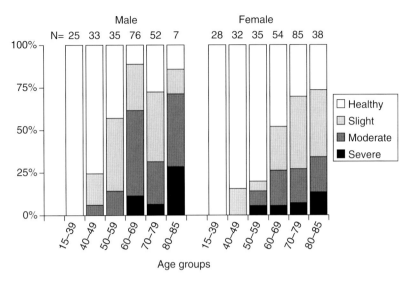

Aging of the spine

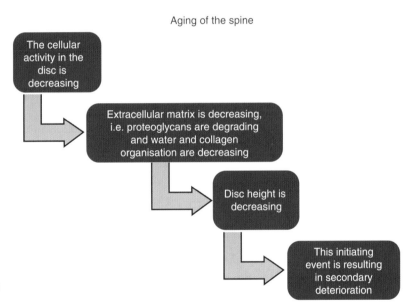

Fig. 2 Aging of the spine – cascade of the intervertebral degeneration (see text)

myelopathy, cauda equina and radicular syndromes and disability. Hence, degeneration alone, or in combination with bone mass reduction by osteoporosis and/or metastatic tumour involvement, contributes – to a different degree – to the development of a variety of lesions and often to a number of painful and invalidating disorders.

From this short introduction it can be concluded that Orthopaedic surgeons and musculoskeletal specialists as well as dedicated spine specialists are going to face huge problems in treating the numbers of patients affected by diseases which are typical for the aging of the musculoskeletal system.

Typical Disorders of the Aging Spine

Typical disorders of the aging spine are:
- Degenerative disease of the disc(s), *osteochondrosis* and *disc prolapse*
- *Degenerative disease of the facet joints* with joint incongruences and arthritis, secondary instability and deformity.
- Degenerative *spondylolisthesis* with or without spinal stenosis and instability.
- *Spinal stenosis*, foraminal stenosis due to a narrowing of the spinal canal following hypertrophy of the ligamentum flavum and the joint capsules and the facet joint by itself.
- *Spinal deformities*: Scoliosis and/or kyphosis and concomitant secondary instability.
- *Osteoporosis* with vertebral compression fractures (VCF) alone or in combination with degenerative defects.
- *Pathological fractures* of the vertebrae due to *metastatic* disease.
- *Infection* of the spine, spondylodiscitis and spondylitis in the elderly.

Disc Degeneration, Osteochondrosis, Disc Herniation

Symptomatic, isolated or multi-level disc degeneration can be seen in the lumbar spine as well as in the cervical spine [13]. The clinically most relevant disc degeneration with subchondral oedema, possible secondary spondylolisthesis and/or translational, rotatory dislocation and consecutive spinal deformity is most frequently seen in the lumbar spine at the level of L3/4 > L2/3 > L4/5 > L1/2. The asymmetrical degeneration may lead to a disc herniation with major or mass dislocation of whole disc fragments (annulus and nucleus parts) leading usually to at least a major neurological complication, such as root compression or cauda compression

with significant radicular pain and/or sensomotor deficit.

This pathology can occur in the context of previous surgery in the lower lumbar spine which led to a fusion or at least poorly mobile spinal segment with an overload and stress arising in the adjacent superior or inferior segment with a rapid degeneration of the disc with potential instability, spinal stenosis and possible extrusion of major disc fragments. This can occur as an acute event in almost all those decompressions of the segment and a stabilisation may become necessary [7, 16, 26].

Asymmetrical degeneration of the disc may lead to a further deterioration of adjacent motion segments and may end with a progressive degenerative scoliosis [4], which may need surgical treatment (see below).

Sometimes it is difficult to differentiate the subchondral bony damage from osteoporotic compression fractures. The precise history and clinical examination may lead to a diagnosis as well as STIR sequences of the MRI, CT-Scan and/or bone scintigraphy.

Symptomatic isolated or multi-level disc degeneration can be seen in the lumbar spine as well as in the cervical spine. This disc degeneration with osteochondrosis and sometimes significant subchondral oedema, as expression of inflammation, and occasionally combined with significant disc protrusion, can occur in elderly people primarily without relevant deformity or instability. This degeneration can start in younger age and can be asymptomatic or can be combined with intermittent back pain affecting people sometimes over years and even decades [13].

For some reason, mostly mechanical, disc degeneration can aggravate and become highly symptomatic, specifically when there is a combination with a segmental instability and osteochondritis (Fig. 3). Since these discs are severely degenerated and dehydrated over many years, a herniation consists almost always of a big, combined annulus and fibrotic nucleus sequestrum. The consequence of this disc degeneration may be a secondary deformity, with typical translatory dislocation of vertebrae in

Fig. 3 Multi-level
degenerated discs with
secondary flat back and
degenerative scoliosis,
spinal stenosis and
mechanical instability in
extension at L2/3 (air
inclusion in the disc)

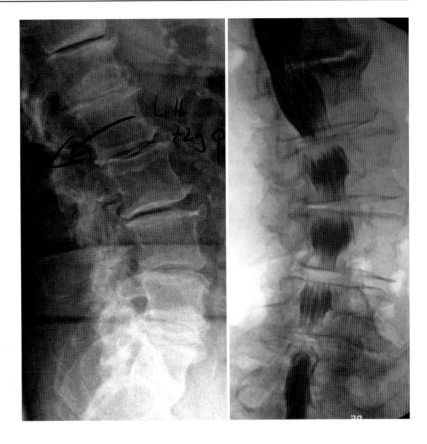

a segment or several segments, rotation and scoliosis and/or kyphoscoliosis [4, 13]. It is also
possible that disc degeneration and facet joint
arthritis can lead to a degenerative spondylolisthesis [27, 32, 38]. As long as the disc degeneration is isolated to one or two or three levels
without a major deformity, a typical axial "instability" pain occurs, mostly in rotational movements or lifting when upright or when turning
in bed during sleep. If conservative treatment
with isometric re-inforcement exercises of the
abdominal and paravertebral muscles is not
successful, surgery may be necessary [32, 33,
37, 39, 42].

There are several surgical options available:
1. Minimally invasive, retroperitoneal anterior,
2. Posterior, as well as
3. Far lateral approach surgery as well as
   combinations.

Anterior surgery with stand-alone cages
(ALIF), fixed with screws is straight forward in
not too adipose patients, and is quite feasible

from L3/4, L4/5 and L5/S1, i. e. in the lower
lumbar spine. In cases where the patient has had
abdominal surgery or is adipose, it is advisable
not to do an anterior surgery, but rather
a posterior surgery with pedicle fixation and
PLIF or TLIF procedure.

In recent years, specifically in elderly people
who are frail and where surgery is only an option
if everything else does not work, surgery should
be limited to a minimum: little blood loss and
little surgical trauma and short anaesthesia time.
A far lateral approach (XLIF) may fulfil these
requirements [6, 21, 25, 34]. However, to avoid
posterior surgery, stand-alone cages need to be
used which can be fixed either by an additional
plate or with the plate incorporated with the cage
(Fig. 4).

However, ALIF and XLIF surgery is contra-
indicated in osteoporotic bone, because there is
a high probability that the cages will sink into the
vertebral bodies [24, 25]. In these cases it is
sometimes necessary to do a posterior pedicle

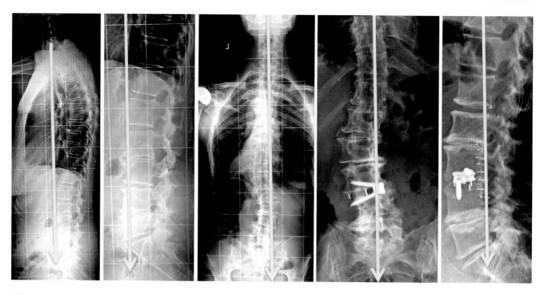

Fig. 4 68 year-old female patient with degenerative sco-liosis and severe motion and activity dependent left leg pain and blocking back pain due to a rapidly progressing osteochondritis and total disc destruction with secondary instability at L3/4 with relatively rigid adjacent segments above and below. Far lateral approach and isolated stabi-lization and partial correction of the segment

screw fixation with cement re-inforcement and even to fill the intervertebral space after remov-ing the disc with cement, i. e., a so-called discoplasty. In some cases where the disc height is significantly reduced and there is significant concomitant facet joint arthritis which partici-pates in the pain generation and if the patient is old with possibly reduced life expectancy and with little demand for physical activity, an interlaminar microsurgical decompression with resection of flavum, capsule and partial arthrectomy, combined with a translaminar facet screw fixation may be sufficient (Fig. 5). This is an atraumatic surgery suitable for very elderly patients with high morbidity and reduced life expectancy and little demand for physical activity, with little blood loss and with one of the major purposes – to control pain – fulfilled by immobilising the facet joints with a screw each.

Spinal Stenosis in the Elderly

Spinal stenosis is a very common condition in the elderly and we have to differentiate between central stenosis, lateral or root canal stenosis, a combination of those two and a combination with or without degenerative spondylolisthesis. There are of course other conditions like the Paget's disease, then degenerative disease, which may cause spinal stenosis with or without neurological complications. There is also second-ary spinal stenosis due to fracture, mostly osteo-porotic fracture, and due to tumour compression of the spinal canal, mostly metastatic disease. Finally, there is iatrogenic stenosis, which can occur as a late result after any spinal surgery at any age. In these cases, spinal stenosis may occur as so-called adjacent segment problem after fusion surgery or be a part of a degenerative deformity (scoliosis and kyphosis) [40].

In most cases, spinal stenosis is due to degen-erative changes and/or a pre-existing narrow canal. These changes can lead to symptoms, how-ever, it must be stressed that so-called stenotic images sometimes are present on imaging studies in a number of symptom-free individuals and that the relationship between degenerative lesions, importance of abnormal images and complaints is still unclear. Lumbar stenosis with a claudication symptomatology is also

Fig. 5 79 year-old
polymorbid, adipous
female patient with
degenerative scoliosis and
spinal stenosis. Because of
the medical risks a very
limited microsurgical
decompression and
localized stabilization at
the apex of the curve has
been done

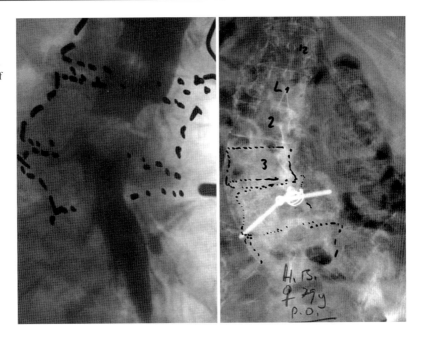

a common reason for decompressive surgery and/or fusion. The investigation of stenotic symptoms should be extremely careful and thorough and should include a choice of technical examinations including vascular investigation. This is of utmost importance, especially if a surgical action is considered, to avoid disappointing results [28].

Surgical management of spinal stenosis can consist of purely decompressive surgery: Here different techniques are available, like classical laminectomy, laminotomy, partial laminectomy, resection of ligamentum flavum and scar tissue, simple foraminal decompression. In recent years it has been suggested in some cases to use a so-called interspinous process distraction. The idea is that with this distraction the foramina are opened and the canal is widened and indirectly decompressed [28, 33]. The interspinous process distraction also unloads the discs as well as the facet joints. The best patients who are fit for this surgery are those with increasing symptoms when doing lumbar extension movements. There is still a quite significant debate whether a decompression needs to be accompanied by instrumentation [28, 33]. Depending on the osteophyte formations in the anterior column as well as the osteoarthritis of the facet joints and in the absence of any "instability", such as

degenerative spondylolisthesis, simple decompression without instrumentation may be sufficient. If there is a need for significant resection of hypertrophic facet joint parts to decompress the dural sac as well as the exiting roots, it may be necessary to stabilise the segment either by simple translaminar/transarticular screw fixation (Fig. 5). This is a less rigid fixation than the alternative with pedicle fixation. The risk of the pedicle fixation in spinal stenosis without any deformity and obvious instability is to generate a rigid spine section with a relevant impact on the adjacent segments, including the discs as well as the vertebral bodies [7, 12, 16, 17, 36]. This increases the risk of fatigue fractures in these vertebral bodies and a disruption of the posterior ligament complex as an expression of the aging of ligaments and muscles (Fig. 6a).

Obviously, in a severely degenerated cervical spine with spinal stenosis, we may deal with compression of the cord with consecutive myelopathy and/or root compression. The spinal stenosis of the cervical spine often goes together with a deformity usually in kyphosis and sometimes in little scoliotic deformity in the frontal plane. In case there is relevant deformity of the cervical spine combined with a narrow spinal canal, diagnostic traction may be applied to

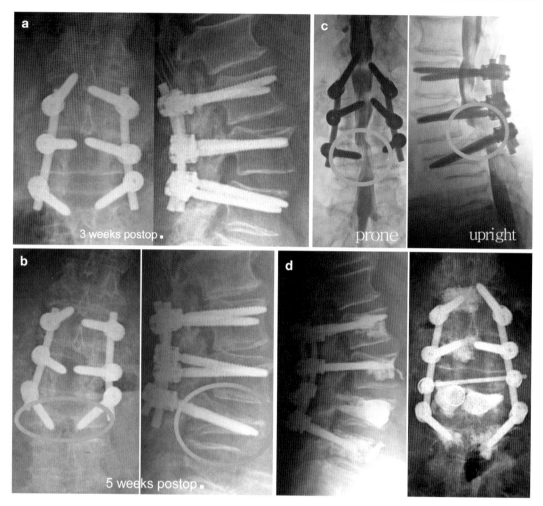

Fig. 6 72 year-old female patient of 101 kg with spinal stenosis at L2/3 and L3/4, here with degenerative spondylosithesis, osteoporosis and massive claudication symptomatology as well as back pain. **a**) She was operated with wide decompression and pedicular stabilization. **b**) For 5 weeks she did very well, then suddenly pain in the back and irradiating into the legs: **c**) compression fracture of L4 with secondary instability in the functional myelogram (supine and upright position) **d**) Reoperation with Fixation from L2 to L5 with cement enhancement of the screws and kyphoplasty with stents of the fracture vertebra L4

explore how far the deformity can be reduced and the cervical spine can be re-aligned. In cases where this is possible, surgery may be done under traction in the reduced position. In this case there is no manipulation to achieve reduction necessary during the surgery but only the decompressive, and if necessary, the stabilisation part.

Again, also in the cervical spine, there are different ways to address the spinal stenosis. It can be done by an anterior surgery, either by multi-level discectomy and resection of the posterior inferior and superior corner of the adjacent vertebra to do a unisegmental anterior decompression. In cases where the compression of the spinal cord is mainly due to disc on several levels, then this technique can be applied on each individual level by maintaining the main part of the vertebral body. The latter is helpful to place intervertebral spacers and to restore the cervical lordosis. In case there is more compression due to relevant osteophytes, extension of the compression beyond the disc space and in case there is concomitant OPLL, one or even two level vertebrectomies may be necessary with an anterior reconstruction with (expandable or rigid) cages or bony struts (fibula or iliac crest) and plate fixation. If this stabilisation seems to be insufficient and specifically is not really restoring lordosis, a combined posterior fixation with tension-banding and re-aligning of the cervical spine in lordosis may be necessary. There is of course the option left of posterior surgery through laminectomy, laminotomy on several levels or laminoplasty. In case there is insufficient physiological lordosis (in fact kyphosis), then a simultaneous fixation of the decompressed cervical spine along with the decompression may be necessary. In this case, today, most of the time lateral mass screws combined with rod systems is the technique of choice. This surgery is combined with a posterolateral fusion, either by bone substitutes or with cancellous bone from the iliac crest. Since the cervical spine surgery is not as invasive as the lumbar spine surgery, also elderly people with significant co-morbidities can be treated specifically by anterior surgery under neuromonitoring, since there is relatively little blood loss to be expected and the surgical trauma is more or less "local", not involving the whole homeostasis of the body as in a surgery of the lumbar spine in prone position over longer time period.

Degenerative Spondylolisthesis

Degenerative spondylolisthesis occurs usually at the level of L4/5, less frequently at the level of L3/4 and L5/S1. Very often, this degenerative spondylolisthesis is combined with spinal stenosis. The spondylolisthesis is a consequence of a disc degeneration and insufficiency of the facet joints to maintain the stability of the segment. In these cases very often the facet joint effusion can be demonstrated, as well as air inclusion in the disc as well as in the facet joints. The spondylolisthesis can also be combined with a facet joint synovial cyst, which may add to the compressive effect of the spondylolisthesis

with a secondary narrowing of the spinal canal. It is still debated whether this pathology needs to be decompressed and stabilised or whether simple decompression is sufficient [1, 27, 32]. If instability can be demonstrated in functional X-rays with maximal bending and maximal extension over a hypomotion of the lumbar spine in supine position and accompanying low back pain in combination with irradiation into the legs, a stabilisation may well be indicated. Here again, there is a debate whether this should be a pedicle fixation alone or in combination with an interbody fusion, like PLIF or TLIF [9, 27, 32, 37, 42].

According to the guidelines of NASS [27], there is very little evidence, whether a spondylolisthesis is to be operated with decompression alone, in combination with fusion with or without implant (screws and cages) and whether a reduction is necessary or not.

Degenerative Deformity (Scoliosis and/or Kyphosis)

The degenerative deformity mainly of the lumbar spine and the thoracolumbar spine is a typical disease of the elderly, specifically women. This is basically a disc disease with the whole cascade described before: disc degeneration as the initial starting point, usually unilateral or asymmetrical, incongruence of the facet joints with subluxation and rotatory deformity, which appears in the AP-view as a translational dislocation, mostly at the level of L2/3 or L3/4 [4]. The deformity in the frontal plane (scoliosis) is practically always combined with a lumbar kyphosis, and this deformity very frequently is combined with recessal or foraminal stenosis, occasionally appearing as a so-called dynamic stenosis, only being clinically relevant when the patient is in upright position or in a certain position while lying or sitting (de novo scoliosis) [4]. The clinical appearance of the degenerative deformity is pain, mostly back pain, with frequent irradiation into the legs, be it a so-called pseudoradicular irradiation or as a real radicular irradiation and claudication symptomatology. Therefore, the clinical problem to be addressed is the progressing deformity, the instability of one or several segments, the neurocompression in the spinal canal, be it centrally or laterally, and very frequently the combination with osteoporosis. These patients are usually unbalanced, not only in the frontal plane but more importantly in the sagittal plane. There is very little substantial non-surgical treatment for these patients. Occasionally, a brace can be tried and a walker or canes may be used to maintain balance.

These patients are generally much better while walking in water, since the water carries them by the buoyant force of the water. The only efficient treatment, however, although tainted by complications and relevant risks, is the surgical treatment.

Surgical treatment is almost always indicated when progression of the curve can be demonstrated over time, and in case of relevant central, recessal and/or foraminal stenosis with significant radicular pain and/or neurological deficit. There is not only a segmental instability, visible in many of these deformities, but there is also a global instability of the spine which means that the spine is collapsing along the sagittal axis which increases the deformity when upright and decreases the deformity when the patient is prone [4].

In general, this surgery is demanding, not only for the patient but also for the surgeon. Since many of these patients are beyond 65 and usually have several risk factors due to polymorbidity, such a surgery needs to be well prepared and thoroughly discussed with the patient and the family, also pointing out risks and consequences in further life. The patients have to understand, together with their family, that such a surgery could finally end up lethally. For this exact reason, a lot has been done in the last few years to facilitate and to reduce the risk of this surgery for these elderly patients. One of the key issues is the blood loss and therefore there are different techniques to be applied to reduce the blood loss, to return the blood with cell saver and to lower the blood pressure as far as possible. Also the staging of the incision during a surgical procedure from the back can help to diminish the blood loss [37],

i.e., the parts of the spine are opened portion by portion, then instrumented and finally corrected and stabilised. This reduces the exposure field of the wound and therefore the potential blood loss. In most of these degenerative scoliosis or deformities, if they need surgery, a pedicle fixation is indicated to develop the power to correct to a certain degree the deformity, specifically in the sagittal plane.

Whether cages need to be placed intervertebrally in these elderly people, usually with concomitant osteoporosis, is certainly a question of debate. By correct restoration of the lordosis and establishing the plumb-line out of C7 behind the hip joint, the force transmission goes through the posterior elements and therefore a disc anterior support with cage may not be necessary. To avoid cage surgery in these elderly patients is a major element to reduce blood loss and surgical risk. As a result, depending on the problem of the patient, the demands of these patients and of course the co-morbidities, different surgical options in terms of invasiveness may be applicable. Again, in recent years, the application of the far lateral trans-psoas approach with selected correction of the most severely involved segments may be a solution to diminish the surgical trauma in these frail patients (Fig. 4) [6, 14, 15, 36].

Vertebral Compression Fractures

In recent years different options have been proposed to treat vertebral compression fractures in elderly people and there is still continuous controversy about these different methodologies. Essentially, several technologies have been developed to augment compressed vertebrae as a consequence of osteoporotic fractures. The simplest one is the so-called vertebroplasty, where transpedicular injection of cement into a fractured vertebral body can stabilise this vertebral body. There is, however no relevant potential to reduce a fracture with this technique, except by positioning of the patient. There are several risks involved in this treatment and there is still an on-going debate whether in randomised clinical trials the surgical augmentation really has a benefit over conservative treatment of these fractures [11, 22]. The major risk of this treatment is cement leak, most relevantly leak of cement into the spinal canal through the posterior wall, less problematically leak to the side or to the front, as long as it is only a small amount of cement. The second relevant risk is that cement can go into the venous sinuses of the vertebral body and from there into the venous system with cement thrombosis and/or embolism in the lung [19]. There has been significant progress in cement technology to diminish cement risk to a minimum. Performance of vertebroplasty includes a third risk, which is the placement of the working tubes through the pedicle into the vertebral body. Obviously, there is the risk that this tube can be placed into the spinal canal or outside the pedicle into the lateral paravertebral area with vascular damage. Just as in pedicle screw placement, however, with today's X-ray technology, percutaneous placement of a cannula into a pedicle has become a standard procedure and it should not be a major obstacle to do this procedure when adhering to the proper recommendations of the technique. The pedicle projection has to be visualized carefully in the AP-view and the guiding K-wire has to be placed in a way that it is projected completely within the oval contour of the pedicle in the frontal plane. The K-wire is slightly convergent towards the mid-line and it can cross the inner wall of the pedicle projection contour when at this point in the lateral view the K-wire tip is already in the vertebral body. Therefore, it is important to observe the forward drilling K-wire in the pedicle projection in the AP-view by checking quickly at each step the lateral view to understand the progress of the tip in the depths of the vertebral body. Once the K-wire is placed properly, the Jamshidi needle or an analogue instrument can be introduced over the K-wire and progressed into the vertebral body. This opens the pedicle for the working tube, which is then introduced after removing the Jamshidi needle. Once the working cannula is positioned properly into the posterior one third of body, the vertebral body can be drilled in preparation of the seat for the balloon

catheter or the cement applicator (in case of simple vertebroplasty). Through this working channel also biopsies can be taken. In case of an additional kyphoplasty, the balloon catheter can be driven into the working cannula and the balloon can be placed in the prepared seat in the vertebral body. The same is true for the balloon catheter, which is armed with a stent, which then is inflated by the balloon and expanded as vertebral body supporter and partial corrector of the compression fracture (Fig. 6d). It is obvious that with the simple vertebroplasty there is almost no correction which can be done directly with the cement. In an early stage of fractures with the kyphoplasty balloon as well as the kyphoplasty balloon combined with a stent, a certain reduction of the impressed end-plate can sometimes be acheived. The introduction of the balloon kyphoplasty and stent kyphoplasty technology has made this procedure of cement augmentation safer. According to some meta-analysis, the morbidity as well as the mortality and the cement complications are significantly lower with kyphoplasty procedure compared to the simple vertebroplasty [19]. The augmentation technology, however, has failed until today to prove superior to conservative treatment in randomised clinical trials [11, 22]; however, there are several flaws in these prospective trials which are basically contradictory to the everyday clinical experience [5]. From prospective case series it has been learned, that this augmentation surgery is very beneficial and successful for patients in severe pain in combination with vertebral body compression fractures. The indication for such augmentation surgery should be primarily pain in still active fractures, i. e., fractures, which are not healed and are represented in the so-called STIR sequences in the MRI as white vertebrae. Usually, the concept is to apply an augmentation surgery not before 6 weeks after the fracture, with all the correct attempts of conservative treatment.

The second benefit, namely the correction of the vertebral body wedge shape and indirect correction of a secondary kyphosis, is less well supported. However, if there are several fractures with wedge deformity of vertebral bodies, it can lead to a significant kyphosis with a significant disturbance of the sagittal balance, which is detrimental in a long term for an elderly patient. In such cases, the surgical treatment with augmentation of the vertebral body to avoid further progression of kyphosis may be extremely beneficial and important for the patient (Fig. 7).

Other Typical Disorders of the Spine in Elderly Patients

As the treatment options for cancer pathology are getting more and more sophisticated with an increase of survival time, there is also a higher probability that elderly patients develop metastases in the spine [3]. Many of those metastases, due to chemotherapy and local irradiation, can be managed today without surgical treatment. However, there are still patients left with significant pain due to metastatic pathological fractures of the spine or compression of the spinal canal due to tumour expansion into the spinal canal. The most frequent tumours are metastasis of breast cancer in women and prostate cancer in men as well as the multiple myeloma disease of the spine [3].

With today's available minimally- invasive technology, there is often a combination possible of so-called augmentation technologies described above with less invasive stabilisation technology, as palliative procedures in this kind of elderly patients who suffer from the consequences of spinal metastasis.

Spinal infections in elderly people are again getting more frequent, too. The spondylodiscitis

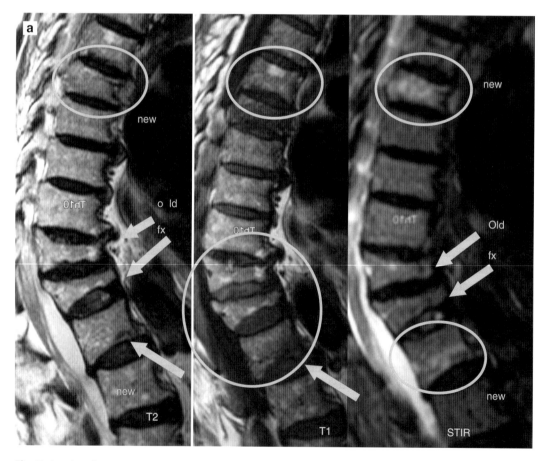

Fig. 7 (continued)

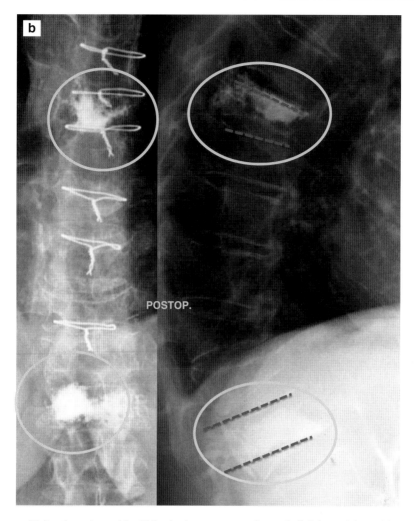

Fig. 7 82 year-old female patient with old kyphosing osteoporotic fractures at Th 11 and Th10 and new fractures at Th 5 and Th12 (6a) with the tendency to collaps in compression and slightly wedging. This spine does not tolerate further kyphosis and the pending collaps needs to be stopped by kyphoplasty at Th 5 and Th12. (6b)

and the spondylitis can be quite a destructive disease with an interruption of the anterior column and secondary kyphosis. The early stage of spondylodiscitis can be treated with antibiotics and partial immobilisation. The indication for surgical treatment is unrelieved pain in spite of proper pain medication, persistent high infection parameters in the blood (CRP, blood sedimentation rate, leucocytes) and increasing secondary deformity and neurological deficit. The procedures are very similar as for tumour surgery. The risks of surgery in frail elderly patients with an infection of the spine, which is mostly a secondary infection of an infection somewhere else in the body (bladder, lungs, lower limbs, skin), is high for septic complications and surgery should only be considered when the above-mentioned criteria are fulfilled.

Summary

Spinal disorders in elderly and usually frail patients with polymorbidity have become a major challenge in spinal surgery. It is not only a major challenge in terms of technical and surgical demands, but also a major challenge in terms of increasing numbers of these patients and the consequences for the treatment. The medical infrastructures are heavily loaded by these pathologies and an interdisciplinary approach to these patients is unavoidable. More and more the surgeon plays here the role of a highly specialised consultant for the specific spinal problem, which needs to be treated in the context of the whole medical care. Therefore, complex spinal problems in elderly patients belong in major medical centres to make sure that these cases can be handled together in an interdisciplinary team.

References

1. Abdu WA, Lurie JD, Spratt KF, et al. Degenerative spondylolisthesis: does fusion method influence outcome? Four-year results of the spine patient outcomes research. Spine. 2009;34(21):2351–60.
2. Adams MA, Roughley PJ. What is intervertebral disc degeneration, and what causes It? Spine. 2006;31 (18):2151–61.
3. Aebi M. Spinal metastasis in the elderly. Eur Spine J. 2003;12 Suppl 2:202–13.
4. Aebi M. The adult scoliosis. Eur Spine J. 2005;14(10):925–48.
5. Aebi M. Vertebroplasty: about sense and nonsense of uncontrolled "controlled randomized prospective trials". Eur Spine J. 2009;18(9):1247–8.
6. Anand N, Baron EM. Minimally invasive approaches for the correction of adult spinal deformity. Eur Spine J. 2013;22 Suppl 2:S232–241.
7. Anandjiwala J, Seo JY, Ha KY, Oh IS, Shin DC. Adjacent segment degeneration after instrumented posterolateral lumbar fusion: a prospective cohort study with a minimum five-year follow-up. Eur Spine J. 2011;20(11):1951–60.
8. Battié MC, Videman T, Parent E. Lumbar disc degeneration: epidemiology and genetic influences. Spine. 2004;29(23):2679–2690. (8a. Heine J. Ueber die arthritis deformans. Virch Arch Pathol Anat. 1926;260:521–663. Cited 8).
9. Battié MC, Videman T, Levälahti E, Gill K, Kaprio J. Genetic and environmental effects on disc degeneration by phenotype and spinal level: a multivariate twin study. Spine. 2008;33(25):2801–8.
10. Bibby SR, Jones DA, Ripley RM, Urban JP. Metabolism of the intervertebral disc: effects of low levels of oxygen, glucose, and pH on rates of energy metabolism of bovine nucleus pulposus cells. Spine. 2005;30(5):487–96.
11. Buchbinder R, et al. A randomized trial of vertebroplasty for painful osteoporotic vertebral fractures. N Engl J Med. 2009;361(6):557–68.
12. Chen BL, Wei FX, Ueyama K, Xie DH, Sannohe A, Liu SY. Adjacent segment degeneration after single-segment PLIF: the risk factor for degeneration and its impact on clinical outcomes. Eur Spine J. 2011;20(11):1946–50.
13. Cheung KM, Samartzis D, Karppinen J, et al. Are "patterns" of lumbar disc degeneration associated with low back pain?: new insights based on skipped level disc pathology (SLDD). Spine. 2012;37(7): E430–8.
14. Cho KJ, Suk SI, Park SR, Kim JH, Choi SW, Yoon YH, Won MH. Arthrodesis to L5 versus S1 in long instrumentation and fusion for degenerative lumbar scoliosis. Eur Spine J. 2009;18(4):531–7.
15. Crawford CH 3rd, Carreon LY, Bridwell KH et al. Long fusions to the sacrum in elderly patients with spinal deformity. Eur Spine J. 2012;21(11): 2165–2169.
16. Ekman P, Möller H, Shalabi A, Yu YX, Hedlund R. A prospective randomised study on the long-term effect of lumbar fusion on adjacent disc degeneration. Eur Spine J. 2009;18(8):1175–86.
17. Harding IJ, Charosky S, Vialle R, Chopin DH. Lumbar disc degeneration below a long arthrodesis (performed for scoliosis in adults) to L4 or L5. Eur Spine J. 2008;17(2):250–4.
18. Horner HA, Urban JP. Volvo Award Winner in Basic Science Studies: effect of nutrient supply on the viability of cells from the nucleus pulposus of the intervertebral disc. Spine. 2001;26(23):2543–9.
19. Hulme PA, Krebs J, Ferguson SJ, Berlenmann U. Vertebroplasty and Kyphoplasty: a systematic review of 69 clinical studies. Spine. 2006;36(17):1983–2001.
20. IIASA/ERD database 2002, International Institute for Applied Systems Analysis, Laxenburg, Austria. www.IIASA.ac.at/research/ERD/. Cited 27th Apr 2003.
21. Isaacs RE, Hyde I, Goodrich JA, et al. A prospective, nonrandomized, multicenter evaluation of extreme lateral interbody fusion for the treatment of adult degenerative scoliosis: perioperative outcomes and complications. Spine. 2010;35(26 Suppl):S322–33.
22. Kallmes DF, et al. A randomized controlled trial of vertebroplasty for osteoporotic spine fractures. N Engl J Med. 2009;361(6):569–79.
23. Kinsella K, Velkoff V. An aging world. U.S. Census Bureau. Washington, DC: U.S. Government Printing Office, series p95/01-1; 2001.
24. Labrom RD, Tan JS, Reilly CW, et al. The effect of interbody cage positioning on lumbosacral vertebral endplate failure in compression. Spine. 2005;30(19): E556–61.
25. Le TV, Baaj AA, Dakwar E, et al. Subsidence of polyetheretherketone intervertebral cages in minimally invasive lateral retroperitoneal transpsoas lumbar interbody fusion. Spine. 2012;37(14):1268–73.

26. Lee CS, Hwang CJ, Lee SW, Ahn YJ, Kim YT, Lee DH, Lee MY. Risk factors for adjacent segment disease after lumbar fusion. Eur Spine J. 2009;18(11):1637–43.

27. NASS edvidence-based clinical guidelines on diagnosis and treatment of degenerative lumbar spondylolisthesis 2008.

28. NASS edvidence-based clinical guidelines on diagnosis and treatment of spinal stenosis 2009.

29. National Center for Chronic Disease Prevention and Health Promotion, CDC. Chronic disease notes and reports, special focus healthy aging 12.3. 1999.

30. Ohshima H, Urban JP. The effect of lactate and pH on proteoglycan and protein synthesis rates in the Intervertebral disc. Spine. 1992;17 (9):1079–82.

31. Pluijm SM, Tromp AM, Smit JH, Deeg DJ, Lips P. Consequences of vertebral deformities in older men and women. J Bone Miner Res. 2000;15(8):1564–72.

32. Resnick DK, et al. Guidelines for the performance of fusion procedures for degenerative disease of the lumbar spine. Part 9: Fusion in patients with stenosis and spondylolisthesis. J Neurosurg Spine. 2005;2:679–91.

33. Resnick DK, et al. Guidelines for the performance of fusion procedures for degenerative disease of the lumbar spine. Part 10:fusion following decompression in patients with stenosis without spondylolisthesis. J Neurosurg Spine. 2005;2:679–91.

34. Rodgers WB, Gerber EJ, Patterson J. Intraoperative and early postoperative complications in extreme lateral interbody Fusion. An analysis of 600 cases. Spine. 2011;36(1):26–32.

35. Roughley PJ. Biology of intervertebral disc aging and degeneration: involvement of the extracellular matrix. Spine. 2004;29(23):2691–9.

36. Schulte TL, Leistra F, Bullmann V, Osada N, Vieth V, Marquardt B, Lerner T, Liljenqvist U, Hackenberg L. Disc height reduction in adjacent segments and clinical outcome 10 years after lumbar 360° fusion. Eur Spine J. 2007;16(12):2152–8.

37. Schwarzenbach O, Rohrbach N, Berlemann U. Segment-by-segment stabilization for degenerative disc disease: a hybrid technique. Eur Spine J. 2010;19(6):1010–20.

38. Sengupta DK, Herkowitz HN. Degenerative spondylolisthesis: review of current trends and controversies. Spine. 2005;30(6 Suppl):S71–81.

39. Suratwala SJ, Pinto MR, Gilbert TJ, et al. Functional and radiological outcomes of 300 fusions of three or more motion levels in the lumbar spine for degenerative disc disease. Spine. 2009;34(10):E351–8.

40. Szpalski M, Gunzburg R. Lumbar spinal stenosis in the elderly: an overview. Eur Spine J. 2003;12 Suppl 2:S170–5.

41. Szpalski M, Gunzburg R, Mélot C, Aebi M. The aging of the population: a growing concern for spine care in the twenty-first century. Eur Spine J. 2003;12 Suppl 2: S81–3.

42. Tsahtsarlis A, Wood M. Minimally invasive transforaminal lumbar interbody fusion and degenerative lumbar spine disease. Eur Spine J. 2012;21(11): 2300–2305.

43. Urban JP, Smith S, Fairbank JC. Nutrition of the intervertebral disc. Spine. 2004;29(23):2700–9.

Infections of the Spine

José Guimarães Consciência, Rui Pinto, and Tiago Saldanha

Contents

J. Guimarães Consciência (✉)
Orthopaedic Department, FCM-Lisbon New University,
Lisbon, Portugal
e-mail: josegconsciencia@yahoo.com

R. Pinto
Orthopaedic Department, S. JoÃo Hospital, Porto,
Portugal
e-mail: ruialexpinto@yahoo.com

T. Saldanha
Giology Department, EGAS Moniz Hospital - CHLO,
Lisboa, Portugal
e-mail: tffaqs@gmail.com

Abstract

Spondylodiscitis, tuberculosis and peri-operative infections are different sub-groups of the same problem that require specific attention. There are patient-related and case-specific risk factors for a spine infection that although well-documented and significant are unfortunately not generally recognized. In each pathological presentation of the disease the relevance of aetiology, epidemiology, diagnostic tools, as well as treatment modalities have to be well-established to clarify the differences between them. The costs of treatment and its failure have to be carefully evaluated. We must emphasise that a spinal infection is usually a treatable condition depending on the patient's immunological defences, the aggressiveness of the infecting agent, elapsed time to diagnosis, and the efficacy of the chosen treatment.

Keywords

Diagnosis, Imaging, Conservative treatment • Discitis/Spondylitis • Infections • Post-operative infection • Spine • Surgical indications • Surgical techniques • Tuberculosis

Introduction

Throughout history the spinal column has undergone changes, making the necessary adaptations to allow us to stand and walk, providing support

G. Bentley (ed.), *European Surgical Orthopaedics and Traumatology*,
DOI 10.1007/978-3-642-34746-7_205, © EFORT 2014

to muscles or ligaments, to protect the neural structures and to facilitate daily living activities [1–3]. Pathological diseases such as spine infection can break this balance producing discomfort, pain and deformity. Also they can really endanger the patients either locally or systemically and thus become an important generalised disease. It is normally recognized that a haematogenous spine infection usually starts in the vertebral endplate area but it can spread from there to either the disc or the vertebral body [4, 5]. Several different infecting agents have been isolated including the most frequent staphylococcus aureus, mycobacterium tuberculosis and even rarely documented fungi. The literature indicates that old age can facilitate disease appearance, that there is no gender difference and also that, in spite of being a treatable condition, it might become a life-threatening situation especially if not properly treated [6, 7]. Diagnosis is often delayed and becomes a real challenge as the patient's symptoms and physical findings are often not severe. So early recognition becomes paramount in decreasing morbidity and mortality rates. For this purpose an exhaustive clinical examination complemented by an appropriate imaging evaluation is essential. As far as imaging is concerned PET scanning has 86 % accuracy and 100 % negative predictive value but MRI, on the other hand, has twice the sensitivity of a plain X-ray and can detect early changes, thus making both quite effective as diagnostic tools [4, 7–9]. The imaging potential of radio-labelled antimicrobial peptides, antibiotic peptides or chemotactic peptides have also been studied and they seem to have some advantage over the classic methods which might increase their role in the near future [10].

Discitis/Spondylodiscitis

Aetiology and Epidemiology

Discitis is an infection of the spine localized in the disc area but also simultaneously in bone and therefore the term "spondylodiscitis" is the most appropriate definition. Percutaneous spread or dissemination through the blood stream is usually the way pathogens reach the infection site. Staphylococcus aureus is often the infecting agent although other very rare organisms such as mucormycosis or even the *Lactococcus garvieae* might be involved [11, 12]. It represents around 2–7 % of all pyogenic osteomyelitis with an incidence reported from 1 per 100,000 to 1 per 250,000 a year [6] which makes it an uncommon condition and about 1 % of all bone infections [13]. It's a very rare in children less than 1 year old (Fig. 1) and although it peaks in childhood it seems to be more common in the elderly and in the lumbar spine rather than the cervical or the thoracic spine. It has been noted that 95 % of these infections involve the vertebral body, while only 5 % reach the posterior area of the spine [14, 15]. An epidural abscess is a possible complication in around 90 % of the cervical cases as well as 33.3 % of thoracic and 23.6 % of lumbar cases and we must bear in mind that it might also present as the primary lesion [5, 16].

Diagnosis

At an early stage of a spinal infection the inconclusiveness of either physical examination or symptoms can make diagnosis difficult (Fig. 2). Nevertheless clinical symptoms usually begin from 4 to 10 weeks before hospital admission and often the time between diagnosis and disease presentation can reach as much as 3 weeks or even 6 months. Therefore the spine surgeon should suspect a spinal infection whenever a patient complains of persistent pain specially if accompanied by systemic features like fever and unexplained weight loss as well as positive laboratory findings like C-reactive protein changes, increased erythrocyte sedimentation rate or raised white cell count [5, 7, 14]. Although many authors would consider these inflammatory parameters very useful others refer to their lack of sensitivity as well as specificity [8]. Therefore percutaneous biopsy remains an effective diagnostic tool in 60 % of all cases, whilst open biopsy is the chosen technique whenever the percutaneous route fails. It is also useful when

Fig. 1 MRI scan in C6-7 spondylodiscitis of 9 month-old child treated conservatively

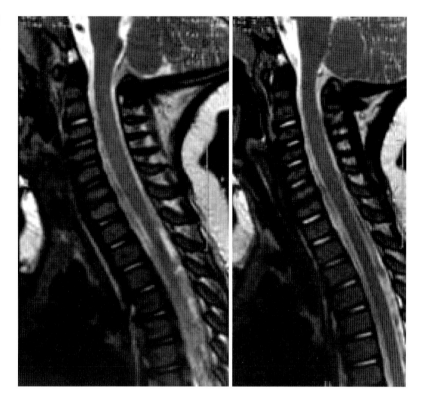

the affected area is otherwise inaccessible without an open approach [14]. For this purpose it is important to note that sometimes histology can in fact produce a diagnosis even when no specific infective agent has been isolated [17] and that a percutaneous biopsy seems to be a more effective tool in diagnosing bacterial rather than fungal infections [18].

Imaging

Knowing that an exhaustive clinical observation as well as an appropriate imaging study can give the correct diagnosis even before microbial confirmation is obtained, the clinician should use a wide variety of laboratory and clinical tests complemented by different types of imaging to confirm the diagnosis. We know that the insignificant anatomical changes inherent to the early stages of the disease significantly reduces the relevance of X-rays, ultrasound, computerized tomography and even sometimes magnetic resonance imaging, but they all become more useful in advanced stages. Nuclear medicine evaluation, which at an early stage allows us not only the visualization of the inflammatory processes, but also the localization or the number of inflammatory foci, becomes much more relevant at that stage (Fig. 3). The radio-isotopic methods also help to detect either physiological or biochemical changes and thus facilitate the differential diagnosis from sterile inflammation [10]. However, they are not always readily available. Since they are expensive and considering that a plain X-ray can give some degree of useful information, although not at a very early stage, we really must define clearly what is the role of MRI or scintigraphy in detecting a spine infection?

MRI is especially important in un-operated cases but is currently of limited value to differentiate between oedema and active infection immediately after a surgical procedure or in the presence of metallic hardware. In fact this is also a problem, even when using nuclear medicine

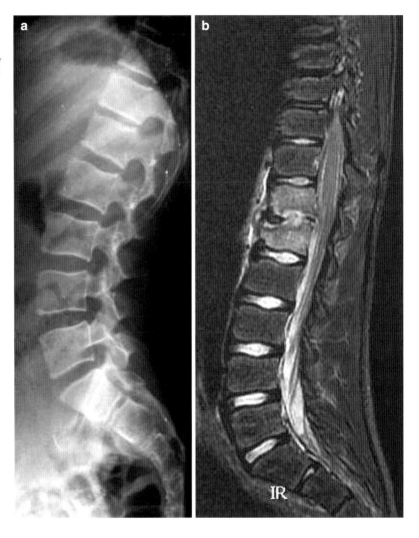

techniques, where specificity also decreases immediately after a surgical approach. One might think that those problems could be overcome using labelled leukocyte scanning. Unfortunately it is useless to evaluate the spine due to high uptake of labelled leucocytes in hematopoietic active bone marrow [8].

PET-scanning, on the other hand, has excellent accuracy providing rapid results and some authors presently consider it the best option especially in difficult cases [8, 9]. There is not a clear option that applies to each and every case so we must realize that different types of image are in fact quite important but they have to be used according to the disease staging or its specific presentation otherwise misdiagnosis may occur.

Treatment

The correct treatment for spondylodiscitis remains a matter of debate. Nevertheless delayed or inappropriate treatment can be quite troublesome leading to widespread sepsis and subsequent organ failure with inherent higher morbidity and mortality. If we can achieve a correct assessment along with an early diagnosis we facilitate an adequate treatment for the disease which is crucial for its effective management. It has been said that spondylodiscitis might sometimes be a self-healing disease but even in such cases the possible remaining bone destruction can produce significant instability requiring further treatment [19]. In the absence of

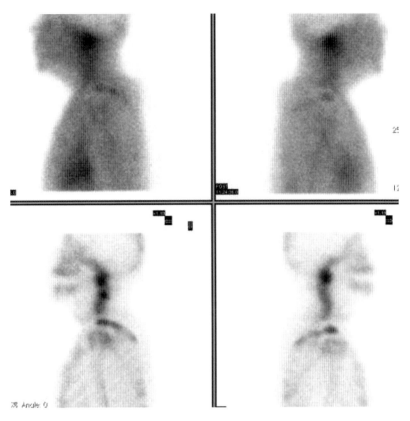

Fig. 3 Scintigram showing significant changes in the upper cervical spine of a patient with C2 infection and large abscess

neurological deficits or progressive symptoms spondylodiscitis will sometimes respond to non-surgical treatment, but otherwise surgery is the option. A wide number of treatment modalities for spinal infection have been suggested, from the non-surgical such as antibiotics and bracing to different types of surgery with anterior, posterior or combined approaches (Fig. 4). As we seldom find a corresponding clear indication for each one of them, at the end of the day the specific features of the cases will probably define treatment strategy. Even so, the option will often be aggressive treatment considering that a spinal infection might be the source of a generalised infection.

Conservative Treatment

When conservative treatment is indicated intravenous antibiotics given for at least 10 weeks, [14] sometimes in association with percutaneous drainage under imaging control, might still be the first option. Nevertheless 43–57 % of the conservatively-treated patients end up needing surgery, and we know that even with appropriate management 14 % may experience late recurrence [7]. On the other hand, we should note that difficult cases will usually require prolonged treatment for sometimes as long as 30 weeks [7] and conservative treatment can only remain an option if there's no neurologic deficits, no significant instability or deformity and no other symptoms. Otherwise, surgery is indicated [4, 5, 7, 16]. When compared with surgically-treated patients, conservatively-treated ones seem to have higher incidence of disabling back pain and worse functional and radiological outcomes. Surgery can in fact be the best option and some would consider that an anterior debridement is a better solution [15] whilst others would claim that a simple direct discectomy or even a transpedicular discectomy are the best techniques. However surgery is definitely the choice whenever we need to reduce deformity or stabilize the spine [20] and then we often also need additional instrumentation which has long been considered controversial in active spine infections.

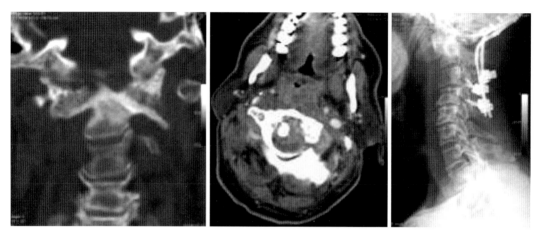

Fig. 4 C2 infection and significant abscess treated with transoral dens removal and occipito-cervical instrumented fusion

Not using instrumentation is not the absolute solution as poor sagittal correction has been reported after non-instrumented fusions [15]. This fact leads many surgeons to clearly recommend instrumented fusion, but the exact role of instruments as well as graft material remains also a matter of debate [4, 19, 21]. Some [5, 13] would support the efficacy of aggressive debridement, anterior bone grafting and posterior stabilization (Fig. 5). If there is not significant vertebral body destruction others would suggest that an anterior titanium mesh cage filled with bone graft and combined with anterior plating is an acceptable solution [15, 20, 22]. In low risk patients there are also favourable reports on the use of PEEK cages without additional instrumentation to treat pyogenic discitis in the cervical spine [22, 23]. But of course the state of the art as far as surgery is concerned is to debride the infected area and stabilize the spine in the best way but always bearing in mind that no matter what operation you perform you will have to employ intravenous antibiotics for no less than 6 weeks [16].

Tuberculosis

Tuberculosis seems to be increasing everywhere and not only in developing countries where nevertheless the problem is definitely more significant. There are approximately 3.8 million new cases reported each year around the world and probably a very significant number not reported or mis-diagnosed. The so called "re-appearance" of the disease might somehow be related not only to the increased immuno-compromised patients but also to the multiple drug-resistant strains and of course different socio-economic factors [24].

Aetiology and Epidemiology

When we consider tuberculosis the Koch bacilli are the infecting agents and the infection can be localized in different body areas as is well-recognized. Coming from either the bloodstream or the lymphatic supply the bacilli may reach the anterior portion of the vertebral body and then, with a high probability, develop spinal tuberculosis. Nevertheless, it will only happen in less than 1 % of all skeletally-infected patients. Especially in uncontrolled patients neurological deficits and deformities such as localized kyphosis are sometimes observed and need to be aggressively addressed. We must realize that even when using histology or culture it is sometimes difficult to differentiate between tuberculosis and a pyogenic infection, in fact it can only be achieved in around 62.2 % of cases [24].

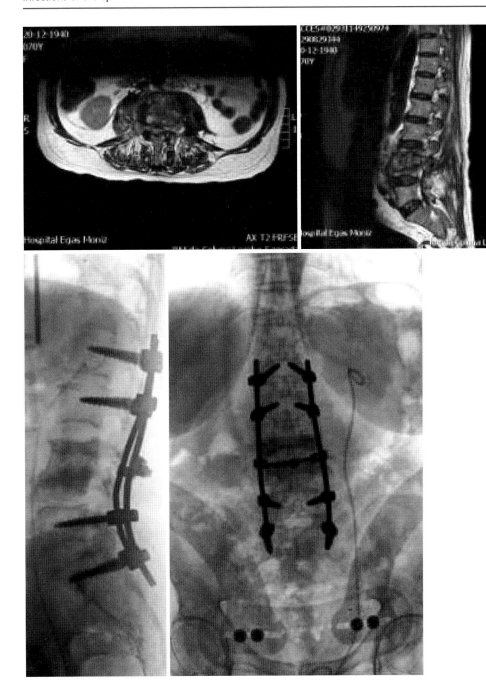

Fig. 5 Lumbar infection and vertebral destruction treated with anterior decompression and fusion associated with long posterior instrumentation

Diagnosis

In spite of only being diagnostic in around 2/3 of the cases, histology and culture are still indispensible as diagnosis is often not an easy task. The delay in diagnosis can become a relevant factor considering shortening of the elapsed time between symptoms and treatment. The physician must carefully identify all the patient's symptoms related to the clinical picture and of course even more so if the patient already has the disease diagnosed else-where. Some authors will claim that even in the presence of a low-virulence pyogenic infection one must suspect co-existent tuberculosis if the disease is not responding as expected to the pre-scribed normal antibiotics, or if the patient is immunocompromised or if a psoas calcification is identified [24].

Treatment

Treatment in spinal tuberculosis is chosen according to the patient's symptoms as well as disease involvement and all this after careful evaluation of any neurological deficits, existent deformity or instability, addressing each one of these problems by itself in an overall perspective, looking for total disease control. At the present time we can usually achieve an early diagnosis and this can make a difference as far as treatment effectiveness is concerned. The new drugs and more effective types of instrumentation allow us also to achieve better results from the prescribed treatments. The assessment of the levels involved, the existence and location of an abscess or bone destruction must be made in selecting adequate treatment. Minor cases can be controlled conservatively with anti-tuberculosis drugs, and this should probably be always a first choice, but more severe cases will definitely need additional surgery and the infection site must of course be thoroughly cleared.

Indications for Surgery

As is well-recognized, surgery is indicated whenever there are significant deformity, major instability, important neurological deficits, large abscesses or failure of conserva-tive treatment leading to either progression of symptoms and signs, or increased bone involvement. There is no single generalized technique for all patients. A wide anterior debridement and fusion, a front and back fusion, either in one or in two procedures and a posterior-alone fusion have all been suggested and all aim to achieve surgical treat-ment goals. These are; controlling the disease

by decompression, exhaustive debridement, re-alignment of the spine, stabilization and fusion. It has been mentioned that a simple posterior decompression and instrumented fusion can effectively solve an early stage, small bone destruction and mild kyphosis case [25]. Nev-ertheless these results seem to be comparable with those obtained after an anterior approach and, even if both approaches can significantly address the kyphosis, both will also allow some degrees of correction loss that has to be taken into consideration. Bezer et al. [26] also dem-onstrated that it was possible to do an anterior decompression and fusion through a posterior approach preventing lumbar kyphosis and maintaining sagittal balance which is quite important considering this is a less aggressive technique. Other authors [27], specifically at L5-S1, also reported good results doing a TLIF (Transforaminac Lumbar Interboy Fusion) to handle patients with failure of con-servative treatment, localized kyphosis, neural compression and limited destruction of the disc as well as adjacent vertebral bodies. So in gen-eral it seems that surgery must be chosen in an individual manner depending on disease specificity, patient characteristics and the surgeon's ability to perform each technique. As with other pathologies our spinal tuberculo-sis patients should be treated with the least aggressive, most effective and long-lasting technique but this, unfortunately, cannot be systematically applied all the time.

Post-Operative Infection

Post-operative infections are sometimes very problematic and troublesome complications of spine surgery. They can be diagnosed immedi-ately after surgery but sometimes even several years later (Fig. 6). We must always be aware of this possibility and take all measures to avoid it by meticulous techniques. We also have to realize that the use of a simple dilute betadine solution can moderately reduce the risk of infection. Meanwhile pursuing an understanding of what can facilitate infection, why some patients are

Fig. 6 Late infection with wound discharge after scoliosis surgery (3 years later)

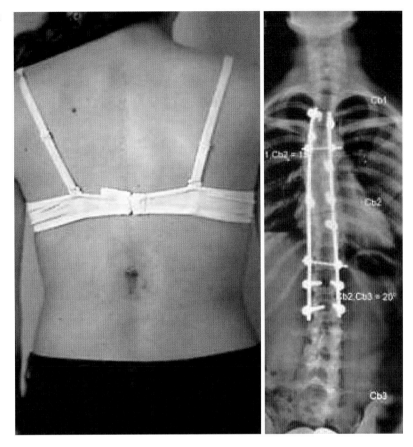

more prone to it as well as how we can prevent it or safely treat it, are crucial steps. We sometimes assume this diagnosis based only on local pain, inflammatory changes or wound discharge and this is not reliable [28].

Aetiology and Epidemiology

Many surgeons would agree that post-operative infections are mainly the result of a surgical wound contamination inside the operating room or in the ward immediately after surgery and that the infecting agent often comes from the patient's own flora. The skin of all individuals accessing the operating room as well as the ward is generally recognised as a main source of all airborne organisms, so the more people we have inside the operating theatre the more organisms will be circulating. The surgical ability and

sterile technique of the team also influence infection rates and this in spite of some reports that question whether post-operative infections are related to the experience of surgical staff [29]. Although we know that staphylococcus aureus or epidermidis are the most common infecting agents a significant number of cases still remain without an isolated agent and of course this creates additional difficulties [30]. Risk factors have to be carefully identified which seem to be multi-factorial and may be case-specific or patient-related ones. Obese people seem to be more prone to infection, wound drainage has a minor role and there is only indefinite evidence suggesting that pre-operative prophylactic antibiotics might improve infection rate even if we are not able to identify the most effective one or the right dosage [31]. Operative time, previous spine surgery, blood loss, tissue damage, diabetes, smoking, old age, rheumatoid arthritis,

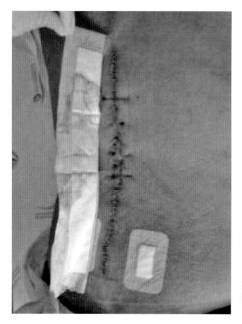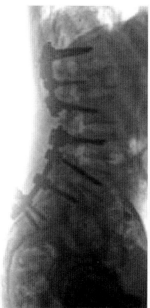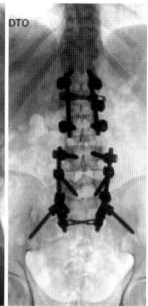

Fig. 7 Early infection and wound discharge after long spine stabilization in trauma patient treated with wide debridement and instruments preservation

steroid use or previous infection are all considered contributory [29, 31–33]. The use of implants might also incur in additional risk of wound infection at the insertion level [34] or even at the level above [35].

Spinal surgery has a higher infection rate then other surgeries such as total hip arthroplasty. However there is a wide variation (0.3–20 %) in reported infection rates after spine surgery [30, 34] and in the incidence of delayed infection which varies from 0.2 % to 6.7 % [28]. So there might be a correspondence between the complexity or increasing number of invasive surgical procedures and higher infection rates. We consider that revision surgery is more prone to infection than implant use and, on the other hand, minimally-invasive surgery is associated with less infection [30], although it takes more operative time. Since the cost of spinal treatments is always increasing, a significant reduction in risk factors would prove valuable, allowing surgeons to carefully identify them and act accordingly. There are inherent differences in hospital rates for per-operative spine infection across teaching and non-teaching hospitals [36]

and that is important, as the consequences of a spinal infection include longer and more expensive hospital stays, a two-fold increase in mortality, a five-fold risk of hospital re-admission, and a 60 % greater chance of intensive care unit admission [29].

Treatment

Usually a post-operative spine infection is treated with multiple wide debridement primary or delayed wound closure and antibiotics for no less than 6 weeks. Different options have been suggested and the use of a vacuum-assisted wound closure is a possibility as it exposes the wound to negative pressures, removes fluid, improves blood supply and stimulates granulation tissue appearance providing good results in association with surgical debridement [37]. In the early stages implant removal is seldom necessary (Fig. 7) since implants can promote fusion and their removal might result in spinal instability and pseudarthrosis [32, 38]. Collins et al. [28] mentioned that there was a confirmed 60 % deep wound infection on subsequent implant removal despite previous long-term antibiotics and wound surgical debridement, so they definitely recommended implant removal and reported 46 % of pain-free stable patients with this technique. When dealing with uncontrolled infection situations, Kim et al. [34] also found that implant removal associated with wide debridement was an effective option as far as controlling infection was concerned. However they also noted the appearance of disc collapse, loss of lordosis or pseudoarthrosis and this has to be taken into consideration. Implant removal has to be carefully evaluated since the advantage of the procedure might in time be overcome by its consequences.

Conclusions

Spinal infections can endanger patients either locally or systemically becoming an important generalised disease. In spite of being treatable conditions they can become life-threatening especially if not properly treated. A wide number of treatment modalities for each spinal infection have been suggested, from the non-surgical such as antibiotics and bracing to different types of surgery with anterior, posterior or combined procedures. Spondylodiscitis, tuberculosis and post-operative infections have to be carefully evaluated, realizing that the specific features of each case will define the best treatment strategy and that the efficacy of all treatments depends not only on the surgeon's ability but also on an early suspicion as well as meticulous handling of the available diagnostic tools.

References

1. Begun DR. African and Eurasian Miocene hominoids and the origins of the hominoid. In: Bonis L, Koufos GD, Andew P, editors. Phylogeny of the neogene hominoid primates of Eurasia. Cambridge: Cambridge University Press; 2001. p. 231–53.
2. Benefit BR, McCrossin ML. Miocene hominoids and hominid origins. Ann Rev Anthropol. 1995;24: 237–56.
3. Richmond BG, Strait DR. Origin of human bipedalism: the knuckle-walking hypothesis revisited. Am J Phys Anthropol. 2001;44:70–105.
4. Hempelmann RG, Mater E, Schön R. Septic hematogenous lumbar spondylodiscitis in elderly patients with multiple risk factors: efficacy of posterior stabilization and interbody fusion with iliac crest bone graft. Eur Spine J. 2010;19:1720–7.
5. Heyde CE, Boehm H, Saghir HE, et al. Surgical treatment of spondylodiscitis in the cervical spine: a minimum 2-year follow-up. Eur Spine J. 2006;15:1380–7.
6. D'Agostino C, Scorzolini L, Massetti AP, et al. A seven-year prospective study on spondylodiscitis: epidemiological and microbiological features. Infection. 2010;38:102–7.
7. Shafafy M, Singh P, Fairbank JCT, et al. Primary non-tuberculous spinal infection; management and outcome. J Bone Joint Surg Br. 2009;91-B(Supp III):478.
8. De Winter F, Gemmel F, De Wiele C, et al. 18-fluorine fluorodeoxyglucose positron emission tomography for the diagnosis of infection in the postoperative spine. Spine. 2003;28:1314–9.
9. Schmitz A, Risse JH, Grünwald F, et al. Fluorine-18 fluorodeoxyglucose positron emission tomography findings in spondylodiscitis: preliminary results. Eur Spine J. 2001;10:534–9.
10. Lambrecht FY. Evaluation of 99mTc-labeled antibiotics for infection detection. Ann Nucl Med. 2011;25: 1–6.
11. Chan JFW, Woo PCY, Teng JLL. Primary infective spondylodiscitis caused by *Lactococcus garvieae* and a review of human *L. garvieae* infections. Infection. 2011;39(3):259–64, Published on line.
12. Chen F, Lu G, Kang Y, et al. Mucormycosis spondylodiscitis after lumbar disc puncture. Eur Spine J. 2006;15:370–6.
13. Schimmer RC, Jeanneret C, Nunley PD, et al. Osteomyelitis of the cervical spine – a potentially dramatic disease. J Spinal Disord Tech. 2002;15(2):110–7.
14. Bettini N, Girardo M, Dema E, et al. Evaluation of conservative treatment of non specific spondylodiscitis. Eur Spine J. 2009;18 Suppl 1:S143–50.
15. Kuklo TR, Potter BK, Bell RS, et al. Single-stage treatment of pyogenic spinal infection with titanium mesh cages. J Spinal Disord Tech. 2006;19:376–82.
16. Hadjipavlou AG, Mader JT, Necessary JT, et al. Hematogenous pyogenic spinal infections and their surgical management. Spine. 2000;25(13):1668–79.
17. Michel S, Pfirmann C, Boos N, et al. CT-guided core biopsy of subchondral bone and intervertebral space in suspected spondylodiskitis. AJR Am J Roentgenol. 2006;186:977–80.
18. Chew F, Kline M. Diagnostic yield of CT-guided percutaneous aspiration procedures in suspected spontaneous infectious diskitis. Radiology. 2001;218:211–4.
19. Hadjipavlou AG, Katonis PK, Gaitanis IN, et al. Percutaneous transpedicular discectomy and drainage in pyogenic spondylodiscitis. Eur Spine J. 2004;13:707–13.

20. Hee HT, Majd ME, Holt RT, et al. Better treatment of vertebral osteomyelitis using posterior stabilization and titanium mesh cages. J Spinal Disord Tech. 2002;15(2):149–56.

21. Spock CR, Miki RA, Shah RV, et al. Necrotizing infection of the spine. Spine. 2006;31:E342–4.

22. Nakase H, Tamaki R, Matsuda R, et al. Delayed reconstruction by titanium mesh–bone graft composite in pyogenic spinal infection – a long-term follow-up study. J Spinal Disord Tech. 2006;19:48–54.

23. Walter J, Kuhn SA, Reichart R, et al. PEEK cages as a potential alternative in the treatment of cervical spondylodiscitis: a preliminary report on a patient series. Eur Spine J. 2010;19:1004–9.

24. Mousa HAL. Concomitant spine infection with *Mycobacterium tuberculosis* and pyogenic bactéria. Spine. 2003;28(8):E152–4.

25. Lee SH, Sung JK, Park YM. Single-stage transpedicular decompression and posterior instrumentation in treatment of thoracic and thoracolumbar spinal tuberculosis – a retrospective case series. J Spinal Disord Tech. 2006;19:595–602.

26. Bezer M, Kucukdurmaz F, Aydin N, et al. Tuberculous spondylitis of the lumbosacral region long-term follow-up of patients treated by chemotherapy, transpedicular drainage, posterior instrumentation, and fusion. J Spinal Disord Tech. 2005;18:425–9.

27. Zaveri GR, Mehta SS. Surgical treatment of lumbar tuberculous spondylodiscitis by Transforaminal Lumbar Interbody Fusion (TLIF) and posterior instrumentation. J Spinal Disord Tech. 2009;22:257–62.

28. Collins I, Wilson-MacDonald J, Chami G, et al. The diagnosis and management of infection following instrumented spinal fusion. Eur Spine J. 2008;17:445–50.

29. Banco SP, Vaccaro AR, Blam O, et al. Spine infections. Spine. 2002;27(9):962–5.

30. Smith JS, Shaffrey CI, Sansur CA, et al. Rates of infection after spine surgery based on 108,419 procedures. Spine. 2011;36:556–63.

31. Schuster JM, Rechtine G, Norvell DC, et al. The influence of perioperative risk factors and therapeutic interventions on infection rates after spine surgery – a systematic review. Spine. 2010;35:S125–37.

32. Ha KY, Kim YH. Postoperative spondylitis after posterior lumbar interbody fusion using cages. Eur Spine J. 2004;13:419–24.

33. Schimmel JP, Horsting PP, De Kleuver M, et al. Risk factors for deep surgical site infections after spinal fusion. Eur Spine J. 2010;19:1711–9.

34. Kim J, Suh KT, Kim SJ, et al. Implant removal for the management of infection after instrumented spinal fusion. J Spinal Disord Tech. 2010;23(4):258–65.

35. Kulkarni AG, Hee HT. Adjacent level discitis after anterior cervical discectomy and fusion (ACDF): a case report. Eur Spine J. 2006;15 Suppl 5:S559–63.

36. Goode AP, Cook C, Gill JB. The risk of risk-adjustment measures for perioperative spine infection after spinal surgery. Spine. 2011;36:752–8.

37. Mehbod AA, Ogilvie JW, Pinto MR, et al. Postoperative deep wound infections in adults after spinal fusion – management with vacuum-assisted wound closure. J Spinal Disord Tech. 2005;18:14–7.

38. Mirovsky Y, Floman Y, Smorgick Y, et al. Management of deep wound infection after posterior lumbar interbody fusion with cages. J Spinal Disord Tech. 2007;20:127–31.

Surgical Management of Spondylodiscitis

Maite Ubierna and Enric Cáceres Palou

Contents

Abstract

Vertebral osteomyelitis or spondylodiscitis is an uncommon, mainly haematogenous, disease that usually affects the adult. The incidence of this condition has steadily risen in recent years because of the increase in spinal surgery and nosocomial bacteraemia, aging of the population and intravenous drug addiction. Pyogenic infection due to *Staphylococcus aureus* is the most frequent form of the disease but tuberculosis is still a common cause of spondylitis. The clinical presentation is non-specific and the diagnosis is often delayed. Magnetic resonance imaging is the most sensitive radiological technique for this disease. Blood cultures are sometimes positive but computed tomography-guided needle biopsy is sometimes required to achieve a microbiological diagnosis. Prolonged antibiotic therapy and occasionally surgery are essential for cure in most patient, and both factors have contributed to a reduction in the morbidity and mortality of the disease in recent years.

Keywords

Anterior • Classification • Clinical features • Diagnosis • Epidemiology • Indications • Medical treatment • Microbiology • Posterior • Pyogenic vertebral osteomyelitis • Radiology and scanning • Results • Spine • Spondylodiscitis • Surgical approaches-anterior and posterior • Techniques • Tuberculosis

M. Ubierna (✉)
Spine Unit, Hospital Germas Trias i Pujol Badalona, Barcelona, Spain
e-mail: Maiteubi8587@gmail.com

E.C. Palou
Department Hospital Vall d'Hebron, Autonomous University of Barcelona, Barcelona, Spain
e-mail: ecaceres@vhebron.net

G. Bentley (ed.), *European Surgical Orthopaedics and Traumatology*,
DOI 10.1007/978-3-642-34746-7_219, © EFORT 2014

Introduction

The spine is the most common site of haematogenous bone infection in adults. At present, the sensitivity and specificity of imaging techniques, the versatility of the spinal instrumentation and decreased surgical morbidity allow healing in these patients. Despite this, diagnosis and treatment remain as major challenges for the Orthopaedic surgeon. Selective antibiotic therapy, early techniques combined with spinal stabilization and biological input if necessary, have reduced mortality from 5 % to 15 % [1].

Epidemiology

Spinal infection represents between 2 % and 5 % of bone and joint infections. Among the risk factors listed are age, obesity, malnutrition, diabetes, immunodeficiency, previous infection and prior surgical procedures. If we compare the epidemiological data of vertebral infection with osteomyelitis in the extremities there are clear differences. The average age of patients with spinal infection is 66 years while that in limb infection is 16 years. The male/female ratio is 1:1–2:1 infection in spine and limbs.

Classification

Classifications are related to the location of the infection and the aetiological organism.

Location

Spondylodiscitis is present when the infection settles in the vertebral body and spreads to the adjacent disc; discitis is a term used for the isolated disc space infection secondary to disc surgery, discography or percutaneous nucleotomy. Currently the existence of isolated hematogenous discitis in children is being discussed because several authors suggest that MRI evidence must

be present in all cases of vertebral body bone involvement [2–5]. Finally, it is very exceptional to see isolated posterior arch involvement, of which there are only16 documented cases in the literature [6].

Micro-Organisms

It is possible to differentiate between bacterial, granulomatous and fungus infections with very different clinical behaviour and histopathological appearances.

The *route of spread* can differentiate between hematogenous, direct inoculation (post-operative) and propagation by continuity (from vascular urological, or gastro-intestinal surgery).

Depending on the age of presentation can speak of spinal infection in children and in adults. The behaviour and the potential consequences are very different.

In the next pages we could will divide the description into two sections , pyogenic vertebral osteomyelitis and secondly vertebral tuberculosis.

Pyogenic Vertebral Osteomyelitis

Pathophysiology of Bacterial Spinal Infection

The haematogenous route is the usual route of infection in the infection of the column from a septic focus such as infection of the skin or soft tissues, urinary tract or respiratory tract, which are among the most common. There are two main theories that could explain haematogenous seeding,
(a) spread via Batson's venous plexus (Fig. 1) or
(b) spread by the venous drainage of the pelvis, which pre-supposes the existence of pressures sufficient to cause retrograde flow to direct the bacteria released from the bowel manipulated in the abdomino-pelvic area to the spinal column.

Currently, most authors seem to favour the arterial system as the route for the transmission of infection. The arteriolar theory described by

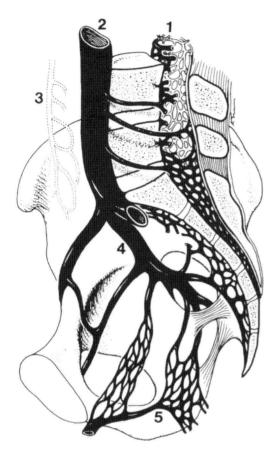

Fig. 1 Batson's paravertebral venous system. It is a set of veins, which anastomose and extra-abdominally communicate with the main intra-abdominal venous system. *1* paravertebral venous plexus, *2* inferior vena cava, *3* inferior mesenteric vessel, *4* iliac vein, *5* pelvic plexus (From Vider et al. 1977 [31])

Wiley and Trueta [7] suggests that bacteria reach the area located in the subchondral vertebral plate arterial anastomosis which form septic thrombus. This triggers a rapid inflammatory response which, together with the lysosomal activity, causes weakening and destruction of the subchondral zone and penetrates the disc and adjacent vertebral body. (Fig. 2). The disc is rapidly destroyed with a sudden loss of intervertberal space height.

In the cervical spine, the prevertebral fascia can spread the infection into the mediastinal space or supraclavicular fossa aggravating the clinical situation. In the lumbar spine infection may go the way of the psoas sheath to the piriform fossa or to the hip area. In some cases the spread of the infection to the spinal canal may cause an epidural abscess. The aggressive osteolytic bone infection causes bone destruction, leading to compression fractures or fracture with neurological or mechanical instability.

In children, the behaviour is different. Vascular channels traversing the end-plate to irrigate the nucleus pulposus allow direct haematogenous spread to the intervertebral disc in this population. Some cases progress rapidly to neurological deterioration. The causes include: the formation of an epidural abscess by posterior common ligament detachment, a bone fragment posteriorlt impinging on the spinal cord or the development of severe deformity due to bone destruction.

Risk factors for neurological injury have been described: diabetes, rheumatoid arthritis, steroid treatment, advanced age and location in the cervical or high thoracic spine [8].

Clinical Features

The mode of presentation of a spinal infection is highly variable. The symptoms depend on host immunity, the aggressiveness of the organism and the duration of the process. The clinical picture can be acute, subacute or chronic. Overall there is a variable interval of time (1–15 months) to reach the diagnosis. This due to the association in elderly patients with common symptoms of spinal pain (degnerative changes and arthritis). MRI imaging early greatly accelerates the diagnostic process.

Always spinal pain is present (90 % of cases). It is an inflammatory pain, not relieved and even accentuated with rest. There is intolerance for sitting. Pain radiating to the extremities can occur when there is root compromise. Fever is only present in 50 % of cases [9].

In advanced stages of the disease with significant bone destruction, segmental mechanical instability clearly increases pain and function of the patient. The most common location is in lumbar spine, around 50 %. while only 10 % are located in the cervical spine.

Neurological involvement appears in between 10 % and 20 % of patients, depending on the different series, in the form of paraesthesiae,

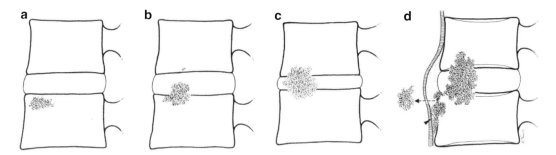

Fig. 2 The most common pathophysiology of spinal infection. Showing septic subchondral bone end-plate. Propagation later to the disc space and adjacent vertebral body

cramps, neurological claudication, motor deficit and even early onset paraplegia [10]. The most common cause is a secondary epidural abscess (27.5 %) followed by inflammatory tissue in 6.1 %.

Microbiology

Staphylococcus aureus remains the most common pathogen (42–55 % in adults and 80–90 % in children [11–15]. Streptococcus occurs in 19.6 % and in the last decade there has been an increased incidence of gram-negative bacilli such as Escherichia coli, Pseudomonas and Proteus microorganisms from the urinary tract, respiratory tract, soft tissue infections or from normal flora in immunocompromised patients. Patients addicted to intravenous drugs have a higher incidence especially Pseudomonas and diabetic patients to anaerobes. Microorganisms like Staphylococcus plasmacoagulase-negative were the cause in 14.7 % of cases in the series published by Hadjipavlou [16–18].

Diagnosis

Diagnostic delay is a characteristic feature of spinal infection despite having tools for identifying pathology with certainty in the short term. We just need to know how to use them and be able to differentiate between: granulomatous infection, bacterial infection, metastases, myeloma, osteoporotic fracture, degenerative disease, and primary neoplasm pseudodiscitis.

It is essential to order appropriate diagnostic and laboratory investigations that will lead to the diagnosis:

History
The patient can come from different medical specialties- rheumatology, Orthopaedics, internal medicine and general surgery because the symptoms are often confusing. In many cases, patients have come to the emergency room on more than one occasion and almost always are labelled "mechanical pain" or "degenerative". Focussed questioning can distinguish the chronic degenerative symptoms from a subacute spinal pain that does not respond to standard treatment and is accompanied by malaise and sometimes gait claudication.

It is important to find a previous infectious in another location, which is responsible for haematogenous sepsis. Sometimes a wound or skin erosion may be the gateway in the immunocompromised patient.

Radiology
Radiological images are often inconclusive during the first 2 or 4 weeks after onset of the disease. The first visible change is usually the loss of disc space height. Then osteolytic lesions appear in the vertebral body adjacent to the end-plate zone may progress to destruction of both vertebral bodies (Fig. 3). In advanced stages of the disease it is easy to see wedge kyphosis deformity, sometimes severe, from destruction of the entire vertebral segment. The soft tissue extension usually is due to prevertebral oedema and inflammation of the

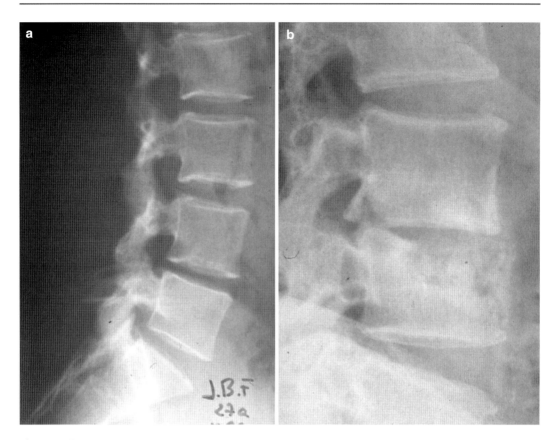

Fig. 3 Differences in behaviour in the initial phase of tuberculosis and bacterial infection. (**a**) Minimal loss of disc space height without visible bone lesion is seen in tuberculous infection. (**b**) Pattern in both aggressive osteolytic vertebral bodies and kyphosis with disc collapse in pyogenic infection

psoas muscle may cause psoas enlargement and detachment in the lower back. A widened mediastinum in the thoracic spine and increased shadow in the retropharyngeal space indicate infection at the thoracic and cervical levels.

Laboratory

Very often laboratory results are non-specific. There is leukocytosis in 13–60 % of cases, however, chronic infections in elderly patients with poor nutrition often have normal blood markers.

The sedimentation rate is increased in 90 % of cases between 50 and 55 mm/h. In the series of 101 cases of bacterial infection collected by Hadjipavlou [16] leukocytosis as statistically significant indicator of epidural abscess, and elevated ESR were associated with a strong tendency to epidural abscess. Both parameters are a "red flag" for possible complications.

CRP is a more sensitive and specific parameter, is increased in most cases in the acute or subacute phase, and returns to normal quickly with effective treatment.

Bone Scanning

Bone scanning is more sensitive than radiography although is not specific to bone infection. It has a role as skeleton tracker to identify septic foci at different levels, a situation described in 3–5 % of occasions. The combined results of the study with 99Tch and Ga 67, provide a sensitivity of 90 % and an efficiency of 85 % for the diagnosis of infection. The specificity of gallium Ga 67 is 85 %, slightly higher than the 99 m Tc Technecio 78 %. Moreover, the Ga 67 can be normalized in a few weeks if the clinical course is favourable, while Tc99m remains positive for about a year.

MRI Scanning

MRI is the technique of choice at present for the diagnosis of infection of the spine. It provides excellent images of the extension of the process in bone, disc, nerve and soft tissue adjacent structures. It provides a very high sensitivity and specificity, 93 % and 96 % respectively in the diagnosis of bone infection [3].

T2-weighted sequences show hyper-intense signal attributable to oedema of the disk and the vertebral body and in T1-weighted images the signal is decreased in both the disk and the vertebral body due to replacement of the fatty tissue of the bone marrow. T1 characteristically shows the loss of boundaries between the disc and the endplate. The paramagnetic contrast injection, gadolinium, is useful in differentiating bone infection of post-surgical origin [19]. MRI allows for the differential diagnosis of bone infection and neoplasia, as the latter does not extend to the intervertebral disc.

CT Scanning

CT scanning has been displaced by the MRI from the point of view of specificity and diagnostic sensitivity. However CT scanning is the best tool to assess the degree of bone destruction and can be of great help in deciding the type surgery that is performed.

Isolation of Aetiologic Bacteria

It is essential to identify the bacteria responsible for spinal infection to confirm the diagnosis. As a protocol, blood and urine cultures are needed in all cases. If fever is present blood culture performance is of greater value.

In patients in whom we have not succeeded in isolating the bacterium, we recommend performing a spinal puncture biopsy. The effectiveness increases if performed by percutaneous CT-guided puncture. The technique increases success if material is referred to microbiology and pathology in all cases. the results are positive in between 70 % and 88 % for the diagnosis of infection [20]. Histopathology can differentiate acute chronic pyogenic infection from granulomatous infection.

In the series of Hadjipavlou et al. they found 24.4 % of negative cultures and suggested three causes: antibiotic therapy before biopsy, insufficient material and a natural ability for healing disc as Fraser had described [21, 22].

Open biopsy is restricted to cases in which the needle biopsy has failed, when the location is inaccessible to closed techniques or when the symptoms of the infection require surgical treatment.

Spinal Tuberculosis

Tuberculous spinal infection is also known as "granulomatous infection". This terminology refers to organisms that cause an immune response in the host characterized by the formation of granulomata. Histologically, these granulomata are chronic inflammatory foci with nodular appearance, with a central area of necrosis surrounded by Langhans giant cells. The most frequent granulomatous infection is caused by *Mycobacterium Tuberculosis* organisms responsible for spinal tuberculosis, described by Sir Percival Pott in 1779.

Epidemiology

Tuberculous spinal infection is the most common form of extrapulmonary Mycobacterium tuberculosis. Its incidence ranges from 1 % in developed countries to 10 % in endemic areas. In the last decade, the incidence has increased in developed countries attributed to increased immunosuppressed patients and bacterial mutations leading to increased virulence and resistance to drug treatment.

An estimated 1.7 billion people, one-third of the population of the earth, are or have been infected with TB. Of all patients with TB, 10 % had musculoskeletal involvement and of these 50 % were of vertebral location.

Pathophysiology

The vertebrae are usually infected secondarily to haematogenous spread from a pulmonary focus.

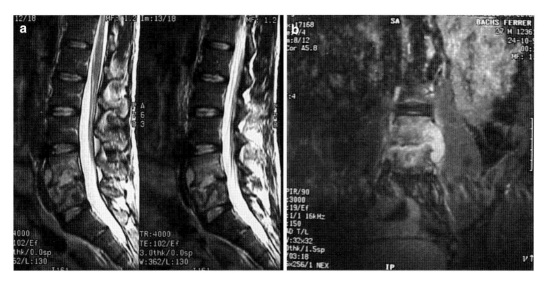

Fig. 4 Formation of paradiscal tuberculosis infection. In the sagittal (**a**) and frontal plane (**b**) the vertebral body involvement and spread to the adjacent vertebra through the anterior common ligament occurs

In some cases it is due to direct expansion or lymphatic spread from a renal focus. Currently, most cases of spinal tuberculosis in adults are silent re-activations of lung foci. Three forms of vertebral involvement are described: paradiscal, anterior and central (Fig. 4). Dobson, in a review of 914 cases, showed 33 % paradiscal, 12 % central and 2 % anterior. Involvement of the posterior structures is less than 10 % [23].

The paradiscal form, the most common, shows haematogenous seeding located at the end-plate. Slowly the infection spreads through the adjacent ,vertebra, the anterior vertebral common ligament in most cases and sometimes through the posterior common ligament. The disc, in incipient forms, is not involved in many cases, unlike pyogenic infection when almost always disc destruction is present. Bone destruction is slow but progressive, with a kyphotic deformity at advanced stages.

The central form affects only the vertebral body, without involvement of the disc and adjacent vertebra. The destruction of bone tissue causes an isolated vertebral body wedging, showing an image that will appear like a fracture or a tumour. The differential diagnosis is more difficult.

Clinical Features

The thoracic location is the most common followed closely by the lumbar location and more infrequent cervical involvement. Multi-segment localization occurs between 1 % and 24 % depending on nutritional status and immunosuppression.

The clinical presentation of tuberculosis infection is much more insidious than the bacterial infection leading to frequent diagnostic delay. According to different publications, there is an interval ranging from between 3 months to 18 from the start of symptoms to diagnosis.

The common onset symptom is slow but progressive spinal pain,. The long duration of symptoms makes the diagnosis at the time associate to other problems: epidural abscess, angular kyphosis deformity and neurological impairment. About 40 % of patients develop sensory-motor déficit more often in the thoracic and cervical location. In the cervical spine there have been reported up to 80 % of cases with neurological deficit. Advanced age and diabetes have been described as risk factors for developing neurological complications.

Paravertebral abscess formation is not rare in large tuberculosis infection. In the cervical region in children retropharyngeal abscess is more common and may displace and compress the trachea and oesophagus. In the thoracic region the abscess causes adhesions between pleura and diaphragm. The abscess located in the lumbar region is more frequent. Large abscesses can descend in the psoas sheath to the region where they present at the adductors muscle site.

The kyphosis deformity at the time of diagnosis is also a characteristic of tuberculosis infection due to severe spinal vertebral destruction. It is accompanied by severe mechanical instability especially in the thoracolumbar junction which often aggravates the already existing neurological instability.

Diagnosis

The diagnostic strategy in TB infection follow the same criteria as described for bacterial infections, with the differences in clinical behaviour and characteristic: slow onset and late diagnosis.

The laboratory studies will include the search for the Koch's bacillus in gastric juice, sputum and urine. Mantoux or PPD testing , which detect active TB or old exposure are useful. Acute phase reactants are still less sensitive than in bacterial infection due to the chronicity of the process. The polymerase chain reaction is a promising technique for the rapid detection of tuberculosis infection.

Radiology can be valuable at the first visit of the patient due to the duration of symptoms. Bone destruction is visible with involvement of two adjacent vertebral bodies. If diagnosed at an early stage the only radiographic sign is loss of disc height since it takes time to see the signs of bone destruction (Fig. 3). Careful examination of the junctional zones, thoracolumbar, lumbosacral and cervicothoracicis necessary since in these áreas, that are difficult to display in standard emergency radiology and destructive infectious lesions, may go unrecognized. The chest X-ray should be part of the study protocol.

The bone scan is less sensitive than in bacterial infections, with up to 40 % false negative Tch 99 and up to 70 % false negative Gallium 67 Ga.

Magnetic resonance imaging is the investigation of choice and probably the most effective. The amplitude of the explored area allows us to obtain complete information on the extent of bone involvement, soft tissue and neurological damage. Signal changes are similar to those described in bacterial infection as opposed to a lesser involvement of the intervertebral disc. The MRI also allow us to differentiate between different types of anatomical involvement (Fig. 2). The use of paramagnetic contrast agent, Gadolinium, allows better visualization of abscesses. If you draw a contrast capture peripheral ring indicating the boundaries of the abscess, and if instead it displays a large mass with contrast enhancement, it is probably tissue granulation.

CT-guided byopsy will give a definitive diagnosis. Microbiological study will be conducted by Loweinstein culture and histopathology for the presence of granulomas that will support the diagnosis and initiate specific treatment pending culture results.

Treatment of Spinal Infection

The goals of treatment of spinal infection are: cure the disease, decrease pain, preserve or improve neurological function and maintain mechanical balance of the spine (sagittal and frontal) and prevent disease recurrence.

Basically the treatment of spinal infection is pharmacological. Surgical treatment is associated with the presence of complications such as neurological deficit, epidural abscess or mechanical disruption in those cases where specific medical treatment can not cure the disease.

Medical Treatment

Pyogenic Infection

Once identified the causative organism should be treated according to the antibiogram. Full doses intravenously should be the choice. This should be maintained between 3 and 6 weeks and then move on to oral if the response has been clinically and biologically positive. PCR repeated during the evolution of the disease reflect the response to treatment. The duration of oral antibiotic therapy will depend on the organism, the immune system of the patient and other factors such as the presence of implants.

Contact orthoses are useful in the lumbar region, while the cervical region may require immobilization with a rigid cervicothoracic halo or brace. Mechanical restraint is intended to relieve pain and prevent deformity.

Prevention and recurrence is important in malnourished hospitalized patients, such as elderly, patients with chronic disease in whom there are increased metabolic needs secondary to fever, severe infection or surgical treatment. The goal is to restore satisfactory nutritional status in the patient. The aim is to achieve a serum albumin >3 g/dl, absolute lymphocyte count >800/ml, blood transferring >1.5 g/l and creatinine excretion in 24 h >10.5 mg in men and 5.8 mg in women [24].

Tuberculosis Infection

Due difficulties in isolating the organism the pharmacological treatment should be long and well-tracked for eradicating the disease and not create drug resistance.

Chemotherapy is the primary treatment for bone tuberculosis eradication. The British Medical Council group has carried out numerous works since 1963 to understand the behaviour and response of bone tuberculosis to various drug treatments. Their results show that specific medical treatment for a period of 6 months is enough to cure bone TB [25]. In the first 2 months, 3 drugs: isoniazid, rifampicin and pyrazinamide are used and in the remaining 4 months, 2 drugs, isoniazid and rifampicin. It is important to monitor the compliance of drug treatment by a TB infection specialist. Changes may be needed depending on treatment resistance or intolerance. However the published results showed that long-term healing of the disease was accompanied by residual kyphosis or lack of fusion in about 40 % [25, 26].

This, today can be improved through the use of specialized surgical techniques to support advances in anesthetics and new instrumentation devices.

Surgical Treatment

At present the surgical treatment in spinal infection has a clear role in promoting bone healing and preventing devastating consequences. There are absolute [27] and relative indications: Among these are absolute indications for surgery are: open abscess drainage not percutaneous drainage; neurological deficit secondary to compression or bone destruction, severe kyphosis that imbalances the spine. Relative indications are: absence of a causative organism, failure of medical treatment to control the symptoms and lack of fusión, pseudarthrosis and segmental pain.

There are considerable risks associated with this surgery. Patients older than 60 years, diabetes, immunosuppression and malnutrition but should not be considered contra-indications. The timing of the surgery will be performed as early as possible from the moment that the patient matches the criteria indicated for surgical treatment.

The type of surgery will depend on the affected segment and the goal of surgery in each case. There are three main surgical techniques required with different clinical situations.

Double Approach Anterior and Posterior

This is the most aggressive but also the safest technique. Preferably it is indicated in cases with: spinal cord compression, and severe kyphotic deformity and psoas abscess. They are usually advanced cases of the disease in which there is severe destruction of the anterior column with or without neurological involvement. Normally, it takes an anterior approach first to allow extensive clearing of the disc-vertebral segment, spinal decompression and reconstruction of

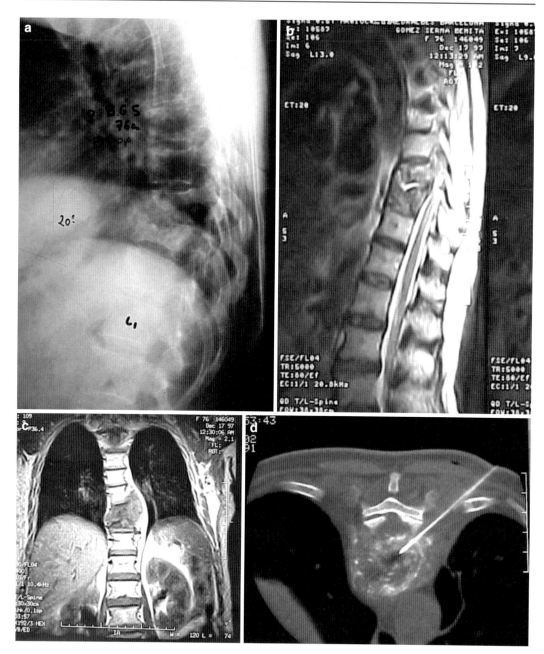

Fig. 5 76 year-old patient with long-standing back pain and paraparesis (Frankel C). (**a**) Radiology with involvement T10-T11 and kyphosis angle of 20°. (**b**) MRI sagittal T2 hyperintense disc and spinal cord compression. (**c**) MRI coronal paravertebral abscess. (**d**) Spinal CT-guided biopsy gave the result- of tuberculosis infection

bone stock from the anterior column by bone grafting as described by the Hong Kong school in 1964 [2].

We recommend using structural autologous graft from iliac crest preferably tri-cortical or pedicled-vascularized rib in the case of the thoracic spine which provides support and immediate vascular supply, resulting in a shorter integration time. Allograft bone will be used rarely in septic processes, as it is associated

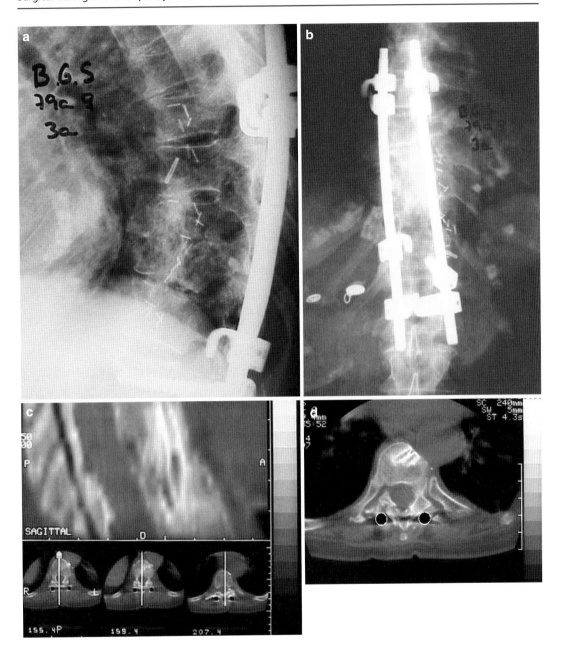

Fig. 6 The same patient was operated on by a double approach with pedicle rib graft and posterior instrumentation. (**a, b**) Radiology infectious focus fusion. (**c, d**) CT reconstruction- previous graft incorporated

with a higher percentage of fracture and delayed union [29]. Recently titanium mesh filled with bone to reconstruct the anterior column has been used. We prefer not to use metal implants unless it is strictly necessary. In the second stage a posterior approach through which correction of the deformity of the posterior column can be stabilized by pedicle instrumentation and posterolateral arthrodesis is performed. Immediate stability is achieved by promoting the incorporation of the graft and the improved fusion rate allows early rehabilitation of the patient. (Figs. 5 and 6). This second approach can be performed in a single procedure or staged at 2-week intervals.

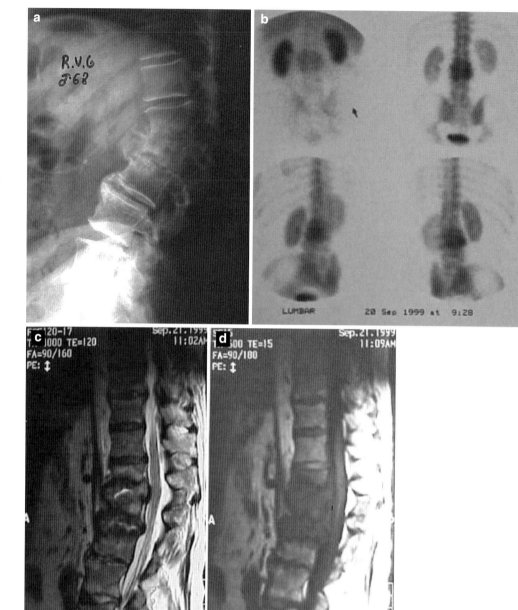

Fig. 7 68 year-old patient diagnosed with vertebral bacterial infection by gram-negative organism. (**a**) Involvement of levels T12-I1-I2 with bone injury and disc space at both levels. Angular kyphosis. (**b**) Positive scintigraphic uptake. (**c**) T2-hyperintense sequence disc. (**d**) T1-weighted sequence shows diagnostic hypo-signal affecting vertebral bodies and disc spaces supporting the diagnosis

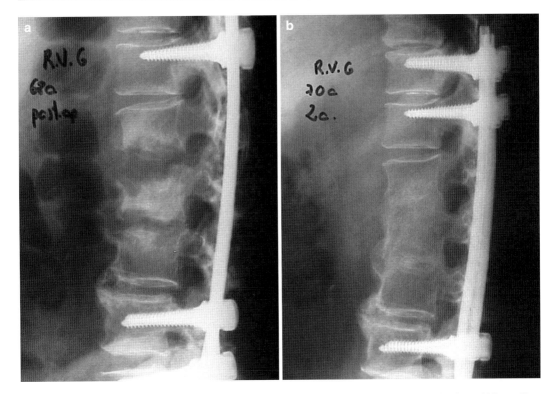

Fig. 8 Same patient who underwent instrumented posterolateral fusion in the absence of complications. (**a**) Immediate post-operative control radiograph. (**b**) 2 years post-operatively showing complete healing of the disease

In cases where there were contra-indications to the anterior approach, costotransversectomy can be used for access to the anterior column and allows radical, clearing and drainage of abscesses.

The double approach is the most commonly used and especially in cases where there is involvement the thoracolumbar junction, because a highly unstable transition area between thoracic kyphosis and lordosis exists. Despite the potential morbidity of this surgery, it has provided excellent results in the literature and this is confirmed by our own experience.

Posterior Approach

This is a common technique using spinal instrumentation with pedicle screws or laminar hooks and provides sagittal deformity correction, moderate posterolateral biological contribution and perhaps most important immediate stabilization

of the infection site. The results have been very satisfactory at intermediate stages of the disease or cases with sequelae without major complications. The technique acts as an internal immobilization system that favours the fusion and reduces the risk of non-union (Figs. 7 and 8). The indication of choice is: the persistence of pain at the end of medical treatment, the tendency to segmental interbody fusion and when there has been no isolation of the pathogen.

Anterior Approach

The isolated anterior approach technique was first described by Hodgson in 1964 for the treatment of tuberculosis infection. Currently performed as an isolated technique is exceptional in the thoracic and lumbar spine. It is most appropriate in rare cases of cervical infection. It can be a valuable in cases where only drainage and bone grafting is sought for the lumbar lordosis.

Yilmaz et al. [30] study showed how infection could be treated by anterior approaches over previous spinal instrumentation, avoiding subsequent second approach. It is imperative to have an intact posterior column to carry on this technique.

In general, surgery is more common in cases of tuberculous spinal infection than in bacterial infection. The clinical behaviour of tuberculosis infection with slow and subacute development. implies that at the time of diagnosis a big imbalance deformity exists or neurological compromise which require more aggressive treatment for healing. In our experience over 50 % of patients with spinal tuberculosis underwent surgical treatment.

Conclusions

Infections are the most common vertebral haematogenous bacterial and tuberculous infections. Early diagnosis and specific medical treatment can cure the disease. Surgery is has specific indications which greatly enhance therapeutic healing. Faced with a poor response to drug treatment or in the presence of complications surgical treatment should not be delayed. The results are excellent in the revised series despite with aggressive surgery and even in elderly patients. Do not forget to maintain a satisfactory nutritional status; it will determine much of the success of treatment.

References

1. Carregee EJ. Pyogenic vertebral osteomielitis. J Bone Joint Surg Am. 1997;79:874–8800.
2. Ring D, Wenger DR. Pyogenic infectious spondylitis in children: the evolution to current Thought. Am J Orthop. 1996;25:342–8.
3. Modic MT, Feiglin DH, Piranio DW, et al. Vertebral osteomyelitis: assessement using MR. Radiology. 1985;157:157–66.
4. Post MJD, Quencer RM, Montalve BM, Katz BH, Eismont FJ, Green BA. Spinal infection: evaluation with MR imaging and intraoperative US. Radiology. 1988;169:765–71.
5. Gorse GJ, Pais MJ, Kusske JA, Cesario TC. Tuberculous spondylitis: a report of six cases and review of the literature. Medicine. 1983;62:178–93.
6. Ergan M, Macro M, Benhamou CL. Septic arthritis of lumbar facet joints: a review of six cases. Rev Rhum Engl Ed. 1997;64:386–95.
7. Wiley AM, Trueta J. The vascular anatomy of the spine and its relationship to pyogenic vertebral osteoyekitis. J Bone Joint Surg Br. 1959;41:796–809.
8. Eismont FJ, Bohlman HH, Soni PL, Goldberg VM, Freehafer AA. Pyogenic and fungal vertebral osteomyelitis with paralysis. J Bone Joint Surg Am. 1983;65:19–29.
9. Torda AJ, Gottlieb T, Bradbury R. Pyogenic vertebral osteomyelitis: analysis of 20 cases and review. Clin Infect Dis. 1995;20:320–8.
10. Emery SE, Chan DP, Woodward HR. Tratment of hematogenous pyogenic vertebral osteomyelitis with anterior debridement and primary bone grafting. Spine. 1989;14:284–91.
11. Hadjipavlou AG, Crow WN, Borowski A, Mader JT, Adesokan A, Jensen RE. Percutaneous transpedicular discectomy and drainage in pyogenic spondylodiscitis. Am J Orthop. 1998;27:188–97.
12. Kemp HBS, Jackson JW, Jeremiah JD, Hall AJ. Pyogenic infections occurring primarily in intervertebral discs. J Bone Joint Surg Br. 1973;55:698–714.
13. Rath SA, Neff U, Schneider O, Ritchter HP. Neurosurgical management of thoracic and lumbar vertebral osteomyelitis and discitis in adults: a review of 43 consecutive surgically treated patients. Neurosurgery. 1996;38:926–33.
14. Sapico F, Montgomerie JZ. Vertebral osteomyelitis. Infect Dis Clin North Am. 1990;4:539–50.
15. Waldvogel FA, Papageorgiou PS. Osteomyelitis: the past decace. N Engl J Med. 1980;303:360–70.
16. Hadjipavlou AG, Mader JT, Necessary JT, Muffoletto AJ. Spine. 2000;25:1668–79.
17. De Witt D, Mulla R, Cowie MR, Mason JC, Davies KA. Vertebral osteomyelitis due to *Staphylococcus epidermidis*. Br J Rheumatol. 1993;32:239–41.
18. Darouchi RO, Hamill RJ, Greenberg SB, Weaathers SW, Musher DM. Bacterial spinal epidural abscess: review of 43 cases and literature survey. Medicine. 1992;71:369–85.
19. Lang IM, Hughes DG, Jenkins JP, St Clair Forbes W, Mc Kenna F. Mr imaging appearances of cervical epidural abscess. Clin Radiol. 1995;50:466–71.
20. Kornblum MB, Wesolowski DP, Fischgrund JS, Herkowitz HN. Computed tomography-guided biopsy of the spine: a review of 103 patients. Spine. 1998;23:81–5.
21. Fraser RD, Osti OL, Vernon-Roberts B. Iatrogenic discitis: the role of intravenous antibiotics in prevention and treatment: an experimental study. Spine. 1989;14:1025–32.
22. Stoker DJ, Kissin CM. Percutaneous vertebral biopsy: a review of 135 cases. Clin Radiol. 1985;36:569–77.
23. Dobson J. Tuberculosis of the spine. An analysis of the results of the conservative treatment and of the factors influencing the prognosis. J Bone Joint Surg Br. 1951;33:517.

24. Tay BKB, Deckey J, Hu SS. Infections of the spine. J Am Acad Orthop Surg. 2002;10:188–97.

25. Medical Research Council Working Party on tuberculosis of the spine. A comparison of 6 or 9 months course regime of chemotherapy in patients receiving ambulatory treatment or undergoing radical surgery for tuberculosis of the spine. Indian J Tuberc. 1989;36(suppl):1.

26. A controlled trial of anterior spinal fusion and debridement in the surgical management of tuberculosis of the spine in patients on standard chemotherapy: a study in Hong-Kong. Br J Surg 1974;61:853–66.

27. Moon MS. Tuberculosis of the spine: controversies and a new challenge. Spine. 1997;22:1791–7.

28. Upadhyay SS, Sell P, Saji MJ, Bell B, Yau AM, Leong CYC. Seventeen year prospective study of surgical management of spinal tuberculosis in children: Hong-Kong operation compared with debridement surgery for short and long term outcome of deformity. Spine. 1993;18:1704–11.

29. Govender S, Parbhoo AH. Support for the anterior column with allografts in tuberculosis of the spine. J Bone Joint Surg Br. 1999;81:106–9.

30. Yilmaz C, Selek HY, Gurkan I, Erdemli B, Korkusu Z. Anterior instrumentation for the treatment of spinal tuberculosis. J Bone Joint Surg Am. 1999;81:1261–7.

31. Vider M, Maruyama Y, Narvaez R. Significance of the vertebral venous (Batson's) plexus in metastatic spread in colorectal carcinoma. Cancer 1977;40:67–71.

Surgical Management of Tuberculosis of the Spine

Ahmet Alanay and Deniz Olgun

Contents

A. Alanay (✉)
Department of Orthopaedics and Traumatology,
Comprehensive Spine Center, Acibadem Maslak
Hospital, Istanbul, Turkey
e-mail: aalanay@hacettepe.edu.tr

D. Olgun
Department of Orthopaedics and Traumatology,
Hacettepe University, Ankara, Turkey
e-mail: aalanay@hacettepe.edu.tr

Abstract

Although an old ancient disease, tuberculosis is still a major public health problem that affects both developing and developed countries. With the increase in immuno-compromised states, it has become a larger problem which is growing ever more difficult to treat. The most common site of extrapulmonary tuberculosiṣ is the spine, and here it causes destruction and deformity which may lead to kyphosis and paraplegia. The natural history of tuberculous spondylitis has been defined in great detail owing to its frequency in the years preceding the advent of anti-tuberculous drugs and effective surgical treatment options. Today the treatment of spinal tuberculosis begins with diagnosis, which can be still a difficult one. This includes a careful history, physical examination, x-rays and, most importantly, MRI.scans However, often, tissue diagnosis is necessary and cultures, though generally reliable, are often slow to yield results. Surgical treatment can commence after obtaining tissue for diagnosis and addresses removal of necrotic tissue at the affected segments, instability and, if it already exists, deformity. The use of implants in tuberculous spondylitis has been shown to be safe, and necessary in specific cases owing to unacceptable kyphosis as an outcome after exclusively conservative treatment. Today, the preferred form of treatment is debridement and instrumented fusion, and depending on the stability of fixation, post-operative

G. Bentley (ed.), *European Surgical Orthopaedics and Traumatology*,
DOI 10.1007/978-3-642-34746-7_36, © EFORT 2014

immobilization. The mainstay of treatment, as it was 50 years ago, is still anti-tuberculous medical therapy.

Keywords

Complications • Diagnosis • Late deformity • Operative techniques • Pathophysiology • Spine • Surgical indications • Tuberculosis

Introduction

Tuberculosis of the spine is one of the most ancient diseases known to mankind, with reports of it dating back 5,000 years [1]. Despite the advances in the previous century, tuberculosis remains an important public health problem with close to ten million new reported cases in 2008 [2]. First characterized by Pott in the late eighteenth century as 'Pott's distemper of the spine', it still represents one third of spinal infections today. Owing to the advent of effective public health measures, anti-tuberculous drugs and, although controversial, the Bacille-Calmette-Guerin vaccine, the incidence of tuberculosis has been declining steadily in the latter half of the twentieth century. However, with the emergence of first the AIDS and then the diabetes epidemics, tuberculosis is back on the rise even in developed countries. Today, patients with co-morbidities make up the bulk of cases, while antibiotic therapy remains the mainstay of treatment. Although spinal tuberculosis remains an uncommon diagnosis, it must yet be kept in mind in patients with spinal complaints whose aetiology is not readily apparent.

Aetiology

Tuberculosis is caused by the pathogen Mycobacterium tuberculosis. It is transmitted mainly through inhalation or ingestion of the bacterium. Less than 10 % of tuberculosis patients have musculo-skeletal involvement, yet 50 % of these have involvement of the spine [3–6]. Neurological deficit at the time of presentation is also common, reported to be between 10 % and 60 % [7].

Extrapulmonary tuberculosis seems to be increasing worldwide [8, 9]. With the increasing number of immune-compromised patients due to AIDS, auto-immune disease, cancer therapy and organ transplantation, the incidence of diseases caused by atypical mycobacteria has also increased. Atypical mycobacteria and fungi constitute a small percentage of the causes of spinal infection, but their clinical and radiologic appearances resemble those of Mycobacterium tuberculosis spondylitis. The most common atypical mycobacterium isolated from vertebral osteomyelitis in one series was found to be mycobacterium avium-intracellular complex [10].

Although anti-tuberculosis drugs provide an effective weapon in the treatment of tuberculous spondylitis, the emergence of multi-drug resistant strains has caused a setback. Tuberculosis treatment is started with four so-called first-line drugs: isoniazid, rifampicin, pyrazinamide and ethambutol. Multi-drug-resistant tuberculosis is defined as that resistant to isoniazid and rifampicin [11–13]. The term "extensively drug- resistant tuberculosis" has been coined by the US CDC and the WHO to describe tuberculosis resistant to at least isoniazid and rifampicin and several second-line drugs [14, 15]. Multi-drug resistant spondylitis has been reported [16, 17]. Multi-drug and extensively drug resistant tuberculosis represent failures of the aforementioned public health measures to control the disease and emphasizes the necessity of a proper drug regimen of appropriate duration and complete patient compliance. The incidence of these problems have been on the rise as well [18].

Before the discovery of anti-tuberculosis drugs and modern surgical techniques, bed-rest and conservative immobilization were the mainstays of treatment of tuberculous spondylitis. This led to an extensive knowledge regarding the natural history of the disease [19, 20]. Untreated tuberculosis of the spine has three stages. The first is the stage of onset, lasting from 1 month to 1 year, the second the stage of destruction which can go on for up to 3 years and the last stage, the stage of repair and ankylosis. Abscess formation and destruction are seen in the second stage, which a third of the patients do not survive, while in the third stage, the joint or spine heals with bony ankylosis or fusion. Non-union is associated with recurrences and super-infections with pyogenic bacteria, generally, an unfavorable outcome. Historic treatments of tuberculosis included bed rest, heliotherapy and sometimes plaster immobilization in order to pre-empt spinal deformity. Despite these measures, kyphosis still was a problem, many times accompanied by paraplegia as described by Pott [20, 21].

Spinal tuberculosis most commonly affects the thoracic or thoraco-lumbar spine, although cervical and lumbo-sacral involvement has been reported [22]. Spinal involvement has been classified by Mehta et al. according to anterior and posterior column involvement into four groups: anterior involvement only, anterior and posterior involvement, anterior or global with thoracotomy presenting grave risk, and posterior involvement only [23]. The most common is anterior involvement with destruction of the disc space and loss of anterior stability, making posterior laminectomy a greater destabilizing factor, should it be chosen as the method for treatment.

Pathophysiology

Tuberculosis reaches the spine either through direct extension through the lungs or haematologic dissemination from a pulmonary or genitorurinary source. Direct extension is rare, whereas the haematologic form of dissemination is far more common. The infection can appear in three distinct patterns: peri-discal, central and anterior [24], the most common of which is peri-discal involvement. The disease begins in the vertebral end-plate adjacent to the disc, extends anteriorly underneath the anterior longitudinal ligament and in this way multiple levels are infected while the intervertebral discs are spared. This presents a contrast to pyogenic spinal osteomyelitis where the disc is involved. Central involvement can lead to deformity. Anterior involvement can lead to spinal abscesses that span many levels. Primary posterior involvement is rare. As in spinal trauma, stability of the spine is lost if two or more columns are affected

[25, 26], but this definition is not as clear-cut as in the case of acute fracture. Inflammation and destruction in tuberculosis co-exist with repair and fibrosis. Yet, the occurrence of a pathologic fracture or global disease affecting posterior elements as well may lead to the loss of stability [27]. With the loss of the support of the anterior column, acute kyphosis develops. Once the disease reaches the healing stage, bony ankylosis is complete and the kyphosis is rigid.

Once the pathogen is safely ensconced in living tissue, the inflammatory response of the immune system causes pus and debris to accumulate, forming abscesses and fluid collection. In contrast to pyogenic infection where proteolytic enzymes cause most of the destruction, in tuberculosis the delayed-type hypersensitivity reaction of the body itself is the culprit [28]. Bone resorption follows. This may take place anterior to the anterior longitudinal ligament, extending downward to the psoas sheath and causing the well-defined psoas-abscesses of Pott's disease. It may also end up in the spinal canal, causing compression of the spinal cord. The neural structures may also be affected directly by tubercle formation, leading to neurologic deficit and even paraplegia. Causes of neurologic deficit include direct involvement of neural structures with the disease, compression by abscess and fluid formation, vascular compromise and compression by bony debris left over from the destructive process.

Diagnosis

The presentation of tuberculosis of the spine can be variable. It depends on the extent of the disease, the nutritional status of the patient and the time that has elapsed since the onset of disease. Back pain is a common presenting symptom. The pain is less severe than in pyogenic infection [24], follows an indolent course, often waxing at night and increases as instability progresses. Pott's paraplegia, the gravest complication of the disease, is a presenting symptom in nearly 10 % of the patients [29, 30]. Constitutional symptoms are also common such as fatigue, malaise, low-grade fever, weight loss and the anaemia of chronic disease. Acute phase reactants such as white blood cell count, sedimentation rate and c-reactive protein may be elevated, but normal values do not rule out the disease. The patient may or may not have a history of pulmonary tuberculosis. Immunosuppression is a risk factor for the development of tuberculous spondylitis. In underdeveloped countries, patients may present with obvious deformity, sinus tract formation and even neurological deficit and paraplegia. Elderly patients are more likely to present with neurologic deficit.

Late-onset paraplegia is defined as new-onset neurologic deficit after the first spinal infection has healed. It can occur many years after soft-tissue and bony healing have been completed. The reasons for late-onset paraplegia are numerous, some of which are re-activation, development of anterior bony ridges and subsequent cord compromise, chronic instability, increase in kyphotic deformity and rarely, degenerative changes in segments adjacent to those that have healed with significant deformity [31].

Radiographs in early disease are most commonly normal. Osteoporosis is the first sign that can be noted in x-ray studies, with loss of definition at the end-plates and only slight narrowing of the disc space [32]. These changes progress to loss of vertebral body height. Disk space is preserved until the disease progresses. Fusiform soft-tissue swelling in the thoracic region and the darkening of the psoas shadow in the lumbar region are other radiological changes that have been previously defined. The destruction of the anterior portions of multiple levels with sparing of the posterior elements will lead to a progressively worsening kyphotic deformity [28]. This kyphosis will progress until the last stage of the disease if it is left untreated. Sinus tract formation can occur during this process, and lead to pyogenic super-infection, which will in turn increase bony destruction and worsen deformity. Plain radiographs usually do not usually indicate the extent of the disease. Further imaging, preferably with MRI, is always necessary.

CT scanning shows bony destruction and can be used for pre-operative planning of complex deformity or, more commonly, as a guide for needle biopsy in order to achieve tissue diagnosis. Bone scanning can be performed but cannot differentiate tuberculous spondylitis from other causes of infectious disease and although it can be helpful in some cases, its use is limited. MRI remains the most helpful imaging modality in the diagnosis of tuberculosis, showing abscess formation, epidural involvement and involvement of the spinal cord as well as bony destruction.

MRI is the modality of choice in vertebral osteomyelitis of any kind as it has very high sensitivity and specificity [33]. Also, MRI is non-invasive and has unequalled resolution for soft, especially neural tissues. MRI is the only modality to distinguish spondylitides of different aetiology [7, 34–37]. The earliest finding is end-plate oedema, which appears as a decreased T1-weighted signal and increased T2-weighted signal. Short-tau inversion recovery images are usually superior to other modalities as they allow the suppression of the bright fat signal of the bone marrow [38]. If the disc space is found to be preserved, the diagnosis of tuberculosis will become more than likely, as it is a pathognomonic finding of this disease. This relative sparing of the disc space is what differentiates it most from pyogenic infection. The infection progresses into the retropharyngeal soft tissue or sub-ligamentously to involve further spinal levels and the paraspinal areas. Abscesses show rim-enhancement with the addition of Gadolinum-containing contrast material, and therefore, cases with suspicion for spinal infection should always be examined with contrast unless otherwise contra-indicated [32]. This abscess wall in tuberculous is thick, and calcifications, though not always present, are also characteristic of the disease.

Tuberculosis is known to mimic other conditions of the spine. One of these is metastatic disease, which can be differentiated from tuberculosis of the spine by the absence of paraspinal and other abscesses. Fungal spondyliitis and spondylitis caused by atypical mycobacteria are far more difficult to differentiate by imaging findings alone and require tissue diagnosis. Radiographic changes may progress with the initiation of medical treatment for more than a year and should not be mistaken for the failure of treatment [39].

Gibbus formation (sharp kyphosis at affected levels), due to anterior column destruction is, seen in late untreated disease and conservatively-treated disease. This deformity may progress despite skeletal maturity and lead to late paraplegia. However, the increase in deformity is not the only cause of late paraplegia in healed disease. Other causes are compression of the spinal cord by bony bridges, calcified caseous material, fibrosis and disease re-activation [28].

Laboratory diagnosis is difficult. Purified protein derivative (PPD) or tuberculin skin testing has lost importance in the passing years. It is especially non-specific in areas where tuberculosis is endemic, BCG vaccination is routine, or the population is frequently exposed to sub-clinical disease [28]. A new blood test measuring interferon-gamma response after in vitro stimulation of the patient's T-cells with tuberculosis antigens is being developed and could replace the less specific tuberculin skin testing and provide a tool for the detection of latent tuberculosis. There are also studies attempting to increase the specificity of the tuberculin skin test [40]. Sputum smears for acid-fast bacilli are one of the primary methods of laboratory diagnosis but are negative in patients without pulmonary tuberculosis and in a significant portion of patients with it. Although mycobacterial culture is quite sensitive, it requires direct tissue sampling in the case of spinal tuberculosis and is slow to yield results. Newer liquid culture systems such as BACTEC have reduced this delay to days rather than weeks with conventional methods and have been found to be more sensitive as well [41]. Diagnostic tests using nucleic acid amplification techniques and polymerase-chain reaction methods have been developed and show high specificity for tuberculosis, yet their cost and requirement for high-technology laboratory facilities coupled with their modest sensitivity have precluded widespread use [40]. Direct visualization of the granulamatous reaction and the presence of intracellular pathogens (acid-fast bacilli) under direct microscopy are the gold standard methods of diagnosis.

Indications for Surgery

Today, the mainstay of treatment for tuberculous spondylitis is medical. Shortened time to disease onset and diagnosis have allowed tuberculous spondylitis to be caught before the development of complex spinal deformity. However, medical therapy alone has been shown to increase healing with kyphosis and deformity in many cases. The addition of bed rest and/or cast or brace immobilization was found to be ineffective in the development of kyphotic deformity in the British Medical Research Council Working Party on Tuberculosis of the Spine reports [42–45].

Multi-drug regimens (three or more drugs) of at least 6 months duration showing good healing responses, and advancement in minimally-invasive techniques to evacuate huge abcessess led to re-definition of surgical indications. These are:
- Lesions not healing after 6 months of anti-tuberculosis therapy
- Lesions developing after 6 months of anti-tuberculosis therapy
- Gross instability of the spine
- New-onset neurologic deficit or worsening of prior neurologic deficit while under anti-tuberculosis therapy
- Unacceptable or impending deformity

Pre-Operative Planning

Once the diagnosis of tuberculosis of the spine has been established, the patient should be started on anti-tuberculous therapy as soon as possible, preferably under the supervision of an infectious diseases specialist. Drug regimens based on isoniazid and rifampicin for at least 6 months have shown good results [46]. According to the recommendations issued by the United States Centers for Disease Control, a four-drug regimen should be used to treat Pott's disease. Rifampin and isoniazid should be administered during the therapy and another first-line drug chosen for the first 2 months along with one second-line drug. The duration of therapy should be at least 6 months, but as studies concerning special circumstances such as neurologic deficit and the involvement of multiple vertebral levels are scanty, some specialists still recommend therapy to last for 9–12 months. In the case of suspicion of multi-drug or extensively drug-resistant tuberculosis, proper consultations should be obtained.

Surgical Techniques

Many approaches to tuberculous spondylitis have been described. Before the advent of effective anti-mycobacterial therapy, surgery carried the quite large risk of sinus tract formation, leading to pyogenic infection and death of the patient. For this reason, indirect operations were favoured in order to increase stability and decrease recurrence, leading to the description of posterior fusion techniques.

After effective anti-tuberculous therapy was shown to heal sinus tracts and ulcers, surgical therapy could directly deal with the problem at hand. Many techniques were described, most of them including radical resection of diseased tissues and massive reconstruction using structural grafts or cages.

Non-Instrumented Posterior Fusion

Posterior fusion was the preferred method of treatment in many centres before anterior spinal surgery was found to be safe and effective. The rationale behind posterior fusion is the achievement of a stable spinal segment in order to hasten healing and decrease the progress of kyphotic deformity. However, results of this technique were disappointing. Kyphotic deformity increased despite posterior fusion and prolonged immobilization, pseudarthrosis was common and healing was not found to be more rapid in several published series [47, 48]. Today, non-instrumented posterior fusion has been abandoned in the treatment of tuberculous spondylitis.

Anterior Radical Resection and Bone Grafting

The "Hong Kong operation" was described by the British Medical Research Council Working Party on Tuberculosis of the Spine. It is the radical removal of all affected tissue until healthy, bleeding bone is encountered and subsequent reconstruction with bone graft with or without internal fixation, a modification of the original technique of Hodgson [49–51]. The reports on the Hong Kong operation, which does not employ instrumentation, are favourable in the long-term with very little loss of correction of kyphosis. However, there is a need for external bracing at least for 3–6 months until bony healing and incorporation of the graft material. On the other hand, it may be difficult to preserve the sagittal plane correction when more than one vertebral level has to be resected and either anterior or posterior instrumentation should be added when reconstruction spans more than one vertebral body. Debridement of all the necrotic and diseased segments and reconstruction of the anterior defect is still the key surgical principle for the treatment of tuberculosis. However, surgeons nowadays prefer to do either anterior or posterior instrumentation in addition to the Hong-Kong procedure to increase stability, preserve the correction in sagittal plane and to obviate the need for external braces (Fig. 1).

Debridement (Anterior or Posterior) and Instrumentation

The study by Oga et al. reporting the lack of glycocalyx capsule formation by tuberculosis bacilli has been a revolutionary step in the surgical treatment of tuberculosis spondylitis [52]. Many studies in the recent years have shown successful use of implants either anteriorly or posteriorly after debridement of necrotic tissues with no recurrence and exacerbation of the infection [50–53].

Both anterior and posterior instrumentation have been used in tuberculous spondylitis with success. Many combinations of the aforementioned approaches exist and should be chosen according to the patient's special features, the resources available and Surgeon preference. Staged operations beginning with anterior debridement and continuing with posterior instrumentation, anterior debridement, posterior instrumentation and subsequent anterior instrumentation, and simultaneous anterior and posterior debridement and instrumentation have been defined and used with success [52, 54].

The thoracic vertebral column can be approached by an anterior trans-thoracic or posterior extra-pleural method. While the transthoracic method is straightforward, it may be associated with pulmonary complications postoperatively. The pulmonary condition of the patient before the operation should be carefully assessed and the risks weighed. The posterior extra-pleural method requires more surgical finesse, but may prevent further deterioration in patients with pulmonary co-morbidity. It also may

be indicated in severe osteoporotic patients where anterior instrumentation may be unsafe and can be an alternative for combined anterior debridement and posterior instrumentation surgery.

The postero-lateral approach as used for posterior vertebral column resection provides adequate exposure and allows the insertion of cages and other anterior struts. This is performed by a posterior approach. The upper and lower end levels are instrumented using pedicle screws. Once this is performed, one rod is inserted in order to prevent accidental movements. On the other side, costo-transversectomy is performed on as many levels as necessary. Nerve roots and intercostal veins are visualized, tied and then cut. Using a periosteal elevator, the exposure is extended to cover the entire circumference of the vertebral body. Once the anterior column is visualized, debridement is commenced. Debridement should remove all necrotic tissue, pus and loose bone fragments, but viable bone is not resected. Tissue sampling should be performed, with

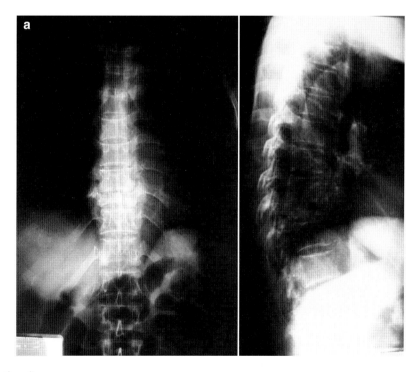

Fig. 1 (continued)

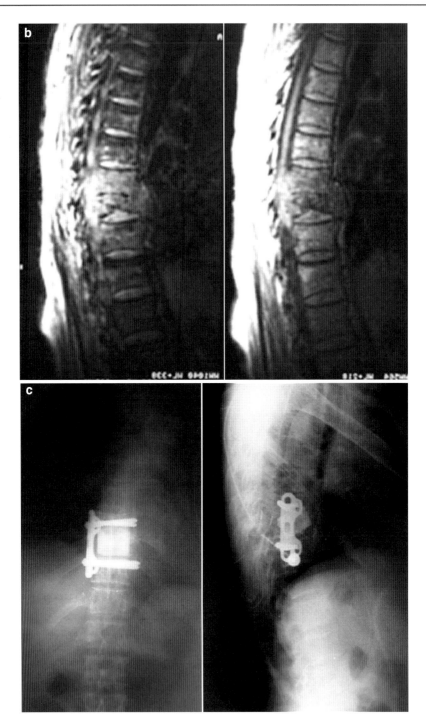

Fig. 1 (**a**) A-P and lateral x-ray of a 42 year-old male patient suffering back pain and neurological symptoms. Patient had a pathologic compression fracture of T9 vertebrae due to tuberculosis. (**b**) Sagittal MRI views demonstrate the abcess at T9 vertebral body and epidural compression due to abcess. (**c**) Follow-up A-P and lateral x-rays. Anterior debridement, reconstruction with allograft and instrumentation was performed

mycobacterial cultures and specimens for patho-logical study. After debridement and decompression anterior structural bone graft is placed and rod is placed on the costo-transversectomy side and pedicle screws are compressed to increase the stability of the anterior graft. Authors have reported good results in tuberculosis as well with this technique [55]. Good results were achieved with the use of the posterior approach alone [53] (Fig. 2).

As deformity is often a result of tuberculous spondylitis, the necessity for instrumentation should be carefully evaluated.

Late Deformity

With recent advances in surgical implants and techniques, the contemporary approach to severe kyphotic deformity includes instrumentation and

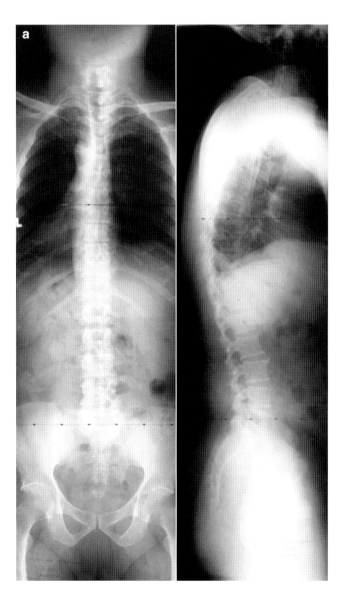

Fig. 2 (continued)

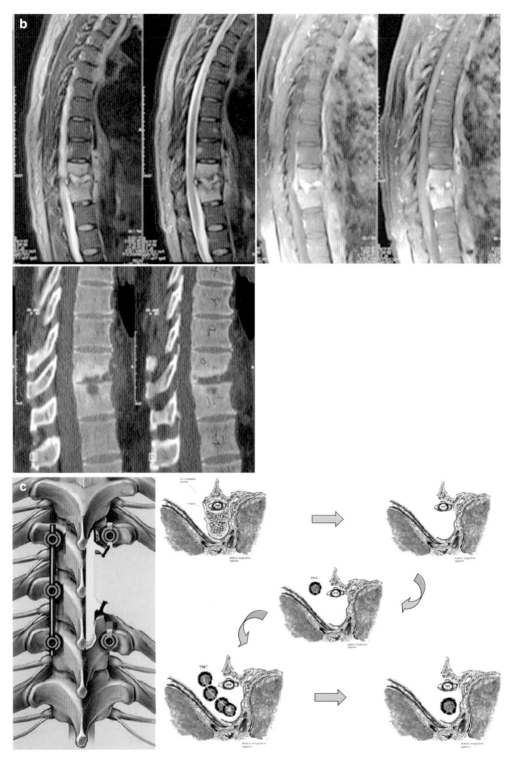

Fig. 2 (continued)

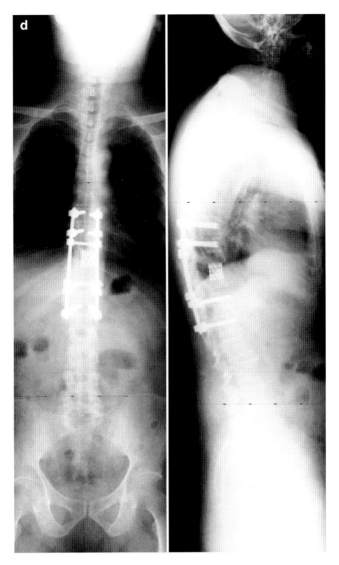

Fig. 2 (a) A-P and lateral x-ray of a 60 year-old male who had tuberculosis at T9 and T10 vertebrae. P. (b) Sagittal MRI scans demonstrating the abcess at T9-T10 vertebral bodies and the disc space. There is also epidural abcess. (c) Figures demonstrating the technical steps of decompression, fusion and instrumentation via a single posterior approach. (d) Follow-up A-P and lateral x-rays (Images and diagrams courtesy of Azmi Hamzoglu, MD)

spinal osteotomy, which can be done in an anterior-posterior-anterior fashion, simultaneous anterior surgery or posterior vertebral column resection (PVCR). These procedures, although challenging and prone to severe complications, have been used successfully for the treatment of late deformity [56–59]. Following spondylectomy, the resulting bone defect is filled with autograft or titanium mesh cages. Pedicle screw instrumentation and vertebral osteotomy are effective in the treatment of most forms of kyphosis, although spondylectomy is more appropriate for sharp, angular kyphosis as occurs following tuberculosis [59]. Previous studies have found that instrumentation of the spine afflicted with tuberculosis is safe [52] and that titanium mesh cages can safely be used in pyogenic infection as well. Fusion rates with any approach are acceptable and deformity correction is best with spondylectomy and pedicle screw instrumentation.

Minimally-Invasive Techniques

Video-assisted thoracoscopic techniques have been described in the treatment of tuberculosis of the spine. They are especially appropriate for the procurement of tissue material for biopsy and culture, and mid-thoracic disease affecting few levels which is unrelated to pulmonary tuberculosis [60, 61].

Complications of tuberculosis of the spine, such as discrete abscesses and collections, can be successfully treated by percutaneous drainage placed under ultrasound or CT guidance [62].

Post-Operative Care and Rehabilitation

The post-operative care for a tuberculosis patient is no different than for any other spine patient, except for the obvious need for anti-tuberculous therapy. Anterior transthoracic approaches are involved with a high degree of pulmonary compromise and may necessitate intensive care and prolonged intubation. Once the patient's general condition permits, the patient may be mobilized according to the rigidity achieved by the instrumentation. Routine immobilization is not required with posterior pedicle screw fixation. Orthoses can be used for 6–12 months in those in whom a spondylectomy has been performed. The physical therapy regimen should follow the standards for spine patients.

Complications

The complications that can be encountered depend on the extent of the disease, previous neurological deficit, the surgical approach selected, the type of graft used and the presence or absence of instrumentation.

In patients with neglected disease, deformity is common. The spine usually heals in a kyphotic position. Kyphotic deformity in excess of 60 is associated with late paraplegia even in healed disease. Pain and cosmetic problems can also be seen.

Kyphosis may increase with age despite fusion. Recurrence and re-activation of the disease if not treated properly with anti-tuberculous medication is also possible. Pyogenic infection may supervene in a spine already de-stabilized by tuberculosis and open to the exterior by sinus tracts.

Complications of surgery include pulmonary complications especially for the anterior approach. Vessel injury and epidural bleeding can also be encountered during debridement due to the ossification and fibrosis of the tissues.

Pedicle screw instrumentation is a safe and effective technique for the treatment of spinal disorders. Complications related to the use of pedicle screws can be related to the mal-positioning and faulty technique. Pull-out in osteoporotic bone has been reported and can be avoided in most cases with careful pre-operative planning. Neurological injury during the placement of pedicle screws is rare but catastrophic. The use of motor and sensory-evoked potential monitoring has been revolutionary in the safety of deformity surgery. Patients presenting with neurological deficit at the time of diagnosis usually have a favourable outcome with decompression and medical therapy.

With better supportive care, intensive-care facilities and the better nutritional status of the patients, post-operative mortality has decreased. Miliary tuberculosis following surgery is rare with concomitant medical therapy.

Non-union and mal-union are uncommon. Fusion rates in surgery for the tuberculosis of the spine have been favourable even in historical reports where instrumentation was not available. Loss of correction is also a minor concern.

Summary

Tuberculosis of the spine is an ancient disease that as a large public health problem has inspired research, the development of many surgical techniques and new drugs. While poor living conditions nurture the disease in developing countries, the falling incidence in developed countries following the discovery of effective anti-tuberculosis drugs has been pre-empted by the appearance of modern epidemics leading to overt or functional immuno-compromise. Starting in the pulmonary system, the disease spreads to the vertebral column via the haematological route and causes significant disability and deformity, and may lead to neurological deficit. Several characteristic radiographic changes point to tuberculosis of the spine, the most notable of which is the early sparing of disk space. MRI is the best imaging modality in the diagnosis of tuberculous spondylitis. Diagnosis often requires tissue biopsy which can be done with minimally-invasive techniques, under CT guidance or during surgery. Treatment of tuberculosis of the spine is with anti-tuberculosis drugs, but drug resistance is becoming a problem. According to the results of a series of studies by the British Medical Research Council on Tuberculosis of the Spine, multi-drug therapy combined with surgical intervention leads to best results. Combined with the advances in surgical technique, anaesthetic procedures and implant technology, the preferred treatment today is debridement, instrumentation and fusion of the spine. While good results are being obtained in patients with tuberculosis of the spine, further support of the public health measures are required in order to obtain eradication.

References

1. Nerlich AG, et al. Molecular evidence for tuberculosis in an ancient Egyptian mummy. Lancet. 1997; 350(9088):1404.
2. World Health Organization. Global tuberculosis control: a short update to the 2009 report (2011), Geneva: World Health Organization.
3. Davidson PT, Horowitz I. Skeletal tuberculosis. A review with patient presentations and discussion. Am J Med. 1970;48(1):77–84.
4. Gropper GR, Acker JD, Robertson JH. Computed tomography in Pott's disease. Neurosurgery. 1982;10(4):506–8.
5. Martini M, Ouahes M. Bone and joint tuberculosis: a review of 652 cases. Orthopedics. 1988;11(6):861–6.
6. Tuli SM. Tuberculosis of the spine. New Delhi/Springfield: Published for the National Library of Medicine, U.S. Dept. of Health, Education, and Welfare available from the U.S. Dept. of Commerce, National Technical Information Service, 1975. xviii, p. 163.
7. Boachie-Adjei O, Squillante RG. Tuberculosis of the spine. Orthop Clin North Am. 1996;27(1):95–103.
8. Kruijshaar ME, Abubakar I. Increase in extrapulmonary tuberculosis in England and Wales 1999–2006. Thorax. 2009;64(12):1090–5.
9. Peto HM, et al. Epidemiology of extrapulmonary tuberculosis in the United States, 1993–2006. Clin Infect Dis. 2009;49(9):1350–7.
10. Petitjean G, et al. Vertebral osteomyelitis caused by non-tuberculous mycobacteria. Clin Microbiol Infect. 2004;10(11):951–3.
11. Pablos-Mendez A, et al. Global surveillance for Antituberculosis-drug resistance, 1994–1997. World health organization-international union against tuberculosis and lung disease working group on anti-tuberculosis drug resistance surveillance. N Engl J Med. 1998;338(23):1641–9.
12. Espinal MA, et al. Global trends in resistance to Antituberculosis drugs. World health organization-international union against tuberculosis and lung disease working group on anti-tuberculosis drug resistance surveillance. N Engl J Med. 2001;344(17): 1294–303.
13. Aziz MA, et al. Epidemiology of Antituberculosis drug resistance (the global project on anti-tuberculosis drug resistance surveillance): an updated analysis. Lancet. 2006;368(9553):2142–54.
14. Holtz TH, Cegielski JP. Origin of the term XDR-TB. Eur Respir J. 2007;30(2):396.
15. Holtz TH. XDR-TB in South Africa: revised definition. PLoS Med. 2007;4(4):e161.
16. Cherifi S, Guillaume MP, Peretz A. Multidrug-resistant tuberculosis spondylitis. Acta Clin Belg. 2000;55(1):34–6.
17. Pawar UM, et al. Multidrug-resistant tuberculosis of the spine–is it the beginning of the end? A study of twenty-five culture proven multidrug-resistant tuberculosis spine patients. Spine. 2009;34(22):E806–10 (Phila Pa 1976).
18. Migliori GB, et al. Multidrug-resistant and extensively drug-resistant tuberculosis in the west. Europe and united states: epidemiology, surveillance, and control. Clin Chest Med. 2009;30(4):637–65.
19. Bailey HL, et al. Tuberculosis of the spine in children. Operative findings and results in one hundred consecutive patients treated by removal of the lesion and anterior grafting. J Bone Joint Surg Am. 1972;54(8): 1633–57.
20. Tuli SM. Tuberculosis of the spine: a historical review. Clin Orthop Relat Res. 2007;460:29–38.
21. Bick EM. Classics of orthopaedics, Series from Clinical orthopaedics and related research 1. Philadelphia: Lippincott; 1976. p. 541. xviii.
22. Hoffman EB, Crosier JH, Cremin BJ. Imaging in children with spinal tuberculosis. A comparison of radiography, computed tomography and magnetic resonance imaging. J Bone Joint Surg Br. 1993; 75(2):233–9.
23. Mehta JS, Bhojraj SY. Tuberculosis of the thoracic spine. A classification based on the selection of surgical strategies. J Bone Joint Surg Br. 2001;83(6): 859–63.
24. Tay BK, Deckey J, Hu SS. Spinal infections. J Am Acad Orthop Surg. 2002;10(3):188–97.

25. Denis F. Spinal instability as defined by the three-column spine concept in acute spinal trauma. Clin Orthop Relat Res. 1984;189:65–76.
26. Jain AK, Sinha S. Evaluation of systems of grading of neurological deficit in tuberculosis of spine. Spinal Cord. 2005;43(6):375–80.
27. Jain AK, Dhammi IK. Tuberculosis of the spine: a review. Clin Orthop Relat Res. 2007;460:39–49.
28. Luk KD. Tuberculosis of the spine in the new millennium. Eur Spine J. 1999;8(5):338–45.
29. Hodgson AR, Skinsnes OK, Leong CY. The pathogenesis of Pott's paraplegia. J Bone Joint Surg Am. 1967;49(6):1147–56.
30. Hodgson AR, Yau A. Pott's Paraplegia: a classification based upon the living pathology. Paraplegia. 1967;5(1):1–16.
31. Luk KD, Krishna M. Spinal stenosis above a healed Tuberculous Kyphosis. A case report. Spine. 1996; 21(9):1098–101 (Phila Pa 1976).
32. Joseffer SS, Cooper PR. Modern imaging of spinal tuberculosis. J Neurosurg Spine. 2005;2(2):145–50.
33. Modic MT, et al. Vertebral osteomyelitis: assessment using MR. Radiology. 1985;157(1):157–66.
34. Jain R, Sawhney S, Berry M. Computed tomography of vertebral tuberculosis: patterns of bone destruction. Clin Radiol. 1993;47(3):196–9.
35. Kim NH, Lee HM, Suh JS. Magnetic resonance imaging for the diagnosis of Tuberculous spondylitis. Spine. 1994;19(21):2451–5 (Phila Pa 1976).
36. Naim Ur R, et al. Neural arch tuberculosis: radiological features and their correlation with surgical findings. Br J Neurosurg. 1997;11(1):32–8.
37. Nussbaum ES, et al. Spinal tuberculosis: a diagnostic and management challenge. J Neurosurg. 1995;83(2):243–7.
38. Stabler A, Reiser MF. Imaging of spinal infection. Radiol Clin North Am. 2001;39(1):115–35.
39. Boxer DI, et al. Radiological features during and following treatment of spinal tuberculosis. Br J Radiol. 1992;65(774):476–9.
40. Pai M, O'Brien R. New diagnostics for latent and active tuberculosis: state of the art and future prospects. Semin Respir Crit Care Med. 2008;29(5):560–8.
41. Cruciani M, et al. Meta-analysis of BACTEC MGIT 960 and BACTEC 460 TB, with or without solid media, for detection of mycobacteria. J Clin Microbiol. 2004;42(5):2321–5.
42. A controlled trial of ambulant out-patient treatment and in-patient rest in bed in the management of tuberculosis of the spine in young Korean patients on standard chemotherapy a study in Masan, Korea. First report of the Medical Research Council Working Party on Tuberculosis of the Spine. J Bone Joint Surg Br. 1973;55(4):678–97.
43. A controlled trial of plaster-of-paris jackets in the management of ambulant outpatient treatment of tuberculosis of the spine in children on standard chemotherapy. A study in Pusan, Korea. Second report of the Medical Research Council Working Party on Tuberculosis of the Spine. Tubercle. 1973;54(4):261–82.
44. A five-year assessment of controlled trials of in-patient and out-patient treatment and of plaster-of-Paris jackets for tuberculosis of the spine in children on standard chemotherapy. Studies in Masan and Pusan, Korea. Fifth report of the Medical Research Council Working Party on tuberculosis of the spine. J Bone Joint Surg Br. 1976;58-B(4):399–411.
45. A 10-year assessment of controlled trials of inpatient and outpatient treatment and of plaster-of-Paris jackets for tuberculosis of the spine in children on standard chemotherapy. Studies in Masan and Pusan, Korea. Ninth report of the Medical Research Council Working Party on Tuberculosis of the Spine. J Bone Joint Surg Br. 1985;67(1):103–10.
46. A 15-year assessment of controlled trials of the management of tuberculosis of the spine in Korea and Hong Kong. Thirteenth Report of the Medical Research Council Working Party on Tuberculosis of the Spine. J Bone Joint Surg Br. 1998;80(3): 456–62
47. Aksoy M, et al. Retrospective evaluation of treatment methods in Tuberculous spondylitis. Hacettepe J Orthop Surg. 1995;5:207–9.
48. Upadhyay SS, et al. The effect of age on the change in deformity after radical resection and anterior arthrodesis for tuberculosis of the spine. J Bone Joint Surg Am. 1994;76(5):701–8.
49. Cavusoglu H, et al. A long-term follow-up study of anterior tibial allografting and instrumentation in the management of thoracolumbar Tuberculous spondylitis. J Neurosurg Spine. 2008;8(1):30–8.
50. Benli IT, et al. The results of anterior radical debridement and anterior instrumentation in Pott's disease and comparison with other surgical techniques. Kobe J Med Sci. 2000;46(1–2):39–68.
51. Benli IT, et al. Anterior radical debridement and anterior instrumentation in tuberculosis spondylitis. Eur Spine J. 2003;12(2):224–34.
52. Oga M, et al. Evaluation of the risk of instrumentation as a foreign body in spinal tuberculosis. Clinical and biologic study. Spine. 1993;18(13):1890–4 (Phila Pa 1976).
53. Guzey FK, et al. Thoracic and lumbar Tuberculous spondylitis treated by posterior debridement, graft placement, and instrumentation: a retrospective analysis in 19 cases. J Neurosurg Spine. 2005;3(6): 450–8.
54. Moon MS, et al. Posterior instrumentation and anterior interbody fusion for Tuberculous Kyphosis of dorsal and lumbar spines. Spine. 1995;20(17):1910–6 (Phila Pa 1976).
55. Sundararaj GD, et al. Extended posterior circumferential approach to thoracic and thoracolumbar spine. Oper Orthop Traumatol. 2009;21(3):323–34.
56. Thomasen E. Vertebral osteotomy for correction of Kyphosis in ankylosing spondylitis. Clin Orthop Relat Res. 1985;194:142–52.

57. Berven SH, et al. Management of fixed sagittal plane deformity: results of the transpedicular wedge resection osteotomy. Spine. 2001;26(18):2036–43 (Phila Pa 1976).

58. Wang Y, et al. Posterior-only multilevel modified vertebral column resection for extremely severe Pott's kyphotic deformity. Eur Spine J. 2009;18(10):1436–41.

59. Macagno AE, O'Brien MF. Thoracic and thoracolumbar Kyphosis in adults. Spine. 2006;31: 161–70 (Phila Pa 1976).

60. Huang TJ, et al. Video-assisted thoracoscopic surgery in managing Tuberculous spondylitis. Clin Orthop Relat Res. 2000;379:143–53.

61. Kapoor SK, et al. Video-assisted thoracoscopic decompression of tubercular spondylitis: clinical evaluationn. Spine. 2005;30(20):E605–10 (Phila Pa 1976).

62. Pieri S, et al. Percutaneous management of complications of Tuberculous spondylodiscitis: short- to medium-term results. Radiol Med. 2009;114(6): 984–95.

Part III

Shoulder

Biomechanics of the Shoulder

David Limb

Contents

Abstract

The shoulder permits a wide range of humeral movement which, coupled with hinge movement at the elbow joint to regulate distance from the body, permits the hand to be placed into an almost spherical potential space. The glenohumeral joint is the articulation that primarily endows the shoulder with its huge range of movement, but this is achieved by trading off inherent stability. The glenohumeral joint itself has to be positioned and stabilised in relation to the trunk by the scapulothoracic joint, which functions by suspension of the scapula from the trunk with a system of muscles. The only synovial joints linking the scapula to the axial skeleton are the acromioclavicular and sternoclavicular joints, at either end of the clavicle. There is a finely-tuned neuromuscular control mechanism that ensures that scapulothoracic and glenohumeral joints work in concert and are protected from injurious forces. However, the glenohumeral joint is more likely than any other joint in the human body to dislocate and the associated rotator cuff tendons almost inevitably degenerate and develop tears if the individual lives long enough. The effects of these pathological changes, and others, are predictable by consideration of natural joint anatomy and biomechanics of the joint.

D. Limb
Chapel Allerton Hospital, Leeds, UK
e-mail: d.limb@leeds.ac.uk

G. Bentley (ed.), *European Surgical Orthopaedics and Traumatology*,
DOI 10.1007/978-3-642-34746-7_58, © EFORT 2014

848 D. Limb

Knowledge of the biomechanics is therefore essential if one is to properly assess and treat shoulder pathology.

Keywords
Anatomy • Biomechanics • Clinical applications • Forces • Kinematics • Shoulder • Stability

Relevant Anatomy

The articulation between the upper limb and the trunk at the human forequarter is referred to as the shoulder, though in reality this is a complex linkage of joints, of which the glenohumeral joint is only one component. The glenohumeral joint is the last link in the chain between trunk and arm and is a ball and socket joint that allows an enormous range of movement between the humerus and scapula, with six degrees of freedom. However, for the joint to work effectively the scapula, which bears the socket, must itself be moved into a complementary position to accept the resultant force vectors from the humerus. Furthermore it must be held in this position with sufficient stability to support forces that can be multiples of body weight, yet be dynamic enough to move rapidly to counter changes in the direction of resultant force. Thus in discussing the shoulder we must not only consider the glenohumeral joint but also the scapulothoracic articulation and the skeletal linkage of the scapula to the trunk, via the clavicle, involving the acromioclavicular and sternoclavicular joints. The functions of the clavicle and its associated joints, however, can be very difficult to elucidate, particularly since some patients with cleidocranial dysostosis have been noted to have gone through life in manual jobs unaware that they were without their clavicles.

Sternoclavicular Joint

The sternoclavicular joint is the only synovial joint connecting the upper limb to the torso but it is clear to see that it is not anatomically adapted to withstanding enormous forces – the two apposed bone surfaces are saddle- shaped (the sternal surface pointing posterior, lateral and upwards) but are separated by an articular disc and observation of any skeleton reveals minimal co-aptation of the reciprocal surfaces. Stability relies in large part on strong ligaments in front, behind, above and below the joint augmented by muscle attachments (Fig. 1).

Above is the interclavicular ligament, which connects the superomedial aspects of both clavicles and is taut when the shoulder is depressed. It shows considerable variation between individuals. Below is the strong, short, costoclavicular ligament, coursing from the medial end of the first rib to the medial clavicle where it attaches at the costal tuberosity. The anterior part of this ligament limits upward movement of the clavicle, whilst the posterior part blends with the posterior sternoclavicular ligament and resists posteroinferior dislocation of the sternoclavicular joint. Anterior and posterior to the joint are the respective sternoclavicular ligaments. The joint allows four movements (elevation, depression, protraction and retraction) and two rotations (upward and downward) [5]. Up to 50° of these axial rotations can occur, facilitated by the articular disc, which attaches peripherally to the capsule that is thickened by the restraining ligaments described above.

Acromioclavicular Joint

The acromioclavicular joint is a plane joint, though the articular surfaces are not perfectly congruent and in childhood there is usually an intra-articular disc, which remains only as meniscus-like remnants extending down from the superior capsule in most adults [6]. The joint is vertically orientated, but often tilted so that the articular surface on the acromion faces somewhat superiorly and anteriorly, or less commonly inferiorly. Reviewing the slope of the joint on plain radiographs can help plan the correct needle insertion trajectory for intra-articular injections.

The capsule of the acromioclavicular joint is thickened superiorly to form the acromioclavicular ligament, which can be preserved in arthroscopic

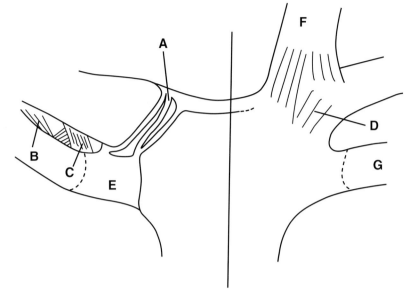

Fig. 1 A diagrammatic representation of the sternoclavicular joint, in cross section on the *left*.
A – articular disc,
B – Subclavius,
C – Costoclavicular ligament, D – Anterior sternoclavicular ligament,
E – First costal cartilage,
F – Sternomastoid,
G – First rib

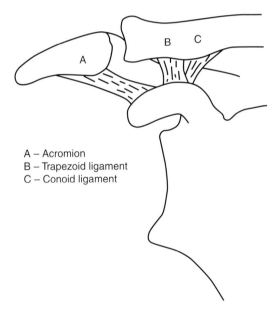

A – Acromion
B – Trapezoid ligament
C – Conoid ligament

Fig. 2 Ligaments attached to the coracoid

excision of the distal clavicle but usually has to be divided in open excision. It merges with the deltotrapezial fascia at the anterosuperior aspect of the joint. The distal clavicle is bound to the coracoid process by the conoid and trapezoid components of the coracoclavicular ligament (Fig. 2). These ligaments limit the range of motion at the acromioclavicular joint, which can therefore

allow the scapula to rotate around the acromioclavicular joint in the anteroposterior plane, the superoinferior plane and around the axis of the clavicle itself [5]. Rotation around the axis of the clavicle is important in elevation of the arm and without it, this movement is limited to about 110° [13]. There is significant variation in the anatomy of the conoid and trapezoid ligaments and there is often a bursa between the two. This bursa can intervene between the horizontal part of the coracoid and the lateral edge of the subclavius attachment to the clavicle, forming an articulation – the coracoclavicular joint [20].

Scapulothoracic Joint

The scapula bears the socket of the glenohumeral joint and is suspended in position, and moved accordingly, by muscle attachments. It does articulate with the clavicle at the synovial acromioclavicular joint, but this can be excised with no alteration in shoulder biomechanics provided that ligaments are preserved. As noted, the coracoid process of the scapula is attached to the clavicle by the conoid and trapezoid components of the coracoclavicular ligament and acute rupture of these, with acromioclavicular dislocation,

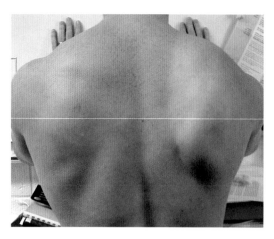

Fig. 3 A patient with right scapular winging secondary to intra-articular pathology of the glenohumeral joint

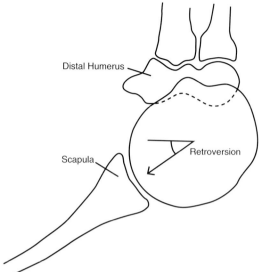

Fig. 4 The glenohumeral joint viewed from above, with the elbow joint seen beyond, in neutral alignment. The retroversion of the humeral head matches the anterior angulation of the scapula on the thoracic cage

does lead to depression of the scapula to a variable degree, which can be misinterpreted as elevation of the clavicle. However, if neuromuscular control of the scapula is retained then very good shoulder function can be maintained.

The muscles that suspend and control the scapula on the axial skeleton are the axoscapular muscles and these are arranged to elevate, depress, protract, retract and rotate the scapula. Proper scapula positioning requires co-ordination of multiple muscles, some contracting isometrically, some concentrically and some eccentrically and the whole under constant flux. It is perhaps not surprising that almost any painful shoulder condition can result in pain inhibition of some of these muscles, leading to slight tilting of the scapula on the chest wall (scapular winging) (Fig. 3). Such winging does not always, therefore, indicate a neurological lesion, such as can occur in long thoracic nerve or accessory nerve palsy, though clinical examination should still rule out such causes.

In the resting position the scapula sits on the chest wall and is rotated anterior to the coronal plane by approximately 30° [18], as viewed from above. This matches the retroversion of the humeral head with respect to the axis of the elbow joint, bringing that axis parallel to the coronal plane when the humeral head directly faces the glenoid (Fig. 4).

The scapula itself gives rise to muscles that provide the motors for arm and forearm movement (the scapulohumeral muscles and biceps/triceps, which cross both glenohumeral and elbow joints), and the axohumeral muscles which span from the torso to the humerus, crossing the scapulothracic and glenohumeral joints. It is perhaps more of a surprise that the neuromuscular control of this arrangement works at all than that it occasionally malfunctions.

Biomechanical analysis of shoulder girdle function has been extensive, but the inroads we have made to a full understanding are limited. Thus we often consider the function of large groups of muscles when discussing clinically relevant biomechanics, such as the scapular stabilisers and the rotator cuff. There is still extensive scope for further work in this complex field.

Glenohumeral Joint

The glenohumeral joint (Fig. 5) is the most extensively studied component of the shoulder

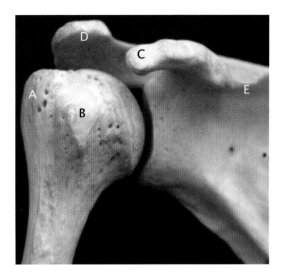

Fig. 5 The glenohumeral joint from in front – *A* – the greater tuberosity, *B* – the lesser tuberosity, *C* – the coracoid process, *D* – the acromion, *E* – the scapular notch

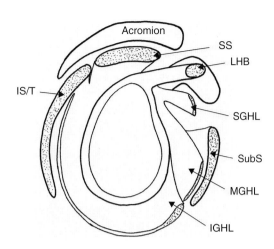

Fig. 6 The glenoid fossa with the humeral head removed. *IST/T* Infraspinatus and teres minor, *SS* Supraspinatus, *LHB* Long head of biceps tendon, *SGHL* superior glenohumeral ligament, *SubS* subscapularis, *MGHL* middle glenohumeral ligament, *IGHL* inferior glenohumeral ligament (*arrow* indicates thicker anterior band)

and for good reason – it is the component that most often causes clinically relevant problems and it is most susceptible to trauma. As noted, it is a ball and socket joint, and a huge range of movement is facilitated at this joint by the significant mis-match between the size of the humeral head and the size of the socket. The glenoid fossa has an area that is typically less than 10 cm^2 yet the humeral head articular cartilage covers typically more than 50 cm^2 – the analogy of a golf ball balancing on a tee is not a bad one and emphasises that the problem associated with this mismatch is that stability is compromised. Ball and socket joints with less of a mis-match, such that the socket encloses more of the ball (as seen in the natural hip) rarely dislocate, whilst the glenohumeral joint is the most commonly dislocated joint in the human body. However this analogy ignores the fact that in the shoulder the 'tee' is significantly deepened by soft tissue structures and the socket of the glenohumeral joint can more correctly be considered to be an osseoligamentous structure, the base of which is formed by the bone of the glenoid fossa.

The glenoid fossa itself has a slight upward tilt with respect to the medial border of the scapula [1].

Compared to a line drawn from the centre of the glenoid to the base of the scapular spine at the medial border of the scapula the glenoid is slightly retroverted in most individuals though the range is considerable amongst individuals, between 12° of anteversion and 14° of retroversion. Furthermore this angle may vary from one part of the glenoid fossa to another [23].

The soft tissue structures that deepen the socket of the glenohumeral joint are the labrum and its attached structures – the shoulder capsule, its thickenings (the ligaments) and the long head of the biceps tendon (Fig. 6). Outside this layer are the rotator cuff tendons, which merge with the capsule laterally. Thus one can see that the socket of the shoulder becomes a dynamic structure and the biomechanics can be influenced by tension and other forces in the ligaments and tendons, which form part of the containment of the humeral head. One does not have to observe many shoulder arthroscopies to realise that the anatomy of the shoulder capsule and ligaments varies enormously between individuals and therefore any study of shoulder biomechanics may not give results that reflect the environment of every shoulder.

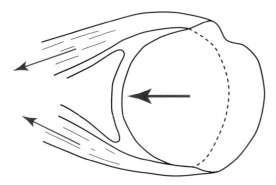

Fig. 7 The rotator cuff contraction compresses the humeral head into the concavity of the glenoid, making translation into a position of subluxation or even dislocation much more difficult. The contracting muscle masses themselves resist displacement of the humeral head away from the glenoid

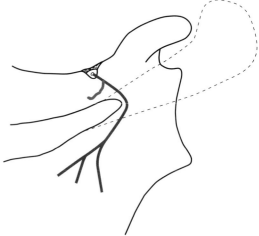

Fig. 8 The suprascapular nerve is susceptible to compression where it passes under the transverse scapular ligament, in which case both supraspinatus and infraspinatus are affected. It can also be compressed where it winds around the base of the scapular spine, at the spinoglenoid notch, resulting in wasting and weakness of infraspinatus alone

The Rotator Cuff

The rotator cuff tendons mentioned above are both biomechanically and clinically important. These tendons form a sleeve that, on contraction of the associated muscle bellies en masse, compresses the humeral head into the glenoid (Fig. 7), being ideally aligned to provide such compression in all shoulder positions [19]. Individually the cuff tendons can internally rotate (subscapularis), abduct (supraspinatus) or externally rotate (infraspinatus and teres minor) the proximal humerus and this forms the basis for clinical tests of cuff integrity. All of the cuff muscles are served by the C5 nerve root and global wasting of all cuff muscles, plus deltoid, occurs in brachial plexus lesions that involve the fifth cervical root. However, the route of nerve fibres to individual cuff muscles varies from muscle to muscle and this may help identify the site of nerve pathology giving rise to localised cuff wasting (Fig. 8).

The suprascaplular nerve is particularly prone to compression and it serves the supraspinatus and infraspinatus. Compression at the scapular notch in relation to the transverse scapular ligament, causes pain and wasting of both supraspinatus and infraspinatus, whilst compression at the spinoglenoid notch (for example by a degenerative cyst connected to the posterior labrum) affects infraspinatus alone. Teres minor is served by the axillary nerve and may be affected by lesions that occur, for example, after shoulder dislocation. The nerve to subscapularis is much less commonly affected by such pathological lesions.

Movements

The shoulder joint, through its constituent linkages, allows an enormous range of humeral movement which, with the elbow modulating distance between the distal radius and the torso, allows the hand to be positioned within an almost spherical field around the glenohumeral joint. Any movements that we care to measure and record are therefore rather artificial descriptions of positioning that do not always give a full picture of the capability or limitations of the shoulder. For convenience we refer to orthogonal planes in relation to the torso to describe shoulder movement – flexion/extension in the sagittal plane, abduction/adduction in the coronal plane and internal/external rotation in the transverse plane. However it is also possible to refer instead to the scapular plane (which is 30–40° forwards of the coronal plane) and describe flexion and abduction in relation to this, as may be reported in basic science research in which the scapula is isolated. Furthermore these planes do not include the direction of movement that the humerus tracks out when reaching overhead, for example. The plane of functional elevation is approximately 30° lateral to the sagittal plane and patients may achieve more in this range than in conventionally measured flexion or abduction. Note that the bone, muscle, tendon and ligament conditions in any position of the arm are affected by how the arm came to be in that position. Codman's paradox describes the observation that if the arm is by the side then the shoulder is fully flexed, the palm ends up facing towards the head but if the arm is abducted fully to the same position the palm is facing away from the head. Essentially the humerus rotates about its long axis by 180° between these movements, emphasising the interdependence of rotations about the glenohumeral joint.

Measurement of Movement

The range of movement is measured in degrees, the zero position being with the arms by the side and palms facing the thigh. Whilst this is satisfactory for flexion, extension, abduction and external rotation, it cannot apply to internal rotation or adduction, as the torso prevents these movements from this starting point. Functionally, therefore, internal rotation is measured as the highest spinal level that can be reached with the ipsilateral thumb (marked restriction means the thumb can reach only the trochanter, buttock or sacro-iliac region, whilst most individuals can usually reach T8 – T6) (Fig. 9a, b). The alternative is to measure in degrees with the arm at 90° of abduction. External rotation can also be measured in this position but the conditions must be specified when the measurement is recorded – external rotation measured with the arm by the side and measured again in 90° of abduction will be different in the same individual.

The same technique can be used to measure adduction, by first flexing the glenohumeral joint to 90° then measuring cross-chest adduction (this being limited in this position by tension in the posterior shoulder capsule).

These movements are not simply glenohumeral movements however – if the scapula is fused to the thoracic wall then significant limitation of 'shoulder' movements occurs. Shoulder movements are a composite of glenohumeral and scapulothoracic movement, the scapula rotating to point the glenoid superiorly in abduction and in flexion. The relative contribution of these two components, and the fluidity with which they are combined, is described by the term 'scapulothoracic rhythm'. Ordinarily both scapulothoracic and glenohumeral movements occur together, though the contribution of the glenohumeral overall is approximately twice that of the scapulothoracic [13, 18, 27]. The relative contributions in the first 30° of elevation appear to vary between individuals and the sexes [7]. Indeed this may even vary within the same individual and with disease. If the glenohumeral joint becomes very stiff, for example in osteoarthritis, the scapulothoracic range may still be preserved. In such patients abduction may be associated with shoulder hunching due to scapular elevation; the relative contributions of the scapulothoracic and glenohumeral joints are reversed – so called reversal of scapular rhythm. Note that this composite movement has been studied in the coronal plane and in the scapular plane. However neither of these reference planes adequately describes the path of the scapula around the chest wall as it both translates and rotates to contribute to elevation of the arm.

The role of the clavicle and its associated joints in shoulder movement is not fully elucidated. As noted, the shoulder can function very well, or even normally, with an incompetent clavicle or without the joints associated with the clavicle. Intuitively the clavicle seems to act as a strut between the scapula and the torso. If this is so, then it is not a significant load-bearing strut as in these circumstances the scapula would collapse in towards the torso with a dislocated AC

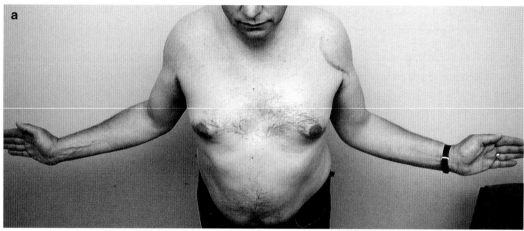

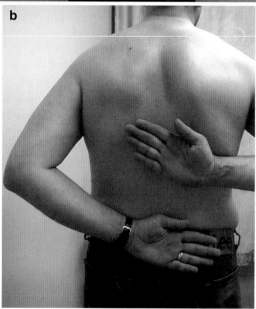

Fig. 9 (**a**) external rotation can be measured with the elbows tucked into the side, using a goniometer to give an angular measurement. Internal rotation (**b**) is more commonly recorded as the highest vertebral level that can be reached with the thumb

joint or un-united clavicle fracture. Instead it may function co-operatively with the scapula suspensory mechanism, perhaps providing proprioceptive feedback into the system. Note that the clavicle rotates around its long axis with arm elevation, particularly in high degrees of elevation. Plates and screws applied in one plane are not good at resisting rotation about an axis parallel to the plate, therefore one must consider when to allow patients to regain full overhead range after internal fixation of the clavicle.

So what movements are possible at the shoulder joint? As is the case in most other joints, there is no 'normal' range. This is quickly confirmed by asking a small group to compare external rotation with the arms held into the torso – it is not uncommon to observe maximal external rotation to vary between 40° and 100° in this situation. Other movements are perhaps less susceptible to variation, largely because the end-points are not determined by soft tissues as is the case with external rotation. Accurate

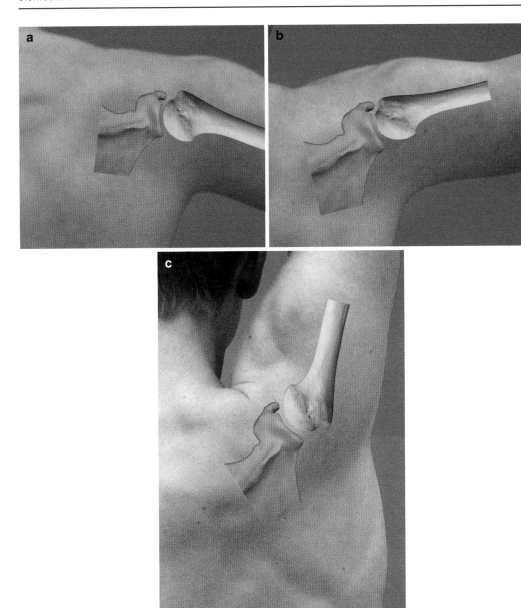

Fig. 10 Shoulder abduction at the glenohumeral joint without humeral rotation is limited to about 80° by impingement of the greater tuberosity (**a**), though scapular rotation increases this to about 120° (**b**). However, external rotation of the humerus clears the greater tuberosity from beneath the acromion and allows full abduction (**c**)

measurement is easily confounded – in the case of flexion the acromion will usually prevent flexion beyond 160° but most individuals can flex until their humerus points directly up, as they lordose the thorax and extend the lumbar spine to tilt the scapula back. Abduction at the glenohumeral joint is limited to about 80° from the zero position described above, as the greater tuberosity and attached supraspinatus impinge against the glenoid. Scapular rotation can allow abduction to around 120° but it is only by external rotation [16], which brings the greater tuberosity away from the glenoid, that allows full abduction of about 180° (Fig. 10a–c). The experimental study of shoulder movement in three dimensions demands that three linear and three angular coordinates are recorded to sufficiently describe the starting and finishing positions where six degrees of freedom exist. The two most commonly described techniques are Eulerian angle and screw displacement methods. Analysis of these is outside the scope of this chapter, though for the upper limb joints the methods are summarised in standard texts [24, 30].

During glenohumeral joint movement the humeral head is retained in the glenoid fossa by the balance of muscle forces (and capsuloligamentous restraining forces at the extremes of range). Although the articulation of the humeral head on the shallow glenoid can incorporate elements of spin, roll and glide, studies suggest that in normal movements of the shoulder the instant centre of rotation varies little from a locus within the humeral head and any translation on the glenoid is limited to a few millimetres.

Stability

As noted, the glenohumeral joint is the most commonly dislocated joint in the human body. As a ball and socket joint, it is characterised by the shallowness of its bony socket and therefore the soft tissues are primarily responsible for keeping the ball in the socket. At rest and under anaesthesia the shoulder does not dislocate, however, so there are static restrains to dislocation that operate even when the patient is paralysed. However these mechanisms are amplified by socalled dynamic factors, which increase the compression force of ball into socket under the influence of muscle contraction.

Static Factors

Glenoid Fossa and Labrum

The glenoid fossa forms a shallow concavity at the base of the osseoligamentous socket of the glenohumeral joint. It was thought that the humeral head could be incongruent with respect to the glenoid fossa, with a radius of curvature

that could be smaller, the same or greater in different people [31]. However it appears that this observation may be attributable to experimental error. The articular cartilage of the glenoid is thinner centrally than peripherally, whist the reverse is true for the humeral head. Recent studies suggest that the humeral head and glenoid are fully congruent in all positions [34], and this facilitates fluid-film adhesion between the two, which enhances stability by generating a negative pressure if there is any attempt to separate the joint surfaces [14, 17]. When this is broken by introducing a needle into the shoulder joint and allowing air to ingress a soft 'pop' is often heard as the fluid film breaks and admits air. Although the humeral head and glenoid cannot be distracted directly apart in the anaesthetised patient this becomes very easy once air or fluid are introduced between the joint surfaces.

The glenoid itself encloses less than one-third of the humeral head articular surface – an arc of about 75° in the coronal plane and 60° in the transverse plane. Saha showed that if the glenoid is relatively small – its vertical height enclosing less than 75 % of the humeral head or its transverse dimension less than 57 % of the humeral head diameter, then the shoulder was more likely to be unstable. Furthermore there is some evidence that the degree of ante- or retroversion of the glenoid fossa can increase the susceptibility to dislocation, those with relative anteversion being more prone to anterior dislocation and vice versa. Again this is an area for investigation and it seems that the glenoid may not be a particularly even-sided cup, the degree of anteversion and retroversion varying within the glenoid depending where it is measured [23].

This shallow fossa is deepened, however, by the glenoid labrum to which the capsule of the shoulder joint and its thickenings – the glenohumeral ligaments – are attached. As the concavity is deepened, the joint is stabilised, but note that if the glenoid labrum were to be detached from the margin of the glenoid then this would abolish the deepening effect and detension the glenohumeral ligaments, significantly compromising their functions. The depth of the glenoid fossa in the transverse plane is only

2.5 mm, but an equivalent depth is added by the labrum. On the whole, however, it is agreed that static constraints related to the shape of the articulation contribute little to the overall stability of the joint, though deficiencies of glenoid bone can permit escape of the humeral head if combined with capsulolabral abnormalities [35]. Although the possibility of abnormal humeral head anteversion has previously been considered as a cause for anterior instability, it is felt to be rarely, if ever, a significant contributory factor [29].

Capsule and Ligaments

The capsule of the glenohumeral joint is thin and elastic with a high type 1 collagen content. It has a volume approximately three times that of the humeral head, which is necessary in order to allow the enormous range of movement described above. Anything that diminishes the volume of the shoulder capsule, such as scarring after trauma or the histological change and contracture that occurs with 'frozen shoulder', causes a restriction of glenohumeral movements.

The ligaments of the glenohumeral joint are very variable, as is demonstrated by observing only a few shoulder arthroscopies. Because the volume of the shoulder capsule is so much greater than the volume of the humeral head it is also true that the ligaments are not under tension, therefore are contributing nothing to stability, except when the humerus is rotated to an extreme position which will put one region of the capsule, and any ligament in that region of capsule, under tension. Thus at rest and in close range movement the glenohumeral ligaments have no role to play in stabilising the shoulder. The patient who subluxes or dislocates whilst in a sling will not be prevented from dislocation by an anterior repair unless this significantly shortens the loose capsule and ligaments, in which case external rotation of the shoulder will be lost. At the end-range of movement, however, the ligaments do come under tension and provide passive restraint to glenohumeral translation over the glenoid margin in the direction of capsular tightening [3].

The only part of the shoulder capsule that is under tension in the erect posture is the superior capsule. Thus the superior glenohumeral ligament (SGHL) and coracohumeral ligament (CHL) have a role to play in preventing inferior subluxation [26]. The SGHL is put under tension by external rotation of the shoulder with the arm by the side. Thus a sulcus sign, indicating inferior subluxation, that disappears on external rotation of the arm indicates that the SGHL is competent. If the sulcus sign persists in external rotation this suggests that the SGHL and its adjacent capsule (the rotator interval capsule and the extra-articular CHL in the same location) are incompetent. The rotator interval capsule also has a role in controlling posterior, as well as inferior, translation [10].

The middle glenohumeral ligament (MGHL) comes under tension with external rotation, particularly in the lower range (less than $45°$) of abduction [26]. At higher degrees of abduction, particularly in external rotation, the inferior glenohumeral ligament (IGHL) is the predominant restraint, as documented in numerous studies [3, 9]. The IGHL forms a hammock-like structure from the inferior glenoid to the humeral head. The posterior and, particularly, the anterior margins of this hammock are thickened. The anterior band of the IGHL comes under tension in full abduction and external rotation. In this position it strongly resists anteroinferior dislocation of the humeral head. If dislocation does occur then a structural alteration occurs – usually avulsion of the anteroinferior labrum, but also stretching of the ligament and/or, less commonly, avulsion of the ligament from its humeral insertion (Humeral Avulsion of the Inferior Glenohumeral Ligament – HAGL lesion).

Muscles

The glenohumeral joint is surrounded by the thick tendons of the rotator cuff, with which the capsule of the joint merges laterally. Indeed, in engineering nomenclature the glenohumeral joint is a force-closed joint, dependant on balanced muscle activity to centre the humeral head in its articulation on the glenoid fossa [21]. The cuff tendons are very thick and, by their very presence around the humeral head, and with their attachments medially to the scapula and laterally to the tuberosities of the humeral head, will resist displacement of the humeral head out of the glenoid fossa. Thus it has been shown experimentally that dividing the rotator cuff tendons in a cadaver significantly reduces resistance to displacement of the humeral head out of the fossa, even if the muscles are not contracting. Contraction of the cuff muscles put the tendons under significant tension, which provides a substantial block to humeral dislocation. Experimentally a 50 % reduction in the force in the cuff muscles results in an almost 50 % increase in displacement of the humeral head in the glenoid in response to external loading [36].

Dynamic Factors

As noted above, the glenoid labrum deepens the socket of the glenohumeral joint and in doing so increases the force required across the face of the glenoid to displace the humeral head towards the joint margins. Any force compressing the humeral head into the glenoid further increases the resistance to lateral translation [21] – in effect the humeral head would have to totally overcome the compressive force to move away from it in order to climb over the glenoid rim. Thus the resultant force in shoulder movement, which should always be directed towards the bony glenoid, acts to deter dislocation. Furthermore the greater the joint reaction force, the greater the force required to overcome this concavity compression effect and create a dislocation (Fig. 11). In effect it is only by creating conditions where the resultant force is no longer directed into the glenoid fossa that dislocation can occur [11].

This simple explanation masks the complexity of the real situation, where the resultant force is achieved by individual contributions from 18 to 26 muscles (depending on how these are counted). Furthermore these are in a constant state of change, accommodating variations in the applied load and executing planned movement whilst responding to unpredictable changes in the resistance met. A very fine system of neuromuscular control is

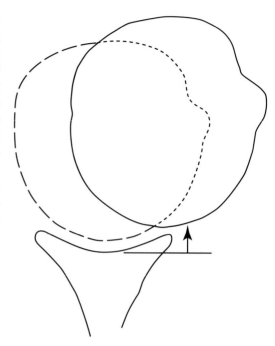

Fig. 11 With an intact bony rim and glenoid, it is necessary to distract the humeral head away from the line of action of the rotator cuff (*arrow*), in addition to translating the head away from the glenoid, to bring about dislocation. Deficiency of the labrum and/or bony glenoid rim means that only translation is needed, without having to provide any distraction against a contracting muscle mass

needed to set the supporting core muscles of the legs and trunk, position the scapula on the torso, and fine tune shoulder girdle muscle tensions to direct the force transmitted through the humeral head directly onto the bone of the glenoid fossa. We are beginning to understand the contributions of neuromuscular control to stability, but 'beginning' is the important word. However this is beginning to shape our concepts of shoulder stability, recognising a triad of interplaying factors – shoulder anatomy that predisposes to instability (laxity, variations in anatomy not resulting from trauma etc.), traumatic structural lesions and neuromuscular control [15].

Concavity compression is also enhanced as the glenohumeral joint moves to an extreme position of movement. As the humeral head rotates towards the limit of motion the capsule and ligaments associated with it become tight. As the humeral head attempts to rotate further the

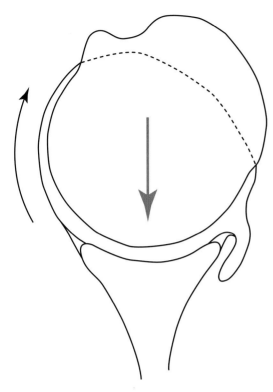

Fig. 12 As the head rotates to the end of the available range of motion the relevant ligament comes under tension, which is countered by increased concavity compression of the humeral head into the glenoid. As the head is forced into further rotation the tension in the ligament increases, effectively increasing the stability of the joint, until ligament failure occurs

tension in the ligaments increases and this is directed to compress the humeral head into the glenoid (Fig. 12). Thus the stability of the joint increases until the tension in the capsule and ligaments can no longer be sustained and soft tissue rupture occurs – the capsule stretches or tears, avulses its attachment to the glenoid or avulses from the humeral head, a predictable range of pathology that is observed in patients after shoulder dislocation.

Forces

We can estimate forces acting across the shoulder girdle, and this suggests that the shoulder transmits the equivalent of body weight, or even multiples of this. However we rely on assumptions and surrogate measurements and still have a lot to learn. For any position of the upper limb it is possible to estimate the force that a muscle is capable of generating, its line of action and the activity of the muscle. From these, the net force across a joint can be computed, remembering that in the case of the glenohumeral joint up to 26 muscles can be involved.

The force a muscle is capable of generating relates to the cross-sectional area of all of the muscle fibres in a muscle (not necessarily therefore the cross-sectional area of the muscle) and the total length of the fibres, and this has been calculated for certain positions of the glenohumeral joint. In abduction and external rotation, for example, the greatest contribution to forces acting across the glenohumeral joint comes from the deltoid, subscapularis, infraspinatus/teres minor, pectoralis major and latissimus dorsi, with contributions declining from the deltoid's 18 % to the 12 % contribution of latissimus [2]. This is a static analysis in one position and simply has not been repeated for most possible positions of the joint. The orientation of the line of action of a muscle may be extremely difficult to define and during a movement the line of action may cross the axis of rotation, completely reversing the action of the muscle [13]. The activity of a muscle can be estimated by EMG studies [32, 33], but these are susceptible to numerous sources of error. We have the ability to derive the order of magnitude of the forces crossing the shoulder and estimate how the force vectors alter with some movements, and this information has informed the development of joint replacements and reconstructive devices. However, it is apparent that we are lacking in detailed knowledge.

Forces Across the Glenohumeral Joint

Most research has been directed to determining the forces acting across the glenohumeral joint – far more is known about this, for example, than the forces in the scapular stabilisers as they rotate the scapula and position it to stabilise the muscles that rotate the humerus in the glenoid. This is driven by need, as it is the glenohumeral

Fig. 13 A simple free-body calculation of the order of magnitude of forces required simply to abduct the arm, with no weight being lifted against resistance. In the loaded arm joint reaction forces can be multiples of body weight

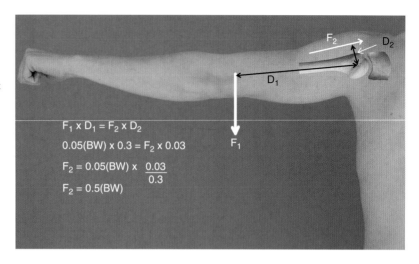

$$F_1 \times D_1 = F_2 \times D_2$$

$$0.05(BW) \times 0.3 = F_2 \times 0.03$$

$$F_2 = 0.05(BW) \times \frac{0.03}{0.3}$$

$$F_2 = 0.5(BW)$$

joint that most commonly develops pathology and the pathology is often amenable to reconstructive surgery. Knowledge of the mechanical environment of the glenohumeral joint is therefore essential not only in developing adequate joint replacement components, but also in designing reconstructive procedures for fractures and soft tissue injuries sufficiently robust to permit the return of joint function.

A simple free-body diagram can be constructed to help calculate forces across the glenohumeral joint. With the arm held in 90° of abduction moments acting to return the arm to the side are a result of the effect of gravity: the weight of the arm through its centre of gravity a fixed distance from the glenohumeral joint (around 30–35 cm). At equilibrium this is balanced by the action of the abductors (deltoid and supraspinatus) whose line of action passes only 2–3 cm from the axis of rotation in the humeral head (Fig. 13). From this it can be estimated that even with no weight in the hand, there is a force equivalent to half body-weight acting through the humeral head onto the glenoid fossa. This multiplies to forces far exceeding body-weight when the hand is significantly loaded, and this includes unexpected loads such as breaking a fall with the outstretched hand – a common scenario for rotator cuff tear.

Free-body diagrams such as this tell us basic information about static events, but dynamic analysis adds important information that is crucial in understanding the long-term behaviour of joint replacements. Although we have stated that the scapular stabilisers rotate the scapula to accept the resultant force from the humerus onto the bony glenoid, this resultant force is not always central in the fossa. It seems that even the straightforward act of initiating a simple movement such as abduction causes significant forces to sweep up and down the glenoid, testing the fixation of any glenoid component in arthroplasty in the short term and threatening it with loosening in the long term. If the abductors contracted to initiate abduction and nothing else occurred, the scapula would be pulled into downward rotation by the weight of the arm and the effort available to abduct the arm would be wasted. The movement pattern of abduction therefore demands that the brain first pre-sets the scapula, fixing it to the trunk. More than this, the trunk itself has to be stable, so activity in the shoulder abductors is in fact preceded, by milliseconds, by contraction of the leg and trunk muscles and scapular stabilisers. The inferior cuff then contracts to pull the humeral head down an instant before the abductors kick in to rotate the humerus up [28] – the result is that the joint reaction force momentarily swings to the inferior glenoid as pre-setting occurs then up to the superior glenoid as deltoid and supraspinatus initiate the upward rotation of the humerus, finally settling in the central glenoid as the humeral abducts and the scapula rotates upwards, contributing the scapulothoracic share to the movement. In the absence of the superior rotator cuff, as occurs with a supraspinatus tear, this cycling of the resultant force from inferior to superior glenoid is magnified and, in the presence of a glenoid replacement, can lead to early loosening of the interface between component and bone – the so called 'rocking horse glenoid'.

If the deltoid is acting alone, or is dominant, then simple consideration of its origin and insertion with respect to the glenoid reveals that shear forces across the glenoid will occur with deltoid contraction. The supraspinatus, however, and indeed the other cuff muscles, acts almost parallel to the scapular plane, the force it generates being directed towards the glenoid with little shear component. With normal muscle-tendon units across the shoulder the shear forces are balanced and the resultant force is directed into the concavity of the glenoid. Loss of any component, and it is most often the superior rotator cuff that is lost, disrupts the normal control mechanism and allows eccentric joint reaction forces that are more difficult for the neuromuscular control mechanisms to contain. However it is clear that some patients develop good compensation, generating appropriate force couples to maintain a well-centred joint reaction force despite apparently significant pathology. Why some patients adapt in this way, with or without physiotherapy to assist, yet others develop significant dysfunction with relatively small cuff tears, is not known.

One advantage that the anatomy of the shoulder presents to the implant designer relates to this discussion on shoulder movements and forces. We have already noted that the centre of rotation of the glenohumeral joint is contained in a relatively small locus only a few mm across. The humeral head itself rotates around a point at the projected centre of a sphere of which it forms a segment. This lies within the metaphysis of the humeral head and consequently the forces acting on a prosthesis push it into a stable position and provide little stress at the fixation interface of the stem. Thus humeral stem loosening is rare (even in uncemented stems that do not have any sort of bio-active coating) and resurfacing prostheses are durable with very few reported complications of humeral component fixation.

Clinical Relevance

An appreciation of the biomechanical environment of the shoulder is essential to the successful management of the range of pathology that can present to the shoulder clinic. The delicate balance of muscle forces and neuromuscular control helps us to understand why instability can easily result from abnormalities in the anatomy of the shoulder or in its controlling mechanism. Anatomical problems can be reconstructed by appropriate ligament or labral repair, or even bony reconstruction, but abnormalities of neuromuscular control could be made worse by the same procedures. The elucidation of the underlying biomechanical cause of instability is key to successful management of the patient with recurrent dislocation or subluxation. Examples of improvements in technique that have resulted from consideration of normal biomechanics include fixation of the labrum onto the face of the glenoid rather than its neck, restoring an anterior buffer, and the realisation that bone defects (the 'inverted pear' glenoid) require bone reconstruction in the way of a Latarjet repair or similar.

Neuromuscular control and the creation of balanced force couples is essential to normal shoulder function. There is much to be learned about how disorders of control can be managed if they occur with no abnormality of the gross shoulder anatomy. However our understanding of neuromuscular control in the face of an obvious anatomical lesion, such as a rotator cuff tear, is also far from complete. The biomechanical analysis that we can perform explains how we can improve the symptoms, range of movement and strength by repairing a rotator cuff tear. However, it is not always clear or explainable why some people with very large tears have excellent function and no pain [22], whilst others have symptoms that improve with non-operative treatment [9]. However, even in those that do not present for treatment, function is poorer and symptoms more significant in the presence of a cuff tear [8]. Furthermore, most patients with a bald humeral head due to a massive rotator cuff tear do go on to develop rotator cuff arthropathy.

The shoulder is a weight-bearing joint – in normal activities loads exceeding body weight are regularly transmitted across the glenohumeral joint. Even simple movements against gravity result in the generation of large forces in the rotator cuff tendons. When shoulder fractures involve the greater and lesser tuberosities it should not be forgotten that during rehabilitation one is aiming for restoration of normal function, which means a normalisation of the forces generated by the cuff muscles and exerted on the tuberosity fragments. Even modern locked-plating systems do not usually provide stable fixation for the tuberosity fragments by screws engaging the plate. Additional fixation, commonly by suture material passing through the plate, is required and one has to be aware of the potentially destructive forces to which the fixation will be subjected.

The same applies to fixation of tuberosity fragments when hemi-arthroplasty is used for the reconstruction of complex fractures and fracture dislocations of the shoulder. One of the commonest reasons for poor results of hemi-arthroplasty for fractures is migration of the greater tuberosity, and one of the most critical steps in surgery is the re-attachment in a position that allows anatomical lines of action for cuff muscles that can withstand physiological forces. Furthermore the biomechanical environment can only be re-created by careful positioning of the prosthesis to re-create the correct length and humeral retroversion. Experimentally it has been shown that mal-positioning of the humeral and/or glenoid components in total shoulder replacement adversely affects the kinematics, range of movement and stability of the shoulder [12].

However this is one situation where knights move thinking has lead to the development of a prosthesis specifically designed to work better when the natural environment of the shoulder cannot be restored. The reverse geometry designs of shoulder prosthesis attach the 'ball', in the form of a glenosphere, to the scapula. The 'socket' is then fixed to the proximal humerus, usually with a stem to stabilise it within the shaft. The centre of rotation becomes the projected centre of the glenosphere rather than the projected centre of a sphere of which a humeral head component is a segment. The result is that the centre of rotation is medialised by 3 cm or so, more than doubling the distance between the line of action of the deltoid muscle and the centre of rotation. Consequently the moment arm of the deltoid is significantly increased and portions of the anterior and posterior deltoid are recruited as abductors. Upward migration of the humerus is prevented by articulation with the glenosphere and indeed the humerus is lowered with respect to the acromion, re-tensioning or increasing tension in the deltoid [4]. As a result the prosthesis is not at all reliant on rotator cuff function, making it suitable for use when the cuff is absent or unreconstructable. Without a working cuff there are significant limitations in both internal and external rotation, and the importance of external rotation to shoulder function has already been noted. This may be addressed by concurrent transfer of latissimus dorsi as a motor for external rotation, though the long-term results of such procedures are not yet available.

Summary

The articulation between the thorax and arm includes scapulothoracic and glenohumeral joints, the clavicle providing a strut between the scapula and thorax through its synovial acromioclavicular and sternoclavicular joints. The scapula is slung on to the axial skeleton by muscles and these control scapular positioning, directing the glenoid fossa to accept the joint reaction force from the humeral head and substantially increasing the range of shoulder movement by its elevation, depression, protraction, retraction and rotation on the ribcage. There is a complex and, as yet, poorly understood system of neuromuscular control which is linked to the system providing core stability to the trunk, providing the platform from which the shoulder can function.

The glenohumeral joint in particular has evolved to allow an enormous range of motion and this is at the cost of inherent stability. Disorders in the natural anatomy or lesions affecting the bone, ligaments, tendons and other soft tissue structures can each, alone or in combination, result in instability. Successful management of instability therefore requires careful history taking and diagnostic skill to identify the responsible lesions. The most successful surgical procedures to treat instability are specifically directed towards restoration of normal anatomy and biomechanics.

Replacement of the glenohumeral joint also requires attention to the restoration of normal anatomy in order to provide the correct length/tension relationships for function of the muscles crossing the articulation. Furthermore the components and fixation techniques must withstand forces exceeding body weight across the joint and, perhaps more importantly, forces of this magnitude which sweep across the face of the glenoid. These rock the component and in the long-term may lead to loosening, particularly if the fixation technique is inadequate or the soft tissues have not been dealt with correctly, leaving eccentric forces acting on the glenoid. Reverse geometry articulations provide a relatively novel solution when a functioning rotator cuff is not available for reconstruction.

The shoulder is very susceptible to disorders of its articular surface or the muscles, tendons and ligaments that contribute to normal function. It is therefore no surprise that the surgeon who does not achieve the best possible reconstruction will be rewarded with poor function in operated patients.

References

1. Basmajian JV, Bazant FJ. Factors preventing downward dislocation of the adducted shoulder joint. J Bone Joint Surg. 1959;41A:1182–6.
2. Bassett RW, Browne AO, Morrey BF, An KN. Glenohumeral muscle force and moment mechanics in a position of shoulder instability. J Biomech. 1990;23(5):405–15.
3. Blasier RB, Goldberg RE, Rothman ED. Anterior shoulder instability: contribution of rotator cuff forces and capsular ligaments in a cadaveric model. J Shoulder Elbow Surg. 1992;1:140–50.
4. Boileau P, Watkinson DJ, Hatzidakis AM, Balg F. Grammont reverse prosthesis: design, rationale and biomechanics. J Shoulder Elbow Surg. 2005;14(1S):147S–61.
5. Dempster WT. Mechanisms of shoulder movement. Arch Phys Med Rehabil. 1965;46A:49–70.
6. De Palma AF. Degenerative changes in the sternoclavicular and acromioclavicular joints in various decades, vol. III. Springfield: Thomas; 1957.
7. Doddy SG, Waterland JC, Freedman L. Scapulohumeral goniometer. Arch Phys Med Rehabil. 1970;51:711–3.
8. Fehringer EV, Sun J, VanOeveren LS, Keller BK, Matsen III FA. Full thickness rotator cuff tear prevalence and correlation with function and co-morbidities in patients sixty-five years of age and older. J Shoulder Elbow Surg. 2008;17(6):881–5.
9. Goldberg BA, Nowinski RJ, Matsen III FA. Outcome of nonoperative treatment of full thickness rotator cuff tears. Clin Orthop. 2001;382:99–107.
10. Harryman III BT, Sidles JA, Clark JM, et al. Translation of the humeral head on the glenoid with passive glenohumeral motion. J Bone Joint Surg. 1990;72A (9):1334–43.
11. Hsu HC, Boardman III ND, Luo ZP, An KN. Tendon-defect and muscle-unloaded models for relating rotator cuff tear to glenohumeral instability. J Orthop Res. 2000;18:952–8.
12. Ianotti JP, Spencer EE, Wnter U, Deffenbaugh D, Williams G. Prosthetic positioning in total shoulder arthroplasty. J Shoulder Elbow Surg. 2005;14(1S):111S–21.
13. Inman VT, Saunders JR, Abbott LC. Observations on the function of the shoulder joint. J Bone Joint Surg. 1944;26:1–30.
14. Inokuchi W, Sanderhoff Olsen B, Sojbjerg JO, Sneppen O. The relation between the position of the glenohumeral joint and the intra-articular pressure: an experimental study. J Shoulder Elbow Surg. 1997;6:144–9.
15. Jaggi A, Lambert S. Rehabilitation for shoulder injuries. Br J Sports Med. 2010;44:333–40.
16. Johnston TB. The movements of the shoulder joint. A plea for the use of the 'plane of the scapula' as the plane of reference for movements occurring at the humero-scapular joint. Br J Surg. 1937;25:252–60.
17. Kumar VP, Balasubramaniam P. The role of atmospheric pressure in stabilising the shoulder; an experimental study. J Bone Joint Surg. 1985;67B:719–21.
18. Laumann U. Kinesiology of the shoulder joint. In: Kölbel R et al., editors. Shoulder replacement. Berlin: Springer; 1987.
19. Lee SB, Kim KJ, O'Driscoll SW, Morrey BF, An KN. Dynamic glenohumeral stability provided by the rotator cuff muscles in the mid-range and end-range of motion. A study in cadavers. J Bone Joint Surg. 2000;82A(6):849–57.
20. Lewis OJ. The coracoclavicular joint. J Anat. 1959;93:296–303.
21. Lippitt SB, Vanderhooft JE, Harris SL, et al. Glenohumeral stability from concavity compression: a quantitative analysis. J Shoulder Elbow Surg. 1993;2:27–35.

22. Matsen III FA. Rotator cuff. In: Rockwood CA, Matsen III FA, editors. The shoulder. Philadelphia: WB Saunders; 1998. p. 755–839.

23. Monk AP, Berry E, Limb D, Soames RW. Laser morphometric analysis of the glenoid fossa of the scapula. Clin Anat. 2001;14(5):320–3.

24. Morrey BF. The elbow and its disorders. 4th ed. Philadelphia: Saunders; 2009.

25. O'Brien SJ, Schwartz RS, Warren RF, Tarzilli PA. Capsular restraints to anterior-posterior motion of the abducted shoulder: a biomechanical study. J Shoulder Elbow Surg. 1995;4:298–308.

26. O'Connell PW, Nuber GW, Mileski RA, Lautenschlager E. The contribution of the glenohumeral ligaments to anterior stability of the shoulder joint. Am J Sports Med. 1990;18:579–84.

27. Poppen NK, Walker PS. Normal and abnormal motion of the shoulder. J Bone Joint Surg. 1976;58A:195–201.

28. Poppen NK, Walker PS. Forces at the glenohumeral joint in abduction. Clin Orthop. 1978;58:165.

29. Randelli M, Gambrioli PL. Glenohumeral osteometry by computed tomography in normal and unstable shoulders. Clin Orthop. 1986;208:151–6.

30. Rockwood Jr CA, Matsen III FA, Lippitt SB, Wirth MA. The shoulder. 4th ed. Philadelphia: Saunders; 2009.

31. Saha AK. Dynamic stability of the glenohumeral joint. Acta Orthop Scand. 1971;42:491–505.

32. Shevlin MG, Lehmann JF, Lucci JA. Electromyographic study of the function of some muscles crossing the glenohumeral joint. Arch Phys Med Rehabil. 1969;50:264–70.

33. Sigholm G, Herberts P, Almstrom C, Kodifors R. Electromyographic analysis of shoulder muscle load. J Orthop Res. 1984;1:379–86.

34. Soslowsky LJ, Flatow EL, Bigliani LU, Mow VC. Articular geometry of the glenohumeral joint. Clin Orthop. 1992;285:181–90.

35. Stevens KJ, Preston BJ, Wallace WA, Kerslake RW. CT imaging and three dimensional recosntructions of shoulders with anterior glenohumeral instability. Clin Anat. 1999;12:326–36.

36. Wuelker N, Korrell M, Thren K. Dynamic glenohumeral joint stability. J Shoulder Elbow Surg. 1998;7:43–52.

Principles of Shoulder Imaging

S. Shetty and Paul O'Donnell

Contents

S. Shetty (✉) • P. O'Donnell
Department of Radiology, Royal National Orthopaedic
Hospital, Stanmore, Middlesex, UK
e-mail: paul.o'donnell@rnohnhs.uk

Keywords

Anatomy • Arthrography • CT and CT arthrography • MR & MR arthrography • Radiographs • Ultrasound

Introduction

Radiographs, fluoroscopy, ultrasound (US), computed tomography (CT) and magnetic resonance imaging (MRI) are the modalities most frequently used in investigating the shoulder. US and MRI are most often used for evaluating the rotator cuff.

The need for imaging of the shoulder, particularly the rotator cuff, has increased over the last few years, probably related to the ageing population and an increase in sport-related injury. The first publication regarding the use of US for the evaluation of the rotator cuff was by Seltzer et al., published in 1979 and for MRI was by Kneeland et al. in 1986. In the ensuing years advances in imaging technology and extensive research have improved understanding of rotator cuff pathology. At present both these modalities still have limitations and a rotator cuff imaging gold standard is yet to be realised. CT and MRI arthrography have significantly improved the imaging of the labrum and ligamentous structures of the gleno-humeral joint. Conventional arthrography is currently not used in isolation for diagnostic purposes. In this chapter we aim to provide the reader with a comprehensive overview of the imaging modalities for investigating shoulder pathology.

G. Bentley (ed.), *European Surgical Orthopaedics and Traumatology*,
DOI 10.1007/978-3-642-34746-7_40, © EFORT 2014

Anatomy

An in-depth knowledge of the anatomy of the shoulder is key to the interpretation of any shoulder imaging. Below is a short overview.

Biceps

The biceps has two heads: the short head of biceps, which arises from the coracoid process, and the long head of the biceps, which arises from the supraglenoid tubercle and superior labrum. The long head of biceps follows an intra-articular, intrasynovial path to descend into the intertubercular groove, between the greater and lesser tuberosities. It is one of the structures in the anterior (rotator) interval of the rotator cuff along with the coraco-humeral ligament and the superior gleno-humeral ligament. The anterior interval is located between the subscapularis and supraspinatus tendons. The biceps tendon inserts into the radial tuberosity of the radius, with an additional aponeurotic insertion into the lacertus fibrosus.

Deltoid

The deltoid arises from the lateral clavicle, the acromion and the lateral scapular spine and inserts into the deltoid tubercle of the humerus.

Rotator Cuff Tendons

Subscapularis
The subscapularis arises from the anterior aspect of the scapula and inserts into the lesser tuberosity of the humerus.

Supraspinatus
The supraspinatus arises in the suprascapular fossa of the scapula and inserts into the superior facet of the greater tuberosity of the humerus.

Infraspinatus
The infraspinatus arises from the medial aspect of the infraspinous fossa of the scapula and inserts onto the middle facet of the greater tuberosity of the humerus.

Teres Minor
The muscle arises from the lateral margin of the scapula and inserts onto the inferior facet of the greater tuberosity of the humerus (Table 1).

Gleno-Humeral Joint

This is the most mobile and the least stable of the joints in the body. This is because the articular surfaces are asymmetrical in size and morphology, with the small and relatively flat glenoid surface, articulating with the large, round articular surface of the humeral head, within a lax joint capsule. This laxity of the capsule allows for a greater range of movement at the shoulder joint, but makes the shoulder inherently unstable and prone to subluxation and dislocation. The fibrocartilaginous labrum at the periphery of the glenoid deepens and widens the shallow glenoid.

The articular surfaces of the humeral head and glenoid are covered by hyaline cartilage. Humeral articular cartilage extends to the anatomical neck, which is also the lateral attachment of the joint capsule. Medially the capsule is attached to the margin of the glenoid just medial to the labrum, posteriorly and inferiorly. Inferiorly, it is lax and this is the weakest part of the capsule. Anteriorly, based on the attachment of the capsule in relation to the glenoid labrum, it is classified into three types:

Type 1. Capsule inserts onto the labrum

Type 2. Capsule inserts onto the scapular neck, within 1 cm of the labrum

Type 3. Capsule inserts onto the scapular neck, greater than 1 cm from the labrum.

Superiorly it extends to the root of the coracoid and contains the supraglenoid origin of the long head of the biceps.

There are two apertures in the capsule, one between the humeral tuberosities, which allows the passage of the biceps tendon, and the other is

Table 1 Anatomy of the rotator cuff muscles

Muscles	Origin	Insertion	Action	Nerve Supply
Subscapularis	Anterior aspect of body of scapula	Lesser tuberosity	Adduction & internal rotation	Upper and lower subscapular nerves
Supraspinatus	Supraspinous fossa of the scapula	Superior facet of the greater tuberosity	Internal rotation & abduction	Suprascapular nerve
Infraspinatus	Infraspinous fossa of the scapula	Middle facet of the greater tuberosity	External rotation	Suprascapular nerve
Teres Minor	Lateral border of the scapula	Inferior facet of the greater tuberosity	External rotation	Axillary nerve
Biceps	Short head: coracoid process Long head: supraglenoid tubercle & superior labrum	Radial tuberosity of the radius and lacertus fibrosus	Supination & flexion	Musculocutaneous nerve
Deltoid	Lateral clavicle, acromion and scapular spine	Deltoid tubercle on the shaft of the humerus	Abduction	Axillary nerve

the subscapularis recess in the sub-corocoid region, which connects the subscapular bursa with the synovial space.

Synovium lines the fibrous capsule and forms a tubular structure around the biceps tendon as it passes through the intertubercular groove, extending to the surgical neck of the humerus. Multiple ligaments (coraco-humeral and the superior, middle and inferior gleno-humeral) re-inforce the capsule. The gleno-humeral ligaments extend from the anterior margin of the glenoid to the lesser tuberosity. These, especially the anterior band of the inferior gleno-humeral ligament, limit external rotation and anterior translation of the humeral head. The coraco-humeral ligament arises from the coracoid and inserts into the lesser and greater tuberosities, re-inforcing the capsule over the biceps tendon.

Acromioclavicular Joint

This joint lies between the medial aspect of the acromion and the lateral aspect of the clavicle. It is a synovial joint and is therefore prone to inflammatory athritis. Osteophytes projecting inferiorly can cause rotator cuff pathology. The joint is re-inforced by strong acromioclavicular ligaments, which limit joint movement, and contains a fibrocartilagenous disc. The coracoclavicular ligament, consisting of the trapezoid component laterally and the conoid component medially also aid in stabilizing the joint.

Sternoclavicular Joint

This joint lies between the medial inferior aspect of the clavicle and the superolateral aspect of the manubrium. It is lined by fibrocartilage and also has a fibrocartilage disc. This joint can be difficult to evaluate with radiographs. Thin section CT or MRI, with the patient prone to stabilise the sternum, provides better quality imaging.

Coraco-Acromial Arch

This is formed by the anterior acromion, the coraco-acromial ligament and coracoid process. The coraco-acromial ligament extends from the anterior acromion to the coracoid process and measures between 2 and 5 mm. in thickness. The subacromial space lies between the coracoacromial arch and the humeral head. The contents of this space are the subacromial bursa, the supraspinatus and infraspinatus tendons and the joint capsule. Thus, any narrowing of this space can cause impingement of the rotator cuff and the other constituents of the subacromial space. Bigliani has classified the under surface of the acromion into three types:

Type 1 (flat), Type 2 (concave) and Type 3 (anterior down slope, or hook, which can narrow the subacromial space).

Radiographs

Despite the advances in imaging technology, standard radiography is still the mainstay of shoulder imaging and is usually the first investigation.

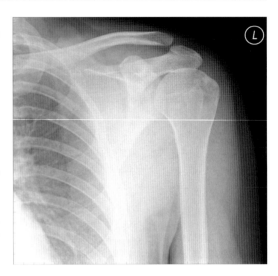

Fig. 1 AP radiograph of the shoulder

Indications

Any acute or chronic shoulder pathology: trauma, including fractures, dislocations (acute or chronic and the resulting bony injury); bony anatomy in chronic shoulder pain (morphological variants that may predispose to dysfunction, extent of arthropathy); radiographic features of rotator cuff disease; calcific tendonosis. Due to the complex anatomy of the scapula, fractures may be poorly demonstrated.

The most frequently used radiographic projections are:

- Anteroposterior (AP) view (Fig. 1)
- Gleno-humeral (GH) view (Fig. 2)
- Lateral (trans-scapular or "Y" view) (Fig. 3); with caudal angulation to show "outlet"
- Axial views (including axillary (Fig. 4) and variants: Stripp [1], Bloom Obata [2]) (Figs. 5, 6)
- Acromioclavicular Joint
- Stryker notch view (Fig. 7a, b)
  See Table 2

Arthrography

Indications

- As a therapeutic (long-acting local anaesthetic agent (LA) combined with corticosteroid) or diagnostic (with long-acting LA only)

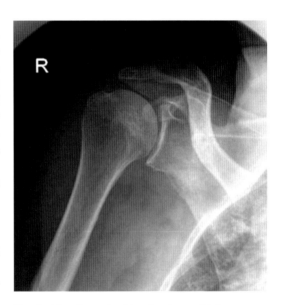

Fig. 2 AP radiograph of the glenohumeral joint

injection. Confirmation of intra-articular injection allows specific assessment of the effect of the injection; alleviation of pain post injection localises the pain to the shoulder joint.

- As part of a CT arthrogram or MR arthrogram with either iodinated contrast (CT) or gadolinium (MRI) injection into the joint.
- Therapeutic hydrodilatation as treatment of adhesive capsulitis. A large volume injection

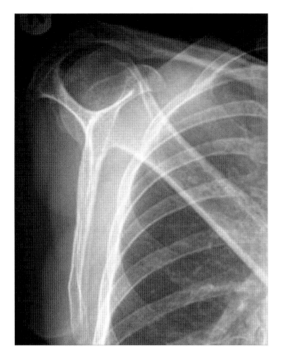

Fig. 3 Lateral scapular "Y view" radiograph

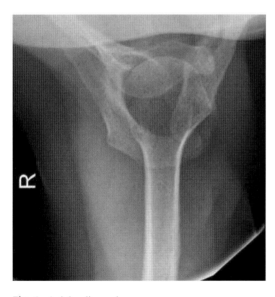

Fig. 4 Axial radiograph

(typically consisting of iodinated contrast, corticosteroid, local anaesthetic and normal saline) is injected under fluoroscopic control to disrupt adhesions in the joint.

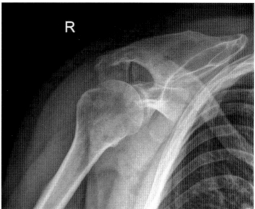

Fig. 5 Stripp (inferosuperior) axial radiograph

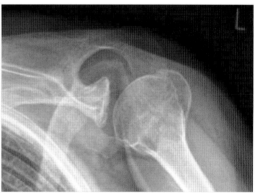

Fig. 6 Bloom Obata (superoinferior) axial radiograph

Anterior Approach

Patient lies supine with arm in external rotation (this moves the biceps tendon lateral to the puncture site and also allows maximum exposure of the humeral articular surface for puncture). The fluoroscopic beam is perpendicular to the table. This is the most common approach used by musculo-skeletal radiologists. The puncture site is variable [3], but usually immediately vertical to the medial cortex of the humeral head, where the skin is marked, cleaned and local anaesthetic administered. A 21 or 22G needle are suitable for joint puncture. The needle is introduced vertically and, when intra-articular, contrast medium is administered to confirm position of the

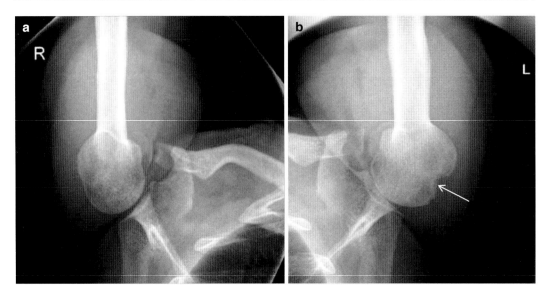

Fig. 7 (**a**) Stryker view (normal) (**b**) Stryker view – Hill-Sachs defect (*arrow*)

needle (Fig. 8). If this is a therapeutic or a diagnostic injection, a mixture of steroid and local anaesthetic or just local anaesthetic respectively is injected into the shoulder joint. If this is part of a CT or MR arthrogram intra-articular contrast medium is administered. A total of 10–15 ml is can be injected, but lax joints will be able to accommodate a larger volume. With adhesive capsulitis, the joint capacity is much reduced.

Posterior Approach

The advantage to this approach is that it prevents inadvertent contamination of the anterior structures by contrast medium.

Patient is in the prone oblique position. A 21G needle is aimed at the inferomedial quadrant of the humeral head.

Ultrasound

Indications

Identification of tendinosis and tears of the rotator cuff (partial and complete tears can be differentiated); tendinosis, rupture and subluxation of the biceps tendon; joint and bursal effusions; muscle, bone and articular cartilage lesions variably demonstrated; paralabral cysts (suggesting possibility of labral tear); suprascapular and axillary nerve pathology; AC and sternoclavicular joint. It also allows for dynamic assessment of impingement and for ultrasound-guided interventional procedures.

Ultrasound (US) has the advantages of being dynamic, with good spatial and contrast resolution, while remaining non-invasive and inexpensive. With good equipment and a skilled examiner, US enables assessment of partial and complete tears of the rotator cuff with high sensitivity and specificity. Many patients prefer US to MRI, aş it is quicker and better tolerated.

Linear ultrasound probes or transducers use a range of high of frequencies, providing high resolution images. Broadband transducers use a spectrum of frequencies, for example 12–5 MHz, rather than a single frequency. High frequency components provide greater spatial resolution but limited depth penetration, whereas low frequency components extend the penetration depth [4]. Other ultrasound functions, which are of use in musculo-skeletal ultrasound, include Doppler, compound imaging, extended field-of-view imaging and beam steering.

Table 2 Radiographic assessment of the shoulder

Radiographic positions	Patient position	Technique/ Centring	Indications
Anteroposterior (AP) view	Patient standing, sitting or supine, with back against film (Fig. 1)	Coracoid process	Acute trauma of shoulder and proximal humerus (less patient discomfort); acromioclavicular joint. Gives an oblique projection of the gleno-humeral joint
Glenohumeral view (true AP of the shoulder joint)	Patient standing, sitting or supine, with back against film. Turn the patient toward the affected side to get the glenohumeral joint in profile (blade of scapula parallel to film) (Fig. 2)	Coracoid process	Chronic (occasionally acute) glenohumeral joint pathology (previous dislocation, arthropathy) demonstrates the gleno-humeral joint in profile
Lateral ("Y") view (posteroanterior)	Patient erect (standing or sitting), affected shoulder rotated 45° anteriorly, placed against the film (blade of scapula perpendicular to film) (Fig. 3)	Humeral head	Subluxation of humeral head; alternative second view in acute trauma
Outlet view (posteroanterior)	As for Y view, with 15° caudal angulation	Glenoid fossa	Contour of coraco-acromial arch, subacromial space
Axial view (superoinferior [SI], inferosuperior [IS])	Patient standing (generally IS), sitting (SI) or supine (IS), film against superior aspect of GH joint (IS) or curved cassette in axilla (SI), with arm abducted. Tube angulation away from (SI) or towards the trunk (IS) (Fig. 4)	Middle of GH joint through axilla	Acute trauma (limited by patient's ability to move); chronic shoulder pain; (Os acromiale)
			Can be performed erect with limited abduction in severe pain/ acute trauma
Stripp Axial (inferosuperior)	The patient sits on a stool with back to the x-ray tube. The x-ray tube is inverted such that the central ray is directed vertically upwards. The cassette placed over the affected shoulder, kept in place by the patient's other hand. The patient leans back slightly (Fig. 5)	Vertical, central ray directed through the axilla	Provides an axial view without the need to abduct the arm in a painful or immobile shoulder
Bloom-Obata Axial (superoinferior)	Patient on stool, leaning back onto table, such that shoulder is vertically above cassette on tabletop. X-ray tube positioned such the central ray directed vertically downwards (Fig. 6)	Vertical, central ray directed to the lateral tip of the clavicle	Provides axial view of the glenohumeral joint. Again useful when abduction is limited
AC Joint	The patient with back to film	Horizontal ray centred at midline at level of head of humerus	Demonstrates subluxations. Both sides on same film for comparison
Stryker (notch) view	Patient supine, hand behind head with shoulder externally rotated and abducted (Fig. 7a, b)	Central ray directed to coracoid process with 10° cranial angulation	Shows humeral head contour (useful in chronic anterior dislocation to show presence of Hill Sachs deformity)

The patient is positioned on a stool with the examiner standing either in front or behind, depending on individual preference. A posterior approach allows for easy access to the US keyboard and the patient's shoulder.

All tendons are examined in their long and short axis, for example, in the following order: the biceps, the subscapularis, the supraspinatus, the infraspinatus and teres minor. A systematic approach, even for

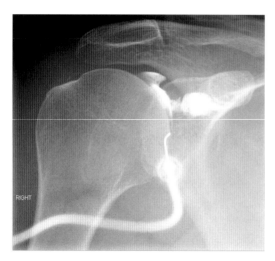

Fig. 8 Fluoroscopy guided needle placement for arthography

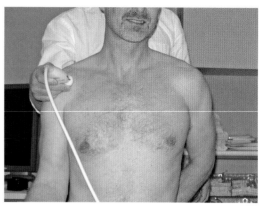

Fig. 9 Position of the probe for examination of the long head of biceps tendon in short axis (elbow flexed to 90°). Turn the probe through 90° to visualise the biceps in the long axis

experienced examiners, will ensure that less obvious findings are not overlooked.

It is important that the US transducer is always orientated perpendicular to the tendon; this avoids the loss of echogenicity, which can simulate a tendon tear. This is apparent hypo-echogenicity of the tendon is called anisotropy and can be overcome by slight rotation/angulation of the transducer. If this is due to real pathology, the hypo-echogenicity will persist. However, if it is due to positioning, the hyper-echoeic tendon fibrils will be visualised again on proper positioning of the transducer perpendicular to the tendon [5].

Ultrasound Examination of the Shoulder

Long Head of Biceps

The normal biceps tendon has a fibrillar appearance. A non-fibrillar appearance is abnormal and would suggest degeneration (tendon tissue still visible) or rupture (tendon not visible). An additional reason for non-visualization of the tendon is subluxation/dislocation from the bicipital groove and the tendon

should always be sought in a more medial location. Tendon (tendonosis, partial and complete tears, instability) and tendon sheath (synovitis, synovial bodies) pathologies should be assessed.

Patient position. The patient is seated comfortably on a stool, with the arm to be examined in the neutral position (arm against trunk, elbow bent to 90°, forearm supinated), or in slight internal rotation (Fig. 9).

The bicipital groove is identified between the lesser and greater tuberosities of the humerus. Within it, the arcuate artery may be identified lateral to the tendon. The biceps tendon is visualised in both the short (Fig. 10) and long axis (Fig. 11). Slight cranial angulation of the probe is usually required in both planes to abolish anisotropy. The myotendinous junction is at the level of insertion of the pectoralis major muscle into the lateral lip of the intertubercular groove. From the neutral position the arm is moved from internal to external rotation to check for subluxation/dislocation.

Rotator Cuff

On US the rotator cuff is variably hyper-echoic when compared to the overlying deltoid muscle. However this echogenicity is age-related and the rotator cuff may not be as hyper-echoeic in older patients.

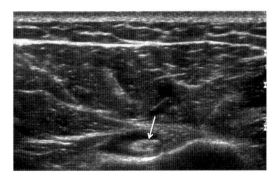

Fig. 10 The long head of biceps – short axis (*arrow*), with a small surrounding tendon sheath effusion

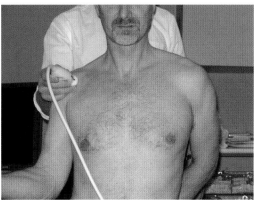

Fig. 12 Position of the probe for examination of the subscapularis tendon in long axis. The patient's shoulder is externally rotated (varying the position allows examination of the whole tendon), the elbow remains against his side. Turn probe through 90° to examine tendon in the short axis

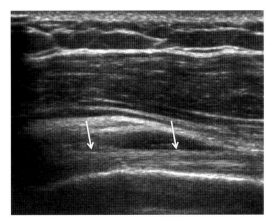

Fig. 11 The long head of biceps – long axis (*arrows*). Note the normal fibrillar pattern

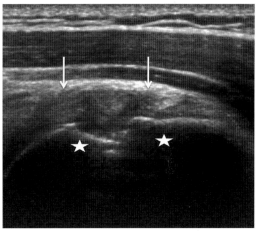

Fig. 13 Short axis view of the multipennate subscapularis tendon (*arrows*). Lesser tuberosity (*asterisks*)

Subscapularis

The patient is then asked to externally rotate the arm (from the neutral position for examination of the biceps tendon), which allows more complete evaluation (Fig. 12). Varying the degree of external rotation allows visualization of the entire tendon.

The short axis view shows the normal multipennate appearance (Fig. 13), which could be mistaken for a tear by the uninitiated. The long axis view demonstrates the insertion into the lesser tuberosity (Fig. 14). Dynamic assessment during internal/external rotation is used for subcoracoid impingement.

Supraspinatus

The patient is then asked to position himself with the arm to be examined behind his back or with the hand in/on his back pocket (Fig. 15). This moves the supraspinatus from under the acromion. In the short axis, the biceps tendon marks the anterior aspect of the supraspinatus tendon in the rotator interval (Fig. 16); extend this view in the same plane (cranial movement of the transducer) to visualise

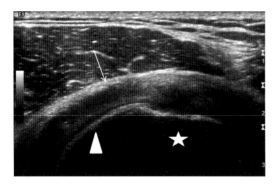

Fig. 14 Long axis view of the subscapularis tendon (*arrow*); lesser tuberosity (*asterisk*). Tendon passes from medial (*on the left*) to lateral (*on the right*) over the humeral head (*arrowhead*)

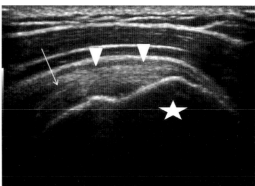

Fig. 17 The supraspinatus tendon – long axis (*arrow*); subacromial bursa (*arrowheads*), greater tuberosity (*asterisk*)

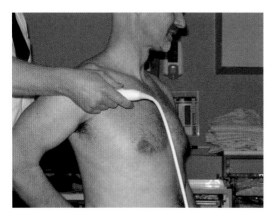

Fig. 15 Position of the probe for examination of the supraspinatus tendon in short axis. The patient's hand is placed over his back pocket

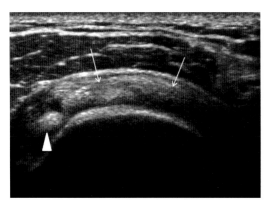

Fig. 16 The supraspinatus tendon – short axis (*arrows*); long head of biceps (*arrowhead*)

the entire tendon in short axis. It is important to visualise the biceps tendon in this view. In the long axis, the insertion into the greater tuberosity is demonstrated (Fig. 17). Partial thickness tears at the bursal surface are identified more clearly, due to abnormal contour of the usually smooth, convex bursal surface of the tendon. Early calcification within the tendon is identified more sensitively than on standard radiographs; evaluation of the subacromial-subdeltoid bursa is possible simultaneously (may be thickened or contain a fluid collection suggesting bursitis).

Infraspinatus
The patient is asked to place the ipsilateral hand on the contralateral shoulder (Fig. 18), allowing better visualisation of the tendon in the short and long axis (Figs. 19, 20). The muscle is examined and fatty atrophy can be clearly seen. The tendon merges posteriorly with teres minor without clear differentiation distally, but the morphology of the muscle belly and separation of the tendons more proximally allows the individual tendons to be evaluated.

Acromio-Clavicular joint AC joint
Examination is also possible in two planes, placing the transducer anteriorly and superiorly over the acromioclavicular joint. Osteophytes, subchondral cysts, synovitis, capsular hypertrophy and ganglia may be seen. The articular disc is

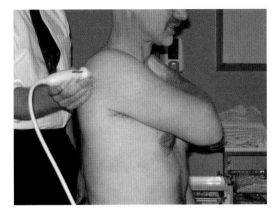

Fig. 18 Position of the probe for examination of the infraspinatus (long axis). The patient's hand is placed on the contralateral shoulder

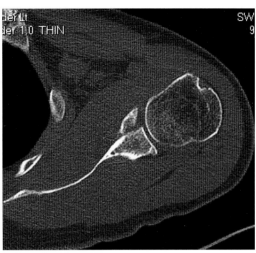

Fig. 21 CT of the shoulder, axial reconstruction. There is an anterior glenoid fracture

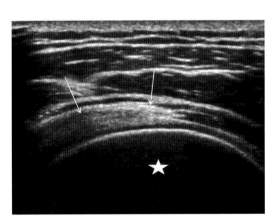

Fig. 19 The infraspinatus tendon – short axis (*arrows*); humeral head (*asterisk*)

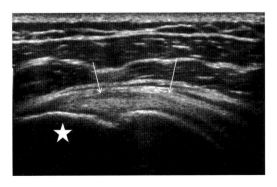

Fig. 20 The infraspinatus tendon – long axis (*arrows*); greater tuberosity (*asterisk*)

particularly well demonstrated in the short axis of the joint (sagittal probe position).

Gleno-Humeral joint

A limited evaluation is possible with ultrasound. The transducer is placed posteriorly over the joint with an increased field of view. Large gleno-humeral joint effusions/synovitis may be seen.

Computed Tomography (CT) and Computed Tomography Arthrography (CT Arthrography)

Indications

Provides high resolution assessment of bone (qualitative, quantitative and morphological) (Fig. 21). Useful for the characterisation of fractures; assessment of the morphology of the glenoid and humeral head, for example humeral torsion, glenoid version; further characterisation of focal bone lesions demonstrated by other imaging techniques (radiographs, MRI), for example the nidus in osteoid osteoma and sequestrum in osteomyelitis; assessment pre- and post- shoulder arthroplasty.

CT arthrography has two parts:

(A) The arthrogram and (B) The CT. The indications are similar to MR arthrography but

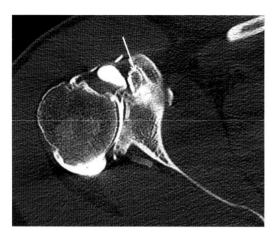

Fig. 22 CT arthrogram, axial reconstruction. There is osteoarthritis, posterior subluxation of the humeral head and an ossified intra-articular body (*arrow*) next to the coracoid process. The glenoid appears retroverted

it can be performed in patients with absolute contra-indications (e.g. pacemaker) and relative contraindications to MRI (e.g. post-arthroplasty). CT arthrography assesses the labrum, articular cartilage, joint capsule, rotator cuff tears and intra-articular bodies.

A. Arthrogram: Refer to the arthrogram section for the procedure. Once the intra-articular position of the needle is confirmed, 10–15 ml of iodinated contrast media is administered to distend the joint (single-contrast arthrography) or 2–3 ml contrast followed by air (double-contrast). Passive movement of the shoulder helps the contrast spread evenly through the joint. The patient should keep the arm close to the body with minimal movement to prevent dissipation out of the joint.

B. CT scan: Multi-planar reconstruction enables full appraisal of the labrum and joint in multiple planes (Fig. 22).

MR and MR Arthrography

Indications

Shoulder MR is used to assess the integrity of the rotator cuff tendons, the muscles of the rotator cuff, with additional arthrography

particularly useful for assessment of articular side partial thickness tears, joint surfaces and intra-articular bodies and the labro-ligamentous complex/capsule. Conventional shoulder MR provides accurate diagnosis of full thickness tears of the rotator cuff, however it is less sensitive in the diagnosis of partial thickness tears. Both US and MRI evaluate cuff tendons accurately, but with full-thickness tears, cuff muscle atrophy (originally studied using CT [6]), crucial in the long-term functional outcome post-surgical repair, can be assessed and graded more easily (and with less operator-dependability) using MRI [7]. MRI also has the advantage of giving a more "global" assessment of the shoulder region.

Normal Anatomical Variants

There are some normal variants in relation to the glenoid labrum that must not be confused with labral tears. If the glenoid articular surface is viewed as the face of a clock most normal variants occur in the 11–3 o' clock position (anterosuperior quadrant) [8].

Sub-Labral Foramen

A localised detachment of the anterosuperior labrum from the glenoid at the 2 o' clock position, anterior to the biceps tendon attachment [9]. It can be difficult to differentiate from an anterosuperior labral tear.

Sub-Labral Recess

A synovial reflection between the cartilage of the glenoid cavity and the superior labrum. It is located at the 12 o' clock position at the site of attachment of the biceps tendon. It can communicate with the sub-labral foramen. This may be misinterpreted as a superior labral anteroposterior (SLAP) tear [9].

Buford Complex

The antero superior labrum is congenitally absent and is associated with a thickened cord like middle gleno-humeral joint. This can simulate an avulsed anterior labral fragment [10].

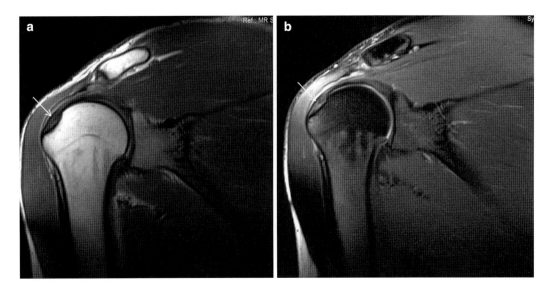

Fig. 23 (**a**) MRI shoulder. Coronal proton density, showing the supraspinatus tendon (*arrow*) (**b**) MRI shoulder. Coronal proton density with fat saturation, showing the supraspinatus tendon (*arrow*)

MR Sequences

Coronal Oblique Images
These are obtained parallel to the supraspinatus tendon, in the coronal oblique plane. Multiple sequences may be used: the authors' preference is proton density (PD) and PD with fat saturation (FS) or inversion recovery sequences (STIR). A high resolution, fluid-sensitive sequence, usually with fat-saturation, gives accurate assessment of full-thickness tears of the cuff (Fig. 23). Fat suppression techniques improve the ability to diagnose full and partial thickness rotator cuff tears [11].

Sagittal Images
These are obtained in a plane perpendicular to the long axis of the supraspinatus tendon. They are useful for assessment of the rotator cuff tendons in short axis, cuff muscle bulk and signal, the subacromial sub- deltoid bursa and the acromioclavicular joint. Useful sequences are proton density (with or without FS) or T2-weighted fast spin echo (Fig. 24).

Axial Images
These evaluate the AC and gleno-humeral joints for arthropathy; useful for visualising the

subscapularis tendon in the long axis, the long head of biceps tendon in the bicipital groove and labral pathology is occasionally seen (better evaluated with intra-articular contrast). Common sequences include T2-weighted gradient echo (T2*) and fat-saturated proton density (Fig. 25).

MR arthrography has been found to be more sensitive than conventional MR for labral tears and is considered to be the imaging gold standard for the detection of labral pathology. It is also better at detection of partial (articular surface) supraspinatus tears, gleno-humeral articular cartilage deficiency and intra-articular bodies than conventional MR. 3 T MRI has recently been shown to improve the demonstration of some of these lesions without contrast injection. MR arthrography is certainly not required in all patients and should be restricted to those with appropriate indications, often instability, in view of the additional time required to perform the arthrogram, the small risk of complications and the limited additional information obtained in some cases.

MR arthrography, similar to CT arthrography, has two components: (A) The arthrogram and (B) MR:

A. Arthrogram: Refer to the arthrogram section for the procedure. Once the intra-articular position of the needle is confirmed using iodinated

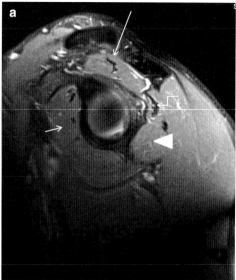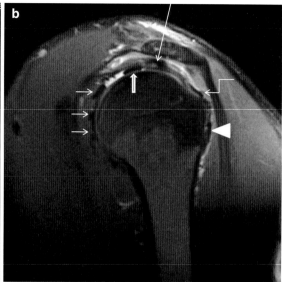

Fig. 24 (**a**) MRI shoulder. Sagittal proton density image with fat saturation at the level of the glenoid, to show cuff muscles and forming tendons. Subscapularis- short arrow, supraspinatus- long arrow, infraspinatus- curved arrow, teres minor- arrowhead (**b**) MRI shoulder. Sagittal proton density image with fat saturation, obtained more laterally for visualisation of the tendons close to their insertions. Subscapularis-short arrows, supraspinatus- long arrow, infraspinatus- curved arrow, teres minor- arrowhead, long head of biceps- block arrow

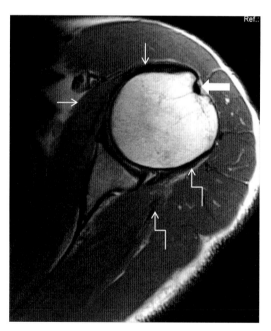

Fig. 25 Axial MR (proton density) image. Subscapularis-*short arrows*, infraspinatus- *curved arrows*, long head of biceps- *block arrow*

contrast, either dilute gadolinium or saline is injected into the shoulder joint. Passive movement of the shoulder helps the contrast spread evenly through the joint. After this the patient should keep the injected arm close to the body with minimal movement to prevent dissipation out of the joint. Care should be taken to avoid injection of even small quantities of air.

B. MRI: The patient then has a shoulder MRI. Depending on whether gadolinium or saline is injected the imaging obtained is either T1-weighted with fat-saturation (with gadolinium) or proton density/T2-weighted. Following injection, MRI should be performed without delay while there is maximal joint distension [12] (Fig. 26).

Indirect MR arthrography is less invasive than direct MR arthrography. This technique involves an intravenous injection of gadolinium, followed by gentle exercise and delayed imaging (15–20 min). This results in contrast in the joint

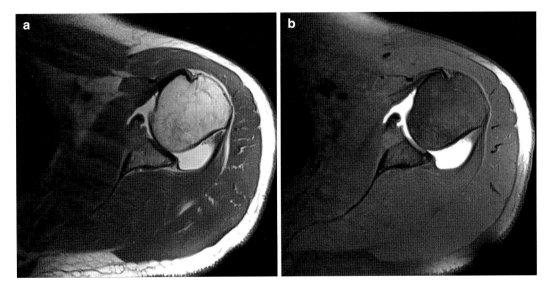

Fig. 26 (**a**) MR arthrogram: axial proton density image (same patient as Fig. 21, anterior glenoid fracture). (**b**) MR arthrogram: axial T1-weighted image with fat saturation (same patient as Fig. 21, anterior glenoid fracture)

secondary to diffusion across the synovium [13]. There is no significant joint distension from injected contrast and intra-articular structures are consequently less well shown – it may be of use if an arthrogram cannot be performed.

Post-Surgical Shoulder

The post-surgical shoulder is imaged using the various imaging modalities previously described (radiographs, ultrasound, CT (+/− arthrogram) and MRI), each of which have advantages and disadvantages.

The challenges to imaging the post-operative shoulder come from the altered anatomy, post-operative scarring and, on CT and MRI, from the artifacts due to ferromagnetic screws, staples and metal shavings. Use of titanium and non-metallic fixation help reduce these artefacts. Also, use of specific sequences such as turbo-spin echo (TSE) and fast-spin echo (FSE), as an alternative to conventional spin-echo and gradient-echo, help reduce the susceptibility artefact. Fat suppression sequences are more prone to disruption and fast-spin echo inversion recovery (STIR)

sequences can be helpful in these situations [14]. MR arthrography can be useful in the post-operative shoulder by distending the joint, which provides improved delineation of the rotator cuff, capsule-labral structures and tendons [15], but CT arthrography is often more appropriate for evaluation of the cuff following shoulder arthroplasty.

References

1. Stripp W. Special techniques in orthopaedic radiography. In: Murray O, Jacobson HG, editors. The radiology of skeletal disorders. 3rd ed. Edinburgh: Churchill Livingstone; 1990.
2. Bloom M, Obata W. Diagnosis of posterior dislocation of the shoulder with use of Velpeau and angle-up roetgenographic view. J Bone and Joint Surg Am. 1967;49A:943–9.
3. Shortt C, Morrison W, Roberts C, Deely D, Gopez A, Zoga A. Shoulder, hip and knee arthrography needle placement using fluoroscopic guidance: practice patterns of musculoskeletal radiologists in North America. Skeletal Radiol. 2009;38:377–85.
4. Whittingham T. Broadband transducers. Eur Radiol. 1999;9 (Suppl 3):S298–303.
5. ESSR Ultrasound Group Protocols. Available at www. essr.org (educational material)

6. Goutallier D, Postel J, Bernageau J, Lavau L, Voisin M. Fatty degeneration in cuff ruptures. Pre and postoperative evaluation by CT scan. Clin Orthop. 1994;304:78–83.

7. Zanetti M, Gerber C, Hodler J. Qualitative assessment of the muscles of the rotator cuff with magnetic resonance imaging. Invest Radiol. 1998;33:163–70.

8. McCarthy CL. Glenohumeral instability. Imaging. 2007;19:201–7.

9. De Maeseneer M, Van Roy F, Lenchik L, et al. CT and MR arthrography of the normal and pathological anterosuperior labrum and labral –bicipital complex. Radiographics. 2000;20:S67–81.

10. Tirman P, Feller J, Palmer W, et al. The Buford complex- a variation of normal shoulder anatomy: MR arthrographic imaging features. AJR Am J Roentgenol. 1996;166:869–73.

11. Reinus W, Sady K, Mirowitz S, Totty W. MR diagnosis of rotator cuff tears of the shoulder: value of using T2-weighted fat saturated images. AJR Am J Roentgenol. 1995;164:1451–5.

12. Andreisek G, Duc S, Froehlich J, Hodler J, Weishaupt D. MR athrography of the shoulder, hip and wrist. Evaluation of contrast dynamics and image quality with increasing injection to imaging time. AJR Am J Roentgenol. 2007;188:1081–8.

13. Bergin D, Schweitzer M. Indirect magnetic resonance arthrography. Skeletal Radiol. 2003;32:551–8.

14. Wu J, Covey A, Katz L. MRI of the postoperative shoulder. Clin Sports Med. 2006;25:445–64.

15. Mohana–Borges AV, Chung CB, Resnick D. MR imaging and MR arthrography of the postoperative shoulder: spectrum of normal and abnormal findings. Radiographics. 2004;24:69–85.

Outcome Scores for Shoulder Dysfunction

Simon M. Lambert

Contents

Keywords
Constant-Murley score • End-result • EQ-5D •
Oxford shoulder score • Shoulder assessment •
Shoulder outcomes • Shoulder score • SPADI •
Subjective shoulder value

Introduction

A compendium of classifications and scores [8] for the shoulder, published in 2006, describes 105 classifications (based on anatomical site, pathological process, surgical intervention) and 22 scores for function (site-dependent and site-independent) and yet admits to being incomplete. A more recent similar compendium, less exhaustive, describes the value of commonly-used measures and instruments for the assessment of shoulder conditions and interventions, and weights the scores helpfully for methodological and clinical utility [17]. An evaluation of the accuracy with which scores are used in shoulder surgery was published from Oxford, UK [9]: 44 scores were evaluated. 22 were clinician-based, 21 patient-based, and 1 used both clinician- and patient-based scoring methodology. This evaluation concluded that patient-related outcome scores (PROMs) were valid, reliable, reproducible, could be conducted remotely and over time, and likely to be the chosen method by which funding bodies could give value to the outcome of interventions in health-care. More recently, still the same group warned against using PROMs as a means to define the level of

S.M. Lambert
The Shoulder and Elbow Service, Royal National
Orthopaedic Hospital, Stanmore, Middlesex, UK
e-mail: slambert@nhs.net

G. Bentley (ed.), *European Surgical Orthopaedics and Traumatology*,
DOI 10.1007/978-3-642-34746-7_57, © EFORT 2014

disability required to access specific heath-care interventions [10]. PROMs are not designed to determine a set of population-based criteria for the level of disability required before intervention could be sanctioned: PROMs are disease- or intervention- specific subjective evaluations which can be followed to determine the value, over time, of an intervention in the specifc population. PROMS, in themselves, do not help a clinician to understand what change to effect for improvement to occur in outcomes for a particular condition. The challenge for the clinician is to match objective data about pre-intervention and post-intervention status, and patient – derived (subjective) data. There is no current system for the shoulder, for any condition or any intervention, that helps the clinician in this way. The multiplicity of scoring systems for function of the shoulder reflects the difficulty of encoding precisely what is important for the outcome of an intervention from the perspective of the patient, the clinician, and the health-care system.

Scores have, historically, been derived from the population set treated by interested clinicians. It is only lately that epidemiologists and biostatisticians have been instrumental in designing tools for understanding outcomes in shoulder conditions. Most simple biological phenomena are more or less normally distributed at population level (e.g., humeral head size) and so can be dealt with using parametric tests for small and large samples. Composite (multi-factorial) or complex (interdependent) phenomena are not necessarily normally distributed so have to be analysed with non-parametric tests: the differences between samples is now more complex with greater chance of overlapping (confounding) factors. Within scoring systems some apparently independent variables may be dependent or surrogate variables: this makes the sensitivity of a score to change less accurate or discriminatory. The AO publication has useful comparisons of methodological evaluations: validity (content, construct, and criterion validity) and reliability (internal consistency, reproducibility, and responsiveness), and clinical utility (patient-friendliness and clinician friendliness, both of which are valued as limited, moderate or strong).

Which Score for Which Purpose?

A relevant and useful study from the Schulthess Klinik, published in 2008 [2], compared the sensitivity to change (responsiveness) of six outcome assessment tools in 153 patients undergoing total shoulder arthroplasty (TSR) for a variety of reasons, but most commonly for osteoarthritis. The Short Form 36 (SF-36), Disabilities of the Arm, Shoulder and Hand questionnaire (DASH), Shoulder Pain and Disability Index (SPADI), American Shoulder and Elbow Surgeons questionnaire (ASES), and the Constant Score (CS) were evaluated before and 6 months after TSR. This study concluded that the CS and SPADI were the most suitable for short, responsive, shoulder-specific assessment, while the SPADI was the most responsive for pain. The subjective (patient-based) part of the ASES questionnaire was considered the most responsive shoulder-function assessment. The authors considered the addition of the DASH or SF-36 to gain a comprehensive assessment of health and quality of life. In summary, scores for pain, function, and overall health status appeared to be best treated separately. Biophysical measures (such as range of motion) may correlate weakly with patients' perception of outcome, but may correlate with some aspects of the functional scores; composite scores (scores which aggregate assessment of pain, function, and biophysical parameters) may be the least useful in terms of responsiveness to change; most scores can differentiate between the outcome of "slightly better" and "slightly worse".

Scores serve several purposes. A shoulder intervention can be assessed from the perspective of the patient, the clinician, and the health-care system. The patient is interested in the likely value, the improvement in quality of life, that he might expect from an intervention; the clinician is interested in the effect of the intervention and how the improvement on quality of life might be explained by the intervention; the health-care system needs to know that it is gaining value for money. To do this the health-care system uses comparators with similar systems or groups of users. There are therefore patho-biomechanical scores of specific diagnoses or interventions (objective clinician-based scores) and subjective patient-based scores both of which aim to distinguish the decrement in function from normal and how closely an intervention restores the shoulder to normal, and biometric quality-of -life scores for the better understanding of the burden of disability due to shoulder problems and for the improved distribution of resources for preventing and treating shoulder problems. Of the latter the SF-36 and the EQ-5D are in common use. The EQ-5D is probably the most useful of these.

Health Status Measures: The EQ-5D

Very few scores for the shoulder fulfill the criteria commonly cited as important for understanding outcomes [14]. Methodological criteria such as reliability, reproducibility, and validity are all relevant but the score should also be easy to administer and simple for the patient to understand: not all scores translate accurately into different languages. The EQ-5D is almost unique in this regard, having been translated from the English into Germanic, Baltic, Central European (Slavic), and Southern European languages while retaining its statistical value. In its present form the EQ-5D method is increasingly used for comparison of interventions in a wide variety of health – related activities, including surgery. The EQ-5D is a score of current health status self-administered by the patient. It comprises five items (mobility, self-care, usual activities, pain/discomfort, and anxiety/depression), with a 3-point categorical response scale (a score of 1 means 'no problems', 2 means 'some/moderate problems', and 3 means 'extreme problems'). A unique score is calculated by a weighted regression-based algorithm, with good reliability, validity, and responsiveness. In addition, overall functional capacity is self-assessed on a linear rating scale. It is simple to administer, and is an effective general health PROM. Users of the EQ-5D are required to register their project with the Euroqol group, which offers support for the project.

Shoulder-Specific General Functional Scores: The Constant Score

The Constant Score was described by Constant and Murley in 1987 [6] and was the result of a survey of the function of the shoulders of a normal population in a provincial market town near Cambridge, East Anglia, Great Britain. The population was skewed towards older people, and showed a decline in function with age. This in itself was not surprising, but the simplicity of the method was attractive. The score is given as a percentage with 100 % being the best score possible, and comprises four domains: pain, function of daily life including sleep and recreation, strength, and range of motion. The value of each domain as a component of the score was 15 %, 20 %, 25 % and 40 % respectively. Since pain was not a common experience in normal shoulders it was afforded only a small proportion of the total (15 %), and is categorised as absent (15 points), mild (10 points), moderate (5 points), and severe (0 points). Pain scores within the CS are often quoted as means with standard deviations and compared to two decimal points. This is not statistically consistent. This categorisation of pain is not compatible with more accepted methods of scoring pain (such as the linear scale or numeric analogue scores). Pain is therefore not discriminated well in the CS. The method of evaluating strength follows a strict definition, in which the arm must be able to be held at the level of the shoulder in the scapular plane (90° abduction): if this position is not possible then by definition the score for strength is zero. This vastly underestimates the value of interventions which give patients pain-free use below shoulder level, such as shoulder replacement in many patients with rheumatoid arthritis, who might rate their shoulder value much higher. To overcome this many observers use what is called a "modified CS", which excludes strength measurement. Whenever a score is modified it becomes invalid. Modification should not be accepted. Strength has been measured with a hand-held "fisherman's" balance, which simply compares the strength of the observer with the subject, and with electronic dynamometry. Both methods have been shown to be comparable [3]. The range of motion at waist level includes "functional internal rotation" in which the thumb is taken as high up the back as possible, giving the spinal level achieved as the functional range. In some conditions, e.g. rheumatoid arthritis, in which many other upper limb joints (particularly the elbow) are affected, the spinal level of achievement may be adversely affected by a joint other than the shoulder. The shoulder score may then be downgraded by the effect of another joint. The subjective component of functional activities of daily living is afforded only 20 points, and gives points for sleep (no disturbance, some disturbance, nightly disturbance), and recreational activities, including sports. The functional score therefore measures 'ability' as opposed to decrement ('disability'), which introduces more problems of subject bias. Since the subjective part of the CS is at best only 35 % of the entire score, the value of this score as a PROM is limited. Over time the CS has been strongly correlated with other scores (i.e., the scores are consistent) and has been found to be reliable and responsive for the detection of improvement after shoulder surgery in a variety of shoulder pathologies [16].

The European Society for Surgery of the Shoulder and Elbow (ESSSE/SECEC) has, for some years, adopted the Constant Score (CS) as the preferred method for reporting outcomes for interventions in the shoulder, excluding those for instability. Attempts have been made to adapt the CS for use as a remotely-administered outcome measure to enable long-term review without the expense of multiple clinic visits, which the current fiscal climate inhibits. These have proven difficult. The scores have been "ponderated" or weighted against age-and gender-matched equivalent normal scores (the so-called "ponderated CS"), and against the contra-lateral shoulder (the "relative CS") which is assumed to be normal.

The essence of the CS is that it measures the decline in function of the rotator cuff over time. For instance, the benefit of total shoulder replacement as measured by the CS is a function of the improvement in the aptitude of the rotator cuff to do work in a joint with less friction, less pain (and so greater muscle strength and better activation), and greater range of motion. It is not a feature of the arthroplasty itself, so unless the biomechanical characteristic of an arthroplasty is very different from another with which it is being compared it is unlikely that the CS will show a substantial difference between two arthroplasties given similar rotator cuff function. Scapular motion is never assessed independently of glenohumeral motion. A shoulder arthrodesis (dependent on scapular motion) may only achieve a moderate CS yet be transformative for the quality of daily life for the patient through pain relief, which is poorly measured by the CS.

Shoulder Pathology: Specific Scores

There are many shoulder-pathology specific scores, such as those for instability (e.g., Walch-Duplay, Rowe, Western Ontario Shoulder Instability index, WOSI), osteoarthritis (e.g., Western Ontario Osteoarthritis of the Shoulder index, WOOS), and rotator cuff disease (e.g., Western Ontario Rotator Cuff index, WORC). These are valuable in the specific pathologies for which they have been designed, but should not be used for other pathological conditions i.e., they are not transferable. The WOSI, WOOS, and WORC have been validated for the conditions they represent, and are therefore the more valuable assessment tools. For a detailed analysis of the application of these tools the reader is directed to references [8, 17].

Shoulder Pain Scores: SPADI, OSS

The SPADI (Shoulder Pain and Disability Index, [15]) was initially derived from a very small group of patients with shoulder pain from a variety of causes, and developed in an iterative manner. It comprises two domains: pain (5 items) and disability (8 items), which are treated equally from a statistical perspective. The index has been used (and validated as a reliable instrument) for patients undergoing non-operative therapy as well as for surgical treatment, and is correlated

The assessment of shoulder dysfunction and the outcome of shoulder interventions should reflect the following:

1. Items essential for Activities of Daily Living (ADL).

This element of a score system should reflect the patient's ability to engage with the internal or personal world space, and the maintenance of independence. This could be expressed as the ability to achieve a "functional triangle" of face (mouth) - opposite axilla - perineum. This is equivalent to a range of motion defined as an "inner cone" of movement in which internal rotation / adduction / low-level flexion and extension motions dominate. Pain will modify this achievement.

2. Items not essential to, but enhancing, ADL.

This element describes the ability to engage with the external world space, and, often, the maintenance of supported locomotion. This is equivalent to a range of motion defined as an "outer cone" of movement in which more external rotation is involved, and high-level flexion is more valued than extension. Pain and weakness will modify this achievement.

3. Items not essential for ADL but which enhance the quality of life.

This reflects the patients' ability to engage in cultural activities e.g. sport, and assesses the impact of the shoulder condition on the quality of daily life interactions. Since emotional, psychological and physical factors are involved, a general health score is relevant: in Europe the EQ-5D is the most universal instrument. This also indirectly indicates the decrement of function as an economic burden to the population as a whole ie what extra resources might be required to permit a patient with shoulder disability to function within their cultural context.

Fig. 1 Hierarchy of information about an individual which might be helpful in understanding decrement of function and response to intervention

1. Pain assessment: SPADI or VAS (or equivalent)
2. Shoulder-specific function: OSS, SPADI (or equivalent)
3. Biophysical assessment (figure 1): ROM
4. General health status: eg. EQ-5D
5. Subjective shoulder assessment: eg. SPONSA

Key

SPADI: Shoulder Pain and Disability Index
VAS: Visual Analogue Score
OSS: Oxford Shoulder Score
ROM: Range of Motion
EQ-5D: see text
SPONSA: Stanmore Percentage of Normal Shoulder Assessment

Fig. 2 The suggested elements of a shoulder scoring system

with changes in active range of motion [4]. In Europe the SPADI has been validated in English, German [1] and Norwegian languages.

The Oxford Shoulder Score (OSS) [7] was developed as a method of evaluating patients' perception of pain following shoulder procedures in a busy University clinic, using an iterative process which was the most statistically precise of any score used in the shoulder at the time. The involvement of statisticians and epidemiologists was a key advantage in this process. The score comprises 12 questions each having 5 responses, from 1 (the best outcome or effect) to 5 (the worst outcome or effect) and was therefore given as a point score in the range 12 (normal) to 60 (completely abnormal). Importantly, the score is not used as a percentage. Latterly, to align the OSS with the Oxford Hip Score and the Oxford Knee Score (currently the preferred PROM scores utilised in the UK National Joint Registry) the range of outcomes has been inverted to give a range from 0 (completely abnormal) to 48 (normal). The questions are independently administered by the patient, and so the OSS can be used as a remote review method. It is quick, requires no special instruments, and universal in that any shoulder condition can be assessed. The sensitivity to change is not understood completely.

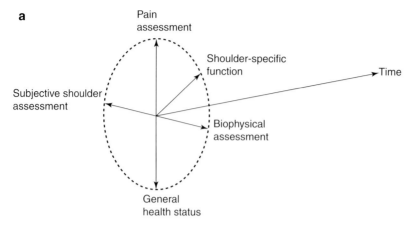

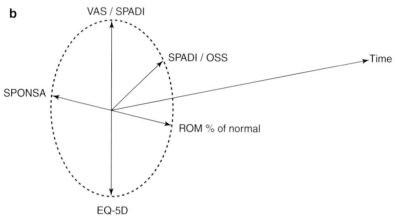

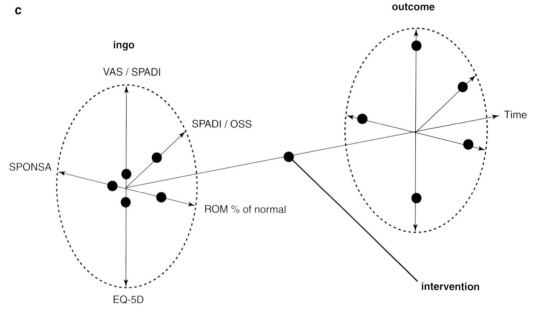

Fig. 3 (continued)

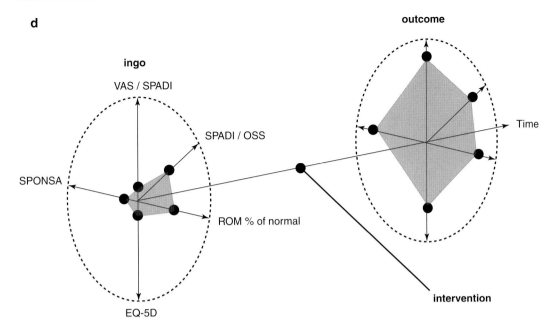

Fig. 3 (**a**) Suggested graphic representation of a shoulder outcome tool. Each radius represents an instrument for measuring an attribute or condition. Better scores occur closer to the perimeter of the area of the shoulder outcome tool. Other scores (more radii) could be added if desired: this might accuracy. (**b**) Graphic representation of shoulder outcome tool with scores. See Fig. 2 for key. (**c**) Graphic representation of shoulder outcome tool for an exemplar patient. (**d**) The change in area represented by the shoulder outcome tool describes the effectiveness (value) of the intervention; the shape of the area describes what each component has contributed to the outcome. In this example case the intervention has contributed by pain relief more than improvement in range of motion, while the subjective shoulder value has greatly improved, contributing to a perceived improvement on general health status

As previously noted it is not an instrument for deciding when 'ability' becomes 'disability' and therefore should not be used to discriminate which patient receives treatment and when. The OSS is not valid for use in patients with glenohumeral instability due to capsulo-labral pathology.

Simple Shoulder Tests: Subjective Shoulder Values

The simple expedient of asking the patient how he/she feels the shoulder is behaving has received increased interest since subjective shoulder scores have been shown to be correlated with both the CS and the OSS [see 13]. The Stanmore Percentage Of Normal Shoulder Assessment (SPONSA, [13]) has been evaluated and shown to be responsive to change, valid, reliable, reproducible, and accurate, while being easier to administer than the CS and as responsive as the OSS. The SPONSA requires the patient to consider the question: *"A normal shoulder is one which, during a normal day, is painfree, with a full range of movement, normal strength and stability, and allows you to do what you feel your shoulder, if normal, should allow you to do. A normal shoulder is scored at 100 % while a completely useless shoulder is scored as 0 %. Overall, where would you rate your shoulder between 0 and 100 % at this present time?"* The question assumes an appreciation of the concept of ratio, percentage or proportion; this does exclude some patients, who find such abstraction difficult. Patient's personal expectations and values are incorporated in this question: the outcome of any intervention is only relevant in the context of patients' concerns, so this way of evaluating outcome is more useful than others as a PROM. The SPONSA can be delivered remotely and is therefore useful for long-term distant review.

Assessing Shoulder Function

All current shoulder scores which attempt to combine biophysical, subjective, and health-related questions have methodological problems (Figs. 1 and 2). A score should measure a specific attribute, and different components of an intervention may require different measurements or scores. Each intervention should therefore be treated as a composite of patient-specific, clinician-specific, and health-status outcomes. Patient-specific outcome and health status can be combined in a subjective evaluation of shoulder function. Factors other than the status of the shoulder (such as cardiac status, metabolic disease, neurological deficit, psychiatric disorder) influence the patient-specific and health-status outcomes. While it is difficult to correlate objective data with subjective data in an attempt to understand the relationship between the specific intervention or problem and the patient's sense of achievement it is important to do so: the value of a procedure may be much underestimated by the subjective assessment [11].

The future for shoulder scores, and other assessments, may be in combinations of analyses, in which several sets of information are combined to give a descriptor of outcome. Bayesian statistics could be used to permit the understanding of how the addition of one or more sets of information influences the accuracy and predictability of outcomes [12]. The elements which might be considered are shown in Figs. 1 and 2. Figure 1 summarises a hierarchy of information about an individual which might be helpful in understanding decrement of function and response to intervention. To measure these attributes a number of tools might be combined (Fig. 2). In this way each individual could be described in a co-ordinate system, one axis of which is time. This is illustrated graphically in Fig. 3.

Summary

Scores are useful, and we should not discard the admonition of Ernest Amory Codman who, in 1913 [5], described the "end-result" model and encouraged the measurement of outcome as the best way of improving outcome. However scores can also be mis-used and mis-interpreted. Scores can also measure apparent or surrogate outcomes, and may not be sensitive enough to accurately describe the value of interventions. Nevertheless we must measure outcome, and therefore we need to know "ingo" i.e., status before intervention or observation, to understand how much difference was gained or lost and how it was achieved. The multiple factors involved in achieving an outcome make a combination of items into a single score unlikely to measure true value. It seems more likely that combinatorial methodologies might provide a mechanism for using different but comparably-valid scoring systems to give useful information about burden of disease, intervention, and improvement (value) of intervention (Fig. 3a–d).

References

1. Angst F, et al. Cross-cultural adaptation, reliability and validity of the German Shoulder Pain and Disability Index (SPADI). Rheumatology (Oxford). 2007;46(1):87–92.
2. Angst F, et al. Responsiveness of six outcome assessment instruments in total shoulder arthroplasty. Arthritis Care Res. 2008;59(3):391–8.
3. Bankes MJ, et al. A standard method of shoulder strength measurement for the constant score with a spring balance. J Shoulder Elbow Surg. 1998;7(2):116–21.
4. Beaton D, Richards RR. Assessing the reliability and responsiveness of 5 shoulder questionnaires. J Shoulder Elbow Surg. 1998;7(6):565–72.
5. Codman EA, et al. Standardisation of hospitals: report of the committee appointed by the Clinical Congress of Surgeons of North America. Trans Clin Cong Surg North Am. 1913;4:2–8.
6. Constant CR, Murley AHG. A clinical method of functional assessment of the shoulder. Clin Orthop Relat Res. 1987;214:160–4.

7. Dawson J, et al. Questionnaire on the perceptions of patients about shoulder surgery. J Bone Joint Surg Br. 1996;78-B(4):593–600.

8. Habermeyer P, et al. Classifications and scores of the shoulder. Berlin/New York: Springer; 2006. ISBN 13 978-3-540-2430-2.

9. Harvie P, et al. The use of outcome scores in surgery of the shoulder. J Bone Joint Surg Br. 2005;87-B: 151–4.

10. Judge A, et al. Assessing patients for joint replacement. Can pre-operative Oxford hip and knee scores be used to predict patient satisfaction following joint replacement surgery and to guide patient selection? J Bone Joint Surg Br. 2011;93-B:1660–4.

11. Kay P. Patient reported outcomes measurement data (PROMs). BON. 2011;49:1–2.

12. Keogh B, Kinsman R. Fifth national adult cardiac surgical database report 2003. The Society of Cardiothoracic Surgeons of Great Britain and Ireland.

13. Noorani A, et al. Validation of the Stanmore percentage of normal shoulder assessment. Accepted for publication, Int J Orth. 2011.

14. Rabin R, de Charro F. EQ-5D: a measure of health status from the EuroQol Group. Ann Med. 2001;33(5): 337–43.

15. Roach KE, et al. Development of a shoulder pain and disability index. Arthritis Care Res. 1991; 4(4):143–9.

16. Roy JS, et al. A systematic review of the psychometric properties of the Constant-Murley score. J Shoulder Elbow Surg. 2010;19(1):157–64.

17. Suk M, et al. Musculoskeletal outcomes measures and instruments, Selection and assessment. Upper extremity, vol. 1. New York: Thieme; 2009. ISBN 978-3-13-141062-7.

Traumatic Lesions of the Brachial Plexus

Rolfe Birch

Contents

R. Birch
War Nerve Injury Clinic at Defence Medical
Rehabilitation Centre, Epsom, Surrey, UK
e-mail: m.taggart@hotmail.co.uk

Abstract

Traumatic lesions of the brachial plexus cause pain, paralysis and loss of sensation. The subclavian-axillary artery is injured in one third of open wounds from knife or missile. Injuries to head, spine, chest or viscera occur in 40 % of closed traction lesions. Whenever possible nerves and arteries should be repaired together at urgent operation. Results of early repair by graft are decisively better. Reconnection to the spinal cord or repair, by transfer, of the avulsed ventral root is possible only in early operations. Pain is usually improved by regeneration and by successful rehabilitation. Rehabilitation is the central core of treatment.

The incidence of birth lesion of the brachial plexus (BLBP) in the UK is 0.42 per 1000 live births. Serious secondary deformities are common. Posterior dislocation or subluxation of the shoulder occurs in about 25 %. Repair is justifiable in severe ruptures of C5 and in preganglionic injuries of the other nerves.

Keywords

Anatomy • Associated injuries • Birth Injuries-aetiology and incidence, prognosis and treatment, indications for surgery, late deformity, posterior gleno-humeral disclocation • Closed injuries-infraclavicular, traction • Examination • Incidence • Indications for surgery • Investigations • Open injuries • Results-relief of pain,functional recovery • Surgical strategies for different injuries • Treatment principles

G. Bentley (ed.), *European Surgical Orthopaedics and Traumatology*,
DOI 10.1007/978-3-642-34746-7_44, © EFORT 2014

Introduction

Rupture of the spinal nerves of the brachial plexus leads to changes in the cell bodies of the ventral horn which culminate in their death. These changes are more extreme when the roots of the spinal nerves are interrupted. *Carlstedt (2007)* [19] estimates that 80 % of motor neurones in the anterior horn disappear by 14 days after avulsion of the ventral root. Cell death in the spinal cord and in the dorsal root ganglia is even more severe in the immature nervous system [33]. These changes are diminished, or even prevented, by urgent reconnection between the cell body and the peripheral tissues, above all, by reconnection with the distal Schwann cell columns. This chapter is based on studies extending for over 45 years of approximately 2,300 cases of lesions of the brachial plexus in the adult including about 1,500 closed injuries to the supraclavicular plexus, and of some 1,800 cases of birth lesion of the brachial plexus.

Anatomy

The spinal nerves leave or enter the cord by ventral, largely motor, roots and dorsal sensory roots. This junction is the weakest mechanical link in the long chain between the central nervous system and the periphery (Fig. 1). The anterior primary rami of the lowest four cervical nerves and most of that of the first thoracic nerve enter the posterior triangle of the neck between scalenus anterior and scalenus medius to unite and branch to form the brachial plexus in the lower part of the neck and behind the clavicle (Fig. 2). The first thoracic nerve passes upward round the neck of the first rib, behind the pleura and behind the vertebral artery and the first part of the subclavian artery. The formation of the *trunks* of the brachial plexus is fairly consistent. C5 and C6 form the upper trunk, the middle trunk is a continuation of C7, the lower trunk from C8 and T1. These lie in front of one another rather than side by side, with the subclavian artery passing antero-medially. The phrenic nerve crosses C5 to pass antero-medially on the

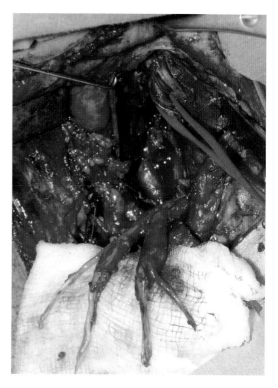

Fig. 1 The 5th, 6th cervical nerves avulsed from the spinal cord. The ventral root is easily distinguishable from the dorsal rootlets. Note the dorsal root ganglion, the dural sleeve merging into the epineurium and the spinal nerve itself. The small pieces of tissue on the proximal ends of the dorsal rootlets (*below*) are probably portions of the spinal cord

surface of scalenus anterior. The transverse cervical and greater auricular nerves wind round the posterior border of the sternomastoid no more than 1 cm. cephalad, the spinal accessory nerve emerges from deep to the sternocleidomastoid about 5 mm. further cephalad. A significant branch from C4 to C5 or to the upper trunk is encountered in between 2 % and 3 % of operated cases.

Three significant nerves pass from the brachial plexus within the posterior triangle:
1. The nerve to serratus anterior is formed by rami from C5, C6 and C7.
2. The dorsal scapular nerve leaves C5 within the foramen lying posterior to the main trunk.
3. The suprascapular nerve passes away from C5, or from the proximal part of the upper

Fig. 2 The right brachial plexus. Note the sequence: the anterior primary rami; trunk; divisions; cord; nerves. Note that the trunks are upper, middle and lower, and that the cords are lateral, medial and posterior from their position in relation to the axillary artery which is, in fact, variable

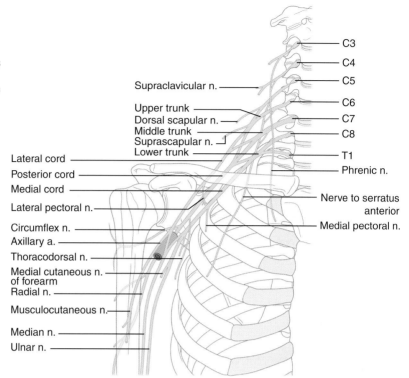

trunk, a finger's breadth above the clavicle passing laterally and then posteriorly through the suprascapular notch.

The *divisions* of the brachial plexus lie deep to the clavicle and their display in a scarred field can be particularly tedious. The posterior division of the upper trunk is consistently larger than the anterior; this is true also for the middle trunk. In some 10 % of cases there is no posterior division of the lower trunk. The formation and relations of the three *cords* are variable and indeed their designations somewhat misleading. Immediately inferior to the clavicle the posterior cord lies *lateral* to the axillary artery, the medial cord *behind*, the lateral cord *in front*. The cords assume their appropriate relations about the axillary artery deep to pectoralis minor.

Open Injuries

The tidy wounds from knife, glass and scalpel are amongst the most rewarding of all nerve injuries to repair. When the opportunity for

repair within hours or days of injury is grasped, the results for C5, C6 and C7 wounds are excellent; better by far than equivalent results even for early repair of more distal nerve trunks ruptured by traction injuries; they are worthwhile for C8 and T1 too. In virtually no other nerve laceration is the harmfulness of procrastination so clearly shown as in the supraclavicular stab wound. On the other hand the nature of the wound is such that other and more pressing problems frequently arise. If the blade or bottle is thrust from above down the lower trunk, subclavian vessels and lung are damaged. When the blade is thrust towards the face or neck the 5th, 6th and 7th cervical with phrenic nerves are damaged: in addition to the jugular and carotid vessels, the trachea and the oesophagus are at risk. The lateral thrust divides the upper and middle trunks, the nerve to serratus anterior and the accessory nerve (Fig. 3).

Penetrating missile wounds commonly involve the viscera, the great vessels, and the spinal cord. Wound contamination is usual.

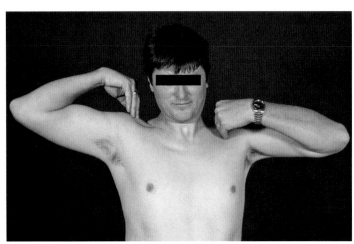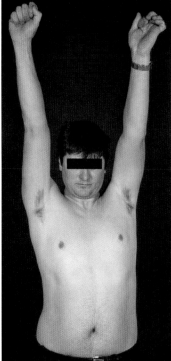

Fig. 3   The outcome 3 years after repair of stab wound of right C5, C6 and C7 and the phrenic nerve

Stewart and Birch (2001) [74] recognised three wound types:

1. Fragment
2. Bullet
3. Bomb blast or close-range shotgun. The lesions were explored in 51 of 58 patients. Correction of false aneurysm or arterio-venous fistula (16 cases) led to dramatic relief of causalgia and improvement in nerve function. Nineteen patients with neurostenalgia, pain arising from an intact nerve which is strangled, compressed, tethered or ischaemic [7] were cured by operation. Main nerves were repaired in 36 patients, results were good or useful in 26 of them, including three repairs of the medial cord or ulnar nerves. The results of repair, although inferior to those seen in tidy wounds, are certainly worthwhile (Fig. 4). *Kline and his colleagues* [42, 43] define indications for operation as : the presence of causalgia or other severe pain; suspected or proven arterial injury or false aneurysm or fistula, and the failure of progression towards recovery for lesions of C5, C6 and C7 or their derivatives.

The Closed Infraclavicular Lesion

Two patterns can be discerned.

The first, which is more common, is caused by violent hyperextension at the shoulder. There is almost always a fracture of shaft of the humerus or injury to the gleno-humeral joint; the axillary artery is ruptured in 30 % of cases, the level of proximal rupture is deep to pectoralis minor which acts as a guillotine on the neurovascular bundle.

The second pattern is even more severe and dangerous. The forequarter is virtually avulsed from the trunk. The subclavian artery is usually torn. There is usually avulsion of the 8th cervical and 1st thoracic nerves which is combined with

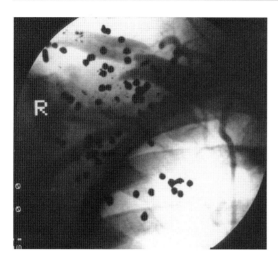

Fig. 4 Shot gun blast to the neck. Bleeding from the first part of the subclavian artery was controlled through the transclavicular exposure

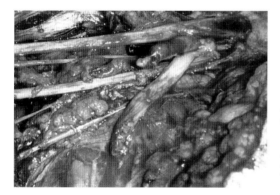

Fig. 5 Rupture of the axillary artery,1, and the radial nerve,2, associated with closed fracture of the upper humerus. Both were repaired (George Bonney 1962)

ruptures of the cords of the plexus more distally. There is, almost always, a phrenic nerve palsy.

The immediate treatment of these limb- and life-threatening injuries includes restoration of ventilation, control of bleeding, stabilisation of the skeleton, repair of the main artery and,if circumstances permit, of the nerves [9,22] (Fig. 5).

The Closed Traction Lesions of the Supraclavicular Brachial Plexus

Perhaps these are the worst of all peripheral nerve lesions because of the frequency of associated injury to the spinal cord and the common

complication of severe pain. In many cases the damage lies between the dorsal ganglion and the spinal cord. To these intradural injuries Bonney (1954) [15] applied the term "preganglionic". The lesion was intradural in about one half of the 7,500 spinal nerves exposed at operation in 1,500 patients since 1966; the incidence of intradural lesion is highest in C7. There are two types of preganglionic injury: intradural *rupture* peripheral to the transitional zone (TZ) and *avulsion* central to it [70]. The lesion may be confined either to the ventral or the dorsal roots, The extent of displacement of the dorsal root ganglion and the level of ruptures of the dura varies. The spinal cord is directly injured in avulsion lesions, an effect worsened by rupture of the subclavian and vertebral arteries. A partial Brown Séquard syndrome was identified in 11.8 % of patients with three or more avulsions [9] (Fig. 6). It is very important to search for even subtle signs of disturbance of the spinal cord at the first and subsequent examinations. Late onset symptoms must be fully investigated to ascertain cause [9, 56].

Incidence – Associated Injuries and Referral Patterns

The 1987 survey by *Goldie and Coates 1992)* [31] uncovered 328 patients with complete or partial lesions. The subclavian artery was ruptured in 5.5 %, and 40 % had other major injuries. *Rosson (1987, 1988)* [66, 67] found an average age of 21 years, injury to the dominant limb in 65 % and severe injuries to the head, the chest, the viscera or other limbs in one half of patients. By one year after injury more than two thirds of patients remained in significant or severe pain and over one third were still unemployed. The severity of the injury may have diminished over the years: 48 from 210 (33 %) patients operated in the years 1966 – 1984 sustained avulsion of C5, compared with 26 from 320 (8 %) operated between 2003 and 2006. Although motor cycle accidents remain the chief cause other mechanisms were responsible for 30 % of the injuries in the most recent group. Severe associated injuries impose delay beyond the ideal time for operation, that is beyond 7 days, in one third of patients. Over the years many patient have been referred urgently. In the 249 patients

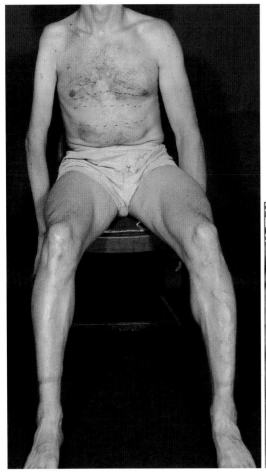
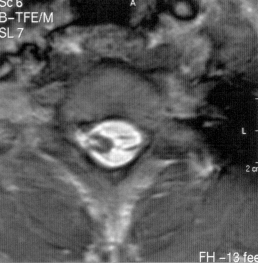

Fig. 6 Wasting of right arm and of muscles in the right lower limb 13 years after preganglionic injury of C7, C8 and T1. Sensory levels marked are (*top to bottom*) warm, cold, pinprick and light touch. The MR scan (*right*) shows deviation of the spinal cord [By courtesy Editor Journal of Bone and Joint Surgery (British)]

operated between 2000 and 2004 nearly 90 % were referred by Orthopaedic surgeons, within 7 days of injury in 98 cases and in another 27 during the second week.

Principles of Treatment

Over the last 40 years we have followed a policy of early exploration and repair especially in arterial injury. An accurate diagnosis is essential in determining prognosis; all reasonable attempts should be made to improve that prognosis. This enables the patient to start the difficult, prolonged, and, at times, painful process of rehabilitation. Potentially life-threatening associated injuries, damage to the spinal column and the spinal cord must take priority over the nerve injury. Fractures of the long bones are not a contra-indication to urgent exploration; arterial injury is a powerful indication.

The proposition that damage to the proximal limb of the axon of the dorsal root ganglion would not affect the distal axon or its myelin sheath was confirmed by studies of the axon reflex *(Bonney 1954)* [14] and by the demonstration of persisting conduction in the afferent fibres of peripheral nerves in cases of preganglionic injury *(Bonney and Gilliat 1958)* [18]. *Bonney (1959)* [16] established that there was no

Table 1 Qualities of pain described by 198 patients 2000–2004

Interval (days)	Burning	Crushing	Electrical	Lightning	Bursting	In a vice	Cold	Total
0–7	65	60	47	34	16	10	1	**233**
8–14	3	3	4	3	1	2		**16**
15–28	4	6	7	4	4	1		**26**
Over 28	11	8	17	14	4	1		**55**
Total	**83**	**77**	**75**	**55**	**25**	**14**	**1**	**330**

1. Many patients describe more than one quality of pain

recovery in nerves which had been avulsed, scarcely any through ruptures and that recovery through less severe lesions in continuity was often complicated by cocontraction. Patients with no recovery experienced intractable pain. This work stimulated a profound and lasting interest in conduction in the central pathways, between the spinal nerve, the spinal cord and the brain. *Jones (1979)* [39] provided the first detailed analysis of peripheral, spinal and cortical sensory evoked potentials. *Landi, Copeland, Wynn Parry and Jones (1980)* [44] compared pre- and intra-operative somatosensory evoked potentials (SSEP's) with surgical findings.

Diagnosis

The History

One common element underlies closed supraclavicular traction lesions and that is the violent distraction of the forequarter from the head, neck and chest so that the angle between the head and shoulder is opened. A description of the shoulder being violently arrested by an object, stone, tree, kerbstone or vehicle whilst the body is flying through the air is associated with severe stretching of the structures in the posterior triangle of the neck.

Severe pain within the paralysed and anaesthetic upper limb indicates serious injury. There is constant crushing, burning and intense pins and needles in the forearm and hand. Two-thirds of conscious patients who experience this pain do so on the day of injury. Superimposed electrical or lightning shoots of pain coursing into the dermatome of a spinal nerve signify preganglionic injury to that nerve. More than one-half of conscious patients experience this pain on the day of injury; in others it becomes apparent at intervals ranging from 14 h to more than 4 weeks after injury (Table 1).

Inspection

One important physical sign is the presence of linear abrasions on the chin and on the face with corresponding abrasions and bruising at the tip of the shoulder. Deep bruising on the point of the shoulder confirms that the limb was violently arrested. Deep bruising in the posterior triangle of the neck suggests rupture of the subclavian artery. An increasing swelling in the posterior triangle of the neck indicates either collection of cerebro-spinal fluid or expanding haematoma or both. Linear bruising in the arm suggests rupture of a nerve trunk or main artery at that level.

Examination

It is very important to conduct a systematic examination of the whole patient. Significant injuries may be missed even in the very best accident department. Rupture of the ipsilateral hemidiaphragm may be confused with phrenic nerve palsy. The severity of an injury to the lung may not be apparent at first examination. An MR scan of the head and of the whole of the spine is advisable when there is the slightest suggestion of upper motor neurone lesion or other abnormality of the central nervous system. It is important also to be on the alert for fractures of the spine and the pelvis.

The patient who is not unconscious will be in pain and distress. Even so it should be possible to find loss of sensation of the skin above the clavicle (C4) which is associated with intradural injury of, at least, the upper nerves, C5 and C6 (Fig. 7). It should be possible to ascertain whether

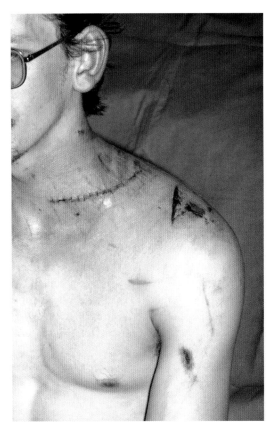

Fig. 7 Linear abrasions in the neck indicate separation of the forequarter from the trunk. The abrasion at the tip of the shoulder marks the point of impact against a road side kerb. Rupture of C5, preganglionic C6 to T1

trapezius and serratus anterior are functioning. Amongst the 72 patients with intradural injury to C5, C6 and C7 operated in the years 2000–2004 serratus anterior was paralysed in 65, 28 had phrenic palsy and C4 was involved in 23. A Bernard Horner sign suggests intradural lesion to C8 and T1 [16].

Tinel's sign is invaluable in the early detection of ruptures. *It should be emphasised that Tinel's sign is detectable in a conscious patient on the day of injury.* It is important to advise the patient that percussion in the posterior triangle of the neck may be painful, and they should be asked to indicate into which regions they experience radiation of intense pins and needles. Rupture of C5 is likely when these sensations extend down the outer

aspect of the arm and the proximal forearm; of C6 when they extend to the lateral aspect of the forearm and the thumb; and of C7 when radiation extends to the dorsum of the hand. Radiation to the outer aspect of the shoulder and the upper part of the arm signifies a lesion of C4. Absence of the sign in a complete, deep lesion accompanied by pain suggests intradural injury (Table 2).

Investigations

The diagnosis of the injury to the nerves is made on clinical grounds. The purpose of supplementary investigations is to clarify that diagnosis but, of even greater importance, to detect associated injuries.

Plain Radiographs
Tilting of the spine away from the side of injury, opening of the intervertebral spaces, avulsion fractures of the vertebral tubercles, and fracture/dislocations of the first rib suggest severe injuries. Some important findings from radiographs of the chest include: a fluid collection at the apex; elevation of the ipsilateral hemi-diaphragm; rib fractures which may be associated with haemo- or haemopneumothorax, and lateral displacement of the shoulder girdle.

Imaging
Early myelography is unpleasant and potentially hazardous in those who have suffered a head injury. *Marshall and de Silva (1986)* [49] showed that computerised tomographic (CT) scanning with contrast enhancement was a good deal more accurate than standard myelography, especially for C5 and C6, findings confirmed by *Nagano et a.l (1989a)* [52], *Carvalho et al. (1997)* [21] and *Oberle et al. (1998)* [57]. The early investigation may detect interruption of a ventral or dorsal root and a residual stump *Tavakazolledah et al. (2001)* [78]. Magnetic resonance imaging (MRI) reveals bleeding within the spinal canal and displacement of the spinal cord. The characteristic features of intradural injury have been summarised by *Hems et al. (1999)* [35]. Digital subtraction, or MR angiography are required when there is suspected arterial injury.

Table 2 Tinel's sign in closed traction lesions of the brachial plexus in 100 adult patients examined and operated 2004–2005

	Tinel sign present (142 nerves). Findings at operation			Tinel sign absent (358 nerves). Findings at operation		
Spinal nerves	Intact	Rupture	Avulsion	Intact	Rupture	Avulsion
C5	1	58	4	0	10	27
C6	0	41	5	10	6	38
C7	0	24	0	40	2	34
C8	0	4	0	45	0	51
T1	0	4	1	52	1	42
Total	**1**	**131**	**10**	**147**	**19**	**192**

Ultrasonography will prove particularly valuable if done early before tissue planes are obliterated by fibrosis.

The Operation

The arguments in favour of urgent operation in cases where rupture or avulsion is suspected include:

1. The biological imperative. The cell bodies of the neurones must be reconnected with the distal Schwann cell columns as soon as possible.
2. It is easier to detect rupture and to resect nerves to a recognisable architecture. This is helped by detecting conduction centrally and distally. Only rarely is it necessary to resect more than 5 mm. of the proximal or distal stump and even less than this when preparing the tips of the ventral roots. Few things are more disheartening than to come to the field where the normal tissue planes are replaced by scar tissue with the consistency of concrete. Accurate diagnosis may be impossible in such cases.
3. The retracted ruptured nerves can be drawn back, so reducing the gap.
4. Repair of avulsed roots, or re-implantation is generally possible only in the early days after injury.
5. It is important always to examine the distal stumps, after pulling them back from their displaced position. Demonstration of the dorsal root ganglion is absolute proof of avulsion but the level of rupture of the ventral root may open the opportunity for direct repair. It is not uncommon to find C6 avulsed whilst the 5th cervical nerve has been sheared from its junction with the trunk.
6. Intra-operative studies of motor and sensory conduction evaluate the central integrity of the proximal stump, enable mapping of the bundles within the distal stump and detect even more distal rupture or ischaemic conduction block. Haematoma causes proximal conduction block. Central conduction studies may not detect intradural injury confined to the ventral roots. It is important to remember during operations performed within 2 or 3 days of injury that avulsion of ventral roots may not be recognised because the spinal nerves continue to conduct. The method is not quantitative (Fig. 8).

Injuries of the spinal nerves are classified in Table 3.

Strategies of Repair

The most important distinction lies between those cases where some spinal nerves are intact or recovering from those where all roots are damaged (Table 4).

Lesion at C5, C6 (C7), intact (C7), C8, T1

This common pattern is most favourable because there is useful hand function and there is usually at least one rupture of the upper nerves. Arterial injury is rare. Urgent repair can produce outstanding results. The situation is more difficult when the upper nerves have been avulsed.

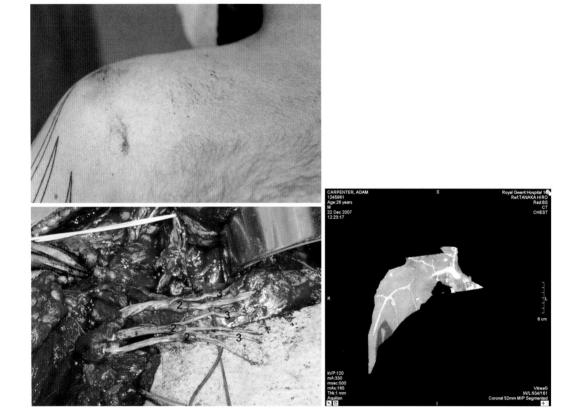

Fig. 8 Ischaemia and conduction. Traction lesion of the brachial plexus was accompanied by rupture of the subclavian artery. There was a weak pulse. At operation, 54 h after injury, stimulation of the avulsed ventral roots of C7, C8 and T1 evoked strong contraction in the relevant muscles distally. This showed that there was neither critical ischaemia within the limb nor that there was a second, more distal, lesion. Strong SSEP's were recorded from the stumps of C5 and C6 (1). The dorsal root ganglia of C7, C8 and T1 (2) and their ventral roots (3) are shown. An extensive repair was done(Case investigated and referred by Mr Tanaka and Mr Shandall, Royal Gwent Hospital)

Intradural C5 and C6. Conventional transfers to the suprascapular and circumflex nerves and to the nerve to biceps are reliable [46] although re-innervation of the avulsed ventral roots using the spinal accessory nerve and one or two bundles within the intact C7 is also effective.

Intradural C5, C and C7 is much more serious because of the deep paralysis of the thoraco-scapular and thoraco-humeral muscles. The loss of cutaneous sensation is extensive and severe pain is usual. C8 usually innervates the radial head of triceps and in about 30 % of cases the extensor muscles of the digits. The ventral root of C5 may be transferred to the spinal accessory nerve, that of C7 onto bundle in C8. Nerve transfer to the nerve to biceps is successful in about 60 % of patients. Intercostal nerves and the medial cutaneous nerve of forearm may be transferred to the lateral root of the median nerve. Extension of the digits and of the wrist is reliably restored by subsequent flexor to extensor transfer (Fig. 9).

Preganglionic C5, C6, C7, C8, intact T1. These patients have extremely poor function. The hand is insensate. Repair of avulsed ventral roots has improved the outlook and significant improvement has been achieved in selected patients by re-implanting the avulsed spinal nerves into the spinal cord.

Table 3 Characteristics of lesions of the spinal nerve

Type of lesion	Tinel's sign	Conduction between spinal nerve and spinal cord	Peripheral conduction	Conduction across lesion	CT Myelography MRI	Appearance
1. Intact	Absent	Intact	Intact	Not applicable – no lesion	Normal	Normal
2. Recovering stretch	Absent or weak	Intact	Intact or diminished	Intact or diminished	Normal	Bundles intact. Epineurium stretched or even torn
3. Rupture	Strong	Intact	Absent	Absent	Normal	Clear separation of stumps (early cases). Good architecture of proximal stump
4. Rupture with intradural component	Present, but weaker than in type 3	Diminished	Absent	Absent	Usually normal	Clear separation of stumps. The proximal stump abnormal, even close to foramen
5. Intradural with no displacement of DRG	Absent	Absent	Sensory conduction preserved	N/A	Separation of roots may be seen	Normal(early). Atrophy, sometimes gray-yellow colour (late)
6. Rupture or avulsion of dorsal or ventral root	Absent	Present if dorsal root intact	Sensory conduction preserved	N/A	Separation of root(s) may be seen	Normal or mild atrophy
7. Intradural with displacement of DRG	Absent	Absent	Sensory conduction preserved	N/A	Clear abnormality with CSF Leak	DRG Visible, with the ventral and dorsal roots

Note The timing of peripheral conduction studies is critical. Motor conduction can be detected for up to 4 days after rupture or intradural injury. Sensory Conduction persists for up to 7-10 days after rupture and indefinitely after intradural injury

Table 4 Patterns of injury in 301 consecutive operated supraclavicular lesions (By number of patients 1989–1993)

Complete lesions: pre-and postganglionic injury.	**148 cases**
Ruptures upper nerves C5 (C6,C7) Intradural lower nerves (C6,C7, C8) T1	83
Ruptures middle nerves (C6) C7 (C8) Intradural above and below	5
Ruptures lower nerves C8, T1 Intradural upper nerves C5, C6, C7	1
Total intradural C5-T1	52
Incomplete lesions: some roots intact.	**153 cases**
Damage C5, C6 (C7) Recovering or intact (C7) C8, T1	117
Damage C6, C7, C8 Recovering or intact C5, T1	23
Damage C7, C8, T1 Recovering or intact C5, C6	13

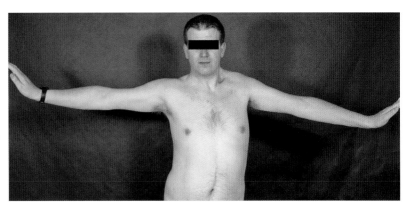

Fig. 9 A 31 year old man: left-sided lesion: rupture C5, preganglionic C6, C7. Operation on the day of injury: accessory to suprascapular, the VR (Ventral root) of C6 and C7 were transferred to the anterior face of proximal C5, the rupture of that nerve was grafted. Function at 28 months

Intact C5 and C6 (C7), C8, T1. These patients are much better off than those with lesions of the upper nerves because function at the thoraco-scapular, glenohumeral, and elbow joints is good, pronosupination and flexion and extension of the wrist is usually preserved and there is good sensation in the thumb, the index and the middle fingers. There are opportunities for palliation by musculo-tendinous transfer. Repair of the lower roots of the plexus is often worthwhile if performed within days of injury.

The Complete Lesion

These are devastating injuries and it is extremely important that the patient is approached in an open and positive manner. It is as bad to give the patient a hopeless prognosis as it is to offer one which is over-optimistic. Every reasonable effort should be made to find proximal stumps of ruptured spinal nerves and to repair these as soon as the patient's condition allows. Return of function is usually only modest and confined to the upper segments of the limb but some patients achieve much more. *Dickson and Biant (2009)* [25] described extensive recovery of function, extending to the hand, in two young adults with complete lesions. The repairs were performed 6 days after injury. In both patients continuing improvement in power, coordination, and cutaneous sensation was detectable for up to 10 years and the rate of recovery was faster in the large myelinated efferent fibres than it was in the A-delta and C fibres (Fig. 10).

(C4), C5-T1 Avulsion

Conventional nerve transfer offers only paltry mitigation in these, the worst cases, and the only realistic prospect for useful function by means of nerve repair lies in reconnection between the avulsed spinal nerves and the spinal cord.

Results

Results are considered by neurological recovery, by relief of pain and by return to work or study.

Neurological Recovery

A good result for repair of a spinal nerve or an element of that nerve means the return of movement against resistance in one axis of a joint of two-thirds or more of normal range. Earlier data has been set out in *Surgical Disorders of the Peripheral Nerves (1998, 2011)* [7, 9]. Recovery of function in 360 patients operated between 1990 and 1996 is summarised in Table 5, and that in 228 patients operated between 2000 and 2004 in Table 6.

Grafts remain the mainstay of repair, nerve transfers supplement them. *Addas and Midha (2009)* [1] point out, in an excellent review of nerve transfers, that surgeons must not turn away from the difficulties of exploring the lesion itself. Some conclusions may be drawn:

1. The outcome is better when repairs are performed within 7 days of injury, especially so in the presence of arterial injury.

Fig. 10 Left sided lesion. Rupture C5, C7, C8 T1, avulsion C6. Function at 96 months after repair in a nurse aged 28 at the time of injury. Wrist extension was regained by transfer of FCU to ECRB

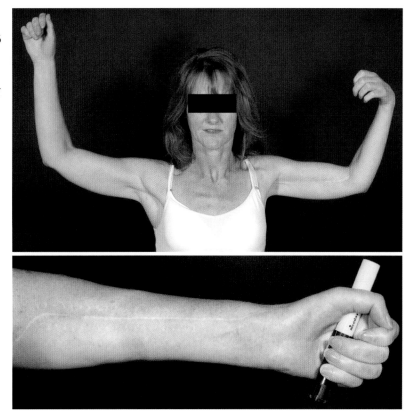

2. Preganglionic lesions exert a depressing effect upon recovery. Good results were recorded in 63 % of repairs in patients without any preganglionic injury compared with 40 % of all repairs in patients with one or more intradural lesion.

3. The decline in outcome with increasing delay is most marked for grafts. Of those performed within 7 days of injury, 52.5 % achieved a good result but the success rate for all grafts was 35.5 %. The success rate for conventional transfers was 42.3 % and 65 % in the ventral root (VR) repairs. However, the average number of function regained through a successful graft was 3.2 compared with 1.9 for the VR repairs and 1.6 for conventional transfers. The admittedly few cases of recovery of useful cutaneous sensation and motor function in the hand followed urgent grafts of ruptured spinal nerves.

4. Lateral rotation at the shoulder and extension of the elbow and wrist was regained in between 30 % and 40 % of grafts compared to 60–70 % of nerve transfers or VR repair.

Conventional Nerve Transfers

The phrenic nerve should not be used. Transfer from the contra lateral brachial plexus is reserved for rare cases of complete bilateral lesion where one limb is so badly damaged that no useful recovery can be anticipated. For these nerve transfers may be used to ease pain in the worst limb. Some conclusions drawn from the study of 958 nerve transfers follow:

1. Transfer of deep divisions of intercostal nerves to the nerve to serratus anterior is the most successful of all nerve repairs with 76 from 92 patients (83 %) regaining powerful protraction of the scapula.

2. Accessory nerve to suprascapular nerve transfer is useful in upper lesions and when

Table 5 Results of repairs, in 360 patients, performed between 1990 and 1996 (By interval and by severity of lesion)

Timing of repair

Functions attributed to the repair	Within 14 days		To 3 months		To 6 months		More than 6 months		Total	
	No	%	No	%	No	%	No	%	No	%
0	8	11.8	10	15.6	8	28.6	20	58.8	46	23.7
1	10	14.7	22	34.3	8	28.8	8	23.5	48	25
2	14	20.6	20	31.2	8	28.8	6	17.6	48	25
3	20	29.4	4	6.2	2	7.2	0	0	26	13.5
4 or more	16	23.5	8	12.5	2	7.2	0	0	26	13.5
Total	68		64		28		34		194	

Complete lesion

	Within 14 days		To 3 months		To 6 months		More than 6 months		Total	
0	15	16.9	18	41.9	8	36.4	8	66.7	49	29.5
1	15	16.9	10	23.2	4	18.2	2	16.6	31	18.6
2	19	21.3	12	27.8	8	36.4	2	16.6	41	24.6
3	23	25.8	2	4.6	2	9.1	0	0	27	16.2
4	6	6.7	1	2.3	0	0	0	0	7	4.2
5	4	4.9	0	0	0	0	0	0	4	2.4
6 or more	7	7.8	0	0	0	0	0	0	7	4.2
Total	89		43		22		12		166	

Overall totals (%)

	Within 14 days		To 3 months		To 6 months		More than 6 months		Total	
0	23	14.6	28	26.2	16	32	28	60.9	95	25.1
1	25	15.9	32	29.9	12	24	10	22	79	20.5
2	33	24.1	32	29.9	16	32	8	17.6	89	22
3 or more	76	48.6	15	13.6	6	12	0	0	97	25.2
	157		107		50		46			

1. This excludes patients with planned, late operations designed to relieve pain.
2. Incomplete lesions: at least one nerve intact or recovering
3. Regeneration did not restore useful function in 91 patients and in 38 of these there was no detectable regeneration

Table 6 Results of repairs in 585 elements in 228 patients operated between 2000 and 2004 – by interval between injury and operation

Interval in days	Number of patients	Results of repairs		Results (excluding ventral root repairs)		Average number of elements repaired in each patient	Average number of functions regained in each patient
		Good/ Total	%	Good/ Total	%		
0–7	52	114/175	65.1	86/40	61	3.4	5.4
8–14	25	41/72	57	21/45	46.7	2.9	3.8
15–28	31	48/87	50.1	34/73	46.6	2.8	3.3
29–56	32	25/74	33.8	21/68	30.1	2.3	1.6
57–84	31	31/67	46.2	30/65	46.2	2.2	1.8
85–112	16	13/35	37.1	12/33	36.4	2.2	1.9
113–182	22	8/34	23.5	7/33	21.2c	1.5	1.1
More than 182	19	12/41	29.3	11/39	28.2	2.2	1
	228	288/585	49.2	222/496	44.8		

1. The average numbers of repairs for each patient was 2.6
2. The average number of functions regained in each patient was 2.9; the total of functions regained was 658

combined with grafts often restores excellent abduction and lateral rotation [60]. From 280 transfers in upper plexus lesions 60 patients (21.5 %) regained abduction of 120° or more and lateral rotation of 40° or more. In 75 (26.8 %) abduction was 60° or better and lateral rotation at least 30°. In 83 patients (29.6 %) either useful abduction or lateral rotation was regained. It is important to exclude rupture of the rotator cuff or damage to the suprascapular nerve.The operation will fail if serratus anterior remains paralysed.

3. Ulnar nerve to nerve to biceps transfer [58] has been used in 103 patients, of whom 45 (43.6 %) regained elbow flexion to MRC Grade 4 and a further 43 (41.7 %) achieved elbow flexion of MRC Grade 3 or 3+. The principle has been extended to re-innervate nerves to the extensor muscles of the wrist, using bundles from the median or the ulnar nerve and also to the repair of the suprascapular nerve or an avulsed ventral root by transfer to a bundle within an adjacent spinal nerve.

4. Just over one half (52 %) of patient with lesions of C5, C6 and C7 regained useful elbow flexion by intercostal transfer. Only one third (34 %) with complete lesions did so, but see *Nagano et al (1989)* [53].

Ventral Root Repair

The roots of the spinal nerves contain far less connective tissue than the peripheral nerves and there is a dense concentration of motor axons in the VR. The specificity of Schwann cells related to the large efferent axons may actively encourages the re-entry of new motor axons [34, 51]. Most repairs were performed within a few days of injury; only then can the dorsal root ganglion be displayed with ease and the ventral root separated from the spinal nerve. The VR may be re-innervated by the spinal accessory nerve, by an adjacent ruptured spinal nerve or by a bundle within an adjacent intact spinal nerve. Interposed grafts are rarely necessary. Since the first repair of a VR in 1992 [7] there have been 111 more in the adult. Results were good in 65 %. Repair of the VR of C7 restored powerful adduction and

medial rotation, with about 20° of forward flexion at shoulder, in 35 of 49 roots. Elbow extension was regained in 29 patients and useful extension of the wrist in 10.

Re-Implantation of Avulsed Spinal Nerves into the Spinal Cord

The first case was operated by George Bonney in 1979 [7]and the method has been greatly developed by Thomas Carlstedt who has described extensive experimental work, indications, contra-indications and results in his important monograph [19].

The method may be considered in cases of complete lesion with four or five avulsions. Operation must not be undertaken in patients with rupture of the subclavian or vertebral arteries, nor in any patient showing any sign of affliction of the spinal cord. Transforaminal endoscopic examination of the cord is helpful: methods of measuring the perfusion of the cervical spinal cord need to be developed. Regeneration into proximal muscle, notably pectoralis major, has been confirmed in all patients. Adduction, medial rotation and forward flexion at the shoulder and flexion and extension at the elbow have been regained in 21 patients. Some have done rather better than this. *Carlstedt et al (2009)* [20] report the case of a 9 year-old boy who sustained complete avulsion of his right brachial plexus and he experienced severe, spontaneous, constant and shooting pain. All five spinal nerves were re-connected by interposed grafts at operation which was performed 4 weeks later. Recovery of muscles at the shoulder girdle was evident by 10 months and at the elbow by 12–15 months by which time his pain had completely resolved. Muscle recovery in the forearm, wrist and hand was apparent by 2 years. He recovered useful function throughout the damaged upper limb and he could grip and carry objects (Fig. 11).

Relief of Pain by Repair

The pain of intradural injury is caused by damage, and subsequent gliosis, in the transitional zone at substantial gelatinosa and by disinhibition and spontaneous firing of cell bodies within the deeper laminae of the dorsal horn of the spinal column [17, 59, 81]. These events occur rapidly [45, 82].

Berman, Taggart and colleagues (1995) [4] studied 116 patients with proven root avulsions, in all of whom nerve transfer or graft had been performed. All patients experienced pain which was severe in 88 % of patients at some time during their course. Pain began within 24 h of the injury in 62 %: pain was at its most intense at, on average, 6 months from injury. Paroxysmal pain was never experienced in the absence of

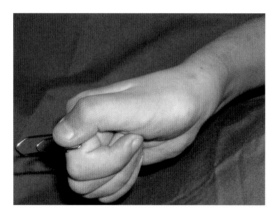

Fig. 11 A 9 year-old boy. Right-sided lesion. Avulsion C5,C,C7,C8,T1. Re-implantation of all five spinal nerves. The hand at 6 years showing useful pinch grip function with some recovery into the small muscles (Courtesy of Thomas Carlstedt)

constant pain. The intensity of pain was closely related to the extent of de-afferentation of the spinal cord [37]. A measurable decrease in pain was noted at a mean time of about 6 months after operation. In 34 % of cases pain remained moderate or severe at 3 years or more. *Berman et al (1998)* [6] went on to show that pain relief coincided with, or preceded by a few days, the return of muscle activity. The correlation between pain relief and the return of function was highly significant; there was no such relation in those patients with poor or no recovery. However, Berman and his colleagues (1996) [5] also found striking pain relief following late intercostal transfer. The mechanism underlying this remains obscure. *Kato and his colleagues (2006)* [41] studied 148 patients. The onset, patterns and important mitigating factors were similar to those recognised in the earlier series. Pain relief was most striking after early operations (Table 7).

The evidence showing that repair offers a good chance of easing pain is strong and the earlier the operation is done the higher the chance of pain relief. These facts provide the strongest indication for operation and repair by one means or another even in the most severe case. Sadly, there are still some patients whose pain remains intractable and for these interventions upon the central nervous system must be considered [9].

Table 7 Improvement in pain against delay before repair. 148 patients studied by Kato et al. (2006) [41]

Interval between injury and repair	Number	Worst pain by visual analogue scale		Final pain by visual analogue scale		Mean of improvement in PNI scale (ranging from 0 to 4 maximum)
		Mean	Median	Mean	Median	
Less than 1 month Group 1	61	8.2 (SD0.3)	9.0 (3–10)	2.6 (SD0.3)	2.0 (0–10)	2.2 (SD 0.1)
From 1 to 3 months Group 2	29	9.1 (SD 0.2)	9.0 (3–10)	3.7 (SD0.4)	3.0 (0–10)	1.8 (SD 0.2)
From 3 to 6 months Group 3	32	8.5 (SD 0.3)	9.0 (3–10)	4.0 (SD0.5)	4.0 (0–10)	1.3 (SD 0.2)
After 6 months Group 4	26	9.0 (SD 0.3)	9.0 (3–10)	5.3 (SD 0.6)	6.0 (0–10)	1.1 (SD 0.2)

The changes were statistically significant taking $p = 0.05$: group 1 and group 3 $p < 0.01$; group 1 and group 4 $p < 0.01$; groups 2 and group 3 $p < 0.05$
Drawn from Kato et al. 2006 [41]

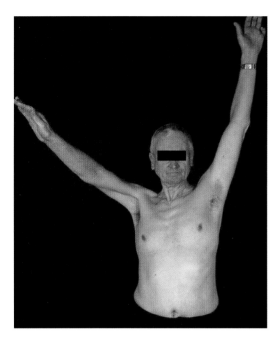

Fig. 12 Right-sided lesion in a 70 year old man. Rupture of C5, C6. Operation at 10 days: accessory to suprascapular, graft of C5 and C6. Function at 15 months

Age

Now is as good a time as any to dispel the notion that nerve injuries will not recover after a certain age. Indeed, the effects of age suggests that there may be increasing vulnerability to pain, because of the diminishing threshold to noxious stimuli [23]. Repairs were performed in 38 patients aged 45 years or more in the years 1988–2004. Useful recovery was observed in 25 (Fig. 12).

The falsity of that assumption that nerve injuries in children do better than in the adult is nowhere better seen than in the outcome of the complete closed traction lesion. The immature neurones are even more vulnerable to proximal axonotomy. The disturbance of growth and deformity provoked by muscular imbalance is particularly severe in the younger child. Recovery of cutaneous sensation is certainly better than in the adult but this may not be true for motor recovery. No child aged less than 15 years complained of the classical pain of avulsion injury, but several developed this as they approached later adolescence.

Table 8 Return to work, retraining, further study, with interval before re-entry. Minimum follow-up of 36 months

Years of study. 1986–1993 – 324 patients		Years of study. 2000-2004 – 238 patients
Same occupation (often with modification)	54	86
Different occupation	195	63
Formal retraining or return to study	81	65
Did not return to work	75	24

Return to Work

The rate of return to work after serious injury to the brachial plexus is encouragingly high but the finding that four out of five patients return to a different job [7] indicates the importance of retraining and information about employment (Table 8). The recent findings from patients operated between 2000 and 2004 appear similarly encouraging but there has been a serious decrease in the rate of return to work since. We attribute this to the collapse of rehabilitation services within the National Health Service with the outstanding exception of certain specialist units. The abolition of the post of Hospital Employment Advisor was a grievous error (Fig. 13).

The Birth Lesion of the Brachial Plexus (BLBP)

The traction and compression forces which are responsible for the birth lesion of the brachial plexus may be less considerable than those causing the most severe injuries in the adult but they are active upon the nerves for several hours during a prolonged and difficult delivery. The response of the neonatal nervous system to injury is profoundly modified by a number of qualities:

1. The density of conducting tissue is higher; so is nerve blood flow which increases the susceptibility to anoxic conduction block.

2. The cell bodies of the neurones in the spinal cord and in the dorsal root ganglion are dependent on neurotrophins for their development,

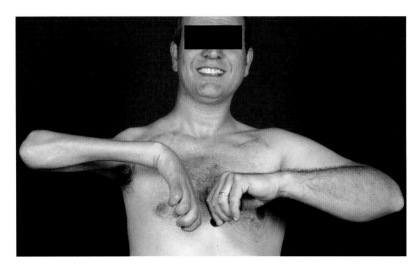

Fig. 13 "Distraction or destruction!" The patient's own motto. Right-sided lesion in a 21 year-old man. Preganglionic injury C5 to T1 with rupture of subclavian artery. Operation at 4 days. There was one branch from C4 passing to the suprascapular nerve and another passing to the nerve to serratus anterior. The subclavian artery was repaired. No nerve repair was performed. He returned to work at 3 months rising to a senior position working with the disabled. Whilst he found the flail arm splint useful he discarded it because it made him feel disabled. Free functioning muscle transfer (latissimus dorsi)- Professor Roy Sanders- was innervated by the accessory nerve

maturation and survival and are more likely to die after proximal axonotomy or avulsion.

3. Interruption of afferent impulses through the somatosensory pathways delays the development of patterns of function and the integration of the injured limb. Change in limb dominance away from the injured side is striking: only 17 % of children with right sided BLPP showed right hand preference [84].

4. Avulsion pain appears to be absent in infants and in young children. It is possible that the absence of a nociceptor associated voltage gated sodium ion channel is contributory [85].

Spontaneous regeneration through lesions in continuity or neuromas is chaotic and disorderly and this contributes to co-contraction between the muscles of the shoulder girdle, which is at times so severe that the gleno-humeral joint acts as an ankylosis. Recovery of the afferent pathways is defective. *Fullerton et al (2001)* [28] noted a selective failure of regeneration of the largest diameter proprioceptive fibres. This contributes to the "clumsiness" of the injured limb which is noticeable even when neurological recovery has been good. However recovery of cutaneous sensibility is far better than in the adult and it is superior to somatic and sympathetic motor recovery [3].

Epidemiology

Incidence

The British Isles census conducted by *Evans-Jones and his colleagues (2003)* [26] found 323 confirmed cases, an incidence of 0.42 per 1,000 live births or 1 in 2300. Fifty-three per cent of the infants were male and there was a slight preponderance of right-sided injury. The injury was partial in 91 % of infants. There were only 10 cases caused by breech delivery. The incidence in the Netherlands may be a little higher [14].

Risk Factors

The direct physical cause of the lesion is the forced separation of the forequarter from the axial skeleton caused by obstruction at the narrowest part of the birth canal. In breech deliveries the upper spinal nerves and the phrenic nerve are particularly at risk and lesions may be bilateral. In difficult cephalic deliveries nerves are stretched, ruptured or avulsed as the angle between the

Table 9 Significant relative risks– 1,060 cases

Dystocia	180.3
Asphyxia	10.8
Gestational diabetes	10
No Caesarean	9
Birth weight > 3.4 kg	8.5
Forceps – assisted delivery	6.9
No episiotomy	5.2
Breech	3.6
Not induced	2.8
Ventouse – assisted delivery	2.6
Age of mother > 30	2
Hypertension	1.4

By kind permission of Adel Tavakkolizadeh, Thesis 2007 [79]

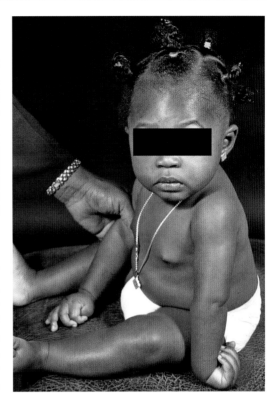

Fig. 14 Lesion of C5, C6 and C7 – Narakas group II

delivered head and the obstructed shoulder widens. In our earlier study [29] the mean birth weight of the babies was 4.5 Kg against the contemporary mean for the North West Thames region, of 3.88 Kg. There was a co-relation between more severe lesions and higher birth weight. Shoulder dystocia was recorded in over 60 % of deliveries. A trend was found towards the mother being heavier and shorter than the national average, and also to excessive maternal weight gain. There was no significant co-relation with social class. The later report, extending to more than 1,060 babies, comes from *Tavakkolizadah (2007)* [79] (Table 9). The older mother, with a high body mass index (BMI) giving birth to a large baby by instrumental delivery, presents the greatest risk. The continuing debate about elective Caesarean section is illuminated by a frequency of LSCS at 2 % in the BLBP group, against the national rate of 18 %.

Diagnosis and Classification

The characteristic posture of the upper limb in the partial injury is caused by injury to C5, C6 and C7 (Fig. 14). The elbow is extended, the forearm pronated and the wrist flexed. In the complete lesion the arm lies flaccid. A Bernard-Horner syndrome suggests serious injury. Discrepancy in the size of the digits is evident from about 6 weeks of age. A lesion of the spinal cord usually passes unnoticed until the child starts to walk, when the parents observe unsteadiness of gait and disparity in the size of the foot.

The differential diagnosis includes: fractures of the clavicle or humerus; neonatal sepsis of the gleno-humeral joint; cerebral palsy; arthrogryposis; ischaemic cord injury and even trigger thumb. Any of these may co-exist with BLBP. Posterior dislocation of the shoulder at, or soon after birth, is frequent.

The Narakas Classification *(1987)* [54] is not applicable to the breech delivery. It is useful at about 4 weeks after birth.

Group 1 (C5,6) There is paralysis of supraspinatus, infraspinatus, deltoid and biceps muscles. The upper limb lies in medial rotation with the elbow extended.

Group 2 (C5,5,7): There is also weakness or paralysis of triceps and of the extensors of the wrists. The hand is clenched into a fist with flexion at the wrist.

Group 3 (C5-T1): The paralysis is virtually complete. There may be some weak flexion of the fingers at, or shortly after, birth.

Table 10 Outcome of 74 children entered into the 12 month National Census (Mean follow-up 32 months)

Narakas group	Full recovery	Persisting defect. No operation	Operation for posterior dislocation of shoulder	Operation on brachial plexus
Group 1 (n =28)	21	4	3	0
Group II (n = 38)	14	5	16	5
Group 111 (n = 5)	4	0	1	1
Group IV (n = 3)	0	0	0	3
Total	39	9	20	9

Drawn from Bisinella and Birch 2003 [10]

Group 4 (C5-T1): The paralysis is complete. The limb is flaccid; there is a Bernard-Horner syndrome.

Neurological recovery is usual in Group 1, it is generally poor in Group 4. We have seen only one example of a lesion confined to C8 and T1.

Natural History

Recovery at 6 months after birth was studied in 276 of the infants entered into the British Isles census. It was "complete" in 143 babies (52 %). Seventy four (26.8 %) of the census cases were followed for a minimum of 2 years in our Unit. Of these recovery was incomplete in just under one half of the children and more than one quarter of them required operation for posterior subluxation or dislocation of the shoulder during the period of study [10] (Table 10). *Pondaag and his colleagues (2004)* [63] studied 1020 articles and concluded that persisting residual defects could be identified in between 20 % and 30 % of children. *Strombeck et al (2007a, b)* [76, 77] studied 70 cases from birth to adolescence or early adult life. One quarter had measurable difficulties in normal daily activities. Strombeck and her colleagues suggest that there is a progressive loss of motor neurones which may explain the deterioration in shoulder function which is so common in late adolescence.

For a full account of the systems used in prospective collection of data the reader is referred to *Birch 2011* [9]. The modified Mallet [48] system is valuable (Fig. 15). The five movements are scored on a scale in range from 1 to 3. A different coloured pencil is used at each attendance and the record is

signed and dated with that colour. This record can be completed in no more than 1 min in most children aged 18 months or above. The Mallet score has proved to be a useful indicator of overall function within the upper limb. *Yang (2005)* [84] found that it strongly correlated with both gross and fine movements. The inferior and posterior scapulo- humeral angles (SHA) detects effects of weakness, of contracture and of bone deformity at the gleno-humeral joint (Fig. 16). Posterior dislocation of the head of the humerus must be suspected when a child presents with a pronated forearm who is unable to supinate even though biceps is strong.

Shoulder and Hand Function in 1,320 Children Studied Prospectively Between 1992 and 2007

1. 252 children were seen only once because their function was so good. The results for the Mallet score against the Narakas grade in the remaining 1,128 children is set out in Table 11. Most children showed a perceptible and, at times significant defect. Just over one-third of all of the children were given the maximum Mallet score of 15 but this does not necessarily signify a normal shoulder.

2. Of the 291 children presenting with complete lesions (Narakas 3 and 4), 89 (30.6 %) went on to exploration and repair of the brachial plexus and 193 (66.3 %) required operations for posterior dislocation of the shoulder whilst 197 (67.7 %) required operations to improve function of the forearm, wrist, and digits.

Fig. 15 The Mallet chart

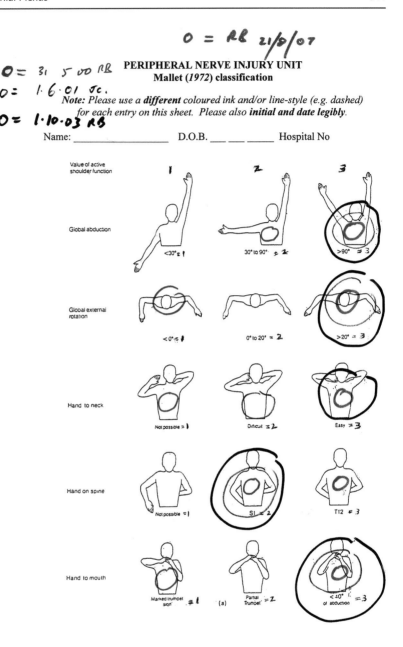

Spontaneous Recovery of Hand Function in the Complete Lesion

Good spontaneous recovery can occur in some infants presenting with a Narakas Type 4 lesion. Of 200 such infants seen in the years 1984–2007 the plexus was repaired in 92 (46 %). Operations were not performed in 108, either because there was recovery or because the children presented too late. Hand function was graded good in 63 of these 108 children and simple musculo-tendinous transfers improved function to a useful level in 28 more. The first signs of recovery included improvement in texture and colour and the temperature of the skin suggesting early recovery of vasomotor tone, changes which usually preceded active movement by some weeks. Neurophysiological investigations suggesting post ganglionic injury for C8 and T1 were consistent favourable findings.

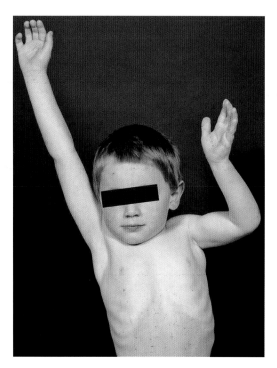

Fig. 16 Both the passive and active inferior scapulo humeral angles were reduced by cocontraction and contracture

Table 11 The initial and final Mallet score in 1,128 children seen in the years between 1992 and 2007. The results are given by median and (mean). The median age at the first record was 13 months. The median and (mean) length of follow-up is given in months

Narakas Group	Number of children	Initial score	Final score	Duration of study
I	249	8 (8.1)	13 (12.8)	43.5 (53.3)
II	518	8.5 (8.6)	13 (12.5)	44 (62.3)
III	217	7 (8)	13 (12.2)	41.5 (51.2)
IV	144	7 (7.3)	11 (10.9)	55.5 (63.3)

Treatment

The first step is to provide the parents with information about the nature and the extent of lesion and of the likely outcome. Parents appreciate a simple diagram showing the brachial plexus and outlining the nature and level of the lesion, which is written out for them by the doctor. This is far preferable to an anonymous "hand out" of printed paper. The parents are advised of the risks of contracture, above all at the shoulder. It is extremely important that all those involved in the care of the child avoid giving conflicting information. After operation, it is for the surgeon to explain what was found, what was done, why it was done and what may follow.

Parents are involved in the treatment of the child from the outset. Regular and gentle exercises may prevent fixed deformity. If gentle stretching movements cause pain then there must be either fracture or posterior dislocation of the shoulder. The role of the therapist and attending doctor is to teach and then to monitor progress. We have seen too many examples of fixed deformity resulting from parents sitting passively at home awaiting the occasional visit by the community physiotherapist. Exercises must be performed, gently, for 2 or 3 minutes before every feed. Both upper limbs are worked simultaneously. For medial and lateral rotation the arms are held against the side, with the elbow flexed to 90°. The forearms are then brought onto the child's body and then moved into full lateral rotation. Then, the upper limbs are brought gently into full elevation. This manoeuvre is repeated with the arms at 90° of abduction. The inferior SHA is maintained by holding the scapula against the chest whilst abducting the arm; the posterior SHA by holding the scapula against the ribs whilst flexing and medially rotating the arm. Much fixed deformity can be prevented by this simple regime. It is essential to warn parents about the significance of pain for this may be the first indication that the gleno-humeral joint is no longer congruent.

Investigations
Neurophysiological Investigations (NPI)
Neurophysiological investigations have been used in nearly 1,000 children since 1980 and they are particularly valuable in partial lesions where recovery of shoulder abduction and elbow flexion is slow and also in apparently unfavourable Group 4 lesions [73].

The clinician using information provided by neurophysiological investigation (NPI) needs to understand the method; their interpretation must always consider clinical findings. Nerve action

Table 12 The clinical interpretation of electrodiagnostic findings

Grade	NAP	EMG	Lesion
A	Normal	No spontaneous activity. Reduced number of normal motor units. Increased firing rates	Conduction block
B favourable	Normal or > 50 % of uninjured side	Relatively good motor unit recruitment. Mixture of normal and polyphasic units suggesting some collateral re-innervation	Modest axonopathy consistent with useful recovery
B unfavourable	Absent or < 50 % of uninjured side	Normal units few or absent. Widespread polyphasia indicating collateral reinnervation. No spontaneous activity	Significant axonopathy. Recovery particularly poor for C5
C	Absent; if present indicative of preganglionic injury	Extensive spontaneous activity. Sometimes poor recruitment of nascent or small polyphasic units	Severe axonopathy consistent with no, or poor, recovery. Preserved NAP suggests preganglionic injury

Drawn from Smith 1998 [73], and from Bisinella Birch and Smith 2003 [11]

potentials are measured from the median and ulnar nerves by stimulating at the wrist and recording at the elbow. The deltoid (C5), biceps (C6), triceps or forearm extensors (C7) forearm flexors (C8) and 1st interosseous (T1) muscles are sampled by EMG. The lesion is graded for each spinal nerve, according to the degree of demyelination and axonopathy (Table 12). A prediction is made about the likely extent of recovery on the basis of the neurophysiological grade.

Some conclusions may be drawn:

1. NPI performed during the first 8 weeks of life may prove unduly pessimistic.
2. Significant axonopathy in C5 is a sure indicator that recovery at the shoulder will be poor.
3. Spontaneous recovery in Type B lesions of C6 and C7 usually matches that seen after successful repair.
4. Proof of post ganglionic injury at C8 and T1 offers a high chance of considerable spontaneous recovery.
5. Pre-operative NPI predictions correlated with the findings at operation. Rupture, avulsion, or a mixture of both was confirmed in 94 % of Type C lesions.
6. The predictions for recovery were matched against the outcome at a mean of 4.3 years in 73 children (199 nerves) in whom operations were not performed even though there

was no recovery of elbow flexion by the age of 3 months. The lesions were graded by NPI as grades A or B and the predictions were confirmed in 92 % of C6 lesions, and in 96 % of C7 lesions. The accuracy of predictions for C5 (78 %) was lower because of the inability to record compound nerve action potentials for this nerve and also by the complication of posterior dislocation. The NPI predictions were accurate in children with congruent shoulders, whereas recovery was good in only 34 % of those with Type A or B lesion but in whom relocation of the shoulder proved necessary.

7. Pre-operative NPI's are more reliable than intra-operative investigations in determining prognosis for the injured nerves; they also inform about the extent of recovery after repair [8].

Imaging

Magnetic resonance imaging has replaced myelography in the diagnosis of avulsion. Ultrasonography in the first few days of life may prove valuable.

The Indications for Operation

These revolve around the cause of the lesion, its extent, and the tempo of recovery.

There are a number of pitfalls lying in wait for those who rely on late return of elbow flexion:

1. Prolonged conduction block underlies prolonged paralysis in as many as 15 % of spinal nerve lesions.
2. The biceps muscle may be damaged or even torn apart during difficult delivery.
3. Shoulder movement is the key to function in the upper limb and poor recovery into the joint is more important than elbow flexion. Too many cases of posterior dislocation have remained undetected for months or even years!

The Toronto scoring system [24, 50] measures recovery at different segments of the upper limb. Combining the scores for return of elbow flexion with extension of the elbow, wrist, thumb and fingers provides an accurate prediction of recovery. *Nehme et al (2001)* [55] showed that the prognosis is reliably predictable by three factors: birth weight, involvement of C7 and the tempo of recovery in biceps.

Our indications have been narrowed by the study of the outcome of repairs in 250 children:

1. Operation should be done as soon as is possible in breech lesions with phrenic palsy and also in those complete lesions where neurophysiological and radiological evidence provides clear evidence of preganglionic injury.
2. Type B Unfavourable or Type C lesions in C5 predict poor recovery at the shoulder.
3. A Type B unfavourable lesion in C6 and in C7 is consistent with useful spontaneous recovery. We no longer believe that repair of a rupture of C6 and C7 materially improves the outlook. Exploration in these nerves is indicated in a Type C lesion.
4. Repair of C8 and T1 is justified only with proof of avulsion.

Principles of Operation

The reader is referred to *Birch 2011* [9] for a full account of methods of exposure and techniques of repair. After induction of anaesthesia, recording electrodes are attached to the skin of the scalp and neck and somatosensory evoked potentials are recorded from the median and ulnar nerves at both wrists. Scarring in the infant neck is often severe, blunt dissection is dangerous. The most serious immediate complication is venous bleeding and superficial veins must be ligated with great care because of the proximity of subclavian vein. Laceration of the phrenic nerve is an extremely serious complication, the nerve must be protected for it is often deviated laterally and involved in the neuroma of the upper and middle trunks. Once the lesion has been exposed further conduction studies are made of the pathway between the spinal nerve and the central nervous system and that traversing the lesion.

The Principles of Repair

1. Repair of ruptures by grafts is the mainstay of repair. Avulsed nerves should always be re-innervated, either from an adjacent postganglionic stump, or by selective graft or transfer to the ventral root and to the dorsal component of the spinal nerve after resection of the dorsal root ganglion.
2. The phrenic nerve should never be used.
3. Hypoglossal nerve transfer leads to unacceptable deficit and poor recovery [13].
4. Transfer of the spinal accessory nerve leads to measurable defect in control and growth of the scapula. Results are inferior to those seen in the adult [12, 64].
5. End-to-side transfer, in which one bundle is sectioned from within an intact nerve either in the neck or from an intact peripheral nerve, such as the ulnar or median is very useful for the suprascapular nerve or the nerves to biceps, triceps, or wrist extensors.
6. In cases of avulsion of C8 and T1 it is preferable always to re-innervate the lower trunk and the ulnar nerve rather than use it as a graft in contra-lateral C7 transfer (Fig. 17).

Results of Repair

The results of 247 spinal nerve repairs in 100 consecutive babies performed between 1990 and 1999 [8] were graded by strict criteria. One-fifth failed. Results were graded good in about

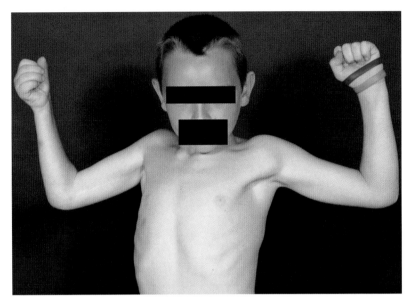

Fig. 17 A 5 year-old boy with a group 4 lesion. At the age of 7 weeks ruptures of C5,6, 7 and C8 were repaired using 16 grafts. The avulsed T1 was repaired by intraplexual transfer and the suprascapular nerve by transfer to accessory nerve. Shoulder 3+,14; elbow 4; hand 4

one-half. The effect of the associated dislocation of the shoulder was severe. The mean Mallet score in children without dislocation was 12.4; it was 10.8 in those children who came to operation for relocation of the shoulder. *Grossman and his colleagues (2003)* [32] are surely right when they recommend re-innervation of the shoulder with correction of any existing shoulder deformity at the same operation. As *Gilbert (2005)* [30] points out secondary operations including musculotendinous transfer can bring about considerable improvement.

Anand and Birch (2002) [3] studied 24 patients with a Narakas Group 4 lesion by quantitative sensory testing and measurement of cholinergic sympathetic function, Recovery of sensibility was far better than somatic and sympathetic motor function. There was accurate localisation in the dermatomes of avulsed spinal nerves which had been re-innervated by intercostal nerves transferred from remote spinal segments.

Deformity

There are four main causes of deformity:

1. Injuries Inflicted During Birth. Parents often describe severe bruising around the shoulder and arm after a difficult delivery. This causes fibrosis of the muscles of the shoulder, especially the subscapularis. The "pseudo-tumour" of the biceps muscle is caused by damage to the muscle at birth [47]. Posterior dislocation occurs at or very shortly after birth in about one case in 4 (Fig. 18).

2. Denervation of the Limb. There is atrophy of the denervated target organs; atrophy of the skin and of the finger nails. Bone growth is impaired in all but the mildest case. Shortening of the clavicle, caused by paralysis of the deltoid, the subclavius and the clavicular head of pectoralis major distorts the posture and development of the scapula.

3. Persisting muscular imbalance is a potent cause of deformity. Poor recovery in C5 leads to an imbalance between the weak lateral and the strong medial rotators at the shoulder and this contributes to many gleno-humeral dislocations. Bad lesions of C7 cause weak medial rotation at the shoulder and supination deformity of the forearm; if C8 is also involved then ulnar deviation at the wrist and thumb-in-palm deformity will ensue [2, 83]. Poor recovery in T1 causes intractable extension deformity at the metacarpophalangeal joints.

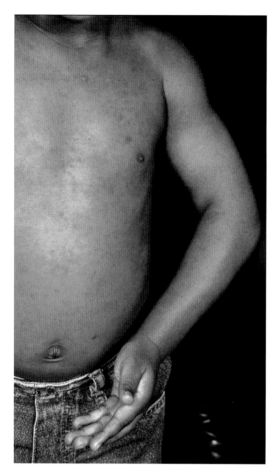

Fig. 18 Biceps "pseudotumour" in 9 year old boy. The shoulder is dislocated

4. Some Deformities are Provoked by Treatment. Overzealous manipulation of the incongruent shoulder damages the head of humerus and glenoid. Incorrect muscle transfers replace one imbalance with another, notably at the shoulder and wrist. Damage to the medial epicondyle during Steindler's elbow flexorplasty leads to dislocation of the elbow. Arthrodesis in the growing skeleton should never be performed until muscular imbalance has been corrected. Joints should be congruent before muscle transfers are performed.

With the exception of posterior dislocation of the shoulder which should be corrected as soon as is reasonable, it seems generally best to defer musculo-tendinous transfer until the age of 5 years by which time regenerating nerves will

have matured and the extent of weakness and cocontraction will be very plain. Careful, prolonged, functional splinting, particularly at the wrist and thumb, enables recovery in many children. These are used in the years before planned muscle transfer and often recovery is good enough for the operation to be cancelled. These splints must be changed regularly and adjusted for comfort and growth. They are reapplied after operation, and retained during the period of post-operative rehabilitation. Only rarely do children reject the splints; in these the matter is not pressed.

Posterior Subluxation (PS) and Posterior Dislocation (PD) of the Gleno-Humeral Joint

More than 500 children with posterior subluxation or dislocation have come to operation since 1986. The finding that dislocation complicates about one quarter of birth palsies suggests that there will be about 70 new cases every year in the British Isles [10] About one quarter of dislocations occur at birth or within the first 12 weeks of life. About one half of cases develop in the first 3 years, the remainder occur after neurological recovery [40].

The ease of clinical diagnosis, the affect of the dislocation upon the posture of the scapula and upon function of the upper limb, and also an explanation for the lack of active supination were all described by Fairbank in 1913 [27]. *Scaglietti (1938)* [69] reporting Putti's work [65] thought that epiphysiolysis was often seen and that it was the: "hallmark of a complicated obstetrical trauma of the shoulder joint". He also described retroversion of the head upon the humeral shaft, one of the most important elements which must be corrected before secure congruent reduction can be achieved.

The deformity is a very complex one. To the violence of delivery is added imbalance between the powerful and active medial rotators and the weak, or paralysed, lateral rotators. The changes in the glenoid occur early [36, 61, 62, 71, 72].

Retroversion of the glenoid improves after relocation of the head of the humerus [38]. The medially-rotated head of humerus is thrust against the posterior and inferior margin of the cartilage of the glenoid which begins to deform so that it becomes convex. The deformity evolves as a double facet or a double socket with the true glenoid lying above and anteriorly and articulating with the lesser tuberosity, and a postero-inferior facet which soon becomes larger. The head of the humerus lies in the postero-inferior facet. The head of the humerus may progress to

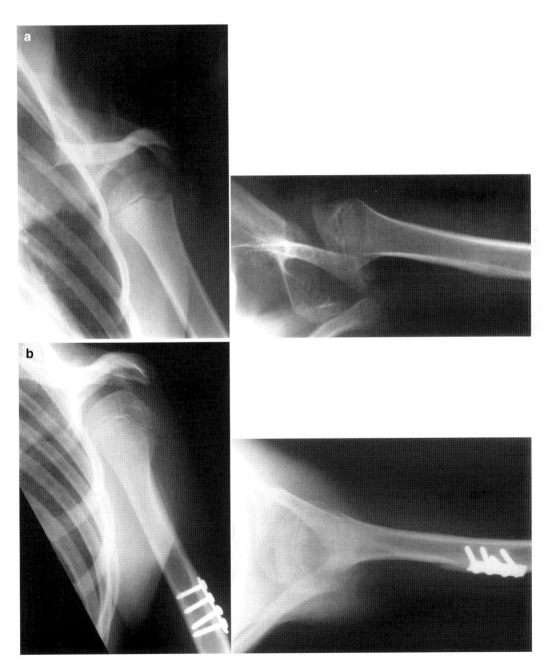

Fig. 19 (continued)

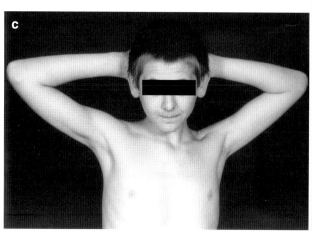
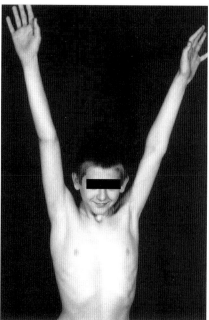

Fig. 19 (**a**) Antero-posterior and axial radiographs show overgrowth of the coracoid and downward displacement of the acromion and lateral clavicle. There is a double facet glenoid and a cone-shaped head. Shoulder scores were 1+, 12. Active forward flexion and abduction was 180°; active lateral rotation was minus 40° and the passive range was minus 20°. Active medial rotation was 90°, the passive range was 110°. Active pronation was 90° and active supination 40°. (**b**) Antero-posterior and axial radiographs taken 5 years after reduction showing remodelling of the head of the humerus and glenoid. The humeral head shows some signs of earlier vascular change. (**c**) Function at 5 years from reduction. The shoulder scores were 5+,15. Active abduction and forward flexion was 170°; active lateral rotation 30°; active medial rotation 90°; and pronation and supination 90°. The posterior scapulo-humeral angle was 90° (By kind permission editor of J. Bone Jt. Surg. 88B: 213–219)

dislocation. In some cases the head of the humerus was never in the glenoid. The displacement of the head of the humerus leads to mal-development of the lateral clavicle and the acromion and even to subluxation or dislocation of the acromioclavicular joint. The abnormal position of the scapula and the dorsal displacement of the coracoid is worsened by the shortening of the clavicle. In a few cases the subscapularis was severely fibrosed suggesting compartment syndrome at birth.

Diagnosis

It is difficult to overstate the requirement for scrupulous clinical examination which is reliable in the detection of early incongruency. Both shoulders must be examined simultaneously, initially with the examiner's eyes closed. Any asymmetry between the shoulders indicates an incongruent joint until proven otherwise. Diagnosis is confirmed by reduction in the passive range of medial rotation measured with both arms adducted to the side. In the older child the posture of the limb and the awkward elevation at the shoulder with fixed medial rotational deformity are characteristic.

Three features are important:

1. The coracoid is nearly always displaced posteriorly, inclined vertically and elongated.
2. The clavicle is shorter on the affected side, by as much as 25 % in the more severe cases.
3. The acromioclavicular joint may be dislocated.

Ultrasound scanning is useful [68]. Radiographs in the antero-posterior, and in the axial plane [75] confirm the diagnosis. MR scanning is reserved for cases of unusual complexity.

Table 13 Results in 183 shoulders treated by reduction by the anterior approach. Retroversion of head of humerus was corrected by medial rotation osteotomy of humeral shaft in 70 cases

Deformity	Number of cases (183)	Number of failures (20)	Pre-operative Mallet score (183 shoulders)	Final Mallet score (183 shoulders)
SS	37	0	10.4	13.4
SD	24	0	7.8	12.4
CS	64	5	9.5	13.2
CD	58	15	9	12.7
Narakas Group				
I	35	3	10.8	13.6
II	110	13	9	13
III	38	4	8.9	12.5

Based on Kambhampati et al. 2006 [40]

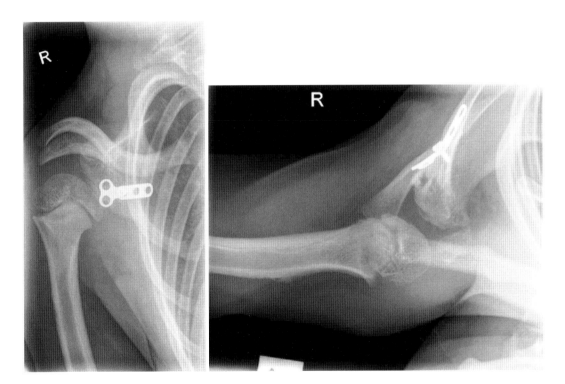

Fig. 20 AP and axial radiographs 24 months after glenoplasty in a 4 year-old child

Treatment

The early onset of glenoid deformity indicates that temporary paralysis of the medial rotator muscles using botulinum is unlikely. *Kambhampati et al (2006)* [40] prospectively studied 183 children in whom an operation was used which corrected the contracted subscapularis, the coracoid deformity and the retroversion of the head but did not address the deformity of the glenoid nor the abnormality of the acromioclavicular arch (Fig. 19a, b, c). Dislocation recurred in 20 children with more advanced bone deformity (Table 13). Currently, glenoplasty is added when the head appears to drop out of the

Fig. 21 Shoulder function 5 years after reduction and glenoplasty on the right side

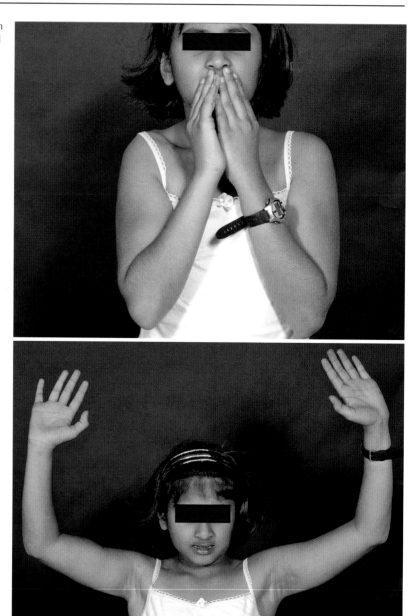

antero-superior true facet into the larger postero-inferior false facet after re-location and de-rotation osteotomy. With the first stage of the operation complete the child is placed prone and the posterior face of the scapula is displayed between the infraspinatus and the teres minor. The relocated head of the humerus leaves behind a mass of redundant capsule which is elevated from the posterior face of the scapula. A radial incision into the capsule permits identification of the posterior labrum and the edge of the hyaline cartilage of the inferior facet. Fine osteotomes elevate the posterior and inferior walls of the glenoid so that it abuts the reduced head of the humerus. The gap is wedged open with the excised coracoid. The flap consists of the posterior and inferior labrum, the inferior (false) socket of the glenoid, the overlying capsule and cortico- cancellous strips petalled from the posterior face of the scapula. In older children the teres major is transferred to infraspinatus because this muscle will have become defunctioned by longstanding dislocation. The early results of this procedure are promising [9, 80] (Figs. 20, 21). The problems caused by the deformity of the acromio clavicular arch and the shortening of the clavicle remain unsolved.

Conclusions

It is clear that nerve repair may improve function in the upper limb in cases of BLBP, particularly so when avulsed nerves are re-innervated. A good shoulder is the foundation for function in the upper limb in a growing child and every reasonable effort must be made to re-innervate the shoulder muscles and to prevent or to treat, medial rotation contracture, posterior subluxation and posterior dislocation as soon as they are detected. Many of these children require review into adult life but hospital admissions and attendances must be kept to an essential minimum to diminish the effects upon the child and the family. Passing the parcel from one "specialist" to another should be avoided.

Acknowledgments The figures and most of the tables are drawn from Surgical Disorders of the Peripheral Nerves, 2nd edition by permission of Springer UK.

References

1. Addas BMJ, Midha R. Nerve transfers for severe nerve injury. In: Spinner RJ, Winfree CJ, editors. Neurosurgery clinics: peripheral nerves: injuries. Philadelphia: Elsevier Saunders; 2009. p. 27–38.
2. Allende CA, Gilbert A. Forearm supination deformity after obstetric paralysis. Clin Orth Rel Res. 2004;426:206–11.
3. Anand P, Birch R. Restoration of sensory function and lack of long-term chronic pain syndromes after brachial plexus injury in human neonates. Brain. 2002;125:113–22.
4. Berman JS, Taggart M, Anand P, Birch R. The effect of surgical repair on pain relief after brachial plexus injuries. Assoc Brit Neurol Proc. 1995;44(abs).
5. Berman J, Anand P, Chen L, Taggart M, Birch R. Pain relief from preganglionic injury to the brachial plexus by late intercostal transfer. J Bone Jointt Surg. 1996;78B:759–60.
6. Berman JS, Birch R, Anand P. Pain following human brachial plexus injury with spinal cord root avulsion and the effect of surgery. Pain. 1998;75:199–207.
7. Birch R, Bonney G, Wynn Parry CB. Surgical disorders of the peripheral nerves. 1st ed. London: Churchill Livingstone; 1998.
8. Birch R, Ahad N, Kono H, Smith S. Repair of obstetric brachial plexus palsy. Results in 100 children. J Bone Joint Surg. 2005;87B:1089–95.
9. Birch R. Surgical disorders of the peripheral nerves. 2nd ed. London: Springer; 2011.
10. Bisinella G, Birch R. Obstetric brachial plexus lesion: a study of 74 children registered with the British Surveillance Unit. J Hand Surg. 2003;28B:40–5.
11. Bisinella G, Birch R, Smith SJM. Neurophysiological predictions of outcome in obstetric lesions of the brachial plexus. J Hand Surg. 2003;28B:148–52.
12. Blaauw G, Slooff ACJM, Muhlig S. Results of surgery after breech delivery. In: Gilbert A, editor. Brachial plexus injuries. London: Martin Dunitz; 2001. p. 217–24.
13. Blaauw G, Sauter Y, Lacroix CLE, Sloof ACJ. Hypoglossal nerve transfer in obstetrical brachial plexus palsy. J Plast Rec Surg. 2006;59:474–8.
14. Blaauw G, Muhlig RS, Vredeveld JW. Management of brachial plexus injuries. Adv Tech Stand Neurosurg. 2008;33:201–31. Review.
15. Bonney G. The value of axon responses in determining the site of lesion in traction lesions of the brachial plexus. Brain. 1954;77:588–609.
16. Bonney G. Prognosis in traction lesions of the brachial plexus. J Bone Joint Surg. 1959;41B:4–35.
17. Bonney G. Causalgia. Brit J Hosp Med. 1973;9:593–6.
18. Bonney G, Gilliatt RW. Sensory nerve conduction after traction lesion of the brachial plexus. Proc Coll Med. 1958;51:365–7.
19. Carlstedt T. Central nerve plexus injury. London: Imperial College Press; 2007.
20. Carlstedt T, Hultgren T, Nyman T, Hansson T. Cortical activity and hand function restoration in a patient after spinal cord surgery. Nat Rev Neurol. 2009;5:571–4.
21. Carvalho GA, Nikkhari G, Mathies C, Penkert G, Samii M. Diagnosis and root avulsion in traumatic brachial plexus: value and computerised tomography myelography and magnetic resonance imaging J. Neurosurgery. 1997;86:69–76.
22. Cavanagh SP, Birch R, Bonney G. The infraclavicular brachial plexus: the case for primary repair. J Bone Joint Surg. 1987;69B:489.
23. Cowen T, Ulfhake B, King RHM. Aging in the peripheral nervous system. In: Dyck PJ, Thomas PK, editors.

Peripheral neuropathy. 4th ed. Philadelphia: Elsevier-Saunders; 2005. p. 483–507. Chapter 22.

24. Curtis C, Stephens D, Clarke HM, Andrews SD. The active movement scale: an evaluation tool for infants with obstetrical brachial plexus palsy. J Hand Surg. 2002;27A:470–8.

25. Dickson J, Biant L. Recovery of hand function after repair of complee lesions of the brachial plexus: a report of two cases. Pers com; 2009.

26. Evans-Jones G, Kay SPJ, Weindling AM, Cranny G, Ward A, Bradshaw A, Hernon C. Congenital brachial palsy: incidence, causes and outcome in the United Kingdom and Republic of Ireland. Arch Dis Fetal Neonatal. 2003;88:F185–9.

27. Fairbank HAT. Subluxation of shoulder joint in infants and young children. Lancet. 1913;I:1217–23.

28. Fullerton AC, Myles LM, Lenihan DV, Hems TEJ, Glasby M. Obstetric brachial plexus palsy: a comparison of the degree of recovery after repair of 16 ventral root avulsions in newborn and adult sheep. Brit J Plas Surg. 2001;54:697–704.

29. Giddins GEB, Birch R, Singh D, Taggart M. Risk factors for obstetric brachial plexus palsies. J Bone Joint Surg. 1994;76B: Orthopaedic Proceedings Supps. II and III:156.

30. Gilbert A. Obstetrical paralysis. In: Tubiana R, Gilbert A, editors. Tendon, nerve and other disorders. Surgery of disorders of the hand and upper extremity series. London/New York: Taylor and Francis; 2005. p. 277–302. Chapter 10.

31. Goldie BS, Coates CJ. Brachial plexus injuries – a survey of incidence and referral pattern. J Hand Surg. 1992;17B:86–8.

32. Grossman JAL, Price AE, Tidwell MA, Ramos LE, Alfonso I, Yaylalli I. Outcome after late combined brachial plexus and shoulder surgery after birth trauma. J Bone Joint Surg. 2003;85B:1166–8.

33. Groves MJ, Scaravilli F. Pathology of peripheral neurone cell bodies. In: Dyke PJ, Thomas PK, editors. Peripheral neuropathy. 4th ed. Philadelphia: Elsevier Saunders; 2005. p. 683–732. Chapter 31.

34. Hall S. The response to injury in the peripheral nervous system. J Bone Joint Surg. 2005;87B:1309–19.

35. Hems TEJ, Birch R, Carlstedt T. The role of magnetic resonance imaging in the management of traction injuries to the adult brachial plexus. J Hand Surg. 1999;24B:550–5.

36. Hoeksma AF, Steeg AMT, Dijkstra P, Nellisen RGHH, Beelen A, Jong BAD. Shoulder contracture and osseous deformity in obstetrical brachial plexus injuries. J Bone Joint Surg. 2003;85A:316–22.

37. Htut M, Misra P, Anand P, Birch R, Carlstedt T. Pain phenomena and sensory recovery following brachial plexus avulsion injury and surgical repair. J Hand Surg. 2006;31B:596–605.

38. Hui JP, Torode IP. Changing glenoid version after open reduction of shoulders in children with obstetric brachial plexus palsy. J Paediatr Orthop. 2003;23:109–13.

39. Jones SJ. Investigation of brachial plexus traction lesion by peripheral and spinal somatosensory evoked potentials. J Neurol Neurosurg Psychiat. 1979;42:107–16.

40. Kambhampati SLS, Birch R, Cobiella C, Chen L. Posterior subluxation and dislocation of the shoulder in obstetric brachial plexus palsy. J Bone Joint Surg. 2006;88B:213–9.

41. Kato N, Htut M, Taggart M, Carlstedt T, Birch R. The effects of operative delay on the relief of neuropathic pain after injury to the brachial plexus. J Bone Joint Surg. 2006;88B:756–9.

42. Kim DH, Murovic JA, Tiel RL, Kline DG. Penetrating injuries due to gunshot wounds involving the brachial plexus. Neurosurg Focus. 2004;16:1–6.

43. Kline DG. Civilian gun shot wounds to the brachial plexus. J Neurosurg. 1989;70:166–74.

44. Landi A, Copeland SA, Wynn-Parry CB, Jones SJ. The role of somatosensory evoked potentials and nerve conduction studies in the surgical management of brachial plexus injuries. J Bone Joint Surg. 1980;62B:492–6.

45. Lawson SN. The peripheral sensory nervous system: dorsal root ganglion neurones. In: Dyck PJ, Thomas PK, editors. Peripheral neuropathy (in two volumes). 4th ed. Philadelphia: Elsevier Saunders; 2005. p. 163–202. Chapter 8.

46. Leechavengvongs S, Witoonchart K, Verpairojkit C, Thuvasethakul P, Malungpaishrope K. Combined nerve transfers for C5 and C6 brachial plexus avulsion injuries. J Hand Surg. 2006;31A:183–9.

47. Mac Namara P, Yam A, Pringle J. Biceps muscle trauma at birth – pseudo tumour formation is a cause of poor elbow flexion and supination. J Bone Joint Surg. 2009;91:1086–9.

48. Mallet J. Paralysie obstétricale du plexus brachiale. Rev Chir Orthop. 1972;58:115–204. Symposium sous le direction de J Mallet. Avec la collaboration de: M Arthris; J Castaing; J Dubousset; R Fayse; Fr Isch; M Lacheretza; P Masse; et P Rigault.

49. Marshall RW, de Silva RD. Computerised tomography in traction lesions of the brachial plexus. J Bone Joint Surg. 1986;68B:734–8.

50. Michelow BJ, Clarke HM, Curtis CG, Zuker RM, Seifs Y, Andrews DF. The natural history of obstetrical brachial plexus palsy. Plast Reconstr Surg. 1994;93:675–80.

51. Mirsky R, Jessen KR. Molecular signalling in Schwann cell development. In: Dyck PJ, Thomas PK, editors. Peripheral neuropathy (in two volumes). 4th ed. Philadelphia: Elsevier Saunders; 2005. p. 341–76. Chapter 16.

52. Nagano A, Ochiai N, Sugioka H, et al. Usefulness of myelography in brachial plexus injuries. J Hand Surg. 1989;14B:59–64.

53. Nagano A, Tsuyama N, Ochiai N, Hara T. Direct nerve crossing with the intercostal nerve to treat avulsion injuries of the brachial plexus. J Hand Surg. 1989;14A(6):980–5.

54. Narakas AO. Obstetrical brachial plexus injuries. In: Lamb DW, editor. The paralysed hand. Edinburgh: Churchill Livingstone; 1987. p. 116.

55. Nehme A, Kany J, Sales-de-Gauzy J, Charlet JP, Dautel G, Cahuzal JP. Obstetrical brachial plexus palsy, predictions of outcome in upper root injuries. J Hand Surg. 2001;27B:9–12.

56. Nordin L, Sinisi M. Brachial plexus avulsion causing Brown Séquard syndrome. J Bone Joint Surg. 2009;91B:88–90.

57. Oberle J, Antoniadis G, Rath SA, et al. Radiological investigations and intra-operative evoked potentials for the diagnosis of nerve root avulsion: evaluation of both modalities by intradural root inspection. Acta Neurochirurgica. 1998;140:527–31.

58. Oberlin C, Beal D, Leechavengvongs S, Salon A, Dauge MC, Sarly JJ. Nerve transfers to biceps muscle using part of ulnar nerve for C5-C6 avulsion of the brachial plexus: anatomical study and report of four cases. J Hand Surg. 1994;19A:232–7.

59. Ovelmen-Levitt J, Johnson B, Bedenbaugh P, Nashold BS. Dorsal root rhizotomy and avulsion in the cat: a comparison of long term effects on dorsal horn neuronal activity. J Neurosurg. 1984;15(6):921–7.

60. Patterson M, Dunkerton M, Birch R, Bonney G. Re-innervation of the suprascapular nerve in brachial plexus injuries. J Bone Joint Surg. 1990;72B:p993.

61. Pearl ML, Edgerton BW. Glenoid deformity secondary to brachial plexus birth palsy. J Bone Joint Surg. 1998;80A:659–67.

62. Pearl ML, Edgerton BW, Kon DS, Darakjian AB, Kosco AE, Kazimiroth PB, Burchette RJ. Comparison of arthroscopic findings with magnetic resonance imaging and arthrography in children with gleno humeral deformities secondary to brachial plexus birth palsy. J Bone Joint Surg. 2003;85A:890–8.

63. Pondaag W, Malessy MJS, van Dijk JG, Thomeer RTWM. Natural history of obstetric brachial plexus palsy: a systematic review. Dev Med Child Neurol. 2004;46:138–44.

64. Pondaag W, de Boer R, van Wijlen-Hempel MS, Hostede-Buitenhuis SM, Malessy MJ. External rotation as a result of suprascapular nerve neurotisation in obstetric brachial plexus palsy. Neurosurgery. 2005;57:530–7.

65. Putti V. Analisi della triada radiosintomatica degli stati di prelussazione. Chir Organi Mov. 1932;XVII:453–9.

66. Rosson JW. Disability following closed traction lesions of the brachial plexus sustained in motor cycle accidents. Hand Surg. 1987;12B:353–5.

67. Rosson JW. Closed traction lesions of the brachial plexus – an epidemic among young motor cyclists. Injury. 1988;19:4–6.

68. Saifuddin A, Heffernan G, Birch R. Ultrasound diagnosis of shoulder congruity in chronic obstetric brachial plexus palsy. J Bone Joint Surg. 2002;84B(1):100–3.

69. Scaglietti O. The obstetrical shoulder trauma. Surg Gynae Obstet. 1938;66:868–77.

70. Schenker M, Birch R. Diagnosis of level of intradural ruptures of the rootlets in traction lesions of the brachial plexus. J Bone Joint Surg. 2001;83B:916–20.

71. Sluisz JA, van Ouwerkerk WJR, de Gast A, Wuisman P, Nollet F, Manoliu RA. Deformities of the shoulder in infants younger than 12 months with an obstetric lesion of the brachial plexus. J Bone Joint Surg. 2001;83B:551–5.

72. Sluijs JA, van Ouwerkerk WJR, de Gast A, Wuisman P, Nollet F, Manoliu RA. Retroversion of the humeral head in children with obstetric brachial plexus lesion. J Bone Joint Surg. 2002;84B:583–7.

73. Smith SJM. Electrodiagnosis. In: Birch R, Bonney G, Wynn Parry C, editors. Surgical disorders of the peripheral nerves. 1st ed. Edinburgh/London: Churchill Livingstone; 1998. p. 467–90. Chapter 19.

74. Stewart M, Birch R. Penetrating missile injuries. J Bone Joint Surg. 2001;83B:517–24.

75. Stripp WJ. Special techniques in orthopaedic radiology. In: Murray RO, Jacobson HG, editors. The radiology of skeletal disorders, vol. 3. Edinburgh: Churchill Livingstone; 1997. p. 1879–940.

76. Strömbeck C, Rehmal S, Krum Linde-Sundholm L, Sejersen T. Long term functional follow up of a cohort of children with obstetric brachial plexus palsy: I; functional aspects. Dev Med Child Neurol. 2007;49(3):198–203.

77. Strömbeck C, Rehmal S, Krum Linde-Sundholm L, Sejersen T. Long term functional follow up of a cohort of children with obstetric brachial plexus palsy: II: neurophysiological aspects. Dev Med Child Neurol. 2007;49(3):204–9.

78. Tavakkolizadah A, Saifuddin A, Birch R. Imaging of adult brachial plexus injuries. J Hand Surg. 2001;26B:183–91.

79. Tavakkolizadeh A. Risk factors associated with obstetric brachial plexus palsy. Dissertation. University of Brighton for degree of M Sc. 2007.

80. Tennant S, Lambert S, Sinisi M Birch R. Complex gleno humeral deformity secondary to obstetrical brachial plexus palsy: bone block or glenoplasty? J.Bone Jt. Surg. Orthopaedic proceedings. 2010;92B:373–73.

81. Wall P, Devor M. The effect of peripheral nerve injury on dorsal root potentials and on transmission of afferent signals into the spinal cord. Brain Res. 1981;209:95–111.

82. Wall PD. In: Swash M, Kennard C, editors. Scientific basis of clinical neurology. Churchill Livingstone, Edinburgh, pp. 163–171; 1985.

83. Yam A, Fullilove S, Sinisi M, Fox M. The supination deformity and associated deformities of the upper limb in severe birth lesions of the brachial plexus. J Bone Joint Surg. 2009;91B:511–6.

84. Yang LJ, Anand P. Limb preference in children with obstetric brachial plexus palsy. Paediatr Neurol. 2005;33:46–9.

85. Yiangou Y, Birch R, Sangeswaram L, Eglen R, Anand P. SNS/PN3 and SNS2/NaN sodium channel like immunoreactivity in human adult and neonate injuries of sensory nerves. FEBS Lett. 2000;467:249–52.

Scapular Dysplasia

Tim Bunker

Contents

T. Bunker
Princess Elizabeth Orthopaedic Centre, Exeter, UK
e-mail: Tim.bunker@exetershoulderclinic.co.uk

Keywords

Apert's syndrome • Dysplasia • Embryology
and genetics • Obstetric brachial plexus palsy •
Posterior-inferior dysplasia • Primary and secondary dysplasia • Scapula • Snapping scapula
• Sprengel's deformity-surgical correction

Introduction

We are just beginning to understand that glenoid
version, depth and shape may have an important
bearing upon shoulder instability, and in particular posterior positional instability, the development of arthritis, and shoulder replacement. On
top of this, primary glenoid dysplasia, secondary
glenoid dysplasia from obstetric brachial plexus
palsy (OBPP) as well as Apert's syndrome,
snapping scapula and finally Sprengel's shoulder
are rare but challenging conditions.

The definition of dysplasia is abnormal
development, growth or absence of a structure.
In order to understand scapula dysplasia we need
to understand the normal development of the
scapula and its constituent parts. Fortunately
recent research in genetics has begun to enlighten
us and bring our understanding of scapula
dysplasia into the twenty-first century. Research
on the genetics and embryology of the scapula
reveals that the blade of the scapula and
the glenoid develop from completely different
tissues. The blade of the scapula seems to be an
ossified muscular attachment whose development is moulded by its environment. The glenoid,

G. Bentley (ed.), *European Surgical Orthopaedics and Traumatology*,
DOI 10.1007/978-3-642-34746-7_81, © EFORT 2014

coracoid and acromion have separate ossification centres, and it is genetics rather than external pressures and forces that determine their eventual morphology.

The scapula differentiates between the 5th and 6th weeks of intra-uterine life as a hyaline cartilage model at the level of the 4th to 6th cervical vertebrae. By the 7th week the shoulder is well formed and the scapula moves caudally to assume its adult position between the second to seventh thoracic ribs.

In Sprengel's shoulder there is failure of descent. There is also failure of remodelling from the short wide scapula to the adult shape of the longer, thinner scapula. Since the scapula is so high it conforms to the shape of the dome of the thoracic cavity, and is therefore more concave on its deep surface than if it had formed in the adult position of T2 to T7.

The *Pax1* gene has been shown to control development of the acromion and scapular spine. Knockout mice lacking the *Pax1* gene are found to have the acromion and part of the scapular spine missing.

The *Emx2* gene controls development of the scapular body. Knockout mice lacking the *Emx2* gene have absence of the body of the scapula and the majority of the ileum, but have a normal acromion that articulates with the clavicle, and a normal glenoid that articulates with the humerus. Pelviscapular agenesis has been recorded in humans.

The Hoxc6 gene controls the development of the coracoid and glenoid. Expanding expressions of Hoxc6 genes in chick embryos results in duplicate coracoid and acromion formation in the chick. This has been seen clinically in humans.

The scapular body forms in a different way and is probably not a skeletal element proper, but an ossifying muscle attachment. This might account for differences in the shape of the scapula from flat to curved according to the underlying thoracic shape that provides the environment around the developing scapula.

Its secondary centres of ossification define post-natal development of the scapula. At birth the body and spine of the scapula have already ossified by intramembranous ossification. The large coracoid base secondary centre appears at 1 year of age and closes at 18–21 years. There are two secondary centres of ossification for the glenoid, the first appears at the base of the coracoid at the age of 10 and fuses at 18. There is a far smaller horseshoe-shaped inferior centre that appears briefly at age 18 and fuses at 19. The acromial apophysis appears at age 15 and usually fuses at age 18–19. Failure of fusion leads to the Os Acromiale that occurs in 4 % of the population and may be associated with some rotator cuff tears.

The scapula can therefore be looked at as a modular bone. It is like a Lego model comprising the glenoid/coracoid block, the spine/acromion block and the blade. These blocks can be assembled in different ways so that the glenoid may be translated forward or backwards on the blade. It can be assembled anteverted or retroverted to the blade. The blade itself can be flat or curved. All these factors combine to create a bone that can be very variable in its shape and this can have implications in terms of pathology, stability and degenerative change.

Primary Glenoid Dysplasia

In 1981 Petterson suggested that glenoid dysplasia might be more common than previously thought. My experience would support this for in 2001 we published 12 cases seen over an 8-year period. There may be minimal symptoms or the condition may be asymptomatic making under-diagnosis inevitable.

The term primary glenoid dysplasia refers to an uncommon condition characterised by incomplete ossification of the lower two-thirds of the cartilaginous glenoid and adjacent neck of the scapula (Fig. 1). The aetiology and inheritance are poorly understood. The pathogenesis appears to be a failure of ossification of the inferior glenoid pre-cartilage. Previous theories concerning a failure of development of the pre-cartilage of the inferior apophysis of the glenoid are not supported by findings on CT arthrography, plain radiography, and arthroscopy, which show that the inferior glenoid

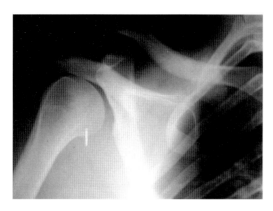

Fig. 1 In primary glenoid dysplasia the glenoid is flat and underdeveloped and the clavicle is bossed

pre-cartilage is present, but unossified. The outline of the glenohumeral joint lines on radiographs demonstrating the 'vacuum phenomenon' also supports the view that the radiological glenoid 'deficiency' compromises unossified cartilage. The underlying cause of this failure of ossification is not established.

Primary glenoid dysplasia often occurs sporadically but there have been reports of familial occurrence consistent with autosomal dominant inheritance. In one of these families, a young woman with normal scapulae had an affected son, daughter and brother. The observation that obligate gene carriers can be clinically unaffected suggests that this gene may have variable penetrance within families. In 2009 I described an affected son and father (and possibly grandfather), providing further evidence that (at least in some cases) this is a single gene disorder with autosomal dominant inheritance. At present the gene is unknown and the linkage analysis (to locate the gene) has so far been precluded by the relatively small number of families reported. It is interesting that this gene seems to have a localised effect on the development of the scapula especially the glenoid fossa.

These familial cases emphasise the importance of taking a family history in this condition. If there is already an affected parent and child within a family, the risk of another child (male or female) inheriting the gene is 50 %. At present it is unknown what percentage of cases of primary glenoid dysplasia are genetically determined and

if so how many are due to errors in the same gene. However it is likely that some apparently isolated cases without a family history (due to new spontaneous mutations) will also be at risk of having an affected child. Definition of the condition at the molecular genetic level will help address these questions in the future.

The clinical findings may be very varied. Most children are asymptomatic, and relatively few symptomatic children have been described. Children are more likely to be diagnosed by serendipity. We found a bi-modal presentation, the first peak at age 12–24 with clicking, instability or pain, and the second group presenting with degenerative changes aged 48–69.

Changes in morphology are always bilateral. If unilateral then another cause should be sort for. The inferior pole of the glenoid is elongated, flattened and medialised and often severely retroverted. There is also bossing of the lateral third of the clavicle and an enlarged and inferiorly pointing acromion.

Shoulder replacement is very difficult in primary glenoid dysplasia as the socket is extremely retroverted and access to ream and prepare this socket is difficult. For this reason the surgeon might be tempted to perform a hemi-arthroplasty, but the Mayo Clinic experience shows this is a disaster for the patients continue to have disabling pain from the socket and most require a second, and more difficult revision to eventually implant a socket. This has also been my experience.

Secondary Glenoid Dysplasia

Obstetric Brachial Plexus Palsy (OBPP)

The lesson of OBPP is that changes in glenoid morphology can be aquired, and this may have relevance when we come to discuss instability. Pearl and Edgerton looked at 25 infants with OBPP. Seven had normal glenoids but 18 had abnormal glenoids, five being flattened, seven bi-concave and six dislocated with a pseudo-glenoid formed posterior to the original glenoid. The severity of glenoid change was proportional to the degree of internal rotation contracture. In another study Waters studied 94 children with OBPP, 42 with persistent weakness were followed with CT and MRI. The bony anatomy of the glenoid was typically normal on the true AP radiographs, but scanning showed the affected side to be 20° more retroverted than the unaffected side, implying that the growth disturbance is an impairment of the cartilaginous development of the posterior glenoid. Ten years later Waters looked at the effect on glenoid development following reconstruction with the QUAD procedure. The QUAD procedure is a transfer of latissimus dorsi and Teres major, release of the contracted subscapularis and pectoralis major plus neurolysis of the axillary nerve. They demonstrated that early and effective surgery could remodel mild to moderate secondary dysplasia. This is confirmation that morphological changes to the socket can be acquired.

Apert's Syndrome

This is an unusual condition of acrocephalosyndactyly. This syndrome is a variant of multiple epiphyseal dysplasia. The skeletal changes show dysplasia of the glenoid, short humeri, elbow dysplasia, syndactyly, hip dysplasia, genu valgum with knee dysplasia and changes in the ribs and spine. These patients may also have subacromial dimples in the skin. Subacromial dimples are also seen in posterior positional dislocation.

Postero-Inferior Glenoid Dysplasia and Instability

Posterior positional instability is being recognised as a common cause of disability in young people. The patient usually presents with a history of shoulder pain. Often there is no true history of dislocation, for in these patients dislocation is both atraumatic and asymptomatic. What the patient may notice is the clunk of relocation that may be asymptomatic, but is often painful. Although subluxation

and dislocation are usually silent the posterior thrust of the humeral head against the inflamed and stretched posterior capsule will cause pain. In posterior positional dislocation the humeral head slips silently backwards when the arm is elevated in the adducted and internally rotated position. This is why patients will present with pain on swimming or with overhead sports and throwing. The patient can often demonstrate re-location (note this is re-location and not dislocation), and when young may even have used this as a party trick. This does NOT mean that they are insane and is not, in itself, an argument for a nihilistic approach to their management. Just because we as doctors have not found an effective and reliable cure for a condition is no excuse for labelling the teenager as abnormal. The condition is entirely separate from muscle patterning where the patient demonstrates dislocation with the elbow at the side effected by active muscle contraction.

Typically the teenager will have joint laxity. This may exhibit as hyperlaxity (external rotation of 85° or more), a positive sulcus sign, positive Gagey sign, and laxity both forwards and backwards on unlocked stoop testing. In other words they have a capacious, high volume "loosy goosy" shoulder. There are two pathognomonic tests of posterior positional instability.

The first is the *Posterior Jerk Test* (Fig. 2). This is a demonstration of the clunk of re-location from the postero-inferiorly subluxed or dislocated position. Elevating the arm in adduction and internal rotation silently dislocates the arm. The humeral head will be felt to thrust out posteriorly. Now the arm is brought from the adducted elevated position out into an abducted elevated position and the humeral head can be felt to reduce with a pop, clunk or snap that is often painful.

The second test is the *Kim Test*. This is a provocative test that thrusts the humeral head in a postero-inferior direction against the inflamed and stretched posterior capsule, eliciting pain and apprehension.

The pathology of posterior positional dislocation is disputed. Some feel that this is a condition

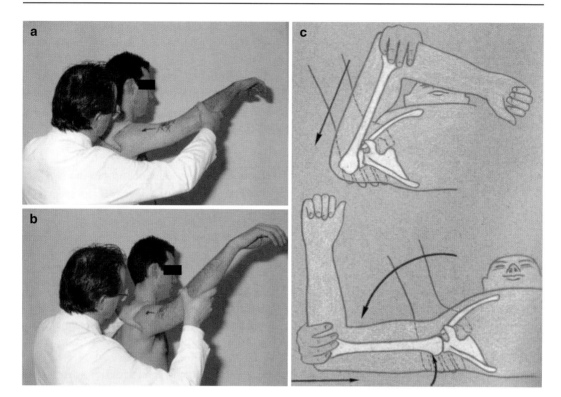

Fig. 2 The posterior jerk test. In posterior positional instability the humerus is elevated in internal rotation (**a**) and thrusts backwards behind the glenoid (**c**) then as the arm is externally rotated (**b**) the head jerks back into joint (**d**)

brought on by a high volume stretched out capsule, implying that treatment should be through a shift, plication or remplissage of the capsule. The other school of thought, championed by Kim, is that this is caused by hypoplasia and retroversion of the postero-inferior bone/cartilage/labrum complex (Fig. 3), implying that treatment should be by correcting the retroversion or increasing the concavity compression containment of the head by moving the labrum so that it acts as a more effective chock-block.

The idea that retroversion of the glenoid may play a significant part in posterior positional instability is not new. Edelson examined 1,150 dried scapulae and found quite a high incidence of postero-inferior hypoplasia of the bone, varying from 19 % amongst the Negev desert Bedouin to 35 % amongst Mexican Indians. He then looked at 300 CT and MRI scans and found that the postero-inferior glenoid was convex rather than concave in 18 %. He termed this the 'lazy J' appearance. Finally he looked at the scans

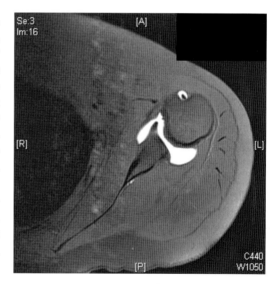

Fig. 3 A J-shaped inferior glenoid with postero-inferior hypoplasia

of 12 patients with posterior dislocation and found that 9/12 had such a deficiency. However the problem has been that methods of

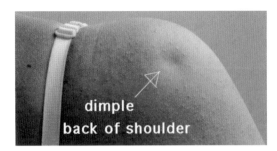

Fig. 4 Some patients with posterior positional instability have a characteristic dimple on the back of the shoulder

measuring retroversion from radiographs have been shown to be invalid. Even measurement from CT and MRI scans can be invalid for the scapula has great variability in terms of its shape. Using the medial border can be unreliable as the glenoid may be translated on the body rather than retroverted, and the scapula blade itself varies from flat to curved.

Accepting these reservations in terms of measurement Innui et al found that there was a significant difference in retroversion between patients with and without posterior dislocation. They also demonstrated differences in surface shape with some glenoids being concave, some flat and some convex.

Interestingly we have described the association of a subacromial dimple with posterior positional instability (Fig. 4), and dimples have also been seen in Apert's syndrome that is known to be associated with glenoid dysplasia.

Kim examined not only the bone shape, but also the combined shape of the bone, cartilage and labrum on MRI scans. What he found was that shoulders with posterior positional instability had greater retroversion of both the bony and chondrolabral portion of the glenoid in the middle and inferior planes. The height of the postero-inferior labrum was decreased and the depth of the labral containment was decreased in patients with instability. At arthroscopy he found that although the postero-inferior labrum looked normal, when it was probed it was found to be torn interstitially. These labral changes could be due to localised chondrolabral hypoplasia, but

of course they could be acquired by recurrent posterior dislocation, just as the changes occur in OBPP.

Chondrolabral containment has been shown in laboratory models to account for 65 % of stability, although in Lazarus and Harryman's study the containment effect of the labrum was more important at the front of the socket than at the back. Based on these findings Kim has devised a procedure of capsulo-labral posterior re-positioning and repair with a 7.5 % recurrence rate.

Snapping Scapula

The snapping scapula is a rare condition that presents as a distressing tactile acoustic phenomenon consisting of medial scapular pain and grating on movement. It was first described in 1867 by Boinnet who described three types of noises, fraissement (gentle friction), frottement (louder friction) and craquement (a pathological snap). In this condition the superomedial corner of the scapula can be more curved than the adjacent rib cage or have a bony nodule on the superomedial corner that is called Lushka's tubercle (Fig. 5). Edelson has described an abnormal protuberance at the inferomedial corner of the scapula that he called the "rhino horn". This rhino horn seems to develop within the origin of Teres Major. Examination of historical bone specimens has shown that the body of the scapula can be flat or markedly angled and it may be that these angled scapulae have taken on the shape of the more angled dome of the thorax and fail to remodel on descent to the adult position. However it is far more difficult to measure this curve or mis-match between the deep surface of the scapula and the thorax in life, than it is in death, and even with 3D CT and MRI scanning it is difficult to quantify this mis-match.

Diagnosis is difficult, and often depends on exclusion of other conditions. Medial scapula pain is far more likely to be referred from the cervical or thoracic spine. Other tactile acoustic phenomena can be caused by osteochondromata

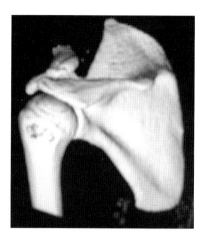

Fig. 5 This patient with snapping scapula has an abnormal shape to the supero-medial angle of the scapula termed the tubercle of Luschka

on the deep surface of the scapula, and even posterior positional dislocation can mimic the clunk of a snapping scapula.

Conservative management is the mainstay of treatment but effectively this means re-assurance and anti-inflammatory analgesia when necessary. Physiotherapy is useful if the patient's posture is abnormal, or if they have scapula dyskinesia or winging that is leading to a secondary snapping phenomenon. Most patients only present to the Orthopaedic surgeon after some years of failed conservative management. Milch wrote, *Even Thoroughly Competent Orthopaedic Surgeons Have Expressed Surprise at the Possibility and Consequences of Surgical Therapy*. In 1933 he described six cases of disabling pain caused by excessive forward curvature of the superior angle of the scapula and stated *"resection resulted in prompt cure"*. More recently Richards and McKee reported on painful scapula thoracic crepitus and an asymmetric scapula on CT in three cases that were successfully treated by surgical excision. Open surgery is relatively straighforward. A short horizontal incision is made over the superolateral scapula, splitting trapezius making sure that the split does not extend more than a centimetre medial to the medial border of the scapula so as to protect the spinal accessory nerve supplying the inferior

trapezius. Supraspinatus is now lifted off the superomedial border and a subperiosteal excision of the superomedial angle of the scapula is performed. The periosteal sleeve remains as an anchor for levator scapula.

Arthroscopic bone resection has been performed, but is fraught with difficulty and is a procedure for experienced experts only. The reason for this is that there are no clear landmarks for the arthroscopic surgeon. The surgery is performed in distended tissue planes rather than true surgical spaces and the spinal accessory nerve, dorsal scapular nerve, suprascapular nerve, brachial plexus and dorsal scapular artery are all at risk. Bell has described a superior portal for resection of the superomedial scapula that is on average 2 cm from the suprascapular nerve in one direction and 3.5 cm from the dorsal scapula nerve in the opposite direction. The results are not as good as the open technique. One study on six patients showed that in none did the pain completely resolve, surgery was abandoned in one patient and another developed a superficial infection.

Sprengel's Deformity

Congenital elevation of the scapula is a rare congenital anomaly. Sprengel (1891) recognized that the deformity was caused by failure of the scapula to descend. In this condition the scapula lies higher than normal, is broad in shape and deeply dished.

The disability is dependent on the severity of the deformity. In mild cases, the scapula is only slightly elevated and smaller than normal with minimal loss of function. In the severe cases it creates an ugly deformity with widening of the base of the neck. Occasionally the scapula can be so elevated that it almost touches the skull. Movement is limited and function poor.

Other congenital anomalies, such as scoliosis, cervical ribs, and anomalies of the cervical vertebrae (Klippel–Feil syndrome), are commonly present; rarely, one or more scapular muscles are partly or completely absent.

Radiographs of the neck should be taken to identify these changes. An omovertebral bone together with a very straight clavicle is found in between a third and half of patients.

Surgery should only be undertaken at a recognised Paediatric Orthopaedic unit, between the ages of 3 and 8 years, and only for severe deformity. The earlier surgery is performed the better the results. In children older than 8 years surgery may seriously stretch and damage the brachial plexus. Limited resection of the prominent superomedial angle may be considered after this age. It must be made clear to the parents that the deformity is never simply elevation of the scapula alone, but always complicated by malformations and contractures of the soft tissues and that the results of surgery may not be all that they were hoping for.

Surgical Technique

Woodward described transfer of the origin of the trapezius muscle to a more inferior position on the spinous processes. This is performed through a mid-line approach from the spinous process of C5 to the T9 vertebra. The patient lies prone and is draped so that the shoulder girdle and arm can be moved freely. The skin and subcutaneous tissues are undermined laterally to the medial border of the scapula. The lateral border of the trapezius is identified distally and separated by blunt dissection from the underlying latissimus dorsi muscle. The origin of the trapezius is released from the spinous processes all the way up to C5. The rhomboids are similarly freed and separated from the muscles of the chest wall. These muscles can be retracted to expose an omovertebral bone or fibrous bands attached to the superior angle of the scapula and these are freed, avoiding injury to the spinal accessory nerve, the nerves to the rhomboids or the transverse cervical artery. The superomedial scapula is often deformed and is excised subperiosteally thus releasing the levator scapulae. The scapula can be displaced inferiorly with the attached sheet of muscles until its spine lies at the same level as that of the opposite scapula. With the scapula in this position,

the aponeuroses of the trapezius and rhomboids are re-attached to the spinous processes at a more inferior level.

A simpler alternative is to lower the scapula by osteotomy. The patient is placed semi-prone with the affected side uppermost. A vertical incision is made over the medial border of the scapula. The scapula is exposed by incising the periosteum along the medial part of the origin of supraspinatus and infraspinatus, which can be swept laterally. An osteotomy is made 1 cm from the vertebral border with an oscillating saw passing through the base of the spine. The superomedial, deformed part of the scapula is excised subperiosteally, allowing removal the omovertebral bone (if present) or any fibrous bands. When the scapula is completely mobile, the lateral portion is rotated downwards and stabilized with sutures passing through the periostium and bone of the medial fragment. Both these procedures run the risk of injury to the brachial plexus, or the spinal accessory nerve and this risk is greater in the more severe deformities.

Summary

The scapula is a complex bone with a variable shape. Understanding the development of the glenoid can help in our understanding of some cases of instability and arthritis as well as in the management of those rare conditions such as primary glenoid dysplasia, snapping scapula and Sprengel's shoulder.

References

1. Capellini T, Vaccari G, Feretti E, et al. Scapula development is governed by genetic interactions of the *Pbx1* gene. Development. 2010;137(15):2559–69.
2. Andrews S, Bunker T. Dominant familial inheritance in primary glenoid dysplasia. Should Elbow. 2009;1(2):93–4.
3. Smith S, Bunker T. Primary glenoid dysplasia; a review of twelve patients. J Bone Joint Surg. 2001;83(B):868–72.

4. Sperling J, Cofield R, Steinman S, et al. Shoulder arthroplsaty for osteoarthritis secondary to glenoid dysplasia. J Bone Joint Surg. 2002;84(4):541–6.

5. Pearl ML, Edgerton BW. Glenoid deformity secondary to brachial plexus palsy. J Bone Joint Surg. 1998;80(5):659–67.

6. Waters PM. Effect of tendon transfers on obstetric brachial plexus palsy. J Bone Joint Surg. 2005;87(2):320–5.

7. Kim SH, Ha K, Yoo J, Noh K. Kim's lesion; an incomplete and concealed avulsion of the postero-inferior labrum. Arthroscopy. 2004;20(7):712–20.

8. Kim SH, Noh KC, Park JS, et al. Loss of chondro-labral containment in atraumatic posteroinferior multi-directional instability. J Bone Joint Surg. 2005;87(1):92–8.

9. Edelson JG. Localized glenoid hypoplasia. Clin Orthop Relat Res. 1995;321:189–95.

10. Van Riebrox A, Campbell B, Bunker T. The association of subacromial dimples with recurrent posterior dislocation of the shoulder. J Shoulder Elbow. 2006;15(5):591–4.

11. Lazarus M, Sidles J, Harryman D. The effect of chondrolabral defects on glenoid concavity and glenohumeral stability. J Bone Joint Surg Am. 1996;78(1):94–102.

12. Edelson JG. Variations in the anatomy of the scapula with reference to the snapping scapula. Clin Orthop Relat Res. 1996;322:111–5.

13. Milch H. The snapping scapula. Clin Orthop. 1961;20:139–50.

14. Bell S, Van Riet PR. The safe zone for arthroscopic resection of the scapula. J Shoulder Elbow Surg. 2008;17(4):647–9.

Snapping Scapula

Roger J. H. Emery and Thomas M. Gregory

Contents

R.J.H. Emery (✉) • T.M. Gregory
St. Mary's Hospital, Imperial College NHS Trust,
London, UK

Department of Mechanical Engineering, Imperial
College, London, UK

European Hospital Georges Pompidou, APHP, University
Paris Descartes, Paris, France
e-mail: roger.emery@o2.co.uk

Keywords

Clinical features • Radiological assessment •
Results • Scapula • Snapping • Treatment-
non-operative, open operative, endoscopic

Introduction

Snapping scapula is an uncommon and largely under-recognised phenomenon that combines a tactile and acoustic clunk localised at the superomedial corner of the scapula. It usually occurs in the third decade and normally only requires treatment if painful. The differential diagnosis is extensive [1–3]. The first description was published in French by Boinet in 1867 [4] and a more comprehensive review was published by Milch and Burman in 1933 [5]. Mauclaire [6] first described surgical treatment of snapping scapula using a muscle transfer technique in 1904. In 1950 Milch et al. [7] reported partial scapulectomy which although modified from its original description is still in current practice. More recently with the development of endoscopy, Ciullo [8] published a series of nine endoscopic resections of the scapulo-thoracic bursa. Although most patients require non-operative treatment, surgical intervention is a proven modality. The most common procedure is resection of the superomedial angle of the scapula. However, painful snapping scapulae are not always associated with scapula supero-medial angle anomalies. Therefore along with a comprehensive knowledge of the anatomy,

G. Bentley (ed.), *European Surgical Orthopaedics and Traumatology*,
DOI 10.1007/978-3-642-34746-7_43, © EFORT 2014

accurate clinical and radiological assessment is essential for choosing the most appropriate procedure among the many described.

This chapter will give insight into the anatomy, the clinical features, the various associated anomalies and radiological presentation of snapping scapula followed by a review of surgical procedures and specific indications.

Anatomy

The superficial muscle layer includes trapezius and latissimus dorsi. Levator scapulae, and major and minor rhomboids that are attached to the supero-medial angle form the middle layer, and the deepest layer includes subscapularis and serratus anterior. There is one constant bursa, the scapulo-thoracic bursa, located between the rib cage and the serratus anterior (Fig. 1, number 2; Fig. 2, number 1). Wallach et al. [9, 10] also identified three inconsistent bursae: the subscapularis bursa, located between the serratus anterior and the subscapularis (Fig. 1, number 1), existing in only 40 % of cases; the scapulo-trapezial bursa, located between trapezius and the scapula blade (Fig. 1, number 3; Fig. 2, number 2); and the third bursa is located between latissimus dorsi and the inferior tip of the scapula (Fig. 2, number 3).

The spinal accessory nerve runs at the deepest aspect of the trapezius, bends over to follow the medial edge of the scapula and along the inferior edge of the trapezius.

The dorsal nerve of the scapula, which has one or two divisions, runs under the levator scapulae and the rhomboids. It is located medially and deep to the spinal accessory nerve. The suprascapular nerve is located in a more lateral position, crossing the supra-clavicular fossa to the spino-glenoid notch.

Clinical Features

Presentation of symptoms ranges from annoying to disabling [2]. Patients describe a tactile and acoustic clunk that can often be voluntarily

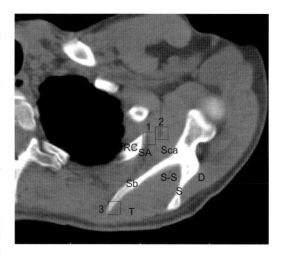

Fig. 1 Axial view of a left shoulder. *RC*, Rib cage; *SA*, Serratus anterior; *Sca*, Subscapularis; *S-S*, Supraspinatus; *T*, Trapezius; *D*, deltoid; *Sb*, Scapula blade; *S*, Spine of the scapula; *1*, Scapulo-thoracic bursa; *2*, Subscapularis bursa; *3*, Scapulo-trapezial bursa

reproduced. A wide range of terms is used to describe it: Single snap, intermittent clunks, continuous grating of muscles, clicking, crunching, and snapping sensations [3, 7, 11–13]. Pain is often difficult to localize but is mostly at the superomedial corner or inferior pole of the scapula [14–16] and is triggered by shoulder motion or shrugging of the shoulders [17, 18]. It can interfere with sports activities, particularly rapid overhead movement (swimming or throwing for example). A history of trauma or less commonly fractures of the scapula and ribs are noted [2, 11, 14, 16, 19–21], although the onset of symptoms is usually gradual. Examination may demonstrate winging of the scapula, an asymmetry of the static position of both shoulders, a spine or rib cage deformity, and sometimes visualisation of the snap is possible. Crepitus at the superomedial angle, the inferior pole of the scapula or along the medial border [3, 16] is palpated in the lateral decubitus position, with the upper limb in neutral whilst pushing the superomedial angle in a cranio-caudal direction [10]. Crepitus is also easily reproduced during abduction, accentuated when the superior angle of the scapula is being pressed against the chest wall [1, 22]. Conversely, lifting the scapula from the rib cage by

Fig. 2 Posterior view of the shoulder: Superficial plane (*D* deltoid, *T* trapezius); deep plane (*LS* levator of the scapulae, *Rm* rhomboid minor, *RM* rhomboid major, *LD* Latissimus dorsi, *S-S* sraspinatus, *I-S* infraspinatus, *TM* terres minor); nerve course (*a* accessory spinal nerve, *b* dorsal scapular nerve, *c* suprascapular nerve); artery course (*d* dorsal scapular artery); Bursae (*1* Scapulo-thoracic, *2* Scapulo-trapezial, *3* bursa between latissimus dorsi and inferior extremity of scapula)

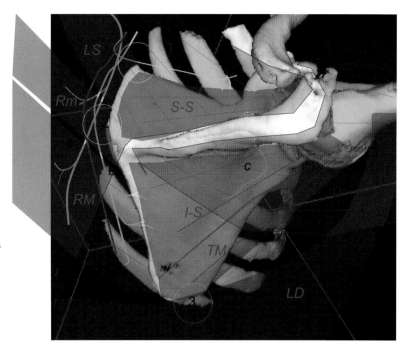

positioning the hand of the affected upper limb on the opposite shoulder decreases pain and snapping [23]. Muscular assessment is essential as well as an examination of the gleno-humeral joint and subacromial space. Bursitis presents with fullness over the bursa and palpation of the bursa elicits pain [2]. Pain can limit shoulder motion or lead to a compensating pseudo-winging of the scapula [1].

Anomalies and Radiological Presentation

Snapping scapulae are due to a disrupted gliding of the concave anterior aspect of the scapula over the convex thorax. A variety of causes have been reported but the condition remains poorly understood.

The causes can be classified as follows [10]: Local due to bursitis, which may be structural or functional. Structural causes include bone anomalies, such as scapular osteochondromata [15, 24] or as bony deformity following either/or scapula and rib fractures. Repetitive micro-trauma mostly described in throwing sports activities can create

bony excrescences; prominent supero-medial tubercle (Luschka's tubercle) or inferior tubercle (Fig. 3). In these patients, the condition is most often located at the infero-medial angle of the scapula. Functional causes are associated with anatomic anomalies: rib or scapula fracture malunion, dorsal spine deformity (scoliosis and kyphosis), and excessive forward curvature of the superomedial border. Other known causes are muscle detachment, serratus calcific tendonitis, malignant or benign (elastofibroma) tumours of the scapulo-thoracic space, and muscle atrophy narrowing the scapula-to-rib cage distance. Extrinsic aetiologies include overuse of the scapulo-thoracic gliding space due to pathology in another joint of the shoulder girdle: acromio-clavicular arthritis, gleno-humeral arthritis or stiffness, or rotator cuff tendinopathy.

Definitive causes are comparatively rare and the majority of patients present with poor posture and sagging of the shoulder girdle such that the superomedial corner descends and impinges on the chest wall. The pain is probably mediated by localized inflammation in the scapulo-thoracic bursa and leads to chronic thickening of the subscapular tissues [25].

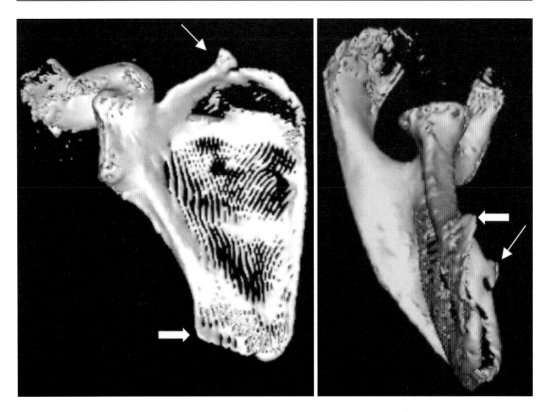

Fig. 3 Anterior view and inferior view of a left scapula responsible for snapping scapula, due to two tubercules, one superior, and the other inferior (*Thin arrow*: superior tubercule, *wide arrow*: inferior tubercule)

Radiological assessment should include plain radiographs of the scapula, especially a carefully positioned lateral view, which will assess the shape of the scapula and exclude an exostosis or obvious bony cause. Plain gleno-humeral or chest radiographs should be included if clinically indicated. Routine CT is of limited value and is difficult to interpret [26]. The radiation exposure of CT must also be considered and is therefore limited to patients with normal radiographs but suspicion of osseous lesions or fractures. Occasionally narrowing between the superomedial corner and the chest wall can be demonstrated when compared to the contralateral side [26, 27]. Modern CT-scan that provides high quality CT 3D reconstruction (Fig. 3) of the scapula and chest is indicated as it shows the accurate location of the snapping site, and superomedial scapula angulation. It is more sensitive than plain radiographs and regular CT-scan [28, 29]. MRI is not recommended, with the exception of defining bursitis or the rare case of tumour. Injection of local anaesthetic is sometimes valuable to confirm clinical interpretation [1, 10]. Differential diagnosis should also consider cardiothoracic diseases, disc protrusion and lung neoplasia.

Treatment

Non-Operative Treatment

Treatment of snapping scapula is usually non-operative, based on careful assessment and correction of abnormal posture plus training of the scapular muscles [16, 30]. The snapping or grating often disappears when the scapula is passively elevated and retracted. This can be demonstrated to the patient and is helpful in

Fig. 4 Chicken-wing position that places the shoulder in a position of extension, external rotation and adduction

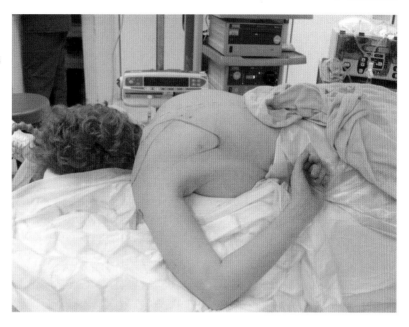

increasing the patient's understanding of the rehabilitation program. Scapula position is responsible for the static positioning of the shoulder girdle. Therefore, endurance training of the scapula musculature is crucial, particularly of the serratus anterior and subscapularis [31]. Postural training is required in the presence of Kyphosis and is based on promoting upright posture and strengthening upper thoracic musculature. To reduce the bursitis, non-operative treatment is often initiated by rest or modification of activities. A course of non-steroidal anti-inflammatory medications can help decrease inflammation [2]. In the presence of uncontrolled pain, corticosteroid injection is warranted [2, 13, 21]. The injection is given with the patient lying prone with the arm in the "chicken-wing position" (Fig. 4), and the hand behind the back. Before abandoning these measures in favour of surgery it is important to consider the natural history and the not infrequent association with psychological disorder. It is interesting to note that very few cases fail to resolve with time, and therefore non-operative treatment must be pursued for at least 6 months to 1 year. Beyond this if symptoms continue to be disabling surgical resection of the scapula may be indicated [3, 19, 22].

Operative Treatment

Open Surgical Technique

An open surgical procedure is a valid option for treating painful, audible and palpable crepitus resistant to non-operative treatment [2]. Neurologic deficit in the limb or wasting of periscapular musculature are contra-indications to surgery [1, 27]. The goal of surgical treatment is to remove the anatomical cause of the clunk, the location of which must be accurately determined pre-operatively [7].

The surgical options vary from open bursectomy (at the superomedial angle and or the inferomedial angle, which are the two most common locations for scapulo-thoracic bursitis) to partial scapulectomy.

Surgery at the inferior bursa is approached through an oblique incision distal to the inferior angle of the scapula. The trapezius and latissimus dorsi are split in line with the muscle fibres to expose the bursa. The bursitis must be thoroughly debrided and ensure all osteophytes on the scapula are removed. For superomedial bursitis, the skin is incised medially to the medial border of the scapula. The trapezius is dissected free and retracted superiorly from the scapular spine. The levator scapulae, subscapularis and suprapinatus are subsequently dissected and retracted proxi-mally through sub-periosteal dissection. The bursa can then be resected and any osteophytes removed. The muscles are re-attached anatomi-cally at the end of the procedure. Bony resection is performed if necessary as determined pre-operatively.

Some authors have suggested [1, 32] when no obvious bony lesion is noted, removal of the medial 2 cm of the scapula allows a more natural articulation of the scapulo-thoracic joint when the muscles are re-attached. However, care must be taken not to disrupt the muscles inserting on the medial border of the scapula. The medial border of the scapula contains the origin of subscapularis, suprapinatus, infraspinatus, serratus anterior, rhomboid and levator scapulae muscles. Significant post-operative disability can be caused by disruption of these muscles through resection of the entire medial border [28, 33]. More recently, authors have published successful treatment of snapping scapula with excision of only the superomedial border, thus avoiding these negative outcomes [1, 2].

To perform the superomedial scapular resec-tion, the patient is placed in the prone position, and an incision over the medial scapular spine is made with dissection through the soft tissue to expose the scapular spine. The perios-teum is incised with subperiosteal elevation of the medial periscapular muscles, including the supraspinatus, subscapularis, rhomboid, and levator scapulae, which are retracted proximally. The trapezius is retracted superiorly. The superomedial angle of the scapula is resected with an oscillating saw in the shape of an equi-lateral triangle extending to the medial base of the scapular spine. Elevated muscles are sutured to the spine of the scapula by drill holes. The affected arm is mobilized during surgery to con-firm relief of the snapping.

Endoscopic Procedure

An endoscopic technique for snapping scapula is an alternative to an open approach for bursectomy and resection of the superomedial corner of scapula, with the same indications and limitations. The morbidity is decreased with

earlier rehabilitation and cosmetic advantages [27, 34–36].

Under general anaesthesia, the patient is positioned in the lateral decubitus position or prone position, with upper limbs free to move. First, the scapulo-thoracic tactile and acoustic clunk is reproduced by positioning the upper limb in maximal internal rotation, with the hand on the back (Fig. 4). The surgeon draws landmarks on the patient's skin: posterior pro-cesses of spine, scapular spine, lateral border of acromion, and inferior border of the trapezius. Three arthroscopic portal sites are also drawn. The entire upper limb is draped. Two portals are placed on the medial border of the scapula approximately 3 cm medial to the border and below the level of the scapular spine [11, 13, 27, 31] to avoid injury to the dorsal scapular nerve and artery, and the accessory nerve (Fig. 5). The superior portal [31] is located one third of the distance from the medial scapular border, between the superior medial angle of the scapula and the lateral border of the acromion, to avoid the neurovascular structures (namely, accessory nerve, suprascapular nerve, dorsal scapular nerve and artery, coursing nearby). One of the medial portals is made first, without prior inflation of the bursa. The scope is pushed forward to the deepest and most anterior aspect of the scapula. Then a second medial portal is made (first instrument portal). The superior por-tal (second instrument portal) is created from inside to out.

The potential complications include penetra-tion of the thoracic cavity, penetration through the serratus anterior muscle into the axillary space or penetration through the scapular blade into the supraspinatus fossa [27, 34, 37]. Cannu-lae are not usually required and a 4.5 mm 30° scope is preferred. Exposure is initially gained by gradual debridement of the bursitis with a shaver or radio-frequency probe. The inflow pressure is set at 50 mm of Hg. Needling is useful to check the position of the scope and instruments [21]. There is no established crite-rion for ensuring a thorough bony resection (Fig. 6). However peri-operative examination combined with arthroscopic visualisation can

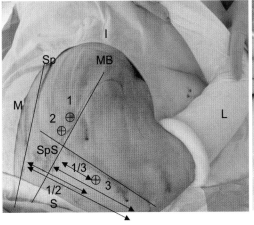
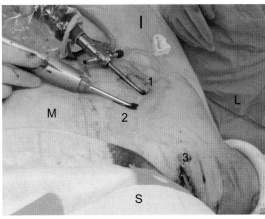

Fig. 5 Endoscopic portals, patient in prone position (Reference plane. *I* inferior, *S* superior, *M* medial, *L* lateral); *Left* figure: Portal skin drawings related to scapula and spine landmarks (*Sp* posterior processes of the spine, *MB* medial border of the scapula, *SpS* spine of the scapula); *Right* figure: Instrumental portals (*1* and *3*) and scope portal (*2*)

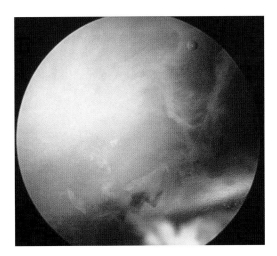

Fig. 6 Endoscopic view of scapulothoracic bursitis shaving

confirm smooth gliding of the scapula against the rib cage and absence of the clunk. Postoperative immobilisation is not required.

Conclusions

The results of non-operative treatment, arthroscopic, and open procedures are difficult to compare, due to the limited population in published series and the wide range of causes associated with snapping scapulae. However, the literature suggests successful non-operative treatment is as high as 80 % [8, 23]. Operative treatment, either arthroscopic or open, is also successful with appropriate pre-operative planning as the aetiology of the clunk is identified and then surgically removed.

Acknowledgments This review article was inspired by the work of Demoisnault et al. and Kuhne et and therefore we would like to give special acknowledgment to these authors.

References

1. Kuhne M, Boniquit N, Ghodadra N, Romeo AA, Provencher MT. The snapping scapula: diagnosis and treatment. Arthroscopy. 2009;25–11:1298–311.
2. Kuhn JE, Plancher KD, Hawkins RJ. Symptomatic scapulothoracic crepitus and bursitis. J Am Acad Orthop Surg. 1998;6–5:267–73.
3. Percy EC, Birbrager D, Pitt MJ. Snapping scapula: a review of the literature and presentation of 14 patients. Can J Surg. 1988;31–4:248–50.
4. Boinet W. Fait clinique. Bull Soc Imp Chir Paris, 2e Sér. 1867;8:458.
5. Milch H, Burman MS. Snapping scapula and humerus varus. Arch Surg. 1933;26:510–85.
6. Mauclaire A. Craquements sous-scapulaires pathologiques traités par l'interposition musculaire

interscapulothoracique. Bull Mem Soc Chir Paris. 1904;30:164–8.

7. Milch H. Partial scapulectomy for snapping of the scapula. J Bone Joint Surg Am. 1950;32-A(3):561–6.

8. Ciullo J. Subscapular bursitis: "Treatment of snapping scapula" or "washboard syndrome". Arthroscopy. 1992;8:412–3.

9. Wallach F. Etude anatomique pour l'abord endoscopique de l'espace scapulo-thoracique. Thèse de Doctorat en médecine, Université Paris VI; 2005.

10. Desmoineaux P, Wallach F, Jouve F, Boisrenoult P. Endoscopic treatment of snapping scapula. Chir Main. 2006;25 Suppl 1:S91–5.

11. Chan BK, Chakrabarti AJ, Bell SN. An alternative portal for scapulothoracic arthroscopy. J Shoulder Elbow Surg. 2002;11–3:235–8.

12. McFarland EG, Tanaka MJ, Papp DF. Examination of the shoulder in the overhead and throwing athlete. Clin Sports Med. 2008;27–4:553–78.

13. Pearse EO, Bruguera J, Massoud SN, Sforza G, Copeland SA, Levy O. Arthroscopic management of the painful snapping scapula. Arthroscopy. 2006;22–7:755–61.

14. Nicholson GP, Duckworth MA. Scapulothoracic bursectomy for snapping scapula syndrome. J Shoulder Elbow Surg. 2002;11–1:80–5.

15. Edelson JG. Variations in the anatomy of the scapula with reference to the snapping scapula. Clin Orthop Relat Res. 1996;322:111–5.

16. Manske RC, Reiman MP, Stovak ML. Nonoperative and operative management of snapping scapula. Am J Sports Med. 2004;32–6:1554–65.

17. Cobey MC. The rolling scapula. Clin Orthop Relat Res. 1968;60:193–4.

18. Kouvalchouk JF, Merat J, Durey A. Subscapular snapping. Rev Chir Orthop Reparatrice Appar Mot. 1985;71 Suppl 2:78–81.

19. Richards RR, McKee MD. Treatment of painful scapulothoracic crepitus by resection of the superomedial angle of the scapula. A report of three cases. Clin Orthop Relat Res. 1989;247:111–6.

20. Daigeler A, Vogt PM, Busch K, Pennekamp W, Weyhe D, Lehnhardt M, Steinstraesser L, Steinau HU, Kuhnen C. Elastofibroma dorsi – differential diagnosis in chest wall tumours. World J Surg Oncol. 2007;5:15.

21. van Riet RP, Van Glabbeek F. Arthroscopic resection of a symptomatic snapping subscapular osteochondroma. Acta Orthop Belg. 2007;73–2:252–4.

22. Milch H. Snapping scapula. Clin Orthop. 1961;20:139–50.

23. Carlson HL, Haig AJ, Stewart DC. Snapping scapula syndrome: three case reports and an analysis of the literature. Arch Phys Med Rehabil. 1997;78–5:506–11.

24. Parsons TA. The snapping scapula and subscapular exostoses. J Bone Joint Surg Br. 1973;55–2:345–9.

25. Sisto DJ, Jobe FW. The operative treatment of scapulothoracic bursitis in professional pitchers. Am J Sports Med. 1986;14–3:192–4.

26. de Haart M, van der Linden ES, de Vet HC, Arens H, Snoep G. The value of computed tomography in the diagnosis of grating scapula. Skeletal Radiol. 1994;23–5:357–9.

27. Harper GD, McIlroy S, Bayley JI, Calvert PT. Arthroscopic partial resection of the scapula for snapping scapula: a new technique. J Shoulder Elbow Surg. 1999;8–1:53–7.

28. Mozes G, Bickels J, Ovadia D, Dekel S. The use of three-dimensional computed tomography in evaluating snapping scapula syndrome. Orthopedics. 1999;22–11:1029–33.

29. Oizumi N, Suenaga N, Minami A. Snapping scapula caused by abnormal angulation of the superior angle of the scapula. J Shoulder Elbow Surg. 2004;13–1:115–8.

30. Tripp BL. Principles of restoring function and sensorimotor control in patients with shoulder dysfunction. Clin Sports Med. 2008;27–3:507–19, x.

31. Pavlik A, Ang K, Coghlan J, Bell S. Arthroscopic treatment of painful snapping of the scapula by using a new superior portal. Arthroscopy. 2003;19–6:608–12.

32. Cameron HU. Snapping scapulae: a report of three cases. Eur J Rheumatol Inflamm. 1984;7–2:66–7.

33. Alvik I. Snapping scapula and Sprengel's deformity. Acta Orthop Scand. 1959;29:10–5.

34. Bell SN, van Riet RP. Safe zone for arthroscopic resection of the superomedial scapular border in the treatment of snapping scapula syndrome. J Shoulder Elbow Surg. 2008;17–4:647–9.

35. Fukunaga S, Futani H, Yoshiya S. Endoscopically assisted resection of a scapular osteochondroma causing snapping scapula syndrome. World J Surg Oncol. 2007;5:37.

36. Lien SB, Shen PH, Lee CH, Lin LC. The effect of endoscopic bursectomy with mini-open partial scapulectomy on snapping scapula syndrome. J Surg Res. 2008;150–2:236–42.

37. Ruland 3rd LJ, Ruland CM, Matthews LS. Scapulothoracic anatomy for the arthroscopist. Arthroscopy. 1995;11–1:52–6.

Fractures of the Scapula

Norbert Suedkamp and Kaywan Izadpanah

Contents

N. Suedkamp (✉) • K. Izadpanah
Department for Orthopedic Surgery and Traumatology,
Freiburg University Hospital, Freiburg, Germany
e-mail: norbert.suedkamp@uniklinik-freiburg.de;
kaywan.izadpanah@uniklinik-freiburg.de

G. Bentley (ed.), *European Surgical Orthopaedics and Traumatology*,
DOI 10.1007/978-3-642-34746-7_242, © EFORT 2014

Keywords

Aetiology • Anatomy • Classification • Clinical features • Complications • Imaging • Results • Scapular fractures • Surgical indications • Techniques • Treatment-conservative, Surgical

General Introduction

Scapular fractures are uncommon injuries and account for only 1 % of all fractures [5], approximately 5 % of all fractures of the shoulder girdle and 3 % of all injuries to the shoulder [41]. Scapular fractures occur preferentially in young males (m/f = 6/49) between 25 and 50 years [3, 40, 60, 66]. 45 % of all scapula fractures occur in the body, 35 % involve the glenoid process (25 % Glenoid neck, 10 % Glenoid cavity), 8 % the acromion and 7 % the coracoid process. Only 10 % of the fractures to the scapular body and the glenoid neck show significant displacement [52].

Scapula fractures are frequently acquired during high-energy trauma and therefore patients suffer a mean of 3.9 associated injuries, predominantly of the chest, the ipsilateral upper extremity and to the skull or brain. All of them are potentially life-threatening. Therefore, patients with scapular fractures should, where possible, be managed in trauma centres.

For a long-time scapular fractures have been treated nearly always conservatively. However, fractures of the scapula have received more consideration in the recent literature and many papers are dealing with specific issues. With increasing knowledge about biomechanics of the upper extremity and invention of modern implants there is evidence that some injuries deserve operative treatment to assure good functional outcome. Therefore, Treatment of scapular fractures belongs in the hands of an experienced Orthopaedic or Trauma surgeon.

This chapter gives a comprehensive overview of current classification systems, standards of treatment and the latest operative techniques for treatment of scapular fractures.

Important biomechanical theories of the scapular suspensory system and simple strategies for decision-making and planning of operative treatment are proposed.

Aetiology and Classification

Eighty to Ninety percent of all scapular fractures occur during high-energy trauma such as motor vehicle collisions or falls from great height [30, 40].

Scapula Body

The majority of scapular body fractures result from direct, blunt trauma. Forces have to be great to cause a fracture of the scapula body due to its great mobility, the thick surrounding deep and superficial muscles layers and the flexibility of the chest wall ("recoil mechanism "of the chest wall) [53].

Some cases report scapular body fractures after electric shock [8, 58] or after seizures with osteodystrophy [38].

Nevertheless, there is a huge variety of fracture patterns existing. The OTA proposed a classification system in two levels. Level 1 as a basic system for all trauma surgeons and Level 2 for specialized Shoulder Surgeons.

In Level 1 the scapula is divided into three regions:

1. The articular segment (Coded F) – which is the area involving the glenoid fossa and the articular rim, limited dorsally by a line joining the dorsal articular rim to the suprascapular notch, distally by the articular rim and medially by a line joining the suprascapular notch to the distal articular rim.

2. The Processes (Coded P) – the coracoid is defined by the dorsal limit of the articular segment, the acromion is lateral to the plane of the glenoid fossa and

3. The Body (Coded B) –the rest of the scapula bone

Articular fractures are subdivided into three groups:

F0 are Fracture of the articular segment, that do not pass through the *fossa glenoidalis*/glenoid rim at all.

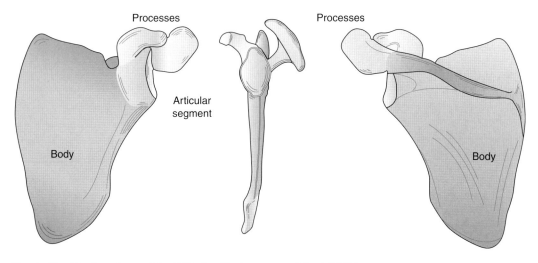

Fig. 1 Classification scheme of the OTA-classification system of the AO/OTA

F1 fractures have a simple articular fragment pattern. They are rim or split fractures that involve the glenoid fossa. Very small fragments less than 2 mm should not be considered for classification. F2 fractures are real multi-fragmentary joint fractures.

Body fractures can be divided into simple indention fractures (B1) with two or less main fragments and complex body fractures (B2) with 3 or more fragments. Fractures of the coracoid process (P1) do not affect the glenoid, as they are articular fractures. Fractures of the acromion are Type A2 fractures and fractures of both processes are A3 fractures. For further details of the level two classification system please see the AO webpage (Figs. 1 and 2).

B		Fx located within the Body
	B1	Simple (Two or less body fracture exits)
	B2	Complex body involvement (Three or more body fracture exits)
P		**Process fracture**
	P1	Coracoid fracture (Separate fracture line not affecting the glenoid fossa nor any part of the body)
	P2	Acromion fracture (Fracture line lateral to the plane of the glenoid fossa)
	P3	Fracture of both coracoid and acromion

F		Fx of articular segment
	F0	Fracture of the articular segment, not through the fossa glenoidalis/glenoid rim
	F1	Simple pattern with two articular fragments: rim or split fracture (Fracture involves the Glenoid Fossa) (Ignore small fragments up to about 2 mm)
	F2	Multi-fragmentary joint fracture (Fracture involves the Glenoid Fossa) (Three or more articular fragments)
	Fx	.1 = without body involvement
		.2 = with simple body involvement
		.3 = with complex body involvement

(*continued*)

Glenoid Neck Fractures

Fractures of the Glenoid neck may be caused by
- impactation of the humeral head against the Glenoid process or
- a blow over the anterior or posterior aspect of the shoulder,
- fall on the outstretched arm, when the humeral had is impacted against the glenoid process or in rare cases by fall on the superior aspect of the shoulder complex [52].

There are three types of glenoid neck fractures [20].

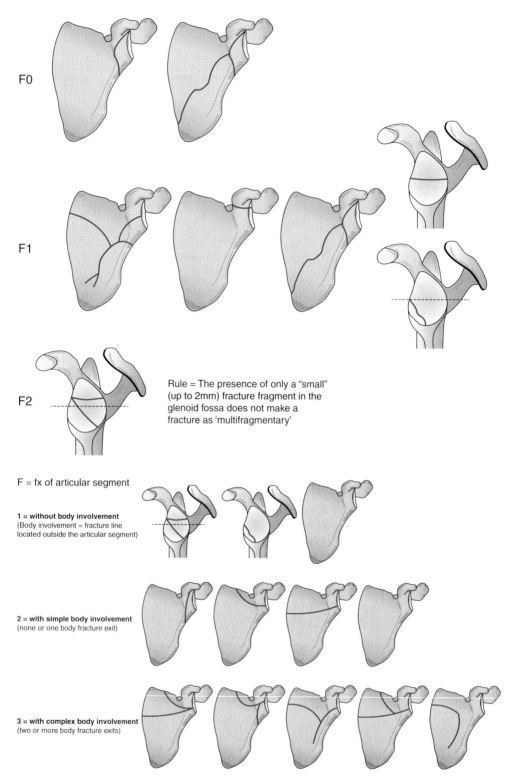

Fig. 2 (continued)

B = Fx located within the Body
(*extra-articular fracture with no Glenoid Fossa involvement*)

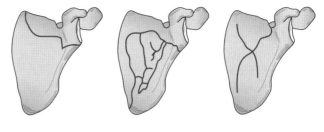

B1 = Simple
(*two or less body fracture exits*)

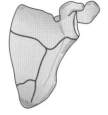

B2 = Complex body involvement
(*Three or more body fracture exits*)

Note this fracture is NOT
a coracoid fracture as it enters
the glenoid fossa

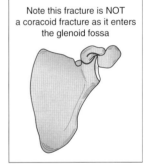

P = Process fracture
(*seperate coding*)

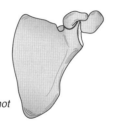

P1 = Corecoid fracture
(*Seperate fracture line not affecting the glenoid fossa not any part of the body*)

P2 = Acromion fracture
(*Fracture line lateral to the plane of the glenoid fossa*)

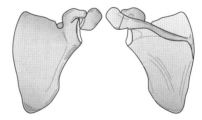

P3 = Fracture of the both coracoid and acromion

Fig. 2 Classification system of scapular fractures according to OTA/AO

One incomplete neck fracture, with the fracture line entering at the inferior border of the glenoid neck, running along the scapular spine and exiting at the medial border. Furthermore there exist two types of complete glenoid neck fractures:

One fracture along the surgical neck and the other along the glenoid neck fractures, anatomic neck.

To be complete the fracture lines have to exit the lateral and the superior border of the scapula.

Fractures of the surgical neck extend medial to the coracoid process and those of the anatomic neck lateral to the coracoid process. A clinical treatment-based classification of glenoid neck fractures is based on the extent of the glenoid fragment dislocation:

Type I Fractures are insignificantly or undisplaced.
Type II fractures are significantly displaced [20].

Zdravkovic and Damholt [69], Nordqvist and Petersson [45] and Ada and Miller [44] defined a major displacement of the glenoid fragment as more than 1 cm or greater than 40° of angulation.

Blauth, Suedkamp and Haas [9] provided a more detailed classification, including the fracture pattern and criteria of stability (Figs. 3 and 4, Table 1).

Combined Glenoid Neck and Clavicle Fractures (Including Floating Shoulder)

Fractures of the clavicle are accompanied with glenoid neck fractures in about 20–50 % [1, 3]. Mechanisms of injury are a fall onto the outstretched arm, a fall onto the shoulder tip or a direct blow [52]. Ganz and Noesberger [15] were the first to describe an altered stability of the glenoid fracture component in cases of additional ipsilateral clavicle fracture. Hersovici and co-workers [28] introduced the term "floating shoulder" for the combination of these fractures. However, biomechanical testing revealed that only an additional disruption of the coraco-acromial or acromio-clavicular ligaments alter the stability of the glenoid. Goss [19] and co-workers therefore introduced the concept of a double disruption of the superior suspensory complex (SSSC) for the definition of a floating shoulder injury.

Glenoid Fossa

Fractures of the *Glenoid rim* are caused by an impact of the humeral head against the periphery of the glenoid cavity [27]. These fractures have to be distinguished from avulsion fractures of the

glenoid rim occurring during dislocation of the humeral head [65]. In the latter, forces meet the peri-articular soft tissue [11]. An avulsion fracture of the glenoid rim results from traction-forces of the surrounding soft tissue. Fractures of the *Glenoid fossa* result from a lateral impact to the humeral head [18], which is then driven into the centre of the glenoid cavity.

A transverse fracture line develops. This mechanism is supported, according to the literature [18, 21] as follows:

1. The concave shape of the glenoid fossa. Therefore, forces concentrate in the centre of the glenoid.
2. The transverse orientation of the subchondral trabeculae. Therefore, forces can spread easily along this orientation.
3. A Crook along the anterior rim, which is a stress-riser. Fractures tend to originate there.
4. The fact that two ossification centres form the glenoid cavity. Therefore, the centre region might remain as a relative "soft spot".

Depending on the sub-direction of the applied force to the humeral head a developing fracture line will propagate. Violent forces can lead to a comminute fracture of the glenoid fossa [18] (Table 2).

Coracoid Process

Ogawa et al. [49] proposed a classification for fractures of the Coracoid process that divides them in two Groups:

Type 1 with the fracture line proximal to the coraco-clavicular ligaments and

Type 2 with the fracture line distal to the coraco-clavicular ligaments.

Type 1 fractures are avulsion fractures that are acquired during indirect trauma. Type 2 fractures can be treated conservatively when not significantly displaced. They are caused either by direct blow or indirectly by a dislocating humeral head. Treatment of Type 1 fractures depends on the concomitant injuries. In cases of an additional alteration

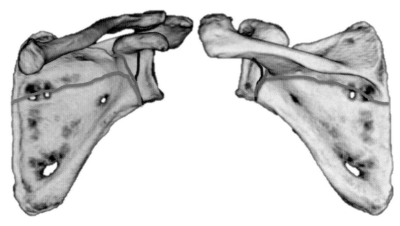

Fig. 3 Illustration depicting three basic fracture patterns involving the glenoid neck: *A* fracture through the anatomical neck, *B* fracture through the surgical neck, and *C* fracture involving the inferior glenoid neck, which then courses medially to exit through the scapular body (this type is managed as a scapular body fracture) (From [20])

of the scapular connection, i.e. the acromio-clavicular joint, an operative refixation is recommended. Isolated injuries can be treated conservatively (see Table 3).

Fractures of the Acromion

Acromial fractures are caused by direct trauma to the acromion or the humeral head directed towards the acromion. Avulsion fractures arise from indirect trauma while tensioning of the coraco-acromial and acromio-clavicular ligaments or the deltoid and trapezeus muscle. Some cases of stress or fatigue fractures have been reported [22]. Kuhn et al. [36] proposed a classification of the Acromion in 1994. Non-displaced Fractures (Type 1) were divided into Avulsion (Type 1a) or Complete (Type 1b) fractures. They can be treated conservatively as no alteration to subacromial space develops. Type 2 fractures of the acromion are displaced but do not reduce the subacromial space. They can predominantly be treated conservatively as well.

If an inferior displacement of the acromion appears (Type 3a) or a combined fracture of the Acromion with a fracture of the glenoid neck (Type 3 b) a narrowing of the subacromial space develops. These fractures should be treated

operatively. However there was a certain criticism to this classification scheme [43, 59] (Table 4).

Scapulo-Thoracic Dissociation

Only exceptional forces can lead to a scapulo-thoracic dissociation (a closed avulsion of the scapula) [13, 50, 70]. This injury is associated with a large spectrum of concomitant osseous, vascular and neurological injuries.

The scapula is dislocated posteriorly from the chest-wall. This can best be diagnosed in coronal CT-Scans of the chest, by determining the distance between the medial border of the scapula and the spinosus process on the healthy and injured side. These patients are always multiple and severely injured. This injury is also called an internal forequarter amputation.

Relevant Applied Anatomy

Anatomy

The *scapula* is a large flat bone. It has a triangular shape and four major processes: the spine, the acromion, the glenoid process and the coracoid process. The scapular body thickness can become less than 2 mm in its central part. The superior, lateral and medial border is thickened as greater muscles insert here. At the base of the coracoid

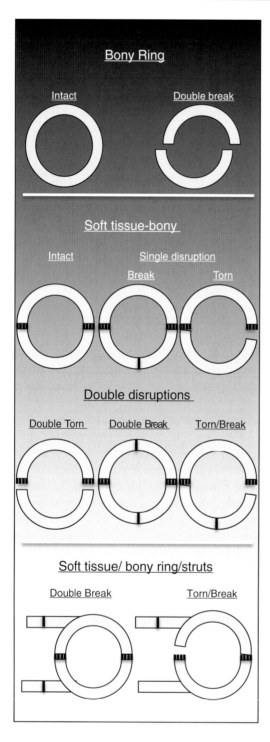

Fig. 4 Illustrations depicting the many possible traumatic ring – strut disruptions (From [19]. é Raven Press, Ltd., New York)

lies the suprascapular notch. The greater scapular notch or spinogelnoidal notch is at the base of the spine. Fractures of the glenoid neck that occur in this notch can be associated with suprascapular nerve palsy. From the *anterior fasciae* of the scapula the subscapularis muscle, the omohyoid and the serratus anterior muscle originate. From the posterior fascia the levator scapulae, the major and minor rhomboid, the supraspinatus and the infraspinatus the latissimus dorsi and the teres major and minor muscles originate (Fig. 11). The coraco-acromial and the transverse scapular ligaments are two ligaments that insert and originate at the same bone, the scapula. The coraco-clavicular the acromio-clavicular, the glenohumeral and the coracohumeral ligaments are the major ligaments of the scapula. The coraco-clavicular ligament is divided into the conoid and trapezoid ligament which form the suspension of the scapula. The surrounding soft tissue offers strong protection and therefore fractures of the scapula body only occur during high-energy traumas.

The *coracoid process* is a hook-like structure, pointing laterally forward. Its base begins between the glenoid process and the anterior margin. It has great clinical relevance as "Surgeon's Lighthouse" during operative procedures. All major neurovascular structures of the upper limb lie medial to this easy-to-identify landmark. Staying lateral to the coracoid process during surgical procedures avoids neurovascular damage.

The pectoralis minor muscle, the biceps brachii and the coracobrachialis muscle originate from the coracoid process. The latter two form the so-called conjoined tendon.

The coraco-acromial and coraco-clavicular ligaments (formed by the conoid ligament and trapezoid ligament.) insert at the coracoid process. The latter participate in the Clavicular–CC-ligamentous-coracoid (C4)-linkage, the major suspension system of the scapula (see below). Anatomic abnormalities of the coraco-clavicular connection have been described in 1 % of all humans, such as a joint or bony connection. There are some cases of coracoid impingement syndrome reported [12, 17, 51].

Table 1 Classification of glenoid neck fractures according to Blauth, Suedkamp and Haas [9]

Classification of scapular neck fractures				
I	**Fractures of the anatomic neck**			
I A	Non-displaced fractures	Medial compression	Stable	Conservative treatment
I B	Displaced fractures	Dist. and lat. glenoidal dislocation	Unstable	ORIF
II	**Fractures of the surgical neck**			
II A	Non-displaced fractures	Clavicle and cor-cor.-lig. not injured	Stable	Conservative treatment
II B	Displaced fractures	Clavicular fracture	Unstable	ORIF of the clavicle
		Ruptured cc-lig. ("Floating shoulder")	Unstable	ORIF of glenoid neck

Table 2 Ideberg classification scheme

Classification of glenoid fractures according to Ideberg/ Goss TP	
I	Fractures of the glenoid rim
I A	Anterior
I B	Posterior
II	Transverse or oblique fracture through the glenoid fossa
II A	Transverse fracture through the glenoid fossa, with an inferior triangular fragment displaced with the subluxated humeral head
II B	Oblique fracture through the glenoid fossa, with an inferior triangular fragment displaced with the subluxated humeral head
III	Oblique fracture through the glenoid exiting at the mid-superior border of the scapula
IV	Horizontal fracture, exciting through the medial border of the blade
V	Combination of type IV with a fracture separating the inferior half of the glenoid
VI	Severe comminution of the glenoid surface

Table 3 Classification system of coracoid fractures according to Ogawa et al.

Classification according to Ogawa [49]	
Type I	Proximal to the coraco-clavicular ligaments
Type II	Distal to the coraco-clavicular ligaments

Table 4 Classification system of acromion fractures

Classification according to Kuhn [36]	
I	**Non-displaced fractures of the acromion**
I a	Avulsion fracture
I b	Complete fracture
II	**Displaced fractures of the acromion, but not reducing the subacromial space**
III	**Displaced fractures of the acromion with reduction of the subacromial space**
III a	Inferior displacement of the acromion
III b	Superiorly-displaced glenoid neck fracture

it bends over anteriorly, forming the summit of the shoulder and overhanging the glenoid cavity.

Moreover the acromion contributes to the acromio-clavicular joint. It is an important component of the superior suspensory complex-forming the acromial strut (see below). An unfused acromion (os acromiale) has to be distinguished from a true acromial fracture. The acromion gives posterosuperior stability to the glenohumeral joint.

The glenoid neck is the portion between the scapular body and the glenoid cavity. From its superior aspect the coracoid process arises. Its stability depends on the osseous connection with the scapular body (1) and its superior suspension through the coracoid process and the coraco-clavicular ligaments (2) to the clavicle–acromioclavicular joint–acromial strut. If, in addition to the scapular body junction, the superior suspension is altered, fractures are defined as unstable or have a high likelihood to dislocate. From the supra-genoidal tubercle the long head of the biceps brachii muscle originates and from the infra-glenoidal tubercle the coracobrachial muscle.

The scapular spine is a bony prominence that starts at the medial margin and ends in the acromion. It gives insertion to the trapezeus muscle and the posterior deltoid muscle originates here. Because of its prominence it gives relevant contribution to the lever arm of these muscles. The acromion is the continuation of the spine and

Superior Suspensory Complex

The glenoid process, the coracoid process, the acromion, the acromio-clavicular joint, the lateral clavicle and the coraco-clavicular ligaments together form the superior suspensory complex. It consists of two bony struts and a bone-soft-tissue ring. The superior strut is the lateral clavicle and the inferior strut is the changeover from the glenoid process to the scapular body. The complex can be sudivided into three further partitions:

- The clavicular- acromioclavicular joint-acromial strut
- The three-process-scapular body junction and last but not least
- The C-4 linkage (Clavicle, coraco-clavicular ligaments and the coracoid process).

The SSSC is of extreme importance with regard to the biomechanics of the shoulder joint. It enables the very limited but crucial movement and changes of the acromio-clavicular joint and the coraco-clavicular distance. The clavicle is the only bony connection of the upper extremity to the skeleton and the scapula is suspended to the clavicle through the coraco-clavicular ligaments (C4 linkage). Goss et al. [19] presented the double disruption concept of the SSSC. Following this very simple idea one can understand the diversity of complex injury combinations of the shoulder girdle and perform correct decision-making even in rarely encountered injuries.

Diagnosis

Scapular fractures are predominantly acquired in high-energy trauma [29]. The primary treating physician should therefore be aware of the frequently associated injuries that can potentially be life-threatening. i.e., thoraco-scapular dissociations are regularly associated with disruptions of the subclavian or axillary vessels [70].

Moreover the treating surgeon should be aware of the complex function of the scapula and its process during arm movement. Diagnosis of scapular fractures should increase awareness of functionally associated injuries, i.e. a fracture

Table 5 Radiographic evaluation of the scapula "Trauma series"

Radiological view	Check for
True anteroposterior (AP)	Glenoid
	Scapula neck
	Scapula body, medial part
	Medial margin
	Scapular spine
Lateral view	Scapular body
True axillary	Acromion,
	AC-joint
	Coracoid process
	Glenoid, anterior and posterior borders

of the coracoid process might indicate prior (sub-) luxation of the glenohumeral joint [14] or, in association with glenoid neck fractures, a double disruption of the superior suspensory complex. Therefore treatment of scapular fractures belongs in the hands of an experienced Orthopaedic surgeon.

Clinical Features

Patients suffering a scapular fracture regularly complain of local pain or tenderness. The relieving posture of a patient presenting in the emergency department is an adduction of the ipsilateral arm, because tenderness and pain increases during arm abduction. Local signs might be crepitus and swelling, however due to the compact surrounding muscles and compartments they may be minor. Before the era of CT-scanning in polytraumatized patients these fractures where overlooked in up to 30 % [60].

Radiographic Evaluation

All scapular fractures can be identified in conventional radiographs. For correct diagnosing of the injury pattern all four processes of the scapula have to be displayed (see Table 5). The complex interaction of the scapula, a careful evaluation of the glenohumeral joint, the acromio-clavicular joint and the scapulo-thoracic articulation have to be performed. Complex injury patterns such as a double disruption of the superior suspensory or alteration to the C4 linkage should be actively excluded in all cases. If any doubts remain weight-bearing AP radiographs of the AC- joint or if available weight-bearing MRI of the shoulder should be performed.

A scapula trauma series should include a true anteroposterior (AP), view a lateral view and a true axillary view of the glenohumeral joint.

McAdams and co-workers did not find an improvement in evaluation of scapular neck fractures by performing a CT-scan [39]. However, they did point out that associated injuries to the SSSC can be detected more easily. The author's belief is that CT-scans should regularly be performed in cases of scapular neck fractures to determine if they are indeed complete and define associated injuries. Using modern post-processing software solutions and 3-D reformatting can provide substantial information of operative planning [2]. Moreover, the use of routine CT-Scans in the diagnostics of polytraumatized patients will probably reduce the former high rates of overlooked scapular fractures [37].

Frequently-Associated Injuries

About 61–88 % of all patients, suffering a scapular fracture, present with associated injuries [37, 54]. Thompson et al. described an average of 3.9 associated injuries [29] per patient. Chest trauma was found to be the most common site of concomitant injury. Rib fractures occurred in 32–45 % [37] and accompanying pulmonary contusion or pneumo-haemato-pneumothorax was found in 15–50 % of these patients [42]. Fractures of the ipsilateral limb can be found regularly: 15–40 % suffer concomitant ipsilateral clavicular fractures and 12 % ipsilateral humeral head fractures. Five to ten percent suffer injuries to the brachial plexus or the subclavian or axillary arteries [13, 23, 46, 61]. Neurovascular Injuries significantly determine the patient's morbidity after treatment. In general morbidity of the patient highly correlates with the

associated injuries [3]. Lantry and co-workers found head injuries to be associated to scapular fractures in 20 % [23, 37]. The presence of scapular fractures in polytraumatized patients correlates with a greater severity score [63] but they are no marker for greater mortality or neurovascular morbidity [56].

Indications for Surgery

Scapular fractures are predominantly acquired during high-energy trauma and are regularly associated with other severe or life-threatening injuries. However, the scapular fracture itself is rarely a surgical emergency except for cases with thoracic penetration or exceptional dislocation of fracture components [10, 24]. Thus, surgical management of the scapular fracture should be performed during "reconvalescence" of the polytraumatized patient. Because of the complex interactions of the scapula and its importance for adequate movement of the whole upper extremity meticulous diagnostics should be performed. An experienced Trauma or Orthopaedic surgeon should decide on surgery or conservative treatment.

A general surgical directive
Surgery is always recommended if there is a relevant alteration to the
1. Scapula suspensory system (SSSC; C4-linkage)
2. Position and integrity of glenoid (articular surface)
3. Lateral column displacement is present
Relevant decision points are
1. Is the SSSC (cor-CCL-clav-ACJ-spine) intact?
2. Is the glenoid fossa in continuity with the SSSC?
3. Is the glenoid fossa intact?
4. Is the lateral column (scapular shape) intact?

Scapular Body Fractures

Isolated fractures of the Scapular body can appear alarming on the x-rays. However, the scapulo-thoracic articulation can largely compensate for deformation of the scapula. The surrounding thick soft-tissue layer prevents further dislocation of the fracture components [31]. Nordquist and Petersson found functional impairment of patients

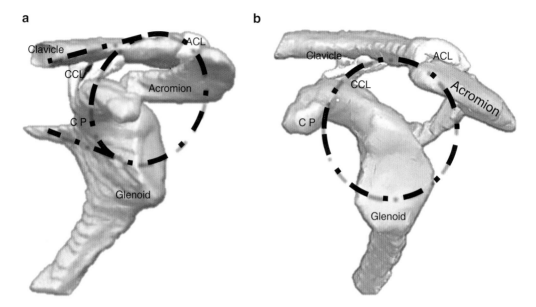

Fig. 5 Illustrations depicting the superior shoulder suspensory complex. (**a**) AP view of the bone – soft tissue ring and the superior and inferior bony struts. (**b**) Lateral view of the bone – soft tissue ring (From [19]. é Raven Press, Ltd., New York)

with fracture-dislocation greater than 1 cm [45]. The authors believe that operative treatment should be considered on a case-based decision with regard to the degree of fracture component dislocation.

In cases of a dissociated suspensory system surgery is always indicated (See Fig. 5 white arrow). In a systematic review of 520 scapula fractures Zlowodki and co-workers [71] found that 99 % of all isolated scapula body fractures were being treated conservatively and in 86 % a good to excellent functional outcome was achieved. It has to be pointed out, that in this review all operatively-treated patients showed excellent functional outcome. Therefore, surgery should not be avoided if indicated. In the literature one case is reported with a fracture spike entering the glenohumeral joint [24] and two cases of intra-thoracic penetration of fracture fragments [10, 26] requiring surgical management.

Glenoid Neck Fractures

Complete glenoid neck fractures cross along the lateral margin of the scapula and the superior margin either lateral (anatomical neck) or medial (surgical neck) to the coracoid process.

Fractures along the anatomical neck occur only occasionally [4, 24] but have to be considered as inherently instable. The glenoid cavity has completely lost it suspension and it is usually displaced distally and laterally, due to the pull of the long head of the triceps muscle. These fractures always need open reduction and internal fixation of the glenoid.

Type 1 glenoid neck fractures of the surgical neck are only minimally displaced (<1 cm) or show angular displacement less than 40°. About 90 % of all scapular neck fracture account for this entity. The management is conservative and good to excellent functional results can be expected.

Type 2 glenoid neck fractures showing significant displacement of the glenoid and require operative stabilization. The glenoid predominantly presents with medialization and long head overturning. This is due to the pull of the long head of the triceps muscle. Significant displacement was described as greater than 1 cm independently by Zdravkovic [69], Nordqist [45] and Ada and Miller [1]. This degree of

Fig. 6 Illustrations depicting a transverse disruption of the glenoid cavity and the factors responsible for this orientation. (**a**) The concave shape of the glenoid concentrates forces across its central region (*arrow*). (**b**) The subchondral trabeculae are oriented in the transverse plane. (**c**) A crook along the anterior rim (*arrow*) is a stress riser where fractures tend to originate. (**d**) Formed from a superior and an inferior ossification centre, the glenoid cavity may have a persistently weak central zone (From [21])

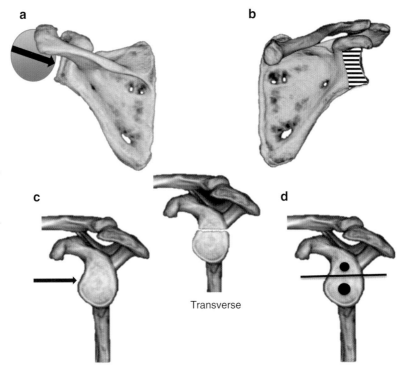

displacement leads to an interference of the humeral head with the coraco-acromial arc during arm abduction [24]. A rotator cuff dysfunction, predominantly of the abduction can be expected, leading to subacromial pain and reduced range of motion. Ada and Miller additionally stated that angular displacement greater than 40° is not tolerable, either in coronal or sagital plane. Inferior angulation greater than 20° was defined as intolerable by van Noort and Kampen [62]. However these angulatory displacements are difficult to detect in conventional radiographs and the authors recommend performing CT-scans for decision-making. In these cases open reduction and internal fixation of the glenoid has to be performed to prevent persistent pain and impaired arm movement.

Combined Glenoid Neck and Clavicle Fractures (Including Floating Shoulder)

Combinations of a glenoid neck with a clavicle fracture can occur with or without a rupture of the coraco-acromial ligaments. Whenever the CC- ligaments are torn internal fixation of the glenoid is indicated. In case of intact CC-ligaments *scapular neck osteosynthesis* is indicated if significant displacement of the glenoid fragment (>2,5 cm medial or >40° dysangulation) is present.

Isolated clavicle osteosynthesis should be performed if only the clavicle is displaced or shortened. If the coraco-clavicular ligaments remain intact repositioning of the moderately-displaced glenoid fracture component through re-positioning of the clavicle might occur [25]. However, reorientation of the glenoid fragment is crucial for the clinical outcome and should be achieved in all cases. Internal fixation of the clavicle and the scapula is recommended if both fractures show significant dislocation (Fig. 6).

Glenoid Cavity Fractures

Glenoid fractures were divided by Goss and Ideberg into glenoid rim fractures (type 1), Glenoid fossa fractures (type 2–5) and comminuted fractures of the glenoid (Type 6) [18] (details see below). Most fractures of the glenoid cavity (90 %) can be treated non-operatively.

Operative treatment is recommended in Type 1 fractures associated with a persisting instability of the glenohumeral joint and all fractures with an intra-articular displacement greater than 5 mm [34]. In Type 1 fractures persisting instability can be assumed in fractures displaced greater than 1 cm or if the posterior rim component is greater than a fourth of its cavity and posterior fracture components. As secondary subluxation or luxation can happen unnoticed Indication for operative treatment should be followed generously. Yamamoto and co-workers [68] suggested that operative stabilization of the glenoid should be performed if the anterior glenoid rim fragment is larger than 20 % of the glenoid length because of the development of an anterior instability.

Type 2 fractures should be treated surgically if an intra-articular gap greater than 5 mm exists or an inferior subluxation of the humeral head is present. These injuries are associated with a significant amount of glenohumeral arthrosis or instability [18].

Type 3 fractures exit medial to the coracoid process. They can be predominantly treated conservatively, if displaced less than 5 mm. However, attention should be drawn to secondary injuries to other parts of superior suspensory complex, C4-linkage or the clavicular-acromioclavicular joint-acromial strut. If they are present operative stabilisation is indicated. A suprascapularis nerve palsy can be present when the fracture line exits the suprascapular notch. In doubtful cases electromyography should be performed and early exploration is recommended [55].

Type 4 and 5 fractures are treated operatively when persisting instability of the glenohumeral joint or an intra-articular displacement greater than 5 mm exists.

Type 6 fractures are treated mainly conservatively as these cases often maintain an adequate secondary congruency. However, surgery carries the danger of disrupting the soft tissue support and often does not allow adequate reduction of the fracture. In rare cases of secondary displacement prosthetic replacement must be performed.

Acromion Fractures

Kuhn et al [36] proposed a classification of acromial fractures that underwent intensive discussion in the literature. They proposed conservative treatment for all fractures with non, minor or superior displacement. Fractures with inferior or major displacement should be treated operatively because of narrowing of the subacromial space and possible development of an impingement syndrome. An os acromiale might complicate evaluation. In these cases CT-scans should be performed to identify the injury to its full extent and distinguish between fractures from os acromiale. Recent work proposes surgical treatment in young patients with high activity level, and the early need for crutches [35].

Coracoid Fractures

Fractures of the coracoid process are divided into fractures of the coracoid base, the coracoid-tip and the inter-ligamental (coracoid ligaments) area. Fractures to the tip of the coracoid appear minimally and largely displaced. However, conservative treatment can be generally performed. In athletes or patients performing heavy manual labour, open reduction and internal fixation can be recommended [48]. Fractures of the inter-ligamental area are regularly acquired during indirect trauma as well. They can be treated conservatively. In case of symptomatic local irritation secondary osteosynthesis should be performed. Again, in athletes or patients performing heavy manual labour, open reduction and internal fixation is recommended.

Fractures of the coracoid base should be treated operatively only when significantly dislocated. However if pain persists or movement is impaired secondary operative procedures lead to gratifying outcomes [48].

Combined Fractures (Some Frequent Combinations)

As a treatment principle combined fractures of the scapula and the shoulder girdle should be primarily analyzed for each injury pattern separately. If operative treatment is indicated, afterwards the impact of the underlying injury combination on the SSSC and the C4 linkage should be evaluated.

Ipsilateral Coracoid and Acromial Fractures

Isolated fractures of the coracoid process or the acromion can be treated conservatively if not displaced significantly (see above). However, combined acromion and coracoid fractures medial to the coraco-clavicular ligaments (Ogawa Type 2) represents a double disruption of the superior suspensory complex (SSSC). For reconstruction of the ring at least one surgery is indicated, usually the coracoid process. If one of the fractures is displaced significantly it should be addressed.

Fractures of the Acromion and Grade 3 Acromio-Clavicular Joint Disruptions

Combination of an acromion fracture and a fracture of the acromio-clavicular-joint creates a free acromial fracture component. To prevent non- or mal-union of the fragment and or the acromio-clavicular-joint the authors recommend surgical treatment of both ACJ and the acromion.

Coracoid Process and Glenoid Neck

A complete fracture of the glenoid neck and a fracture of the coracoid process medial to the coracoclavicular ligaments denotes a separation of the glenoid fracture component to the C4 linkage. Secondary displacement of glenoid is very likely and surgery is indicated. Open reduction and internal stabilization of the glenoid fracture should be performed. Reduction of the coracoid process should only be performed if significantly displaced.

Coracoid Process and Distal Third of the Clavicle

Fractures of the distal third of the clavicle, lateral to the coraco-clavicular ligaments in combination with a fracture of the base of the coracoid process can lead to a significant dislocation of the coracoid process if the coraco-clavicular ligaments stay

intact, due to the pull of the trapezius muscle. Operative stabilization of the coracoid process is indicated. If disruption of the coraco-clavicular ligaments is present only displaced fractures of either the clavicle or the coracoid process have to be fixed. In cases of a combined clavicle fracture, medial to the coraco-clavicular ligaments and a coracoid process base fracture surgery is only indicated in displaced fractures.

Fracture	Indications for surgery
Isolated body fracture	Displacement greater than 1 cm [45]
	Dissociated suspensory system
Surgical glenoid neck	Displacement greater than 1 cm
	Angular displacement greater than 40° in coronal or sagital plane
	Inferior angulation greater than 20°
Anatomic glenoid neck	All fractures of the anatomic neck have to be considered as inherently instable and should be treated operatively
Glenoid cavity	Type 1 fractures associated with a persisting instability of the glenohumeral joint
	All fractures with an intra-articular displacement greater than 5 mm [34]
Type 3 Glenoid Cavity	With associated alteration of the SSSC
	With nerve palsy of the suprascapular nerve
Acromial fractures	Fractures with inferior or major displacement or accompanied ACJ disruptions grade 3 (Rockwood) or higher.
Coracoid tip-interligamental area	Athletes or patients performing heavy manual labour- open reduction and internal fixation is recommended
Coracoid base	When significantly dislocated or symptomatic

Pre-Operative Preparation and Planning

Scapular fractures are generally acquired during high-energy traumata and patients are often polytraumatized. Before planning operative treatment all concomitant injuries have to be identified and patients should be stabilised.

If surgery is indicated precise radiological evaluation of all fracture patterns is essential for successful treatment. A true anterior and posterior, a trans-axillary and a lateral scapular view should be taken as minimum. Glenoid displacement in the coronal and sagittal plane has to be evaluated. In case of a scapular neck or glenoid fracture additional CT-scans and 3-D reconstructive views enable measurements of the degree of displacement and fracture size. This is crucial information for the surgeon to choose the right surgical approach and operative technique.

Approaches

There are 4 standard approaches to the scapula: Anterior, posterior, superior, and lateral.

Selection of the appropriate approach should be based on the fracture morphology.

The authors recommend an anterior approach for treatment of: Ideberg Ia fractures (bony Bankart fractures) Ideberg III fractures with clavicular fractures and a posterior approach in cases of Ideberg Ib fractures Ideberg II-V fractures, scapula neck and scapula body fractures. In cases of a coracoid or an acromion fracture a superior approach is indicated. The lateral approach is well suited for fractures of the lateral Margin and inferior aspects of the glenoid [65].

Anterior Approach
There is a choice of anterior approaches to the scapula:
- A delto-trapezoideal approach and
- An anterior deltoid split (superior extension to the delto-trapezoideal approach).

Anterior Deltoid Split
The incision is performed above the glenohumeral joint from the superior to the inferior margin of the humeral head. The deltoid muscle is exposed and split in line with its fibres

above the coracoid process. The conjoined tendon should be retracted medially and the deltoid muscle laterally. The subscapularis muscle is exposed and its tendon incised 2 cm medial to biceps groove. Tendon and glenohumeral capsule are separated and the latter is turned back medially after incision about 5 mm medial to the humeral neck. The whole glenohumeral cavity and the anterior rim of the glenoid can be inspected now. One has to take care of the axillary nerve passing nearby.

Posterior Approach
Extended posterior approaches should be chosen only if truly necessary because extensive tissue scarring can be expected. Especially the dorsal approach from Judet is hardly used apart from tumour surgery or scapular body fractures with relevant displacement of the medial margin of the scapula or the scapular spine.

Rockwood (Basic Posterior) Approach
The patients are placed in prone position with the arm at 90° abduction [67]. The incision is performed from the posterior aspect of the acromion over the lateral third of the scapular spine and then down distally in the mid-lateral line for 2.5 cm. The deltoid muscle is dissected sharply off the acromion and the scapular spine and than split along its fibres for about 5 cm. After separation of the deltoid muscle from the underlying infraspinatus and teres minor muscles the musculotendinous units are retracted downwards. Any further operative development should carefully protect the closely-related axillary and suprascapular nerves. The infraspinatus tendon is incised along its superior and posterior borders and dissected from the underlying posterior glenohumeral capsule. After incision of the capsule the entire glenoid cavity can be inspected. Alternatively the interval between the infraspinatus and teres minor muscle can be exposed. After detachment of the long head of the triceps muscle the inferior aspect of the glenoid process and the lateral border of the scapular body can be exposed.

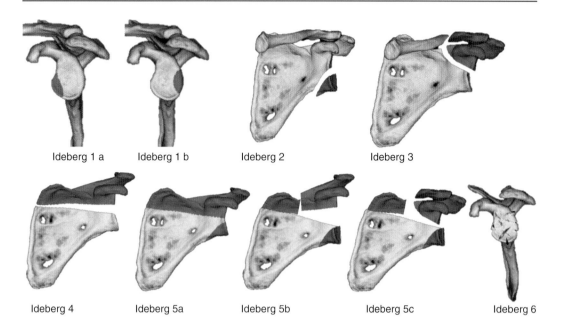

Ideberg 1 a   Ideberg 1 b   Ideberg 2   Ideberg 3

Ideberg 4   Ideberg 5a   Ideberg 5b   Ideberg 5c   Ideberg 6

Fig. 7 Ideberg classification scheme for fractures of the glenoid cavity (From [18])

Extended Judet Approach

The patient is placed in a prone position [6, 33]. A "boomerang" skin incision along the scapular spine and along the medial margin of the scapular body is performed (see Fig. 7). The deltoid is than dissected off from the scapular spine. Afterwards the infraspinatus muscle is reflected proximally after careful mobilization. One has to carefully avoid damage to the neurovascular bundles while mobilizing the infraspinatus muscle in the spinoglenoid notch.

Superior Approach

In cases where it is difficult to stabilize a superior glenoid fragment a superior approach can be performed or added to a posterior or anterior approach. If needed either incision can be extended over the tip of the shoulder. The superior aspect of the clavicle and the AC- Joint and the acromion are exposed. The trapezius muscle and the supraspinatus muscle underneath are split along their fibres between the clavicle and the acromion. Depending whether one aims at the ventral or posterior aspects of the upper glenoid the supraspinatus muscle is prepared more ventral or dorsal.

The superior aspect of the coracoid process is identified. Here one has to take care and avoid injury to the suprascapular nerve and accompanying vessels medial to the coracoid process. The scapular notch should always be identified to avoid injury to the suprascapular nerve.

Lateral Approach

The lateral approach is less popular but very suitable for treatment of fractures of the lateral margin and inferior aspects of the glenoid.

The Patient is placed in the prone position and with the arm abducted at 90°. The incision is starts in the mid-line but slightly caudal of the scapular spine. It runs parallel to the ribs along the muscle fibres of the infraspinatus muscle and the teres minor muscle to the lateral margin of the scapula. With preparation cranial along the margin one can identify the inferior border of the glenoid. During preparation one has to identify and avoid injury to the axillary nerve. Now the axillary recesses can be exposed and the glenohumeral joint can be opened to expose the dorso-inferior aspects of the glenoid.

Operative Technique

Scapular Body Fractures

Surgical management of a scapular body is performed through a posterior approach (see Fig. 8). The extent of exposure has to be chosen depending on the fracture type. However, the limited window technique should be favoured, whenever possible. Using limited windows fractures at the lateral border, the acromial spine, and the vertebral border can be accessed. Whenever there are more than three exit points of the fractures in the scapular ring extensive exposure might be indicated to gain full control of these complex fracture patterns. There exist no specific reduction tools for the scapular body. The authors preferably use small pointed reduction clamps. Fracture reduction and osteosynthesis should be applied at the scapular ring if possible as the bone is thicker here. 2.7-mm and 3.5-mm dynamic, compression plates are used for definitive fixation.

Glenoid Neck Fractures (incl. "Floating Shoulder")

The glenoid neck is best reached through a posterior approach. As with scapular body fractures the smallest possible approach should be favoured. Van Noort and Obremskey described modifications of posterior approaches for open reduction and internal fixation of the glenoid neck fractures [32, 47]. The interval between the infraspinatus and the teres minor muscle is entered to expose the lateral scapular border as well as the postero-inferior aspects of the glenoid neck. In difficult to control cases, of superior fracture components, an extension to a superior approach can be performed. 2.7 mm and 3.5 mm malleable reconstruction plates are particularly helpful to constitute firm stabilization. Additionally lag screws can be placed. In case of severe comminution of the scapular neck and body, making plate fixation impossible, k-wire or lag screw fixation can be used.

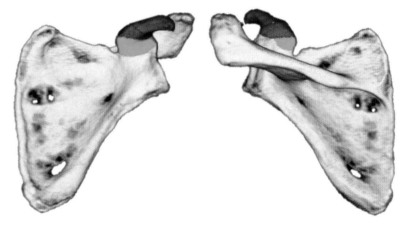

Fig. 8 Classification scheme of coracoid fractures according to Ogawa et al. Type 1 fractures include the coracoid base and Type 2 fractures the coracoid tip [49]

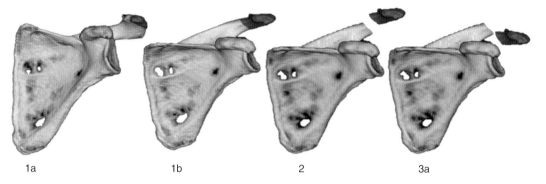

1a   1b   2   3a

Fig. 9 Classification scheme of acromion fractures according to Kuhn et al. (From [36])

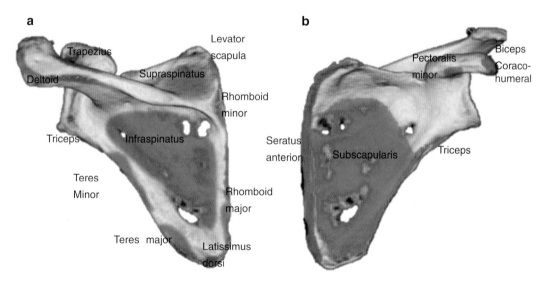

Fig. 10 Anatomy of the scapula with insertion points of the originating muscles (Modified from: http://img.medscape.com/pi/emed/ckb/orthopedic_surgery/1230552-1263076-111.jpg)

In case of an additional ipsilateral clavicle fracture osteosynthesis of the scapular neck should be performed if significant displacement (>1 cm) or dysangulation (>40°) is present. In case of an additional disruption of the C4-linkage. reduction might be achieved by reduction-fixation of the glenoid neck. However, if not achieved additional osteosynthesis should be performed (see Fig. 9).

Glenoid Cavity Fractures

Glenoid cavity fractures are treated surgically if an articular step >1 cm or persistent instability of the humeral head is present. Type 1a fractures are approached anteriorly or arthroscopally [7, 57]. The displaced fragment is fixed, if large enough, with two cannulated interfragmentary compression screws to guarantee rotational

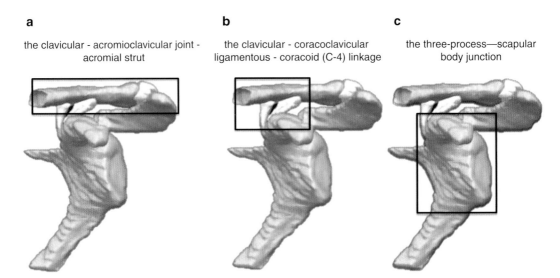

a
the clavicular - acromioclavicular joint - acromial strut

b
the clavicular - coracoclavicular ligamentous - coracoid (C-4) linkage

c
the three-process—scapular body junction

Fig. 11 The three components of the superior shoulder suspensory complex: (**a**) the clavicular – acromioclavicular joint – acromial strut; (**b**) the clavicular – coracoclavicular ligamentous – coracoid (C-4) linkage; (**c**) the three-process – scapular body junction

stability. Type 1b fractures are approached posteriorly and treated in the same way. If fracture components are comminuted but glenoid cavity defect demands operative treatment, a tri-cortical graft harvested from the iliac crest can be used to fill the defect (Fig. 10).

Type 2 Fractures are treated using a posterior approach. The inferior fragment is exposed through the infraspinatus-teres minor interval. Reconstruction plates or cannulated compression screws are used for internal fixation after reduction (see Fig. 11).

Type 3 fractures can be treated either by an anterior, posterior or arthroscopic approach. For an anterior approach the rotator interval has to be incised. In case of an additional injury of the superior suspensory complex (SSSC) this injury might be reduced by reduction of the glenoid fragment (see below). If secondary reduction cannot be achieved additional open reduction and internal fixation of the injury has to be performed.

For surgical treatment of Type 4 an anterosuperior or a combined anterior and posterior approach should be chosen. A K-wire placed into the superior fracture component can be used as a handle and after successful reduction

of the glenoid the k-wire is then driven across the fracture and can be used to place a cannulated screw.

Type 5a fractures are treated as type 2 fractures and Type 5b and c fractures as Type 3 fractures. Type 6 fractures are rarely treated surgically.

Surgical approaches to glenoid fractures
Anterior approach:
Ideberg I Fractures (bony Bankart Fractures)
Ideberg III Fractures with Clavicular Fractures
Posterior approach:
Ideberg II-V Fractures
Basic posterior approach (extended posterior approach (Judet))
Arthroscopic approach:
Ideberg I Fracture (bony Bankart Fx)
Ideberg III Fracture

Acromion Fractures

Acromial fractures are treated surgically if significantly displaced or inferior displacement occurs. Distal disruptions are treated with tendon band construct. Proximal fractures can be treated using a dorsal radial plate fixation (regular or angle-stable).

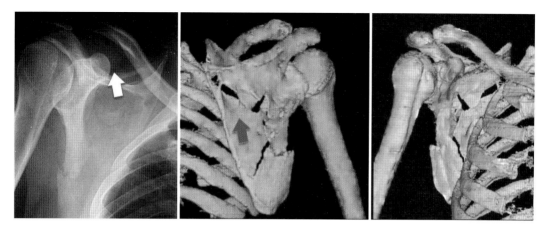

Fig. 12 Operative treatment of the scapular body fracture is indicated due to an alteration of the scapular suspensory system (*white arrow*) and significant fracture dislocation in a multi-fragmentary situation (*blue arrow*)

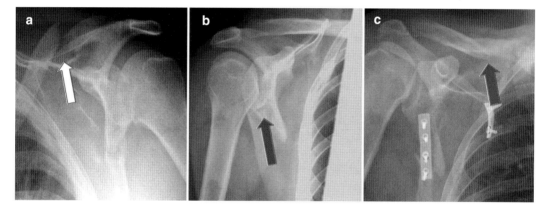

Fig. 13 Case of a combined glenoid neck (*blue arrow head*) and clavicle fracture (*white arrow head*). Because of significant dislocation of the glenoid fragment a scapular osteosynthesis was performed

Coracoid Fractures

An anterior deltoid-splitting approach is used in all coracoid fractures. In cases of Ogawa Type 1 fracture the rotator interval is opened if needed. Compression screw- fixation is performed. Type 2 Ogawa fractures are treated surgically if the bony fragment is dislocated significantly or becomes symptomatic [16]. An anterior approach is performed and whenever the bony fragment is large enough cannulated 3.5-mm or 4.0-mm compression screws are used for refixation of the fragment. In comminuted fractures a suture fixation of the conjoined tendon is performed (see Fig. 12).

Principles of Post-Operative Treatment/Conservative Treatment

All operative procedures and fractures treated conservatively should be protected from physiological stress. Early motion is of crucial importance to prevent shoulder stiffness. After post-operative

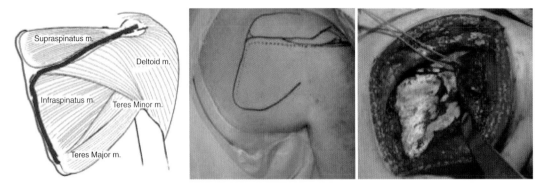

Fig. 14 Stages of the extended posterior approach after Judet. A" boomerang" incision is performed (**a, b**). The infraspinatus muscle is mobilized an retracted laterally. Careful attention has to be performed to avoid suprascapular nerve damage

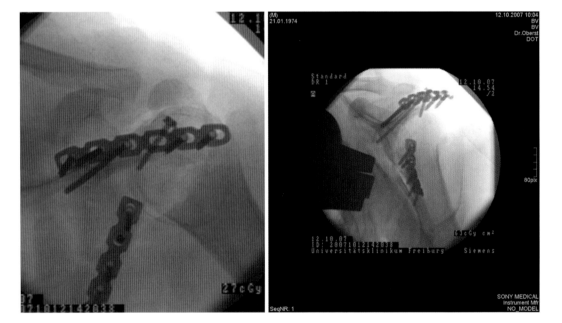

Fig. 15 Open reduction and internal fixation of a scapular body fracture using 3.5-mm dynamic compression plates

pain has subsided it is the aim to achieve a good range of motion, if tolerable for the patient.

Continuous passive motion (CPM) therapy should be applied additionally.

All patients should be encouraged to fulfill easy activities of daily living. Lifting of weights should not be performed until bony healing has occurred (12 weeks). Patients with associated brachial plexopathy need special treatment. They might benefit from additional operative strategies such as brachial plexus exploration and nerve grafting.

Glenoid fractures with or without anterior instability acquire an after-treatment comparable to that of operations for shoulder instabilities.

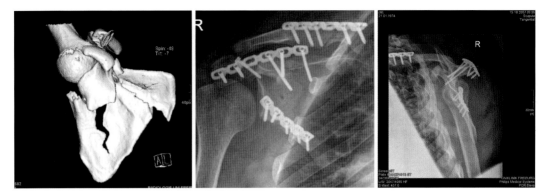

Fig. 16 Complex scapular body and neck fracture with an associated clavicle fracture. Both clavicle and scapular neck fracture are significantly displaced and therefore treated operatively using 3.5 mm LCPDCP malleable plates

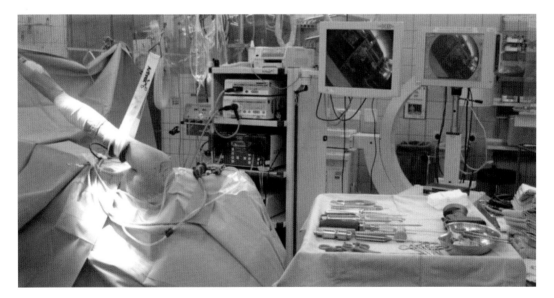

Fig. 17 Operative set up for arthroscopic treatment of glenoid rim fractures

Complications

Lantry and co-workers presented a meta-analysis (of 212 scapular fractures) and described a mean of 4,2 % of post-operative infections being the most common complication [37].

Many infections can be treated successfully with antibiotics and superficial drainage. Post-operative injuries of neural structures appeared in 2,4 %. In one case heterotopic ossification led to a nerve palsy. Implant failure occurred in 7.1 %. Post-traumatic arthritis developed in 1.9 %

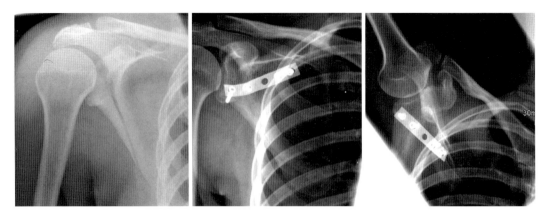

Fig. 18 Operative treatment of an Ideberg 2 glenoid cavity fracture using a 2,5 mm reconstruction plate using a posterior approach

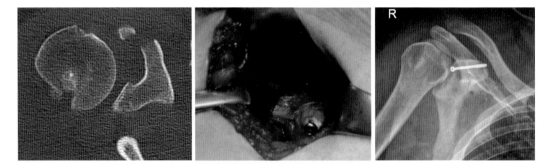

Fig. 19 Surgical management of an coracoid fracture (Ogawa Type 2) because of significant fracture displacement. The bony fragment is fixed using a cannulated 3,5 mm compression screw. Additionally a suture fixation of the conjoined tendon is performed

Summary

Fractures of the scapula are uncommon injuries resulting predominantly from high-energy trauma. Patients suffering a scapular fracture should be treated where possible at a trauma centre, because they are possibly associated with life-threatening injuries to the head, chest or large vessels. Treatment of scapular fractures can be performed during early recovery of the patient, as they are rarely surgical emergencies themselves. About 90 % of all scapular fractures can be treated conservatively. However surgical treatment is indicated if there is significant displacement or damage to the scapula suspensory system (SSSC; C4-linkage), the position or integrity of the glenoid fragment (articular surface) or if the lateral column is displaced.

References

1. Ada JR, Miller ME. Scapular fractures. Analysis of 113 cases. Clin Orthop Relat Res. 1991;269:174–80.
2. Armitage BM, Wijdicks CA, Tarkin IS, et al. Mapping of scapular fractures with three-dimensional computed tomography. J Bone Joint Surg Am. 2009;91(9): 2222–8.
3. Armstrong CP, Van der Spuy J. The fractured scapula: importance and management based on a series of 62 patients. Injury. 1984;15(5):324–9.
4. Arts V, Louette L. Scapular neck fractures; an update of the concept of floating shoulder. Injury. 1999;30(2):146–8.

5. Baldwin KD, Ohman-Strickland P, Mehta S, Hume E. Scapula fractures: a marker for concomitant injury? A retrospective review of data in the National Trauma Database. J Trauma. 2008;65(2):430–5.

6. Bartonicek J, Tucek M, Lunacek L. Judet posterior approach to the scapula. Acta Chir Orthop Traumatol Cech. 2008;75(6):429–35.

7. Bauer T, Abadie O, Hardy P. Arthroscopic treatment of glenoid fractures. Arthroscopy. 2006;22(5):569 e561–566.

8. Beswick DR, Morse SD, Barnes AU. Bilateral scapular fractures from low-voltage electrical injury. Ann Emerg Med. 1982;11(12):676–7.

9. Blauth M, SN, Haas N. Knöcherne Verletzungen von Schlüsselbein und Schulterblatt vol 10. München/Wien/Baltimore: Urban&Schwarzenberg; 1991.

10. Blue JM, Anglen JO, Helikson MA. Fracture of the scapula with intrathoracic penetration. A case report. J Bone Joint Surg Am. 1997;79(7):1076–8.

11. De Palma A. Surgery of the shoulder. 3rd ed. Philadelphia: JB Lippincott; 1983.

12. Dines DM, Warren RF, Inglis AE, Pavlov H. The coracoid impingement syndrome. J Bone Joint Surg Br. 1990;72(2):314–6.

13. Ebraheim NA, Pearlstein SR, Savolaine ER, Gordon SL, Jackson WT, Corray T. Scapulothoracic dissociation (closed avulsion of the scapula, subclavian artery, and brachial plexus): a newly recognized variant, a new classification, and a review of the literature and treatment options. J Orthop Trauma. 1987;1(1):18–23.

14. Eyres KS, Brooks A, Stanley D. Fractures of the coracoid process. J Bone Joint Surg Br. 1995;77(3):425–8.

15. Ganz R, Noesberger B. Treatment of scapular fractures. Hefte Unfallheilkd. 1975;(126):59–62.

16. Garcia-Elias M, Salo JM. Non-union of a fractured coracoid process after dislocation of the shoulder. A case report. J Bone Joint Surg Br. 1985;67(5):722–3.

17. Gerber C, Terrier F, Zehnder R, Ganz R. The subcoracoid space. An anatomic study. Clin Orthop Relat Res. 1987;215:132–8.

18. Goss TP. Fractures of the glenoid cavity [Current Concepts Review]. J Bone Joint Surg Am. 1992;74(2):299–305.

19. Goss TP. Double disruptions of the superior shoulder suspensory complex. J Orthop Trauma. 1993;7(2):99–106.

20. Goss TP. Fractures of the glenoid neck. J Shoulder Elbow Surg. 1994;3(1):42–52.

21. Goss TP. Fractures of the shoulder complex. In: Pappas AM, editor. Upper extremity injury in the athlete. New York: Churchill Livingston; 1995. p. 268.

22. Hall RJ, Calvert PT. Stress fracture of the acromion: an unusual mechanism and review of the literature. J Bone Joint Surg Br. 1995;77(1):153–4.

23. Halpern AA, Joseph R, Page J, Nagel DA. Subclavian artery injury and fracture of the scapula. JACEP. 1979;8(1):19–20.

24. Hardegger FH, Simpson LA, Weber BG. The operative treatment of scapular fractures. J Bone Joint Surg Br. 1984;66(5):725–31.

25. Hashiguchi H, Ito H. Clinical outcome of the treatment of floating shoulder by osteosynthesis for clavicular fracture alone. J Shoulder Elbow Surg. 2003;12(6):589–91.

26. Heatly MD, Bredk LW, Higinbotham NL. Bilateral fracture of the scapula. Am J Surg. 1946;71:256–9.

27. Heggland EJ, Parker RD. Simultaneous bilateral glenoid fractures associated with glenohumeral subluxation/dislocation in a weightlifter. Orthopedics. 1997;20(12):1180–3 discussion 1183–1184.

28. Herscovici Jr D, Fiennes AG, Allgower M, Ruedi TP. The floating shoulder: ipsilateral clavicle and scapular neck fractures. J Bone Joint Surg Br. 1992;74(3):362–4.

29. Ideberg R, Grevsten S, Larsson S. Epidemiology of scapular fractures. Incidence and classification of 338 fractures. Acta Orthop Scand. 1995;66(5):395–7.

30. Imatani RJ. Fractures of the scapula: a review of 53 fractures. J Trauma. 1975;15(6):473–8.

31. Jeanmaire E, Ganz R. [Treatment of fractures of the scapula. Surgical indications]. Helv Chir Acta. 1982;48(5):585–94.

32. Jones CB, Cornelius JP, Sietsema DL, Ringler JR, Endres TJ. Modified Judet approach and minifragment fixation of scapular body and glenoid neck fractures. J Orthop Trauma. 2009;23(8):558–64.

33. Judet R. Surgical treatment of scapular fractures. Acta Orthop Belg. 1964;30:673–8.

34. Kavanagh BF, Bradway JK, Cofield RH. Open reduction and internal fixation of displaced intra-articular fractures of the glenoid fossa. J Bone Joint Surg Am. 1993;75(4):479–84.

35. Kim DS, Yoon YS, Kang DH. Comparison of early fixation and delayed reconstruction after displacement in previously nondisplaced acromion fractures. Orthopedics. 2010;33(6):392.

36. Kuhn JE, Blasier RB, Carpenter JE. Fractures of the acromion process: a proposed classification system. J Orthop Trauma. 1994;8(1):6–13.

37. Lantry JM, Roberts CS, Giannoudis PV. Operative treatment of scapular fractures: a systematic review. Injury. 2008;39(3):271–83.

38. Mathews RE, Cocke TB, D'Ambrosia RD. Scapular fractures secondary to seizures in patients with osteodystrophy. Report of two cases and review of the literature. J Bone Joint Surg Am. 1983;65(6):850–3.

39. McAdams TR, Blevins FT, Martin TP, DeCoster TA. The role of plain films and computed tomography in the evaluation of scapular neck fractures. J Orthop Trauma. 2002;16(1):7–11.

40. McGahan JP, Rab GT, Dublin A. Fractures of the scapula. J Trauma. 1980;20(10):880–3.

41. McGinnis M, Denton JR. Fractures of the scapula: a retrospective study of 40 fractured scapulae. J Trauma. 1989;29(11):1488–93.

42. McLennan JG, Ungersma J. Pneumothorax complicating fracture of the scapula. J Bone Joint Surg Am. 1982;64(4):598–9.

43. Miller ME. Letter to the editor. J Orthop Trauma. 1994;8:14.

44. Miller ME, Ada JR. Injuries to the shoulder girdle. Philadelphia: WB Saunders; 1992.

45. Nordqvist A, Petersson C. Fracture of the body, neck, or spine of the scapula. A long-term follow-up study. Clin Orthop Relat Res. 1992;283:139–44.

46. Nunley RL, Bedini SJ. Paralysis of the shoulder subsequent to a comminuted fracture of the scapula: rationale and treatment methods. Phys Ther Rev. 1960;40:442–7.

47. Obremskey WT, Lyman JR. A modified judet approach to the scapula. J Orthop Trauma. 2004; 18(10):696–9.

48. Ogawa K, Ikegami H, Takeda T, Watanabe A. Defining impairment and treatment of subacute and chronic fractures of the coracoid process. J Trauma. 2009; 67(5):1040–5.

49. Ogawa K, Yoshida A, Takahashi M, Ui M. Fractures of the coracoid process. J Bone Joint Surg Br. 1997;79(1):17–9.

50. Oreck SL, Burgess A, Levine AM. Traumatic lateral displacement of the scapula: a radiographic sign of neurovascular disruption. J Bone Joint Surg Am. 1984;66(5):758–63.

51. Paulson MM, Watnik NF, Dines DM. Coracoid impingement syndrome, rotator interval reconstruction, and biceps tenodesis in the overhead athlete. Orthop Clin North Am. 2001;32(3):485–93, ix.

52. Rockwood CJ, Matsen III FA. The shoulder, vol. 1. 4th ed. Philadelphia: Saunders Elsevier; 2009.

53. Rowe CR. Fractures of the Scapula. Surg Clin North Am. 1963;43:1565–71.

54. Scavenius M, Sloth C. Fractures of the scapula. Acta Orthop Belg. 1996;62(3):129–32.

55. Solheim LF, Roaas A. Compression of the suprascapular nerve after fracture of the scapular notch. Acta Orthop Scand. 1978;49(4): 338–40.

56. Stephens NG, Morgan AS, Corvo P, Bernstein BA. Significance of scapular fracture in the blunt-trauma patient. Ann Emerg Med. 1995;26(4):439–42.

57. Sugaya H, Kon Y, Tsuchiya A. Arthroscopic repair of glenoid fractures using suture anchors. Arthroscopy. 2005;21(5):635.

58. Tarquinio T, Weinstein ME, Virgilio RW. Bilateral scapular fractures from accidental electric shock. J Trauma. 1979;19(2):132–3.

59. Taylor J. Letter to the editor. J Orthop Trauma. 1994;8:359.

60. Thompson DA, Flynn TC, Miller PW, Fischer RP. The significance of scapular fractures. J Trauma. 1985; 25(10):974–7.

61. Tomaszek DE. Combined subclavian artery and brachial plexus injuries from blunt upper-extremity trauma. J Trauma. 1984;24(2):161–3.

62. van Noort A, van Kampen A. Fractures of the scapula surgical neck: outcome after conservative treatment in 13 cases. Arch Orthop Trauma Surg. 2005;125(10): 696–700.

63. Veysi VT, Mittal R, Agarwal S, Dosani A, Giannoudis PV. Multiple trauma and scapula fractures: so what? J Trauma. 2003;55(6):1145–7.

64. Wiedemann E. Skapulafrakturen. In: Haber- Meyer P, editor. Schulterchirurgie. München: Urban & Fischer; 2002. p. S453–468.

65. Wiedemann E. [Fractures of the scapula]. Unfallchirurg. 2004;107(12):1124–33.

66. Wilber MC, Evans EB. Fractures of the scapula. An analysis of forty cases and a review of the literature. J Bone Joint Surg Am. 1977;59(3):358–62.

67. Wirth MA, Butters KP, Rockwood Jr CA. The posterior deltoid-splitting approach to the shoulder. Clin Orthop Relat Res. 1993;296:92–8.

68. Yamamoto N, Itoi E, Abe H, et al. Effect of an anterior glenoid defect on anterior shoulder stability: a cadaveric study. Am J Sports Med. 2009;37(5):949–54.

69. Zdravkovic D, Damholt VV. Comminuted and severely displaced fractures of the scapula. Acta Orthop Scand. 1974;45(1):60–5.

70. Zelle BA, Pape HC, Gerich TG, Garapati R, Ceylan B, Krettek C. Functional outcome following scapulothoracic dissociation. J Bone Joint Surg Am. 2004;86-A(1):2–8.

71. Zlowodzki M, Bhandari M, Zelle BA, Kregor PJ, Cole PA. Treatment of scapula fractures: systematic review of 520 fractures in 22 case series. J Orthop Trauma. 2006;20(3):230–3.

Scapulothoracic Arthrodesis

Deborah Higgs and Simon M. Lambert

Contents

Keywords

Shoulder arthrodesis • Long thoracic nerve • Muscular dystrophy • Nerve palsy • Scapular winging • Scapulothoracic

Introduction

The most common manifestation of scapulothoracic dysfunction is symptomatic scapular winging (scapulothoracic instability). Most cases can be treated with physiotherapy, using subscapular injection of steroid and local anaesthetic to facilitate therapy when needed. Persistent painful scapular dyskinesia may require scapulothoracic arthropexy (soft tissue stabilization or augmentation) for partial palsy or limited winging, but scapulothoracic arthrodesis (fusion) is a reliable and safe intervention when indicated for irreversible neuromuscular disease.

Classification

Scapulothoracic instability is classified as traumatic structural (type I), atraumatic structural (type II), and neuromuscular (type III), using the same concept as described for glenohumeral instability. Three common patterns of instability are seen in clinical practice: superior polar, medial border, and inferior polar. Complex combinations of these are seen with glenohumeral instability, and patterns of scapoluthoracic instability may vary in ascent

D. Higgs (✉)
Royal National Orthopaedic Hospital, Stanmore, Middlesex, UK

S.M. Lambert
The Shoulder and Elbow Service, Royal National Orthopaedic Hospital, Stanmore, Middlesex, UK
e-mail: slambert@nhs.net

G. Bentley (ed.), *European Surgical Orthopaedics and Traumatology*,
DOI 10.1007/978-3-642-34746-7_261, © EFORT 2014

and descent of the arm at the shoulder. The commonest causes include injury to the dorsal scapular nerve (to the rhomboid muscles), the long thoracic nerve (to serratus anterior) or the spinal accessory nerve (to trapezius) singly or in combination. Scapular fractures, scapular tumours, rib fractures or chest wall deformity can also cause scapular winging. Glenohumeral joint pathology, particularly posterior glenohumeral instability and large rotator cuff tears are often associated with scapular instability. The commonest indication for arthrodesis of the scapulothoracic joint at the Royal National Orthopaedic Hospital, UK is primary neurological or muscular disease, including sporadic and familial fascioscapulohumeral dystrophy and muscular dystrophies (Duchenne and Spinal Muscular Atrophy)

Aetiology

The spinal accessory nerve is a small nerve (2 mm in diameter), which crosses the posterior triangle of the neck. It is vulnerable to injury by inadvertent division during neck dissection, by irradiation, and by traumatic laceration. Scapular instability is due to injury of this nerve if surgery has been undertaken previously.

The natural history of facioscapulohumeral dystrophy has only recently been studied prospectively [1, 2]. Genetic transmission is autosomal dominant with variable expression and penetrance, but can be sporadic. Initially it involves the muscles of the face, shoulder girdle and upper limb. Involvement is bilateral but often asymmetrical. Typically there is asymmetrical involvement of serratus anterior, rhomboids, trapezius, teres major and minor muscles. The pectoralis minor and major, the biceps, and triceps, are also often involved. Deltoid is usually spared, and becomes the principle muscle that moves the shoulder. It appears to be slowly progressive and may include the lower limbs with eventual wheelchair dependence in up to 19 % of patients [3]. It has been hypothesized that the pathology is related to calcium regulation in the muscle cells and that calcium antagonists such as

diltiazem may be effective in delaying progression [4]. Initial studies looking at prednisolone to halt or retard the muscle weakness were unsuccessful [5] however some benefit was seen with albuterol, a beta-2-adrenergic agonist [6] and this may prove to be useful following surgery.

Biomechanics of Scapulothoracic Motion

The nomenclature of scapular instability is variable in literature. No more than $120°$ of abduction is possible at the glenohumeral joint, and further abduction at the shoulder joint requires the scapula to rotate. Scapular rotation tilts the glenoid fossa forward and upwards. After the initial $30°$ of abduction, which occurs without scapular rotation, abduction occurs due to a combination of glenohumeral joint motion and scapular rotation, at a ratio of 2–1 (Fig. 1).

Injury to the long thoracic nerve results in paradoxical movement of the scapula away from the chest wall, because of the unopposed action of trapezius, levator scapulae, and the rhomboid muscles. The scapula assumes a higher position, the inferior angle of the scapula rotates towards the midline and the medial border of the scapula becomes more prominent. The biomechanical result is to reduce the arc of motion available to the glenohumeral joint because of loss of the mechanical advantage of the deltoid and rotator cuff.

Injury to the spinal accessory nerve results in the scapula sitting lower, with rotation of the inferior pole laterally and the upper medial pole medially, due to the paralysis of trapezius and unopposed action of serratus anterior. This places the rhomboids and, to a lesser extent, the levator scapulae at a biomechanical disadvantage, so that whilst elevation above the horizontal plane is possible, the force generated is compromised.

Injury to the dorsal scapular nerve (levator scapulae and rhomboids) can result in winging that is milder but similar in pattern to that seen with trapezius muscle paralysis.

In fascioscapulohumeral dystrophy the deltoid becomes the principle muscle that moves the shoulder. The effect of the cantilever of the arm

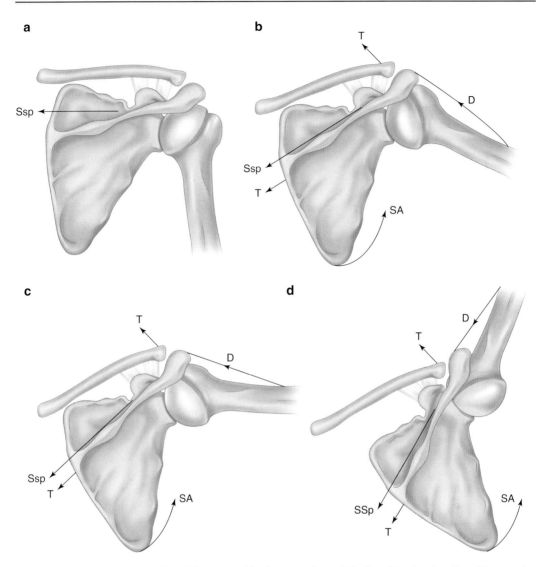

Fig. 1 Abduction of the shoulder joint, a combined glenohumeral joint motion and scapular rotation (**a–c**). At 120° (**d**) the greater tuberosity impinges on the lateral acromion and further abduction is achieved by scapular rotation. *Ssp* supraspinatus, *T* trapezius, *D* deltoid, *SA* serratus anterior

and unopposed use of deltoid along with the loss of the scapular stabilisers causes winging of the scapula and a reduction in forward flexion and abduction.

Diagnosis

The position of the winged scapula depends on the specific nerve injury and the resulting pattern of muscle paralysis as described.

In serratus anterior weakness patients often simply complain of pain and/or weakness affecting activities of daily living. Pain is often located over the scapula. There may be symptomatic impingement in the subacromial space. Muscle atrophy is not usually a feature. At rest the scapula may lie in a winged position. In neuralgic amyotrophy the patient may present with a history of pain, a fever, and then weakness of one or more muscles around the shoulder. The 'scapula stabilisation test' can be used to predict the value of physiotherapy or whether scapulothoracic arthrodesis might improve the patient's function. This is performed by stabilising the scapula against the chest wall with one hand, and providing counter-pressure over the coracoid with the other hand. If there is improved range of movement and symptomatic relief during active forward elevation then scapulothoracic arthrodesis should be predictably beneficial.

An electromyographic study should be performed to help establish the diagnosis, but not all patients with obvious winging secondary to serratus anterior dysfunction will have abnormal electromyographic findings. A period of conservative treatment (generally up to 1 year) should be allowed for nerve recovery before considering scapulothoracic arthrodesis.

In patients with scapular winging due to paralysis of trapezius there is drooping of the shoulder and limited active shoulder movements. If the spinal accessory nerve has been divided the patient usually has severe pain in the shoulder girdle.

Patients with fascioscapulohumeral dystrophy present with bilateral weakness, which may be asymmetrical, with restricted shoulder movement and marked winging of the scapula, in association with the classic facies.

Scapulothoracic Arthrodesis

Surgical Technique

In our preferred technique, the patient is positioned prone, on a padded Montreal mattress with particular care of the skin overlying the prominent bones of the pelvis. The arms are placed in elevation supported on a transverse arm board. The patient is prepared and draped so that the mid-line is exposed together with the entire shoulder on the affected side. The posterior superior iliac spine from which autologous graft is to be taken (usually the same side) is left exposed. The skin is incised at $20°$ to the midline in line with the posterior angle of the ribs (Fig. 2).

The infraspinatus is elevated from the medial scapular border as a strip about 1.5 cm wide. The medial extent of the spine of scapula is burred to allow seating of the re-inforcing plate (see below). The subscapularis and serratus anterior are elevated from the deep surface of the medial border and partially excised. The posterior angle of the second or third to sixth ribs are exposed sub-periosteally and the external surface partially decorticated with a burr. Four or five 12G stainless steel or titanium cables are passed sub-coastally (Fig. 3) and through the scapula supported on its dorsal surface by a nine or ten-hole stainless steel one-third semi-tubular plate. The scapula is then brought to its desired position and the cables provisionally tensioned. Cancellous bone, harvested from the posterior iliac crest, is packed under the medial border and the cables sequentially and definitively tensioned to achieve stability (Fig. 4). The operative site is then filled with crystalloid solution to detect any tears in the pleura, followed by a layered closure over a suction drain.

A thoracobrachial spica is applied post-operatively with the shoulder in neutral rotation and $20°$ abduction and $20°$ internal rotation. Post-operative radiographs are taken to assess scapula and implant position, and a chest radiograph to assess for pneumothorax.

Post-Operative Management

The shoulder is supported in the spica for 3 months, at which point the spica is replaced by a bolster cushion, and physiotherapy with hydrotherapy instituted.

In the literature other authors have described rigid bracing [7], immobilisation with sling and swathe [8, 9], bandaging the elbow against the body for 2 months [10], simple sling and early movement [11], and figure-of-eight bandaging. We advocate relative immobilisation in a spica cast for 12 weeks. The fusion surfaces are narrow and any movement of the arm produces a substantial rotational force at the fusion site [12–15].

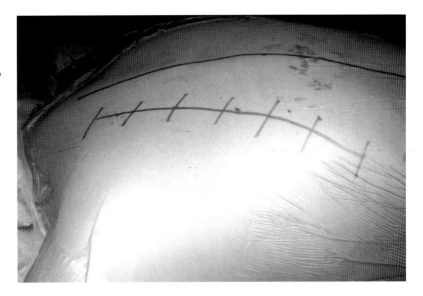

Fig. 2 Prone patient with mid-line and skin incision marked for left scapulothoracic arthrodesis. The head is to the *left* of the photograph

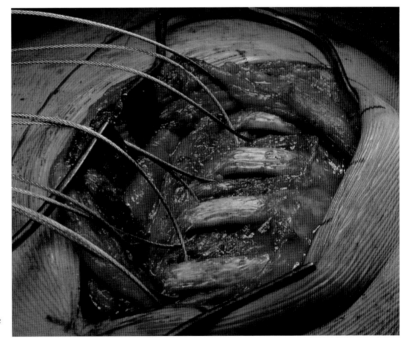

Fig. 3 Sub-costal positioning of the cables around the partially decorticated ribs. Note the posterior angle of the ribs, used as a guide to the angle of fusion

Complications

Scapulothoracic arthrodesis has been associated with a variety of complications including haemothorax [16], pneumothorax, rib fractures, brachial plexopathy [17] and other neurovascular complications [18].

Krishnan et al. [7] reported on 24 scapulothoracic fusions in 22 patients with various clinical disorders. Of these, 20 patients reported their pain had improved following surgery. However they reported a complication rate of over 50 % including pulmonary complications, "hardware" failure, pseudarthrosis, and persistent pain. We have not

Fig. 4 The plate and cables after definitive tensioning

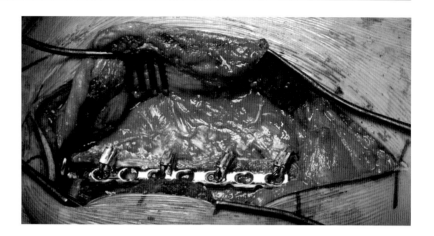

experienced any of these with the surgical technique described in this chapter.

There is a theoretical risk of reduced respiratory function in cases of bilateral fusion due to reduced chest expansion. One study demonstrated a reduction of forced vital capacity by 21 % [19]. Other studies however have shown little or no change in respiratory function [8, 9, 12, 15, 20].

Progressive deltoid weakness is a potential cause for concern in patients with fascioscapulohumeral dystrophy. In 4 out of 20 cases reported by Diab et al. deltoid weakness developed. However others found no loss in achieved function and deltoid strength; Bunch and Seigel [15], after 23 years, Copeland et al. [12] after 20 years and Letournel et al. [8] after 6 years. Twyman et al. [19] found maintenance of achieved range of motion and increased deltoid strength.

Summary

The aim of performing a scapulothoracic arthrodesis is to stabilise the scapula in an appropriate position so that it can provide a stable fulcrum against which the abductors can work. Whilst this can result in an improvement in function and periscapular pain, the loss of scapulothoracic movement by arthrodesis means that function is not that of a normal shoulder.

References

1. A prospective, quantitative study of the natural history of facioscapulohumeral muscular dystrophy (FSHD): implications for therapeutic trials. The FSH-DY Group. Neurology. 1997;48(1):38–46.
2. Personius KE, Pandya S, King WM, Tawil R, McDermott MP. Facioscapulohumeral dystrophy natural history study: standardization of testing procedures and reliability of measurements. The FSH DY Group. Phys Ther. 1994;74(3):253–63.
3. Lunt PW, Harper PS. Genetic counselling in facioscapulohumeral muscular dystrophy. J Med Genet. 1991;28(10):655–64.
4. Lefkowitz DL, Lefkowitz SS. Facioscapulohumeral muscular dystrophy: a progressive degenerative disease that responds to diltiazem. Med Hypotheses. 2005;65(4):716–21.
5. Tawil R, McDermott MP, Pandya S, King W, Kissel J, Mendell JR, Griggs RC. A pilot trial of prednisone in facioscapulohumeral muscular dystrophy. FSH-DY Group. Neurology. 1997;48(1):46–9.
6. Kissel JT, McDermott MP, Mendell JR, King WM, Pandya S, Griggs RC, Tawil R. Randomized, double-blind, placebo-controlled trial of albuterol in facioscapulohumeral dystrophy. Neurology. 2001;57(8):1434–40.
7. Krishnan SG, Hawkins RJ, Michelotti JD, Litchfield R, Willis RB, Kim YK. Scapulothoracic arthrodesis: indications, technique, and results. Clin Orthop Relat Res. 2005;435:126–33.
8. Letournel E, Fardeau M, Lytle JO, Serrault M, Gosselin RA. Scapulothoracic arthrodesis for patients who have facioscapulohumeral muscular dystrophy. J Bone Joint Surg Am. 1990;72(1):78–84.
9. Diab M, Darras BT, Shapiro F. Scapulothoracic fusion for facioscapulohumeral muscular dystrophy. J Bone Joint Surg Am. 2005;87(10):2267–75.

10. Berne D, Laude F, Laporte C, Fardeau M, Saillant G. Scapulothoracic arthrodesis in facioscapulohumeral muscular dystrophy. Clin Orthop Relat Res. 2003;409:106–13.

11. Ketenjian AY. Scapulocostal stabilization for scapular winging in facioscapulohumeral muscular dystrophy. J Bone Joint Surg Am. 1978;60(4):476–80.

12. Copeland SA, Howard RC. Thoracoscapular fusion for facioscapulohumeral dystrophy. J Bone Joint Surg Br. 1978;60-B(4):547–51.

13. Jeon IH, Neumann L, Wallace WA. Scapulothoracic fusion for painful winging of the scapula in nondystrophic patients. J Shoulder Elbow Surg. 2005;14(4):400–6.

14. Kocialkowski A, Frostick SP, Wallace WA. One-stage bilateral thoracoscapular fusion using allografts. A case report. Clin Orthop Relat Res. 1991;273:264–7.

15. Bunch WH, Siegel IM. Scapulothoracic arthrodesis in facioscapulohumeral muscular dystrophy. Review of seventeen procedures with three to twenty-one-year follow-up. J Bone Joint Surg Am. 1993;75(3):372–6.

16. Ziaee MA, Abolghasemian M, Majd ME. Scapulothoracic arthrodesis for winged scapula due to facioscapulohumeral dystrophy (a new technique). Am J Orthop. 2006;35(7):311–5.

17. Wolfe GI, Young PK, Nations SP, Burkhead WZ, McVey AL, Barohn RJ. Brachial plexopathy following thoracoscapular fusion in facioscapulohumeral muscular dystrophy. Neurology. 2005;64(3):572–3.

18. Mackenzie WG, Riddle EC, Earley JL, Sawatzky BJ. A neurovascular complication after scapulothoracic arthrodesis. Clin Orthop Relat Res. 2003;408: 157–61.

19. Twyman RS, Harper GD, Edgar MA. Thoracoscapular fusion in facioscapulohumeral dystrophy: clinical review of a new surgical method. J Shoulder Elbow Surg. 1996;5(3):201–5.

20. Jakab E, Gledhill RB. Simplified technique for scapulocostal fusion in facioscapulohumeral dystrophy. J Pediatr Orthop. 1993;13(6):749–51.

21. Demirhan M, Uysal M, Onen M. The use of the cable-grip system in the treatment of winged scapula caused by post-traumatic combined nerve injury: a case report. Acta Orthop Traumatol Turc. 2002;36(2): 162–6.

22. Szomor ZL, Fermanis G, Murrell GA. Scapulothoracic fusion for a stroke patient with Achilles tendon allograft. J Shoulder Elbow Surg. 2000;9(4):342–3.

23. Bizot P, Teboul F, Nizard R, Sedel L. Scapulothoracic fusion for serratus anterior paralysis. J Shoulder Elbow Surg. 2003;12(6):561–5.

24. Giannini S, Ceccarelli F, Faldini C, Pagkrati S, Merlini L. Scapulopexy of winged scapula secondary to facioscapulohumeral muscular dystrophy. Clin Orthop Relat Res. 2006;449:288–94.

Sternoclavicular Joint and Medial Clavicle Injuries

Alistair M. Pace and Lars Neumann

Contents

A.M. Pace (✉)
York Teaching Hospital NHS Foundation Trust,
York, UK
e-mail: alistairpace@hotmail.com

L. Neumann
Nottingham University Hospitals, Nottingham, UK
e-mail: larsneumann@me.com

Keywords

Aetiology • Anatomy • Classification • Clinical signs • Imaging • Instability-Sterno-Clavicular joint, medial clavicle • Mechanism of injury • Medial clavicle fractures • Physeal injuries • Results and complications • Treatment-closed and surgical

Introduction

Traumatic and atraumatic pathology of the sternoclavicular joint (SCJ) is rare. It is difficult to achieve useful plain imaging of this joint and as a result an accurate diagnosis is often missed in Accident and Emergency departments. The treatment may include non-operative or surgical interventions. The operative techniques involved are technically difficult with a high risk of complications. When mismanaged however, SCJ pathology can produce significant morbidity and mortality.

Anatomy

The clavicle forms from two primary centres of ossification that fuse in utero, making the clavicle amongst the first long bones to become radiologically visible [1]. The two ossification centres subsequently fuse leaving a medial epiphysis. It is the last bone in the body to have its epiphysis close at a mean age of 25 years. Hence there is a potential for traumatic Salter-Harris type fractures involving the physis at the medial clavicle up to this age [2].

G. Bentley (ed.), *European Surgical Orthopaedics and Traumatology*,
DOI 10.1007/978-3-642-34746-7_50, © EFORT 2014

The sternoclavicular joint is the only real joint connecting the arm to the axial skeleton. It is a true synovial joint with both the sternal and clavicular sides of the joint being lined by fibrocartilage. It has been described as the most incongruous joint in the body [3].

The sternoclavicular joint is a saddle-shaped diathrodal double-plane joint with the clavicular end being bulbous in shape and the clavicular notch of the sternum being curved. In 2.5 % of cases there is an additional small facet on the inferior aspect of the clavicle that forms a joint with the superior aspect of the first rib [4].

Movement at the joint can occur passively in three planes and is usually produced by transmission of movements of the scapula on the chest wall. During abduction of the shoulder the sternoclavicular joint can elevate 35° in the coronal plane and has a range of movement of 70° around neutral in the antero-posterior plane [5]. Biomechanical studies have documented significant motion in the SCJ with shoulder activities. Indeed the SCJ allows 35° of flexion and extension and 45° of rotation around its longitudinal axis when the arm is elevated. Most of the SCJ motion occurs between the articular disc and the clavicle [6]. The stability of joint relies on both bony and soft tissue structures. The sternoclavicular joint is shallow and has very little bony stability due to the paucity of contact between the sternal and clavicular sides of the joint making the joint incongruent. The stability of the joint is thus highly dependant on the surrounding ligaments, the intra-articular disc and the subclavius muscle.

1. The intra-articular disc absorbs energy on impact to the shoulder and is a thick fibrous structure dividing the joint into two separate compartments. The disc may be incomplete in 6 % of individuals. It is attached from the postero-superior aspect of the medial clavicle at the junction of the first rib to the sternum and usually blends in with the capsular ligaments. Occasionally this disc may be perforated. The disc's role is to act as a soft tissue cushion as well as preventing the clavicle displacing medially.

2. The rhomboid ligament is also vital to the stability of the joint. It is composed of two fasiculi (anterior and posterior bands) and has an interlaced appearance. It is attached to the upper surface of the first rib and to the impression on the inferior aspect of the medial end of the clavicle. The anterior fasiculus of the ligament allows for stability in upward rotation and lateral displacement of the clavicle and the posterior fibres resist downward rotation and medial displacement.

3. The interclavicular ligament binds the superomedial aspects of both clavicles with the upper margin of the sternum. They aid the capsular ligaments in holding up the shoulder girdle.

4. The capsular ligament is composed of the anterior and posterior portions and covers the anterosuperior and posterior aspects of the joints. It represents a thickening of the capsule and is the strongest ligament supporting the joint, resisting superior displacement of the medial clavicle together with the intra-articular disc when the lateral clavicle is pulled inferiorly. The ligament is attached to the epiphysis of the medial clavicle and is vital in maintaining normal shoulder poise [7] (Fig. 1).

The sternoclavicular joint is subcutaneous and the thoracic inlet lies posteriorly. The great vessels of the superior mediastinum, trachea, oesophagus, vagus and phrenic nerves lie very close to the joint. Posterior dislocation of the SCJ can damage these structures causing serious injury. The proximity of these structures to the joint also places them at risk during surgery [8] (Fig. 2).

Epidemiology

Dislocations of the sternoclavicular joint are far less common than the glenohumeral and acromioclavicular joint. They comprise 1 % of all joint dislocations in the body and 3 % of upper limb dislocations. They frequently occur in active

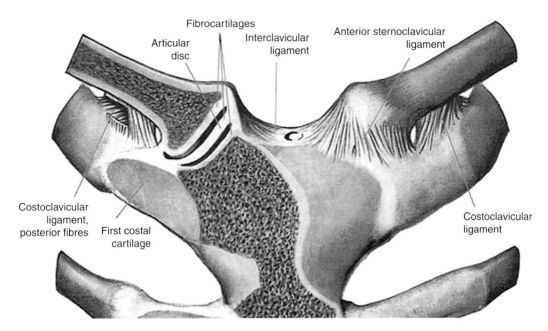

Fig. 1 Diagram illustrating the anatomy of sternoclavicular joint and surrounding stabilizing structures including the rhomboid, interclavicular and capsular ligaments. The rhomboid ligament has two bands that are attached from the first rib to the medial clavicle. The interclavicular ligaments bind the superomedial aspects of both clavicles with the upper margin of the sternum

young males and as a result of high energy injuries [9]. Minor sprains and medial physeal injuries are more common but rarely do patients seek medical advice for these conditions.

Mechanisim of Injury

In spite of the sternoclavicular joint being a small and incongruent joint, the ligamentous structures are strong and hence it rarely dislocates. The sternoclavicular joint most commonly disloclates either anteriorly or posteriorly although superior and inferior dislocation of the joint has been described. When it does, it usually follows a high energy force and this may be directly onto the sternoclavicular joint region such as when a force is applied to the clavicle in an anterior-posterior direction or indirectly to the shoulder joint by a fall on a outstretched hand [10]. The most common causes of sternoclavicular joint dislocation are motor vehicle accidents and sports injuries.

Classification of Sternoclavicular Joint Injuries

The joint may become partially incongruent with some of the joint surface remaining in contact(subluxation) or fully incongruent when there is no contact remaining between the two joint surfaces (dislocation). These injuries may be classified according to the anatomic position of dislocation or the cause of dislocation.

Anatomic Classification

Anterior Dislocation
This is the most common type with the medial end of the clavicle being displaced anteriorly or anterosuperiorly to the margin of the sternum. This usually results from a direct lateral blow to the shoulder with the shoulder retracted [1].

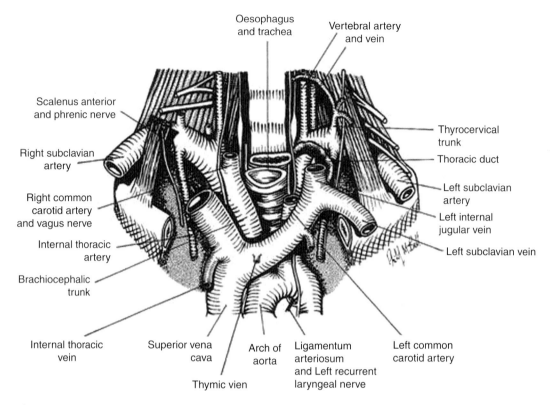

Fig. 2 Diagram illustrating the mediastinal structures in close proximity to the sternoclavicular joint and at risk of injury. Posterior dislocation of the sternoclavicular joint can compress the aorta as well as subclavian artery and vein

Posterior Dislocation

This is less common with the medial clavicle displacing posteriorly or postero-superiorly with respect to the sternum. The ratio of anterior to posterior dislocation is 20:1 [11]. Posterior dislocation most commonly results from indirect forces imparted to the shoulder girdle with the shoulder adducted and protracted. The force is applied laterally and indirectly, transmitted along the long axis of the clavicle. The force can be applied by a lateral blow to the ipsilateral shoulder. Alternatively, force applied to the contralateral shoulder can yield the same effect when the ipsilateral shoulder is braced against an immobile object. Less commonly the joint may be dislocated posteriorly with posteriorly directed blow to the medial clavicle [12].

The direction of the dislocation depends on the relation of the acromion to the manubrium at the time of impact. If the acromion is anterior then a posterior dislocation will occur as the clavicle is levered out by a posteriorly-directed force. If the acromion is posterior to the manubrium at the critical point of impact then the joint dislocates anteriorly. The acromion is usually situated posteriorly relative to the manubrium explaining why anterior dislocations are more common. Moreover the posterior capsule is much more substantial than the anterior capsule further increasing the propensity to anterior dislocation [13, 14].

Aetiology

Traumatic
Sprain
When the joint is sprained, the stabilizing ligaments are damaged but there is no instability and the joint remains congruent. This may be mild, moderate or severe with increasing damage to the stabilising ligaments [12].

Subluxation

With further damage to the stabilizing structures of the joint, relative movement between the joint surfaces may occur, however the joint usually spontaneously reduces. The joint sufaces may sublux so that the joint surfaces are temporarily out of place and non-congruent. The patient may experience a clicking sensation resulting from the abnormal joint surface movements or from an associated intra-articular meniscal tear.

Acute Dislocation

If the capsular and intra-articular ligaments are completely disrupted a full joint dislocation can occur and the joint surfaces lose contact and remain in a dislocated position. The joint may dislocate anteriorly or posteriorly. In some cases the costoclavicular ligaments may simply be stretched and not completely disrupted. Full dislocations need to be distinguished from very medial fractures and epiphysiolysis particularly in young adults.

Recurrent Dislocation

In these patients there is a history of an acute dislocation when, after reduction, the ligament damage does not heal and subsequently dislocations may occur with minimal or no trauma. These recurrent dislocations may be painless or painful and associated with clicking as the joint dislocates recurrently.

Atraumatic

These occur particularly in children and adolescents and the natural history and results of treatment are quite different to the traumatic cases. These may be of two types.

Spontaneous Subluxation and Dislocation

In this type of subluxation and/or dislocation there is no history of injury.

These patients are usually young or middle-aged females presenting with a palpable deformity over the medial clavicle. Clinically patients usually have features of generalized joint laxity and the episodes of dislocation typically occurs on the dominant side.

There can be a painless subluxation of one or both joints during overhead activities however there is usually no danger to mediastinal structures [15] Spontaneous posterior dislocation may occur but this is very rare and can be treated similarly to a traumatic dislocation [3].

Congenital Subluxation or Dislocation

This has been reported as far back as 1841. There is usually loss of bone stock of the medial clavicles causing instability with subluxation or dislocation. The condition can also occur in patients with severe scoliosis causing anterior displacement of the shoulder girdle and hence posterior dislocation of the strernoclavicular joint. The condition is usually hereditary and are treated conservatively unless the dislocation is posterior [16].

Physeal Injuries

Salter-Harris type epiphyseal fractures may involve the medial clavicle and they are often difficult to distinguish from simple dislocations. As the medial clavicle epiphysis is the last physis to close at around the age of 25 years, this diagnosis must be considered in a patient below this age who present with traumatic pathology of the medial clavicle. The principles of managing these injuries differs from simple sternoclavicular joint dislocations. Most of these injuries have the potential to remodel and hence surgical intervention is rarely indicated. The ability for these injuries to remodel is illustrated by several case reports in the literature [17]. However some authors have argued that significantly displaced physeal injuries should be treated operatively as the potential for remodelling in these cases is limited.

Whilst conservative treatment is advocated with anterior physeal injuries, it is vital that patients with posterior physeal injuries are investigated radiologically to assess any potential compression of mediastinal structures. Only once this has been excluded can these injuries be safely treated conservatively. If there is evidence of compromise the injury must be reduced. This may be achieved by closed methods or operatively if this fails [18].

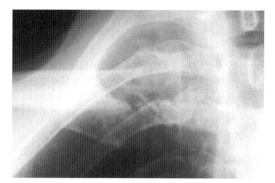

Fig. 3 Antero-posterior radiograph of the proximal clavicle showing fractured medial end of the right clavicle

Fractures of the Medial Clavicle

Fractures of the medial third of the clavicle are rare, accounting for between 2 % and 9.3 % of all clavicular fractures (Fig. 3). These fractures are often sustained in high-speed motor-vehicle collisions, and seat belt use, while life-saving, may have a role in the production of these injuries [19].

Typically, patients with a fracture of the medial third of the clavicle also have severe thoracic injuries including pneumothorax and/or pulmonary contusion, with respiratory failure occurring in nearly half of the patients. Other injuries include rib fractures, head injuries, and cervical spine and other upper-extremity injuries. The mortality rate is as high as 19 % for patients with these fractures [20]. The fractures are classified according to their configuration, with transverse and comminuted fractures presenting most commonly. Non-operative treatment is most often recommended, but an open fracture is an indication for operative fixation. Many patients have residual pain, and the non-union rate may approach 15 %. Some authors have reported success with surgical reduction and internal fixation [21].

Signs and Symptoms

If the sternoclavicular joint has suffered a sprain then the stabilising ligaments of the joint are structurally intact and the patient complains of varying amounts of pain around the area with movement of the upper limb girdle. There may

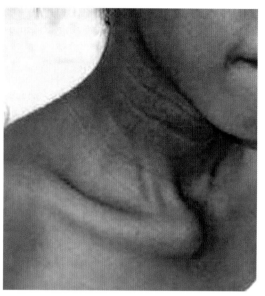

Fig. 4 Clinical photograph demonstrating a patient with an right anterior sternoclavicular joint dislocation. The anterior bulge is the medial clavicle end

be swelling and tenderness but no evidence of instability as the joint surfaces remain continually in congruous contact. In more severe types of injury when the stabilizing ligaments have been damaged, swelling and pain with movement is usually more marked and there may be subluxation or instability, when the joint is stressed. In patients with ligamentous laxity and multidirectional instability, there may be no history of injury but the patient may be aware of a painful or painless lump presenting intermittently at the sternoclavicular joint as the medial clavicle translates in and out of the joint (Fig. 4).

When the capsular and disc-stabilising ligaments of the joint have been disrupted the medial clavicle end may displace anteriorly or posteriorly. The patient complains of severe pain exacerbated by movement of the arm particularly when the shoulders are pressed together by a bilateral force. The patients may protectively take the weight of the affected arm by supporting it across the chest. The discomfort may be worse on lying flat. The neck may be be tilted toward the dislocated side to minimize the painful traction on the clavicle provided by the sternocleidomastoid muscle [22].

If the dislocation is chronic, the patient may be pain-free. Clinically, there is shortening and protraction of the shoulder with tilting of the head towards the affected side. A common pitfall lies in diagnosing an anterior SCJ dislocation because of a palpable, tender swelling at the medial clavicle when in fact it is posterior. This may simply be from palpating the swollen joint capsule, which can be prominent even if the displacement is posteriorly [23]. Chronic anterior instability is a rare problem and usually presents with pain, clicking, crepitus or popping with shoulder motion. There may be limitation in use when attempting activities away from body or overhead.

In anterior dislocation the medial end of the clavicle is very prominent and may be palpated anterior to the sternum. The dislocation may be fixed or reducible. Patients with posterior dislocations are often in more pain than those with an anterior dislocation. In these patients the medial end of the clavicle may be felt to be located posteriorly and the anterior margin of the sternum may be easily palpated. The medial end of the clavicle may compress the large veins of the neck causing venous congestion or decreased circulation. There may be anterosuperior fullness of the chest. If the respiratory system is compressed the patient may show signs of breathlessness, choking or shortness of breath. The patient may have difficulty swallowing or he/she may be complaining of a tight feeling in the throat. It is thus vital that patients presenting with SCJ pathology are thoroughly assessed. The pulses should be palpated, the upper extremity neurologically tested and the venous return assessed [24].

In patients where the diagnosis of sternoclavicular joint subluxation is not obvious the joint may be assessed by placing a finger or a hand on the joint anteriorly whilst the patient circumducts and extends the shoulder. In cases of subluxation, displacement of the medial clavicle may cause a simple click or abnormal movement may be felt as the joint is axially loaded.

Sternoclavicular joint dislocations are usually high energy injuries and there may be associated haemothorax or pneumothorax. Worman and Leagus have reported that 16 out of 60 patients they reviewed with posterior dislocation of the sternoclavicular joint had complications of the trachea, oesophagus or great vessels. The majority of these complications were noted at the time of injury but later complications including thoracic outlet syndrome, subclavian artery compression, exertional dyspnea and fatal sepsis after the development of a tracheo-oesophageal fistula have been recorded [25]. Other authors have reported mediastinal injuries in 30 % of cases. It must be emphasised that these complications are rare but when they do occur are serious and require the expertise of a cardiothoracic surgeon usually necessitating a thoracotomy [26].

Radiographic Evaluation

Radiographic evaluation of the sternoclavicular joint can be difficult due to its anatomy as well as its relationship to overlying and adjacent structures. A chest radiograph may occasionally reveal asymmetrical clavicle lengths and abnormal joints but these finding are usually subtle. A number of dedicated radiographic views for the sterno-clavicular joint have been developed as the standard clavicle diaphyseal radiographs often fail to reveal the necessary detail. Heinig proposed a tangential radiograph of the SCJ with the patient supine and the cassette placed behind the opposite shoulder. The beam is angled in the coronal plane, parallel to the longitudinal axis of the opposite clavicle, providing a profile of the affected sternoclavicular joint [27]. Hobbs has proposed a 90° cephalocaudal lateral, taken with the patient seated and flexed over a table. The cassette is placed on the table, against the chest wall, and the beam is directed through the cervical spine [28] (Fig. 5). The "serendipity" view proposed by Rockwood involves the cassette being placed behind the chest and the radiographic beam angled at 40° cephalad centred on the sternum, allowing for the visualisation of both SCJs. In cases of anterior dislocation, the affected clavicular head will appear superiorly compared with the unaffected side. Conversely, with posterior displacement, the medial clavicle will appear inferior [29] (Figs. 6 and 7).

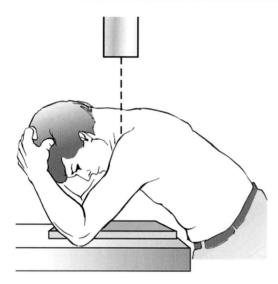

Fig. 5 Patient positioning when performing the Hobb's radiographic view of the sternoclavicular joint. A 90° cephalocaudal lateral, taken with the patient seated and flexed over a table. The cassette is placed on the table, against the chest wall, and the beam is directed through the cervical spine

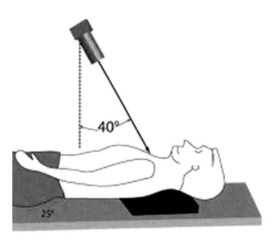

Fig. 6 Patient positioning when performing the "Serendipity" radiographic view of the sternoclavicular joint. involves the cassette being placed behind the chest and the radiographic beam angled at 40° cephalic centered on the sternum, allowing for the visualisation of both SCJs. In cases of anterior dislocation, the affected clavicular head will appear superiorly compared with the unaffected side

It must be emphasized that there are reported cases of reducible dislocations, which are difficult to visualize with plain radiology. Therefore, if a disruption is clinically suspected despite

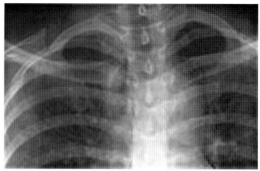

Fig. 7 Rockwood's "Serendipity" radiographic view illustrating clearly the sternoclavicular joint

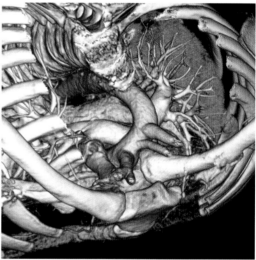

Fig. 8 Three dimensional CT scan demonstrating posterior dislocation of left sternoclavicular joint. This image is particularly useful for assessing how much clavicle displacement is present and which structures are being compressed by the clavicle

unremarkable plain views, then computed tomography should always be performed.

Three-dimensional computer-aided tomography is now being increasingly used and improved resolution helps distinguish different SCJ injuries including physeal fractures and true dislocations (Fig. 8). In patients with a past history of trauma or long history of joint instability, swelling at the sternoclavicular joint may be related to degenerative changes rather than subluxation or dislocation of the joint. Swelling in this area may more commonly be related to degenerative joint

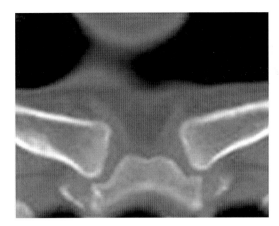

Fig. 9 CT scan demonstrating normal sternoclavicular joint

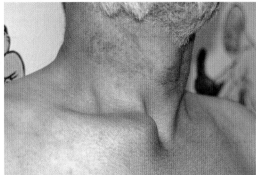

Fig. 11 Clinical photograph demonstrating an old fracture/dislocation of the right sternoclavicular joint

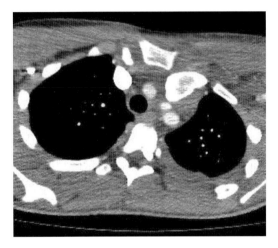

Fig. 10 CT scan demonstrating right posterior dislocation of the right sternoclavicular joint

disease, medial clavicle osteitis, joint sepsis or aseptic inflammatory reaction of the joint. The CT scan is particularly useful in distinguishing these different pathologies (Figs. 9, 10 and 11). Concomitant angiography should be performed if obstruction of the thoracic outlet or vascular injury is suspected. MRI may also be useful in assessing associated soft tissue damage after injury. Some authors also recommend the use of stress views to exacerbate the deformity on plain radiographs and others suggest the use of ultrasound to assess bony displacement and associated soft tissue injury. However both these modalities are not widely used [30].

Treatment Principles

Traumatic Injuries

Mild Sprain

In this injury the joint is stable but painful. These are treated conservatively with rest, analgesia and ice packs alternating with heat packs. The shoulder is rested in a sling for 5–7 days and then gradual mobilization is commenced.

Subluxation

This injury is also treated like a soft tissue sprain injury with ice and heat. The subluxation may occasionally need to be reduced by manipulating the shoulder girdle. A clavicle strap may be applied to aid maintainence of the reduction and a sling to prevent excess arm movement. This should be kept on for 6 weeks. DePalma suggests the use of plaster figure-of-eight dressings [31] whilst Allman prefers the use of a soft figure-of-eight bandage with a sling [32]. In cases where the subluxation cannot be reduced or improved by conservative treatment open reduction and subsequent repair of the ligaments and stabilization by internal fixation using sternoclavicular wires across the joint has been suggested. The use of wires across this joint however are fraught with risk and possible complications most notably wire migration. However in most cases the patient may simply chose to ignore the pathology particularly if painless and prefer it to be treated by physiotherapy [33].

Dislocations

A number of principles guide the treatment of SCJ fracture-dislocations:

1. The time from initial injury. Non-operative or surgical treatment options must be considered depending on the chronicity of the injury. A chronically dislocated joint may be treated non-operatively particularly if painless. An acutely posterior dislocated sternoclavicular joint however may require emergency surgery particularly if it compresses the mediastinum.
2. Anterior dislocations may produce little in terms of pain or functional compromise. Posterior dislocations however are more serious and can result in life-threatening complications.
3. The risks and benefits of the interventions must be considered in relation to the severity of symptoms
4. Patient expectations. In elderly patients with minimal demands, an acutely dislocated sterno-clavicular joint may be accepted and treated non-operatively. In high demand patients, particularly athletes, a dislocated stenoclavicular joint may result in persistent pain and disability if not addressed surgically.

Spontaneous Subluxation and Dislocation

Rockwood and Oder have suggested the benign course of this condition and treatment including patient education and reassurance usually occurs in an unaltered lifestyle with little discomfort. Rarely the condition however may be painful enough to restrict activities. The problem may be secondary to condensing osteitis affecting the medial clavicle [3].

Closed Treatment of Anterior Dislocation

Closed treatment of sternoclavicular joint dislocations is usually only effective in the acute stage. In the chronic stage the joint scars and develops a contracture making closed reduction difficult. In these circumstances there should be a low threshold for open reduction and reconstruction of the joint [34]. Anterior dislocations are usually unstable and should be reduced under general anaesthesia if diagnosed early. This is simply achieved by direct pressure over the medial portion of the clavicle of a supine patient with a solid pad placed between the shoulders. Successful reduction has been reported up to 5–10 days after dislocation however early reduction within 72 hrs is advocated. The patient should be immobilized in an arm sling for 3–6 weeks and physiotherapy commenced thereafter. Pure sternoclavicular dislocations often are stable once reduced in a closed fashion. The fracture-dislocation pattern of the injury, however is inherently unstable, because the high energy imparted to the shoulder girdle had stripped the majority of the soft tissues that normally would stabilize the clavicle once reduced [35]. The long-term success of closed reduction is limited and a proportion of patients may have chronic anterior dislocation due to incomplete capsular healing. Nettles reported on 14 cases of acute anterior dislocation treated with early closed reduction. In 3 cases there was persistent instability of the joint [7]. Moreover Eskola reported on a series of eight patients treated by closed reduction and five had recurrent dislocation. Recurrent anterior instability following an acute anterior dislocation rarely results in functional deficit. Moreover, some anterior dislocations are irreducible and in both cases these can be accepted and treated with physiotherapy and slings [36]. According to Miller the surrounding shoulder muscles including trapezius and sternocleidomastoid compensate for maintaining shoulder poise [37]. A study by Savastano and Stutz reported the results of 12 patients treated closed and open. They concluded that reduction and stability of the SC joint is not necessary to ensure normal function of the involved limb. They also found that residual prominence of the medial portion of the clavicle does not cause pain and does not interfere with function of the shoulder. Operative intervention in these cases should be considered only if there is persistent pain and functional disability. In young patients a substantial degree of remodelling may occur during growth and the functional deficit with "skillful" neglect is often minor [38].

Closed Treatment of Posterior Dislocation

This can be achieved by abducting the arm and applying traction whilst the shoulder is moved into an extended position. If this fails or the dislocation is more than 48 h old then an anteriorly directed traction may be applied to the medial clavicle with sterile reduction forceps clipped percutaneously into the bone. Alternatively, reduction may be achieved by adducting the arm at the affected side and to apply traction to the arm at the same time as applying a posteriorly directed pressure on the glenohumeral joint. The procedure should be performed under anaesthesia both to provide pain relief and muscle relaxation, but also to allow an EUA (examination under anaesthesia) to be performed and hence assess the stability of the joint after reduction and the likelihood of re-dislocation (Fig. 12). In all cases of closed relocation, the patient should be admitted to hospital and monitored for signs of mediastinal obstruction. The arm should be immobilized after reduction in a sling. Posterior dislocations are usually stable once reduced unlike anterior dislocations. This results from the more substantial posterior sternoclavicular joint stabilising structures as compared to the anterior structures. These thick stabilising ligaments are only mildly stretched and only rarely disrupted with a posterior dislocation. Anterior dislocations unlike posterior dislocations frequently disrupt the anterior less rigorous structures and hence the joint is not as stable when reduced. Posterior dislocations may be accepted and treated conservatively but late thoracic outlet syndrome, exertional dyspnoea and chronic vascular insufficiency have been described as has pain arising from

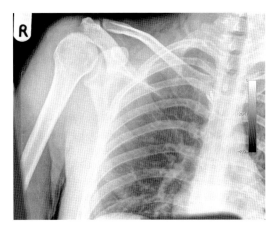

Fig. 12 Post-operative radiograph demonstrating the anchors utilized in achieving stabilization of the sternoclavicular joint using the technique described by Frostick et al

a chronically dislocated degenerate joint [39]. Reconstruction of a chronically dislocated sternoclavicular joint is usually more technically difficult to perform and the risks are greater than an acute joint reconstruction. Buckerfield and Castle reported successful closed reduction of a traumatic posterior sternoclavicular dislocation or a posterior physeal fracture- dislocation in six of seven patients ranging from 13 to 26 years of age. Their technique involved retraction of the shoulders with caudal traction on the adducted arm with an interscapular bolster supporting the patient. 1 patient with persistent post-reduction instability was treated by holding the shoulders in full retraction with a figure-of-8 clavicular strap [40]. Lafosse recently reported that in a series of closed early reduction of posterior dislocations only half were successfully reduced [41]. Rockwood et al. have also reported similar findings. In their series one patient underwent successful reduction 10 days following injury which suggests that in some cases, it may be still possible to reduce these injuries even after 10 days [42]. The use of external splints, figure-of-eight bandages and local pressure dressings only provide symptomatic support and have not been proven to have any influence in preventing redisplacement of unstable reductions.

Open Treatment of Anterior and Posterior Sternoclavicular Joint Dislocation

This may be required in patients where closed reduction of anterior and posterior dislocations has failed or when there is persistent painful instability of the joint possible, or if there is risk of skin compromise in an anterior dislocation. The latter may follow trauma or occur in individuals with generalized joint laxity. A number of studies have reported the outcome of treatment of acute dislocation [43]. The proximity of the adjacent vessels dictates that a cardiothoracic surgeon should always be present in theatre when open surgical treatment of a posterior dislocation is attempted. Approximately 30 cases of iatrogenic lesions of the heart, lungs or large mediastinal vessels (thoracic aorta, pulmonary artery, brachiocephalic vessels) have been reported in the French-, English-, and German-language literature. A skin crease incision is made centred on the joint and forceful traction may need to be applied to the abducted shoulder to reduce the clavicle from the retrosternal position under direct vision. Reduction may be facilitated using a reduction forceps on the medial end of the clavicle [44]. If open reduction of the joint on the table is not stable then double breasting of the anterior or posterior capsule (open reduction and capsulorraphy) and re-inforcing it with sutures passed through the bone and fixed either with anchors on one side or through drill holes on both sides has been described. This is usually all that is required in the acute situation [45]. In cases of recurrent instability or persistent dislocation, various surgical procedures have been suggested in the literature. These include open reduction and stabilization with wires, k- wires, plates, screw fixation, external fixator, reconstruction with fascial loops and tendon grafts (fascia lata, Palmaris longus and semi-tendinosus tendon), tenodesis, stabilization with Polydioxonone (PDS) cord and excision of the medial end of the clavicle (medial clavicular resection arthroplasty) and arthrodesis of the joint. The use of pins across the sterno-clavicular joint is not recommended because of the serious complications that can occur with this technique. There is a risk of migration of intact or broken wires into the heart, pulmonary artery, innominate artery or aorta. Seven deaths and three near deaths have been reported in the literature from complications of transfixing the sternoclavicular joint with Kirschner wires or Steinmann pins [46]. The use of more stable implants such as Balser plates have been advocated although not widely used or tested. These plates allow early mobilization but require removal at about 3 months post-operatively. The series presented on 10 patients had a Constant score of 90.2 +/− 6.6 with no ongoing instability [44]. Although these implants also are at risk of breakage and loosening with subsequent migration this complication was not reported. Brinker et al. reported the use of two large-bore cannulated screws in conjunction with open reduction to stabilize an unstable sternoclavicular joint. The patient was immobilized post-operatively and the metalwork was removed after 3 months [47]. Suture anchors and capsulorrhapy, as described by Frostick et al., does not involve exposure of the first rib and 7 year results have been reported with good stability. The technique is simple, anatomic and has low complication rates. This technique is the preferred method of sternoclavicular joint reconstruction by the senior author. The technique is particularly useful in patients with subtle instability and clicking [48] (Fig. 12). Tendon grafts are usually looped through drill holes in the manubrium and medial clavicle. The soft tissue reconstruction is then secured and augmented with strong non-absorbable sutures. The results of stabilization using ligament substitution have been mixed with a high prevalence of soft-tissue complications and failure of the reconstruction resulting in recurrence of the deformity. The best outcomes were shown with the use of a semi-tendinosis graft configured in a figure-of-eight arrangement through two pre-drilled holes in the clavicular head and manubrium [49] (Fig. 13). Synthetic material has been used in reconstructing the sternoclavicular joint but results have been poor with erosion and

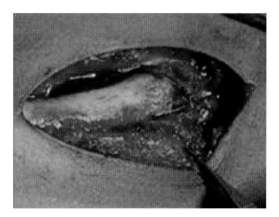

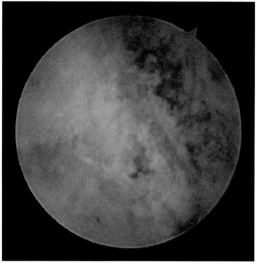

Fig. 13 Peri-operative picture of the right sternoclavicular joint being stabilized using a semi-tendinosis graft. The picture shows the semitendinosis graft channeled as a figure of 8 through intraosseous drill holes in the medial end of clavicle and sternal end stabilizing the joint

Fig. 15 Peri-operative arthroscopic picture of the sternoclavicular joint following resection. The degenerative meniscus has been resected and the medial end of the clavicel shaved by about 10 mm with an arthroscopic shaver allowing an excision arthroplasty to be created (Acknowledgments to Mr. G. Tytherleigh-Strong. Consultant Orthopaedic Surgeon)

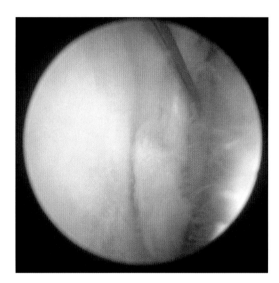

Fig. 14 Peri-operative arthroscopic picture of a torn degenerate intra-articular meniscus of the sternoclavicular joint. The degenerative medial end of the clavicle is to the left of the picture and the degenerative sternal end to the right. The arthroscopic hook in the background is in contact with the pathological fibrocartilage meniscus (Acknowledgments to Mr. G. Tytherleigh-Strong. Consultant Orthopaedic Surgeon)

non-union of the first rib. Carbon fibre ligament has been used to reconstruct the sternoclavicular joint together with Kirschner wire temporary fixation. Dacron has also been used as a suture material but there are reports of bone erosion [50]. Rockwood et al. have described good results

using a procedure involving decompression of the mediastinum by excision of the medial clavicle. The residual clavicle was then stabilized to the costo-clavicular ligament and the periosteum of the first rib [51]. Eskola et al. however has reported poor results in patients treated with resection for old traumatic dislocations and reported good results with tendon grafts and fascial loops [36]. Medial resection arthroplasty (1–2 cm) is mostly indicated in the setting of bony changes and joint arthrosis or if a ligament reconstruction cannot be performed because of absent residual soft tissue attachments. It is important that the remaining medial clavicle is stabilized by ligamentous repair or augmentation of the costo-clavicular ligaments as the results of resection arthroplasty are poor without this soft tissue stabilization. Arthroscopic sternoclavicular joint resection can be indicated in degenerate sternoclavicular joints. The technique is developing but excellent results have been reported [52] (Figs. 14 and 15). Arthrodesis is contra-indicated due to the marked restriction in shoulder movements it produces [53].

References

1. Macdonald PB, Lapointe P. Acromioclavicular and sternoclavicular joint injuries. Orthop Clin North Am. 2008;39(4):535–45, viii. Review.

2. Robinson CM, Jenkins PJ, Markham PE, Beggs I. Disorders of the sternoclavicular joint. J Bone Joint Surg Br. 2008;90(6):685–96. Review.

3. Bicos J, Nicholson GP. Treatment and results of sternoclavicular joint injuries. Clin Sports Med. 2003;22(2):359–70. Review.

4. Renfree KJ, Wright TW. Anatomy and biomechanics of the acromioclavicular and sternoclavicular joints. Clin Sports Med. 2003;22(2):219–37. Review.

5. Bontempo NA, Mazzocca AD. Biomechanics and treatment of acromioclavicular and sternoclavicular joint injuries. Br J Sports Med. 2010;44(5):361–9.

6. Ludewig PM, Phadke V, Braman JP, Hassett DR, Cieminski CJ, LaPrade RF. Motion of the shoulder complex during multiplanar humeral elevation. J Bone Joint Surg Am. 2009;91:378.

7. Nettles JL, Linscheid RL. Sternoclavicular dislocations. J Trauma. 1968;8(2):158–64.

8. Chakarun CJ, Wolfson N. Adult male with right shoulder pain. Posterior sternoclavicular joint dislocation. Ann Emerg Med. 2009;53(6):714–45.

9. Jarrett PM. Sternoclavicular dislocations. J R Soc Med. 2002;95(9):476–7.

10. Lemos MJ, Tolo ET. Complications of the treatment of the acromioclavicular and sternoclavicular joint injuries, including instability. Clin Sports Med. 2003;22(2):371–85. Review.

11. Pensy RA, Eglseder WA. Posterior sternoclavicular fracture-dislocation: a case report and novel treatment method. J Shoulder Elbow Surg. 2010;19(4):e5–8. Epub 2010 Mar 19.

12. Stewart DP, Van Klompenberg LH. Posterior dislocation of the clavicle at the sternoclavicular joint. Am J Emerg Med. 2008;26(1):108.e3–4.

13. Jaggard MK, Gupte CM, Gulati V, Reilly PJ. A comprehensive review of trauma and disruption to the sternoclavicular joint with the proposal of a new classification system. J Trauma. 2009;66(2):576–84. Review.

14. Bahk MS, Kuhn JE, Galatz LM, Connor PM, Williams Jr GR. Acromioclavicular and sternoclavicular injuries and clavicular, glenoid, and scapular fractures. Instr Course Lect. 2010;59:209–26. Review.

15. Hiramuro-Shoji F, Wirth MA, Rockwood Jr CA. Atraumatic conditions of the sternoclavicular joint. J Shoulder Elbow Surg. 2003;12(1):79–88. Review.

16. Hoekzema N, Torchia M, Adkins M, Cassivi SD. Posterior sternoclavicular joint dislocation. Can J Surg. 2008;51(1):E19–20.

17. Laffosse JM, Espié A, Bonnevialle N, Mansat P, Tricoire JL, Bonnevialle P, Chiron P, Puget J. Posterior dislocation of the sternoclavicular joint and epiphyseal disruption of the medial clavicle with posterior displacement in sports participants. J Bone Joint Surg Br. 2010;92(1):103–9.

18. Hecox SE, Wood II GW. Ledge plating technique for unstable posterior sternoclavicular dislocation. J Orthop Trauma. 2010;24(4):255–7.

19. Groh GI, Wirth MA. Management of traumatic sternoclavicular joint injuries. J Am Acad Orthop Surg. 2011;19(1):1–7.

20. Fenig M, Lowman R, Thompson BP, Shayne PH. Fatal posterior sternoclavicular joint dislocation due to occult trauma. Am J Emerg Med. 2010;28(3):385.e5–8.

21. Panzica M, Zeichen J, Hankemeier S, Gaulke R, Krettek C, Jagodzinski M. Long-term outcome after joint reconstruction or medial resection arthroplasty for anterior SCJ instability. Arch Orthop Trauma Surg. 2010;130(5):657–65. Epub 2009 Jun 10.

22. Chien LC, Hsu IL, Tsai MC, Lo CJ. Bilateral anterior sternoclavicular dislocation. J Trauma. 2009;66(5):1504.

23. Johnson MC, Jacobson JA, Fessell DP, Kim SM, Brandon C, Caoili E. The sternoclavicular joint: can imaging differentiate infection from degenerative change? Skeletal Radiol. 2010;39(6):551–8. Epub 2009 Oct.

24. Little NJ, Bismil Q, Chipperfield A, Ricketts DM. Superior dislocation of the sternoclavicular joint. J Shoulder Elbow Surg. 2008;17(1):e22–3.

25. Shuler FD, Pappas N. Treatment of posterior sternoclavicular dislocation with locking plate osteosynthesis. Orthopedics. 2008;31(3):273.

26. Armstrong AL, Dias JJ. Reconstruction for instability of the sternoclavicular joint using the tendon of the sternocleidomastoid muscle. J Bone Joint Surg Br. 2008;90(5):610–3.

27. Gobet R, Meuli M, Altermatt S, Jenni V, Willi UV. Medial clavicular epiphysiolysis in children: the so-called sterno-clavicular dislocation. Emerg Radiol. 2004;10(5):252–5. Epub 2004 Feb 3.

28. Hobbs DW. Sternoclavicular joint: a new axial radiographic view. Radiology. 1968;90(4):801.

29. Garretson III RB, Williams Jr GR. Clinical evaluation of injuries to the acromioclavicular and sternoclavicular joints. Clin Sports Med. 2003;22(2):239–54.

30. Hudson VJ. Evaluation, diagnosis, and treatment of shoulder injuries in athletes. Clin Sports Med. 2010;29(1):19–32.

31. Marinelli M, de Palma L. The external rotation method for reduction of acute anterior shoulder dislocations. J Orthop Traumatol. 2009;10(1):17–20. Epub 2009 Jan 8.

32. Allman Jr FL. Fractures and ligamentous injuries of the clavicle and its articulation. J Bone Joint Surg Am. 1967;49(4):774–84.

33. Lee SU, Park IJ, Kim YD, Kim YC, Jeong C. Stabilization for chronic sternoclavicular joint instability. Knee Surg Sports Traumatol Arthrosc. 2010;18(12):1795–7. Epub 2010 Sep 18.

34. Higginbotham TO, Kuhn JE. Atraumatic disorders of the sternoclavicular joint. J Am Acad Orthop Surg. 2005;13(2):138–45. Review.

35. Buckley BJ, Hayden SR. Posterior sternoclavicular dislocation. J Emerg Med. 2008;34(3):331–2. Epub 2007 Sep 10.

36. Eskola A, Vainionpää S, Vastamäki M, Slätis P, Rokkanen P. Operation for old sternoclavicular dislocation. Results in 12 cases. J Bone Joint Surg Br. 1989;71(1):63–5.

37. Turman KA, Miller CD, Miller MD. Clavicular fractures following coracoclavicular ligament reconstruction with tendon graft: a report of three cases. J Bone Joint Surg Am. 2010;92(6):1526–32.

38. Savastano AA, Stutz SJ. Traumatic sternoclavicular dislocation. Int Surg. 1978;63(1):10.

39. Salgado RA, Ghysen D. Post-traumatic posterior sternoclavicular dislocation: case report and review of the literature. Emerg Radiol. 2002;9(6):323–5. Epub 2002 Nov 9.

40. Buckerfield CT, Castle ME. Acute traumatic retrosternal dislocation of the clavicle. J Bone Joint Surg Am. 1984;66(3):379–85.

41. Taam SA, Molinier F, Chaminade B, Puget J. Orthop Traumatol Surg Res. 2010;96(3):314–8. Epub 2010 Apr 15.

42. Wirth MA, Rockwood Jr CA. Acute and chronic traumatic injuries of the sternoclavicular joint. J Am Acad Orthop Surg. 1996;4(5):268–78.

43. Baumann M, Vogel T, Weise K, Muratore T, Trobisch P. Bilateral posterior sternoclavicular dislocation. Orthopedics. 2010;33(7):510. doi:10.3928/01477447-20100526-19.

44. Fenig M, Lowman R, Thompson BP, Shayne PH. Fatal posterior sternoclavicular joint dislocation due to occult trauma. Am J Emerg Med. 2010;28(3):e5–8.

45. Gove N, Ebraheim NA, Glass E. Posterior sternoclavicular dislocations: a review of management and complications. Am J Orthop (Belle Mead NJ). 2006;35(3):132–6. Review.

46. Franck WM, Jannasch O, Siassi M, Hennig FF. Balser plate stabilization: an alternate therapy for traumatic sternoclavicular instability. J Shoulder Elbow Surg. 2003;12(3):276–81.

47. Brinker MR, Bartz RL, Reardon PR, Reardon MJ. A method for open reduction and internal fixation of the unstable posterior sternoclavicular joint dislocation. J Orthop Trauma. 1997;11(5):378–81.

48. Abiddin Z, Sinopidis C, Grocock CJ, Yin Q, Frostick SPJ. Suture anchors for treatment of sternoclavicular joint instability. J Shoulder Elbow Surg. 2006;15(3):315–8.

49. Castropil W, Ramadan LB, Bitar AC, Schor B, de Oliveira D'Elia C. Sternoclavicular dislocation–reconstruction with semitendinosus tendon autograft: a case report. Knee Surg Sports Traumatol Arthrosc. 2008;16(9):865–8. Epub 2008 Apr 17.

50. Burri C, Neugebauer R. Carbon fiber replacement of the ligaments of the shoulder girdle and the treatment of lateral instability of the ankle joint. Clin Orthop Relat Res. 1985;196:112–7.

51. Groh GI, Wirth MA, Rockwood Jr CA. Treatment of traumatic posterior sternoclavicular dislocations. J Shoulder Elbow Surg. 2011;20(1):107–13. Epub 2010 Jun 26.

52. Tavakkolizadeh A, Hales PF, Janes GC. Arthroscopic excision of sternoclavicular joint. Knee Surg Sports Traumatol Arthrosc. 2009;17(4):405–8. Epub 2008 Dec 17.

53. Elhassan B, Chung ST, Ozbaydar M, Diller D, Warner JJ. Scapulothoracic fusion for clavicular insufficiency. A report of two cases. J Bone Joint Surg Am. 2008;90(4):875–80.

Fractures of the Shaft of the Clavicle

Iain R. Murray, L. A. Kashif Khan, and C. Michael Robinson

Contents

I.R. Murray
Department of Trauma and Orthopaedics, The University
of Edinburgh, Edinburgh, UK
e-mail: Iain.Murray@ed.ac.uk

L.A.K. Khan • C.M. Robinson (✉)
The Edinburgh Shoulder Clinic, Royal Infirmary of
Edinburgh, Edinburgh, UK
e-mail: kashkhan@doctors.org.uk;
c.mike.robinson@ed.ac.uk

G. Bentley (ed.), *European Surgical Orthopaedics and Traumatology*,
DOI 10.1007/978-3-642-34746-7_48, © EFORT 2014

Keywords

Classification • Clavicle • Clinical signs • Complications-non-union, mal-union, neurovascular • Epidemiology • Floating shoulder • Imaging • Shaft • Technique • Treatment-non-operative, surgical

Introduction

The traditional view that the vast majority of mid-shaft clavicular fractures heal with good functional outcomes following non-operative treatment is now contested. While there is a general concensus that undisplaced fractures are best treated non-operatively, there is growing evidence of a higher rate of non-union and poorer functional shoulder outcome in subgroups of patients with clavicular fractures. These fractures can no longer be viewed as a single clinical entity which should always be treated non-operatively, but as a spectrum of injuries with diverse functional outcomes, each requiring individualized assessment and treatment.

Epidemiology

The clavicle is one of the most commonly fractured bones, accounting for 2.6–4 % of adult fractures and 35 % of injuries to the shoulder girdle [1–3]. The incidence of clavicular fractures is estimated to be between 29 and 24 per 100,000 population per year [1, 3, 4]. The majority of clavicular fractures (69–82 %) occur in the shaft, where typical compressive forces on the point of the shoulder combine with the narrow bone cross-section result in failure [2, 3, 5, 6]. Distal third fractures are the next most common type (20 %), with medial third fractures rarest (5 %) [7–12]. Shaft fractures occur most commonly in young adults, whereas lateral and medial-end fractures are more common in the elderly [1, 3, 4]. The majority of shaft fractures are displaced, unlike most lateral end fractures [3].

The first and largest peak incidence of clavicular fractures is in males under 30 years of age (Fig. 1). These fractures tend to result from a direct force applied to the point of the shoulder during sport [6]. Equestrian sports and cycling account for a large number of injuries, when, as a result of inertia when the horse or bicycle stops suddenly, the rider is thrown forward and lands on the unprotected shoulder. High-energy clavicular fractures with comminution, displacement, and shortening are increasing [1]. A second, smaller peak of incidence occurs in elderly patients (over 80 years of age), with a slight female predominance. The majority of these are related to osteoporosis, sustained during low-energy falls in the home.

Clinical and Radiological Assessment

The history should explore standard demographic information and the mechanism of injury. A clavicle fracture which results from a simple fall is unlikely to be associated with other significant injuries. However, fractures occurring in the context of high velocity road-traffic accidents should prompt a thorough search for concomitant injuries. The majority of fractures result from direct force to the point of the shoulder, although fractures can also result from a traction injury [13]. These injuries often occur in industrial settings such as where the arm becomes entangled in machinery and is pulled from the body. If the clavicle fractures with minimal force, the possibility of pathologic fractures secondary to metabolic processes and tumours must be considered. Information that may influence the risk/benefit analysis when considering surgery should also be sought when taking a history [13].

Mid-shaft clavicular fractures typically produce swelling and bruising at the fracture site with displaced fractures resulting in obvious deformity. An abrasion over the point of the shoulder is suggestive of a direct blow, with abrasions over the mid-line indicating a shoulder strap or seatbelt injury [14]. There is often downward displacement of the lateral fragment and elevation of the medial fragment [15]. A droopy, medially-driven, and shortened

Fig. 1 The incidence of clavicular fractures in relation to age and sex cohorts (Reproduced with modification, with permission and copyright © of the British Editorial Society of Bone and Joint Surgery [Robinson CM. Fractures of the clavicle in the adult. Epidemiology and classification. J Bone Joint Surg [Br] 1998;80-B:476-484])

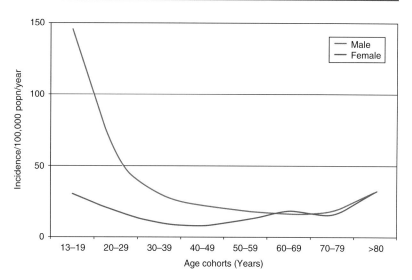

shoulder in completely displaced fractures has been described as shoulder 'ptosis' [16, 17]. Prominence of the displaced fracture fragments, which 'button-hole' through the platysma muscle can occur with severely angulated or comminuted fractures [18]. Despite the superficial position of the clavicle, open fractures or soft-tissue tenting sufficient to produce skin necrosis are uncommon [3]. Shortening of the clavicle should be measured clinically. The difference between the involved and normal shoulder girdle can be calculated by measuring the distance between the suprasternal notch and the palpable ridge of the AC joint.

A thorough examination should be performed to exclude co-existing injuries, particularly as a result of high-energy trauma. Fracture-dislocations of the AC and SC joints and physeal injuries in younger patients should be excluded. The entire limb distal to the fracture should be assessed to exclude brachial plexus or vascular injury. Any deficit not noted pre-operatively may be falsely blamed on surgery with significant prognostic and medico-legal implications [13]. The risk of neurovascular injury increases with high-energy trauma and marked fracture displacement or comminution. Generally, deficits result directly from displaced fracture fragments or by stretch or blunt injuries associated with overall injury of the arm [19–21]. A blood pressure discrepancy

between upper extremities is suggestive of vascular injury. Duplex scanning and arteriography should be undertaken when the diagnosis is in any doubt [22, 23].

The diagnosis is usually made radiographically on the basis of a single anteroposterior (AP) view (Fig. 2) [18]. In an urgent trauma setting the diagnosis is often made on a chest radiograph, which can also be used to evaluate the deformity relative to the normal side. Radiographs should be taken in the erect position where gravity will demonstrate maximal deformity of the clavicle, particularly when considering surgery. Some authors advocate the use of a 15° posteroanterior (PA) radiograph to assess the degree of shortening [24]. Three per cent of patients [25] have an associated chest injury requiring radiological investigation, such as a pneumothorax or haemothorax. These injuries are almost universally associated with multiple rib fractures [26]. Evidence of an ipsilateral shoulder girdle injuries including a double disruption of the superior shoulder suspensory complex [27], should be sought on the initial trauma series radiographs.

Computed tomography (CT) scanning of midshaft clavicular fractures can demonstrate the complex three-dimensional deformity that affects the shoulder girdle with clavicular fractures but is rarely performed as a primary investigation.

Fig. 2 Plain radiograph of
a displaced, comminuted
mid-shaft clavicular
fracture (**a**). This fracture
was treated with open
reduction and plate
fixation (**b**)

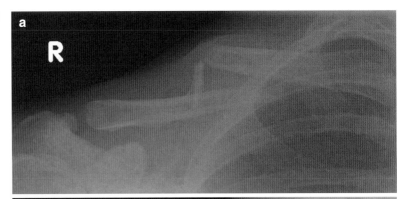

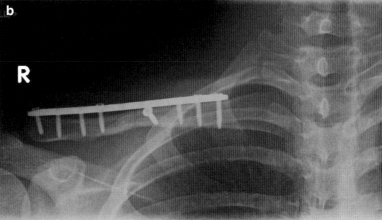

CT is useful for delineating associated glenoid neck fractures in cases of 'floating shoulder' [28–30]. Spiral CT with three-dimensional reconstruction allows the best assessment of displacement and can be useful in evaluating fracture union (Fig. 3).

Classification

A number of classification systems have been described that delineate mid-shaft fractures of the clavicle. The classification proposed by Allman [5] is based solely on the anatomic location of the fracture and numbered according to fracture incidence (mid-shaft I, lateral II, medial III). Recognising that this basic system does not consider factors influencing treatment and prognosis such as fracture pattern and shortening, further classifications have been refined to include other variables. The classification system

of the Orthopaedic Trauma Association separates diaphyseal clavicular fractures into three types: 06-A (simple), 06-B (wedge) and 06-C (complex) [31]. Each type is further divided into three groups.

The Robinson Classification [3] is based on an analysis of 1,000 clavicular fractures, and was the first system to sub-classify shaft fractures according to their displacement and degree of comminution (Fig. 4). Mid-shaft clavicular fractures are divided into type 2A (cortical alignment fracture) and type 2B (displaced fracture). Further division is made into sub-group types 2A1 (nondisplaced), 2A2 (angulated), 2B1 (simple or wedge comminuted), and 2B2 (isolated or comminuted segmental) fractures. These guide treatment and prognosis. These parameters are independently predictive of non-union after operative treatment [32]. The Robinson Classification has been shown to have acceptable levels of interobserver and intra-observer variation [3].

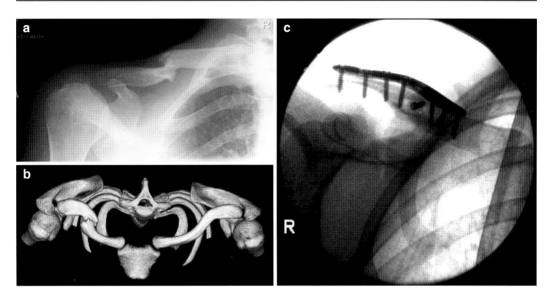

Fig. 3 Hypertrophic non-union following a fracture of the mid-shaft of the clavicle seen on AP plain radiograph (**a**), computed tomography (**b**) and following open reduction and plate fixation (**c**)

Surgical and Applied Anatomy

The clavicle is the first bone to ossify at 5 weeks gestation [14], with initial growth arising from the ossification centre in the central portion of the clavicle up to age five. Further growth then occurs at the medial and lateral epiphyseal plates [14]. The medial growth-plate accounts for the majority of longditudinal growth and is generally the only plate seen radiographically. It is also the last physis to close, between ages 22 and 25 [14]. The clavicle is 'S' shaped with a cephalad-caudad curvature [33, 34]. It is relatively thin, and is widest at its medial and lateral expansions where it articulates with the sternum and acromion. The bone in the relatively thin diaphysis is typically hard cortical bone best suited for cortical screws, unlike the softer bone in the medial and lateral expansions where larger pitch cancellous screws are more suitable. The clavicle articulates medially with the sternum and is securely fixed to the first rib by the costoclavicular ligaments, subclavius and the intra-articular sternoclavicular (SC) joint cartilage. The clavicle articulates laterally with the acromion, where it is held by the acromioclavicular (AC) and coracoclavicular ligaments. The superior shoulder suspensory complex (SSSC) is analogous to the pelvic ring and comprises the laterally-placed structures in the shoulder girdle – the glenoid neck, the lateral clavicle, coracoid and acromion and the ligaments which connect them.

The clavicle lies subcutaneously, with only the supraclavicular nerves crossing the bone superiorly. A number of fascial layers, muscles and ligaments attach to the clavicle and are responsible for the predictable deformities associated with fracture [14]. Sternocleidomastoid is attached to its medial border and pulls proximal fragments superiorly and posteriorly. On the lateral side, part of the deltoid and pectoralis major muscles are attached. Due to the weight of the upper extremity and the pull of pectoralis on the humerus, distal fragments tend to sag forward and rotate inferiorly.

The mid-shaft of the clavicle forms a transition zone between the flattened lateral part and the tubular-to-triangle medial pole [35]. The relatively thick and strong medial

Fig. 4 The Robinson classification of clavicular fractures (Reproduced with modification, with permission and copyright © of the British Editorial Society of Bone and Joint Surgery [Robinson CM. Fractures of the clavicle in the adult. Epidemiology and classification. J Bone Joint Surg [Br] 1998;80-B:476-484])

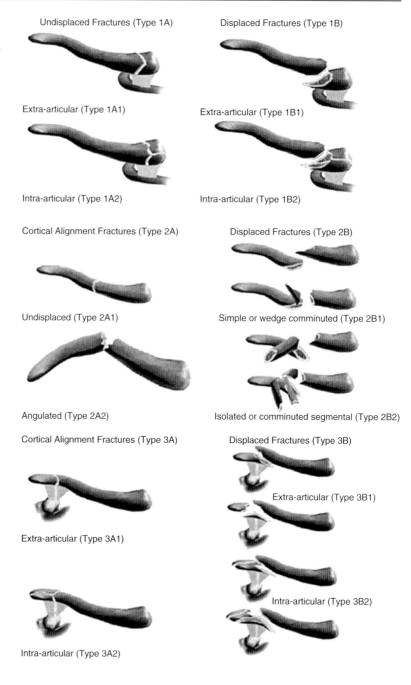

clavicle protects the underlying neurovascular structures. The area of biomechanical weakness lies laterally, protecting these structures during fracture [36]. Cadaveric studies have demonstrated that the axillary vein and artery lie under the apex of the anterior curve of the S-shaped clavicle and travel from superomedial to inferolateral [35]. The neurovascular bundle is further protected by the subclavius muscle and the costocoracoid membrane, lying on the inferior surface of the clavicle.

Management

There is currently considerable debate about the most appropriate treatment for midshaft clavicular fractures. Undisplaced fractures of the diaphysis (Robinson Type 2A) have a high rate of union and are associated with good functional outcomes when treated non-operatively. Until relatively recently, even displaced fractures were rarely stabilised operatively. Early studies evaluating complications in clavicular fractures managed non-operatively reported a rate of non-union of <1 % [6, 25, 37–40], higher than after primary open reduction and internal fixation [25, 39]. A number of other early studies have reported high levels of patient satisfaction after non-operative treatment [37, 38, 41]. However, more contemporary studies have demonstrated increased rates of non-union and poorer functional outcomes after non-operative treatment, with results of primary operative reduction and fixation improving considerably (Table 1) [31, 57, 59].

Compliant patients in the 16–60 age group, who have physically-demanding occupations or active physical lifestyles are candidates for primary operative repair if they are medically fit and have completely displaced fractures with good bone quality [51, 57, 60–62]. Drug and alcohol abuse, untreated psychiatric conditions, homelessness and uncontrolled seizure conditions are associated with non-compliance and fixation failure and are therefore considered as contra-indications for primary operative repair of clavicle fractures [53].

Non-Operative Treatment

The simple sling and 'figure-of-eight bandage' (Fig. 5) are the most widely-used methods of conservative treatment, although many immobilising techniques have been described [63]. Neither technique reduces a displaced fracture [37]. The risk of axillary pressure sores, neurovascular compromise secondary to compression, and non-union are higher in patients treated with the figure-of-eight bandage [24, 37, 40, 64–67]. Better patient satisfaction with the simple sling was demonstrated in a comparative study, but with identical functional and cosmetic results [37]. The sling can normally be discarded once the acute pain has subsided, with patients encouraged to undertake normal activities as far as pain allows. If the fracture heals, range of motion and shoulder function are restored rapidly. Patients rarely require supervised physiotherapy, and generally progress well with self-directed range-of-motion and strengthening exercises.

Primary Operative Treatment

There is growing evidence to support early operative treatment of displaced clavicular fractures, with an increasing number of studies demonstrating benefit when compared with non-operative management [25, 32, 53, 68–70]. In a retrospective clinical series of 52 displaced fractures treated non-operatively, initial shortening of $\geq$20 mm was associated with a greater risk of non-union and a poor clinical outcome [71]. Another study reporting patient-centred outcome measures in fractures treated non-operatively demonstrated significant deficits in shoulder strength and endurance in those with initial displacement [59]. A large multi-centre trial comparing non-operative treatment with primary plate fixation in 138 patients with displaced fractures reported better functional outcomes, lower rates of mal-union and non-union, and a shorter time to union in those undergoing plate fixation [57]. Although, the operative group had a complication rate of 34 % and a high re-operation rate (18 %), the majority of these were for hardware removal. Significant benefits in functional scores were demonstrated with plate fixation ($p = 0.001$ for the Constant score [72] and $p < 0.01$ for the Disabilities of the Arm, Shoulder and Hand [DASH] score [73]). These results must be interpreted with caution, as a minority of outlying patients with poor scores due to non-union may have contributed to the poorer overall scores in the non-operative group. The authors of this trial support the use of primary plate fixation of displaced fractures in

Table 1 Results of acute fixation of clavicle shaft (Edinburgh Type 2) fractures with reported rates of complications and functional results[a]

Technique	Authors	Method of fixation	Number treated	Nonunions (%)	Complications	Functional results
Wiring Techniques	Ngamukos et al. [42]	K wires	99	0 (0)	3 wire migration	Not given
	Total		**99**	**0 (0)**		
Nailing techniques	Grassi et al. [43]	2.5 mm threaded intramedullary pin	40	2 (5)	3 refractures, 2 pin breakage	Mean Constant score 82.9, 75 % 'satisfied with treatment'
	Chu et al. [44]	Knowles pin	75	1 (1.3)	Pin migration	70/75 (93.3 %) good/excellent (constant>80)
	Jubel et al. [45]	Titanium nail	58	1 (1.7)	12 hardware removals	Mean Constant score 97.9
	Meier et al. [46]	Elastic nailing	14	0 (0)	1 secondary fracture displacement	Mean Constant score 98 at 6 months
	Lee et al. [47]	Knowles pin	32	0 (0)	20 hardware removals	Mean Constant score 85
	Strauss et al. [48]	Hagie pin	14	0 (0)	3 skin breakdown, 2 breakages	93 % symptom free
	Kettler et al. [49]	Titanium nail	87	2 (2.3)	4 nail migration, 2 revisions for poor position	Mean Constant score 81
	Mueller et al. [50]	Titanium nail	32	0 (0)	8 nail migration, 2 nail breakage, 29 nail removal	Mean Constant score 95
	Total		**352**	**6 (1.7)**		
Plating techniques	Poigenfurst et al. [51]	Plate fixation[b]	110	5 (4.5)	2 deep infections, 4 refracture	Not given
	Faithfull et al. [52]	Plate fixation	18	0 (0)	14 plate removal	'Full range of movement'
	Bostman et al. [53]	Plate fixation	103	2 (1.9)	5 deep infections, 3 plate loosening, 3 plate failures, 1 refracture	Not given
	Shen et al. [54]	Plate fixation	251	7 (2.8)	1 deep infection, 171 hardware removals	94 % 'satisfied'
	Coupe et al. [55]	Reconstruction/ DCP plates	62	0 (0)	1 deep infection, 19 plates removed	Not given
	Collinge et al. [56]	Plate fixation[c]	42	1 (2.4)	1 fixation failure, 3 infections, 2 removal of metalwork	American Shoulder and Elbow Score 93
	Lee et al. [47]	Plate fixation[b]	30	1 (3.3)	22 hardware removals	Mean Constant score 84
	COTS [57]	Plate fixation[d]	62	2 (3.2)	3 wound infections, 5 metalwork removal, 1 mechanical failure	Mean Constant score 98

(*continued*)

Table 1 (continued)

Technique	Authors	Method of fixation	Number treated	Nonunions (%)	Complications	Functional results
	Russo et al. [58]	Mennen plate fixation	43	2 (4.7)	10 hypothesia	Mean Constant score 96
	Total		**721**	**20 (2.7)**		

COTS Canadian Orthopedic Trauma Society

[a]Only English-language studies, or studies with an English-language translation, appearing in peer-reviewed journals during the last 20 years are shown

[b]Plates used included one-third-tubular, reconstruction (2.7 and 3.5 mm), semitubular and dynamic compression

[c]Plates used included 3.5 mm reconstruction, dynamic compression or fibular composite

[d]Plates used included low-contact dynamic compression, 3.5 mm reconstruction, or precontoured

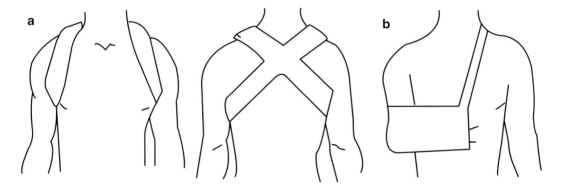

Fig. 5 The figure-of-eight bandage (**a**) and simple sling (**b**) are the most widely-used methods of non-operative management for mid-shaft clavicle fractures

active adults on the basis of this evidence. Interestingly, number-needed-to-treat analysis reveals that operative fixation of nine fractures would be required to prevent one non-union, and fixation of 3.3 fractures would be required to prevent one symptomatic mal-union or non-union [74]. The results of other ongoing randomised controlled trials are eagerly awaited.

Potter et al. [75] demonstrated no significant difference in DASH scores when they compared acute operative treatment with delayed treatment of established non-unions and mal-unions of mid-shaft fractures. A significant difference ($p = 0.05$) was evident in only one of the six strength and endurance variables studies [75]. Although, there was a significant difference ($p = 0.02$) of 6 points in the Constant score, all patients reported a high level of satisfaction.

There is no current agreement on which displaced fractures should be treated operatively.

Increasing numbers of young, active patients are seeking operative treatment in the hope that better functional outcome and an earlier return to contact sports can be achieved. Following adequate counselling about the risks of surgery and likely outcomes, we believe that these patients should be offered the option of operative treatment. In such cases, there are a wide variety of methods available for the operative fixation of shaft fracture including plate fixation, intramedullaryfixation and Kirschner wires [25, 42–58, 70, 76–78].

Plate Fixation

Open reduction and plate fixation enables immediate absolute stability, controlling pain and facilitating early mobilization [60, 68, 71, 79–81]. With displaced mid-shaft fractures, the skin is typically bruised and swollen. It may be advantageous to delay operative intervention until the surrounding tissue is more amenable to surgery – this can be up to 2 weeks. A pre-operative plan should be carefully made taking into consideration displacement, degree of comminution and the location of the main fracture line [13]. Three dimensional reconstruction of computed tomography images has greatly facilitated this for complex cases.

The plate is most commonly implanted on the superior surface of the clavicle with the patient in the 'beach-chair' position. Biomechamical studies support the use of a superiorly positioned plate in providing more secure fixation, especially in the presence of inferior cortical comminution [82]. This approach is associated with an increased risk of injury to the underlying neurovascular structures during drilling and fracture manipulation. Prominence of superiorly-placed plates may necessitate removal, particularly in thin individuals. An anterior-inferior approach to allow inferior implantation of the plate was developed in an attempt to address these problems. Inferior implantation was associated with a low complication rate in a series of 58 patients [56]. However, it is technically more demanding and biomechanically less secure than superior implantation.

The most frequently used implants are dynamic compression and locking plates. Reconstruction plates are susceptible to deformation at the fracture site, leading to mal-union, and are now less popular. Clavicle-specific locking plates have been introduced that are less prominent after healing and are less likely to require removal once the fracture has united [34, 57]. Locking screws have improved fixation of fractures that occur in elderly patients with osteoporotic bone. These implants are yet to be fully evaluated in comparative clinical studies.

Surgical Technique: Superior Fixation of Pre-Contoured Plate for Displaced Mid-Shaft Clavicle Fractures

The patient is positioned in the 'beach-chair' position with the head held on a dedicated support. The anaesthetic endotracheal tube is deflected and secured to the contralateral side. A rolled towel can be usefully placed underneath the operative shoulder to improve manoeuvreability around the

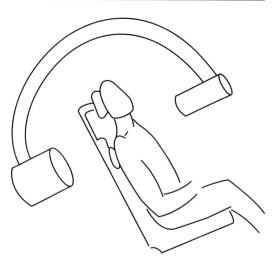

Fig. 6 'Beach-chair' position for open reduction and plate fixation of the clavicle. A roll behind the affected shoulder elevates the clavicle into the operative field. The C-arm of the image intensifier should be placed to allow multi-planar images to be taken while not compromising the surgeon's access to the operative field

clavicle. The arm can be secured to the patient's side and does not require to be mobile. The shoulder girdle is prepared and draped exposing the entire length of the clavicle, acromion and upper half of the scapula. The surgical draping should not interfere with the image intensifier that should be positioned such that the clavicle can be imaged in multiple planes (Fig. 6).

An oblique incision, centred over the fracture site is made along the superior border of the clavicle. The subcutaneous tissue and platysma are dissected as one layer with care taken to identify and protect any larger branches of the supraclavicular nerve. The myofascial layer that covers the clavicle is incised and deflected. It is imperative that every attempt is made to preserve soft tissue attachments to the clavicle while the fracture site is identified and exposed for haematoma and fracture debris. The fracture configuration may warrant fixation of a free fragment to either the distal or proximal portion with a lag screw. This simplifies the fracture pattern and aids reduction.

Reduction of the main fracture line can be assisted using pointed reduction forceps and K-wires (Fig. 7). An interfragmentary lag screw secures the reduction but is not always

Fig. 7 Superior fixation of pre-contoured plate for displaced mid-shaft clavicle fractures (**a**) Reduction of the main fracture line can be assisted using pointed reduction forceps. (**b**) An interfragmentary lag screw secures the reduction and is desirable but not always achievable. (**c**) A pre-contoured plate is then placed on the superior aspect of the reduced clavicle and secured with bicortical screws

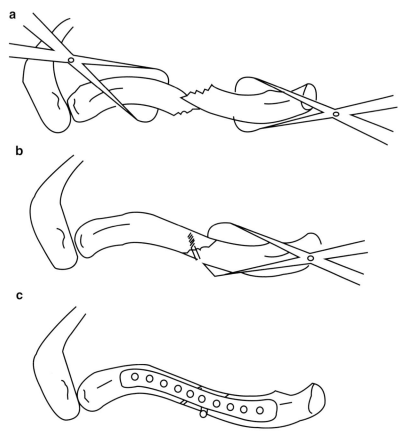

achievable. The size of the pre-contoured plate is then confirmed and placed on the superior aspect of the reduced clavicle being secured with bi-cortical screws. Ideally three bi-cortical screws on either side of the fracture are inserted. Locking screws are only required if the bone is very osteoporotic Great care must be taken to protect the structures in the subclavicular space, particularly while drilling and tapping. Compression holes can be used in stable transverse and short oblique fracture patterns to apply interfragmentary compression. The quality of the reduction, plate placement and screw lengths should be assessed intra-operatively with fluoroscopy. Following irrigation, the soft tissue layers are closed with interrupted sutures with subcuticular sutures used for final skin closure.

Formal post-operative radiographs should be taken in the recovery area. The neurovascular status of the limb post-operatively must be documented. A standard sling is used for comfort with only simple pendulum exercises permitted in the early post-operative period. The patient should be reviewed in clinic at 10–14 days where the wound is inspected, further radiographs obtained and the sling discarded. At this stage unrestricted range of motion is permitted with resisted exercises reserved until 6 weeks following the procedure. Patients should be counselled that contact sports should be avoided until at least 12 weeks although compliance in this young active group of patients is variable. This procedure is increasingly being done on a day-case basis.

Intramedullary Fixation

Intramedullary (IM) pinning of clavicular shaft fractures confers a number of benefits, although this technique has not been as successful in the clavicle as in the femur or tibia [15, 43, 45, 83, 84]. The clavicle's sigmoid shape poses specific problems in the use of intramedullary devices. The implant must be narrow and flexible enough to pass through the medullary canal and curvature of the clavicle, yet strong enough to withstand the forces acting over the fracture until it unites [25, 33, 85]. Static locking is currently not possible with the implants that are available. Biomechanical studies suggest that plate fixation provides a stronger construct than intramedullary fixation [86].

Implants can be inserted antegrade, through an anteromedial entry point in the medial fragment, or retrograde, through a posterolateral entry portal in the lateral fragment. The medullary canal of the clavicle is very narrow and therefore, the fracture site is usually opened through a separate incision to expose the proximal and distal parts of the canal to assist implant insertion. The use of a number of different devices, including Knowles pins [70, 78], Hagie pins, Rockwood pins, and minimally-invasive titanium nails, has been described [45].

Results of intramedullary fixation have been more varied than those after plate fixation [43, 70, 78]. Shortening, particularly with comminuted fractures, can occur due to an inability to statically lock implants [18]. Significant rates of implant failure, brachial plexus palsy, and skin breakdown over the insertion site have also been reported [48, 87]. Intramedullary fixation has therefore been used less commonly than open reduction and plate fixation techniques. However, It has been argued that the less invasive approach is advantageous in patients with multiple injuries or other shoulder girdle injuries [45].

Surgical Technique: Retrograde Intramedullary Fixation

The patient is positioned in the 'beach-chair' position in a similar manner to that for plate fixation. The image intensifier should be positioned such that multi-planar views of the clavicle can be obtained, while minimising disruption to the operating field. An incision is made around two centimetres medial to the AC joint, at the posterolateral corner of the clavicle.

An appropriately-sized drill for the pin is used to penetrate the posterior wall of the clavicle and enter the medullary canal (Fig. 8). The pin or k-wire can then used to manoeuvre ('joystick') the fracture into a reduced position together with a percutaneous reduction clamp secured to the medial fragment [13]. A small incision over the fracture site can be made to assist reduction, particularly in comminuted fractures. This also allows accurate correction of rotation and length through direct vision of the intramedullary device as it is inserted across the fracture site. The medullary canal can then be prepared to accept the intramedullary device. The surgeon should be aware of the potential for the fracture to be distracted when the pin engages the medullary wall of the proximally-situated fragment. Available intramedullary devices include partially-threaded pins or screws, headed pins and cannulated screws. The pin ends can be left flush to bone minimising disruption to soft tissues, or left in a more prominent position for ease of removal. Bone graft or bone graft substitute can be added at the fracture site in an attempt to shorten the time to union. Following thorough irrigation the soft tissue layers are closed with interrupted absorbable sutures. The post-operative protocol is similar to that for plate fixation.

Other Techniques

External fixation is generally suggested only for open fractures or infected non-unions [88]. Kirschner wires and smooth pins have also been used to hold reduction. A number of complications arising from wire breakage and migration of implants have been reported with catastrophic consequences [80, 89]. The use of these implants in the management of acute closed clavicular fractures is therefore strongly discouraged.

The Floating Shoulder

The term 'Floating shoulder' has been used to define an ipsilateral mid-shaft fracture of the clavicle and a fracture of the scapular neck.

Fig. 8 Retrograde intramedullary fixation with a headed, distally-threaded, pin. A drill is used to penetrate the posterolateral corner of the clavicle to prepare the medullary canal (**a**). Whilst using pointed reduction forceps to control the proximal fragment, the pin or a wire can be used as a 'joy stick' to aid reduction (**b**). The device can then be secured across the fracture site and bone graft or bone graft substitute added in an attempt to shorten the time to union

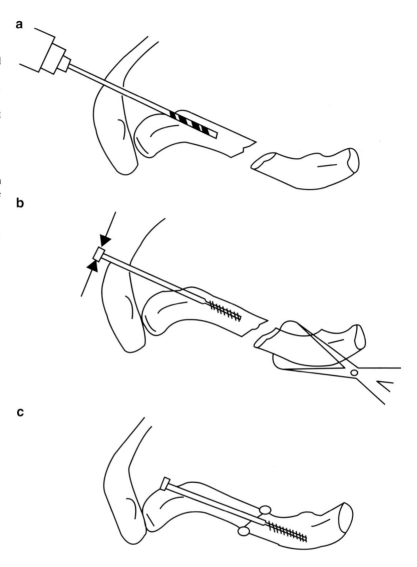

Goss [27] described a floating shoulder as a double disruption of the superior suspensory shoulder complex. However, this has been contested by other authors who argue that as the clavicular mid-shaft is not part of the SSSC, this injury does not represent a double disruption. Furthermore, biomechanical studies have demonstrated that ipsilateral fractures of the scapular neck and the clavicular shaft do not produce a floating shoulder without additional disruption of the coracoacromial and acromioclavicular ligaments [90].

Ipsilateral fractures of the scapular neck and shaft of the clavicle are rare and occur in approximately 0.1 % of all fractures [91]. This combination of injuries is almost always associated with high energy trauma, usually in association with other injuries such as head injury, rib fractures, haemo-pneumothorax, pulmonary contusions, long-bone fractures and cervical spine fractures [92].

No specific classification system exists for this combination of injury, with both fractures classified individually. Scapular neck fractures can be divided into two types [27]: in type A the fracture line runs to the superior border of the scapula lateral to the coracoid process (anatomical neck), and in type B fractures the fracture line runs to the superior border of the scapula medial to the corcacoid process (surgical neck). Over 90 % of scapular fractures are type B (surgical neck).

Although the diagnosis of floating shoulder is often made on plain radiographs alone, three-dimensional CT reconstruction views offer more accurate assessment of the fracture configuration, displacement and angulation.

Despite widespread acceptance that this pattern of injury is unstable, considerable controversy remains over the most appropriate treatment for these injuries [13]. There is a lack of prospective randomised trials evaluating treatment methods, with current literature including only a number of small retrospective studies. Possible strategies include non-operative management, clavicular fracture fixation in isolation, or fixation of both the clavicle and scapular fractures. However, due to a lack of prospective studies with adequate numbers, it is not possible to recommend uniform methods of treatment for ipsilateral clavicle shaft and fractures of the scapular neck.

Good functional results with non-operative management have been reported by a number of authors. Egol et al. [28] demonstrated comparable functional outcome scores for patients treated non-operatively and operatively. Furthermore, operatively treated shoulders were found to be weaker in certain movements. Edwards et al. [93] reported excellent or good results in 20 patients managed non-operatively, including five with severe displacement (>5 mm) of the glenoid neck. In a retrospective multi-centre study, Van Noort et al. [94], showed that in the absence of caudal glenoid displacement, non-operative management resulted in good functional outcomes in 28 patients.

A number of authors have recommended fixation of the clavicle only. Herscovici et al. [91] reported results on nine patients: seven patients who were treated operatively achieved excellent functional scores. Of those treated non-operatively, one achieved good functional scores with the other scoring poorly. A number of authors argue that fixation of the clavicle neutralizes forces applied to the shoulder, stabilizing the scapular neck and precluding the need for

scapular fixation [95]. Hashiguchi and Ito [96] reported satisfactory outcome after fixation of the clavicle alone in five patients, although recommended this method for minimally-displaced fractures of the scapula neck, type B (surgical neck) fractures and those without involvement of the coracoclavicular ligaments, recommending that these more problematic injuries be treated with fixation of both the clavicle and scapula. Leung and Lam reported good or excellent results in 14 patients treated with fixation of both the clavicle and scapula, recommending this approach to prevent poor shoulder function resulting from fracture displacement in non-operatively treated fractures [92].

Complications of Mid-Shaft Clavicular Fractures

Non-Union

Although non-union was traditionally considered to be rare (reported prevalence of <1 % following non-operative treatment) [25], recent studies report a higher rate of non-union (up to 15 %; eight of 52) in adults with displaced fractures [3, 25, 32, 38, 39, 67, 69–71, 97]. In a meta-analysis of all series of displaced mid-shaft fractures from 1975 to 2005, Zlodowski et al. [62] found that, for completely displaced mid-shaft fractures of the clavicle, the non-union rate with non-operative treatment was 15.1 %, while the non-union rate following operative treatment was 2.2 %. Increasing age, female sex, shortening of greater than 2 cm, complete fracture displacement, and comminution are thought to increase the risk of non-union [3, 32]. As most clavicular fractures occur in a young, predominantly male population [1–3, 32], the majority of non-unions occur in patients of this demographic. Accurately predicting which patients will develop non-union occur is difficult, although an assessment of risk can be made on the basis of known independently predictive risk factors for non-union (Table 2) [3, 32, 98].

Non-unions of the clavicular shaft are usually symptomatic in active individuals. There are

Table 2 The calculated probability of a non-union at 24 weeks after a clavicle shaft fracture, based upon age, gender, comminution and displacement in a study of 581 fractures (Reproduced with permission from Khan LA et al. [159])

Age (years)	Not displaced, not comminuted		Displaced, not comminuted		Comminuted, not displaced		Displaced and comminuted	
	Males	Females	Males	Females	Males	Females	Males	Females
20	<1 %	2 %	8 %	16 %	2 %	7 %	18 %	30 %
30	<1 %	3 %	10 %	20 %	4 %	9 %	20 %	35 %
40	1 %	5 %	13 %	26 %	5 %	12 %	25 %	38 %
50	2 %	6 %	18 %	28 %	6 %	13 %	29 %	40 %
60	2 %	7 %	19 %	30 %	8 %	15 %	31 %	44 %
70	4 %	10 %	21 %	37 %	9 %	18 %	35 %	49 %

reports in the literature of pain [39, 67, 80, 99, 100], a clicking sensation on movement [39, 67], restriction of shoulder movement [67, 80, 100], weakness [39, 67, 100], cosmetic deformity [39, 67, 99], neurological symptoms [80, 99, 101], thoracic outlet syndrome [67, 80, 99, 102], and subclavian vein compression. Patients may complain of an inability to perform manual work, driving difficulty, withdrawal from normal sporting activities, sleep disturbance, and reduced libido secondary to pain [99]. Non-union is suspected clinically with mobility or pain on stressing of the fracture. Radiographic examinations demonstrate an absence of bridging callus [32, 103]. If the diagnosis is in doubt, the presence or absence of bridging callus across the fracture site can be assessed accurately with three-dimensional reconstructions of computed tomography scans.

Treatment

A number of operative techniques have been described to treat shaft non-unions (Table 3).

Plate fixation is the most widely-used technique to treat shaft non-unions (Fig. 3) [30, 55, 60, 67, 79–81, 83, 97, 99, 104–119], providing secure fixation and enabling early mobilization of the shoulder, with a high rate of union and low risk of complications [80, 104, 105, 107, 111, 116, 118–120]. Reconstruction [97, 107, 112], dynamic compression [81, 107, 116, 118], and low-contact compression plates [60, 81] have all been used. The 'foot-printed' under-surface of low-contact dynamic compression plates optimally preserve the blood supply to the underlying

bone fragments with potentially beneficial effects on healing over traditional plates [60, 81]. Reconstruction and semi-tubular plates are prone to deformation or failure when used to treat non-unions. The use of wave-plates has been advocated for clavicular non-unions to reduce hypertrophic callus formation, which may result in thoracic outlet obstruction [105]. Pre-contoured locking plates specifically manufactured for the clavicle may also be employed for non-unions, although results are yet to be published to our knowledge.

Autologous bone-grafting is widely used and may shorten the time to union following operative treatment of a clavicular non-union [81, 105, 116]. Iliac crest bone is the most widely used graft to restore length, when non-union is associated with clinically important shortening and bone loss through comminution [80]. Vascularized fibular [121, 122] and medial femoral condylar [123, 124] grafts have also been advocated in revision cases.

Surgical Technique: ORIF Mid-Shaft Non-Union of the Clavicle

Patient positioning, draping and positioning of the image intensifier are similar to that of plate fixation for acute clavicle fractures with the addition of contra-lateral iliac crest site preparation if autologous grafting is expected. The clavicle is approached in the same way as for acute fractures with dissection of the soft tissues to expose the ends of the non-union. The sclerotic ends and excess callus are cleared back to bleeding bone and the medullary canal re-established with a drill. Any removed callus is saved to be

Table 3 Results of English language reports of the treatment of non-union after clavicle shaft fractures (Edinburgh Type 2) with reported complications and functional outcomes[a]

Technique	Authors	Method of fixation	Number treated	Persistent nonunions after treatment (%)	Bone graft	Complications	Functional results
Plating techniques	Mullaji and Jupiter [60]	Limited contact - dynamic compression plate	6	0 (0)	All cases	2 scar sensitivity	6/6 (100 %) full range of motion
	Pedersen et al. [104]	4 hole semi-tubular	12	Not given	All cases	6 failures	9/12 (75 %) 'good result
	Olsen et al. [105]	Plate fixation	16	1 (6.3)	All cases	1 screw loosening	11/16 (68.7 %) full range of motion
	Bradbury et al. [79]	Plate fixation	15	1 (6.7)	All cases	2 screw cut outs requiring plate removal	mean Constant score 87
	Bradbury et al. [79]	Reconstruction plate	17	2 (11.8)	All cases	delayed infection	mean Constant score 82
	Davids et al. [97]	Reconstruction plate	14	0 (0)	All cases	1 deep infection	all 'normal range of motion'
	Boyer and Axelrod [106]	Plate fixation	7	Not given	All cases		all 'normal range of motion'
	Ebraheim et al. [107]	Plate fixation	16	1 (6.3)	All cases	1 removal of hardware for cosmesis	all 'normal range of motion'
	Wu et al. [108]	Dynamic compression or semitubular plate	11	2 (18.2)	All cases	1 deep infection	Not given
	Ballmer et al. [109]	Plate fixation	32	2 (6.3)	65 %	1 wound infection, 23 plate removals	86 % full range of motion
	Laursen et al. [110]	Plate fixation	16	0 (0)	All cases		11/12 (91.7 %) constant >70 (good/excellent)
	Der Tavitian et al. [99]	Plate fixation	9	0 (0)	All cases	1 plate breakage (semitubular plate)	9/9 (100 %) 'full use'
	Marti et al. [111]	Wave plate	9	1 (11.1)	All cases	2 delay in wound healing, 2 infections	7/7 (100 %) Constant score >80 good/excellent
	Marti et al. [111]	Plate fixation	19	0 (0)	All cases	1 infection, 4 brachialgia	10/13 (76.9 %) Constant score>80 good/excellent.

	Kabak et al. [81]	Plate fixation	16	2 (12.5)	'Selected' cases	implant failure, 8 plate removals	mean DASH score 14.8
	Kabak et al. [81]	Limited contact - dynamic compression plate	17	0 (0)	'Selected' cases	1 plate removal	mean DASH score 6.7
	O'Connor et al. [112]	Reconstruction/dynamic compression plate	22	2 (9.1)	All cases	6 plate removals, 1 deep infection	AAOS DASH Mean 55
	Coupe et al. [55]	Reconstruction/dynamic compression	19	1 (5.3)	Not stated	1 plate breakage	Not given
	Rosenberg et al. [30]	Reconstruction/dynamic compression	11	0 (0)	Not stated		5/11 (45.5 %) constant>80
	Khan et al. [113]	Locking plate	9	0 (0)	4 cases	1 infection, 1 reflex sympathetic dystrophy	mean DASH score 24
	Total		**293**	**15 (5.1)**			
Intramedullary techniques	Boehme et al. [83]	Hagie intramedullary pin	21	1 (4.8)	All cases	17 pin removals for pain	Not given
	Capicotto et al. [114]	Steinman pin	14	0 (0)	All cases	2 refractures, all hardware removed	12/14 (85.7 %) 'painless range of motion'
	Wu et al. [108]	Steinman or Knowles pin	18	2 (11.1)	All cases		Not given
	Der Tavitian et al. [99]	Knowles pin	2	0 (0)	All cases		2/2 (100 %) 'full use'
	Hoe-Hanson et al. [115]	Intramedullary cancellous screw	6	0 (0)	All cases	1 screw removal	5/6 (83.3 %) Constant score >80 good/excellent
	Total		**61**	**3 (4.9)**			

aOnly English-language studies, or studies with an English-language translation, appearing in peer-reviewed journals during the last 20 years are shown
AAOS - American Academy of Orthopaedic Surgeons
DASH - Disabilities of the Arm, Shoulder and Hand

morsellized and inserted around the fracture site at the end of the procedure. Reduction is achieved by drawing the two fracture ends together with reduction forceps attempting to restore the anatomical shape and natural superior bow of the clavicle. The use of an interfragmentary lag screw can help to secure a reduced fracture as the plate is applied. Alternatively, the reduction can also be held temporarily with k-wires. As the fracture configuration and lag screw position often interfere with the placement of central screws, a plate with at least eight holes is advocated. In short oblique or transverse fracture patterns the first screws on either side can be used in compression mode. The wound is irrigated thoroughly and the prepared morsellized graft inserted into the fracture site. The majority of non-unions are atrophic and therefore often require addition of autologous iliac crest graft or bone substitute. Wound closure and post-operative protocol are the same as for acute fractures.

Other Methods

Intramedullary fixation [83, 99, 100, 108, 114, 115, 125] and external fixation [88, 120] produce more cosmetically acceptable incisions and disturb the soft-tissue envelope less [83, 114], but provide less rigid fixation [70, 80, 116]. Papineau's technique [126] of external fixation has been utilized rarely to treat infected pseudoarthroses [61].

Severe bone loss may occur with infection and multiple failed operative procedures. In such circumstances the most radical option is partial or complete excision of the clavicle [15, 127, 128]. Given the clavicle's pivotal role in providing support for the upper extremity this must only considered a salvage procedure in the most extreme circumstances [13].

Mal-Union

Although the majority will be asymptomatic, it is inevitable that all displaced clavicular fractures treated non-operatively will heal with some degree of mal-union due to angulation or shortening [129, 130]. Traditionally, it was thought that mal-union was of radiographic interest only, with success in the clinical setting equating to fracture union [13]. However, it is now accepted that mal-union may be associated with intrusive symptoms [30, 31, 73] secondary to both anteroposterior angulation and overlapping of bone ends [129]. Shortening of the muscle tendon units over the site of mal-union may cause weakness and increase fatigue, and pseudo-winging of the scapula [13]. Angular deformity and shortening may also alter the orientation of the glenoid, changing the shoulder dynamics [131]. Bony encroachment into the thoracic outlet often results in numbness and paraesthesia that may be exacerbated by overhead activities and is usually noted in a C8-T1 nerve root distribution. Patients may also complain of discomfort when wearing bags and with shoulder straps on clothes.

The factors that predispose to symptomatic mal-union are unclear. Hill et al. [132] reported an association between shortening of over 2 cm, poor outcome and dissatisfaction with other studies also supporting this finding. A number of authors have doubted the clinical relevance of shortening, despite its frequency following fracture [133, 134]. In a prospective study evaluating risk factors for long-term functional problems, initial displacement, and increasing age were independently predictive of symptomatic mal-union [103]. In this series, shortening was not associated with poor outcomes.

Treatment

Patients with symptomatic mal-union despite strengthening physiotherapy can either accept the disability or undergo a further operative procedure that aims to improve their symptoms [13]. Young, healthy patients with good bone quality should be considered for surgery. The patient should have sufficiently intrusive symptoms specific to their clavicular mal-union to warrant surgery without any guarantee of benefit [13]. Corrective osteotomy and plate fixation has been shown to improve function in patients with neurovascular compression, discomfort and weakness, or cosmetic deformity [30, 59, 130, 131, 135]. An intramedullary device for stabilisation has also been described [20].

Although restoration of the normal shoulder contour and function has been reported in the literature, there is only limited information available on the treatment of symptomatic post-traumatic shortening in the absence of neurovascular compression [60, 131, 135–137].

Surgical Technique: ORIF Mid-Shaft Mal-Union of the Clavicle

Clinical and radiological measurement of the deformity are essential pre-operatively to assess the success of surgery. Patient positioning and surgical approach are similar to those used for acute fracture fixation [59]. Having cleared the non-union site, marks are made proximally and distally to enable measurement of any lengthening to be made. The original fracture plane is usually identifiable because of the typical pattern of the fracture ends relative to each other, with the osteotomy performed through this plane. In cases where the original fracture line is not easily recognised, an oblique sliding osteotomy can be performed [138]. The medullary canal is re-established with a drill to restore blood supply to the osteotomy site. Any lengthening can be determined by re-measuring the distance between the original marks. The pre-contoured clavicular plate is then applied over the osteotomy on the postero-superior surface. Adjuvant autologous bone-grafting can be used in some cases. There is limited literature available on the timing of treatment, although corrective osteotomy performed within 2 years of the fracture appears to produce better results than when performed a long time after fracture healing [139].

Neurovascular Complications

Although acute nerve compression may result from displacement of fracture fragments, most neurovascular injuries result from excessive traction [13]. Classically, the clavicular fragments are distracted rather than shortened in these injuries. Angiograms can confirm the presence of vascular injury and can potentially be therapeutic if interventional techniques are available.

Operative decompression of the brachial plexus by reduction and fixation of the clavicular fracture is indicated in the presence of direct neurological injury [19, 53, 140–143].

Chronic mal-union or non-union associated with hypertrophic callus formation, subclavian pseudoaneurysm, or scar constriction (delayed type) may result in a more insidious onset of neurovascular symptoms [19, 20, 101, 141, 142, 144–149]. This condition has been described as thoracic outlet syndrome, costoclavicular syndrome, and fractured clavicle-rib syndrome [146, 150]. Typically, the medial cord of the brachial plexus is impinged by callus around the fracture site superiorly and by the first rib inferiorly (costoclavicular space), producing predominantly ulnar nerve symptoms. Hypertrophic non-union or mal-union predispose patients to this condition [19, 80, 101, 142]. The diagnosis is subjective, and the prevalence of this condition is therefore poorly defined. In 1968, Rowe [25] reported late neurovascular sequelae after 0.3 % (two) of 690 fractures, although prevalences of between 20 % and 47 % in series of between 15 and 52 patients have been reported in more recent studies [57, 71, 99, 147].

The diagnosis should be made only when a patient has a suggestive history with supportive evidence on electrophysiological testing [20], arteriography or venography [21, 23], and specialized imaging. Treatment should be directed toward correction of the underlying cause – generally the mal-union or non-union – to re-establish the dimensions of the pre-injury thoracic outlet [19, 20, 101, 142, 149]. Attempts to simply remove the 'bump deformity' at the mal-union site or the first rib have a high failure rate as the condition results from the change in dimensions of the thoracic outlet from the displaced fracture segment rather than local impingement [13].

Re-Fracture

Re-fracture of the clavicle has been reported following fractures treated operatively and non-operatively. Recognised risk factors include an early return to contact sports, epilepsy and alcoholism [151]. Further trauma with implants in situ may result in fractures at the end of plates, or implant breakage or bending [13, 55, 99, 114]. Fractures occurring following plate removal may occur through the original fracture site. Osteoporosis below the plate and the stress riser effect at the empty screw holes may contribute to re-fracture risk [51, 53, 152]. Internal fixation is often required following re-fracture because of the high risk of non-union [18]. Fractures occurring at the end of a stable implanted diaphyseal plate generally require fixation that should ideally span the area of bone previously repaired in addition to fixing the fresh fracture [13].

Other Complications of Operative Treatment

A feared potential intra-operative complication is injury to the subclavian artery or vein at the time of fracture immobilization or from drill penetration [18]. The risk of this complication is low, but if it occurs is potentially catastrophic necessitating vascular or cardiothoracic surgical intervention. Plate failure [53], hypertrophic or dysaesthetic scars [153], implant loosening [53, 152], have been reported and may require revision surgery.

Infection

The use of peri-operative antibiotics, selective operative timing to optimize soft tissue conditions, improved soft tissue handling, two-layer soft tissue closure, and biomechanically superior fixation have all been shown to decrease the high rate of deep infection reported in early series [15, 39, 51, 57, 58, 76, 78, 154–156]. Superficial infection rates of 4.4 %, and deep infection rates of 2.2 % have been reported in a large meta-analysis [62]. Superficial infections with a bacterologically-proven growth of pathogenic organisms generally resolve with antibiotic

therapy. Deep infections may occur early or as a delayed phenomenon, as with any implant- related infection. Early sepsis with a stable implant should be treated with a protocol of repeated debridement and irrigation with a prolonged parenteral and then oral antibiotic therapy. More radical debridement and metalwork removal may be required to eradicate persisting infection. Immediate reconstruction with plating, bone grafting, and local antibiotics may be considered in healthy patients. Alternatively, antibiotic-impregnated beads or bone substitute can be inserted as a temporizing measure with reconstruction performed at a later date. Skin and soft tissue loss may occur in these patients requiring plastic surgical input with soft-tissue flap coverage [157, 158].

Conclusions

It is widely accepted that undisplaced fractures of the mid-shaft of the clavicle are best treated non-operatively. Although good outcomes have been reported after operative treatment of acute diaphyseal fractures, it is difficult to predict which patients should be offered primary operative reconstruction and which technique should be used. Factors associated with a poor prognosis with non-operative treatment include displacement (especially shortening), comminution and an increased number of fracture fragments. Operative reconstructions of diaphyseal non-unions have good outcomes, and the large number of case series documenting consistently good outcomes after plate fixation lends support to the use of this technique as the treatment of choice. Randomized studies are required to refine the indications for primary operative repair and to establish the most appropriate method of treatment.

References

1. Nordqvist A, Petersson C. The incidence of fractures of the clavicle. Clin Orthop. 1994;300:127–32.
2. Postacchini F, Gumina S, De Santis P, Albo F. Epidemiology of clavicle fractures. J Shoulder Elbow Surg. 2002;11(5):452–6.

3. Robinson CM. Fractures of the clavicle in the adult. Epidemiology and classification. J Bone Joint Surg Br. 1998;80(3):476–84.

4. Nowak J, Mallmin H, Larsson S. The aetiology and epidemiology of clavicular fractures. A prospective study during a two-year period in Uppsala, Sweden. Injury. 2000;31(5):353–8.

5. Allman Jr FL. Fractures and ligamentous injuries of the clavicle and its articulation. J Bone Joint Surg Am. 1967;49(4):774–84.

6. Stanley D, Trowbridge EA, Norris SH. The mechanism of clavicular fracture. A clinical and biomechanical analysis. J Bone Joint Surg Br. 1988;70(3):461–4.

7. Goldberg JA, Bruce WJ, Sonnabend DH, Walsh WR. Type 2 fractures of the distal clavicle: a new surgical technique. J Shoulder Elbow Surg. 1997;6(4):380–2.

8. Robinson CM, Cairns DA. Primary nonoperative treatment of displaced lateral fractures of the clavicle. J Bone Joint Surg Am. 2004;86-A(4):778–82.

9. Rokito AS, Zuckerman JD, Shaari JM, Eisenberg DP, Cuomo F, Gallagher MA. A comparison of nonoperative and operative treatment of type II distal clavicle fractures. Bull Hosp Jt Dis. 2002;61(1–2):32–9.

10. Seo GS, Aoki J, Karakida O, Sone S. Nonunion of a medial clavicular fracture following radical neck dissection: MRI diagnosis. Orthopedics. 1999;22(10):985–6.

11. Throckmorton T, Kuhn JE. Fractures of the medial end of the clavicle. J Shoulder Elbow Surg. 2007;16(1):49–54.

12. Webber MC, Haines JF. The treatment of lateral clavicle fractures. Injury. 2000;31(3):175–9.

13. McKee MD. Clavicle fractures. In: Bucholz RW, C-BCHJTP, editors. Rockwood and greens fractures in adults. 7th ed. Oxford: Lippincott Williams and Wilkins; 2009. p. 1106–43.

14. Jeray KJ. Acute midshaft clavicular fracture. J Am Acad Orthop Surg. 2007;15(4):239–48.

15. Craig EV. Fractres of the clavicle. In: Rockwood Jr CA, Matsen III FA, editors. The shoulder. Philadelphia: WB Saunders; 1990. p. 367–412.

16. Owens BD, Goss TP. The floating shoulder. J Bone Joint Surg Br. 2006;88(11):1419–24.

17. Rikli D, Regazzoni P, Renner N. The unstable shoulder girdle: early functional treatment utilizing open reduction and internal fixation. J Orthop Trauma. 1995;9(2):93–7.

18. Khan LA, Bradnock TJ, Scott C, Robinson CM. Fractures of the clavicle. J Bone Joint Surg Am. 2009;91(2):447–60.

19. Barbier O, Malghem J, Delaere O, Vande BB, Rombouts JJ. Injury to the brachial plexus by a fragment of bone after fracture of the clavicle. J Bone Joint Surg Br. 1997;79(4):534–6.

20. Chen CE, Liu HC. Delayed brachial plexus neurapraxia complicating malunion of the clavicle. Am J Orthop. 2000;29(4):321–2.

21. Yates DW. Complications of fractures of the clavicle. Injury. 1976;7(3):189–93.

22. Lusskin R, Weiss CA, Winer J. The role of the subclavius muscle in the subclavian vein syndrome (costoclavicular syndrome) following fracture of the clavicle. A case report with a review of the pathophysiology of the costoclavicular space. Clin Orthop. 1967;54:75–83.

23. Penn I. The vascular complications of fractures of the clavicle. J Trauma. 1964;27:819–31.

24. Sharr JR, Mohammed KD. Optimizing the radiographic technique in clavicular fractures. J Shoulder Elbow Surg. 2003;12(2):170–2.

25. Rowe CR. An atlas of anatomy and treatment of midclavicular fractures. Clin Orthop. 1968;58:29–42.

26. Dugdale TW, Fulkerson JP. Pneumothorax complicating a closed fracture of the clavicle. A case report. Clin Orthop. 1987;221:212–14.

27. Goss TP. Double disruptions of the superior shoulder suspensory complex. J Orthop Trauma. 1993;7(2):99–106.

28. Egol KA, Connor PM, Karunakar MA, Sims SH, Bosse MJ, Kellam JF. The floating shoulder: clinical and functional results. J Bone Joint Surg Am. 2001;83-A(8):1188–94.

29. Ramos L, Mencia R, Alonso A, Ferrandez L. Conservative treatment of ipsilateral fractures of the scapula and clavicle. J Trauma. 1997;42(2):239–42.

30. Rosenberg N, Neumann L, Wallace AW. Functional outcome of surgical treatment of symptomatic nonunion and malunion of midshaft clavicle fractures 6. J Shoulder Elbow Surg. 2007;16(5):510–13.

31. McKee MD, Pedersen EM, Jones C, Stephen DJ, Kreder HJ, Schemitsch EH, et al. Deficits following nonoperative treatment of displaced midshaft clavicular fractures. J Bone Joint Surg Am. 2006;88(1):35–40.

32. Robinson CM, Court-Brown CM, McQueen MM, Wakefield AE. Estimating the risk of nonunion following nonoperative treatment of a clavicular fracture. J Bone Joint Surg Am. 2004;86-A(7):1359–65.

33. Andermahr J, Jubel A, Elsner A, Johann J, Prokop A, Rehm KE, et al. Anatomy of the clavicle and the intramedullary nailing of midclavicular fractures. Clin Anat. 2007;20(1):48–56.

34. Huang JI, Toogood P, Chen MR, Wilber JH, Cooperman DR. Clavicular anatomy and the applicability of precontoured plates. J Bone Joint Surg Am. 2007;89(10):2260–5.

35. Galley IJ, Watts AC, Bain GI. The anatomic relationship of the axillary artery and vein to the clavicle: a cadaveric study. J Shoulder Elbow Surg. 2009;18(5):e21–5.

36. Harrington Jr MA, Keller TS, Seiler III JG, Weikert DR, Moeljanto E, Schwartz HS. Geometric properties and the predicted mechanical behavior of adult human clavicles. J Biomech. 1993;26(4–5):417–26.

37. Andersen K, Jensen PO, Lauritzen J. Treatment of clavicular fractures. Figure-of-eight bandage versus a simple sling. Acta Orthop Scand. 1987;58(1):71–4.

38. Eskola A, Vainionpaa S, Myllynen P, Patiala H, Rokkanen P. Outcome of clavicular fracture in 89 patients. Arch Orthop Trauma Surg. 1986; 105(6):337–8.

39. Neer CS. Nonunion of the clavicle. JAMA. 1960;172:1006–11.

40. Sankarankutty M, Turner BW. Fractures of the clavicle. Injury. 1975;7(2):101–6.

41. Nordqvist A, Petersson CJ, Redlund-Johnell I. Midclavicle fractures in adults: end result study after conservative treatment. J Orthop Trauma. 1998;12(8):572–6.

42. Ngarmukos C, Parkpian V, Patradul A. Fixation of fractures of the midshaft of the clavicle with Kirschner wires. Results in 108 patients. J Bone Joint Surg Br. 1998;80(1):106–8.

43. Grassi FA, Tajana MS, D'Angelo F. Management of midclavicular fractures: comparison between nonoperative treatment and open intramedullary fixation in 80 patients. J Trauma. 2001;50(6):1096–100.

44. Chu CM, Wang SJ, Lin LC. Fixation of mid-third clavicular fractures with knowles pins: 78 patients followed for 2–7 years. Acta Orthop Scand. 2002;73(2):134–9.

45. Jubel A, Andermahr J, Schiffer G, Tsironis K, Rehm KE. Elastic stable intramedullary nailing of midclavicular fractures with a titanium nail. Clin Orthop. 2003;408:279–85.

46. Meier C, Grueninger P, Platz A. Elastic stable intramedullary nailing for midclavicular fractures in athletes: indications, technical pitfalls and early results. Acta Orthop Belg. 2006;72(3):269–75.

47. Lee YS, Lin CC, Huang CR, Chen CN, Liao WY. Operative treatment of midclavicular fractures in 62 elderly patients: knowles pin versus plate. Orthopedics. 2007;30(11):959–64.

48. Strauss EJ, Egol KA, France MA, Koval KJ, Zuckerman JD. Complications of intramedullary Hagie pin fixation for acute midshaft clavicle fractures. J Shoulder Elbow Surg. 2007;16(3):280–4.

49. Kettler M, Schieker M, Braunstein V, Konig M, Mutschler W. Flexible intramedullary nailing for stabilization of displaced midshaft clavicle fractures: technique and results in 87 patients 7. Acta Orthop. 2007;78(3):424–9.

50. Mueller M, Burger C, Florczyk A, Striepens N, Rangger C. Elastic stable intramedullary nailing of midclavicular fractures in adults: 32 patients followed for 1–5 years. Acta Orthop. 2007; 78(3):421–3.

51. Poigenfurst J, Rappold G, Fischer W. Plating of fresh clavicular fractures: results of 122 operations. Injury. 1992;23(4):237–41.

52. Faithfull DK, Lam P. Dispelling the fears of plating midclavicular fractures. J Shoulder Elbow Surg. 1993;2(6):314–16.

53. Bostman O, Manninen M, Pihlajamaki H. Complications of plate fixation in fresh displaced midclavicular fractures. J Trauma. 1997; 43(5):778–83.

54. Shen WJ, Liu TJ, Shen YS. Plate fixation of fresh displaced midshaft clavicle fractures. Injury. 1999;30(7):497–500.

55. Coupe BD, Wimhurst JA, Indar R, Calder DA, Patel AD. A new approach for plate fixation of midshaft clavicular fractures 4. Injury. 2005;36(10):1166–71.

56. Collinge C, Devinney S, Herscovici D, DiPasquale T, Sanders R. Anterior-inferior plate fixation of middle-third fractures and nonunions of the clavicle. J Orthop Trauma. 2006;20(10):680–6.

57. Canadian Orthopaedic Trauma Society. Nonoperative treatment compared with plate fixation of displaced midshaft clavicular fractures. A multicenter, randomized clinical trial. J Bone Joint Surg Am. 2007;89(1):1–10.

58. Russo R, Visconti V, Lorini S, Lombardi LV. Displaced comminuted midshaft clavicle fractures: use of Mennen plate fixation system. J Trauma. 2007;63(4):951–4.

59. McKee MD, Wild LM, Schemitsch EH. Midshaft malunions of the clavicle. J Bone Joint Surg Am. 2003;85-A(5):790–7.

60. Mullaji AB, Jupiter JB. Low-contact dynamic compression plating of the clavicle. Injury. 1994; 25(1):41–5.

61. Vidal J, Buscayret C, Connes H, Melka J, Orst G. Guidelines for treatment of open fractures and infected pseudarthroses by external fixation. Clin Orthop Relat Res. 1983;180:83–95.

62. Zlowodzki M, Zelle BA, Cole PA, Jeray K, McKee MD. Treatment of acute midshaft clavicle fractures: systematic review of 2144 fractures: on behalf of the Evidence-Based Orthopaedic Trauma Working Group. J Orthop Trauma. 2005;19(7):504–7.

63. Lester CW. The treatment of fracures of the clavicle. Ann Surg. 1929;89:600–6.

64. Hanby CK, Pasque CB, Sullivan JA. Medial clavicle physis fracture with posterior displacement and vascular compromise: the value of three-dimensional computed tomography and duplex ultrasound. Orthopedics. 2003;26(1):81–4.

65. Hoofwijk AG, van der Werken C. Conservative treatment of clavicular fractures. Z Unfallchir Versicherungsmed Berufskr. 1988;81(3):151–6.

66. Mullick S. Treatment of mid-clavicular fractures. Lancet. 1967;1:499.

67. Wilkins RM, Johnston RM. Ununited fractures of the clavicle. J Bone Joint Surg Am. 1983;65(6):773–8.

68. Neer CS. Fractures of the distal third of the clavicle. Clin Orthop Relat Res. 1968;58:43–50.

69. Wick M, Muller EJ, Kollig E, Muhr G. Midshaft fractures of the clavicle with a shortening of more than 2 cm predispose to nonunion. Arch Orthop Trauma Surg. 2001;121(4):207–11.

70. Zenni Jr EJ, Krieg JK, Rosen MJ. Open reduction and internal fixation of clavicular fractures. J Bone Joint Surg Am. 1981;63(1):147–51.

71. Hill JM, McGuire MH, Crosby LA. Closed treatment of displaced middle-third fractures of the clavicle

gives poor results. J Bone Joint Surg Br. 1997;79(4):537–9.

72. Constant CR, Murley AH. A clinical method of functional assessment of the shoulder. Clin Orthop Relat Res. 1987;214:160–4.

73. Hudak PL, Amadio PC, Bombardier C. Development of an upper extremity outcome measure: the DASH (disabilities of the arm, shoulder and hand) [corrected]. The Upper Extremity Collaborative Group (UECG). Am J Ind Med. 1996;29(6):602–8.

74. Jenkins PJ, Huntley JS, Robinson CM. Primary fixation of displaced clavicle fractures: unanswered questions. www.ejbjs.org/cgi/eletters/89/1/1#3652. 2007. Ref Type: Generic

75. Potter JM, Jones C, Wild LM, Schemitsch EH, McKee MD. Does delay matter? The restoration of objectively measured shoulder strength and patient-oriented outcome after immediate fixation versus delayed reconstruction of displaced midshaft fractures of the clavicle. J Shoulder Elbow Surg. 2007;16(5):514–18.

76. Ali Khan MA, Lucas HK. Plating of fractures of the middle third of the clavicle. Injury. 1978;9(4):263–7.

77. Geckeler EO. Fractures of the clavicle in adults; Kirschner wire fixation (Murray method). Am J Surg. 1951;81(3):333–5.

78. Neviaser RJ, Neviaser JS, Neviaser TJ, Neviaser JS. A simple technique for internal fixation of the clavicle. A long term evaluation. Clin Orthop. 1975;109:103–7.

79. Bradbury N, Hutchinson J, Hahn D, Colton CL. Clavicular nonunion. 31/32 healed after plate fixation and bone grafting. Acta Orthop Scand. 1996;67(4):367–70.

80. Jupiter JB, Leffert RD. Non-union of the clavicle. Associated complications and surgical management. J Bone Joint Surg Am. 1987;69(5):753–60.

81. Kabak S, Halici M, Tuncel M, Avsarogullari L, Karaoglu S. Treatment of midclavicular nonunion: comparison of dynamic compression plating and low-contact dynamic compression plating techniques. J Shoulder Elbow Surg. 2004;13(4):396–403.

82. Iannotti MR, Crosby LA, Stafford P, Grayson G, Goulet R. Effects of plate location and selection on the stability of midshaft clavicle osteotomies: a biomechanical study. J Shoulder Elbow Surg. 2002;11(5):457–62.

83. Boehme D, Curtis Jr RJ, DeHaan JT, Kay SP, Young DC, Rockwood Jr CA. Non-union of fractures of the mid-shaft of the clavicle. Treatment with a modified Hagie intramedullary pin and autogenous bone-grafting. J Bone Joint Surg Am. 1991;73(8):1219–26.

84. Fann CY, Chiu FY, Chuang TY, Chen CM, Chen TH. Transacromial Knowles pin in the treatment of Neer type 2 distal clavicle fractures. A prospective evaluation of 32 cases. J Trauma. 2004;56(5):1102–5.

85. Thumroj E, Kosuwon W, Kamanarong K. Anatomic safe zone of pin insertion point for distal clavicle fixation. J Med Assoc Thai. 2005;88(11):1551–6.

86. Golish SR, Oliviero JA, Francke EI, Miller MD. A biomechanical study of plate versus intramedullary devices for midshaft clavicle fixation. J Orthop Surg. 2008;3(1):28.

87. Ring D, Holovacs T. Brachial plexus palsy after intramedullary fixation of a clavicular fracture. A report of three cases. J Bone Joint Surg Am. 2005;87(8):1834–7.

88. Schuind F, Pay-Pay E, Andrianne Y, Donkerwolcke M, Rasquin C, Burny F. External fixation of the clavicle for fracture or non-union in adults. J Bone Joint Surg Am. 1988;70(5):692–5.

89. Lyons FA, Rockwood Jr CA. Migration of pins used in operations on the shoulder. J Bone Joint Surg Am. 1990;72(8):1262–7.

90. Williams Jr GR, Naranja J, Klimkiewicz J, Karduna A, Iannotti JP, Ramsey M. The floating shoulder: a biomechanical basis for classification and management. J Bone Joint Surg Am. 2001;83-A(8):1182–7.

91. Herscovici Jr D, Fiennes AG, Allgower M, Ruedi TP. The floating shoulder: ipsilateral clavicle and scapular neck fractures. J Bone Joint Surg Br. 1992;74(3):362–4.

92. Leung KS, Lam TP. Open reduction and internal fixation of ipsilateral fractures of the scapular neck and clavicle. J Bone Joint Surg Am. 1993;75(7):1015–18.

93. Edwards SG, Whittle AP, Wood GW. Nonoperative treatment of ipsilateral fractures of the scapula and clavicle. J Bone Joint Surg Am. 2000;82(6):774–80.

94. van Noort A, te Slaa RL, Marti RK, van der Werken C. The floating shoulder. A multicentre study. J Bone Joint Surg Br. 2001;83(6):795–8.

95. Herscovici Jr D, Sanders R, DiPasquale T, Gregory P. Injuries of the shoulder girdle. Clin Orthop Relat Res. 1995;318:54–60.

96. Hashiguchi H, Ito H. Clinical outcome of the treatment of floating shoulder by osteosynthesis for clavicular fracture alone. J Shoulder Elbow Surg. 2003;12(6):589–91.

97. Davids PH, Luitse JS, Strating RP, van der Hart CP. Operative treatment for delayed union and nonunion of midshaft clavicular fractures: AO reconstruction plate fixation and early mobilization. J Trauma. 1996;40(6):985–6.

98. Brinker MR, Edwards TB, O'Connor DP. Estimating the risk of nonunion following nonoperative treatment of a clavicular fracture. J Bone Joint Surg Am. 2005;87(3):676–7.

99. Der Tavitian J, Davison JN, Dias JJ. Clavicular fracture non-union surgical outcome and complications. Injury. 2002;33(2):135–43.

100. Johnson Jr EW, Collins HR. Nonunion of the clavicle. Arch Surg. 1963;87:963–6.

101. Kay SP, Eckardt JJ. Brachial plexus palsy secondary to clavicular nonunion. Case report and literature survey. Clin Orthop. 1986;206:219–22.

102. Chen CH, Chen WJ, Shih CH. Surgical treatment for distal clavicle fracture with coracoclavicular ligament disruption 7. J Trauma. 2002;52(1):72–8.

103. Nowak J, Holgersson M, Larsson S. Can we predict long-term sequelae after fractures of the clavicle based on initial findings? A prospective study with nine to ten years of follow-up. J Shoulder Elbow Surg. 2004;13(5):479–86.

104. Pedersen M, Poulsen KA, Thomsen F, Kristiansen B. Operative treatment of clavicular nonunion. Acta Orthop Belg. 1994;60(3):303–6.

105. Olsen BS, Vaesel MT, Sojbjerg JO. Treatment of midshaft clavicular nonunion with plate fixation and autologous bone grafting. J Shoulder Elbow Surg. 1995;4(5):337–44.

106. Boyer MI, Axelrod TS. Atrophic nonunion of the clavicle: treatment by compression plate, lag-screw fixation and bone graft 2. J Bone Joint Surg Br. 1997;79(2):301–3.

107. Ebraheim NA, Mekhail AO, Darwich M. Open reduction and internal fixation with bone grafting of clavicular nonunion. J Trauma. 1997;42(4):701–4.

108. Wu CC, Shih CH, Chen WJ, Tai CL. Treatment of clavicular aseptic nonunion: comparison of plating and intramedullary nailing techniques. J Trauma. 1998;45(3):512–16.

109. Ballmer FT, Lambert SM, Hertel R. Decortication and plate osteosynthesis for nonunion of the clavcle 7. J Shoulder Elbow Surg. 1998;7(6):581–5.

110. Laursen MB, Dossing KV. Clavicular nonunions treated with compression plate fixation and cancellous bone grafting: the functional outcome. J Shoulder Elbow Surg. 1999;8(5):410–13.

111. Marti RK, Nolte PA, Kerkhoffs GM, Besselaar PP, Schaap GR. Operative treatment of mid-shaft clavicular non-union. Int Orthop. 2003;27(3):131–5.

112. O'Connor D, Kutty S, McCabe JP. Long-term functional outcome assessment of plate fixation and autogenous bone grafting for clavicular non-union. Injury. 2004;35(6):575–9.

113. Khan SA, Shamshery P, Gupta V, Trikha V, Varshney MK, Kumar A. Locking compression plate in long standing clavicular nonunions with poor bone stock. J Trauma. 2008;64(2):439–41.

114. Capicotto PN, Heiple KG, Wilbur JH. Midshaft clavicle nonunions treated with intramedullary Steinman pin fixation and onlay bone graft. J Orthop Trauma. 1994;8(2):88–93.

115. Hoe-Hansen CE, Norlin R. Intramedullary cancellous screw fixation for nonunion of midshaft clavicular fractures. Acta Orthop Scand. 2003;74(3):361–4.

116. Eskola A, Vainionpaa S, Myllynen P, Patiala H, Rokkanen P. Surgery for ununited clavicular fracture. Acta Orthop Scand. 1986;57(4):366–7.

117. Karaharju E, Joukainen J, Peltonen J. Treatment of pseudarthrosis of the clavicle. Injury. 1982;13(5):400–3.

118. Manske DJ, Szabo RM. The operative treatment of mid-shaft clavicular non-unions. J Bone Joint Surg Am. 1985;67(9):1367–71.

119. Pyper JB. Non-union of fractures of the clavicle. Injury. 1978;9(4):268–70.

120. Nowak J, Rahme H, Holgersson M, Lindsjo U, Larsson S. A prospective comparison between external fixation and plates for treatment of midshaft nonunions of the clavicle. Ann Chir Gynaecol. 2001;90(4):280–5.

121. Erdmann D, Pu CM, Levin LS. Nonunion of the clavicle: a rare indication for vascularized free fibula transfer. Plast Reconstr Surg. 2004;114(7):1859–63.

122. Krishnan KG, Mucha D, Gupta R, Schackert G. Brachial plexus compression caused by recurrent clavicular nonunion and space-occupying pseudoarthrosis: definitive reconstruction using free vascularized bone flap-a series of eight cases. Neurosurgery. 2008;62(5 Suppl 2):ONS461–9.

123. Choudry UH, Bakri K, Moran SL, Karacor Z, Shin AY. The vascularized medial femoral condyle periosteal bone flap for the treatment of recalcitrant bony nonunions. Ann Plast Surg. 2008;60(2):174–80.

124. Fuchs B, Steinmann SP, Bishop AT. Free vascularized corticoperiosteal bone graft for the treatment of persistent nonunion of the clavicle. J Shoulder Elbow Surg. 2005;14(3):264–8.

125. O'Rourke IC, Middleton RW. The place and efficacy of operative management of fractured clavicle. Injury. 1975;6(3):236–40.

126. Papineau LJ. Excision-graft with deliberately delayed closing in chronic osteomyelitis. Nouv Presse Med. 1973;2(41):2753–5.

127. Crenshaw A. Fractures of the shoudler girdle. In: Willis CC, editor. Campbell's Opertive Orthopaedics. 8th ed. St Louis: Mosby; 1992. p. 989–995.

128. Wood VE. The results of total claviculectomy. Clin Orthop Relat Res. 1986;207:186–90.

129. Edelson JG. The bony anatomy of clavicular malunions. J Shoulder Elbow Surg. 2003;12(2):173–8.

130. McKee MD, Wild LM, Schemitsch EH. Midshaft malunions of the clavicle. Surgical technique. J Bone Joint Surg Am. 2004;86-A(Suppl 1):37–43.

131. Chan KY, Jupiter JB, Leffert RD, Marti R. Clavicle malunion. J Shoulder Elbow Surg. 1999;8(4):287–90.

132. Hill JM, McGuire MH, Crosby LA. Closed treatment of displaced middle-third fractures of the clavicle gives poor results. J Bone Joint Surg Br. 1997;79(4):537–9.

133. Nordqvist A, Redlund-Johnell I, von Scheele A, Petersson CJ. Shortening of clavicle after fracture. Incidence and clinical significance, a 5-year follow-up of 85 patients. Acta Orthop Scand. 1997;68(4):349–51.

134. Oroko PK, Buchan M, Winkler A, Kelly IG. Does shortening matter after clavicular fractures? Bull Hosp Jt Dis. 1999;58(1):6–8.

135. Bosch U, Skutek M, Peters G, Tscherne H. Extension osteotomy in malunited clavicular fractures. J Shoulder Elbow Surg. 1998;7(4):402–5.

136. Simpson NS, Jupiter JB. Clavicular nonunion and malunion: evaluation and surgical management. J Am Acad Orthop Surg. 1996;4(1):1–8.

137. Wilkes RA, Halawa M. Scapular and clavicular osteotomy for malunion: case report. J Trauma. 1993;34(2):309.

138. Hillen RJ, Burger BJ, Poll RG, de Gast A, Robinson CM. Malunion after midshaft clavicle fractures in adults. Acta Orthop. 2010;81(3):273–9.

139. Hillen RJ, Eygendaal D. Corrective osteotomy after malunion of mid shaft fractures of the clavicle. Strategies Trauma Limb Reconstr. 2007;2(2–3): 59–61.

140. Della SD, Narakas A, Bonnard C. Late lesions of the brachial plexus after fracture of the clavicle. Ann Chir Main Memb Super. 1991;10(6):531–40.

141. Fujita K, Matsuda K, Sakai Y, Sakai H, Mizuno K. Late thoracic outlet syndrome secondary to malunion of the fractured clavicle: case report and review of the literature. J Trauma. 2001;50(2):332–5.

142. Howard FM, Shafer SJ. Injuries to the clavicle with neurovascular complications. A study of fourteen cases. J Bone Joint Surg Am. 1965;47(7):1335–46.

143. Rumball KM, Da SV, Preston DN, Carruthers CC. Brachial-plexus injury after clavicular fracture: case report and literature review. Can J Surg. 1991; 34(3):264–6.

144. Bargar WL, Marcus RE, Ittleman FP. Late thoracic outlet syndrome secondary to pseudarthrosis of the clavicle. J Trauma. 1984;24(9):857–9.

145. Bateman JE. Neurovascular syndromes related to the clavicle. Clin Orthop. 1968;58:75–82.

146. Chen DJ, Chuang DC, Wei FC. Unusual thoracic outlet syndrome secondary to fractured clavicle. J Trauma. 2002;52(2):393–8.

147. Connolly JF, Dehne R. Nonunion of the clavicle and thoracic outlet syndrome. J Trauma. 1989; 29(8): 1127–32.

148. Kitsis CK, Marino AJ, Krikler SJ, Birch R. Late complications following clavicular fractures and their operative management. Injury. 2003; 34(1):69–74.

149. Miller DS, Boswick Jr JA. Lesions of the brachial plexus associated with fractures of the clavicle. Clin Orthop Relat Res. 1969;64:144–9.

150. Gelberman RH, Leffert RD. Thoracic outlet syndrome. In: Gelberman RH, editor. Operative nerve repair and reconstruction. Philadelphia: Lippincott; 1991. p. 1177–95.

151. Flinkkila T, Ristiniemi J, Lakovaara M, Hyvonen P, Leppilahti J. Hook-plate fixation of unstable lateral clavicle fractures: a report on 63 patients 1. Acta Orthop. 2006;77(4):644–9.

152. Bronz G, Heim D, Pusterla C, Heim U. Osteosynthesis of the clavicle (author's transl). Unfallheilkunde. 1981;84(8):319–25.

153. Kuner EH, Schlickewei W, Mydla F. Surgical therapy of clavicular fractures, indications, technic, results. Hefte Unfallheilkd. 1982;160:76–83.

154. Fowler AW. Treatment of fractured clavicle. Lancet. 1968;1(7532):46–7.

155. Kloen P, Sorkin AT, Rubel IF, Helfet DL. Anteroinferior plating of midshaft clavicular nonunions. J Orthop Trauma. 2002;16(6):425–30.

156. Schwarz N, Hocker K. Osteosynthesis of irreducible fractures of the clavicle with 2.7-MM ASIF plates. J Trauma. 1992;33(2):179–83.

157. Tarar MN, Quaba AA. An adipofascial turnover flap for soft tissue cover around the clavicle. Br J Plast Surg. 1995;48(3):161–4.

158. Williams GR, Koffler K, Pepe M, Wong K, Chang B, Ramsey M. Rotation of the clavicular portion of the pectoralis major for soft-tissue coverage of the clavicle. An anatomical study and case report. J Bone Joint Surg Am. 2000;82-A(12):1736–42.

159. Khan LA et al. Fractures of the clavicle. J Bone Joint Surg [Am] 2009;91:447–460.

Acromioclavicular Injuries

Jonas Franke and Lars Neumann

Contents

Keywords

Acromioclavicular joint • Aetiology and classification • Anatomy • Chronic injuries-weaver Dunn and "Surgilig" techniques • Complications • Diagnosis • Injuries • Operative techniques-acute injuries • Rehabilitation • Results • Surgical indications

Introduction

Injuries to the acromioclavicular joint are common. They are usually caused by a direct fall on to the top of the shoulder and are more common in younger adults than in children and elderly. The contentious issue about conservative or surgical treatment for these injuries seem to be a never- ending debate within the Orthopaedic community. The majority of these injuries can be treated conservatively and usually with very good results. However, for the more severe injuries with greater displacement, surgery is usually recommended early. For those with chronically painful and unstable joints, surgical treatment may be required at a later stage.

Already Hippocrates realized that there would be a "tumefaction" or deformity from such an injury "for the bone cannot be properly restored to its natural situation" but he also stated that no impediment, whether small or great, will result from such an injury. This statement, as Rockwood has commented, "Apparently was, has been and will be received by the Orthopaedic community as a challenge" [1].

J. Franke (✉) • L. Neumann
Nottingham Shoulder and Elbow Unit, Nottingham University Hospitals, Nottingham, UK
e-mail: jonas.franke@aol.se; larsneumann@me.com

G. Bentley (ed.), *European Surgical Orthopaedics and Traumatology*,
DOI 10.1007/978-3-642-34746-7_256, © EFORT 2014

There are numerous arthroscopic and open procedures described in the literature. We will focus on one method for the acute open repair and two slightly different techniques for coracoclavicular ligament repair of the chronically symptomatic dislocations; a modified Weaver-Dunn procedure and a repair using an artificial ligament, the Nottingham "Surgilig".

Anatomy and Function

The acromioclavicular joint is the diarthrodial joint between the lateral end of the clavicle and the medial facet of the acromion. There is considerable variation in topography of the acromioclavicular joint from subject to subject. Bosworth has stated that the average size of the acromioclavicular joint surface is 9×19 mm [2]. The inclination of the joint, when viewed from the front, may be almost vertical or inclined diagonally from medially inferiorly to more lateral superiorly and thus with the clavicle over-riding the acromion with an angle sometimes as large as $50°$. The majority of movement taking place in the joint is rotation in the long axis of the clavicle. However, the degree of rotational movement in the joint as such is fairly limited ($5°$–$8°$) since there is simultaneous rotation of the scapula – synchronous scapular rotation.

The acromioclavicular joint is stabilized by the acromioclavicular (intra-articular) and coracoclavicular (extra-articular) ligaments as well as the deltoid and trapezius muscles. The coracoclavicular ligaments are divided into the conoid and trapezoid ligaments. The relationship of the clavicular and the acromial component of the joint is kept rather stable throughout its range of movement. It has been suggested that the anteroposterior stability is provided by the acromioclavicular ligaments and that the superoinferior stability is supplied by the coracoclavicular ligaments [3]. The conoid and trapezoid ligaments run obliquely from the coracoid to the clavicle in opposing directions and are analogous to the cruciate ligaments of the knee,

providing stability throughout the range of movement of the joint [4]. Several authors are also emphasizing the importance of the deltotrapezius muscle fascia for the overall stability of the joint. There is a fibrocartilagenous diskc(meniscus) in the joint with great variation in shape and size. Injuries to the stabilizing structures can result in instability and subsequently in various degrees of dislocation of the joint. With the joint dislocated the clavicle will, to some extent, lose its function as a strut and the whole of the shoulder girdle will subsequently be somewhat destabilised.

Aetiology and Classification

It has been suggested that as many as 40 % of shoulder injuries affect the AC-joint and that AC-joint dislocations accounts for 8 % of all joint dislocations in the body [5–8]. It is more common in males and in the age group under 35 and it is commonly a sports injury predominantly associated with horse riding, alpine skiing, snowboarding, ice hockey, rugby etc. [6, 9–12].

Injuries to the AC-joint are most often caused by a fall on to the point of the shoulder with the arm adducted [13]. The AC-joint separation is caused as the direct force of the blow drives the acromion and shoulder girdle inferiorly, whereas the clavicle remains in its anatomical position [13, 14]. Once the stabilizing structures are damaged, the joint is left unstable and the remaining displacement is a result of the force of gravity on the affected arm causing vertical displacement and the tractional force of the trapezius causing posterior displacement.

The severity of an injury to the AC-joint is determined by the preservation, or loss of structural integrity of the acromioclavicular and coracoclavicular ligaments and by the degree of damage to the muscular attachment of the Deltoid and Trapezius [14–17]. In a more severe lesion with subluxation or displacement of the joint, the periosteum is torn away from its attachment to the inferior surface of the clavicle. This explains the frequent radiographic finding of subperiostial new bone formation, inferior to the clavicle, following these injuries (Fig. 1a). With increasing force the deltoid and trapezius muscles and the clavipectoral fascia, and its condensations are torn from a lateral to a medial direction. The miniscus usually maintains its attachment to the acromial side of the joint in the complete dislocations [4].

After the early works of Cadenet, describing this sequential patho-anatomy, and previous classifications by Allman, Tossy and Bannister, Rockwood and colleagues came up with the classification most widely used today [18–20].

These six classifications of AC joint dislocations are based on the patho-anatomy and clinically determined by the degree and direction of displacement of the clavicle (Fig. 2).

The Rockwood type I injury is a sprain, or incomplete injury to the acromioclavicular ligaments, with no involvement of the coracoclavicular ligaments. The joint is still completely stable.

The type II injuries constitute a complete injury to the acromioclavicular ligaments and an incomplete injury to the coracoacromial ligaments.

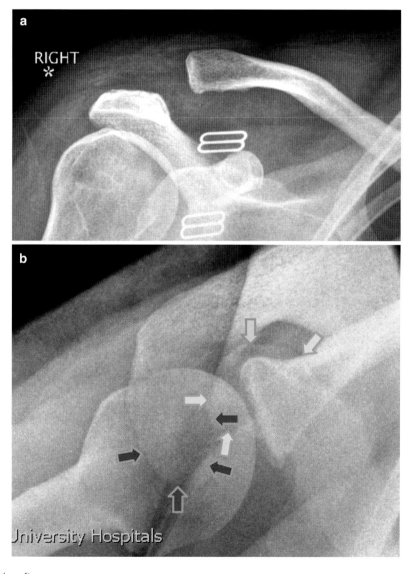

Fig. 1 (continued)

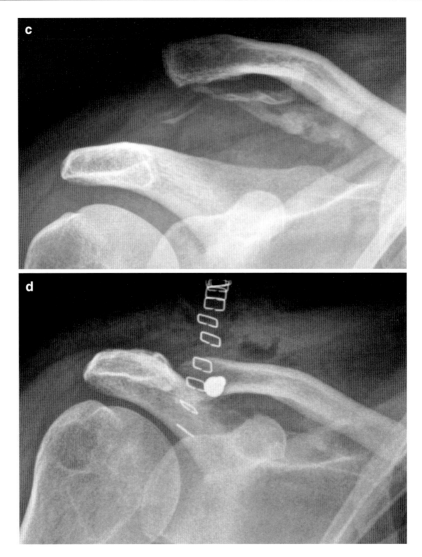

Fig. 1 (**a**) A shoulder AP view of a grade V dislocation in a 30 year-old woman. (**b**) Axial view x-ray clearly displaying posterior displacement in the same patient. *Blue arrows* indicate clavicle and *red* the acromion. (**c**) Pre-operative films of the same patient as in (**a**) and (**b**) 4 months after trauma, showing ossification inferior to the clavicle due to the detachment of the inferior periosteum. (**d**) The same patient as in Fig. 1a–c after "Surgilig" procedure and removal of inferior osteophytes on the clavicle. Note the clips on the strap incision

There might be some widening of the joint but only very slight, if any, step deformity in the joint.

In type III injuries both the acromioclavicular and coracoclavicular ligaments are torn completely, always resulting in instability and usually also significant, but not severe displacement of the joint, mainly restricted to the sagittal plane with the clavicle positioned higher than the acromion.

Type IV injuries are defined by an additional posterior displacement of the clavicle, the lateral end of the bone may even penetrate posteriorly through the trapezius.

The type V injury represents a superior displacement of the clavicle, which is significantly more than in a type III injury, due a more extensive to loss of the muscular attachments of the deltoid and trapezius muscles on the clavicle.

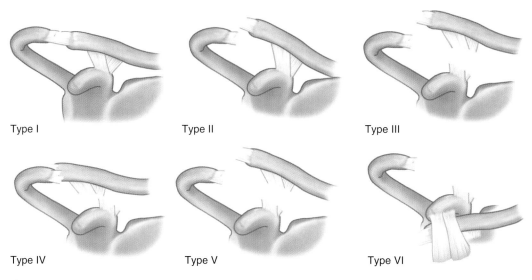

Type I   Type II   Type III

Type IV   Type V   Type VI

Fig. 2 The six classifications of AC-joint injuries according to Rockwood

A type VI injury constitutes a clavicle displaced inferiorly to the acromion or even under the coracoid process.

Diagnosis

The diagnosis of an acromioclavicular joint dislocation is primarily clinical and radiological, although other methods have been tried [21–26]. The patient will typically describe a traumatic onset with a fall on to the top of the shoulder and complain of pain localised over the AC-joint, sometimes extending medially along the clavicle. In more chronic cases, particularly when there is no large displacement present, the pain is usually fairly localised and the patients often point with their finger to the joint when describing the pain source, "The finger sign". With a careful history taking and a good clinical examination, x-rays will but confirm the clinical diagnosis.

A clinical examination will, as for all joints, consist of inspection, palpation and movement. There will be weakness on flexion and abduction, particularly above 90° in milder cases, a decrease in range of movement with regards to flexion and abduction, tenderness on palpation over the joint and loading of the joint will trigger indirect pain. Pain is localised to the joint and will be triggered by the cross-body adduction test when the arm is in 45° of elevation and adducted across the chest. The cross body test can trigger pain also in impingement cases but it thus tends to be localised more laterally and subacromial. Sometimes it is also possible in this manoeuvre that the highly unstable clavicle will slide over the cranial surface of the acromion.

In a case with large displacement the diagnosis is obvious, but with milder cases applying downwards, traction to the arm may reveal the instability, as if gravity alone does not manage to displace the unstable joint, adding the extra force may do so.

To reduce the joint one must push the arm upwards whilst stabilizing the clavicle with one's opposite hand. To obtain reduction it may be necessary to direct the upward push slightly posteriorly and to add an anteriorly-directed force to the clavicle if there is significant posterior dislocation. It is usually not possible to reduce the dislocation simply by pushing the clavicle downwards. It is rather the arm that is displaced inferiorly as described earlier not the clavicle that is lifted.

As with any musculoskeletal injury, radiographs must be obtained in two planes, anteroposterior and lateral. An AP view of the shoulder alone is not sufficient since this does not provide a clear view through the AC-joint and there will be overlying shadows from other structures, typically the scapular spine. The correct AC-joint AP view is obtained with a 30° cranial tilt of the x-ray beam and this should be routinely used. With a correct AP view there is good visualisation not only of the AC-joint as such but also of the coracoid, and the coracoclavicular distance can consequently be measured to estimate the degree of vertical displacement of the clavicle. The lateral, or axial, views are most important to detect any horizontal and posterior displacement and thus differentiating type III and IV injuries, whereas the AP views will uncover any supero-inferior translocation. Furthermore, because there is a significant variation between individuals in normal AC-joint anatomy, the contra lateral joint should consequently always be imaged (Fig. 1a–d).

Stress views can be used to indicate the integrity of the coracoclavicular ligaments and have proven to unmask grade III injuries in patients with relatively normal plain x-rays [27]. However, it is generally not suggested as a routine due to its low yield. About 5 kg of weights are suspended by loops of webbing round the wrist. Holding the weight in the hand prevents total relaxation of the muscles around the shoulder and might hinder coracoclavicular separation.

A patient with a type I injury usually has only mild to moderate pain localised distinctly on the AC-joint. Pain is triggered or enhanced with loading of the joint. There is no displacement clinically and x-rays are normal also when compared to the other side.

The type II injury is characterised by pain and moderate swelling over the joint and x-rays can reveal a widening of the acromioclavicular joint, but no significant vertical displacement should be present. If stress X- rays are made there is no increase in the coracoclavicular distance, since the damage to the coracoclavicular ligaments is not complete.

A patient with a type III AC-joint injury will often keep the arm adducted and supported to relieve pain. The shoulder complex will typically be depressed as mentioned with the lateral end of the clavicle prominent and seemingly lifted above the level of the acromion. AP-view X-rays will, for the type III injury, usually reveal displacement with an increased coracoclavicular distance, but it can sometimes be necessary to conduct stress views as discussed above.

In type IV injury the posteriorly-displaced clavicle can sometimes protrude through the trapezius muscle and be clearly palpated subcutaneously (Fig. 3). X-rays and particularly the lateral view will confirm the posterior displacement and hence the diagnosis.

It is sometimes difficult, however important, to clinically differentiate the type III lesion from the type V, where the superior displacement is significantly larger. The latter will leave the patient in considerably more pain, not rarely continued medially because of the damage to the insertion of the deltoid and trapezius muscles and the periosteum further medial on the clavicle. Again x-rays will provide support for the diagnosis and may show a very marked increase (up to two to three times normal or more) of the coracoclavicular distance. A comparison with the other side will define the normal coracoclavicular distance for the particular patient.

The rare type VI injuries are usually the result of high energy injuries and are not rarely associated with concomitant injuries such as clavicular and rib fractures and vascular and brachial plexus injuries. The complexity and severity of this injury will frequently necessitate other investigations such as CT-scans and/or MRI's.

Management and Indications for Surgery

The correct management for the acute acromioclavicular injuries will depend on the classification type of the injury and on patient factors. The conservative management of Rockwood type I and II lesions is fairly unchallenged historically and in modern literature [28, 29].

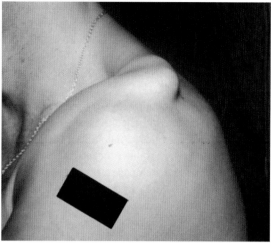
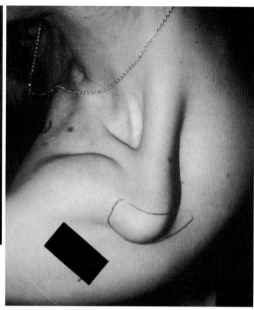

Fig. 3 Severe posterior dislocation in a grade V injury. The clavicle is penetrating trough the trapezius muscle posteriorly and can clearly be seen to over-ride the acromion

The patient suffering a type 1 injury requires no treatment and symptoms will usually subside within a couple of weeks, even though prolonged symptoms up to 6 months have been reported. It is also believed that type 1 injuries and even undiagnosed type 1 injuries will occasionally cause later post-traumatic AC-joint osteoarthritis.

For the patient with a type II injury the arm is kept in a sling until pain is under control and early mobilization is encouraged, not loading the arm or returning to sports or heavy manual labour for usually 6–8 weeks. An almost full recovery can generally be expected [13]. However later AC-joint osteoarthritis or arthropathy could result from this injury [30].

There is a widespread agreement that the Rockwood type IV, V and VI injuries should be subjected to surgical repair [29]. Hence the controversy concerns the type III lesions where the debate is vivid and good scientific evidence still scarce and somewhat contradictory [5, 29, 31–40].

Multiple studies have reported that even patients with reasonably large residual deformities may very well have good functional results [39, 41–43]. However, a considerable number of patients do not become pain-free, and are left with discomfort around the shoulder, weakness, and inability to pursue demanding physical activities, particularly throwing and overhead sports. Furthermore surgery and anatomical restoration of the joint does not always relieve symptoms completely [34, 40, 44–48]. However, It has also been suggested that the results from early surgical treatment exceed those of the delayed therapy for chronic symptoms [49]. No study has to our knowledge successfully delineated a group of patients who would definitely, with statistic significance, benefit from an early operation. By offering all early surgical treatment however, some would undoubtedly have an unnecessary operation.

The difficulty thus lies in selecting the right candidates for surgery after an acute type III injury. It is generally argued that surgical repair for the acute type III injury should be considered in the younger, more athletic individuals and heavy manual workers, especially those involved in overhead activities. Other factors in favour for early surgery are injuries to the dominant side and a highly unstable joint. The patient must be trusted to comply with the post-operative programme and, as always, surgical treatment should be strongly questioned in the unreliable patient with alcohol or drug abuse or with a considerable mental disorder. It is also important not to underdiagnose the more unstable type V injuries as type III injuries since the patients with the more severe injury, particularly if younger or heavy manual workers will probably be best helped by being treated early.

Chronic Injuries

For the chronically symptomatic AC-joint injuries the decision-making, is more straightforward. In the case of persistent pain, i.e. secondary osteoarthritis or post-traumatic arthropathy after a type I or II injury, where the coracoclavicular ligaments are preserved and the joint is still stable, a resection of the lateral clavicle according to Mumford is usually quite successful [50]. However for the chronic type III to VI injuries with unstable AC-joints a clavicular resection as above should always be accompanied by a stabilization of the clavicle [50, 51].

Pre-Operative Preparation and Planning

It is important to have x-rays of the contra lateral AC-joint as part of the pre- operative planning. As mentioned there are large variations in anatomy and in some individuals the normal AC-joint can have a vertical step with the lateral end of the clavicle at a higher level than the acromion. It is important to consider this to avoid over-correcting the displacement with a too- tight repair.

It is furthermore important when dealing with the chronically symptomatic injuries to have fairly recent x-rays. Even if the diagnosis as such can be based on clinical examination and on previous x-rays it is not rarely the

case that additional calcifications has formed in the meantime, often inferior to the clavicle or along the torn coracoclavicular ligaments (Fig. 1c). Other abnormalities, such as osteolysis of the lateral clavicle, may also have developed.

The neurovascular status of the affected arm should be thoroughly checked and clearly noted pre-operatively since concomitant damage to these structures may have occurred at the time of the trauma or developed over time and because of the close proximity of the neurovascular bundle to the coracoid process and the surgical field and the risk of iatrogenic damage.

We use for all our AC-joint procedures the "deck-chair" position with the patient's head slightly tilted away from the affected shoulder (Fig. 4). We generally do not use image intensifiers but this could of course be considered at the surgeon's discretion in particular cases. The arm and shoulder is scrubbed and draped.

Operative Techniques

There is an abundance of methods described in the literature for the treatment of both acute and chronic dislocations [17, 52–74]. This in itself probably indicates that none of them are entirely satisfactory. Historically a great variety of operations has been performed and modern techniques, whether open or arthroscopic, use a combination of a few basic principles: acromioclavicular repair and fixation, coracoclavicular repair and fixation and resection of the lateral clavicle. Acromioclavicular fixation can be achieved with pins, screws, suture wires, plates etc and can be performed with or without acromioclavicular and/or coracoclavicular ligament repair. Coracoclavicular fixation can be achieved with a screw, wire, fascia, conjoined tendon, synthetic sutures or implants and can be performed with or without acromioclavicular and coracoclavicular ligament repair or reconstruction.

The original Weaver Dunn procedure which was described in 1972 uses a transfer of the

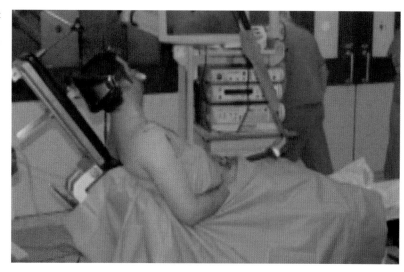

Fig. 4 Set-up of the patient for a right shoulder "Surgilig" procedure in the "deck-chair" position with the head slightly tilted to the left. The procedure is performed under local block anaesthesia

coracoacromial ligament to the clavicle to restore coracoclavicular stability (Fig. 5) [51]. Bosworth used a screw to achieve coracoclavicular stability under local anaesthesia without exploring either the acromioclavicular joint or ligaments nor the coracoclavicular ligaments [75]. A more recently-described technique suggests the use of a semitendinosus allograft instead to reconstruct the ligament [76]. Other authors use Hook plates to achieve acromioclavicular stability [77]. Good results have also been reported simply by closed reduction and percutaneuos pinning under image intensifier. Several authors have recently reported on successful series of arthroscopic repairs [57, 60, 78, 79]. Boileau et al. used a double-button in their arthroscopic technique whereas others have used suture anchors to achieve coracoclavicular stability [57, 80].

Surgical Treatment for Acute AC-Joint Displacement

In the case of surgery for an acute dislocation, the aim is to restore a functioning anatomy as close to normal as possible. We recommend an open technique for repair of an acute AC-joint dislocation. We believe that it is important to restore the anatomical position and integrity of the joint and its capsular ligaments and if

possible of the intra-articular disk. We do not believe that a direct repair of the coroacoclavicular ligaments is necessary since it requires further dissection and since good enough stability has been proven to occur by direct healing following acromioclavicular repair and fixation alone. All other ruptured structures including the acromioclavicular ligaments as well as the deltoid and trapezius muscles insertions should of course be repaired as well.

By using K-wires for temporary transfixation of the AC joint it is possible to correct both the horizontal and vertical dislocation with great accuracy and thus to achieve a correct reduction of the joint. We believe that this is not as easily achieved neither with coracoclavicular fixation, be it with a Bosworth screw or wires or sutures, nor with the use of the hook plate. Again, since, in the acute case, the aim is to restore the joint without any resection of the clavicle, it is important that exact reduction is reached.

Authors' Preferred Method

The patient is set up in a "deck-chair" position (Fig. 4) with the head slightly tilted to the contra-lateral side. A 5–7 cm strap incision is made

Fig. 5 Post-operative
x-rays after a Weaver-Dunn
procedure where the
displacement of the clavicle
has been over-corrected

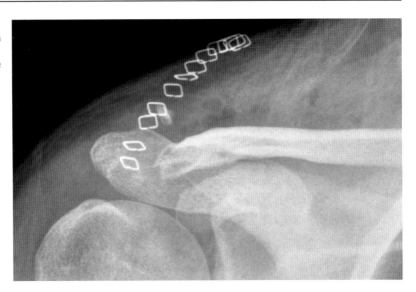

starting 2 cm posterior to the clavicle and 1 cm medial to the AC-joint (Fig. 6). The skin is undermined. The AC-joint together with the deltotrapezius muscle fascia and lateral clavicle is exposed (Fig. 7). Usually the deltotrapezius muscle fascia is at least partially ruptured by the trauma, but if not it should be incised horizontally over the lateral 5 cm of the clavicle and the muscles should be mobilized accordingly. The joint is then reduced and the capsule and the acromioclavicular ligaments are tagged with untied sutures.

Two 2.5 mm k-wires are used to transfix the joint in the correct anatomical position. It is recommended that these wires are double pointed and introduced in the acromion articular surface and pulled out posterolaterally through the skin before again being "backed" medially into the clavicle. However, it is not always possible to access the acromion this way and alternatively the wires can be introduced from lateral through the skin over the acromion first.

We recommend that the wires are directed slightly obliquely towards the posterior aspect of the acromion since the bone is usually thicker here which makes it easier to stay in the bone since the anterior part of the acroimion can sometimes be rather thin (Fig. 9). We also believe that there is a mechanical advantage with this diagonal placement of the wires.

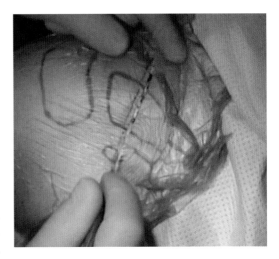

Fig. 6 Strap incision

Furthermore, the medial end of the wires will with this technique penetrate the clavicle more anterosuperiorly, which is safer with regard to the neurovascular bundle inferior to the bone. In the case of fracture and migration the wires will also most probably penetrate through the skin anteriorly before they have a chance to escape to anywhere else. It is also important that the "far" cortex of the clavicle anterior-superiorly is penetrated and that the wire is then not drilled back and forwards which may unnecessarily widen the hole which could increase the risk of wire loosening and migration.

Fig. 7 "Figure of 7" – incision of the deltoid, with the use of the bipolar diathermy

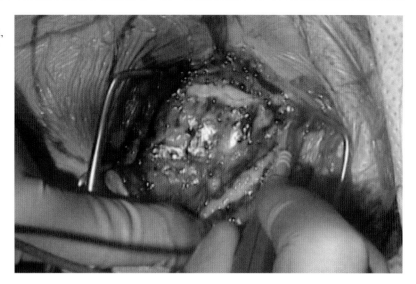

The sutures in the capsule and acromioclavicular ligaments are then tied with particular attention to restoring the position of the intra-articular disk. However if it is severely damaged or degenerated it should rather be removed. The deltotrapezius muscle fascia and the muscle insertions are then carefully restored with heavy absorbable sutures. The K-wires are then cut and bent laterally. We tend to leave the wires bent over the skin which clearly facilitates the removal of them but they could of course be left subcutaneously under the skin if preferred. Finally, routine subcutaneous and skin closure of the wound is performed.

Surgical Treatment for Chronic AC-Joint Displacement

For the case of a stable but symptomatic chronic type I or II injury with possible arthritis we, as other authors, recommend an arthroscopic AC-joint excision. This procedure is described elsewhere.

However, for the unstable chronic type III or higher grade injuries we use a modified Weaver Dunn procedure where additional temporary support and stabilization is achieved through multiple absorbable sutures tied around the coracoid and the clavicle. The aim of this procedure is to restore a stable link between the scapula and the clavicle eliminating direct contact between the coracoid and the acromion and avoiding impingement between the coracoid and the clavicle. We strongly believe in the use of multiple absorbable sutures for temporary coracoclavicular stability as this will give a good enough stability initially during the healing but will eliminate the possible late problem of non-absorbable sutures eroding into the clavicle. The need for a second procedure to remove screws or other implants is also eliminated by this technique. Alternatively when the coracoclavicular ligament is absent or of poor quality or in the rare event of a re-do stabilization we use the Nottingham Surgilig artificial ligament.

Whatever technique is used it is important to achieve enough resection of the clavicle. Great care must be taken not to resect too much bone. Too little resection will result in painful impingement between the acromion and lateral end of the clavicle. Too much resection will jeopardise stability.

If calcifications or osteophytes are present in the torn coracoclavicular ligaments or inferiorly along the clavicle they should be removed not to hinder reduction or cause coracoclavicular contact and impingement. It is probably better, for the same reason, to accept a slight step deformity, and not fully correct the vertical dislocation than to overcorrect the displacement. If only the vertical displacement of the clavicle is corrected and not the posterior, there is a risk of the posterior corner of the clavicle meeting the acromion even if a good bone resection has been performed which may result in painful impingement. Adequate reduction of the posterior displacement can sometimes be hindered by the shortened clavicular fibres of the trapezius muscle and a thorough release of the muscle is therefore necessary. It is occasionally also needed to divide even the acromial fibres of the muscle since they cause direct pressure on the clavicle and thus hinder reduction.

Authors' Preferred Method

The patient is set up in a "deck-chair" position with the head slightly tilted to the contra-lateral side. A 7–10 cm strap incision is made starting 2 cm posterior to the clavicle and 1 cm medial to the AC-joint continued forwards to the level of the tip of coracoid process. The skin is undermined. The displaced lateral end of the clavicle and the deltotrapezius muscle fascia is identified. The deltoid muscle incision is made as a figure of seven (Figs. 7 and 8): the muscle is split along its fibres from just over the tip of the coracoid and onto its insertion on the clavicle. The deltoid and trapezius fasciae are then divided along the clavicle and the periosteum is lifted to both sides and the trapezius and deltoid insertions are mobilised. A triangular flap of the deltoid muscle is thus made and retracted laterally with a stay suture in the superomedial corner. This gives a very good access to the coracoid process and the coracoacromial ligament. As mentioned it is crucial to do a good release of the trapezius muscle insertion, as otherwise a complete reduction of the posterior horizontal displacement of the clavicle would not be possible. Once the muscles have been mobilized the clavicle can be lifted using a bone clamp to allow any inferior osteophytes and calcifications to be cleared.

The AC-joint is by now well exposed and about 0.5–1 cm of the lateral clavicle is excised, leaving a gap of 1–1.5 cm in the reduced joint. If the patients arm can be elevated above 90° with the surgeon's index finger in the reduced

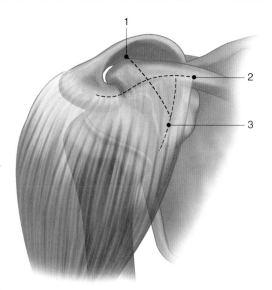

Fig. 8 Deltoid muscle incision

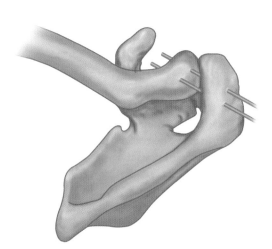

Fig. 9 Correct placement of K-wires for Ac-joint transfixation

AC-joint not getting squeezed there is usually an adequate gap.

The medullary canal of the clavicle is curetted and two 2 mm holes are drilled through the superior cortex, 1 cm medial to the resected joint surface of the clavicle, into the medullary canal. The coracoacromial ligament is released by mobilising its insertion with a bone chip from the acromion. Two heavy non-absorbable sutures, No 2 Ethibond, are sown into the

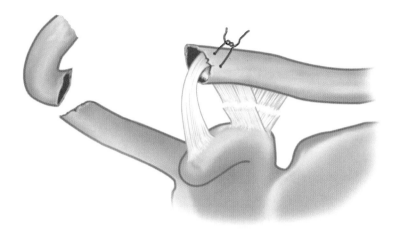

mobilised ligament in a Kessler fashion. Should the ligament be too short to reach the medullary canal of the clavicle it can be lengthened somewhat by detaching the anterior part of its coracoid insertion. No less than 6–8 strands of No 2 Vicryl absorbable sutures are then passed with a suture passer around the coracoid from medial to lateral and around the clavicle. The non-absorbable sutures from the acromioclavicular ligament are passed into the medullary canal of the clavicle and through the superior drill holes (Fig. 10). The AC-joint is then reduced by lifting the arm rather than depressing the clavicle. The eight absorbable sutures are tied individually over the clavicle while the clavicle is held reduced in the correct position. A coracoclavicular distance of about 1 cm should be the aim. A finger or instrument of suitable size between the coracoid and the clavicle facilitates this manoeuvre and prevents over-correction. The sutures from the coracoclavicular ligament are then tied pulling the ligament with its bone chip into the clavicle. The deltoid split and the deltotrapezius interval are carefully repaired over the clavicle with heavy interrupted absorbable sutures. As the reduction usually has caused a considerable change of the position of the clavicle in an anterior direction, it is not rare that the deltotrapezius interval no longer lies on top of the clavicle but more posteriorly. Interrupted subcutaneous and intracutaneous skin sutures for wound closure.

Alternative Method with Use of the Artificial Ligament, the Nottingham "Surgilig"

Should the coracoacromial ligament be absent or of poor a quality we instead use the Surgilig ligament, a polyester implant specifically designed for this purpose [81–83] (Fig. 11). The incision and approach is the same as mentioned above but of course the coracoacromial ligament is not detached from the acromion. Instead of passing absorbable sutures around the coracoid the introducer for the implant, a measuring gauge is passed around the bone from medial to lateral. The brachial plexus is close and it is important that the introducer is kept close to bone. The metal tip of the combined lead and length-measuring gauge for the Surgilig is then passed through the introducer on the lateral side of the coracoid and pulled around it. The combined lead and gauge is then looped into itself and tightened around the coracoid before being passed posteriorly to the clavicle, around and over it, to the front. After reduction of the clavicle the length of the required implant is measured using the markings on the gauge. The correct final implant is then "daisy-chained" to the measuring gauge and pulled around the coracoid. It is then looped into itself and tightened around the coracoid before it, in the same fashion, is passed behind

Fig. 11 The "Surgilig" artificial ligament in position on a skeleton: pulled around the coracoid, looped around itself and then continued posterior to the clavicle and over it to anterior where it is secured with a bicortical screw

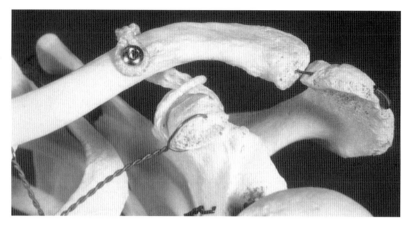

and over the clavicle. The Surgilig is finally secured to the clavicle with a 3.5 mm bicortical screw placed horizontally from anterior to posterior. Muscle repair and closure is the same as above.

Post-Operative Care and Rehabilitation

Acute repairs with K-wires are kept in a 45° abduction splint for 6 weeks at which stage the K-wires are removed. During this time the patient is allowed to do pendular motions with the arm out of the splint after 2 weeks and after 6 weeks full range of motion is allowed not loading the arm. Returning to sport or heavy labour is not allowed for 3 months.

Chronic dislocations treated with a Weaver Dunn repair are kept in a sling at all times for 4 weeks and then seen in the out-patient clinic with a check x-ray prior to allowing gentle mobilization but not lifting the arm above 90° of flexion and abduction for another 4 weeks. At 8 weeks hence full mobilization is allowed but no heavy weight-bearing or return to sports is allowed for 3 months.

When the Surgilig artificial ligament is used the patient is only kept in the sling for 2 weeks where after full mobilization is allowed but heavy lifting or demanding physical activities are avoided for 3 months post-operatively.

Results

It is generally argued that excellent results can be expected from the conservative treatment of grade I and II injuries. However one study reveals that only 52 % of patients remained asymptomatic, that the majority showed late radiological pathology and that 27 % required subsequent surgery thus indicating that the long-term effects of these injuries, and the risk of post-traumatic osteoarthritis, might be underestimated [84].

Several authors have reported generally good results for the conservative treatment of type III injuries [32, 39, 85]. Some authors have reported better results for surgically-treated type III injuries [32, 86]. However, many others have failed to prove any improvement from surgery or even found the outcome worse in the surgically-treated [13, 36, 38, 85, 87].

Other authors have reported good results with acromioclavicular repair and temporary joint transfixation using techniques similar to the one described here [33, 88]. The outcome of the Weaver Dunn procedure, and modifications thereof, has been widely documented [51, 77, 89].

Our unit has recently presented a comparative study with a non-randomised follow up of 55 patients operated with our modified Weaver Dunn procedure ($n = 31$) and the Surgilig artificial ligament ($n = 24$) showing good results in both groups with the Surgilig patients returning to work significantly earlier. No major complications where noted in any of the groups in this series [90].

Complications

Acromioclavicular injuries may be associated with other injuries around the shoulder. Reports of concomitant fractures to the clavicle itself, the coracoid process and ribs are reported in the literature. Neurological injuries to the brachial plexus are rare but can occur early or late [91, 92].

Coracoclavicular ossification is commonly associated with these injuries whether treated operatively or conservatively [93, 94]. Osteoarthritis of the AC-joint or even osteolysis of the lateral clavicle may follow the acute type I or II injury or be the result of repeated micro-trauma it can also affect the acutely repaired joint after a grade III injury.

The surgical treatment of these injuries can apart from the general post operative complications such as infection, nerve damage and recurrence, result in erosion of the clavicle from sutures or metal, migration and/or fracture of pins or wires and unsightly scars (Fig. 12c).

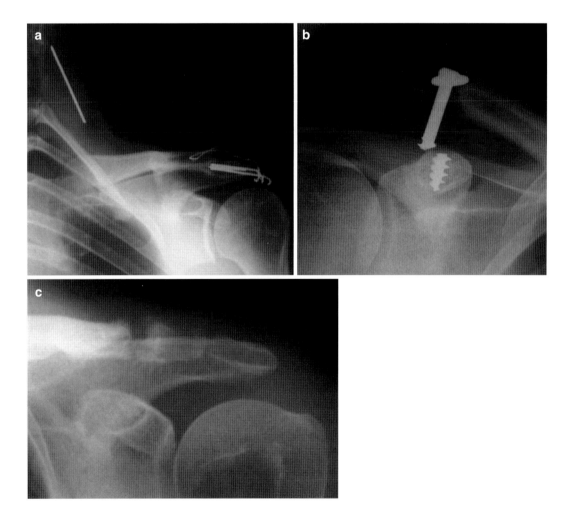

Fig. 12 (**a**) X-ray showing known possible complication to fixation with k-wires: fracture of the wire and migration. (**b**) Fracture of a screw (Bosworth) used for coracoclavicular fixation. (**c**) X-rays showing complication of non-absorbable sutures used for coracoclavicular fixation with the sutures cutting through the clavicle

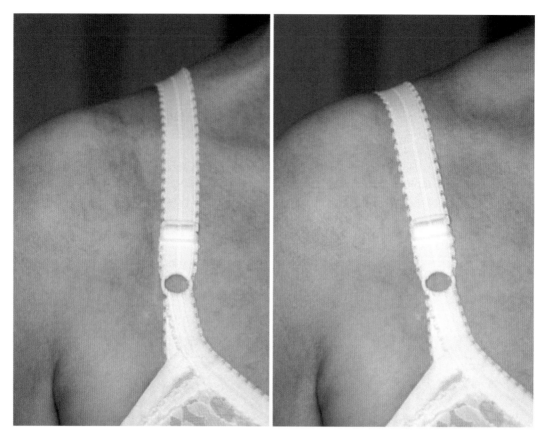

Fig. 13 The strap incision hardly visible (*right*)and also well-positioned and easily hidden under the bra. strap (*left*)

The strap incision used follow the lines of Langerhans which reduces the risk of a wide scar and it can also easily be hidden under a bra strap (Fig. 13).

The temporary transfixation with k-wires we use for the acute repair will to some extent damage the joint surface and we therefore believe it is important to only pass the wires through the joint once to limit the damage (Fig. 9). To avoid loosening, migration and fracture of the wires it is important that they are removed at 6 weeks and that the patient is not allowed elevation above 90° prior to this. If late osteoarthritis occurs, which it will in some patients no matter what kind of initial surgical treatment is used, a simple arthroscopic Mumford procedure is recommended if the joint is still stable. This does not seem to de-stabilise a joint that has been previously successfully repaired with temporary transfixation and ligament repair.

It has repeatedly been proven that too rigid or too weak coracoacromial fixations will often fracture or fail (Fig. 12a–b). This is the reason for us not using screws or non-absorbable materials for this fixation. With the use of multiple absorbable sutures it seems as if good enough stability is achieved to allow good healing yet without the long term risks of sutures cutting through the clavicle or fracture of screws and without the need for a second operation to remove fixation.

The Surgilig ligament does not seem to cause erosion of the clavicle in the way previous ligament implants did and we believe this is because it only comes around from posterior. As the clavicle rotates, on elevation of the arm, it slacks the ligament instead of tightening it, as an implant going around from anterior as well would do. The implant will move with the bone instead of sawing and cutting through it. There has to our knowledge been no case with the Surgilig implant eroding through the clavicle. In a few cases patients have been troubled by the screw protruding under the skin. It has then easily been removed and this will not de-stabilised the clavicle.

To avoid calcifications and ossification along the ligaments after surgery several authors have suggested that patients should be put on indometacin postoperatively. In our experience however this has not been a common problem and we are therefore not routinely using this prophylaxis.

Summary

It is clearly the case that most AC-joint injuries can be treated conservatively with good results. However it is also without doubt not rare that some patients are left with considerable symptoms if left untreated. It is our task to classify these injuries acutely and to try to carefully select the right candidates for acute surgical repair. The acute surgical repair should only be considered in the younger patients with high demands. We argue that the acute repair should aim at stability and restoration of the joint which is best achieved through acromioclavicular repair and temporary transfixation of the joint.

For those left with chronic problems the arthroscopic joint resection is the treatment of choice, whenever the joint is still stable. The resection must be combined with some kind of stabilising procedure should the joint be unstable. In these cases the aim of surgery is a stable link between the scapula and the clavicle without restoration of the joint without direct contact between the clavicle and the acromion or the underlying coracoid. This is best achieved we believe with a modified Weaver Dunn coracoacromial ligament transfer and temporary coracoclavicular fixation or by using the Nottingham Surgilig.

We have provided some short descriptions of our preferred methods for doing this surgery which are but modifications of already described procedures. This could hopefully, together with the references mentioned, act as a platform from where the reader could then develop his or hers own modification of these basic principles.

References

1. Rockwood Jr CA, Matsen FA, Wirth MA, Lippitt SB. The shoulder, vol. 1. 3rd ed. Philadelphia: Saunders; 2004.
2. Bosworth B. Complete acromioclavicular dislocation. N Engl J Med. 1949;241:221–5.
3. Urist MR. Complete dislocation of the acromioclavicular joint. J Bone Joint Surg Am. 1963;45:1750–3.
4. Copeland S. Operative shoulder surgery, vol. 1. Edinburgh: Churchill Livingstone; 1995.
5. Rollo J, Raghunath J, Porter K. Injuries of the acromioclavicular joint and current treatment options. Trauma. 2005;7:217–23.
6. Nordqvist A, Petersson C. Incidence and causes of shoulder girdle injuries in an urban population. J Shoulder Elbow Surg. 1995;4:107–12.
7. Cave E. Fractures and other injuries. Chicago: Year Book; 1961.
8. Riand N, Sadowski C, Hoffmeyer P. Acute acromioclavicular dislocations. Acta Orthop Belg. 1999;65:393–403.
9. McCall D, M Saffran. Br J Sports Med . 2009;43(13):987–92.
10. Daly PH SF, Simonet WT. Ice hockey injuries: a review. Sports Med. 1990;10:122–31.
11. Dias JJ GP. Acromioclavicular joint injuries in sport: recommendations for treatment. Sports Med. 1991;11:125–32.
12. Rowe CR. Acute and recurrent dislocation of the shoulder â . In Symposium on surgical lesions of the shoulder; 1962.
13. Jakobsen BW. Acromioclavicular dislocation. Conservative or surgical treatment? Ugeskr Laeger. 1989;151(4):235–8.
14. Cadenet F. The treatment of dislocations and fractures of the outer end of the clavicle. Int Clin. 1917;1:145–69.
15. Allman FJ. Fractures and ligamentous injuries of the clavicle and its articulation. J Bone Joint Surg Am. 1967;49:774–84.
16. Tossy J, Mead N, Sigmond H. Acromioclavicular separations: useful and practical classification for treatment. Clin Orthop. 1963;28:111–9.
17. Lizaur A, Marco L, Cebrian R. Acute dislocation of the acromioclavicular joint. Traumatic anatomy and the importance of deltoid and trapezius. J Bone Joint Surg Br. 1994;76(4):602–6.

18. Rockwood CJ. Injuries to the acromioclavicular joint. In: Fractures in adults, 1. 2nd ed. Philadelphia: JB Lippincott; 1984. p. 860–910.

19. Bannister G, et al. A classification of acute acromioclavicular dislocation: a clinical, radiological, and anatomical study. Injury. 1992;23:194–6.

20. Tossy JD, Mead NC, Sigmond HM. Acromioclavicular separations: useful and practical classification for treatment. Clin Orthop Relat Res. 1963;28:111–9.

21. Holst AK, Christiansen JV. Epiphyseal separation of the coracoid process without acromioclavicular dislocation. Skeletal Radiol. 1998;27(8):461–2.

22. Alyas F, et al. MR imaging appearances of acromioclavicular joint dislocation. Radiographics. 2008;28(2):463–79. quiz 619.

23. Nguyen V, Williams G, Rockwood C. Radiography of acromioclavicular dislocation and associated injuries. Crit Rev Diagn Imaging. 1991;32(3):191–228.

24. Heers G, Hedtmann A. Correlation of ultrasonographic findings to Tossy's and Rockwood's classification of acromioclavicular joint injuries. Ultrasound Med Biol. 2005;31(6):725–32.

25. Antonio GE, et al. Pictorial essay. MR imaging appearance and classification of acromioclavicular joint injury. Am J Roentgenol. 2003;180(4):1103–10.

26. Kock HJ, et al. Standardized ultrasound examination for classification of instability of the acromioclavicular joint. Unfallchirurgie. 1994;20(2):66–71.

27. Bossart PJ, et al. Lack of efficacy of 'weighted' radiographs in diagnosing acute acromioclavicular separation. Ann Emerg Med. 1988;17(1):20–4.

28. Ref to other book??

29. Bradley JP, Elkousy H. Decision making: operative versus nonoperative treatment of acromioclavicular joint injuries. Clin Sports Med. 2003;22(2):277–90.

30. Cox JS. The fate of the acromioclavicular joint in athletic injuries. Am J Sports Med. 1981;9(1):50–3.

31. Fremerey RW, et al. Surgical treatment of acute, complete acromioclavicular joint dislocation. Indications, technique and results. Unfallchirurg. 1996;99(5):341–5.

32. Gstettner C, et al. Rockwood type III acromioclavicular dislocation: surgical versus conservative treatment. J Shoulder Elbow Surg. 2008;17(2):220–5.

33. Leidel BA, et al. Consistency of long-term outcome of acute Rockwood grade III acromioclavicular joint separations after K-wire transfixation. J Trauma. 2009;66(6):1666–71.

34. Ceccarelli E, et al. Treatment of acute grade III acromioclavicular dislocation: a lack of evidence. J Orthop Traumatol. 2008;9(2):105–8.

35. Sehmisch S, et al. Results of a prospective multicenter trial for treatment of acromioclavicular dislocation. Sportverletz Sportschaden. 2008;22(3):139–45.

36. Hootman JM. Acromioclavicular dislocation: conservative or surgical therapy. J Athl Train. 2004;39(1):10–1.

37. Fremerey RW. Acute acromioclavicular joint dislocation – operative or conservative therapy? Unfallchirurg. 2001;104(4):294–9.

38. Phillips AM, Smart C, Groom AF. Acromioclavicular dislocation. Conservative or surgical therapy. Clin Orthop Relat Res. 1998;353:10–7.

39. Rawes ML, Dias JJ. Long-term results of conservative treatment for acromioclavicular dislocation. J Bone Joint Surg Br. 1996;78(3):410–2.

40. Bannister GC, et al. The management of acute acromioclavicular dislocation. A randomised prospective controlled trial. J Bone Joint Surg Br. 1989;71(5):848–50.

41. Soni RK. Conservatively treated acromioclavicular joint dislocation: a 45-years follow-up. Injury. 2004;35(5):549–51.

42. Cresswell TR. Spontaneous reduction of an inferior acromioclavicular joint dislocation. Injury. 1998;29(7):567–8.

43. Mulier T, Stuyck J, Fabry G. Conservative treatment of acromioclavicular dislocation. Evaluation of functional and radiological results after six years followup. Acta Orthop Belg. 1993;59(3):255–62.

44. Li BC, et al. Postoperative complications of acromioclavicular joint dislocation of Tossy III. Zhongguo Gu Shang. 2009;22(2):95–7.

45. Boldin C, et al. Foreign-body reaction after reconstruction of complete acromioclavicular dislocation using PDS augmentation. J Shoulder Elbow Surg. 2004;13(1):99–100.

46. Broos P, et al. Surgical management of complete Tossy III acromioclavicular joint dislocation with the Bosworth screw or the Wolter plate. A critical evaluation. Unfallchirurgie. 1997;23(4):153–9.

47. Colosimo AJ, Hummer 3rd CD, Heidt Jr RS. Aseptic foreign body reaction to Dacron graft material used for coracoclavicular ligament reconstruction after type III acromioclavicular dislocation. Am J Sports Med. 1996;24(4):561–3.

48. Habernek H, Walch G. Secondary wire migration following percutaneous bore wire fixation of acromioclavicular dislocation. Aktuelle Traumatol. 1989;19(5):218–20.

49. Rolf O, et al. Acromioclavicular dislocation Rockwood III-V: results of early versus delayed surgical treatment. Arch Orthop Trauma Surg. 2008;128(10):1153–7.

50. Mumford E. Acromioclavicular dislocation. J Bone Joint Surg Am. 1941;23:709–802.

51. Weaver J, Dunn HK. Treatment of acromioclavicular injuries, especially complete acromioclavicular separation. J Bone Joint Surg Am. 1972;54:1187–97.

52. Pavlik A, Csepai D, Hidas P. Surgical treatment of chronic acromioclavicular joint dislocation by modified Weaver-Dunn procedure. Knee Surg Sports Traumatol Arthrosc. 2001;9(5):307–12.

53. Wang S, et al. A modified method of coracoid transposition for the treatment of complete dislocation of

acromioclavicular joint. Chin J Traumatol. 2002;5(5):307–10.

54. Luis GE, et al. Acromioclavicular joint dislocation: a comparative biomechanical study of the palmaris-longus tendon graft reconstruction with other augmentative methods in cadaveric models. J Orthop Surg Res. 2007;2:22.

55. Law KY, et al. Coracoclavicular ligament reconstruction using a gracilis tendon graft for acute type-III acromioclavicular dislocation. J Orthop Surg (Hong Kong). 2007;15(3):315–8.

56. Jiang C, Wang M, Rong G. Proximally based conjoined tendon transfer for coracoclavicular reconstruction in the treatment of acromioclavicular dislocation. Surgical technique. J Bone Joint Surg Am. 2008;90(Suppl 2 Pt 2):299–308.

57. Boileau P, et al. All-arthroscopic Weaver-Dunn-Chuinard procedure with double-button fixation for chronic acromioclavicular joint dislocation. Arthroscopy. 2010;26(2):149–60.

58. Cirstoiu C, et al. Acroplate–a modern solution for the treatment of acromioclavicular joint dislocation. J Med Life. 2009;2(2):173–5.

59. Li X, et al. Repair of acromioclavicular dislocation with clavicular hook plate internal fixation and coracoacromial ligament transposition. Zhongguo Xiu Fu Chong Jian Wai Ke Za Zhi. 2009;23(6):654–6.

60. Murena L, et al. Arthroscopic treatment of acute acromioclavicular joint dislocation with double flip button. Knee Surg Sports Traumatol Arthrosc. 2009;17(12):1511–5.

61. Tischer T, Imhoff AB. Minimally invasive coracoclavicular stabilization with suture anchors for acute acromioclavicular dislocation. Am J Sports Med. 2009;37(3):e5.

62. Zvijac JE, Popkin CA, Botto-van BA. Salvage procedure for chronic acromioclavicular dislocation subsequent to overzealous distal clavicle resection. Orthopedics. 2008;31(12):1235.

63. Shin SJ, Yun YH, Yoo JD. Coracoclavicular ligament reconstruction for acromioclavicular dislocation using 2 suture anchors and coracoacromial ligament transfer. Am J Sports Med. 2009;37(2):346–51.

64. Ejam S, Lind T, Falkenberg B. Surgical treatment of acute and chronic acromioclavicular dislocation Tossy type III and V using the Hook plate. Acta Orthop Belg. 2008;74(4):441–5.

65. Wellmann M, et al. Biomechanical evaluation of minimally invasive repairs for complete acromioclavicular joint dislocation. Am J Sports Med. 2007;35(6):955–61.

66. Wellmann M, Zantop T, Petersen W. Minimally invasive coracoclavicular ligament augmentation with a flip button/polydioxanone repair for treatment of total acromioclavicular joint dislocation. Arthroscopy. 2007;23(10):1132 e1–5.

67. Jiang C, Wang M, Rong G. Proximally based conjoined tendon transfer for coracoclavicular reconstruction in the treatment of acromioclavicular

dislocation. J Bone Joint Surg Am. 2007;89(11):2408–12.

68. Lafosse L, Baier GP, Leuzinger J. Arthroscopic treatment of acute and chronic acromioclavicular joint dislocation. Arthroscopy. 2005;21(8):1017.

69. Rolla PR, Surace MF, Murena L. Arthroscopic treatment of acute acromioclavicular joint dislocation. Arthroscopy. 2004;20(6):662–8.

70. Tienen TG, Oyen JF, Eggen PJ. A modified technique of reconstruction for complete acromioclavicular dislocation: a prospective study. Am J Sports Med. 2003;31(5):655–9.

71. Wolf EM, Pennington WT. Arthroscopic reconstruction for acromioclavicular joint dislocation. Arthroscopy. 2001;17(5):558–63.

72. Monig SP, et al. Treatment of complete acromioclavicular dislocation: present indications and surgical technique with biodegradable cords. Int J Sports Med. 1999;20(8):560–2.

73. Guy DK, et al. Reconstruction of chronic and complete dislocations of the acromioclavicular joint. Clin Orthop Relat Res. 1998;347:138–49.

74. Kutschera HP, Kotz RI. Bone-ligament transfer of coracoacromial ligament for acromioclavicular dislocation. A new fixation method used in 6 cases. Acta Orthop Scand. 1997;68(3):246–8.

75. Bosworth B. Acromioclavicular separation: new method of repair. Surg Gynecol Obstet. 1941;73:866–71.

76. Tauber M, et al. Semitendinosus tendon graft versus a modified Weaver-Dunn procedure for acromioclavicular joint reconstruction in chronic cases: a prospective comparative study. Am J Sports Med. 2009;37(1):181–90.

77. Bostrom Windhamre HA. Surgical treatment of chronic acromioclavicular dislocations: a comparative study of Weaver-Dunn augmented with PDS-braid or hook plate. J Shoulder Elbow Surg. 2010;19(7):1040–8.

78. DeBerardino TM, et al. Arthroscopic stabilization of acromioclavicular joint dislocation using the AC graftrope system. J Shoulder Elbow Surg. 2010;19(2 Suppl):47–52.

79. Elhassan B, et al. Open versus arthroscopic acromioclavicular joint resection: a retrospective comparison study. Arthroscopy. 2009;25(11):1224–32.

80. Somers JF, Van der Linden D. Arthroscopic fixation of type III acromioclavicular dislocations. Acta Orthop Belg. 2007;73(5):566–70.

81. Wood TA, Rosell PA, Clasper JC. Preliminary results of the 'Surgilig' synthetic ligament in the management of chronic acromioclavicular joint disruption. J R Army Med Corps. 2009;155(3):191–3.

82. Bhattacharya R, Goodchild L, Rangan A. Acromioclavicular joint reconstruction using the Nottingham Surgilig: a preliminary report. Acta Orthop Belg. 2008;74(2):167–72.

83. Jeon IH, et al. Chronic acromioclavicular separation: the medium term results of coracoclavicular ligament

reconstruction using braided polyester prosthetic ligament. Injury. 2007;38(11):1247–53.

84. Mouhsine E, et al. Grade I and II acromioclavicular dislocations: results of conservative treatment. J Shoulder Elbow Surg. 2003;12(6):599–602.

85. Bathis H. Conservative or surgical therapy of acromioclavicular joint injury – what is reliable? A systematic analysis of the literature using "evidence-based medicine" criteria. Chirurg. 2000;71(9):1082–9.

86. Hack U, Bibow K. Dislocation of the acromioclavicular joint – conservative or surgical therapy? Zentralbl Chir. 1988;113(14):899–910.

87. Calvo E, Lopez-Franco M, Arribas IM. Clinical and radiologic outcomes of surgical and conservative treatment of type III acromioclavicular joint injury. J Shoulder Elbow Surg. 2006;15(3):300–5.

88. Leidel BA, et al. Mid-term outcome comparing temporary K-wire fixation versus PDS augmentation of Rockwood grade III acromioclavicular joint separations. BMC Res Notes. 2009;2:84.

89. LaPrade RF, et al. Kinematic evaluation of the modified Weaver-Dunn acromioclavicular joint reconstruction. Am J Sports Med. 2008;36(11):2216–21.

90. Garg S, Elzein I, Lawrence T, Manning P, Neumann L, Wallace WA, Reconstruction of chronic ACJ dislocation using a braided polyester prosthetic ligament (surgilig) and the modified weaver dunn (WD) procedure – a comparative study. Bess 21st annual scientific meeting Oxford 2010, Oxford; 2010.

91. Meislin RJ, Zuckerman JD, Nainzadeh N. Type III acromioclavicular joint separation associated with late brachial-plexus neurapraxia. J Orthop Trauma. 1992;6(3):370–2.

92. Docimo Jr S, et al. Surgical treatment for acromioclavicular joint osteoarthritis: patient selection, surgical options, complications, and outcome. Curr Rev Musculoskelet Med. 2008;1(2):154–60.

93. Smola O. Ossification of the coracoclavicular and acromioclavicular ligaments as adaptation to trauma. Acta Chir Orthop Traumatol Cech. 1972;39(1):38–40.

94. De Sousa A, Veiga A. Ossification of the coracoclavicular ligament following acromioclavicular dislocation. J Med (Oporto). 1951;18(453):515–8.

The Fibrous Lock (Skeleton) of the Rotator Cuff

Olivier Gagey

Contents

Abstract

MRI and anatomical studies of shoulder muscles provide evidence of a deep strong fibrous organization. The rotator cuff has a strong deep fibrous frame that emphasizes the most important functional areas. The acromial belly of the deltoid is also multipennate therefore the most powerful.

Keywords

Clinical applications-torn subscapularis, shoulder arthroplasty • Constituent muscles • Rotator cuff-fibrous skeleton (lock)

Introduction

MRI studies of the shoulder show evidence of an anatomical organisation of the muscles especially regarding the presence inside the muscle bellies of strong deep fibrous bands.

This structure involves all the muscles of the rotator cuff and includes the deltoid.

These fibrous structures are of great importance since they modify the mechanical properties of the muscles. A pennate or multi-pennate muscle has a shorter contraction but, on the other hand, a stronger force. In addition if the fibrous tissue is abundant the muscle has special visco-elastic properties.

O. Gagey
Orthopaedic Department, Paris-South University, Paris, France
e-mail: Olivier.gagey@bct.ap-hop-paris.fr

G. Bentley (ed.), *European Surgical Orthopaedics and Traumatology*,
DOI 10.1007/978-3-642-34746-7_47, © EFORT 2014

The Subscapularis Muscle

Anatomical studies have demonstrated that the two upper thirds of its humeral attachment contain a thick and strong tendon whereas the distal third has no tendon and is attached directly to the lesser tuberosity. Inside the muscle belly, at the level of the tendon, there are 4–5 strong fibrous digitations that prolong the tendon inside the muscle. The most superior digitation is like a 6–8 mm. thick tendon coursing 6–8 cm. along the superior border of the muscle. These digitations are intercalated with the digitations originating from the spinal border of the scapula. These structures are obvious on MRI views (Fig. 1).

Then the subscapularis in a multipennate muscle.

Regarding the "superior tendon" it should be emphasized that during abduction with external rotation this tendon is in strong contact with the vertical part of the coracoïd process through a bursa. The coracoïd process acts on the subscapularis like a pulley giving to the muscle an important role of fixation of the humeral head and strong internal rotation during the throwing movement [1].

The Supraspinatus Muscle

A strong fibrous band exists inside the anterior part of the supraspinatus [2]. This band is attached at the level of the anterior part of the tendon that is thicker than the rest of the tendon (Fig. 2).

The Infraspinatus Muscle

There is also a deep fibrous band within the superior part of the muscle according the same pattern as for the supraspinatus.

The Fibrous Frame of the Rotator Cuff

These fibrous structures provide the rotator cuff with an amazing deep fibrous frame. This frame indicates the most solid areas of the cuff which is

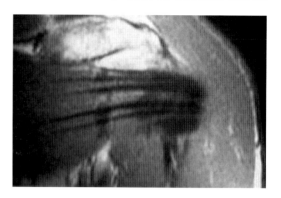

Fig. 1 MRI view (coronal plane) of the subscapularis showing the fibrous bands (*black lines*) inside the muscle belly

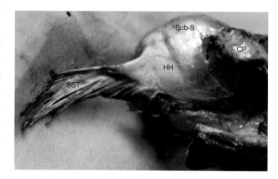

Fig. 2 Supraspinatus muscle, all the muscles bundles have been removed leaving the fibrous part only

the area transmitting the maximum applied forces (Figs. 3, 4 and 5).

Considering the fibrous structures it appears that a special area of the rotator cuff is gathering an amazing concentration of fibrous structures [3]. Located in an anterosuperior position there are:

i. The anterior part of the supraspinatus tendon,
ii. The superior tendon of suscapularis,
iii. The longer part of biceps brachialis,
iv. The coracohumeral ligament, and
v. The superior gleno-huméral ligament.

We proposed to name this area the "anterosuperior fibrous lock of the rotator cuff". Basically the fibrous lock is located just around the Rotator interval.

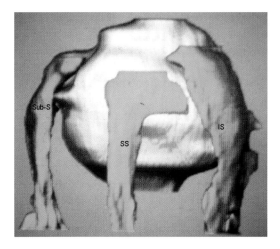

Fig. 3 Upper view of the fibrous frame of the rotator cuff: this view presents the deep fibrous structures inside the rotator muscles bellies. Reconstructions obtained from high-resolution MRI

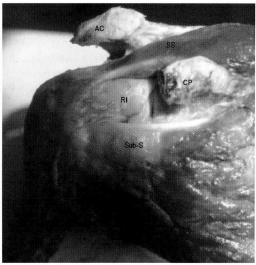

Fig. 5 Anterior view of the fibrous lock of the cuff. *AC* acromion, *SS* supraspinatus, *S-Scap* subscapularis, *CP* coracoïd process, *RI* rotator interval. Coracohumeral ligament and superior glenohumeral ligament are not visible on this view

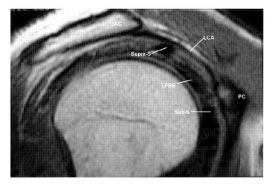

Fig. 4 Shoulder MRI in sagittal plane evidencing the main components of the fibrous lock: *Sub-S* upper tendon of subscapularis, *LCA* coracoacromial ligament, *LPBB* tendon of the long head of Biceps, *AC* acromion, *PC* coracoïd process, *Supra-S* supraspinatus

The Deltoid Muscle

Our anatomical work [4] has established that the deltoid is divided into three totally different parts not only according their bony attachment (clavicule, acromion and scapular spine) but also because of strong differences regarding the deep structure (Fig. 6). The acromial part of the deltoid is the sole part of the muscle with tendious attachment on the acromion. This part contains five fibrous digitations attached on the acromion

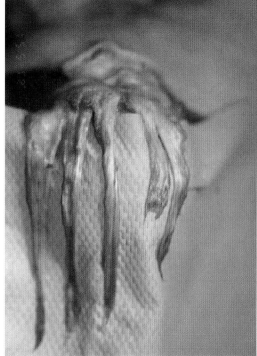

Fig. 6 Middle deltoid after removal of all the muscle bundles leaving only the fibrous frame of the muscle

and intercalated with five distal fibrous bands originating from the distal muscle tendon. There are no bands inside the clavicular or spinal portions of the muscle. This suggests that the acromial part of the deltoid is the most powerful and consequently the main engine providing humeral elevation in the scapulo-humeral joint. Interestingly this part is orientated to provide elevation in the plane of the scapula.

Clinical Applications

The Delto-Pectoral Approach

This approach is the most used for shoulder surgery; this doesn't mean that it is a totally safe approach. The surgeon has to keep in mind that this approach may weaken the fibrous lock either by cutting the subscapularis (that should be carefully repaired especially in its superior tendon) or by weakening the supraspinatus at the time of dislocation or when inserting the prosthesis in the humerus.

Shoulder Arthroplasty

A good illustration of the importance of the fibrous lock is given by prosthetic surgery of the shoulder. In case of failure of the repair of the fibrous lock the main complication would be the anterosuperior migration of the humeral head.

Rotator Interval Syndrome

The rotator interval syndrome is not related to a virtual weakness of the anatomical area, since we demonstrated that this area is especially strong. Overuse of the superior part of the subscapularis during overhead sports may lead to degenerative and micro-traumatic lesions of the subscapularis (upper tendon and attachment as well). It may also create middle glenohumeral ligament lengthening. These both lesions may progressively lead to a anterosuperior shoulder instability.

Traumatic Tear of the Subscapularis

The most frequent traumatic lesion of the cuff is the tear of the upper third of the subscapularis tendon. The trauma is highly specific: the patient tries to stop a fall, being suddenly suspended by his upper limb. The functional importance of the subscapularis tendon justifies the necessity for a surgical repair.

References

1. Colas F, Nevoux J, Gagey O. The subscapular and subcoracoid bursae: descriptive and functional anatomy. J Shoulder Elbow Surg. 2004;13(4): 454–8.
2. Gagey NF, Gagey OJ, Bastian D, Lassau JP. The fibrous frame of the supraspinatus muscle. Correlations between anatomy and MRI findings. Surg Radiol Anat. 1990;12(4):291–2.
3. Gagey OJ, Arkache J, Welby F. Le squelette fibreux de la coiffe des rotateurs. La notion de verrou fibreux. Rev Chir Orthop. 1993;79(4):452–5.
4. Lorne E, Gagey O, Quillard J, Hue E, Gagey N. The fibrous frame of the deltoid muscle. Its functional and surgical relevance. Clin Orthop. 2001;386: 222–5.

Rotator Cuff Tears-Open Repair

Tim Bunker

Contents

T. Bunker
Princess Elizabeth Orthopaedic Centre, Exeter, UK
e-mail: Tim.bunker@exetershoulderclinic.co.uk

G. Bentley (ed.), *European Surgical Orthopaedics and Traumatology*,
DOI 10.1007/978-3-642-34746-7_76, © EFORT 2014

Keywords

Anatomy • Arthroscopy • Clinical signs • Investigations-ultrasound • MRI • Open cuff repair-indications • Rotator cuff tears • Shoulder • Subscpularis tears • Tear patterns • Techniques

Anatomy

Supraspinatus is not as most textbooks show it. In fact it has a strong tendon that passes from the centre of the muscle belly to insert at the very front edge of the greater tuberosity, and sometimes even in front of the biceps pulley (Fig. 1). This anterior column is very strong and it is this feature that accounts for where tears start, how they progress, and how we can repair them.

Nakajima [1] showed that the central tendon is markedly denser and stronger than the rest of the tendon on histological preparations of the supraspinatus tendon. They demonstrated how the central thick tendon migrates towards the anterior margin of the tendon as you move towards its insertion. Nakagaki et al. [40] and Bigliani et al. confirmed this work and provided correct illustrations of the nature of the tendon. Gagey et al. introduced the concept of the fibrous frame of the rotator cuff. These workers performed three-dimensional reconstruction of MRI scans and demonstrated the deep fibrous re-inforcement of the supraspinatus that is the central oblique tendon. They showed how supraspinatus has one tendon, whereas subscapularis is multipennate and they show how the single tendon of supraspinatus inserts into the anterior extremity of the greater tuberosity. This pattern of migration of the central oblique tendon has been confirmed by Roh et al. Over a 20-year period the chapter author (TDB) has made the observation on ultrasound scanning and at surgery that this central oblique tendon (that we will term the *anterior column*), being the strongest part of supraspinatus, remains intact when all the tendinous tissues around it fail. In effect it acts as a *firebreak* and determines the

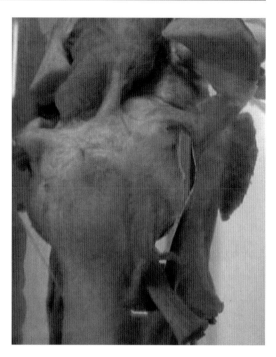

Fig. 1 The true anatomy of the cuff, showing the central oblique tendon of supraspinatus

pattern of postero-superior rotator cuff tearing. From these observations a hypothesis was developed that there is a definite and progressive pattern of cuff tear extension that is determined by the special anatomy of this tendon. Understanding this pattern allows the surgeon to predict which structures are contracted and need to be released, and to develop a plan to close the defect using fundamental surgical techniques such as rotationplasty, rather than treating each surgery as a "magical mystery tour".

Aetiology of Cuff Tears

For many years we have had a simplistic idea of why cuff tears occur. It is time for this simplistic 'Intrinsic or extrinsic' theory to be challenged. Codman championed the idea of intrinsic degeneration of the cuff tissue (Fig. 2) as the main cause of rotator cuff tearing. Forty years later Neer suggested that tears occurred not through intrinsic damage, but because of extrinsic

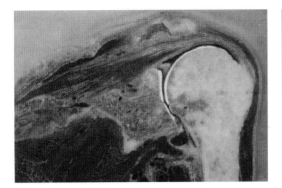

Fig. 2 The footprint of insertion of supraspinatus

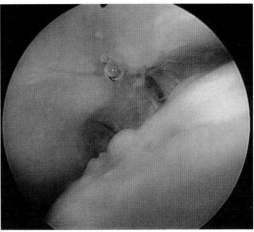

Fig. 3 An arthroscopic view of the rim rent lesion

damage due to continuing repetitive abutment of the anterior acromion upon the superior bursal side of the cuff. Neer's views held sway for 30 years, and his protégé, Bigliani, said there were morphological differences in the acromion (the hooked acromion) that accounted for this impingement and tearing. The hooked shape of the acromion has now been shown to be reactive, and so. although impingement does occur, it is usually secondary to intrinsic cuff failure and not the primary cause of cuff tearing.

There are two instances where extrinsic cuff compression from the acromion may be the primary event. The first is the 50 year-old with a large cuff tear and a mobile Os Acromiale. The second is the rare patient who is shown to have a bursal-side partial cuff tear with no evidence of a partial thickness articular surface tear or rim rent lesion.

However intrinsic cuff failure is the initiating event in the majority of people. This is why the rim rent lesion (Fig. 3), or partial thickness artic-ular surface tear is so commonly seen in patients with the earliest symptoms and signs of cuff dis-ease undergoing arthroscopy. This rim rent lesion may be caused by repetitive tensile overload with work, daily living or sport, or sudden overload as in a fall. It may also be caused by shear of the articular margin against the glenoid rim that occurs in the elevated position, either repetitively with work or sport, or suddenly with a fall.

Carr's work showed that genetics plays a part, for cuff tears are twice as common in close rela-tives of patients undergoing cuff repair as in those

partners they live with. We also know that they occur with age, Sher's classic work on MRI scan-ning of asymptomatic individuals showing that cuff tears are rare under the age of 60. In their study no-one under 40 had a cuff tear, between 40 and 60, 4 % did, but of those over 60, 26 % had a full thickness tear.

So cuff tears are complex, there is a genetic element, an ageing element a functional element due to tensile or shearing overload, leading to cuff dysfunction and secondary extrinsic impingement and compressive overload. Add micro- or macro-trauma into the mix and a cuff tear results.

Pattern of Cuff Tearing-Anatomical Factors

Repeated tensile, shear or compressive overload can cause changes within the ageing rotator cuff. Macroscopically this leads to the initiating event, which is the rim-rent lesion. The rim-rent lesion can be demonstrated by ultrasound or by arthros-copy. This lesion is constantly situated 7 mm. behind the biceps pulley just posterior to the insertion of the anterior column. Gradually the rim-rent peels further back off its footprint of insertion into the superior facet of the greater tuberosity. As it does so, secondary reactive changes occur on the bone, which becomes

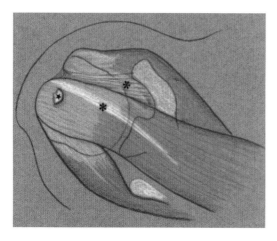

Fig. 4 The small tear starts just behind the anterior pillar

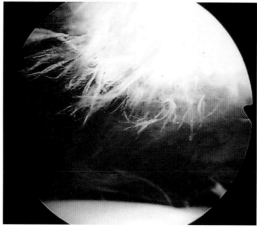

Fig. 5 The impingement lesion

sclerotic and nodular. These nodules appear on radiographs as tiny sclerotic rings and are often misreported as cysts, although tiny true cysts can also occur. Eventually the deep surface rim-rent will peel so far back that it emerges on the bursal side as a pinhole full thickness tear (Fig. 4). This gradual enlargement of the deep surface partial thickness tear may take years to evolve. During this time the supraspinatus is weakened and its normal centring effect is lost. The head subluxes upward and secondary impingement occurs between the bursal surface of the cuff and the acromion.

These secondary reactive changes can be seen by placing an arthroscope into the bursa. The bursa becomes fibrillated, and then wears through and the bursal surface of the cuff becomes damaged and fibrillates, this is the impingement lesion of Neer. Reactive changes will occur on the acromion (Fig. 5) and have been classified into four grades by Uhtoff:

- Firstly, there is a loss of areolar tissue under the acromion.
- Then, the coraco-acromial ligament and the fibrous pad that represents its footprint of insertion into the acromion thicken.
- Thirdly, there is fibrillation of the insertion of the coraco-acromial ligament.
- Finally, there is eburnation of the undersurface of the acromion and loss of the footprint of insertion of the coraco-acromial ligament.

Meanwhile the cuff tear extends, either slowly, or it may suddenly tear with even mild trauma. Knowledge of the normal morphology of the tendon explains the pattern of tear exposed at surgical repair. Knowledge of the morphology of the capsule explains the contractures that occur, and which will need to be released during surgical reconstruction. We must always remember that the tendon and capsule merge and blend towards their combined insertion, and that for a full thickness tear to occur, both capsule and tendon must have dis-inserted. The tendon retracts, but the capsule contracts.

As the small tear extends into a moderate tear the anterior column, being so strong, acts as a firebreak and resists extension, and so instead of becoming a larger crescentic tear, the tear becomes asymmetric or L-shaped (Fig. 6). At the same time the superior capsule, having dis-inserted, contracts back towards the glenoid, pulling the cuff, with which it is merged, along with it. The coraco-humeral ligament re-inforces the superior capsule and, as this powerful thickening of the capsule contracts, it pulls the anterior column with it, towards the coracoid. This determines the releases that will be necessary for a small to moderate tear.

Now a singular event happens, at 3–5 cms. the tear extends over the North Pole of the humeral head, causing a button-hole (boutonniere) situation. Just as in the PIP joint of the finger when

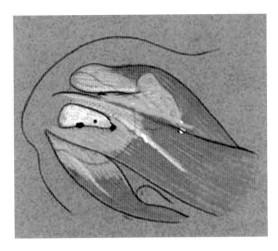

Fig. 6 The small tear extends to a moderate U-shaped or L-shaped tear

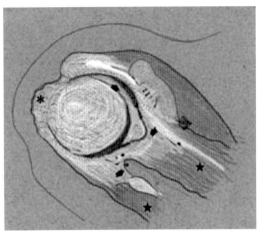

Fig. 8 The tear progresses to a massive fixed tear

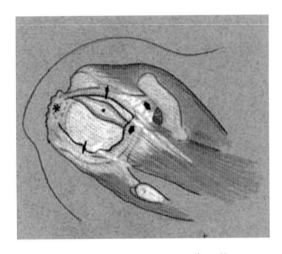

Fig. 7 As the tear progresses a Boutonnière effect occurs

a boutonniere lesion occurs the joint button-holes up through the tear and the lateral slips sublux around the joint (Fig. 7). In the case of the shoulder the lateral slips are the anterior column to the front, and infraspinatus to the rear. Because the infraspinatus has subluxed backwards and cannot be retrieved from under the acromion at surgery the surgeon may erroneously think that it too has torn, but this is hardly ever the case. The capsule at the junction of the supra- and infra-spinatus contracts severely and it is the release of this *junctional scar* that allows advancement of

supraspinatus in large cuff tears. This *junctional scar* is hidden under the acromion and the suprascapular nerve runs underneath the spinoglenoid ligament just medial to this contracture. Long head of biceps hypertrophies and may start to fray. The capsule continues to contract. The muscle bellies, being de-functioned, waste away.

Finally the tear continues to extend and retracts right back to the edge of the glenoid rim (Fig. 8). The anterior column may still be intact, although now very stretched. Finally the anterior column uproots, uncovering long head of biceps, which now becomes painful, frays further, and can sublux or rupture. As the biceps pulley fails the superior margin of subscapularis may tear and the humeral head now subluxes forward as well as upward. The capsule contracts further. Infraspinatus subluxes further back yet, contrary to popular opinion, rarely tears although the tendon is stretched out and the wasted muscle belly has no function. The junctional scar becomes even thicker. This is the classic 'bald head tear'.

Arthritic change may now occur between the North Pole of the humerus and the acromion, as well as the surfaces of the humerus and superior pole of the acromion, which are maintained in a subluxed position. This arthritic change is called 'cuff tear arthropathy' (Fig. 9) and is the

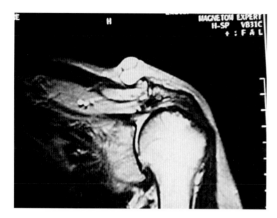

Fig. 9 Cuff tear arthropathy

end-stage of the spectrum of cuff disease. 2 % of the population over the age of 80 will have cuff tear arthropathy.

Symptoms and Signs

Codman described the symptoms and signs of the patient with a full thickness tear of the rotator cuff 70 years ago. This portrayal still cannot be bettered. He gave 18 features that are classically present in such a patient. A manual labourer, aged over 40, with a previously normal shoulder, has an injury, with immediate pain, followed by a lucid interval, with severe pain coming on that night, a loss of power, eased by stooping, with a faulty rhythm, a tender point, a palpable sulcus, and eminence, which causes a jog and a wince, and crepitus on elevation, which re-appears on descent, with a normal radiograph.

A manual labourer. In fact the first patient Codman wrote up in 1911 was a woman who was beating her carpets clean in her back garden. Men do get full thickness tears more commonly. We have already stated how manual labour is implicated in the aetiology of cuff tears. Full thickness tears occur rarely under the age of 40. Most shoulder surgeons can count on the fingers of one hand how many cuff tears they have seen in patients under the age of 40!

The shoulder may be previously normal, but this is not always the case. Often the patient will have had a rim-rent tear for some time that will cause intermittent shoulder pain on reaching, particularly if sustained or repeated.

The injury may be relatively trivial, often elevating the arm against resistance (lifting the garage door, putting a case in the overhead locker). The injury can be severe, and dislocation of the shoulder over the age of 40 is a common cause of cuff tear.

The injury gives immediate pain. Yet it is followed by a lucid interval. This confuses the emergency room doctor the following day for, lacking in knowledge, they can not understand how anything serious could have happened if the patient continued working during the afternoon following the injury.

That night *severe pain* comes on, which is the reason the patient goes to the emergency room in the following morning, where a radiograph is taken, which is always normal.

The patient has *a loss of power.* This may be quite subtle in a small tear, but in the large tears there is a pseudoparalysis. As supraspinatus is powered up against resistance the tear is put under tension and this hurts. Stooping, the arm can be swung forwards passively, or the patient can cheat and swing the arm forwards using deltoid alone.

There is a *faulty rhythm to elevation* as pain through the mid-arc makes the patient protective and slows down the velocity of ascent. During ascent supraspinatus is contracting concentrically, but as the arm descends supraspinatus contracts eccentrically, which is weaker, and thus the faulty rhythm is even more apparent and protective coming down. The patient may actually lock the glenohumeral joint through the painful arc, and the scapula pseudo-wings.

On palpation there is a *tender point* over the insertion of supraspinatus. In the thin patient a defect can be felt in the cuff (*the sulcus*), and as the finger slides down the empty footprint of insertion it then bumps up against the greater tuberosity (*the eminence*).

As the arm is elevated the patient hesitates as the tear passes under the anterior edge of the acromion causing *a jog*, which is so painful as to make the patient screw their eyes up and *wince*.

The torn edges of the cuff rub against the acromion causing crepitus, and all these features re-appear, often more exaggerated on descent.

Examination and Investigation

The Poster-Superior Cuff (Supraspinatus)

Neer's Sign
This is the classic painful arc. Movement into the first 70° of flexion is easy and pain-free, but then as the footprint of the supraspinatus passes under the acromion, from 70° to 120°, there is impingement between the surfaces and pain, and motion slows. As the footprint clears the undersurface of the acromion, from 120° to full abduction, pain eases and motion speeds up once more.

Neer's Test
Neer's test is to inject some local anaesthetic into the bursa, bathing the bursal side of the footprint of cuff insertion. This abolishes the impingement and the normal pattern of movement is restored.

Hawkins's Sign
The arm is elevated in the scapular plane to 90°. Now the elbow is flexed to a right angle and the arm is internally, and then externally rotated. Pain is seen to occur on internal rotation as the footprint of supraspinatus impinges against the anterior acromion. The sensitivity and specificity for Hawkins sign is 75 %. It is one of the most useful tests of the posterosuperior cuff. Beware that passive limitation of internal rotation nullifies this test.

Jobe's Sign
The arm is brought up in the scapular plane with the elbow extended and the arm fully internally rotated so that the thumb points to the ground. (The Australians call this the 'empty tinny test' for it is the position in which you test that your can of beer is finally empty). The patient is asked to hold this position against resistance from the examiner. If there is damage to the supraspinatus insertion then pain will register with the patient.

If there is a tear of supraspinatus the arm will be weak. The accuracy of Jobe's sign is 58 %. It is another good test.

If either Neer's, Hawkins's or Jobe's signs are positive then ultrasound examination is essential. The ultrasound will show whether there is a tear, give its exact position and a measure of its dimension; it is worth a great number of eponymous tests. However there are many other tests of the posterosuperior cuff and it is pertinent to test for them.

Lag Signs
Lag signs depend on weakness of a segment of the cuff. They are the modern equivalent of the '*drop arm sign*'. The drop arm sign was a particularly unpleasant way of examining a patient with a massive supraspinatus tear. The examiner elevated the arm to 120° in the full knowledge that, without a functioning cuff, the patient will find it impossible to maintain this position. The examiner then let go and the arm dropped to the side! Patients feel severe pain.

The External Rotation Lag Sign
The external rotation lag sign demonstrates that there is a significant tear in supraspinatus. Like the "drop arm" sign this depends on placing the arm into a position that needs a strong supraspinatus and then letting go. The examiner takes the affected elbow and supports the weight of the upper arm with the shoulder in 90° of scapular elevation. Now, using his other arm, the examiner externally rotates the forearm into full external rotation. Maintaining this position against gravity depends upon an intact supraspinatus. Now the examiner lets go of the forearm. If the cuff is intact this position can be maintained by the patient, but if the cuff is torn then the forearm will drop by about 30°, the external rotation lag. There are problems with the test. The examiner must understand exactly what he is doing, as must the patient. Pain may interfere with the test. Stiffness will render it null and void. There is difficulty between assessing how much movement is recoil and how much is lag. It is poorly reproducible. It has a specificity of 63 % and a sensitivity of 80 %. It has been superseded by portable ultrasound.

Hornblower's Sign

This is another lag sign. All military hornblowers must assume an identical position when blowing their horns. This position is with the hand at the lips and the elbow as high as it will go so that the arm, and forearm are parallel to the ground. This position can be maintained even with a torn rotator cuff. However if the examiner now takes the hand, and fully externally rotates the forearm so that the forearm is now perpendicular to the ground we now have a position that can only be maintained with an intact cuff. Let go of the hand now and the forearm will drop, or lag, by 30°. This test suffers from the same problems as the external rotation lag sign. It has been superseded by portable ultrasound.

The Antero-Superior Cuff (Subscapularis)

Tears of the anterosuperior cuff (subscapularis and biceps) are less common than those of the posterosuperior cuff. These tears start around the biceps pulley and the superior part of the insertion of subscapularis into the lesser tuberosity. Subscapularis has a multipennate tendon of insertion into the lesser tuberosity.

The "belly Press" Sign (Napoleon's Sign)

This is the single most useful test of subscapularis function. The patient is asked to place the palm of the hand upon their abdomen. Now they are asked to keep the hand where it is and bring the elbow forward as far as it will go. If there is a complete tear of the subscapularis they will not be able to bring the elbow forwards. If they can pull the elbow forwards they are then asked to press the hand hard into the belly. If there is a partial tear of subscapularis they elbow will drop back (a lag sign). Beware; if the shoulder is stiff a false "belly press" sign occurs, for instance in patients with limited internal rotation from arthritis. Beware, patients can cheat; in this case they flex the wrist pulling the elbow forwards, producing a false- negative "belly press" sign. They must keep the wrist in a neutral position or the test is null and void. Finally biceps problems can mimic subscapularis problems confounding the "belly press" sign.

The Lift off Test

The lift off test is similar to the "belly press" sign, but is performed in more internal rotation. This means that the wrist must be placed on the small of the back, rather than on the abdomen. Now the patient is asked to actively increase the internal rotation by lifting the wrist away from the skin. The problem with this test is pain. Patients with cuff problems do not like placing the hand into internal rotation, and pain nullifies the test. Stiffness will also nullify the test.

Internal Rotation Lag Sign

This is a modification of the lift off test. The arm is placed with the wrist on the small of the back. The examiner now takes the wrist and pulls it 5 cms. away from the skin. With an intact subscapularis, and no pain or stiffness, the patient should be able to maintain this position. However if subscapularis is torn then the wrist will drop (lag) back onto the skin of the small of the back. Once again it is difficult to discriminate between recoil and lag, and has the same problems of pain and stiffness.

The Biceps

There is no good test for biceps! Biceps shape is important. All medical students know the 'Popeye sign' of a ruptured long head of biceps. However you can have a complete intra-articular rupture of long head of biceps without a Popeye sign when the hypertrophied tendon jams in the sulcus, like a cork in a bottleneck. Between these two extremes the biceps can adopt subtle changes in shape.

Lafosse Sign

This test is designed to isolate biceps by asking the patient to supinate the forearm against resistance. The examiner cradles the elbow with the shoulder held at about 40° of scapular elevation. The examiner grips the patient's wrist and pronates the forearm, asking the patient to resist (supinate) this force.

O'Brien's Test

This is designed to detect a SLAP (Superior Labrum antero-posterior) tear. It is performed similarly to the Jobe test, but with the arm held at 20° inside the neutral position (across the body) and at 90° elevation, and full internal rotation. The patient is then asked to resist the attempts of the examiner to push the arm towards the ground.

Yergason only described his test in one patient, yet this test has been copied from textbook to textbook. Speed's test also has a low sensitivity and specificity.

Ultrasound

Medical ultrasound uses wavelengths of 2.5–14 MHz. The higher the wavelength the better the definition of the returning echoes, but more sound is attenuated, meaning you can't see as deeply through the tissues. Fortunately the rotator cuff is reasonably superficial so 8–10 MHz linear array probes can be used that give good definition, indeed the pictures captured on a good machine are so good as to show histology rather than morphology. The problems come with extremely fat or well-muscled individuals where the definition falls off dramatically.

The linear array probe is made of a series of crystals that vibrate as electricity is applied to them (the piezo-electric effect) producing sound waves. In this case ultrasound waves. The crystals are arranged in a row, much like the keys of a piano. Each crystal in turn produces a tiny blip of sound and then waits for the echoes to return as they are reflected by the interfaces between tissues. The echoes causes the crystal to vibrate and this is turned into an electrical impulse, amplified and displayed as a two-dimensional picture of the tissues.

In the clinic, time is important, so an abbreviated study is permitted, scanning in only three planes, as opposed to the 12 planes recommended in most radiological texts. An axial scan is first used to demonstrate the lesser tuberosity,

subscapularis, biceps sulcus and long head of biceps tendon. Secondly an oblique coronal (or longitudinal) view is used to show the greater tuberosity and the supraspinatus. Finally a saggittal oblique (transverse) view is used demonstrating the greater tuberosity and supraspinatus tendon, rotator interval and biceps. All findings are recorded in detail at the time. In each of the three planes a record is made of the articular appearance (normal, positive cartilage reflection sign, osteophytes), the bone (normal, irregular, calcification, fracture line), the collagen (normal, heterogeneous, hypertrophic), presence of a defect (rim-rent, cleft, de-lamination, focal absence, absent cuff), and the presence of an effusion (nil, effusion, flattening of bursa, bursal concavity). A firm diagnosis of the state of the rotator cuff and biceps is then recorded. A full thickness tear is diagnosed on sonography if the tendon is absent, or if there is a focal deficit. A combination of one or more indirect signs such as a bursal concavity, an effusion around the biceps, bony irregularity or a positive cartilage reflection sign allow a judgement to be made by the surgeon on the presence of a supraspinatus tear.

Ultrasound has been shown to be an effective tool for determining the presence of a full thickness tear in the hands of trained radiologists with an accuracy of 81–95 %. Errors in detection and measurement are small in the hands of experienced radiologists Teefey [41]. Errors are often clinically irrelevant such as a grading error, mistaking a deep partial thickness tear for a pinhole full thickness tear, or a small measurement error, mistaking a large tear for a massive tear due to inability to follow the retracted tendon under the acromion. Such errors would not change the clinical management of the patient. Inter-observer error between experienced radiologists is low with full agreement on categorization in 92 % of scans Middleton [39]. However referral to a radiologist for ultrasound scanning inevitably leads to a delay for the patient and a journey that involves three attendances, the first to see the surgeon, the second for the scan and the third to return to the surgeon for the result to be discussed and a treatment strategy to be agreed. The delay from first contact to agreement of

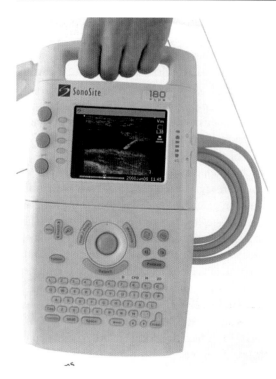

Fig. 10 Portable ultrasound

a plan of treatment may vary from a few days to several months depending on the efficiency of the department of radiology. The new generations of back-pack portable high-resolution and relatively inexpensive ultrasound machines (e.g., Sonosite 180 plus) allow for an ultrasound scan to be performed by the surgeon wherever he first meets the patient (Fig. 10). Al Shawi & Bunker [38] showed such a scan performed by a surgeon was sufficiently accurate (96.3 % sensitivity and 94.3 % specificity for full thickness tears), compared to previously published radiology studies, to allow a one-stop clinic where the patient is seen by the surgeon, has the ultrasound performed by the surgeon and a treatment plan agreed at the first encounter.

Magnetic Resonance Imaging (MRI) and MR Arthrography (MRA)

MRI has revolutionised the field of imaging in the shoulder, because it can image the soft tissues.

Unlike ultrasound MRI can image through the bone, and it can image the bone, and it can image to depths of tissue that cannot be reached by high frequency ultrasound. It is therefore the imaging modality of choice for instability, as it will demonstrate labral abnormalities. Visualisation of SLAP tears and Bankart tears are improved by MRA using gadolinium enhancement.

MRI is the imaging modality of choice for large rotator cuff tears where the degree of retraction under the acromion, and the degree of wasting and fatty infiltration of the muscle belly will determine whether the tear should be repaired, or whether repair is a forlorn hope. MRA is useful in demonstrating articular side partial tears.

However MRI is not without problems. The equipment is extremely expensive and far from portable! Patients do not like MRI. It is claustrophobic, noisy and patient unfriendly. One third of patients will not have a second MRI scan. It will demonstrate morphology, but not histology. It suffers from a phenomenon called the 'magic angle effect' that can produce false positive results. MRI is very bad at showing calcific deposits as these are dark, as is the tendon, so there is no contrast difference between the calcium and the tendon.

MRA suffers from the problem that it is invasive. Intra-articular injection of gadolinium is usually done under image intensifier control and local anaesthetic. This increases the degree of difficulty, often needing two radiology suites, careful timing, transfer from room to room and the time of a skilled radiologist. Additionally, patients do not like invasive diagnostic procedures.

Arthroscopy

Shoulder arthroscopy remains the gold standard forensic investigation for the shoulder. Not only can the inside of the gleno-humeral joint be appreciated (Fig. 11), but also the outside view of the rotator cuff from within the subacromial bursa. An essential pre-amble to arthroscopy is examination under anaesthetic.

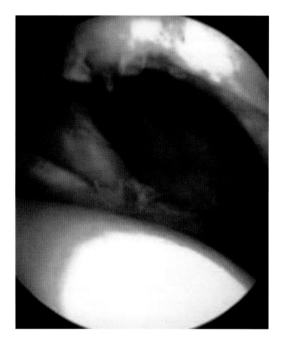

Fig. 11 Arthroscopic view of a moderate cuff tear

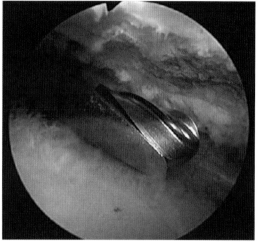

Fig. 12 Arthroscopic subacromial decompression

Open Treatment of Posterosuperior Rotator Cuff Tears

We have demonstrated how there is a spectrum of advancing pathology, from cuff dysfunction leading to impingement, through partial thickness cuff tears, to small full thickness tears and on through moderate to large, to massive tears of the rotator cuff. Treatment must be tailored to fit the symptoms from which the patient is suffering and the pathology causing the symptoms.

Impingement

The patient is usually aged 40–50 and has mild rotator cuff symptoms. These will include pain on reach and exercise, difficulty getting to sleep, but little awakening, a painful arc on elevation that interferes with recreation but the patient continues in their normal work routine. The pain is relieved by subacromial injection of local anaesthetic (Neer's Test).

Conservative treatment involves turning the dysfunctional cuff into a functional cuff again. Two facets need to be addressed, pain and function. The pain can be eased by injection of cortisone (in any form) into the subacromial bursa, and refraining from those activities that aggravate the condition (reaching, sport, and overhead work). Therapists can then supervise muscle re-training, starting with scapular control, and then working on to glenohumeral control.

Indications for surgery are failure of proper conservative treatment, in the patient aged over 40 who has true impingement, which has been abolished temporarily by subacromial injection of local anaesthetic.

The surgical procedure of choice is arthroscopic subacromial decompression. Dr. Harvard Ellman who published his results in 1987 pioneered this technique and now this is the benchmark throughout the advanced world. In the properly selected patient arthroscopic subacromial decompression (Fig. 12) should give excellent or good results in 88 % of patients. These days there is no place for open decompression except as a method of exposure for open cuff repair. However this does not mean that lessons cannot be transferred from the era of open surgery. Open acromioplasty evolved from Neer's first description where a wedge of anterior acromion was removed using an osteotome, and ended with the two stage Rockwood acromioplasty. In this technique the first stage is to remove the full thickness of the acromion that extends anterior to the acromioclavicular joint. The second stage is to remove a wedge of anterior acromion extending from the initial cut and exiting the inferior surface of the acromion 1.5 cms. (three burrs-breadths) posterior to the anterior cut. This technique is now copied arthroscopically.

Partial Thickness Tears

There is great debate over how partial thickness tears should be treated. Some authorities advocate decompression alone, but more these days advocate excision and repair. This is the area where arthroscopic repair with anchors or arthroscopic tacks is of increasing importance. Small tears (<1 cm.) can be dealt with in the same manner, either arthroscopically or through the 'mini-open' technique.

Surgical Treatment of Moderate, Large and Massive Tears

The surgical repair of larger tears remains a difficult undertaking for surgeon, patient and therapist. Difficulties for the surgeon include the surgical approach, retraction of the tendon, contraction of the capsule, degenerate tendon, poor healing, soft bone and weak muscles. Problems for the patient include pain, protection of the repair and frustration due to the long time-course for healing. Problems for the therapist include weak muscles that have lost their control, adaptive muscle patterning and posture and the psychology of protracted recovery. With all these difficulties to overcome it is not surprising that re-tear rates vary from 15 % to 50 % in the massive tears.

Conservative treatment should be tried before recourse is taken to surgery. The only exception to this is the acute massive tear following trauma where surgery is far better immediately and before the tendon retracts. However most large cuff tears present as a chronic problem or an acute-on-chronic problem. In these cases an injection of cortisone should be given to relieve pain and therapy started to regain control of the scapula and then the glenohumeral joint.

Specific Indications for Surgery

The indication for surgery is a proven rotator cuff tear, demonstrated by ultrasound or MRI, in the patient aged over 40 yet under 70, who has symptoms which interfere with daily life, or awaken at night. Weakness up to the point of pseudo paralysis may or may not be present. The patient should have failed a proper course of conservative treatment.

There are six *principles of surgery*:
1. Assess the cuff tear
2. Release the capsular contractures
3. Re-introduce healing biology
4. Re-attach the tendon to its anatomical footprint
5. Protect the repair
6. Regain movement and its control

Assessing the cuff tear means exposing it such that the front, the medial retracted edge and the rear of the tear can be seen. This is best done arthroscopically. However this is not always easy. The bursa may be thickened so much that it mimics cuff tissue; de-lamination makes assessment tricky; the bursa is often inflamed with quite an aggressive nodular synovitis; and the assessment must be performed rapidly before swelling occurs. The size and pattern of the tear, the state of long head of biceps, and subscapularis must be assessed. The degree of retraction and the mobility of the tendon edges can be seen by inserting a grasper and pulling. The quality of the cuff should be noted as to whether it is an acute or chronic tear, whether the adjacent cuff tissue is malacic or de-laminated.

Contractures must be released so that the tendon can be brought without tension to its anatomical position. For moderate tears this means releasing the capsule in the paralabral gutter just as one would for a contracted (frozen) shoulder. For large tears the coracohumeral ligament and rotator interval also need to be released. For massive tears the junctional scar must be released. In all cases the bursa needs to be freed of scar tissue.

Re-introducing healing biology. Most cuff tears are chronic and any attempts to heal have long ago been abandoned by the local cells. They need to be re-awakened by decorticating the greater tuberosity so that blood and, with it, fibroblasts, can actively engage in repair. In the future it may be possible to stimulate repair using synthetic growth factors.

The tendon must be *re-attached* to its anatomical insertion point, its footprint, over as wide an area as possible. This is where the skill of the surgeon is paramount and will be described in greater detail below.

Finally the *repair must be protected* against forces of a magnitude that would re-tear it during the healing phase (6 weeks) and the strengthening phase (3 months). The patient or the therapist, in error or in ignorance, may apply these forces. Protocols must be adhered. Unfortunately in this area ignorance is widespread.

Recovery is a team effort. The team consists of the surgeon, the anaesthetist (who gives the scalene block and controls post-operative pain) the patient, the nursing teams in theatre, on the wards and in outpatients, and in particular the therapist.

Re-Attaching the Tendon

There are three *technical objectives* for the surgeon:
- Adequate exposure
- Sufficient release
- Secure hold

Exposure must be extensile. There are six stages to the extensile exposure. These are:
- All-arthroscopic repair
- Arthroscopic subacromial decompression and mini-open repair
- Matsen deltoid-on with two stage Rockwood modification of Neer's acromioplasty
- Plus acromio-clavicular excision
- Plus trapezius take down (Wiley extension)
- Plus oblique acromial osteotomy (Grammont Osteotomy)

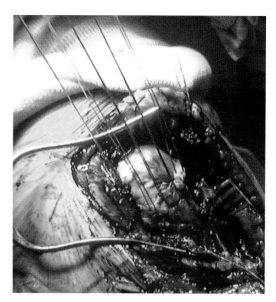

Fig. 13 Exposure of the cuff tear with stay sutures inserted

All-arthroscopic repair is beginning to come of age for small, mobile tears, in the hands of an expert. However it is a difficult procedure with a long learning curve. In 5 years time it will probably become the standard treatment for small and moderate tears. Presently it should be restricted to expert shoulder arthroscopists only.

The Matsen deltoid-on approach is a deltoid split that meets the front of the acromion half way across its anterior surface. Medial and lateral flaps are created in line with the split in deltoid lifting the periosteum from the top surface of the acromion, and then if necessary splitting the trapezius in the same line. Thus two flaps are raised which consist of deltoid-periosteum-trapezius; much like the direct lateral approach to the hip this technique lifts intact fascio-periosteal flaps off the bone. In this manner the acromion is exposed, yet the flaps can be closed side-to-side with no weakening of deltoid. The problem with this approach is that the periosteum over this part of the acromion is very thin; particularly in women, and can easily tear. For this reason this author splits the deltoid so that the split exposes the acromio-clavicular joint. The superior acromio-clavicular ligament is divided much as the periosteum would be with the true Matsen deltoid-on approach, but it is five times as thick as the periosteum and much easier to repair.

If the tear is too big to be seen through a deltoid-on approach with an acromioplasty then the first extension is made, excising the acromio-clavicular joint. One third of the bone is taken from the acromion, and two-thirds from the clavicle, leaving a 1.5–2 cms. gap. This now allows the fat pad to be raised off the belly of supraspinatus and exposure is increased.

If the whole tear still cannot be seen, stay sutures are placed in the edges of the tear, and the humeral head extended and rotated to see if the whole tear can be seen (Fig. 13). If it cannot then the next extension is made. This is the trapezius take-down, which allows an excellent view of the suprascapular fossa and the belly of supraspinatus.

If at this point the whole tear cannot be seen,the full time shoulder surgeon now has a choice, to perform an oblique scapular osteotomy or to perform tendon transposition or augment. The results of tendon transfers (deltoid flap or latissimus transfer) are to improve the shoulder from a Constant score (CS) of 30 to a CS of 60. The alternative is the Grammont osteotomy of the spine of the scapula. This gives a fantastic view of the rotator cuff, and is re-assembled with a small locking plate but is beyond the limits of this text.

Release of Contractures

The second technical objective is to release the capsular contractures. Now an understanding of the sequence and pattern of tearing will turn the course of the operation from a "pot pourri" to a controlled predictable experience.

Small tears (less than 1 cm.) will not have any contractures, the capsule has not retracted enough and so no releases will be needed.

Moderate tears may have enough capsular retraction for stiffness to set in. Here the contraction will be similar in extent to contracted (frozen) shoulder, and the same release (along the paralabral gutter) will need to be performed. This can be done arthroscopically or open.

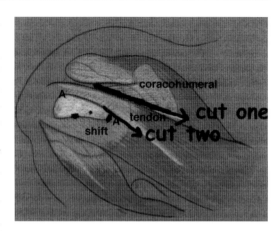

Fig. 14 An extension is made behind the central oblique tendon and A is rotated to A

Large and massive tears have additional scarring at the front of the tear and at the back. At the front the coracohumeral ligament contracts and tethers the anterior pillar. At the back the junctional scar develops at the base of the spine of the scapula. This plane between the supraspinatus and infraspinatus needs to be released, but care must be taken not to damage the adjacent suprascapular nerve.

Rotationplasty or Margin Convergence?

Even with all the contractures released a large to massive chronic tear may have such a loss of tendon material that the tidied-up edge of the tendon cannot be advanced on to the prepared bony footprint. Now what can be done? The alternatives are to lash the front of the tear to the back (margin convergence), perform a rotator interval slide (which is now condemned as a poor procedure), perform a rotationplasty, or give up the idea of direct repair and either augment or perform a tendon transfer.

Margin convergence is the preferred method for the arthroscopist. This is because it is relatively easy and it will work for a tear that is not extensive from front to back. It will not work for a tear that is extensive in both directions.

In the rotator interval slide the only remaining strong attachment of the supraspinatus, the anterior column is detached, this allows the anterior column to be re-attached further back and what is acheived is to close the back of the defect by opening up the front. This actually makes things far worse, for now the head will escape through the anterior defect, decreasing cuff function.

If the tear is extensive in both directions then basic plastic surgical techniques must be adapted to close the defect, and this means a rotation flap (Fig. 14). The remaining anterior column and its attachment should be protected. If the tear pattern is an anterior L-shape, then an extension is made along the back of the central oblique tendon and the cuff is rotated clockwise to close the defect. If the shape is a posterior L-shape then the extension is between supra- and infraspinatus (through the junctional scar) and the cuff is rotated anticlockwise to fill the defect. Sometimes if the tear is massive then both extensions are required and the block of posterior cuff is advanced.

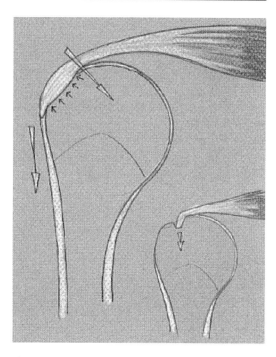

Fig. 15 Two row repair gives a stronger and better footprint than one row

Secure Repair. Eliminating the Weakest Link

The final technical objective is to gain a secure repair to the de-corticated and bleeding surface of the greater tuberosity, over as large a footprint area as possible, for long enough for biological union to occur. Most surgeons will use a *two-row technique* in order to attach the tendon to as great an area of footprint as possible. Two-row arthroscopic repair was first devised by DeBeer from Cape Town (2002). However, open two-row repair came first. By 1992 it was our favoured method of open repair and we first published and illustrated this in our textbook ((Fig. 15) Bunker and Schranz: Challenges in Orthopaedic Surgery; the Shoulder) in 1997. Two-row repair involves attaching the cuff to both extremities of the de-corticated tuberosity. The two-row repair has been made more secure by over-sewing the cuff, joining the proximal and distal rows using such techniques as the *suture bridge* (Fig. 16).

Any method of linking tendon to bone has a potential to separate wherever there is a *weak*

link in the chain. In rotator cuff repair there are five linkage points:
- Tendon to suture
- The suture itself
- The knot
- Suture to anchor
- Anchor to bone

A great deal of effort has gone in to overengineering all these linkages to prevent failure. Some of the weak points are under the surgeon's control, but the quality of the tendon and the quality of the bone are not.

The Suture-Tendon Junction

Decades of effort by generations of hand surgeons have seen the grasping core suture become the method of choice for flexor tendon repair. Gerber and Schneeberger showed experimentally how grasping sutures remain secure under load when simple sutures cut out. They found that the best grasping suture was the Mason Allen grasping suture, closely followed by the modified Kessler. Grasping sutures are extremely difficult to perform arthroscopically, so it was with

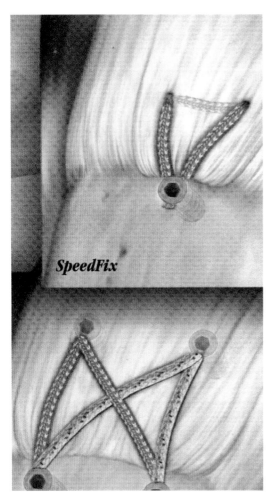

Fig. 16 Suturebridge technique

concernthat experienced shoulder surgeons saw the arthroscopic pioneers performing cuff repairs with simple sutures, a technique that they knew from observation failed at open surgery. However White & Bunker showed that the strength at this interface might be proportional to the number of passes of the suture through the tendon rather than the pattern of passage. Thus two mattress sutures (four passes) are as strong as one Mason-Allen suture (three passes). The Mason Allen suture is easy and quick to perform open and remains the gold standard.

The Suture

Properties of the suture depend upon the material, whether it is monofilament or braided and the diameter of the suture. Theoretically one could over-engineer the suture just by increasing its diameter so that its breaking strain was far greater than the original tendon, but the thicker the thread the more difficult it becomes to knot, so a compromise needs to be made. Any suture thicker than number 2 knots poorly. The breakthrough with sutures has been in materials. New sutures such as orthocord and fibrewire are almost unbreakable.

The Knot

All knots have a breaking strain of half the suture itself. Clearly it is a weak link. All knots rely upon friction between the two suture ends. One of these is designated the post and the other the loop. Friction is increased by reversing the post for alternate half hitches, and by increasing the number of half hitches performed. The surgeons knot is the strongest knot and better than sliding knots of whatever variety.

Because the knot is a weak link surgeons have tried to get rid of them using knotless techniques. Most of these involve trapping the knot within the anchor using a pop-rivet technique.

Suture to Anchor

The sutures have been linked to the anchor with an eyelet. The eyelet has been a real problem as early anchors had sharp metal edges where the eyelet had been drilled or formed in the anchor. This sharp edge used to cut the anchor. Gerber and Schneeberger modelled arthroscopic repair and found that the weakest point was always the eyelet. Better anchor manufacture and the new unbreakable super-sutures have eliminated the eyelet problem.

The Anchor

The original descriptions of rotator cuff repair by the pioneers such as McLaughlin and Neer described attaching the suture to the bone using bone tunnels, because they had nothing else. These days we have suture anchors and suture screws. Whereas a bone tunnel of 1 cm. in length will fail with a low force of 16 N, suture anchors will take 280 N to pull out. Anchors are not only stronger but also easier and quicker to use.

Bone tunnels are still used by some because anchors are expensive. Gerber has tried to overcome the weakness of bone tunnels by using a titanium plate to augment the sutures and Bunker has used a metaphyseal screw or post with a pull-out strength of 900 N. For the last decade anchors have been so secure compared to all the other links in the chain that failure was unheard of. However the new generation of super-sutures have removed the weakest link and recently failure by anchor pull-out has been described.

Results of Rotator Cuff Repair

The Panacryl Study appears to give the most honest appraisal of the results of surgery for rotator cuff repair. This was a British multi-centre prospective controlled study of rotator cuff repair. 159 patients were analysed from 15 UK centres. 17 % of the tears were small and closed with side-to-side sutures, 83 % were closed with modified Mason-Allen suture technique. Patients were assessed by Constant scores pre-operatively, at 6 months and at 1 year. They were also followed by real-time dynamic ultrasound scanning performed by experienced consultant ultrasonographers.

The Constant pain scores improved following surgery from 6/15 to 12/15 at 6 months where 15 is no pain at all. Total Constant scores improved from 46/100 to 66/100 at 6 months.

The re-tear rate was 26 % overall at 6 months, but varied from 15 % in tears less than 5 cms. in diameter to 51 % in massive tears. Despite the high re-tear rate there is still a good effect from the surgery with statistically significant improvements in most parameters of the Constant score, including pain and total scores.

Subscapularis Repair

Ruptures of the anterior cuff are far less common than postero-superior tears. They are often consequent on transient or locked dislocation in the elderly patient. However they may follow on from expanding pulley lesions or medial biceps dislocations. They are almost impossible to repair through a superior approach. An MRI must be performed before surgery to assess the wasting and degree of fatty atrophy of the muscle belly, because if this is marked then repair should not be undertaken.

The surgical approach should be the standard deltopectoral approach to the shoulder. Often the tendon will have retracted under the conjoined tendon. This means that the musculo-cutaneous nerve should be identified and a pre-drilled coracoid osteotomy performed. Subsequently a 360° release of the subscapularis tendon should be performed taking care not to damage the posterior cord of the brachial plexus that is scarred on to the anterior surface of subscapularis and always closer than the surgeon has estimated. The lesser tuberosity is now de-corticated and a two-row repair of the mobilised tendon is performed using the techniques that have just been given for supraspinatus repair.

Biceps is always damaged with a substantial subscapularis tear. Biceps will need to be tenotomised close to its origin and an extra-articular tenodesis performed.

Tendon Transfers

Pectoralis Major Transfer

This transfer is reserved for inoperable subscapularis tears. The aim of surgery is to replace the absent subscapularis with a local muscle tendon unit that can cover the defect, thus containing the humerus and increasing the power of internal rotation. The sternal head of pectoralis major has all these attributes.

Surgery is affected through a standard deltopectoral approach. The combined heads of pectoralis major, or just the sternal head are harvested from their insertion on to the humeral shaft. They are then transferred to cover the anterior defect and are attached to the prepared lesser tuberosity using suture anchors. There is some theoretical advantage to using the sternal head and taking it under the conjoined tendon so that it replicates the line of pull of subscapularis more accurately. However this is more difficult and great care must be taken to identify and protect the musculocutaneous nerve.

Early results with this transfer show that it is the method of choice for irreparable tears of subscapularis.

Latissimus Dorsi Transfer

The primary repair of massive postero-superior rotator cuff tears is extremely difficult and is associated with prolonged rehabilitation and a high re-tear rate. This then raises the question, is there an alternative surgical solution to the problem of pain and weakness in this situation? The latissimus dorsi transfer has long been used in children with brachial plexus palsy, where it goes by the name of the L'Episcopo procedure. The effect of this transfer in children with C5 plexus palsy (effectively causing a suprascapular nerve palsy) is to give them external rotation at the shoulder. The idea behind latissimus dorsi transfer is to affect the same result in the elderly patient with a massive cuff tear. The aim of the operation is two-fold, to contain the humeral head against upward subluxation, and to increase the power of external rotation. It has been found that two criteria must be satisfied for this transfer to work. The first is that deltoid must be functional, and the second that subscapularis is intact. The results of latissimus transfer in the face of a tear extending into subscapularis are so poor that it should not be attempted.

At surgery the patient is placed in lateral decubitus so that both the front and the back of the shoulder are available to the surgeon. A single posterior incision or the classic two incision approach can be used. The first is a standard superior approach to supraspinatus and the main incision runs along the lateral margin of the latissimus. Care is taken to protect the axillary nerve where it exits the quadrilateral space, and the tendon of latissimus is identified and traced to its insertion on the humerus. The radial nerve and the profunda brachia vessels pass below the tendon insertion through the triangular space

and these must be protected as well. The muscle belly is now cautiously released taking care not to damage the neurovascular supply. The tendon is now whip-stitched and a tunnel developed under deltoid and the acromion so that the tendon can be passed from the posterior incision through to the anterior incision where it is attached to infraspinatus stump, or if possible the supraspinatus stump on the anterior facet of the greater tuberosity of the humerus.

Early clinical results of latissimus transfer, in well-selected patients, operated upon by good surgeons have shown promise. Time will tell how acceptable this technique will become.

Conclusions

Surgeons are only just beginning to understand rotator cuff disease. Our understanding has been helped by examining the precise anatomy of the supraspinatus tendon, and by recent advances in comprehending the aetiology of this disease, as well as advances in investigation such as ultrasound, MRI and arthroscopy. We are beginning to understand the natural history of rotator cuff dysfunction and tearing, and the pattern of cuff tears and capsular contractures. Principles for surgery and technical objectives are now understood and the techniques for surgery are beginning to be worked out. Despite all of this, surgery remains difficult for the surgeon, painful and frustrating for the patient and demanding of the therapist. We have a long way to go before we have all the answers for this extremely common, yet extremely disabling, degenerative disease of the shoulder.

References

1. Nakajima F. Histological and biomechanical characteristics of the supraspinatus tendon. J Shoulder Elbow Surg. 1994;3:79–87.
2. Urwin M, Symmons D, Allison T. Estimating the burden of musculoskeletal disease in the community. Ann Rheum Dis. 1998;57:649–55.
3. Bonger PM. Leader. BMJ. 2001;322:64–5.

4. Moseley H, Goldie I. The arterial pattern of the rotator cuff of the shoulder. J Bone Joint Surg Br. 1963;45(B): 780–9.
5. Walch G, Nove JL. Tears of the supraspinatus tendon associated with hidden lesions of the rotator interval. J Shoulder Elbow Surg. 1994;3:353–60.
6. Gerber C, Hersche O, Forra A. Isolated rupture of subscapularis. J Bone Joint Surg Br. 1996;78: 1015–23.
7. Neer C. Anterior acromioplasty for chronic impingement lesions of the shoulder. J Bone Joint Surg Br(A). 1972;54:41–50.
8. Neer C. Impingement lesions. Clin Orthop. 1983;173: 70–7.
9. Nicholson GP, Goodman DA, Flatow EL, Bigliani LU. The acromion; morphological and age related changes. J Shoulder Elbow Surg. 1996;5:1–11.
10. Edelson JG, Taitz C. Anatomy of the coracoacromial arch. J Bone Joint Surg Br. 1992;74(B):589–94.
11. Wang JC, Shapiro MS. Changes in acromial morphology with age. J Shoulder Elbow Surg. 1997;6:55–9.
12. Hyvonen P, Lohi S. Open acromioplasty does not prevent the progression of an impingement syndrome to a tear. J Bone Joint Surg Br. 1998;80:813–6.
13. Bunker T, Esler C, Leach W. Rotator cuff tear of the hip. J Bone Joint Surg Br. 1997;79B:618–20.
14. Shah NN, Bayliss NC, Malcolm A. Shape of the acromion; congenital or aquired? J Shoulder Elbow Surg. 2001;10:309–16.
15. Codman EA. The shoulder. Boston: Thomas Todd; 1934.
16. Ozaki J, Fujimoto S, Nakagawa Y, Mashura K, Tamai S. Recalcitrant chronic adhesive capsulitis of the shoulder. J Bone Joint Surg Br. 1989;71A: 1511–5.
17. Budoff J, Nirschl R. Debridement of partial thickness tears. J Bone Joint Surg Am. 1998;80:733–48.
18. DePalma AF. Surgery of the shoulder. Philidelphia: J.B. Lipincott; 1973.
19. Ozaki J, Fujimoto S, Nakagawa Y, Mashura K, Tamai S. Tears of the rotator cuff associated with pathological changes in the acromion. J Bone Joint Surg Br. 1988;70A:1224–30.
20. Sher U. Abnormal findings on MRI of asymptomatic shoulders. J Bone Joint Surg Br. 1995;77A:10–5.
21. Frost P, Andersen JH. Occupational factors in shoulder pain. Occup Environ Med. 1999;56:494–8.
22. Walch G, Boileau P. Impingement of the deep surface of the supraspinatus tendon. J Shoulder Elbow Surg. 1992;1:238–45.
23. Habermeyer, Anterosuperior impingement. Presented at SECEC 2001.
24. Uhtoff H, Loehr J. The pathogenesis of rotator cuff tears. Proceedings of the 3rd International Conference on Surgey of the Shoulder, 1986 Oct 27; Fukuora, Japan; 1986.
25. Cyriax J. Textbook of orthopaedic medicine. London: Bailliere; 1982.
26. Kolbel R. The bow test for subacromial impingement. J Shoulder Elbow Surg. 1994;3:254–5.
27. MacDonald PB, Clark P, Sutherland K. Impingement signs. J Shoulder Elbow Surg. 2000;9(4):299–301.
28. Hertel R, Ballmer FT, Lambert S, Gerber C. Lag signs in the diagnosis of rotator cuff rupture. J Shoulder Elbow Surg. 1996;5:307–13.
29. Teefey SA, Middleton WD, Yamaguchi K. Ultrasonography of the rotator cuff. J Bone Joint Surg Br. 2000;82:498–504.
30. Ellman H, Kay S, Wirth M. Arthroscopic treatment of rotator cuff. Arthroscopy. 1993;9:195–200.
31. Gleyze P, Thomazeau H, Flurin PH, Lafosse L, Gazielly DF, Allard M. Arthroscopic rotator cuff repair. Rev Chir Orth. 2000;86:566–74.
32. Matsen FA. In Rockwood CA, Matsen FA editors. The shoulder. Philidelphia: WB Saunders; 1998. p. 668.
33. Ha'eri GB, Wiley AM. An extensile exposure for subacromial derangements. Can J Surg. 1980;23(5): 458–61.
34. Gerber C, Schneeberger AG, Beck M, Schlegel U. Mechanical strength of repairs of the rotator cuff. J Bone Joint Surg Br. 1994;76:371–80.
35. McLaughlin H. Lesions of the musculotendinous cuff of the shoulder. J Bone Joint Surg Br. 1944;26:31–51.
36. Barber F, Herbert M, Click JN. Update on internal fixation strength. Arthroscopy. 1997;13:355–62.
37. Panacryl study. Presented at SECEC 2001.
38. Al-Shawi A, Badge R, Bunker T. The detection of full thickness rotator cuff tears using ultrasound. J Bone Joint Surg Br. 2008;90(7):889–92.
39. Middleton WD, Teefey SA, Yamaguchi K. Sonography of the rotator cuff; Analysis of interobserver error. AJR Am J Roentgenol. 2004;183(5):1465–8.
40. Nakagaki K, Ozaki J, Tomita Y, Tamai S. Fatty degeneration in supraspinatus after rotator cuff tear. J Shoulder Elbow Surg. 1996;5(3):194–200.
41. Teefey SA, Middleton WD, Payne WT, Yamaguchi K. Detection and measurement of rotator cuff tears; analysis of diagnostic errors. AJR Am J Roentgenol. 2005;184(6):1768–73.

Partial Rotator Cuff Ruptures

Antonio Cartucho

Contents

Abstract

Degenerative partial-thickness tears are an important part of pathology of the rotator cuff, that occur mainly on the supraspinatus tendon. More recently a more thorough assessment of the subscapularis during arthroscopy led to better understanding of the potential role that this tendon may play as a cause of anterior shoulder pain and biceps instability.

The supraspinatus footprint has a very particular microscopic anatomy that contributes to create differential shear stress within the tendon.

Symptoms arise from mechanical impairment with adaptative response of the shoulder girdle, from inflammatory changes and involvement of the long head of the biceps.

Progression of the tear is more frequent in symptomatic patients and regression was found in less than 10 % of the cases.

With tear progression, clinical cure by conservative measures may be impossible to obtain.

The decision for surgical treatment depends on the type of rupture, the age and level of activity of the patient and of the degree of pain and functional impairment.

Keywords

Shoulder arthroscopy • Rotator cuff • Partial rupture

A. Cartucho
Orthopaedic Department, Hospital Cuf Descobertas,
Lisbon, Portugal
e-mail: a.cartucho@netcabo.pt

G. Bentley (ed.), *European Surgical Orthopaedics and Traumatology*,
DOI 10.1007/978-3-642-34746-7_45, © EFORT 2014

Introduction

Partial rotator cuff ruptures are not rare and occur mainly on the supraspinatus tendon and may extend to the infraspinatus. Isolated lesions of the infraspinatus and teres minor tendons are rare. Isolated ruptures of the, but rarely to, the subscapularis tendon had a 30 % incidence in cadaveric studies [52]. Partial ruptures usually occur before the sixth decade of life and can be a cause of unexplained pain in the shoulder, giving considerable disability.

Anatomy of the Supraspinatus Footprint

Gross Anatomy

In order to classify and to grade partial rotator cuff ruptures we must be aware of the characteristics of supraspinatus insertion on the humerus. The mean antero-posterior dimension of the supraspinatus insertion is 25 mm. The mean superior to inferior thickness at the rotator interval is 11.6 mm, 12.1 at mid-tendon and 12 mm at the posterior edge. The distance from the articular cartilage margin to the bony tendon insertion ranges between 1.5 to 1.9 mm, with a mean of 1.7 mm. This being said, articular partial-thickness tears with more than 7 mm of exposed bone lateral to the articular margin should be considered significant tears, approximating 50 % of the tendon substance [51].

The superficial tendon fibres run longitudinally, while the deep fibres run obliquely. The supraspinatus tendon fuses with the infraspinatus tendon approximately 15 mm proximal to their insertion on the greater tuberosity. They are not visualised as two individual tendons and cannot be separated by blunt dissection in this region [9]. In direct communication with the supraspinatus is the deep projection of the coraco-humeral ligament which runs perpendicular and deep to the supraspinatus tendon but superficial to the joint capsule.

Microscopic Anatomy

The tendons of the rotator cuff are composed primarily of water (55 % of net weight) and type I Collagen (85 % of dry weight). Additional constituents include other collagens (III and XII), PGs. abd GAGs., elastin and fibroblasts. The collagen bundles of the cuff tendons are confluent and form a hood over the humeral head [40].

Near the insertions of the supraspinatus and infraspinatus tendons into the greater tuberosity, a five-layer complex has been described that details the density and organisation of collagen and its associated elements. Layer one is the superficial coraco-humeral ligament. Layer two represents the main portion of the tendon complex with large closely-packed fascicles. Layer three is also dense, but with smaller fascicles running in a less uniform direction. Layer four is loose connective tissue with thick collagen fibres running perpendicular to the primary fascicle orientation. This layer contains the deep coraco-humeral ligament. Layer five is the true joint capsule. It has been suggested that this intra-tendinous variation of collagen fiber density and orientation may produce shearing forces within the layers during active movement and produce intra-substance tears [22, 58].

Blood Supply to the Rotator Cuff

The rotator cuff receives its blood supply from several different branches of the axillary artery. The rotator cuff tendons are not encased by a true synovial sheath or paratenon [5]. They are supplied by the above-named branches that send smaller branches through the periosteum, across the musculotendinous junction, and via the overlying bursa. A 'critical zone' has been described in the supraspinatus tendon, within 1 cm. of its insertion into the greater tuberosity [45]. Arm position has been shown to affect the tenuous blood flow pattern in this region with abduction causing compression of the supraspinatus against the humeral head, squeezing the vessels in this critical region [50]. The bursal surface blood flow in the supraspinatus tendon is more robust than its corresponding articular surface [38].

Although less robust in some areas, this vascular pattern may be adequate to meet the metabolic needs of a healthy rotator cuff, as corresponding histological evidence of hypoperfusion has not been demonstrated [7]. Therefore, the existence of a true critical zone, and its significance relative to pathological changes occurring within the rotator cuff remains in question.

Histologic, immunohistochemical and intra-operative Doppler flowmetry analysis have reported relative hyperperfusion at the area of the critical zone [17, 28]. The hypervascularity in such cases is thought to come from proliferation in the subsynovial layer in response to injury.

Local Biomechanics

Variation in fibre orientation within the cuff/capsule complex from superficial to deep affects its biomechanical properties. The bursal side of the supraspinatus tendon has been demonstrated to have a lower modulus of elasticity with a higher ultimate strain and stress, compared with the articular side of the tendon. This finding suggests that the articular portion of the supraspinatus may be more susceptible to mechanical failure in tension. Indeed, articular-sided tears have been more commonly reported [59].

The bursal layers are composed primarily of tendon bundles which may elongate with a tensile load and are resistant to rupture, whereas the joint-side layers, a complex of tendons, ligaments, and joint capsule, do not stretch and tear easily. This suggests that intratendinous lamination is caused by differential shear stress within the supraspinatus tendon.

In addition, with a simulated partial-thickness tear in one portion of the tendon, the remainder of the tendon demonstrated increased strain. This reflects the supraspinatus tendon's interconnected five-layer complex and helps to explain why partial-thickness tears may propagate into large full-thickness tears [4]. Other studies support the view that partial thickness tears could potentially propagate in the transverse plane, especially in >50 % thickness partial tears. From biomechanical data, bursal sided tears of over 50 % thickness should warrant more concern to the surgeon. As the results from this studies may imply tear propagation in the transverse plane in the antero-posterior direction [54].

Rotator cuff tears disrupt the force balance in the shoulder and the gleno-humeral joint in particular resulting in compromised arm elevation torques. This dynamic instability contributes to further structural damage aggravating the initial lesion.

Definition and Classification

A partial-thickness tear is considered to be a definite disruption of the fibers of the tendon and is not simply fraying, roughening or softening of the surface. The degree of tearing is better defined by the depth involved in the thickness of the tendon than by the area of the tear. There are three sub-types described for the supraspinatus:

1. A bursal-side tear (BT) which is confined to the bursal surface of the tendon
2. An intratendinous tear (IT) which is found within the tendon; and
3. A joint-side tear (JT) which is present on the side of the tendon adjacent to the joint.

Ellman [13] proposed a classification which included the site and extention of the partial tear, whether its location was adjacent to the articular or bursal surface or whether it was intra-tendinous. The grade was defined in terms of the depth as measured arthroscopically by a probe:

Grade-I tears had a depth of less than 3 mm,

Grade II of 3–6 mm and

Grade III, involvement of more than half of the thickness of the tendon.

More recently Habermeyer [25] described a 2-dimensional classification of articular-sided supraspinatus tendon tears in the coronal plane as well as the sagittal plane, with regard to the origin of articular-sided partial tears at the tendon insertion. The authors described three types of ruptures regarding the sagital plane:

Type A tear: tear of the coraco-humeral ligament continuing into medial border of supraspinatus tendon

Type B tear: isolated tear within the crescent zone and

Type C tear extending from the lateral border of the pulley system over the medial border of supraspinatus tendon up to the crescent zone.

This classification completes the classifications of Snyder [56] and Ellman that lack anatomic landmarks with reference to the localisation of the tear at the insertion of the tendon, especially at the border of the tendon insertion, at the rotator cable, or within the crescent zone.

The subscapularis partial ruptures can be classified in tree different types according to Lafosse [36]:

Type1 – partial superior third,
Type II – Complete superior third,
Type III – Complete superior two-thirds.

Incidence

The incidence of partial tears of the supraspinatus is difficult to access, because most lesions can only be identified during arthroscopy, and MRI may demonstrate partial tears in asymptomatic individuals [55]. Cadaver studies have consistently shown that partial-thickness are more common than full-thickness tears [63]. Among the three sub-types of partial tear, JTs. are two to three times more common than BTs. Intrasubstance tears are less frequent, comprising 7.9–13.6 % in the series of Fukuda et al. [16, 18]. Most of the earlier reports did not include intra-tendinous lesions. The apparent lack of the last in published series is due to the difficulty of the diagnosis [19, 33, 44, 48].

According to some authors [30, 52] the incidence of partial ruptures of the subscapularis is more than 30 %. This fact led many to a more thorough assessment of the subscapularis during arthroscopy and appreciation of the potential role that this tendon may play as a cause of anterior shoulder pain and biceps instability.

Pathogenesis

Probably, rotator cuff tendinopathy is secondary to multiple factors. Combinations of intrinsic and extrinsic factors are responsible in the development pathology on the rotator cuff. Pathologic changes in tendons can lead to reduced tensile strength and a predisposition to rupture [26]. Intrinsic tendinopathy and/or enthesopathy due to changes in vascularity of the cuff or other metabolic alterations associated with aging, may lead to degenerative tears. Extrinsic factors produce lesions to the rotator cuff through compression of the tendons by bony impingement or direct pressure.

More recently a postero-superior impingement due to repetitive interaction between the undersurface of the supraspinatus tendon and the postero-superior glenoid was found responsible for JT partial tears [59].

The injured tendon has inflammatory changes. Oxidative stress, tissue remodelling and apoptosis are all important parts of this pathological process [28].

The loss of dynamic, fine-tuned control, due to rotator cuff pathology leads to numerous adaptative changes on a regional and broader scale. Increase of effective moment arms through connections to other tendon sub-regions tend to overload the last [37]. On a broader scale there are modifications on the shoulder muscle firing patterns namely the upper trapezius and an increase of scapular contribution to arm elevation [43].

The loss of normal shoulder kinematics leads to further stress not only on the injured tendon but in all rotator cuff tendons and scapular muscles [48]. This fact may contribute to further aggravation of the structural injury, of the functional problem and of the clinical presentation.

All these inflammatory, degenerative and mechanical factors, contribute to the onset, stabilisation, propagation and aggravation of the partial rotator cuff rupture (Fig. 1).

Natural History

Determining the natural history of partial rotator cuff ruptures is essential to decision-making on treatment strategies. Studies of anatomical findings according to age have established that degenerative rotator cuff tears are exceedingly

Fig. 1 Propagation and aggravation of the partial rotator cuff rupture

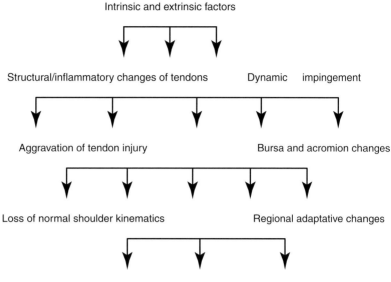

Intrinsic and extrinsic factors

Structural/inflammatory changes of tendons   Dynamic   impingement

Aggravation of tendon injury   Bursa and acromion changes

Loss of normal shoulder kinematics   Regional adaptative changes

Further aggravation of the structural injury

rare before the age of 40 and that both their prevalence and their extention increase with advancing age. Thus, partial-thickness tears usually occur in the sixth decade of life, full-thickness tears in the seventh decade, and involvement of multiple tendons in the elderly patients [2]. These data support clinical experience regarding the progression of degenerative rotator cuff pathology.

Not all partial tears are symptomatic but more than 50 % of patients with partial rotator cuff tears become symptomatic over the years [63], especially on a context of a symptomatic contralateral tear.

Although anatomical damage fails to correlate with clinical manifestations, tear progression may be more common in patients with symptoms. Nevertheless, half the patients with symptoms experienced no progression. Pain was far more closely correlated to subacromial bursitis and long biceps tendinopathy than to tear size or site [65].

From the clinical and histological aspects, spontaneous healing of partial tears appears to be unlikely except on rare occasions. Various untoward factors involved in the healing of the torn tendon include ageing, separation of the tear caused by muscular contraction and the

weight of the arm, hypovascularity, inflammatory changes, oxidative stress, augmented apoptosis, shear stress within the tendon, and subacromial impingement. In the same way any process that impairs tissue healing, like smoking, will also contribute to cuff disease and a less effective healing response [28].

Clinical Presentation

There have been few data on the characteristics of asymptomatic rotator cuff tears such as their size, location, involvement of the biceps tendon and bursal or gleno-humeral effusion. Asymptomatic tears are typically limited to the supraspinatus tendon and are very uncommon in subjects younger than the age of 60 but the prevalence increases with age [44].

The physical signs and symptoms of rotator cuff disease can be separated in two categories. The ones from mechanical impairment due to the structural damage with the adaptative response of the shoulder girdle and others resulting from inflammatory changes and involvement of the long head of the biceps.

Pain especially at night is the most disturbing symptom. There is evidence that the pain is

Fig. 2 Hawkins sign

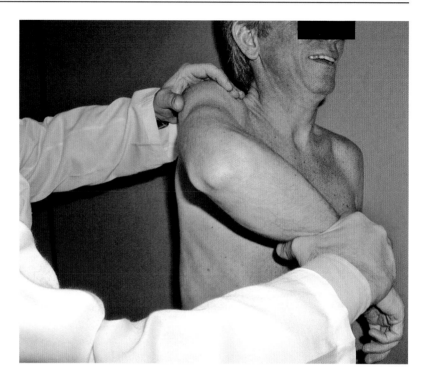

proportional to the degree of subacromial bursi-tis, not to the depth or extent of the tear [23]. Impingement signs, painful arc and a positive procaine test are the result of tendon and bursal inflammatory status. The consequences of the tendon rupture are muscle atrophy, muscle weak-ness, lack of dynamic control ("drop-arm" sign), crepitus, changes on muscle activation patterns with an early activation of the upper trapezius and changes in the shoulder rhythm with elevation of the scapula in the initial two- thirds of movement [34, 43]. Differential shoulder muscle firing pat-terns in patients with rotator cuff pathology may play a role in the presence or absence of symp-toms. Asymptomatic patients have increased fir-ing of the subscapularis whereas symptomatic subjects continue to rely on torn rotator cuff tendons and periscapular muscle substitution resulting in compromised function. Increased scapular contribution to arm elevation may allow function at a higher level and can be con-sidered a positive adaptation [34]. At present it his not possible to confirm the direction of these effects in order to be able to design rehabilitation programs to optimise scapular mechanics.

The Neer and Hawkins (Fig. 2) tests have good sensitivity but low specificity for subacromial impingement syndrome to diagnose supraspinatus or infraspinatus tears, the Jobe sign and the "full-can" test shows similar perfor-mance characteristics to the Patte test and resisted external rotation with the elbow at the side flexed at 90° [3].

Clinical assessment of the subscapularis should include the lift-off test [20], belly-press test [21], Napoleon and bear-hug test [1] to opti-mise the chance of detecting and predicting the size of a subscapularis tear.

The lift-off test (Fig. 3) is performed by plac-ing the hand of the affected arm on the back (at the position of the midlumbar spine) and asking the patient to internally rotate the arm to lift the hand off of the back. The test is considered positive if the patient is unable to lift the arm off the back.

The belly-press test (Fig. 4) is performed with the arm at the side and the elbow flexed to 90°, by having the patient press the palm of the hand into the abdomen by internally rotating the shoulder. The active internal rotation force against the patient's belly is assessed and quantified.

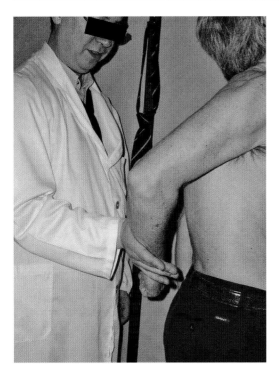

Fig. 3 Lift off test

The test is considered positive if the patient showed a weakness in comparison to the opposite shoulder.

The Napoleon test, a variation of the belly-press test, is performed by placing the hand on the stomach in the same position in which Napoleon Bonaparte held his hand for portraits. The Napoleon test is considered negative if the patient is able to push the hand against the stomach with the wrist straight, and positive if the wrist was flexed to 90° to push against the stomach.

The bear-hug test (Fig. 5) is performed with the palm of the hand involved side placed on the opposite shoulder and the elbow positioned anterior to the body. The patient is then asked to hold that position (resisted internal rotation) as the physician tries to pull the patient's hand from the shoulder with a force applied perpendicular to the forearm. The test is considered positive if the patient can not hold the hand against the shoulder.

A positive bear-hug and belly-press tests suggest a tear of at least 30 % of the subscapularis, whereas a positive Napoleon test indicates that more than 50 % of the subscapularis is torn. A positive lift-off test is not seen until at least 75 % of the subscapularis is involved.

Diagnostic Imaging

Although it is possible to use shoulder arthrography for the diagnosis of partial rotator cuff tears MRI and ultrasonography are the most commonly used. Arthrography of the shoulder allows evaluation of the integrity of the undersurface of the rotator cuff. However, its value in diagnosing JTs remains uncertain with an accuracy ranging from 15 % to 83 %.

There has been substantial improvement of ultrasound technology in recent years which enables higher spatial resolution and superior image quality with modern, high-frequency probes. Recent studies [61] found comparable accuracy for ultrasonography and MRI in the detection of partial tears, with MRI having slightly superior rates regarding sensitivity in intrasubstance ruptures (Fig. 6).

MRI arthrography has been considered superior in detecting rotator cuff pathology, especially partial tears [14, 33]. Ultrasound scan, unlike MRI, is a dynamic examination that enables the examiner to repeat and re-scan the suspected area. In addition; relationships with other tendons and the presence of secondary signs of impingement may aid correct diagnosis.

MRI should be reserved for doubtful cases and in patients with involvement of multiple anatomical structures on the gleno-humeral joint like the capsule-labral complex.

Diagnosis at Surgery

The use of arthroscopy permits a very effective inspection of the cuff. Nevertheless it is essential to correlate the arthroscopic findings with the clinical presentation in order to understand if the structural change present is responsible for

Fig. 4 The belly-press test

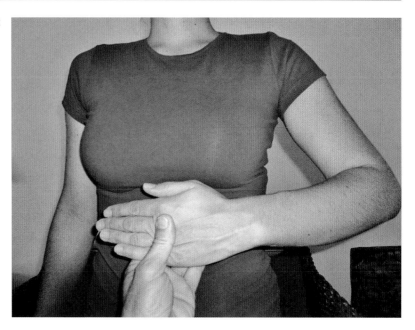

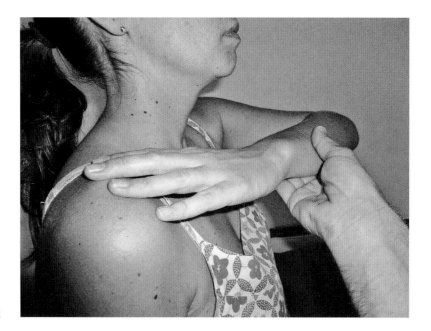

Fig. 5 The bear-hug test

the patient's complaints. For confirmation of the diagnosis a systematic inspection and palpation of the joint and bursal sides of the cuff should be performed. Joint side fraying should be debrided, the extention of the lesion measured and a suture marker passed. Inspection of the bursal side should follow by carefully performing a boursectomy while assessing the qaulity of the tendon. If an intratendinouse lesion is suspected the surgeon must look for thinning or

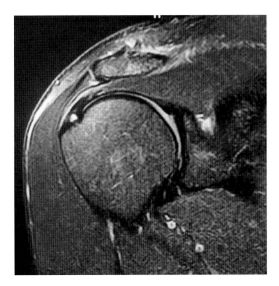

Fig. 6 Intra-substance ruptures

bulging of the cuff and then, using a shaver, the leasion can be put in sight. Also using a probe while performing elevation and rotation of the arm, can locate the lesion [42].

Treatment Options and Indications

It is important to recognise that the choice of treatment depends on the exact cause of the lesion. Treatment of most symptomatic partial tears should be directed towards a primary diagnosis such as an impingement syndrome or instability, with treatment of the partial tear itself being considered a part of a broader problem. Nevertheless in traumatic lesions the rotator cuff lesion is the cause of the dynamic impairment and consequently of the secondary inflammatory process and the repairment of the structural problem is the key.

The goal is to achieve a clinical cure. If the signs and symptoms of inflammation are alleviated, and if those due to the mechanical deficiency of the torn cuff are compensated for, by the residual cuff muscles and prime movers, the patient becomes asymptomatic. Then the benefits of an operation should be carefully accessed, taking in to consideration the possibility of tear

progression and of new onset of symptoms based on the quality of the mechanical balance achieved by conservative treatment.

Conservative Treatment

Patients with degenerative partial-thickness tears due to impingement are treated similarly to those with rotator cuff tendinopathy and subacromial bursitis. Time, local rest, application of cold or heat, massage, non-steroidal anti-inflammatory medication for a short period of time, modification of activities, gentle exercises for anterior and posterior capsular stretching, and later, muscle-strengthening for the rotator cuff and the peri-scapular musculature to restore the mechanical balance [35]. Subacromial or intra-articular corticosteroid injections can also be used judiciously, depending on the location of the tear for those patients with persistent symptoms unresponsive to other means of pain reduction. Classically no more than two or three injections should be administered but there is no data to support the view that patients that do not respond to an injection and the described conservative methods, would benefit from the use of more injections.

Fukuda [17] found no evidence of healing occurring in histological sections obtained from partial-thickness tears. Yamanaka [64] followed 40 articular-sided tears treated non-operatively during a 2-year period and found tear progression in 80 % of patients. A decrease in tear size occurred in only 10 %, and complete disappearance of the tear occurred in another 10 %. Therefore, tear progression is the greater concern during non-operative management.

Pain and loss of active elevation have been identified as poor prognostic factors for successful conservative treatment [62]. Most BTs respond poorly to conservative treatment [27]. Once the round circle of subacromial impingement has been established and/or the tear is deep, conservative treatment is rarely helpful. Early surgical intervention should be considered when the severe clinical manifestations and positive imaging suggest a BT diagnosis [11].

Fig. 7 Assessment and debridement of the supraspinatus

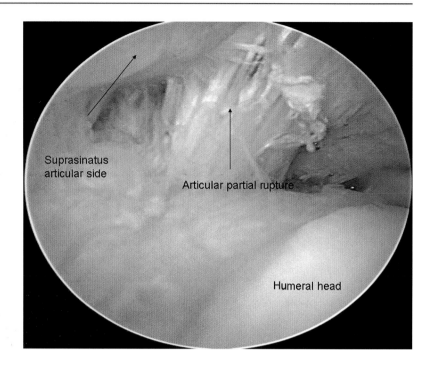

In most cases, 3 months of conservative treatment are sufficient to assess the clinical gains achievable without surgery. A rapid therapeutic response predicts better outcomes. Among the components of the clinical presentation, strength failed to improve [6, 31]. In contrast, conservative treatment consistently alleviated the pain and improved the range of motion.

Operative Treatment

The timing of surgical intervention has to be established according to the age and activity of the patient, type of rupture (degenerative/traumatic), the presence of associated pathology and the response to conservative measures.

The surgical management of partial-thickness supraspinatus tears basically involves one of three options:

1. Arthroscopic debridement of the tear,
2. Debridement with acromioplasty, or
3. Rotator cuff repair with or without acromioplasty.

Surgery may be performed open, arthroscopically-assisted with mini-open approach,

or entirely arthroscopically. Although, there is not sufficient data to support one technique over the other in the management of partial-thickness tears, arthroscopy permits the evaluation of the articular and bursal side of the cuff which represents a major advantage over an open surgical procedure especially in articular partial tears.

Arthroscopic Assessment

Arthroscopy can be performed on a "beach chair" or lateral decubitus position depending on the training and preferences of the surgeon. Through a posterior portal an articular side inspection is performed.

The quality of the supraspinatus should be assessed, fraying should be debrided and the presence of associated lesions should be noted (Fig. 7).

Very often a superior labrum lesion is present. Normally a Snyder type one lesion resulting from vertical dynamic instability of the humeral head and only a debridement should be considered (Fig. 8).

In other rare cases with type two or three "slap" lesions, the stability of the fragments and of the long head of the biceps should be assessed

Fig. 8 Snyder type one lesion

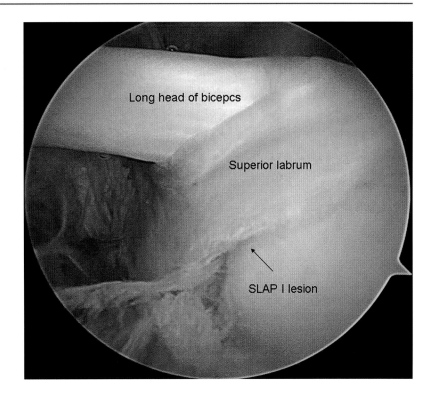

in order to decide whether to repair the lesion or perform a biceps tenodesis.

After debriding the lesion, the extent of the lesion should be measured. Using a bent, preferably calibrated arthroscopic probe, the amount of bone footprint undercovered should be measured and a monofilament suture marker should be passed through the tendon (Fig. 9). Care should be taken to assess the integrity of the biceps posterior pulley and biceps stability (Fig. 10).

Through the same posterior portal the arthroscope is directed to the subacromial space. A careful but complete bursectomy should be performed and the suture marker identified (Fig. 11). The quality of the tendon on the bursal side should be assessed and any indirect signs of impingement, such as fraying of the coraco-acromial arch, should be noted (Fig. 12).

Palpation of the cuff tissue to assess tissue integrity and the injection of saline into the area in question can be used to diagnose intra-tendinous tears.

At this point the surgeon must decide according to his or her experience and depending on the type of rupture, if an all arthroscopic technique, a mini-open technique or an open procedure is should be performed.

Visualisation of the subscapularis tendon and its footprint on the lesser tuberosity is best performed through a posterior viewing portal. Positioning the arm in abduction and internal rotation, the subscapularis insertion and footprint can be easily visualized.

Because of the close proximity of subscapularis and the superior gleno-humeral ligament/coraco-humeral ligament complex on the humeral side, when the subscapularis is detached from the lesser tuberosity, the superior gleno-humeral ligament/coraco-humeral ligament complex is also torn but a portion of it remains attached to the superolateral corner of the subscapularis tendon producing the "comma sign" [29].

In addition, tearing of the superior gleno-humeral ligament/coraco-humeral ligament

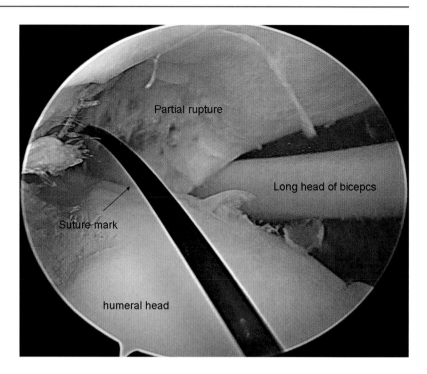

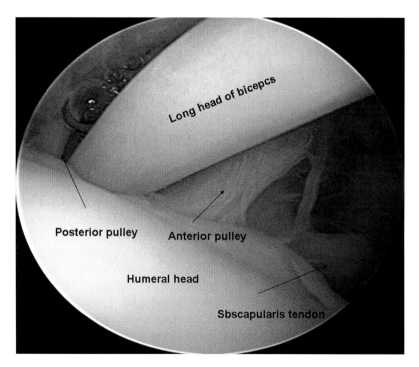

complex disrupts the medial sling of the bicipital sheath predisposing the biceps tendon to subluxation (Fig. 13). Stability can be dynamically evaluated by rotating the arm into internal and external rotation. The long head of the biceps should be also assessed for degeneration, and the amount of partial tearing is estimated by pulling of the biceps tendon intra-articularly [30, 36].

Fig. 11 Identification of the suture mark on the bursal side

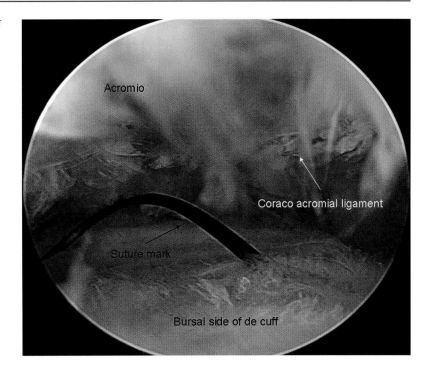

Fig. 12 Fraying of the coraco-acrominal arch

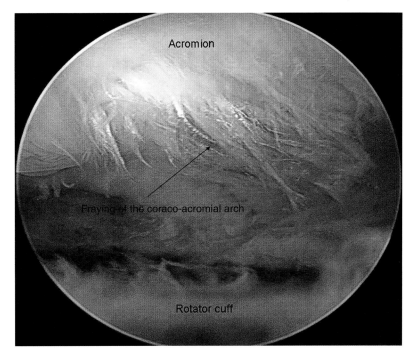

Arthroscopic Debridement Alone

Budoff [8] evaluated 79 shoulders with partial-thickness cuff tears treated with arthroscopic debridement alone with a mean follow-up of 58 months and using the (UCLA) Shoulder Rating Scale, found the results of debridement alone were good to excellent in 89 % in the group of patients with less than 5 years of

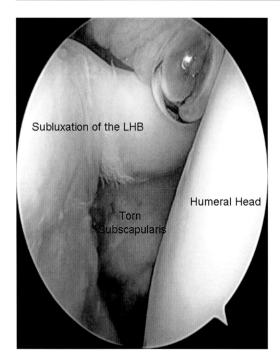

Subluxation of the LHB

Humeral Head

Torn
Subscapularis

Fig. 13 Biceps tendon subluxation

follow-up and decreased to 81 % in those with more than 5 years.

Arthroscopic Debridement and Subacromial Decompression

Release of the coraco-acromial ligament and debridement of the undersurface of the acromion with a high-speed burr to remove any acromial or acromioclavicular spurs (co-planing) have been recommended by some authors for the older patient with either articular-side or bursal-side tears due to external cuff impingement [46, 53].

Snyder [57] in a retrospective study of 31 patients with partial thickness tears treated with debridement and decompression reported 84 % good to excellent results. However, 13 of the 31 patients did not undergo subacromial decompression and no significant difference was found in the outcome, regardless of whether decompression was performed. This fact gives special importance to the mechanical imbalance produced by the injured tendon as a major prognosis factor.

Another study [11] evaluated the clinical outcome of arthroscopic acromioplasty and debridement in 162 patients with normal cuffs and impingement syndrome or partial-thickness tears of the rotator cuff. There was no difference in outcome between those with partial-thickness tears less than 50 % of tendon thickness compared with those without any tears. However, an increased failure rate in patients with grade 2B (bursal-sided tears) even affecting less than 50 % of tendon thickness was detected.

Arthroscopic debridement should be performed in ruptures that involve less than 50 % of the tendon in the articular side. The age and level of activity of the patient should be taken in to account. Bursal side, Ellman type B2 ruptures, should be repaired at an early phase. Subacromial decompression should be performed if there is evidence of an anterior acromial or acromioclavicular spur.

Cuff Repair

The critical decision is to know which patients will benefit from a repair and the ones that should be managed otherwise. Regarding he supraspinatus, once a decision for a repair is made, another decision to be made is whether to do a transtendon repair or to remove the remaining tissue and treat the rupture as a complete rupture. Some authors believe that the cuff material that remains in the immediate area is of poor quality which increases the possibility of post-operative pain and re-rupture [49]. Besides a 5 mm anchor should pass the remnant tissue and the correct positioning can be difficult to achieve. The procedure implies an articular vision and working through the subacromial space to pass the sutures in the cuff (Fig. 14). After this step the previously "cleaned" subacromial space is accessed in order to collect and tie the sutures (Fig. 15).

In a recent work in cadavers from Lomas [39], in situ trans-tendon repair was biomechanically superior to tear completion in articular-sided supraspinatus tears. If a completion of the rupture is decided upon the configuration of the fixation should be designed according to the extent of the rupture, the tissue quality and elasticity. If a single-row technique is used, the sutures of a double-loaded anchor can be passed in a mattress or in a modified Matsen-Allen stitch. If more stability and footprint coverage is necessary, a double-row

Fig. 14 Passing the
sutures

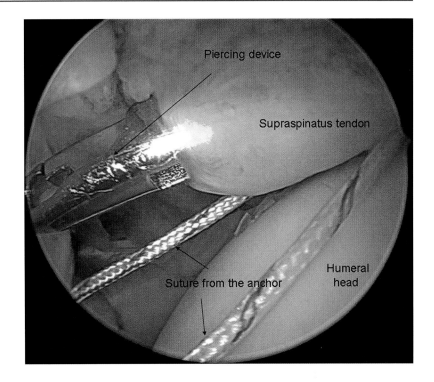

Fig. 15 Passed sutures on
the bursal side

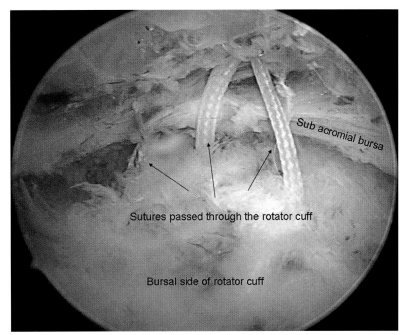

or a suture-bridge configuration should be considered (Fig. 16). The former can be useful especially on poor quality tendons that won't support the outer stitch. For a double-row repair, medial anchors are placed at the medial margin of the rotator cuff footprint just lateral to the articular surface, and the lateral anchors are placed at the lateral margin of the footprint.

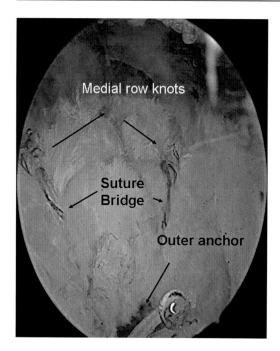

Fig. 16 Suture bridge configuration

On bursal-side ruptures, if maintenance of the articular tissue is decided upon, a fairly external position of the suture anchor is a good solution to achieve a good position of the tendon on the footprint (Fig. 17).

If an intra-tendinous tear is identified, it should be opened on the bursal surface, while viewing from the subacromial space. All non-viable tissue is debrided, with care taken not to disrupt the articular surface attachment of the cuff. Through an accessory anterior working portal multiple vertical mattress No. 2 non-absorbable sutures are passed from anterior to posterior along the entire length of the tear.

The results of surgical treatment of partial thickness supraspinatus ruptures have been presented by several authors [10, 15, 32, 41, 47, 49, 58, 60]. Park compared the results of arthroscopic repair of patients who had partial-thickness rotator cuff tears with those of patients who had full-thickness tears. Evaluation showed that 93 % of all patients had good or excellent results, and 95 % demonstrated satisfactory outcome with regard to pain reduction and

functional outcome. A pre-operative assessment of the acromio-clavicular joint as a potential source of pain was recommended in patients with arthritic changes of this joint. Porat, in a retrospective study of 51 patients with a minimum follow-up of 2 years, reported 83 % of excellent/good results and recommends completion of full thickness tears with an all arthroscopic repair technique.

Regarding the subscapularis, the surgical approach can also be open or athroscopic. In the open technique a delto-pectoral approach should be preferred. After identification of the long head of the biceps the torn subscapularis tendon lying medially to this structure should be free and mobilised from the scarring adhesions. Doing so, the surgeon must be aware of neurovascular structures lying medially to the conjoint tendon. Once the tendon is mobile, the lesser tuberosity should be prepared as well as the bicipital groove if a tenodesis of the long head of the biceps is to be performed. Trans-osseous sutures or suture anchors are used to securely fix the tendon and the biceps to the lesser tuberosity and to the groove.

Arthroscopic repair can be performed viewing from a standard posterior portal in type I and II ruptures but frequently in type III an antero-lateral viewing portal (Fig. 18) is used in order to permit a complete intra- articular and extra-articular assessment of the rupture. The tendon edge is identified after debridement of the middle gleno-humeral ligament from the posterior aspect of the subscapularis and of the subdeltoid and subcoracoid adhesions. In more retracted ruptures the use of a traction suture (Fig. 19) can be helpful. After, the lesser tuberosity is prepared for anchor placement. The author prefers the use of metallic anchors that should be placed along the anterior border of the bicipital groove in order to achieve an anatomic footprint repair. The sutures are passed through the subscapularis tendon with use of a bird-beak suture-passer (Fig. 20). Reconstruction of the footprint should be performed from the most inferior aspect of the torn tendon progressing superiorly in the direction to the rotator interval.

Fig. 17 External position of the suture anchor

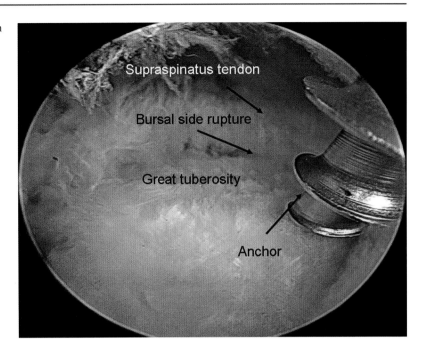

Supraspinatus tendon

Bursal side rupture

Great tuberosity

Anchor

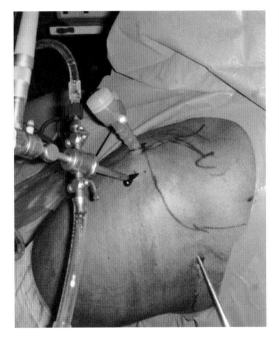

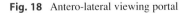

Fig. 18 Antero-lateral viewing portal

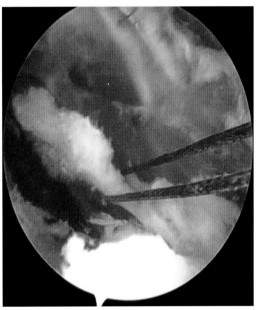

Fig. 19 Traction suture of the subscapularis

According to the works of Edwards [12] and Lafosse [36] open and arthroscopic repair of subscapularis isolated tears can yield marked improvements in shoulder function and pain reduction.

Biceps Tenodesis/Tenotomy

As said previously in this chapter symptoms are most dependent on the inflammatory changes and involvement of the long head of the biceps. For this reason a careful assessment of biceps

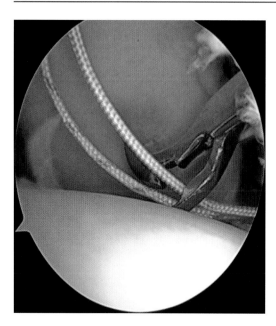

Fig. 20 Passing the sutures through the subscapularis

integrity and stability is mandatory [12]. Our indications for biceps tenodesis/tenotomy include degeneration involving 50 % of the thickness of the tendon or biceps tendon instability due to disruption of the anterior (subscapularis) or posterior (supraspinatus) pulley.

We perform an arthroscopic biceps tenodesis to the bicipital groove using a suture anchor or a simple tenotomy in low function-demanding patients.

Repairing subscapularis tears, with associated biceps dislocation, and trying to preserve and relocate the biceps and stabilise it within the bicipital groove, failed secondary to redislocation of the biceps and should not be recommended [30].

Conclusions

Degenerative partial-thickness tears are an important part of pathology of the rotator cuff with unknown incidence. This condition occurs more often in the population aged over 40 years. Traumatic ruptures occur in a younger and more active population.

Functionally they produce mechanical imbalance responsible for an impingement syndrome. Morphologically, they can be placed between subacromial bursitis/tendinitis, and the full-thickness tear.

Symptoms arise from mechanical impairment with adaptative response of the shoulder girdle and from inflammatory changes and involvement of the long head of the biceps.

The diagnosis is difficult even with MRI and ultrasonography.

With progression of the tear, clinical cure by conservative measures may be impossible to obtain. Surgical treatment with the correct indications has consistent results. The choice of the surgical treatment depends on the type of rupture, the age and level of activity of the patient and of the degree of pain and functional impairment.

In the future, better understanding of injury mechanism, natural history and risk of tear progression, the fine tuning of indications for operative intervention, based on prospective, randomised clinical trials and finally the use of growth factors to stimulate healing [24], as has been applied to other areas of sports Medicine, may contribute to optimise the treatment of this condition.

References

1. Bart JRH, Burkhart SS, de Beer JF. The bear hug test for diagnosing a subscapularis tear. Arthroscopy. 2006;22(10):1076–84.
2. Beaudreil J, Bardin T, Orcel P. Natural history or outcome with conservative treatment of degenerative rotator cuff tears. Joint Bone Spine. 2007;74:527–9.
3. Beaudreuil J, Nizard R, Thomas T, Peyre M, Liotard JP, Boileau P, Marc T, Dromard C, Steyer E, Bardin T, Orcel P, Walch G. Contribution of clinical tests to the diagnosis of rotator cuff disease: a systematic literature review. Joint Bone Spine. 2009;76:15–9.
4. Bey MJ, Ramsey ML, Soslowsky LJ. Intratendinous strainfields of the supraspinatus tendon: effect of a surgically created articular-surface rotator cuff tear. J Shoulder Elbow Surg. 2002;11(6):562–9.
5. Blevins FT, Djurasovic M, Flatow EL, et al. Biology of the rotator cuff tendon. Orthop Clin North Am. 1997;28(1):1–16.

6. Bokor DJ, Hawkins RJ, Huckell GH, Angelo RL, Schickendantz MS. Results of nonoperative management of full-thickness tears of the rotator cuff. Clin Orthop Relat Res. 1993;294:103–10.

7. Brooks CH, Revell WJ, Heatley FW. A quantitative histological study of the vascularity of the rotator cuff tendon. J Bone Joint Surg Am. 1992;74B(1):151–3.

8. Budoff JE, Nirschl RP, Guidi EJ. Debridement of partial-thickness tears of the rotator cuff without acromioplasty: long-term follow-up and review of the literature. J Bone Joint Surg Am. 1998;80:733–48.

9. Clark JM, Harryman II DT. Tendons ligaments, and capsule of the rotator cuff. J Bone Joint Surg Am. 1992;74A(5):713–25.

10. Conway JE. Arthroscopic repair of partial-thickness rotator cuff tears and SLAP lesions in professional baseball players. Orthop Clin North Am. 2001; 32:443–56.

11. Cordasco FA, Backer M, Craig EV, Klein D, Warren RF. The partial thickness rotator cuff tear: is acromioplasty without repair sufficient? Am J Sports Med. 2002;30:257–60.

12. Edwards BT, Walch G, Sirveaux F, Molé D, Noveé-Josserand J, Boulahia A, Leyton L, Szabo I, Lindgren B. Repair of tears of the subscapularis. J Bone Joint Surg Am. 2005;87A:725–30.

13. Ellman H. Diagnosis and treatment of incomplete rotator cuff tears. Clin Orthop. 1990;254:64–74.

14. Ferrari FS, Governi S, Burresi F, Vigni F, Stefani P. Supraspinatus tendon tears: comparison of US and MR arthrography with surgical correlation. Eur Radiol. 2002;12:1211–7.

15. Fukuda H. The management of partial- thickness tears of the rotator cuff. J Bone Joint Surg Am. 2003;85-B (1):2–11.

16. Fukuda H, Craig EV, Yamanaka K. Surgical treatment of incomplete thickness tears of rotator cuff: long-term follow-up. Orthop Trans. 1987;11:237–8.

17. Fukuda H, Hamada K, Nakajima T, Tomonaga A. Pathology and pathogenesis of the intratendinous tearing of the rotator cuff viewed from en bloc histologic sections. Clin Orthop Relat Res. 1994;304: 60–7.

18. Fukuda H, Mikasa M, Ogawa K, Yamanaka K, Hamada K. The partial thickness tear of the rotator cuff. Orthop Trans. 1983;7:137.

19. Gartsman GM, Milne JC. Articular surface partial-thickness rotator cuff tears. J Shoulder Elbow Surg. 1995;4:409–15.

20. Gerber C, Krushell RJ. Isolated rupture of the tendon of the subscapularis muscle. Clinical features in 16 cases. J Bone Joint Surg Br. 1991;73:389–94.

21. Gerber C, Hersche O, Farron A. Isolated rupture of the subscapularis tendon. J Bone Joint Surg Am. 1996; 78:1015–23.

22. Gohlke F, Essigkrug B, Schmitz F. The pattern of the collagen fiber bundles of the capsule of the glenohumeral joint. J Shoulder Elbow Surg. 1994; 3:111–28.

23. Gotoh M, Hamada K, Yamakawa H, Inoue A, Fukuda H. Increased substance P in subacromial bursa and shoulder pain in rotator cuff diseases. J Orthop Res. 1998;16:618–21.

24. Gulotta VL, Rodeo SA. Growth factors for rotator cuff repair. Clin Sports Med. 2009;28:13–23.

25. Habermeyer P, Krieter C, Tang K, Lichtenberg S, Magosch P. A new arthroscopic classification of articular-sided supraspinatus footprint lesions: a prospective comparison withSnyder's and Ellman's classification. J Shoulder Elbow Surg. 2008;17:909–13.

26. Hashimoto T, Nobuhara K, Hamada T. Pathologic evidence of degeneration as a primary cause of rotator cuff tear. Clin Orthop Relat Res. 2003;415: 111–20.

27. Hawkins RH, Dunlop R. Nonoperative treatment of rotator cuff tears. Clin Orthop. 1995;321:178–88.

28. Yadav H, Nho S, Romeo A, MacGillivray JD. Rotator cuff tears: pathology and repair. Knee Surg Sports Traumatol Arthrosc. 2009;17:409–21.

29. Lo IK, Burkhart SS. The comma sign: an arthroscopic guide to the torn subscapularis tendon. Arthroscopy. 2003;19:334–7.

30. Ian K, Lo Y, Burkhart SS. The etiology and assessment of subscapularis tendon tears: a case for subcoracoid impingement, the roller-wringer effect, and TUFF lesions of the subscapularis. Arthroscopy. 2003;19:1142–50.

31. Itoi E, Tabata S. Conservative treatment of rotator cuff tears. Clin Orthop Relat Res. 1992;275:165e73.

32. Itoi E, Tabata S. Incomplete rotator cuff tears: results of operative treatment. Clin Orthop. 1992;284:128–35.

33. Kassarjian A, Bencardino JT, Palmer WE. MR imaging of the rotator cuff. Radiol Clin North Am. 2006;44:503–23, vii–viii.

34. Kelly BT, Williams RJ, Cordasco FA, Backus SI, Otis JC, Weiland DE, Craig EV, Wickiewicz DE, Warren RF. Differential patterns of muscle activation in patients with symptomatic and asymptomatic rotator cuff tears. J Shoulder Elbow Surg. 2005; 14:165–71.

35. Kuhn JE. Exercise in the treatment of rotator cuff impingement: a systematic review and a synthesized evidence based rehabilitation protocol. J Shoulder Elbow Surg. 2009;18:138–60.

36. Lafosse L, Jost B, Reiland Y, Audebert S, Toussaint B, Gobezie R. Structural integrity and clinical outcomes after arthroscopic repair of isolated subscapularis tears. J Bone Joint Surg Am. 2007;89:1184–93.

37. Langenderfer JE, Patthanacharoenphon C, Carpenter JE, Hughes RE. Variation in external rotation moment arms among subregions of supraspinatus, infraspinatus, and teres minor muscles. J Orthop Res. 2006;24(8):1737–44.

38. Lohr JF, Uhthoff HK. The microvascular pattern of the supraspinatus tendon. Clin Orthop. 1990;254:35–8.

39. Lomas G, Kippe MA, Brown GD, Gardner TR, Ding A, Levine WN, Ahmad CS. In situ transtendon repair outperforms tear completion and repair for

partial articular-sided supraspinatus tendon tears. J Shoulder Elbow Surg. 2008;17:722–8.

40. Malcarney HL, Murrell GAC. The rotator cuff – biological adaptations to its environment. J Sports Med. 2003;33(13):993–1002.

41. Matava MJ, Purcell DB, Rudzki JR. Partial-thickness rotator cuff tears. Am J Sports Med. 2005;33:1405–17.

42. McConville OR, Ianotti JP. Partial-thickness tears of the rotator cuff: evaluation and management. J Am Acad Orthop Surg. 1999;7:32–43.

43. Mell AG, Lascalza S, Guffey P, Ray J, Maciejewski M, Carpenter JE, Hughes RE. Effects of rotator cuff pathology on shoulder rhythm. J Shoulder Elbow Surg. 2005;14:58S–64.

44. Moosmayer S, Smith J, Tariq R, Larmo A. Prevalence and characteristics of asymptomatic tears of the rotator cuff. J Bone Joint Surg Br. 2009;91-B:196–200.

45. Moseley HF, Goldie I. The arterial pattern of the rotator cuff and the shoulder. J Bone Joint Surg Br. 1963;45B:780–9.

46. Olsewski JM, Depew AD. Arthrscopic subacromial decompression and rotator cuff debridement for stage II and stage III impingement. Arthroscopy. 1994;10:61–8.

47. Park JY, Chung KT, Yoo MJ. A serial comparison of arthroscopic repairs for partial- and full-thickness rotator cuff tears. Arthroscopy. 2004;20:705–11.

48. Perry SM, Getz CL. Soslowsky alterations in function after rotator cuff tears in an animal model. J Shoulder Elbow Surg. 2009;18:296–304.

49. Porat S, Nottage WM, Fouse MN. Repair of partial thickness rotator cuff tears: a retrospective review with minimum two-year follow-up. J Shoulder Elbow Surg. 2008;17:729–31.

50. Rathbun JB, Macnab I. The microvascular pattern of the rotator cuff. J Bone Joint Surg Br. 1970;52B:540–53.

51. Ruotolo C, Fow JE, Nottage WM. The supraspinatus footprint: an anatomic study of the supraspinatus insertion. Arthroscopy. 2004;20(3):246–9.

52. Sakurai G, Ozaki J, Tomita Y, Kondo T, Tamai S. Incomplete tears of the subscapularis tendon associated with tears of the supraspinatus tendon: cadaveric and clinical studies. J ShoulderElbow Surg. 1998;7:510–5.

53. Seitz WH, Froimson AI, Sordon TL. A comparison of arthroscopic subacromial decompression for full thickness versus partial thickness rotator cuff tears. Paper #36, ASES Specialty Day, Anaheim, CA; March 1991.

54. Yang S, Park HS, Flores S, Levin SD, Makhsous M, Lin F, Koh J, Nuber J, Zhang LQ. Biomechanical analysis of bursal-sided partial thickness rotator cuff tears. J Shoulder Elbow Surg. 2009;18:379–85.

55. Sher JS, Uribe JW, Posada A, Murphy BJ, Zlatkin MB. Abnormal findings on magnetic resonance images of asymptomatic shoulders. J Bone Joint Surg Am. 1995;77-A:10–5.

56. Snyder SJ, editor. Arthroscopic classification of rotator cuff lesions and surgical decision making. In: Shoulder arthroscopy. 2nd ed. Philadelphia: Lippincott Williams & Wilkins; 2003. p. 201–7.

57. Snyder SJ, Pachelli AF, Del Pizzo W, Friedman MJ, Ferkel RD, Pattee G. Partial thickness rotator cuff tears: results of arthroscopic treatment. Arthroscopy. 1991;7:1–7.

58. Soslowsky LJ, Carpenter JE, Bucchieri JS. Biomechanics of the rotator cuff. Orthop Clin North Am. 1997;28(1):17–30.

59. Walch G, Boileau P, Noel E, Donell ST. Impingement of the deep surface of the supraspinatus tendon on the posterosuperior glenoid rim: an arthroscopic study. J Shoulder Elbow Surg. 1992;1:238–45.

60. Weber SC. Arthroscopic debridement and acromioplasty versus mini-open repair in the treatment of significant partial-thickness rotator cuff tears. Arthroscopy. 1999;15:126–31.

61. Vlychou M, Dailiana Z, Fotiadou A, Papanagiotou M, Fezoulidis IV, Malizos KN. Symptomatic partial rotator cuff tears: diagnostic performance of ultrasound and magnetic resonance imaging with surgical correlation. Acta Radiol. 2009;1:101–5.

62. Yamaguchi K, Tetro MA, Blam O, Evanoff BA, Teefey SA, Middleton WD. Natural history of asymptomatic rotator cuff tears: a longitudinal analysis of asyntomatic tears detected sonographically. J Shoulder Elbow Surg. 2001;10(3):199–203.

63. Yamanaka K, Fukuda H. Pathological studies of the supraspinatus tendon with reference to incomplete thickness tear. In: Takagishi N, editor. The shoulder. Tokyo: Professional Postgraduate Services; 1987. p. 220–4.

64. Yamanaka K, Matsumoto T. The joint side tear of the rotator cuff: a follow-up study by arthrography. Clin Orthop Relat Res. 1994;304:68–73.

65. Zeitoun-Eiss D, Brasseur JL,Goldmard JL. Corrélations entre la sémiologie échographique et la douleur dans les ruptures transfixiantes de la coiffe dês rotateurs. In: BlumA, Tavernier T, Brasseur JL, et al., editors. Une approche pluridisciplinaire. Montpellier: Sauramps médical; 2005. p. 287e94.

Arthroscopic Management of Full-Thickness Rotator Cuff Tears

Jean-François Kempf, Aristote Hans-Moevi, and Philippe Clavert

Contents

Abstract

Objective Regain shoulder function and freedom of pain through arthroscopic fixation of the torn rotator cuff using anchors and tension bands.

Indications Indications have increased these recent years, with the tremendous technical progress of arthroscopic surgeons. They are:

1. Isolated full-tendon rupture of the supraspinatus.
2. All full-tendon tears of the supraspinatus, the infraspinatus or the teres minor, in cases of moderate retraction.
3. Incomplete tears affecting the superior part of the subscapularis, either isolated or associated with a rupture of the supraspinatus.
4. For lesions of the long head of the biceps: tenodesis for patients <60 years of age or for manual workers; tenotomy in all other instances.

Contra-indications Fatty infiltration of infraspinatus and subscapularis of stages 3 and 4.

Frozen shoulder in the active phase.

Narrowing of the subacromial space (<7 mm).

Relative contra-indications: Patients ≥65 years.

Surgical Technique Subacromial bursoscopy and glenohumeral arthroscopy.

Repair of the tendons using a posterior portal and an inside-out anterior portal, associated

J.-F. Kempf (✉) • A. Hans-Moevi • P. Clavert
Centre de Chirurgie Orthopedique et de la Main, Illkirch-Graffenstaden, France
e-mail: jean-francois.kempf@chru-strasbourg.fr

G. Bentley (ed.), *European Surgical Orthopaedics and Traumatology*,
DOI 10.1007/978-3-642-34746-7_46, © EFORT 2014

with one or two additional anterolateral portals.

Attachment with a single row or double row anchors.

Tenotomy/tenodesis of long head of biceps, if indicated.

Keywords

Arthroscopy • Repair • Rotator cuff • Shoulder • Surgical technique

Introduction

Shoulder arthroscopy was developed in the USA in the 1980s [1, 17, 27, 39, 40, 67] and introduced subsequently in Europe. The surgical technique has improved over the years due to better material and equipment [50, 51].

Tears of the rotator cuff vary, not only in respect to their location but also to their degree of disruption. It is well known that normal tendons never tear and that pre-existing conditions decrease the tensile strength of the tendon. Two mechanisms have been discussed:

1. Intrinsic factors [4, 18, 41, 55, 61]: age-related changes that take place in a more or less well-vascularized tendon lead to a weakening of the tendons' mechanical properties.
2. Extrinsic factors: these factors are mechanical and responsible of an impingement that either leads to a progressive attrition or to a sudden traumatic failure at the level of the enthesis of the tendon. The most common is the subacromial impingement, according to Neer, [53] that results in a subacromial abrasion of the bursal layers of the supraspinatus. During forward elevation and abduction of the arm the coraco-acromial arch exerts a friction on the tendon. A second location of impingement is found between the subscapularis and the coracoid process, also known as subcoracoid impingement [32, 36]. A third site has been described posterosuperiorly between the articular surface of the supra- and infraspinatus and the posterosuperior edge of the labrum [37, 38, 63, 64]. Tears at these sites occur mostly in middle- aged persons and manual workers.

All ruptures undergo a progressive deterioration accompanied by a medial retraction of the musculotendinous stump. The muscle loses its elasticity and becomes the site of a fatty infiltration. Ruptures not only affect the active range of motion but also the relationship between humeral head and glenoid. In instances of supraspinatus tears, a superior translation of the humeral head occurs in abduction and forward elevation caused by the absence of the depressor effect of this muscle.

This upward displacement is compensated by an increased depressor action of the subscapularis and the infraspinatus.

The abnormal movements may eventually lead to glenohumeral osteoarthritis and to a progressive loss of the centric position of the humeral head.

Disruption of the subscapularis can influence the anteroposterior stability, particularly when its distal part is involved.

Surgical Principles and Objective

Arthroscopy of the shoulder, inspection of the glenohumeral joint and the subacromial space. Fixation of the torn tendon with suture anchors using the tension band principle to achieve restitution of function and relief of pain.

Advantages of the Arthroscopic Procedure

- Less damage to peri-articular structures, in particular to the acromial insertion of the deltoid, in comparison to open procedures.
- Decreased risk of infection.
- Shorter hospital stay, in general 24–48 h, or out-patient surgery.
- Increased patient comfort.
- Shorter functional recovery period.
- Absence of displeasing scars.

Indications

- Complete cuff tears in active patients <65 years of age.
- In older patients the indications depend on the state of the tendon, the clinical and radiologic findings, and the patient's motivation.

- Partial tears affecting >50 % of the tendon thickness [66].
- For subscapularis tears the indication is open to discussion given the technical difficulties.

Therefore, we personally limit the indications to incomplete tears affecting the superior part, either isolated or associated with rupture of the supraspinatus.

For Associated Lesions of the Long Head of the Biceps

- Tenodesis in patients <60 years of age or in manual workers, tenotomy in all other instances.

Contra-Indications

- Poor prognosis of repairs, and technical limitation [5, 21, 65].
- Fatty infiltration of infraspinatus and subscapularis of stages 3 and 4 [34].
- Frozen shoulder in the active phase.
- Narrowing of the subacromial space (<7 mm). As shown by Walch [62], good clinical result after repair may be obtained only when the remaining subacromial space is greater than 7 mm. It is always the case for an isolated and distal supraspinatus tear.
- Poor compliance expected during rehabilitation.
- Complete tear of the posterosuperior cuff reaching the teres minor.
- Complete tear of the subscapularis (relative).
- Patients ≥65 years (relative).

Patient Information

- General surgical risks such as thrombophlebitis, embolism, infection, injury to neurovascular structures.
- Explain in simple terms the pathological condition of the shoulder, preferably with the help of a plastic shoulder model.
- Inform the patient that spontaneous healing cannot be expected, that the prognosis without surgery is not favourable, and that in the absence of repair the eventual outcome may be osteoarthritis of the glenohumeral joint.
- Surgery will result in an almost normal function and will decrease pain. For this to be achieved, the torn tendon will be re-attached to bone [33].

Explain principles of arthroscopy and the possible need for open surgery.

- Enumerate possible complications such as recurrence of the tear, reaction to sutures, or injury to articular cartilage.
- Insist on the need for post-operative physiotherapy and explain the basic methods to be used.
- Expected absence from work: 4–6 months.
- If possible, a relevant patient's educational media explaining the procedure and post-operative care should be supplied.

Pre-Operative Work-Up

- For the proper patient selection for arthroscopic repair, a detailed history, a full physical examination and complementary examinations (CT arthrogram, arthro-MRI) are necessary. Only thereafter, a decision can be made as to whether an arthroscopic repair is indicated. The patient's history should include kind of work, dominant side, onset and kind of symptoms, work-related accident, previous treatments, and limitation of function.
- Advanced age, an accident at work or an occupational disease constitute factors contributing to a poor prognosis. Compliance of the patient is very important, as a perfect operation without proper post-operative rehabilitation will lead to a poor result.
- Physical examination includes inspection of the shoulder to detect possible muscle atrophy. Atrophy in the absence of a tear may indicate involvement of the suprascapular nerve. Check for possible rupture of long head of biceps. Inspection is followed by palpation with the purpose to find the site of maximum pain. The degree of active and passive motion should be recorded. Various shoulder-specific tests should be executed (Neer, Hawkins and Yocum tests, relocation test, palm-up test, Speed test, Yergason test).

Specific tests of the subscapularis include the lift-off and press belly test [29], for the supraspinatus the Jobe test, and for the infraspinatus the external rotation against resistance with the elbow at the side [46, 56].

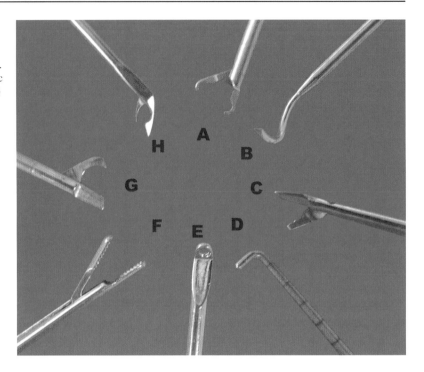

Fig. 1 Different arthroscopic surgical instruments. (**a**) Suture retriever. (**b**) Suture Hook. (**c**) Punch. (**d**) arthroscopic hook. (**e**): Knot pusher. (**f**) Grasper. (**g**) Scissor. (**h**) Bird Peak

- Complimentary examinations include plain radiographs in the scapular plane with true anteroposterior view in internal, neutral and external rotation and a supraspinatus outlet view [49]. The subacromial space must be measured.
- To define the lesion of the rotator cuff in detail, we recommend a CT arthrogram or arthro-MRI. These examinations allow the determination of the degree of fatty infiltration of the subscapularis and the infraspinatus based on the classification of Goutallier et al. [23, 34, 35], as well as the degree of muscular atrophy involving supraspinatus.

Surgical Instruments and Implants

- Pressure-monitoring fluid-pumping system.
- Electrocautery.
- Motorized shaving system with suction.
- Arthroscopic instruments (Fig. 1): forceps to grasp suture, hook for suture passage, arthroscopic scissors, arthroscopic hook, knot pusher, grasping forceps, "Bird Beak®" forceps.

- Anchors and sutures:
  - We choose from a wide variety of anchors available, including metallic anchors with eyelets [3], bioabsorbables anchors
  - We prefer non-resorbable sutures such as Ethibond® 3–0 (Ethicon, Somerville, NJ, USA, Johnson and Johnson) or re-inforced sutures as Fiberwire® 2–0 (Arthrex) or Orthocord® (Mitek).

Anaesthesia and Positioning

- Interscalene nerve block supplemented by light sedation [26] or more often general anaesthesia. A catheter can be used for post-operative pain relief.
- "Beach-chair" position on a Maquet table avoids very often the need for traction. The head is placed in a head support. Care must be taken to have a free access of the posterior part of the shoulder.
- Free draping of arm for easy manipulation.
- Slight flexion of knees. This position is comfortable for the patient. The entire positioning

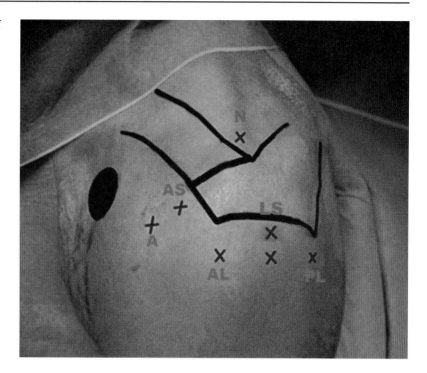

Fig. 2 Anterior views of arthroscopic portals

allows conversion to an open procedure without the need for repositioning of the patient.

Surgical Technique

Portal Placements for Glenohumeral Joint

Primary posterior portal (P): 2 cm distal and 1 cm medial to the posterolateral border of the acromion passing between infraspinatus and teres minor. A blunt trocar is inserted in the direction of the coracoid process permitting to enter the Superior part of the joint. This position is checked with the camera before opening the irrigation (Figs. 2 and 3).

Postero-inferior portal (not shown): the entry point lies 2 cm inferior to the posterior portal. This portal is used to access the postero-inferior capsule pouch.

Anterior portal (A): this access is created by the inside-out technique under arthroscopic control through the posterior portal to avoid injury to the musculocutaneous nerve. Using the outside-in technique, a spinal needle is passed through the rotator interval that is limited medially by the anterosuperior portion of the glenoid, superiorly by the long head of the biceps, and inferiorly by the subscapularis muscle. The skin incision is located next to the needle, and a Wissinger rod is advanced into the joint. A cannula is then passed over the rod.

Anterosuperior portal (AS): this additional portal is placed 1–2 cm in front of the acromioclavicular joint. It must be lateral and superior to the coracoid process to avoid injury to the musculocutaneous nerve. The position of the spinal needle used is checked with the arthroscope.

Superior portal (N; Neviaser): the entry point is located between the posterior margin of the distal end of the clavicle and the medial border of the acromion. To avoid damage to the suprascapular nerve, the patient's head should be inclined to the opposite side.

The spinal needle must pass behind the insertion of the long head of the biceps.

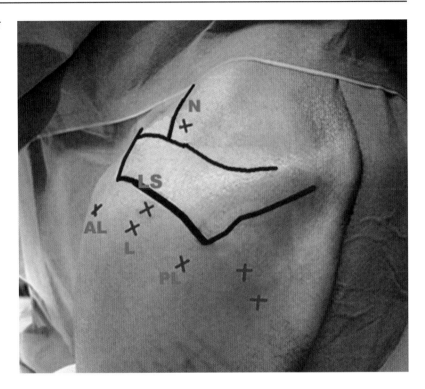

Portal Placements for the Subacromial Bursoscopy

In addition to the already described anterior (A) and posterior (P) portals, the posterolateral (PL), the anterolateral (AL), the lateral (L), and the laterosuperior (LS) portals can be used.

The posterolateral portal is placed 2 cm distal to the posterolateral angle of the acromion. The entry point to the anterolateral portal is found 2 cm distal to the anterolateral angle of the acromion. The lateral portal is placed 1 or 2 cm lateral to the acromion and 2 cm behind its anterior border. The entry point to the laterosuperior portal is placed 1–2 cm above the lateral portal under the lateral border of the acromion.

How to Pass Sutures Through Tendons: Tips and Tricks

Many Tools are available to pass sutures through tendons. Whatever our choice, some rules must be respected.

The Tools
A Needle

The cheapest tool is a simple spinal needle! You can deform it, adjust its curvature, in order to adapt the needle and pass a rigid suture such as a PDS which will be used as shuttle relay to place the definitive suture through the tendon (Fig. 4).

Others Solutions (More Expensive)

A suture-passer such as the Banana Lasso (Fig. 5) or others suture-passers with various curved tip configurations can be used for arthroscopic Bankart, SLAP & rotator cuff repairs.

Others Suture-passers such as "bird Peak" allow fast tissue penetration and suture retrieval (Fig. 6).

Retrievers are designed for atraumatic suture retrieval and manipulation

The Crochet Hook (Spectrum Suture-Passer®-Linvatec) (Figs. 7 and 8) will offer surgeons an easy suture passing, with the possibility to choose between crescent hook ([45] right or left hook, or more).

Fig. 4 The cheapest tool: a needle

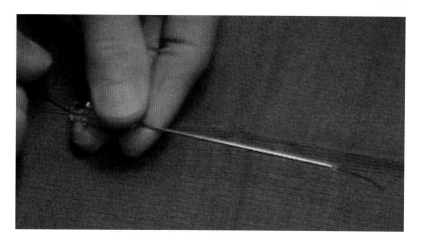

We recommend to use at the same time of a grasper to maintain the tendon stable and facilitate the passage of the PDS suture through the tendon.

The Suture Pinchers

The combination of a grasper and a suture passing pinch combine the need for precision and speed of arthroscopic surgery. Their design allows for one-handed surgery (and one shot!) (Fig. 9).

Many companies offer this kind of device, allowing the surgeon to pass sutures through soft tissue in a single step, for instance EXPRESSEW™ (Mitek), the Scorpion® or the Viper® (Arthrex).

Which Kind of Suture?

The easiest suture is the simple stitch (Fig. 10)

The most common is the mattress suture

The strongest is the Mason-Allen modified by Gerber [30], but difficult to do arthroscopically
1. The simple stitch:
   Could be enough in some simple cases
2. The mattress suture (Fig. 11):
   • Simple
   • The Lasso Loop described by Lafosse [47].
   • The Haubannage (Mattress-Tension-Band (Boileau) [6, 7] easy to do with a "crochet hook".

Arthroscopic Knots

A wide variety of arthroscopic knots exists [42]. Fingers needed to make these knots are represented. The dark thread is wrapped around the red thread (the post) that is held by three fingers: thumb; index and middle finger. We use the following sliding knots: SMC [43, 44], Roeder, MCK, MSK, Duncan, and Nicky. They have the advantage of not being too bulky and also are easy to lock. Before tying the knot, one has to verify that the suture slides easily. If it does not, a standard knot, with two half hitches thrown in the same direction, should be followed by five half-hitches alternated in direction (Fig. 12).

For the last two half-hitches, the post should be alternated.

Irrespective of the type of sliding knot used, the knot must be backed up by three half-hitches to be secured! [60]. Mastery of the technique is mandatory [14, 15, 17, 54].

The Different Suture Techniques

Two main options: the single row technique and the double row [52].

Double-row rotator cuff repair techniques incorporate a medial and lateral row of suture anchor in the repair configuration. Clinical studies, however, have not demonstrated

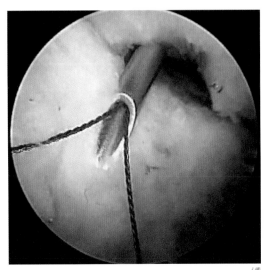

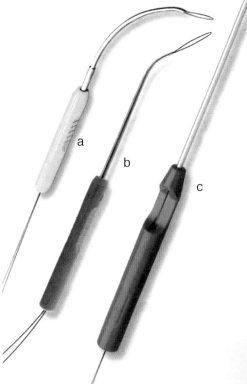

Fig. 5 Example of a suture passer with a lasso: The Banana lasso®

a substantial improvement over single-row repair with regard to either the degree of structural healing or functional outcomes! [24].

Arthroscopic Suture Techniques of the Supraspinatus: Single Row Technique

Before proceeding with a rotator cuff repair, an exploration of the glenohumeral joint is imperative. This is achieved through the posterior portal, and an assessment of all intra-articular structures, including the long head of the biceps, is carried out. The tear is visualized and its size and morphology are assessed. The tendon stumps are retracted. The 'scope is then introduced into the subacromial space through the posterior portal. The anterior portal is placed by an inside-out technique. Careful debridment of the subacromial space with a motorized shaver introduced through a lateral portal is performed. If the acromion is prominent, an acromioplasty is performed with a motorized burr at the beginning of the procedure to enlarge the subacromial space.

With the forceps introduced through the lateral portal the stump of the tendon is grasped and pulled toward the greater tuberosity. This allows determining whether a re-insertion is possible or not.

A juxtaglenoid capsulotomy with a hooked electrocautery may allow added mobilization of the tendon. Two situations are possible:
1. The tendon can be sufficiently mobilized and re-inserted.
2. The tendon is retracted and thus prevents its suture to the greater tuberosity requiring the margin convergence technique, as described by Burkhart [10–16] (see Fig. 13).

If re-insertion is possible, multiple anchors inserted at the Lateral Superior surface of the greater tuberosity are used. Their number depends on the size of the tear. They are spaced every 5–8 mm (Fig. 14).

Although several techniques have been described, we describe the authors' preferred method. The technique using one row of anchors, also known as tension-band technique, described by Boileau [6–8] (Fig. 15).

A Suture Hook® (Linvatec) is used to facilitate suture passage through the tendon. Its use involves the initial passage of a small-diameter monofilament-type PDS® suture or of a suture

Fig. 6 Different others tools to pass the suture through the tendon: the "Bird Peak"

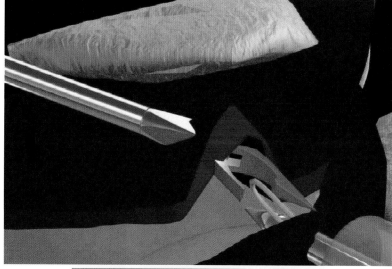

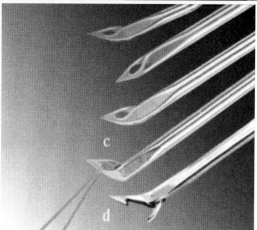

Relay® Shuttle (Linvatec). The Suture Hook® with its hook pointing to the right for the right shoulder and to the left for the left shoulder is introduced through the anterior or anterolateral portal or – less often – through the lateral portal for very posterior ruptures. By this way the relay suture is passed through the tendon 1 cm medial from its free end and allows a good purchase in the tendon. The free end of the PDS suture is grasped with a forceps and the definitive non-absorbable suture (or number 5 Orthocord®, Mytek, or a number 5 Fiberwire®, Arthrex) is tied to the PDS® or placed in the loop of the shuttle Relay. The non-absorbable

suture is then shuttled back through the tendon by withdrawing the PDS® (or the Shuttle Relay®). The anterior suture is withdrawn with the suture forceps through the lateral portal in order to get the two sutures through the lateral portal.

This technique allows making U-stitches that have a better purchase in the stump than simple stitches. Moreover, it allows a perfect and uniform approximation of the tendon stump to the freshened bony surface thanks to the tension-band effect.

The knot pusher or the suture forceps is slid down each suture to assure absence of tissue

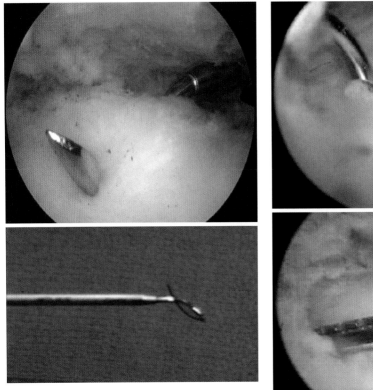

Fig. 7 A suture passer: the Spectrum® (Livatec)

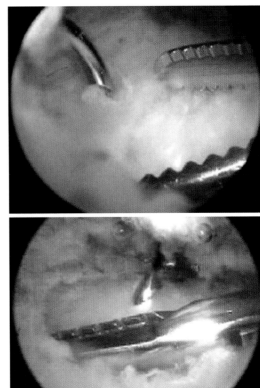

Fig. 8 Simultaneus use of a grasper and the Crochet Hook

tangling. To facilitate suturing, the arm is placed in abduction. The sliding knot is fashioned over the post and pushed down with a knot pusher under direct visualization. Once in contact with the tendon and locked, three half-hitches complete and secure the knot.

The sutures are cut at 5 mm from the knot with the arthroscopic scissors or a suture cutter. The other stitches are placed using the same technique.

Boileau report good results with this simple technique [6]. He reported 65 consecutive shoulders with a chronic full-thickness supraspinatus tear which were repaired arthroscopically with the use of a tension-band suture technique. Patients ranged in age from 29 to 79 years. The average duration of follow-up was 29 months. Fifty-one patients had a computed tomographic arthrogram, and fourteen had a magnetic resonance imaging scan, performed between 6 months and 3 years after surgery. All patients were assessed with regard to function and the strength of the shoulder elevation. Results: The rotator cuff was completely healed and watertight in 46 (71 %) of the 65 patients and was partially healed in 3. Although the supraspinatus tendon did not heal to the tuberosity in 16 shoulders, the size of the persistent defect was smaller than the initial tear in 15. Sixty-two of the sixty-five patients were satisfied with the result. The Constant score improved from an average (and standard deviation) of 51.6 ± 10.6 points pre-operatively to 83.8 ± 10.3 points at the time of the last follow-up evaluation ($p < 0.001$). The average strength of the shoulder elevation was significantly better ($p = 0.001$) when the tendon had healed (7.3 ± 2.9 kg) than when it had not (4.7 ± 1.9 kg). Factors that were negatively associated with tendon healing were increasing age

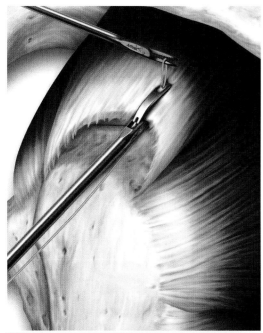

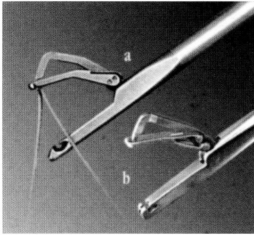

Fig. 9 2 examples of suture Pinches: the Scorpion® or The Viper® (Arthrex)

and associated delamination of the subscapularis or infraspinatus tendon. Only 10 (43 %) of 23 patients over the age of 65 years had completely healed tendons ($p < 0.001$). The author concludes that arthroscopic repair of an isolated supraspinatus detachment commonly leads to complete tendon healing. The absence of healing of the repaired rotator cuff is associated with inferior muscle strength. Patients over

the age of 65 years ($p = 0.001$) and patients with associated delamination of the subscapularis and/or the infraspinatus ($p = 0.02$) have significantly lower rates of healing.

A French multicentric study of the SFA found the same conclusions [22].

The Double-Row Technique

Re-establishment of the native footprint during rotator cuff repair has been suggested to be important for optimizing fixation strength and healing potential. However, the complexity of most double-row repairs and the added surgical time remains a concern.

In this repair method, 2 rows of anchors are used to fix the cuff (Fig. 16), one along the articular cartilage margin and the other at the lateral ridge of the greater tuberosity. This technique increases the strength of repair by increasing the number of sutures passed through the tendon, as well as increasing the area of contact between the tendon and bone [46].

For many cases (small or medium tears), it is possible to do a double row with only two anchors, using the two strands (of various colours) of the first suture of the medial anchor to do a "bar" and then a Haubannage with the two strands of the second suture fixed laterally with a second impacted anchor (Fig. 17). In this situation, we don't need to tie knots inside the joint, as described by Boileau [8]. The technique, termed mattress-tension-band (MTB), is performed with 1 screwed anchor inserted medially at the articular margin and an impacted anchor inserted laterally on the greater tuberosity. An extra-corporeally-tied knot figure-of-8 forms the mattress suture medially, whereas a knotless tension-band is placed laterally. The mattress-tension-band technique restores the rotator cuff footprint anatomy in a simple, quick, and reproducible manner, thus reducing operative time. The main advantages are that there is no need to tie any knot inside the joint and that the only knot, tied extra-corporeally, cannot slip, thereby improving initial strength and stiffness of the repair.

An other possibility, the suture bridge technique (Fig. 18), involves using a medial row anchors with sutures passed and tied through the

Fig. 10 Different kind of sutures

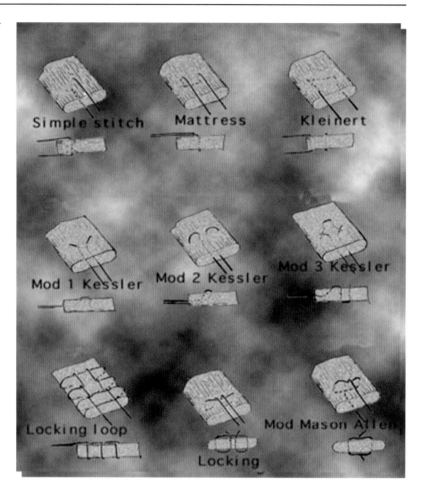

tendon medially, after which the suture tails are draped over the remaining lateral cuff tendon and fixed laterally. This repair configuration has been shown to increase the contact area and has an « Haubannage « effect (=tension-band technique + medial mattress suture).

Discussion: What Type of Suture: Single or Double Row?

Snyder [57, 58] recently recommend a single row of suture anchors with two or three sutures per Anchor associated with multiple perforations placed through the cortical bone of the greater tuberosity into the bone marrow space, laterally to the sutures. He commonly observed on MRI

post-operative follow-up examinations that the footprint of the rotator cuff completely regenerates to cover the greater tuberosity (« Crimson Duvet ») despite having been completely debrided of all soft tissues at the time of the repair.

According to Dines [19], we agree that biomechanical studies of double-row repair showed increased load to failure, improved contact areas and pressures and decreased gap formation at the healing enthesis [46]. A double row of suture anchors increases the tendon-bone contact area, reconstituting a more anatomical configuration of the rotator cuff footprint.

The authors recruited 60 patients. In 30 patients, rotator cuff repair was performed with a single-row suture anchor technique (group 1).

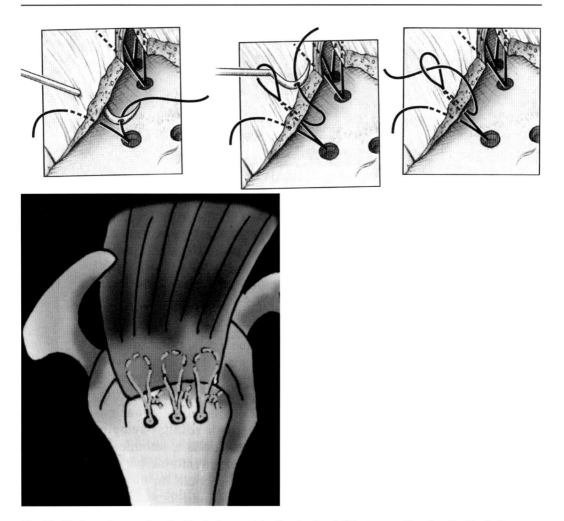

Fig. 11 The Lasso loop as described by Lafosse and the Tension Band ("Haubannage") as described by Boileau

In the other 30 patients, rotator cuff repair was performed with a double-row suture anchor technique (group 2).

Results: Eight patients (4 in the single-row anchor repair group and 4 in the double-row anchor repair group) did not return at the final follow-up. At the 2-year follow-up, no statistically significant differences were seen with respect to the University of California, Los Angeles score and range of motion values. At 2-year follow-up, post-operative magnetic resonance arthrography in group 1 showed intact tendons in 14 patients, partial-thickness defects in 10 patients, and full-thickness defects in 2 patients. In group 2, magnetic resonance arthrography showed an intact rotator cuff in 18 patients, partial-thickness defects in 7 patients, and full-thickness defects in 1 patient. The authors concluded that single- and double-row techniques provide comparable clinical outcome at 2 years. A double-row technique produces a mechanically superior construct compared with the single-row method in restoring the anatomical footprint of the rotator cuff, but these mechanical advantages do not translate into superior clinical performance.

According to the potentially increased implant costs and surgical times associated with the double-row rotator cuff repair, we recommend this sophisticated technique for retracted or extended

Fig. 12 Differents Knots

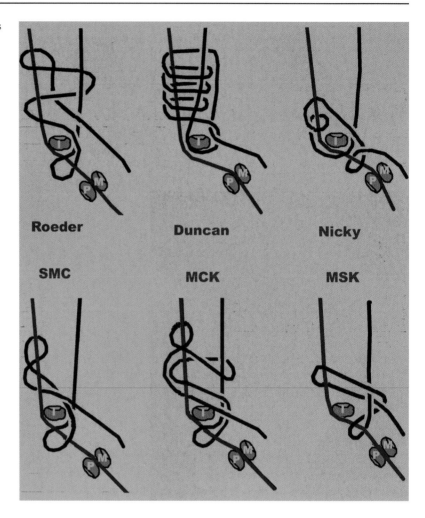

tears, and we prefer a single row (Tension-Band) for distal tears of the supraspinatus. A systematic review of the rate of structural healing of rotator cuff repair (single versus double-row) done by Duquin [20] concluded recently that double-row repair methods lead to significantly lower re-tear rates when compared with single-row methods for tears greater than 1 cm!

Tenotomy/Tenodesis of the Long Head of the Biceps

A tenotomy of the long head of biceps is always done in instances of tears of the subscapularis.

In case of a tear of the postero-superior cuff (supraspinatus and infraspinatus), a tenotomy is done in the presence of pathological changes of the long head of biceps.

The tenodesis is performed only in young, active patients, particularly if they are manual workers. The tenodesis is done at the upper portion of the bicipital groove [28]. The arthroscope is inserted through the posterior portal and an out-side-in antero-superior portal is created at the level of the groove to insert a cannula for instrumentation. With the arm in forward elevation and internal rotation an anchor with to sutures is employed to fix the tendon at the upper portion of the groove (Fig. 19), using a lasso-loop technique [47] with

Fig. 13 Margin convergence

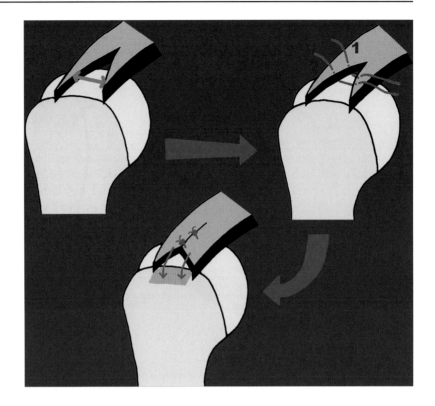

the help of a sliding knot. Tenotomy medially to the knot and resection of the proximal intra-articular stump are then performed.

Another technique [2], using interference screws [9] (Fig. 20), is a little more difficult but offers a stronger fixation!

Arthroscopic Suture of a Subscapularis Tear

We perform an arthroscopic repair when the tear is limited to the superior intra-articular aspect of the tendon (authors' preferred option). If the tear extends further distally, a conventional open repair is indicated.

The arthroscope is inserted into the glenohumeral joint through a posterior portal. The anterosuperior portal is created from the inside out as already described. The visualization of the torn edge is sometimes difficult and the use of a 70° arthroscope should be considered.

Placement of the arm in 30° of abduction and in internal rotation helps to visualize the upper aspect of the subscapularis insertion on the lesser tubercle. The superior glenohumeral ligament is often avulsed together with the superolateral portion of the tendon.

The distal aspect of the ligament acts as a landmark to identify the proximal point of re-insertion.

With the help of a motorized burr the insertion zone of the tendon is freshened. A PDS® suture is placed in the superolateral part of the tendon stump with a Bird Beak® or a Suture Hook® (a). The suture permits traction on the tendon stump. Instrumentation through an anterolateral portal may be required to mobilize the retracted tendon from the anterior glenoid (Fig. 21).

The rupture of the upper part of the subscapularis is often accompanied by a medial subluxation of the long head of the biceps. For this reason we always proceed with a tenotomy of the long head of biceps or with a tenodesis.

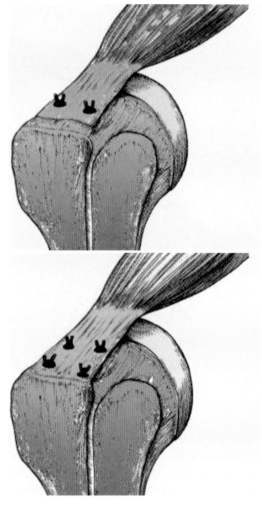

Fig. 14 Single and double rows

Some authors, as Lafosse [48], repair all the types of lesions, except the type V (complete and retracted tear with fatty infiltration stage 3 or 4).

Post-Operative Management

Rehabilitation after rotator cuff repair is done in two stages [25]:

1. The first stage is started on post-operative day 1 and lasts for 6 weeks. During this time the arm is placed in a sling. The position of the arm depends on the quality and the tension put on the tendon.

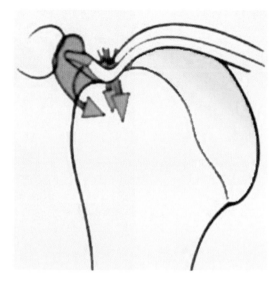

Fig. 15 Tension-band suture technique (Haubanage)

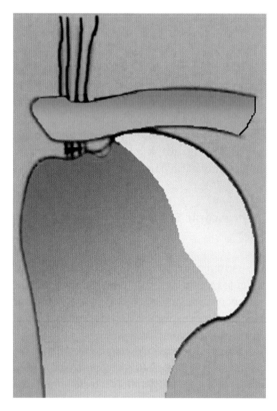

Fig. 16 Double row

Fig. 17 Double row technique with a « bar » : mattress-tension-band (MTB)

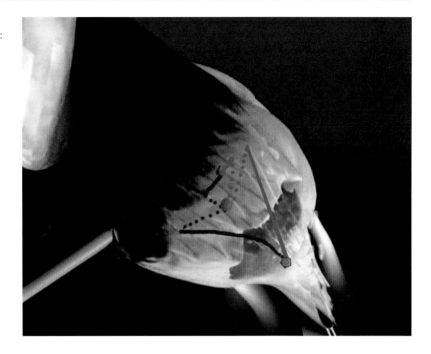

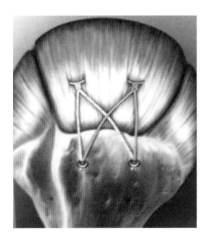

Fig. 18 The Suture bridge technique

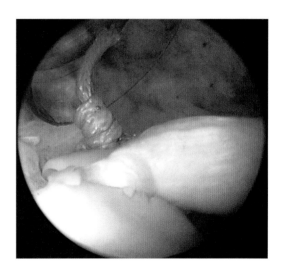

Fig. 19 Tenodesis of the Long Head of Biceps with suture Anchor

Most of the time, the arm is immobilized with the elbow at the side to take advantage of the tension-band effect of the U-stitches. Daily pendulum and passive range of motion exercises are done under the control of a physiotherapist and consist of flexion and abduction above the level of the sling. Passive external rotation is only done if the subscapularis tendon was not torn, and is usually limited to 20–30°.

2. The second stage begins after 6 weeks, and is ideally carried out in an out-patient rehabilitation specialized department. It includes active mobilization preferably started in a

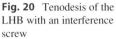

Fig. 20 Tenodesis of the LHB with an interference screw

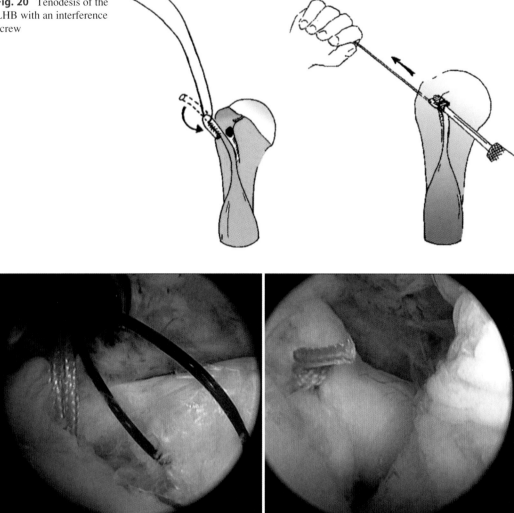

Fig. 21 Suture of the upper part of the subscapularis left shoulder

pool, and is associated with a progressive increase in the range of motion. Strengthening or active-resisted exercise of the short rotator muscles should be avoided for at least 12 weeks post-operatively, until the bone-tendon Healing is almost, but not quite, mature [59].

Errors, Hazards, Complications

- Infection seldom occurs and is usually caused by Staphylococcus aureus. A swab for culture and sensitivity should be taken, and should include a search for Propionibacterium acnes. Appropriate treatment for infection may then be initiated.

- Nerve injuries: rare, involve the axillary nerve, the musculocutaneous nerve, or the suprascapular nerve.

- The axillary nerve can be injured when the posterior or lateral portals are placed too distally. The musculocutaneous nerve is at risk when the anterior portal is placed too medially. The suprascapular nerve can be injured when the posterior portal is placed too medially.

- Neurapraxia: transient, most commonly affects the musculocutaneous nerve. Its incidence has been reduced since we adopted the "beach-chair" position. It remains, however, a complication to be feared when significant and prolonged traction is used with the patient in the lateral decubitus position.
- Reflex sympathetic dystrophy: the most frequent complication of arthroscopic surgery, leads to shoulder stiffness. The treatment being essentially medical is protracted and difficult and follows well-accepted principles.
- Oedema of peri-articular tissues: due to the use of the pump and caused by irrigating fluid seeping into the surrounding tissues. If present, Steri-Strips should be used for skin closure to allow drainage. No compartment syndrome has been reported.
- Breakage of instruments: more frequent in the past, its occurrence is now rarely seen. All instruments used during arthroscopy must be inspected carefully and if breakage has occurred, care must be taken to remove all fragments from the operative site.
- Avulsion of suture anchors [31]: this complication is seen mostly in the presence of an osteoporotic greater tuberosity or the presence of a cystic cavity. The anchor usually remains attached to the tendon and may lead to symptomatic subacromial impingement.

The anchor must be removed arthroscopically.

References

1. Andrews JR, Carson WG. Shoulder joint arthroscopy. Orthopedics. 1983;6:1157–62.
2. Ahrens PM, Boileau P. The long head of biceps and associated tendinopathy. J Bone Joint Surg Br. 2007;89(8):1001–9.
3. Barber AF, Herbert MA, Click JN. The ultimate strength of suture anchors. Arthroscopy. 1995;11:21–8.
4. Bigliani LU, Morrison DS, April EW. The morphology of the acromion and its relationship to the rotator cuff-tears. Orthop Trans. 1986;10:10–228.
5. Bjorkenheim JM, Paavolainen P, Ahuvo J, et al. Surgical repair of the rotator cuff and surrounding tissues. Factors influencing the results. Clin Orthop. 1988;236:148–53.
6. Boileau P, Brassart N, Watkinson DJ, Carles M, Hatzidakis AM, Krishnan SG. Arthroscopic repair of full-thickness tears of the supraspinatus: does the tendon really heal? J Bone Joint Surg - Series A. 2005;87(6):1229–40.
7. Boileau P, Chuinard C, Brassard N, Trojani C. The tension Band Suture Technique for arthroscopic rotator cuff repair. Tech Shoulder Elbow Surg. 2007;8(1):47–52.
8. Boileau P, Brassard N, Roussanne Y. The Mattress-Tension-Band Technique: a knotless double-row arthroscopic rotator cuff repair. In: Boileau P, editor. Shoulder concept 2008. Arthroscopy & Arthroplasty. Montpellier: Sauramps Medical; 2008. p. 245–52.
9. Boileau P, Neyton L. Arthroscopic tenodesis for lesions of the long head of the biceps. Oper Orthop Traumatol. 2005;17:601–23.
10. Burkhart SS. Arthroscopic treatment of massive rotator cuff tears. Clin Orthop. 1991;267:45–56.
11. Burkhart SS. Margin convergence: a method of reducing strain in massive rotator cuff tears. Arthroscopy. 1996;12:335–8.
12. Burkhart SS. Partial repair of massive rotator cuff tears: the evolution of a concept. Orthop Clin North Am. 1997;28:125–32.
13. Burkhart SS, Nottage W, Ogilvie-Harris D, et al. Partial repair of irreparable rotator cuff tears. Arthroscopy. 1994;10:363–70.
14. Burkhart SS, Wirth MA, Simonich M. Loop security as a determinant of tissue fixation security. Arthroscopy. 1998;14:773–6.
15. Burkhart SS, Wirth MA, Simonich M. Knot security in simple sliding knots and its relationship to rotator cuff repair: how secure must the knot be? Arthroscopy. 2000;16:202–7.
16. Burkhart SS. Arthroscopic repair of massive rotator cuff tears: concept of margin convergence. Tech Shoulder Elbow Surg. 2000;1:232–9.
17. Caspari RB. Shoulder arthroscopy: a review of the present state of the art. Contemp Orthop. 1982;4:523–5.
18. Cofield RH. Current concepts review: rotator cuff disease of the shoulder. J Bone Joint Surg Am. 1985;67:974–9.
19. Dines JS, Bedi A, ElAttrache NS, Dines DM. Single row versus double-row rotator cuff repair: techniques and outcomes. J Am Acad Orthop Surg. 2010;18:83–93.
20. Duquin TR, Buyea C, Bisson LJ. Which method of rotator cuff repair leads to the highest rate of structural Healing. A systematic review. Am J Sports Med. 2010;38(4):835–41.
21. Ellman H, Hanker G, Bayer M. Repair of the rotator cuff. End result study of factors influencing reconstruction. J Bone Joint Surg Am. 1986;68:1136–44.
22. Flurin PH, Landreau P, Gregory T, et al. Reparation arthroscopique des ruptures transfixiantes de la coiffe

des rotateurs: etude retrospective multicentrique de 576 cas avec contrôle de la cicatrisation. Rev Chir Orthop. 2005;91(S8):32–42.

23. Fuchs B, Weishaupt D, Zanetti M, et al. Fatty degeneration of the muscles of the rotator cuff: assessment by computed tomography versus magnetic resonance imaging. J Shoulder Elbow Surg. 1999;8:599–605.

24. Franceschi F, Ruzzini L, Longo UG, Martina FM, Beomonte Zobel B, Maffulli N, Denaro V. Equivalent clinical results of arthroscopic single-row and double-row suture anchor repair for rotator cuff tears: a randomized controlled trial. Am J Sports Med. 2007;35(8):1254–60.

25. Galatz LM, Griggs S, Cameron BD, et al. Prospective longitudinal analysis of postoperative shoulder function: a ten-year follow-up study of full thickness rotator cuff tears. J Bone Joint Surg Am. 2001;83:1052–6.

26. Gaertner E, Mahoudeau G. Le bloc interscalenique. Le praticien en anesthesie-reanimation. 1998;2:131–5.

27. Gartsman GM, Khan M, Hammermann SM. Arthroscopic repair of full-thickness tears of the rotator cuff. J Bone Joint Surg Am. 1998;80:832–40.

28. Gartsman GM, Hammerman SM. Arthroscopic biceps tenodesis: operative technique. Arthroscopy. 2000;16:550–2.

29. Gerber C, Krushell RJ. Isolated tears of the tendon of the subscapularis muscle. Clinical features in sixteen cases. J Bone Joint Surg Br. 1991;73B:349–94.

30. Gerber C, Schneeberger A, Beck M, Schlegel U. Mechanical strength of repairs of the rotator cuff. J Bone Joint Surg Br. 1994;76-B:371–9.

31. Gerber C, Meyer DC, Nyfeler RW, et al. Failure of suture material at suture anchor eyelets. Arthroscopy. 2002;18:1013–9.

32. Gerber C, Sebesta A. Impingement of the deep surface of the subscapularis tendon and the reflection pulley on the anterosuperior glenoid rim: a preliminary report. J Shoulder Elbow Surg. 2000;9:483–90.

33. Gleyze P, Thomazeau H, Flurin PH, et al. Arthroscopic rotator cuff repair: a multicentric retrospective study of 87 cases with anatomical assessment. Rev Chir Orthop Reparatrice Appar Mot. 2000;86:566–74.

34. Goutallier D, Postel JM, Bernageau J, et al. Fatty muscle degeneration in cuff ruptures: pre and post operative evaluation by CT-scan. Clin Orthop. 1994;304:78–83.

35. Goutallier D, Postel JM, Lavau L, et al. Influence de la degenerescence graisseuse des muscles supraepineux et infraepineux sur le pronostic des reparations chirurgicales de la coiffe des rotateurs. Rev Chir Orthop. 1999;85:668–76.

36. Habermeyer P, Magosch P, Pritsch M, et al. Anterosuperior impingement of the shoulder as a result of pulley lesions: a prospective arthroscopic study. J Shoulder Elbow Surg. 2004;13:5–12.

37. Jobe CM, Sidles J. Evidence for a superior glenoid impingement upon the rotator cuff. J Shoulder Elbow Surg. 1993;2:19. abstract.

38. Jobe CM. Posterior superior glenoid impingement: expanded spectrum. Arthroscopy. 1995;11:530–7.

39. Johnson LL. Arthroscopy of the shoulder. Orthop Clin North Am. 1980;11:197–204.

40. Johnson LL. Diagnostic and surgical arthroscopy. The knee and other joints. 3rd ed. St. Louis: Mosby; 1986.

41. Kannus P, Kozsa L. Histopathological changes preceding spontaneous rupture of a tendon. J Bone Joint Surg Am. 1991;73:1507–25.

42. Kempf JF, Clavert P. Arthroscopic knots: tips and tricks. In: Boileau P, editor. Shoulder arthroscopy and arthroplasty: current concept. Montpellier: Sauramps; 2004. p. 175–86.

43. Kim SH, Ha KI. The SMC knot: a new slip knot with locking mechanism. Arthroscopy. 2000;16:563–5.

44. Kim SH, Ha KI, Kim JS. Significance of the internal locking mechanism for loop security enhancement in the arthroscopic knot. Arthroscopy. 2001;17:850–5.

45. Kim KC, Rhee KJ, Shin HD. Arthroscopic double-pulley suture-bridge technique for rotator cuff repair. Arch Orthop Trauma Surg. 2008;128:1335–8.

46. Kulwicki KJ, Kwon YW, Kummer FJ. Suture Anchor loading after rotator cuff repair: effects of an additional lateral row. J Shoulder Elbow Surg. 2010;19:290–9.

47. Krishnan SG, Hawkins RJ, Bokor DJ. Clinical evaluation of shoulder problems. In: Rockwood CA, Matsen FA, Wirth MA, et al., editors. The shoulder. 3rd ed. Philadelphia: Saunders; 2004. p. 145–85.

48. Lafosse L, Brozska R, Toussain B, Gobezie R. The outcome and structural integrity of arthroscopic rotator cuff repair with use of the double row suture technique. J Bone Joint Surg Am. 2007;89:1533–41.

49. Lafosse L. Traitement arthroscopique des lesions de la coiffe des rotateurs. EMC-Tech Chir Orthop Traumatol. 2007;2:44–284. doi:10.1016/S0246-0467(07)39544-5.

50. Liotard JP, Cochard P, Walch G. Critical analysis of the supraspinatus outlet view: rationale for a standard scapular Y-view. J Shoulder Elbow Surg. 1998;7:134–9.

51. Lo IKY, Burkhart SS. Current concepts in arthroscopic rotator cuff repairs. Am J Sports Med. 2003;31:308–24.

52. Mazzocca AD, Millett PJ, Guanche CA, Santangelo SA, Arciero RA. Arthroscopic single-row versus double-row suture anchor rotator cuff repair. Am J Sports Med. 2005;33(12):1861–8.

53. Murray TF, Lajtai G, Mileski RM, et al. Arthroscopic repair of medium to large full-thickness rotator cuff tears: outcome at 2 to 6 year follow-up. J Shoulder Elbow Surg. 2002;11:19–24.

54. Neer II CS. Impingement lesions. Clin Orthop. 1983;173:70–7.

55. Nottage WM, Lieurance RK. Arthroscopic knot tying techniques. Arthroscopy. 1999;15:515–21.

56. Ozaki J, Fujimoto S, Nakagawa Y, et al. Tears of the rotator cuff of the shoulder associated with pathological changes in the acromion. J Bone Joint Surg Am. 1988;70:1224–30.

57. Samilson RL. Congenital and developmental anomalies of the shoulder girdle. Orthop Clin North Am. 1980;11:219–31.

58. Snyder SJ, Burns J. Rotator cuff Healing and the bone marrow « Crimson Duvet » from clinical observations to science. Tech Shoulder Elbow Surg. 2009;10(4):130–7.

59. Tauro JC. Arthroscopic rotator cuff repair: analysis of technique and resultsat 2 and 3 year follow-up. J Shoulder Elbow Surg. 2002;11:19–24.

60. Sonnabend DH, Howlett CR, Young AA. Histological evaluation of repair of the rotator cuff in a primate model. J Bone Joint Surg Br. 2010;92B:586–94.

61. Trimbos JB. Security of various knots commonly used in surgical practice. Obstet Gynecol. 1984;64:274–80.

62. Uhthoff HK, Löhr J, Sarkar K. The pathogenesis of rotator cuff tears. In: Takagishi N, editor. The shoulder. Tokyo: Professional Postgraduate Services; 1990. p. 211–2.

63. Walch G, Marechal E, Maupas J, Liotard JP. Traitement chirurgical des ruptures de la coiffe des rotateurs. Facteurs pronostiques. Rev Chir Orthop. 1992;78:379–88.

64. Walch G, Boileau P, Noel E, et al. Impingement of the deep surface of the supraspinatus tendon on the posterosuperior glenoid rim: an arthroscopic study. J Shoulder Elbow Surg. 1992;1:238–45.

65. Walch G, Liotard JP, Boileau P, et al. Le conflit glenoidien postero-superieur: un autre conflit de l'epaule. Rev Chir Orthop. 1991;77:571–4.

66. Wilson F, Hunov V, Adams G. Arthroscopic repair of full-thickness tears of the rotator cuff: 2 to 14 year follow-up. Arthroscopy. 2002;18:136–44.

67. Wolf EM, Bayliss RW. Arthroscopic rotator cuff repair: clinical and arthroscopic second-look assessment. In: Gazielly DF, Gleyze P, Thomas T, editors. The cuff. Paris: Elsevier; 1999. p. 319.

Inverse/Reverse Polarity Arthroplasty for Cuff Tears with Arthritis (Including Cuff Tear Arthropathy)

Alexander Van Tongel and Lieven De Wilde

Contents

Keywords

Biomechanics • Complications • Indications • Inverse/reverse polarity arthroplasty • Rotator cuff-deficient arthritic shoulder • Surgical Technique • Shoulder

History

The first total shoulder replacement is widely credited to Dr. Jules Emile Péan in 1893. However, in his original report Péan refers to the work of Themistocles Gluck as being the inspiration for his shoulder prosthesis, a fact understated if not completely overlooked during the last 100 years. Themistocles almost certainly designed the first shoulder arthroplasty in the late 1800's although he never published on the implantation of his shoulder designs in humans [1, 2]. Arthroplasty played a limited role in the treatment of shoulder problems until in 1955 when Neer reported the use of a proximal humerus arthroplasty for fractures with good results [3]. In 1974, Neer subsequently described the use of his proximal humeral arthroplasty for the treatment of glenohumeral osteoarthritis [4].

But the arthritic shoulder with irreparable massive cuff deficiency remained difficult and a challenging issue in shoulder practice.

In the 1970's, the idea of reversing the prosthesis emerged because of difficulties encountered in implanting an anatomical glenoid implant large enough to stabilize the prosthesis and prevent

A. Van Tongel (✉) • L. De Wilde
Department of Orthopaedic Surgery and Traumatology, Ghent University Hospital, Ghent, Belgium
e-mail: alexander.vantongel@uzgent.be;
Lieven.dewilde@ugent.be

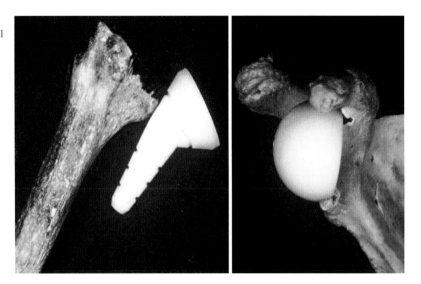

proximal migration [5]. Early in the 1970s Neer designed three variations of a constrained reversed shoulder prosthesis. These prostheses created a foundation for reverse shoulder arthroplasty. But dislocation and scapular fixation remained a concern with these implants [2]. In 1973 Kessel described a reversed prosthesis that was fixed to the glenoid by a large central screw. In the same year, the Bayley-Walker system made advances in both design and fixation compared to the Kessel design by coating the large central screw with hydroxyapatite and increasing the screw thread diameter [6]. These design changes were made in an attempt to achieve secure glenoid fixation without a concomitant increase in loosening. During the next years several other semi-constrained and constrained prosthesis were designed. Unfortunately, all these prostheses so far described resulted in only marginal functional improvement or were largely abandoned as failures [5].

It was not until the work of Grammont that a reliable solution for the treatment of rotator cuff arthropathy was achieved. In the early 1980s, he advocated a medialized centre of rotation to improve the biomechanics of the deltoid muscle by restoring length and increasing the lever arm. The Ovoid arthroplasty was tried in 1983. It had an egg-shaped head on the humeral side. The centre of rotation was medialized but, due to the ovoid shape, the deltoid muscle was maintained in the lateral position to improve

abduction. Range of motion was improved, but instability was a concern. Grammont therefore moved to a reverse design with a large hemisphere on the glenoid side to place the centre of rotation at the bone–implant interface. His first reverse design was the "trumpet" prosthesis in 1985 (Fig. 1). The humeral component was all polyethylene, and the glenoid component was a ball made of metal or ceramic and two- thirds of a sphere with a 42-mm diameter. Both components were cemented. Preliminary results of eight cases were published 1987 [7]. Four of these were revisions of failed anatomic arthroplasties. Results varied, but in three patients the elevation was more than 100°. The implant was further redesigned into the Delta 3 arthroplasty (DePuy International, Ltd), available in 1991 [8, 9]. In the first generation, the metaglenoid was a circular plate with a central peg for press-fit impaction. It was fixed with divergent 3.5 mm screws superiorly and inferiorly in order to resist the shearing forces. The glenosphere was screwed directly onto the peripheral edge of the plate. This concept of peripheral screwing of the glenosphere had to be abandoned because of secondary loosening of the screws. In the second generation the periphery of the metaglenoid was conical and smooth with a Morse-Taper effect. The metaglenoid was coated with hydroxyapatite on its deep surface to improve bony fixation. The centre of the metaglenoid was hollow in order to allow locking of the glenosphere with a central securing screw. The humeral component was a monobloc with a cup of standard thickness. The third generation became available in 1994 with the new features pertaining to the humeral component. Because the cup was of insufficient size, it rapidly deteriorated as a result of medial impingement. It was therefore replaced by a lateralized cup available in two diameters of 36 and 42 mm [5].

Reverse total shoulder arthroplasties (RTSA) today vary in certain design details, although their intrinsic design remains based on Grammont's principles. The variables in the current prostheses have been developed to address concerns that have arisen with reverse shoulder arthroplasty [2]. These problems and their possible solutions will be discussed extensively in the section on biomechanics and complications.

Biomechanics

Moment Arm, Stability and Loading

Grammont's system focusses on four keys features [2]:

1. The prosthesis must be inherently stable;
2. The weight-bearing part must be convex, and the supported part must be concave;
3. The centre of the sphere must be at or within the glenoid neck;
4. The centre of rotation must be medialized and distalized.

Concerning the first two features, RTSA can restore the joint stability by reversing the envelope of the joint contact forces and by changing the critical articulating surface [10]. The half-spherical glenoid fixation provides a large surface reacting to the increased shear forces. Also the use of large ball offers more stability than a small ball. The critical stability region is now the area of the humeral cup where the depth determines the maximum dislocating shear force. In addition, the humeral cup follows the direction of the deltoid force and the high shear forces are well constrained within the cup rim. Because the

supported part is concave, also the concavity compression mechanism makes the shoulder more stable.

Concerning the third feature, the centre of rotation was lateralized and outside the glenoid bone in the old designs of RTSA. This created a high stress on the fixation of the glenoid component, resulting in aseptic loosening. By using a small lateral offset (absence of neck), the centre of rotation is directly placed in contact with the glenoid surface and this reduces the torque at the point of fixation of the glenoid component [11–13].

Concerning the last point, bringing the centre of rotation more medial and distal creates a mechanical advantage for the deltoid muscle, increasing its lever arm and allowing for a greater recruitment of deltoid fibres during active shoulder motion. Portions of the deltoid initially medial to the native glenohumeral joint centre of rotation become active abductors and elevators in their new lateral position. Distalization further increases the efficiency of the deltoid during shoulder motion through elongation and an associated increase in its resting tension [10, 14, 15].

Scapular Impingement

The biomechanics of rotation of the reverse prosthetic glenohumeral joint differ from the anatomic prosthetic joint because of the hinging (rotation around a lateral axis/point) instead of spinning (rotation around a central axis/point) movement. As a result of the prosthesis hinging in the adducted position, a contact between the humeral component and the body of the scapula can occur and thereby limit the range of motion [16]. This mechanical contact between the metaphyseal implant and scapula is called scapular impingement and it is related to the design of the prosthesis. This can cause a mechanical block. This repetitive mechanical abutment can also be a reason for glenoid neck erosion. This erosion is known as scapular notching. Most commonly the impingement is inferiorly during adduction of the arm. But also anterior

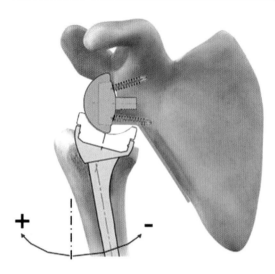

Fig. 2 Notch angle

and posterior scapular impingement is possible. This may restrict internal and external rotation.

The clinical relevance of inferior scapular notching is controversial in the literature, with some authors reporting no impact on post-operative function [11, 17, 18] and overall outcome and others describing a negative correlation between a scapular notch and the results after RTSA [19, 20].

Inferior scapular impingement can be evaluated with the notch angle (Fig. 2). This is the adduction angle in the scapular plane between the humerus and a vertical line parallel to the glenoid plane, which is the plane formed by the rim of the inferior quadrants of the glenoid, when a contact between the polyethylene cup and the scapular pillar occurs. A positive value means that contact occurs before the humerus reaches the vertical position. A negative value means that the humerus can be adducted further than the vertical position [21].

Several solutions have been described to overcome the problem of scapular notching.

Prosthetic overhang creates the biggest gain in notch angle (Fig. 3) [21–23]. This can be achieved by low positioning of the glenosphere (flush to the inferior glenoid rim). This effect can be enlarged with the use of a glenosphere with increase radius. Also downward glenoid inclination [21, 24] and a change in cup depth

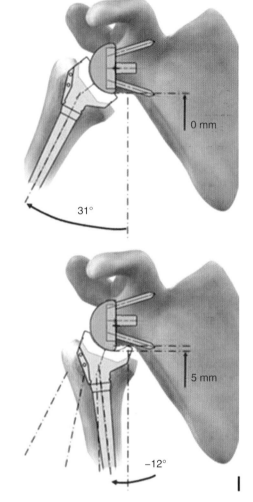

Fig. 3 Influence of inferior prosthetic overhang on the notch angle

(a decrease in prosthetic contact area) [21] results in a gain in notch angle. Reducing the humeral component neck-shaft angle [21, 25] results also in increased gain. However, this also results in reduced stability and therefore is not recommended [26, 27]. Also increasing the offset of the glenosphere and/or baseplate can cause less scapular impingement [21, 28, 29]. But there is a disadvantage of increasing torque or shear force applied to the glenoid component and potentially increasing the risk of glenoid loosening [11].

Concerning the anterior and posterior scapular impingement, Simovitch et al. found a significant correlation of posterior notching with increased external rotation at 0° of abduction [19]. Stephenson et al. described the optimal version for the humeral component in Grammont-style prostheses which appears to be between 20° and 40° of retroversion, giving a potential for impingement-free ROM from 28°–44° external rotation to 83°–99° internal rotation, with the arm in adduction [30]. Karelse et al. found that an increase in the divergence angle, which corresponds to a decrease in humeral component retroversion, correlates with an increase in radiographically-measured passive internal rotation with the arm adducted [16]. They described that a divergence angle of 30°–35° gives a good equilibrium between external and internal rotation.

Indication

RTSA is indicated in patients with rotator cuff–deficient arthritic shoulder (RCDA). RCDA is not one unique pathologic entity but it is a common end-stage of several disease processes such as rheumatoid arthritis, "Milwaukee shoulder" syndrome and rotator cuff tear arthropathy. All these pathologies have a unique clinical feature which is a painful arthritic shoulder with a massive, irreparable rotator cuff defect. RCDA is one of the most difficult and challenging issues in shoulder practice, due to the combination of severe articular and peri-articular soft tissue damage.

In RCDA large and massive defects in the rotator cuff tendons lead to a loss in the centreing of the humeral head. Loss of a fixed centre of rotation for the humeral head results in decreased power of the deltoid [31]. At the end-stage the patient presents with a clinically symptomatic, irreparable rotator cuff tear associated with an irrecoverable pseudoparesis of anterior elevation and/or abduction [26].

Rheumatoid arthritis (RA) is a common cause of RCDA. The incidence of radiographic glenohumeral joint affection of the rheumatoid shoulder varies from 48 % to 64 %. About 24 % of those having glenohumeral arthritis have a simultaneous rotator cuff tear [32].

Superimposed on the aforementioned changes are severe osteopenia, erosions of the entire glenoid without osteophyte formation, and medialization of the glenohumeral joint [33].

Apatite-associated destructive arthropathy, also known as the "Milwaukee shoulder" syndrome was originally described by McCarty in 1981 [34]. It is a degenerative disorder affecting predominantly elderly women, characterized by dissolution of the fibrous rotator cuff and destruction of the glenohumeral joint [35]. It consists of a massive rotator cuff tear, joint instability, bony destruction, and large blood-stained joint effusion containing basic calcium phosphate crystals, detectable protease activity, and minimal inflammatory elements.

Cuff tear arthropathy (CTA) is the extreme end result of a massive rotator cuff tear.

Robert Adams first described the clinical findings of CTA in 1857 [36], however it was not until 1977 that Charles Neer coined the term "cuff tear arthropathy." Neer et al. went on to provide the first detailed description of CTA in 1983 [37]. CTA encompasses a condition characterized by a massive rotator cuff tear, proximal migration of the humerus resulting in femoralization of the humeral head and acetabularization of the acromion, glenoid erosion, loss of glenohumeral articular cartilage, osteoporosis of the humeral head and eventually humeral head collapse [37].

To date, the only attempts to classify RCDA have been based on radiographic classifications. In the literature three different classifications have been described, each focussing on a specific part of the pathology.

Seebauer et al. described a biomechanical classification of cuff tear arthropathy. It targets the superior migration of the humeral head and its containment within the coraco-acromial (CA) arch [38].

The Hamada classification system characterizes the structural changes associated within the CA arch [39].

Favard et al. proposed a classification that focusses on the glenoid erosion [20]. The study of Iannotti et al. demonstrated that there was a fair to poor agreement based on these three

x-ray classification systems [40]. One of the reasons is the fact that discrete grades of
a continuous spectrum of the pathology makes it
difficult for different observers to agree on
a reading of an image. The inter-rater reliability
for surgical recommendations was low and
was not improved with the addition of clinical
information, which indicates disagreement on
how to use this information to make a surgical
recommendation. Middernacht et al. also
described that a conventional antero-posterior
radiograph cannot provide any predictive information on the clinical status of the patient [41].

The reverse ball-and-socket arthroplasty relies
on the deltoid muscle for function; therefore, the
function of the axillary nerve and deltoid muscle
must be checked before surgery. The easiest way
to evaluate the function is by asking the patient to
elevate the arm while the examiner places his or
her fingers over the anterior third of the deltoid
muscle. If contraction is felt, the function of
the muscle is satisfactory. If it is difficult to
clinically determine the function of the deltoid
muscle, electromyography or electroneurography
can be used.

Also pre-operative testing of the teres minor
muscle with the "hornblower" sign [41, 42] and
the exorotation lag signs [41, 43] because the
integrity of teres minor, is essential for the recovery of external rotation and significantly
influenced the post-op Constant score [20].

Surgical Technique

Every surgical procedure starts with a good pre-
operative plan.

Pre-operatively a strict AP in neutral position
and axillary shoulder X-ray is performed. With
the available templates it is possible to determine
the size and the alignment of the humeral component. A template for the glenoid component is
not used because of the use of polyaxial screws.
We also perform a CT-scan in a standardized
fashion, as described previously [44]. In the
supine position, a thoracobrachial orthosis is
applied to position the arm adducted in the coronal plane and the forearm flexed in the sagittal

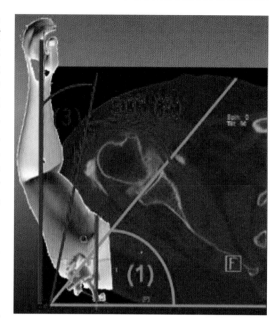

Fig. 4 90° – axis of glenoid component (*1*), 30° (divergence angle), (*2*), axis of the humeral component (*3*)

plane of the body. This represented the shoulder
in neutral rotation approximating the neutral
shoulder orientation in the surgical position. The
coronal plane parallel with the back of the patient
is the X-plane. A measurement of the axis of the
glenoid component is performed. This axis is
defined, on the level of the centre of the glenoid
component, as the line drawn along the bony
surface of the metaglene and is measured as an
angle made with the X-plane [16].

As described, a divergence angle (the angle
between the axes of the glenoid and humeral
components) of 30° gives a good equilibrium
between the external and internal rotation.
This means the optimal axis of the humeral
component = 90° – 30° (divergence
angle) – axis of the glenoid component (Fig. 4).

Per-operatively the patient is positioned in the
"beach chair" position and, before sterile draping,
a check is mage for good extension and
adduction.

An RTSA is performed via a deltopectoral or
a superolateral approach. In the largest currently
available multcentre study, that of 527 RTSAs for
massive rotator cuff tear, both approaches had

Fig. 5 Visualization of
humeral head through
superolateral approach

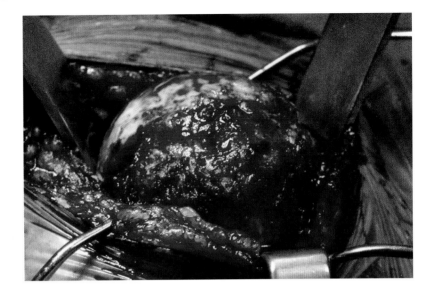

statistically significant advantages and disadvantages [45]. A superolateral approach was found to be much better than a deltopectoral approach in terms of post-operative instability and was better in terms of preventing fractures of the scapular spine and the acromion. A deltopectoral approach afforded better preservation of active external rotation as well as better orientation of the glenoid component, glenoid loosening, and inferior scapular notching.

In our department a superolateral approach is used if this approach has been used previously for rotator cuff repair, if there is an os acromiale, when the shoulder is not stiff or in patients with posterosuperior CTA (Fig. 5). We do not use this approach in revision surgery or for late sequelae post-traumatic surgery. The deltopectoral approach is used when this approach was used before, in stiff shoulders, in patients with anteroposterior CTA or in late sequelae post-traumatic surgery. Also for revision surgery we use the deltopectoral approach and if necessary a clavicular osteotomy as described by Redfern and Wallace is performed to gain an excellent access to the shoulder [46].

Afterwards complete anterior and posterior digital humeral release is performed. Concerning the subscapularis, in the deltopectoral approach it is necessary to detach the tendon to obtain good access. We perform a tenotomy at the attachment of the bone. In the superolateral approach a partial detachment of the subscapularis may be performed when the superior dislocation of the humerus is difficult to obtain.

If the biceps is still in place a soft-tissue tenodesis is performed.

The humeral resection guide is inserted into the entry point in line with the long axis of the humerus (Fig. 6) and with the aid of a jig the humeral head is resected, preserving the greater and lesser tuberosities. At that time the retroversion of the humeral component can be adapted as calculated pre-operatively on the CT. It is important to not over-resect the head. The resection is adequate if plane of it corresponds to inferior glenoid. Afterwards a protecting plate can be used while preparing the glenoid.

The next step is a very important step. It is necessary to have a perfect visualization of the glenoid before the positioning of the base plate (Fig. 7). The biceps remnant and the labrum can be excised and the capsule needs to be detached (but not excised). A complete 360° capsular release is needed. Inferiorly, the tendon of the long head of the triceps is released under protection of the axillary nerve.

The guide-wire for the glenoid reamer must be positioned so that the glenoid baseplate is as low as possible. This means in the centre glenoid circle formed by the outer edge of the inferior

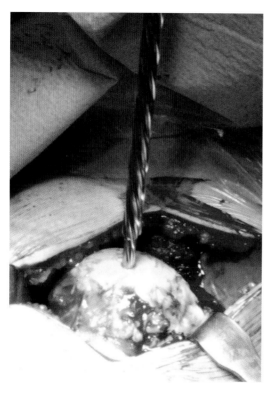

Fig. 6 Insertion of humeral resection guide into the entry point in line with the long axis of the humerus

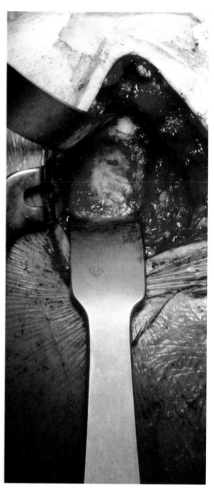

Fig. 7 Perfect visualization of the glenoid before the positioning of the base plate

glenoid quadrants (Figs. 8 and 9). The inferior border of the baseplate should not be proximal to the inferior glenoid rim, so that the glenoid component eventually overlaps the inferior border of the glenoid [21].

An inferior tilt may favour notching if reaming is performed far medially. With a glenoid reaming level-checker the adequate reaming can be checked. Locking screws are used to provide primary stability. They are usually anchored in the lateral pillar of the scapula and in the base of the coracoid. If necessary, locking or non-locking screws can be used in the anterior or posterior holes for compression.

Concerning the humeral component, this can be cemented or non-cemented and modular or monobloc. A modular component can be helpful when there is an anterior cortical contact. In these cases a component with posterior offset can be necessary.

The humerus is then broached, and the humeral trial is inserted.

An appropriate-size glenoid hemisphere (i.e., glenosphere) is then mounted on the baseplate. Current results suggest that larger glenospheres are associated with less pain and better strength and less notching [20, 21] but it may not be possible to use a large implant in a small individual.

After inserting a humeral cup a trial reduction is performed. The implanted prosthesis is relocated by pushing the concave humeral cup downward rather than by pulling on the arm. Seating of the prosthesis is easiest in approximately neutral rotation and slight anterior

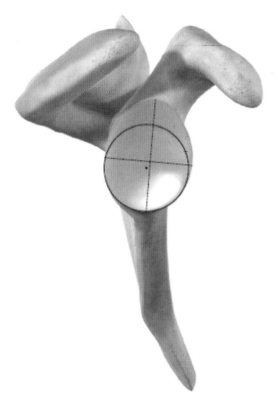

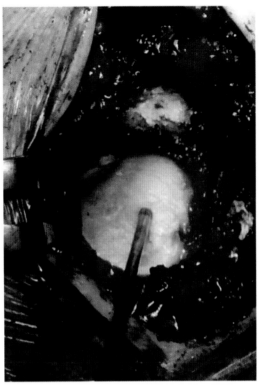

Fig. 8 Position of guide-wire in the centre glenoid circle formed by the outer edge of the inferior glenoid quadrants

Fig. 9 Status after reaming glenoid with the use of a concave reamer

elevation [26] (Fig. 10). While testing prosthetic mobility, no detectable separation between prosthetic components should be seen. At that time correct soft tissue tension and passive range of movement should be tested. Be aware of any soft tissue and osseous contact or instability problem and correct it if necessary. Stability is tested with the arm in abduction and internal rotation.

This is the position that patients use to get out of bed or out of a chair, and it represents the most frequent position of anterior dislocation. When anterior dislocation occurs with the arm in abduction and internal rotation, the antetorsion of the humerus must be increased, and the surgeon has to ascertain that the glenoid component was not implanted with anteversion.

With the arm at the side, anterior opening during external rotation is checked for posterior impingement. If there are during evaluation signs of superior bony impingement, it is necessary to

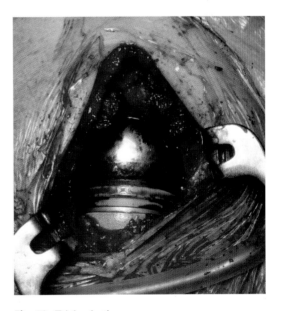

Fig. 10 Trial reduction

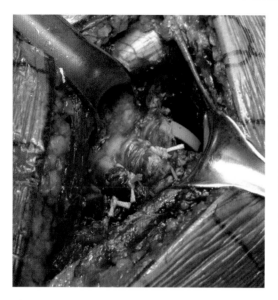

Fig. 11 Status after closure of remnants of remaining cuff

remove the superior part of the glenoid. With subcoracoidal impingement, the use of an eccentric glenosphere or removal of the greater tuberosity and/or subcoracoidal release can improve the ROM. The height of the polyethylene component should be such as to lengthen the arm (i.e., tip of the acromion to the elbow) by approximately 2–3 cm with a very snug fit after relocation [26].

While positioning the definitive glenoid hemisphere, it is essential to check that no soft-tissue is between the baseplate and the hemisphere to prevent early loosening of the component [47].

The definitive humeral component is inserted and a final check with a trial humeral cup is done. After evaluation of the proper positioning and stability, the definitive humeral cup is inserted and the shoulder is reduced.

At the end of the procedure the subscapularis is re-attached with non-absorbable sutures (Fig. 11) and in a superolateral approach the deltoid is also re-attached.

Post-operatively a sling is used only for comfort and is discontinued as soon as possible. Active and active-assisted ranges of motion exercises are started immediately. No passive stretching exercises should be performed. Specific anterior and posterior deltoid exercises in

neutral position are taught. The arm can be used immediately for daily activities such as brushing teeth or eating. During the first 6 weeks strengthening exercises of the external rotator muscle are performed in neutral position. If the patient is able to gain active external rotation in 90° of abduction, he can start to do exercises of the external rotator muscles also in this position.

Results

Reverse total shoulder arthroplasty has been shown to be effective in treating RCDA, with numerous studies demonstrating improvements in shoulder motion and patient satisfaction [8, 18, 20, 45, 48–62].

Sirveaux et al. published the first large outcome study reporting the results of Dr. Grammont's reverse prosthesis in 2004. These authors reported on 80 patients with a mean follow-up of 3.6 years [20]. The procedure was associated with good pain relief in 96 % of the patients, mean active elevation increased from 73° to 138°, and Constant scores improved from 22 to 65 points.

In 2007 a French multi-centre study described the results in 484 patients after a minimum of 24 months. At the latest follow-up the Constant score had increased from 24 points pre-operatively to 62 points post-operatively, pain increased from 3.7 to 12.6 points (15 points represents freedom from pain), and elevation increased from 71° to 130°. At 52 months postoperatively, 90 % of the patients were very satisfied or satisfied with their shoulder [37].

Concerning the survival rate, Sirveaux et al. found 91.3 % implant survival rate at 5 years [20]. Also Guery et al. found 91 % implant survival at a minimum follow-up of 5 years but there was a substantially better survival rate in those patients with arthropathy associated with a massive cuff tear (MCT) than other indications [57].

The study of Favard et al. showed that the need for revision of reverse shoulder arthroplasty was relatively low at 10 years, but Constant-Murley score and radiographic changes deteriorated with time. They conclude that therefore caution must be exercised when recommending reverse shoulder arthroplasty, especially in younger patient [63].

It is also reported that the results are dependent on the indication for which type of RCDA a reversed shoulder prosthesis is used, and that functional outcome and complication rates are distinctly different in primary versus revision cases [26].

The best results have been shown in patients with CTA. Reversed shoulder prosthesis has been shown to reliably restore overhead elevation in patients [18, 28, 45, 57] (Table 1).

In patients with rheumatoid arthritis, the most important pre-requisite is appropriate glenoid bone stock. When this is compromised by medial and superior erosion of the glenoid cavity, hemi-arthroplasty may remain the least unsatisfactory treatment [26]. For the patient with sufficient glenoid bone stock, however, RTSA has shown encouraging short-term results, with good pain relief and a significant improvement in Constant score [50, 53, 60, 62]. However, the scores are slightly inferior to some that have been reported in patients with cuff tear arthropathy [50].

To our knowledge, there is no literature concerning the use of RTSA in patients with "Milwaukee shoulder" syndrome.

Another important factor is the integrity of teres minor. It is reported that the functional results of reversed shoulder prosthesis are inferior when the posterior rotator cuff muscles are absent or are deficient because of atrophy and fatty infiltration of the teres minor muscle [26, 45, 64]. Post-operatively these patients still have a loss of active external rotation in abduction. This loss has a dramatic impact on activities of daily living. Latissimus dorsi ± teres major tendon transfer have been described through one [65] or two incisions [66], both with good results.

It is important to know that in evaluation the result of reversed shoulder prosthesis, positive patient ratings of satisfaction may not necessarily be evidence of positive outcomes. A study of Roy et al. suggests 93 % of the subjects were satisfied even though some of the satisfied

patients had less than 50° of shoulder elevation, no active external rotation, moderate to severe pain and post-operative complications [67].

Complications

Scapular Notching

Scapular notching is described as glenoid erosion caused by repetitive mechanical abutment of the humeral component with the scapular neck (Fig. 12). The most commonly used classification of Sirveaux describes the erosion according to the size of the defect as seen on the anteroposterior radiograph [20].

Notching is present in almost half of the cases using the Grammont-type reverse shoulder system (49.8 %) [68], but no cases of notching were reported using the lateralized prosthetic shoulder system [28]. Whether or not scapular notching progresses over time continues to be debated in the Orthopaedic literature. In the clinical studies reported by Werner et al. [18] and Simovitch et al. [19], the extent of the scapular notch appeared to plateau over time. However, another study has demonstrated that the extent of scapular notching after reverse TSA can increase with the length of follow-up [17].

There is also still some discussion as to whether scapular notching affects the patient's final outcome. In the study of Sirveaux et al. the presence of the notch significantly affected the Constant score when the notch was either over the screw or extensive [20]. This was also confirmed by the study of Simovitch et al. [19]. These results are in contrast with the study of some other authors where no clinical effect was found between notching and the post-operative function [11, 17, 18].

In our opinion, although notching is not yet a proven precursor of loosening, it should not be considered a harmless and unavoidable phenomenon of RTSA.

As discussed in the biomechanical section above, several solutions have been described to try to overcome the problem of scapular notching [21–25].

Table 1 Summary of reports of clinical outcomes following reversed shoulder prosthesis in patients with RCDA

	Year	Indication	Number	Mean follow-up (months)	Mean CS pre-op	Mean CS postop	Mean ASES pre-op	Mean ASES postop	Mean AAE pre-op	Mean AAE postop
Baulot et al. [8]	1995	CTA	16	27	14	69			60°	114°
Boileau et al. [11]	2005	CTA- failed SA - FS	45	40	17	58			55°	121°
Boileau et al. [61]	2011	CTA- failed RCR - FS	42	28	34	75			86°	146°
Cuff et al. [58]	2008	CTA – failed RCR – failed SA – FS	112	27.5			30	77.6	63.5°	118°
Ekelund et al. [50]	2010	RA	27	18	13	52			33°	115°
Favard et al. [63]	2011	CTA – MRCT	331	<60		62.8				130.1°
	2011	CTA – MRCT	148	>60		61.53				128.6°
	2011	CTA – MRCT	69	>84		59.9				124.9°
	2011	CTA – MRCT	41	>108		56.7				124.1°
Frankle et al. [28]	2005	CTA	60	33			34.3	68.2	55°	105.1°
Holcomb et al. [60]	2010	RA	21	36			28	82	52°	126°
Jacobs et al. [52]	2001	CTA	7	26	17.9	56.7			<90°	>90°
Molé et al. [45]	2007	CTA – MRCT	484		24	62			71°	130°
Rittmeister et al. [53]	2001	RA	8	54.3	17	63				
Sayana et al. [48]	2009	CTA – failed RCR	19	30	14.8	60.9				145°
Seebauer et al. [55]	2005	RCDA	46	18.2	37	67				
Sirveaux et al. [20]	2004	CTA	80	44	22.6	65.6			73°	138°
Vanhove et al. [54]	2004	CTA	14	29.5		60				
Werner et al. [18]	2005	CTA – failed RCR- failed SA	58	38	29	64			42°	100°
Woodruff et al. [62]	2003	RA	13	87.5		59				

AAE active anterior elevation, *ASES* American Shoulder and Elbow score, *CS* Constant-Murley score, *CTA* cuff tear arthropathy, *FS* fracture sequelae, *RA* reumatoid arthritis, *RCR* rotator cuff repair, *SA* shoulder arthroplasty, *MRCT* massive rotator cuff tear

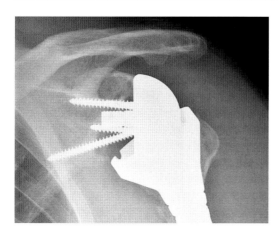

Fig. 12 Scapular notching

Aseptic Loosening

Lucent lines around the glenoid are rare in the Grammont-type reverse shoulder system and are almost twice as frequent in the prosthetic shoulder system with a lateralized centre of rotation. Until now no clinical effect has been reported but premature mechanical failure due to loosening is a concern. This is confirmed by the fact that aseptic glenoid loosening is twice as frequent in the studies using the lateralized prosthetic shoulder system than in the studies using the Grammont-type reverse shoulder arthroplasty system (5.8 % vs. 2.5 %) [68].

Infection

There is a incidence of deep infection after RSA of 3.8 % [68]. This is lower than previously described [45] and is comparable with anatomic arthroplasties but it is still higher than in other shoulder procedures. There is an increased rate of infection in the revision group compared with the primary group (5.8 % vs. 2.9 %) [68]. Most infections occur early and can be treated with lavage and antibiotics; some occur after 3 months and appear to respond poorly to débridement and prosthesis retention [45]. Recently two clinical types of infections have been distinguished:

1. Patients with a painful stiff shoulder.
2. Patients with good shoulder function but with a chronic fistula. The latter can be uneventfully treated with a one-stage revision [69].

Instability

Instability is a common post-operative complication with an incidence of 4.7 %. Instability is more frequent after revision of a previous hemi- or total shoulder arthroplasty (9.4 %) than in the primary arthroplasty group (4.1 %) The deltopectoral approach was used in 97.3 % of the shoulders with subsequent instability [68]. Instability is always anterior and occurs with the arm in extension and internal rotation [26]. It is difficult to analyze the causes of instability. However, the complete release of the subscapularis, including the inferior and middle glenohumeral ligament at the glenoid insertion site, may predispose to weakened anterior restraints. Another potential cause of instability is loss of tension of the deltoid [68]. Preventive measures are focused on using a superolateral approach, avoiding retroversion of the humeral component, avoiding anteversion of the glenoid component, and establishing optimal length of the humerus.

To prevent dislocation, it is important to create room around the glenosphere to enable the prosthesis to hinge. We also advise to use a "standard" polyethylene insert instead of an insert with less contact area (high-mobility insert). Combined with an optimal prosthetic tensioning, these steps can prevent the creation of an opening wedge between the polyethylene and the glenosphere over the full range of movement. Early dislocations can easily be treated with closed reduction under general anaesthesia and an abduction pillow in the first weeks postoperatively [70].

Other Problems

Intra-operative fractures may occur on the humeral side at the time of exposure in

Fig. 13 Post-operative
fracture of the acromion

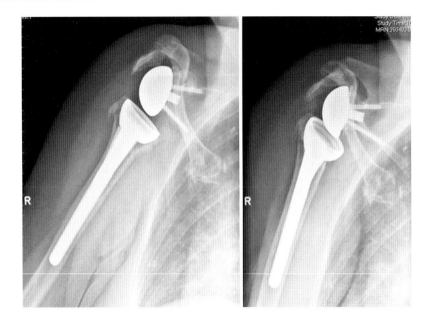

patients with severe pre-operative stiffness and
osteopenia, especially in the revision setting.
The proximal humerus may also be fractured
by retractors and at the time of glenoid
exposure; it is recommended not to complete
the humeral preparation until the glenoid
component is implanted to protect the proximal
humeral bone stock.

Glenoid fractures may occur during
preparation of the glenoid, especially reaming,
and may prevent component implantation
[68, 71].

Post-operative fractures of the acromion are
rare and should be treated conservatively with
immobilization (Fig. 13).

Postoperative fractures of the scapular spine
lead to poor functional outcome and may require
osteosynthesis [72, 73].

Glenosphere disengagement has been described in literature and this can be partial or
complete [47]. The presence of partial
disengagement of the glenosphere was not
associated with a difference in clinical outcome
but close follow-up is necessary.

Axillary nerve palsy is fortunately very rare
[18, 49].

Conclusions

Reverse total shoulder arthroplasty has been
shown to be effective in treating rotator
cuff-deficient arthritis with numerous studies
demonstrating initial improvements in shoulder
motion and patient satisfaction. Long term
results shows that Constant-Murley score
and radiographic changes can deteriorate with
time and therefore caution must be exercised when recommending reverse shoulder
arthroplasty in the younger patient. Scapular
notching is not yet a proven precursor of
loosening, but it should not be considered
a harmless and unavoidable phenomenon of
reverse total shoulder arthroplasty. Prosthetic
overhang is the most effective way to overcome
the problem.

References

1. Bankes MJ, Emery RJ. Pioneers of shoulder replacement: themistocles Gluck and Jules Emile Pean.
   J Shoulder Elbow Surg. 1995;4(4):259–62.

2. Flatow EL, Harrison AK. A history of reverse total shoulder arthroplasty. Clin Orthop Relat Res. 2011;469(9):2432–9.

3. Neer II CS. Articular replacement for the humeral head. J Bone Joint Surg Am. 1955;37(2):215–28.

4. Neer II CS. Replacement arthroplasty for glenohumeral osteoarthritis. J Bone Joint Surg Am. 1974;56(1):1–13.

5. Katz D, O'Toole G, Cogswell L, Sauzieres P, Valenti P. A history of the reverse shoulder prosthesis. Int J Should Surg. 2007;1:108–13.

6. Ahir SP, Walker PS, Squire-Taylor CJ, Blunn GW, Bayley JI. Analysis of glenoid fixation for a reversed anatomy fixed-fulcrum shoulder replacement. J Biomech. 2004;37(11):1699–708.

7. Grammont P, Trouilloud P, Laffay J, Deries X. Design and manufacture of a new shoulder prosthesis. Rhumatologie. 1987;39:407–18.

8. Baulot E, Chabernaud D, Grammont PM. Results of Grammont's inverted prosthesis in omarthritis associated with major cuff destruction. Apropos of 16 cases. Acta Orthop Belg. 1995;61 Suppl 1:112–19.

9. Grammont PM, Baulot E. Delta shoulder prosthesis for rotator cuff rupture. Orthopedics. 1993;16(1):65–8.

10. Kontaxis A, Johnson GR. The biomechanics of reverse anatomy shoulder replacement – a modelling study. Clin Biomech (Bristol, Avon). 2009;24(3):254–60.

11. Boileau P, Watkinson DJ, Hatzidakis AM, Balg F. Grammont reverse prosthesis: design, rationale, and biomechanics. J Shoulder Elbow Surg. 2005;14(1 Suppl S):147S–61.

12. Severt R, Thomas BJ, Tsenter MJ, Amstutz HC, Kabo JM. The influence of conformity and constraint on translational forces and frictional torque in total shoulder arthroplasty. Clin Orthop Relat Res. 1993;292:151–8.

13. Harman M, Frankle M, Vasey M, Banks S. Initial glenoid component fixation in "reverse" total shoulder arthroplasty: a biomechanical evaluation. J Shoulder Elbow Surg. 2005;14(1 Suppl S):162S–7.

14. De Wilde LF, Audenaert EA, Berghs BM. Shoulder prostheses treating cuff tear arthropathy: a comparative biomechanical study. J Orthop Res. 2004;22(6):1222–30.

15. De Wilde L, Audenaert E, Barbaix E, Audenaert A, Soudan K. Consequences of deltoid muscle elongation on deltoid muscle performance: a computerised study. Clin Biomech (Bristol, Avon). 2002;17(7):499–505.

16. Karelse AT, Bhatia DN, De Wilde LF. Prosthetic component relationship of the reverse Delta III total shoulder prosthesis in the transverse plane of the body. J Shoulder Elbow Surg. 2008;17(4):602–7.

17. Levigne C, Boileau P, Favard L, Garaud P, Mole D, Sirveaux F, et al. Scapular notching in reverse shoulder arthroplasty. J Shoulder Elbow Surg. 2008;17(6):925–35.

18. Werner CM, Steinmann PA, Gilbart M, Gerber C. Treatment of painful pseudoparesis due to irreparable rotator cuff dysfunction with the Delta III reverse-ball-and-socket total shoulder prosthesis. J Bone Joint Surg Am. 2005;87(7):1476–86.

19. Simovitch RW, Zumstein MA, Lohri E, Helmy N, Gerber C. Predictors of scapular notching in patients managed with the Delta III reverse total shoulder replacement. J Bone Joint Surg Am. 2007;89(3):588–600.

20. Sirveaux F, Favard L, Oudet D, Huquet D, Walch G, Mole D. Grammont inverted total shoulder arthroplasty in the treatment of glenohumeral osteoarthritis with massive rupture of the cuff. Results of a multicentre study of 80 shoulders. J Bone Joint Surg Br. 2004;86(3):388–95.

21. De Wilde LF, Poncet D, Middernacht B, Ekelund A. Prosthetic overhang is the most effective way to prevent scapular conflict in a reverse total shoulder prosthesis. Acta Orthop. 2010;81(6):719–26.

22. Nyffeler RW, Werner CM, Gerber C. Biomechanical relevance of glenoid component positioning in the reverse Delta III total shoulder prosthesis. J Shoulder Elbow Surg. 2005;14(5):524–8.

23. Nicholson GP, Strauss EJ, Sherman SL. Scapular notching: recognition and strategies to minimize clinical impact. Clin Orthop Relat Res. 2011;469(9):2521–30.

24. Gutierrez S, Levy JC, Lee 3rd WE, Keller TS, Maitland ME. Center of rotation affects abduction range of motion of reverse shoulder arthroplasty. Clin Orthop Relat Res. 2007;458:78–82.

25. Gutierrez S, Levy JC, Frankle MA, Cuff D, Keller TS, Pupello DR, et al. Evaluation of abduction range of motion and avoidance of inferior scapular impingement in a reverse shoulder model. J Shoulder Elbow Surg. 2008;17(4):608–15.

26. Gerber C, Pennington SD, Nyffeler RW. Reverse total shoulder arthroplasty. J Am Acad Orthop Surg. 2009;17(5):284–95.

27. Roche C, Flurin PH, Wright T, Crosby LA, Mauldin M, Zuckerman JD. An evaluation of the relationships between reverse shoulder design parameters and range of motion, impingement, and stability. J Shoulder Elbow Surg. 2009;18(5):734–41.

28. Frankle M, Siegal S, Pupello D, Saleem A, Mighell M, Vasey M. The reverse shoulder prosthesis for glenohumeral arthritis associated with severe rotator cuff deficiency. A minimum two-year follow-up study of sixty patients. J Bone Joint Surg Am. 2005;87(8):1697–705.

29. Valenti P, Boutens D, Nerot C. Delta 3 reversed prosthesis for osteoarthritis with massive rotator cuff tear: long term results (>5 years). In: Walch G, Boileau P, Molé D, editors. Shoulder prosthesis. Montpellier: Sauramps Medical; 2001. pp. 253–259.

30. Stephenson DR, Oh JH, McGarry MH, Hatch GF, 3rd, Lee TQ. Effect of humeral component version on impingement in reverse total shoulder arthroplasty. J Shoulder Elbow Surg. 2011;20(4):652–8.

31. Macaulay AA, Greiwe RM, Bigliani LU. Rotator cuff deficient arthritis of the glenohumeral joint. Clin Orthop Surg. 2010;2(4):196–202.

32. Lehtinen JT, Kaarela K, Belt EA, Kautiainen HJ, Kauppi MJ, Lehto MU. Relation of glenohumeral and acromioclavicular joint destruction in rheumatoid shoulder. A 15 year follow up study. Ann Rheum Dis. 2000;59(2):158–60.

33. Lehtinen JT, Belt EA, Kauppi MJ, Kaarela K, Kuusela PP, Kautiainen HJ, et al. Bone destruction, upward migration, and medialisation of rheumatoid shoulder: a 15 year follow up study. Ann Rheum Dis. 2001;60(4):322–6.

34. McCarty DJ, Halverson PB, Carrera GF, Brewer BJ, Kozin F. "Milwaukee shoulder" – association of microspheroids containing hydroxyapatite crystals, active collagenase, and neutral protease with rotator cuff defects. I. Clinical aspects. Arthritis Rheum. 1981;24(3):464–73.

35. Epis O, Caporali R, Scire CA, Bruschi E, Bonacci E, Montecucco C. Efficacy of tidal irrigation in Milwaukee shoulder syndrome. J Rheumatol. 2007;34(7):1545–50.

36. Adams R. A treatise on rheumatic gout or chronic rheumatic arthritis of all the joint. London: John Churchill & Sons; 1873.

37. Neer C, Craig E, Fukuda H. Cuff-tear arthropathy. J Bone Joint Surg Am. 1983;65(9):1232–44.

38. Visotsky JL, Basamania C, Seebauer L, Rockwood CA, Jensen KL. Cuff tear arthropathy: pathogenesis, classification, and algorithm for treatment. J Bone Joint Surg Am. 2004;86 Suppl 2:35–40.

39. Hamada K, Fukuda H, Mikasa M, Kobayashi Y. Roentgenographic findings in massive rotator cuff tears. A long-term observation. Clin Orthop Relat Res. 1990;254:92–6.

40. Iannotti JP, McCarron J, Raymond CJ, Ricchetti ET, Abboud JA, Brems JJ, et al. Agreement study of radiographic classification of rotator cuff tear arthropathy. J Shoulder Elbow Surg. 2010;19(8):1243–9.

41. Middernacht B, de Grave PW, Van Maele G, Favard L, Mole D, De Wilde L. What do standard radiography and clinical examination tell about the shoulder with cuff tear arthropathy? J Orthop Surg Res. 2011;6:1.

42. Walch G, Boulahia A, Calderone S, Robinson AH. The 'dropping' and 'hornblower's' signs in evaluation of rotator-cuff tears. J Bone Joint Surg Br. 1998;80(4):624–8.

43. Hertel R, Ballmer FT, Lombert SM, Gerber C. Lag signs in the diagnosis of rotator cuff rupture. J Shoulder Elbow Surg. 1996;5(4):307–13.

44. De Wilde LF, Berghs BM, VandeVyver F, Schepens A, Verdonk RC. Glenohumeral relationship in the transverse plane of the body. J Shoulder Elbow Surg. 2003;12(3):260–7.

45. Mole D, Favard L. [Excentered scapulohumeral osteoarthritis]. Rev Chir Orthop Reparatrice Appar Mot. 2007;93 Suppl 6:37–94.

46. Redfern TR, Wallace WA, Beddow FH. Clavicular osteotomy in shoulder arthroplasty. Int Orthop. 1989;13(1):61–3.

47. Middernacht B, De Wilde L, Mole D, Favard L, Debeer P. Glenosphere disengagement: a potentially serious default in reverse shoulder surgery. Clin Orthop Relat Res. 2008;466(4):892–8.

48. Sayana MK, Kakarala G, Bandi S, Wynn-Jones C. Medium term results of reverse total shoulder replacement in patients with rotator cuff arthropathy. Ir J Med Sci. 2009;178(2):147–50.

49. Boileau P, Watkinson D, Hatzidakis AM, Hovorka I. Neer Award 2005: the Grammont reverse shoulder prosthesis: results in cuff tear arthritis, fracture sequelae, and revision arthroplasty. J Shoulder Elbow Surg. 2006;15(5):527–40.

50. Ekelund A, Nyberg R. Can reverse shoulder arthroplasty be used with few complications in rheumatoid arthritis? Clin Orthop Relat Res. 2011;469(9): 2483–8.

51. De Wilde L, Mombert M, Van Petegem P, Verdonk R. Revision of shoulder replacement with a reversed shoulder prosthesis (Delta III): report of five cases. Acta Orthop Belg. 2001;67(4):348–53.

52. Jacobs R, Debeer P, De Smet L. Treatment of rotator cuff arthropathy with a reversed Delta shoulder prosthesis. Acta Orthop Belg. 2001;67(4):344–7.

53. Rittmeister M, Kerschbaumer F. Grammont reverse total shoulder arthroplasty in patients with rheumatoid arthritis and nonreconstructible rotator cuff lesions. J Shoulder Elbow Surg. 2001;10(1):17–22.

54. Vanhove B, Beugnies A. Grammont's reverse shoulder prosthesis for rotator cuff arthropathy. A retrospective study of 32 cases. Acta Orthop Belg. 2004;70(3):219–25.

55. Seebauer L, Walter W, Keyl W. Reverse total shoulder arthroplasty for the treatment of defect arthropathy. Oper Orthop Traumatol. 2005;17(1):1–24.

56. Frankle M, Levy JC, Pupello D, Siegal S, Saleem A, Mighell M, et al. The reverse shoulder prosthesis for glenohumeral arthritis associated with severe rotator cuff deficiency. A minimum two-year follow-up study of sixty patients surgical technique. J Bone Joint Surg Am. 2006;88(Suppl 1 Pt 2):178–90.

57. Guery J, Favard L, Sirveaux F, Oudet D, Mole D, Walch G. Reverse total shoulder arthroplasty. Survivorship analysis of eighty replacements followed for five to ten years. J Bone Joint Surg Am. 2006;88(8):1742–7.

58. Cuff D, Pupello D, Virani N, Levy J, Frankle M. Reverse shoulder arthroplasty for the treatment of rotator cuff deficiency. J Bone Joint Surg Am. 2008;90(6):1244–51.

59. Grassi FA, Murena L, Valli F, Alberio R. Six-year experience with the Delta III reverse shoulder prosthesis. J Orthop Surg (Hong Kong). 2009;17(2):151–6.

60. Holcomb JO, Hebert DJ, Mighell MA, Dunning PE, Pupello DR, Pliner MD, et al. Reverse shoulder arthroplasty in patients with rheumatoid arthritis. J Shoulder Elbow Surg. 2010;19(7):1076–84.

61. Boileau P, Moineau G, Roussanne Y, O'Shea K. Bony increased-offset reversed shoulder arthroplasty: minimizing scapular impingement while maximizing glenoid fixation. Clin Orthop Relat Res. 2011;469(9): 2558–67.

62. Woodruff MJ, Cohen AP, Bradley JG. Arthroplasty of the shoulder in rheumatoid arthritis with rotator cuff dysfunction. Int Orthop. 2003;27(1):7–10.

63. Favard L, Levigne C, Nerot C, Gerber C, De Wilde L, Mole D. Reverse prostheses in arthropathies with cuff tear: are survivorship and function maintained over time? Clin Orthop Relat Res. 2011;469(9):2558–67.

64. Simovitch RW, Helmy N, Zumstein MA, Gerber C. Impact of fatty infiltration of the teres minor muscle on the outcome of reverse total shoulder arthroplasty. J Bone Joint Surg Am. 2007;89(5):934–9.

65. Boileau P, Rumian AP, Zumstein MA. Reversed shoulder arthroplasty with modified L'Episcopo for combined loss of active elevation and external rotation. J Shoulder Elbow Surg. 2010;19 Suppl 2:20–30.

66. Gerber C, Pennington SD, Lingenfelter EJ, Sukthankar A. Reverse Delta-III total shoulder replacement combined with latissimus dorsi transfer. A preliminary report. J Bone Joint Surg Am. 2007;89(5):940–7.

67. Roy JS, Macdermid JC, Goel D, Faber KJ, Athwal GS, Drosdowech DS. What is a successful outcome following reverse total shoulder arthroplasty? Open Orthop J. 2010;4:157–63.

68. Zumstein MA, Pinedo M, Old J, Boileau P. Problems, complications, reoperations, and revisions in reverse total shoulder arthroplasty: a systematic review. J Shoulder Elbow Surg. 2011;20(1):146–57.

69. Beekman PDA, Katusic D, Berghs BM, Karelse A, De Wilde L. One-stage revision for patients with a chronically infected reverse total shoulder replacement. J Bone Joint Surg Br. 2010;92-B(6):817–22.

70. De Wilde L, Boileau P, Van der Bracht H. Does reverse shoulder arthroplasty for tumors of the proximal humerus reduce impairment? Clin Orthop Relat Res. 2011;469(9):2489–95.

71. Sanchez-Sotelo J. Reverse total shoulder arthroplasty. Clin Anat. 2009;22(2):172–82.

72. Walch G, Mottier F, Wall B, Boileau P, Mole D, Favard L. Acromial insufficiency in reverse shoulder arthroplasties. J Shoulder Elbow Surg. 2009;18(3): 495–502.

73. Hattrup SJ. The influence of postoperative acromial and scapular spine fractures on the results of reverse shoulder arthroplasty. Orthopedics. 2010;33(5):302.

Glenohumeral Instability – an Overview

Pierre Hoffmeyer

Contents

Keywords

Glenohumoral Instability • Epidemiology • Clinical features-special tests • Imaging • Patho-anatomy • Classification-anterior, posterior, multi-directional, voluntary, chronic • Treatment-closed, surgical stabilisation, complications

Introduction

Glenohumoral dislocation is defined as a complete loss of contact between the glenoid and the humeral head. The dislocation may be traumatic, non-traumatic or voluntary. It may be uni-directional, anterior-posterior or inferior, or multi-directional. Subluxation implies a partial loss of contact between the joint surfaces. Instability is an impression expressed by the patient. Objectively it may range from fleeting episodes of subluxation to outright dislocation. Laxity is a clinical finding where more than "normal" passive motion or translation may be generated during the physical examination [1].

Most anterior dislocations are of traumatic origin. The circumstances of the dislocation will give useful indications as to the extent of the damage inflicted upon the joint. Usually the dislocation is caused by a fall on the outstretched hand. In some areas a high prevalence of sports injuries of a specific type is found. Mountainous and Nordic regions will see winter sports-related dislocations while in other areas the injury-producing activities

P. Hoffmeyer
University Hospitals of Geneva, Geneva, Switzerland
e-mail: Pierre.Hoffmeyer@hcuge.ch;
pierre.hoffmeyer@efort.org

G. Bentley (ed.), *European Surgical Orthopaedics and Traumatology*,
DOI 10.1007/978-3-642-34746-7_49, © EFORT 2014

will be soccer or rugby. Interestingly shoulder dislocations at the workplace are relatively uncommon.

Age is an important factor: Younger patients tend to have higher recurrence rates for antero-inferior dislocations than older patients. Young patients tend to dislocate a previously healthy shoulder in a high energy trauma causing carti-laginous and capsuloligamentous damage while older patients will dislocate after low energy falls because of a pre-existing degenerative changes or torn rotator cuff.

The first episode of dislocation is usually due to a memorable traumatic event but the following tend to occur with decreasing amounts of trauma, some patients reporting dislocations after turning in bed. The patient must be questioned as to the frequency of unstable or dislocating events. This information is useful, in assessing the amount of ligamentous insuffi-ciency, for example. High energy injuries such as rugby tackles or high speed ski falls are more likely to produce fractures of the glenoid than a countered overhand pass [2]. Patients with an accompanying fracture of the greater tuberosity tend not to recur.

It is imperative to know whether the patient has been able to reduce the dislocation by himself or whether he had to be reduced in a hospital setting under anaesthesia. It is also important to have the patient precisely describe the events leading to the dislocation. This will often not be possible for patients that are victims of seizures; the origin of which needs careful appraisal.

Family history is important; other family mem-bers may have had episodes of shoulder disloca-tions or recurrent sprains of other joints indicating familial laxity, congenital malformations or even Marfan's syndrome [2, 3].

The examiner must question the patient atten-tively as to the existence of apprehension. Some patients may come to fear that even raising the arm above shoulder level will cause dislocation. This is important information before proceeding with the physical examination, an iatrogenic dislocation in the examining room is a particularly embarrassing situation!

Clinical Examination of the Post-Traumatic Unstable Shoulder

In the non-acute setting *inspection* of the seated patient's shoulder will reveal global muscular atrophy, a tell-tale sign of upper extremity dis-use, due to the apprehension associated with multiple of dislocations. Deltoid atrophy will indicate an axillary nerve injury. The position of the humeral head should be noted and in case of a prominent coracoid and a posterior fullness a posterior dislocation may be suspected. An anterior fullness and a subacromial depres-sion are pathognomonic of a chronic anterior dislocation. Atrophy of the supraspinatus and infraspinatus fossae are indicative of a rota-tor cuff tear or supraspinatus nerve injury and fullness all around the joint represents an effusion.

Strength in internal and external rotation, abduction, antepulsion and retropulsion should be assessed isometrically with the arm at the side. At the same time the examiner observes the contractions of the different muscles. Loss of strength in a particular direction may signal a tendinous or neurological injury.

Range of motion is first tested actively. Lim-itations may be linked to an underlying glenohumeral or subacromial disorder. The onset of *apprehension* signals the limits of pas-sive range of motion testing. In cases of insta-bility the range of motion of the shoulder should not be limited except for the apprehension that occurs in abduction and external rotation with the arm above the horizontal. Generally in the normal situation, elevation does not exceed 170° and if so laxity is suspected. External rota-tion with the arm at the side exceeding 85° is certainly indicative of capsular laxity. *Gagey's sign* is positive when abduction is unilaterally greater than 90° with a blocked scapula [4, 5]. An *anteroposterior drawer test* is then performed to evaluate laxity [6]. Usually it is not possible to subluxate the shoulder anteriorly but posteriorly the compressive abduction-adduction test may cause a "clunk" accompanied by pain or discomfort. *Jobe's apprehension re-location test* is most informative and assesses inflammation or scarring of the anterior capsule-labro-ligamentous complex [7, 8]. The shoulder of the supine patient is brought to 90° of abduction and maximal external rotation. At some point, the patient will feel a painful sensation. The examiner then presses his palm on the humeral head, chasing it posteriorly; this produces immediate relief and external rotation can be maximized painlessly. *O'Brien's test* explores the labrum, the bicipital insertion and the AC joint. The physician standing behind the patient applies a downward pressure on the maximally-internally rotated and pronated upper extremity in 90° of elevation and 10°–15° of adduction. The provoked pain should disappear when the pressure is applied to the arm in the same position with the arm in external rotation with the extremity maximally supinated [9].

The rotator cuff and acromioclavicular joint are checked clinically for integrity and stability [1, 2].

Always keep in mind that an acutely dislocated shoulder may be accompanied by severe collateral injuries. Stretching or tearing of the brachial plexus or axillary nerve occurs especially in the elderly or after high energy injuries. The axillary artery or vein may be torn with the ensuing well-known problems if not diagnosed at an early time. Erecta type dislocations may entail a passage of the humeral head through the ribs into the thorax and even into the abdomen. Caution must be exercised in this situation. With these possible additional injuries in mind, a careful neurological and vascular examination must be undertaken for every patient presenting with a shoulder dislocation [1, 11].

Investigations

Because clinical evaluation and tests are not always reliable or diagnostic, imaging modalities will be necessary to assess the existing lesions [11].

Standard X-Rays

The investigation of the painful and unstable shoulder includes standard X-rays, and specialized studies. AP and axillary views are mandatory to evaluate the joint space, the glenoid and the humeral head. Bony Bankart lesions are best seen on the AP view and Hill-Sachs lesions are evaluated on the axillary view. Other standard views developed the pre-CT era such as the Y view, the transthoracic view, the Westpoint view or the Bernageau views all still retain their usefulness to delineate glenoid rim or humeral head defects [1, 12–14].

Computed Tomography

CT scan will allow accurate description of any bony abnormalities (Hill-Sachs, reverse Hill-Sachs or bony Bankart lesions of the antero-inferior glenoid). Arthro-CT will outline cartilage defects, labral fissures or tearing and capsular stretching by delineating the intervening pouches.

Magnetic Resonance Imaging

MRI and athro-MRI will be used to image capsulolabral lesions as well as cartilage defects. The rotator cuff is also well delineated. Muscle atrophy or changes are well highlighted by both CT and MRI [15].

In case of clinical suspicion vascular studies as well as electroneurological studies might prove necessary to fully evaluate the patient's condition.

Patho-Anatomy of Shoulder Instability

Unstable shoulders present a multitude of capsuloligamentous and bony lesions identified by plain X-ray, MRI, CT or by direct observation, either arthroscopic or open.

In many cases of antero-inferior instability a bony trough in the posterior-superior region of

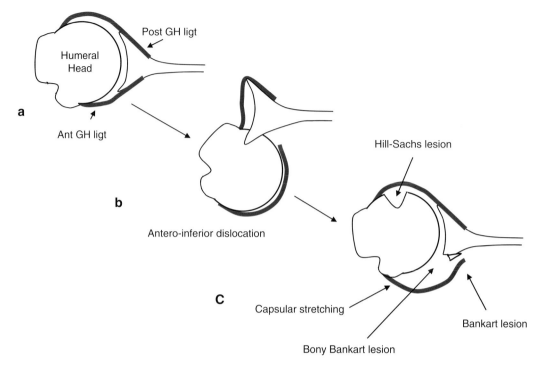

Fig. 1 Mechanism of sequellar lesions leading to recurrence of anterior dislocations (**a**–**c**). Pre-dislocation situation (**a**). Dislocation: Impaction of the humeral head against the glenoid or Hill-Sachs lesion, bony and ligamentous Bankart lesions due forceful passage of the humeral head (**b**). Sequellar lesions: Capsular stretching and loss of glenohumeral ligamentous and/or bony integrity responsible for recurrence (**c**)

the head may be caused by the impaction of the humeral head against the glenoid rim which if violent enough can fracture off the greater tuberosity: The *Hill-Sachs lesion*. With MRI bony oedema without actual fracture may be seen at the antero-inferior glenoid and in the posterosuperior head region, corresponding to impacts and spongiosa oedema without fracture (Fig. 1). In rare cases a fracture of the coracoid may be seen in association with a dislocation usually after a seizure. An isolated *coracoid fracture* should always prompt the question: Was this due to a self- reduced dislocation? Appropriate measures and investigations should be undertaken.

The *Bankart lesion* is defined as an avulsion of the antero-inferior labrum from the anterior rim of the glenoid with a disrupted periosteum. Bony lesions are also frequent with the *bony Bankart* lesion involving a fracture of the antero-inferior glenoid due to the violent passage of the head during an episode of dislocation. Multiple passages may also erode the glenoid to give it a rounded appearance. A defect of the glenoid may thus appear and augment giving rise in some cases to an "*inverted pear*" appearance. The *Perthes lesion* is an antero-inferior labral avulsion continued by a peeling off of the intact periosteum from the anterior glenoid neck. The anterior labrum periosteal sleeve avulsion (*ALPSA*) is an avulsion of the antero-inferior labrum that is displaced and rolled over medially. The humeral avulsion of the glenohumeral ligament (*HAGL*) is a peeling off of the inferior glenohumeral ligament on its insertion on the humeral neck. The superior labral tear from anterior to posterior (*SLAP*) represents various levels of avulsion of the proximal attachment of the long head of the biceps on the glenoid which may be associated with glenohumeral

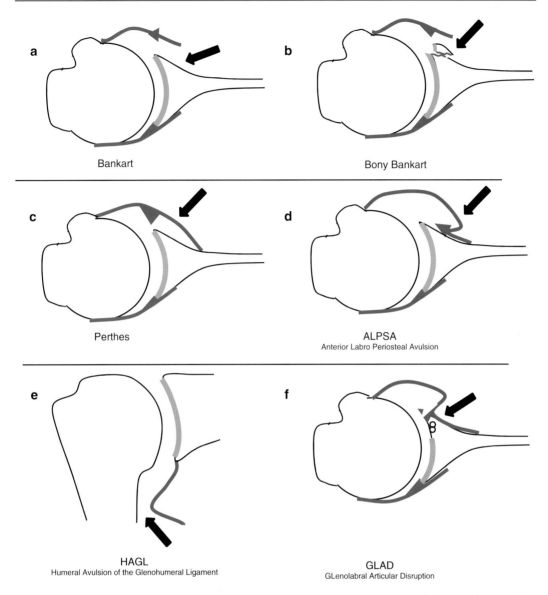

Fig. 2 Patho-anatomy of traumatic instability (**a–f**). *Bankart* lesion (*Arrow*) (**a**). *Bony Bankart* lesion (*Arrow*) (**b**). *Perthes* lesion (*Arrow*) (**c**). *ALPSA* Anterior labrum periosteal sleeve avulsion (*Arrow*) (**d**). *HAGL* Humeral avulsion of the glenohumeral ligament (*Arrow*) (**e**). *GLAD* GLenolabral articular disruption (*Arrow*) (**f**)

dislocations. Shoulders with multi-directional instability will present large and distended capsular pouches. The lesion glenolabral articular disruption (*GLAD*) was first described by Neviaser as a superficial tear of the antero-inferior labrum with an associated injury of the adjacent glenoid articular cartilage. As a rule this lesion is not associated per se with instability but is the cause of shoulder pain [9, 12, 14, 16–21] (Fig. 2).

Dislocation and Instability Types

Anterior Dislocation

This is usually related to sports activities (soccer, skiing etc.) or falls. Recurrence rates are high in patients below 20 years (up to 90 %), between 20 and 40 years 60 %

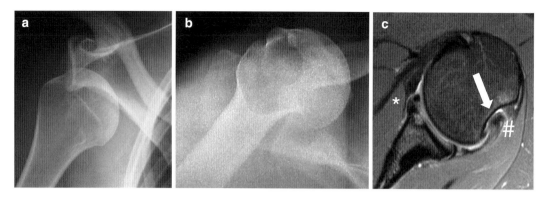

Fig. 3 Anterior dislocation (**a**, **b**). Anteroposterior (**a**) and axillary view (**b**). MRI (**c**) depicting a Hill-Sachs lesion (*arrow*) and a GLAD lesion (*) (For definition see text). A partial avulsion of the infraspinatus is also present (#)

recurrence rates, above 40 years 10 %. These numbers vary depending on the authors but trends remain [1, 2, 22].

Clinical examination is dominated by apprehension in abduction and external rotation. Signs of generalized laxity are often present: Anteroposterior drawer, inferior sulcus sign, joint hyperlaxity (fingers, thumb, and elbow).

In acute cases plexular or axillary nerve injury occurs in 5 % of patients. Imaging involves AP and axillary views (Fig. 3). Arthro-CT scans delineate precisely bony morphology of fractures; Hill-Sachs lesions, glenoid brim fractures or rounding-off are well visualized. MRI may be helpful to image the rotator cuff and the capsulolabral soft tissue lesions but demonstrate poorly bony lesions.

Closed reduction techniques for acute antero-inferior dislocations abound and should only be performed after precise neurovascular testing: Care-axillary nerve! (Fig. 4). Some of the more popular techniques are briefly described below:

Hippocrates: With the patient under general anaesthesia, traction is exerted on the arm in slight abduction and elevation with the operator's heel simultaneously pushing in the axilla or better with an aide pulling on a folded bed sheet placed around the axilla). This manoeuvre is traumatic should only be performed when other non- traumatic techniques have failed [23].

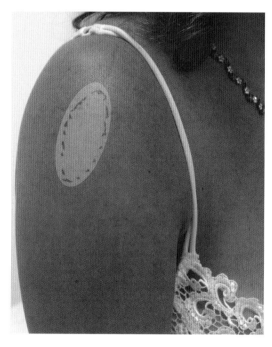

Fig. 4 Axillary nerve injury. Area of cutaneous sensate deficit or numbness on the lateral aspect of the shoulder after an axillary nerve neurapraxia following an anterior glenohumeral dislocation. This zone may be quite small and its identification requires meticulous assessment

Stimson: Patient lies prone with arm left hanging down; 1–3 kg weights are taped to the wrist for traction [24, 25].

Saha: In this technique a slow elevation in the plane of the scapula is performed [26].

Kocher: This is a classical technique but seen by many as dangerous. It consists in adducting the dislocated arm in internal rotation followed by abduction in external rotation [23]).

Davos (*Boss-Holzach-Matter method*): The patient in sitting position hands locked by intertwining his fingers around his ipsilaterally flexed knee with elbows extended is then instructed to let himself gradually lean backwards [27].

All of these techniques may be facilitated by an intra-articular injection of lidocaïne or equivalent [25].

Post-reduction treatment includes, after neurovascular testing, immobilisation in internal rotation or in an external rotation splint. The rationale for the external rotation immobilisation is to force the Bankart lesion to stay fixed to the anterior glenoid rim pressured in place by the subscapularis [28, 29]. Immobilisation should be 2–4 weeks followed by strengthening exercises [24].

Caution

Closed reduction manoeuvres after an *inaugural* episode should be approached with caution. A fracture may be associated and it is prudent to obtain an X-ray before embarking on manoeuvres that could have disastrous results. Beware of interpositions of the labrum, subscapularis, rotator cuff, biceps tendon or other structures that may result in a widened joint space on the post-reduction X-ray [30].

Surgical Stabilisation

Indications for surgical stabilisation of recurrent antero-inferior dislocations include one episode of dislocation too many, or severe apprehension. Techniques include capsuloplasty, Bankart lesion re-fixation and bony augmentation if there is severe rounding-off or fracture of the glenoid rim. Open or arthroscopic techniques are both suitable. Balg and Boileau have delineated the conditions where open repair is more suitable than arthroscopic repair. Factors such as patient age less than 20 years, competitive or contact sports, forced overhead activity, shoulder hyperlaxity, a Hill-Sachs lesion present on an anteroposterior radiograph of the shoulder in external rotation with loss of the sclerotic inferior glenoid contour, all tend to indicate open repair with a bone block (Latarjet-Bristow) according to these authors [31, 32]. Closed arthroscopic techniques are advocated in traumatic Bankart lesions, open techniques are recommended in cases of capsular stretching or of large Hill-Sachs lesions. Recurrence rates range between 5 % and 30 % depending on the type of technique used, solidity of reconstruction and patient compliance.

Patients are immobilized from 3 to 6 weeks in internal rotation; rehabilitation emphasizes muscular strengthening in the first weeks followed by range of motion exercises. Patients are advised to avoid contact sports for a year following stabilisation [33–41].

Posterior Dislocation

Posterior dislocation is relatively rare; less than 5 % of all instabilities. Falls on the outstretched hand, epileptic seizures or electrical shocks are the main causes of posterior dislocations. Aprehension can be elicited in adduction and internal rotation in posterior instability. When dealing with locked or chronic posterior dislocation one has to be beware of the diagnosic difficulties: The cardinal signs are active and passive limitation of external rotation, fixed abduction and limitation of supination.

AP shoulder X-rays and especially axillary views are the mainstay of the diagnosis. On the AP view the diagnosis may be missed by the unwary even though the joint space is not visible because of overlapping with the glenoid rim. The axillary view is *always* diagnostic. Scapular Y views and transthoracic views are often misinterpreted. In case of doubt a CT scan will solve the issue (Cadet, [13, 42–44]).

If a small (i.e. less than 10 % of head surface) reverse Hill-Sachs impaction fracture is present, gentle traction will generally reduce the shoulder which should then be immobilized in an external rotation splint for 3–6 weeks. Rowe has suggested keeping the affected arm at the side in neutral rotation fixed with a wide tape across the back [45]. A rehabilitation programme should follow with muscle strengthening and range of motion exercises.

Indications for surgical stabilisation of a posterior dislocation are an irreducible dislocation or recurring dislocations. When no major reverse Hill-Sachs lesion is present an open posterior approach with a cruciate capsulorraphy and fixation of the reverse Bankart lesion may be performed. A bone graft taken from the spine of the scapula or of the iliac crest may be necessary if a bony defect is present [46, 47]. Arthroscopic stabilisation is also an option in experienced hands [48].

If a larger reverse Hill-Sachs lesion is present, a McLaughlin procedure will be necessary and if insufficient an adjunct posterior procedure may be required. The McLaughlin operation consists in suturing the subscapularis tendon into the reverse Hill-Sachs defect. This creates an adequate barrier for any recurrence. Neer has modified the technique where the lesser tuberosity is osteotomized along with the subscapularis attachment and screwed into the defect. The shoulder is then immobilized in neutral, or slightly external, rotation for 6 weeks followed by a rehabilitation programme [47, 49, 50] (Fig. 5).

Multi-Directional Instability

This is a clinical entity formally identified by Neer and Foster [51]. The patient complains of a loose and unstable shoulder in multiple positions such as external rotation and abduction, adduction and internal rotation. Frequently, patients report pain, discomfort, apprehension and even paraesthesiae in the hand especially when carrying loads with the arm at the side. On clinical examination, external rotation is more than 90° both in the R1 (Arm at the side) or in the R2 position (Arm at 90° of abduction). Further clinical tests include the inferior sulcus test; the patient expresses discomfort as the examiner pulls down the arm held at the side

creating a subacromial sulcus. For these signs indicative of laxity to be clinically relevant, they must provoke patient discomfort [51–53] (Fig. 6).

Standard X-rays, arthro-CT or MRI will delineate the existing lesions. Surgery is indicated only after 1 year of serious muscle strengthening physiotherapy and exercises [51, 54].

The most commonly accepted operation is Neer's capsular shift which may be performed through an anterior deltopectoral approach but in certain cases may need an adjunct posterior approach. The axillary nerve must be protected during this demanding and complex intervention. Six weeks of immobilisation in neutral (handshake) position is necessary which should be followed by a muscle- strengthening programme. In experienced hands arthroscopic techniques may be used [51, 54, 55].

Voluntary Dislocation

This is usually encountered in adolescents and young adults who have found a way to dislocate their shoulder joint posteriorly. This is used by the patient to relieve psychic tensions (Tic), to show off to their friends and family or both. Treatment should consist of re-assurance and counselling to avoid dislocating the joint as this augments capsular laxity. Physiotherapy may be helpful. Sometimes psychiatric help may be needed. Surgery should be avoided at all costs because of the near 100 % recurrence rate.

Some patients will evolve to involuntary dislocation after a period of voluntary dislocation. This is due to excessive capsular stretching. Physiotherapy and re-harmonization exercises should be started. If not effective, an operative intervention consisting of a capsular tightening procedure such as a capsuloplasty (Described below), may be advocated. The surgeon must be certain however that the voluntary aspects of the dislocation have disappeared.

Positional dislocation may be falsely diagnosed as voluntary dislocation. Some patients will dislocate their shoulder posteriorly only in a certain

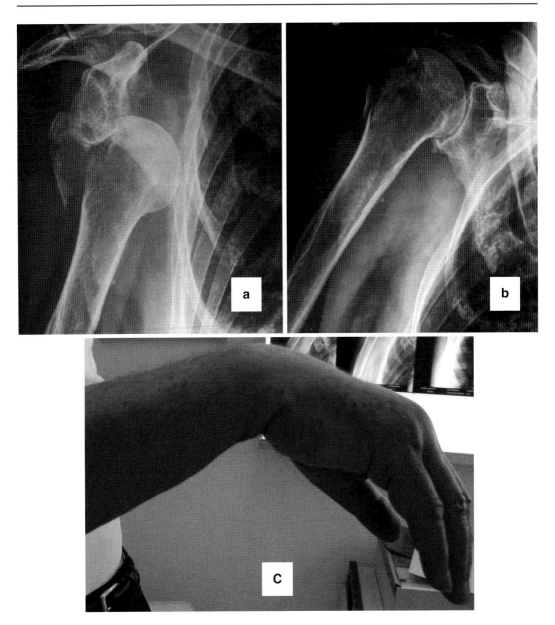

Fig. 5 Anterior fracture dislocation associated with neurological injury (**a–c**). Anterior dislocation with an associated fracture of the greater tuberosity (**a**). Reduction (**b**). Associated paraesthesiae and loss of strength due a radial nerve injury causing a wrist drop (**c**)

position usually in 90° of forward flexion, slight adduction and internal rotation. In this position with a lax capsule combined with a glenoid defector hypoplasia, the humeral head will tend to dislocate. Again after thorough investigation and adequate physiotherapy a stabilizing capsuloplasty procedure may be performed [56].

Recurrent Dislocation in the Elderly Patient

Often these dislocations are associated with minor trauma. A massive rotator cuff tear is the usual cause. If repairable the supra- and infraspinatus lesions should be repaired. If not repairable the

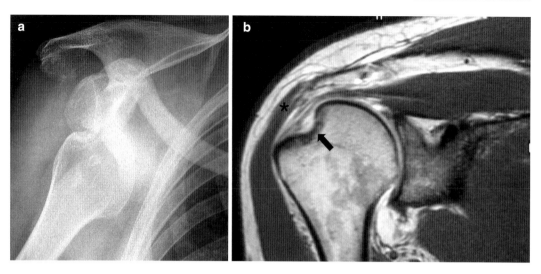

Fig. 6 (AB) Anterior dislocation (**a**), with resulting rotator cuff tear (*) and Hill-Sachs impaction (*arrow*) in an elderly patient (**b**)

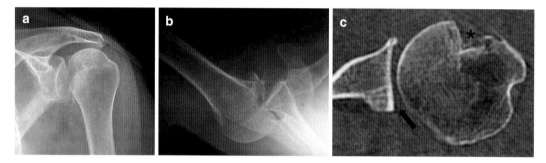

Fig. 7 Posterior dislocation (**a**–**c**). Anteroposterior (**a**) and axillary view (**b**). The CT (**c**) depicts dislocation sequellae: Reverse Hill-Sachs fracture impaction (*) and glenoid impaction (*arrow*)

reverse prosthesis may be an option and if not glenohumeral fusion may have to be performed [57] (Fig. 7).

Chronic Dislocation

This condition is usually seen in debilitated, neglected or epileptic patients. The dislocation may be anterior or posterior. Closed reduction is usually not successful and attempts at reduction may even be dangerous after some weeks in a chronically dislocated shoulder. In many cases the best option may be no treatment, the patient adapting to the situation. It is often surprising to see how much mobility is preserved.

In cases of a *chronic antero-inferior* dislocation with pain and discomfort, open reduction with a rotator cuff repair and glenoid augmentation procedure using a coracoid transfer or an iliac bone graft, may be attempted. A prosthetic replacement may also be used. It is prudent to use a bigger head than usual in a little more retroversion. Some authors advocate the reverse prosthesis but the danger of post-operative dislocation remains a high risk.

In cases of *chronic posterior* dislocation a McLoughlin procedure is indicated whereby, after open reduction, the detached subscapularis is fixed into the reverse Hill-Sachs impaction fracture, the Neer variation involves osteotomizing the lesser tuberosity and fixing it into the anterior

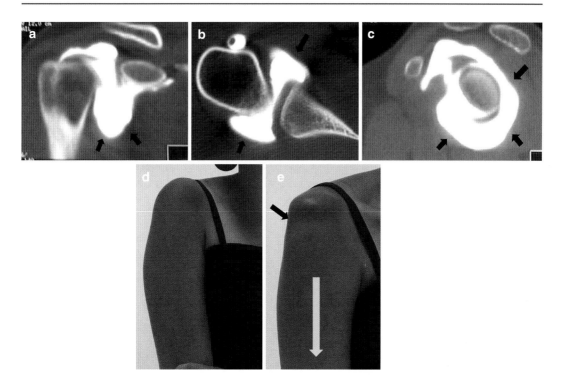

Fig. 8 Multi-directional instability (**a–e**). Arthro-CT demonstrates a large capsular pouch (*arrows*) seen in the transverse (**a**), frontal (**b**) and sagittal (**c**) cuts. Normal contour (**d**), Sulcus sign produced by pulling down on the arm held at the side (**e**)

impaction area with screws. When the head impaction is too large, i.e. more than 30 % or 50 % of the head surface, a hemi-prosthesis can be inserted. A larger head with a little less anteversion is a wise choice. Some authors advocate a reverse prosthesis but the risk of dislocation is significant. In cases of major instability with avulsed rotator cuff tendons a shoulder fusion may be contemplated [47, 58, 59].

Complications of Glenohumeral Dislocations

Neurovascular complications are common; most pertain to infra-clinical lesions of the axillary nerve. Plexular lesions may occur and are more frequent in elderly patients. Rarely vascular lesions may occur after a dislocation with the axillary artery being either sectioned (rarely) and more frequently presenting intimal tears leading to arterial occlusion. Post-immobilisation

or post- operative stiffness can occur in patients not following the rehabilitation regimen. Late-onset post-dislocation arthritis of varying intensity may occur in a fair number of patients up to 100 %. In most instances this radiographic finding is clinically irrelevant but it may become symptomatic, needing specific treatment [60–65] (Fig. 8).

References

1. Matsen FA, Lippitt S, Bertlesen A, Rockwood CA, Wirth MA. Glenohumeral instability. In: Rockwood CA, Matsen FA, Wirth MA, Lippitt SB, editors. The shoulder. 4th ed. Philadelphia: Saunders/Elsevier; 2009. p. 617–770.
2. Hovelius L, Augustini BG, et al. Primary anterior dislocation of the shoulder in young patients. A ten-year prospective study. J Bone Joint Surg Am. 1996;78(11):1677–84.
3. O'Driscoll SW, Evans DC. Long-term results of staple capsulorrhaphy for anterior instability of the shoulder. J Bone Joint Surg Am. 1993;75(2):249–58.

4. Gagey OJ, Gagey N. The hyperabduction test. J Bone Joint Surg Br. 2001;83(1):69–74.

5. Beaudreuil J, Nizard R, Thomas T, Peyre M, Liotard JP, Boileau P, Marc T, Dromard C, Steyer E, Bardin T, Orcel P, Walch G. Contribution of clinical tests to the diagnosis of rotator cuff disease: a systematic literature review. Joint Bone Spine. 2009;76(1):15–9.

6. Gerber C, Ganz R. Clinical assessment of instability of the shoulder. With special reference to anterior and posterior drawer tests. J Bone Joint Surg Br. 1984;66(4):551–6.

7. Hamner DL, Pink MM, Jobe FW. A modification of the relocation test: arthroscopic findings associated with a positive test. J Shoulder Elbow Surg. 2000;9(4):263–7.

8. Parentis MA, Glousman RE, Mohr KS, Yocum LA. An evaluation of the provocative tests for superior labral anterior posterior lesions. Am J Sports Med. 2006;34(2):265–8.

9. O'Brien SJ, Pagnani MJ, Fealy S, McGlynn SR, Wilson JB. The active compression test: a new and effective test for diagnosing labral tears and acromioclavicular joint abnormality. Am J Sports Med. 1998;26:610–3.

10. Warner JJ, Micheli LJ, et al. Patterns of flexibility, laxity, and strength in normal shoulders and shoulders with instability and impingement. Am J Sports Med. 1990;18(4):366–75.

11. Calvert E, Chambers GK, Regan W, Hawkins RH, Leith JM. Special physical examination tests for superior labrum anterior posterior shoulder tears are clinically limited and invalid: a diagnostic systematic review. J Clin Epidemiol. 2009;62(5):558–63.

12. Bankart A. The pathology and treatment of recurrent dislocation of the shoulder. Br J Surg. 1938;26:23–9.

13. Goud A, Segal D, Hedayati P, Pan JJ, Weissman BN. Radiographic evaluation of the shoulder. Eur J Radiol. 2008;68(1):2–15.

14. Sanders TG, Zlatkin M, Montgomery J. Imaging of glenohumeral instability. Semin Roentgenol. 2010;45(3):160–79.

15. Schreinemachers SA, van der Hulst VP, Jaap Willems W, Bipat S, van der Woude HJ. Is a single direct MR arthrography series in ABER position as accurate in detecting anteroinferior labroligamentous lesions as conventional MR arthography? Skeletal Radiol. 2009;38(7):675–83.

16. Bui-Mansfield LT, Banks KP, Taylor DC. Humeral avulsion of the glenohumeral ligaments: the HAGL lesion. Am J Sports Med. 2007;35(11):1960–6.

17. Melvin JS, Mackenzie JD, Nacke E, Sennett BJ, Wells L. MRI of HAGL lesions: four arthroscopically confirmed cases of false-positive diagnosis. Am J Roentgenol. 2008;191(3):730–4.

18. Neviaser TJ. The GLAD lesion: another cause of anterior shoulder pain. Arthroscopy. 1993;9(1):22–3.

19. Neviaser TJ. The anterior labroligamentous periosteal sleeve avulsion lesion: a cause of anterior instability of the shoulder. Arthroscopy. 1993;9(1):17–21.

20. Yiannakopoulos CK, Mataragas E, Antonogiannakis E. A comparison of the spectrum of intra-articular lesions in acute and chronic anterior shoulder instability. Arthroscopy. 2007;23(9):985–90.

21. Yin B, Vella J, Levine WN. Arthroscopic alphabet soup: recognition of normal, normal variants, and pathology. Orthop Clin North Am. 2010;41(3):297–308.

22. Pagnani MJ, Dome DC. Surgical treatment of traumatic anterior shoulder instability in American football players. J Bone Joint Surg Am. 2002;84-A (5):711–5.

23. Sayegh FE, Kenanidis EI, Papavasiliou KA, Potoupnis ME, Kirkos JM, Kapetanos GA. Reduction of acute anterior dislocations: a prospective randomized study comparing a new technique with the Hippocratic and Kocher methods. J Bone Joint Surg Am. 2009;91(12):2775–82.

24. Cofield RH, Kavanagh BF, Frassica FJ. Anterior shoulder instability. Instr Course Lect. 1985;34:210–27.

25. Miller SL, Cleeman E, Auerbach J, Flatow EL. Comparison of intra-articular lidocaine and intravenous sedation for reduction of shoulder dislocations: a randomized, prospective study. J Bone Joint Surg Am. 2002;84-A(12):2135–9.

26. Saha AK. The classic. Mechanism of shoulder movements and a plea for the recognition of "zero position" of glenohumeral joint. Clin Orthop Relat Res. 1983;173:3–10.

27. Ceroni D, Sadri H, Leuenberger A. Anteroinferior shoulder dislocation: an auto-reduction method without analgesia. J Orthop Trauma. 1997;11(6):399–404.

28. Itoi E, Hatakeyama Y, Sato T, Kido T, Minagawa H, Yamamoto N, Wakabayashi I, Nozaka K. Immobilization in external rotation after shoulder dislocation reduces the risk of recurrence. A randomized controlled trial. J Bone Joint Surg Am. 2007;89(10):2124–31.

29. Siegler J, Proust J, Marcheix PS, Charissoux JL, Mabit C, Arnaud JP. Is external rotation the correct immobilisation for acute shoulder dislocation? An MRI study. Orthop Traumatol Surg Res. 2010;96(4):329–33.

30. Stern R, Brigger A, Hoffmeyer P. Pseudo-reduction of an acute anterior dislocation of the shoulder-a case report. Acta Orthop. 2005;76(6):932–3.

31. Hovelius L, Sandstrom B, Saebö M. One hundred eighteen Bristow-Latarjet repairs for recurrent anterior dislocation of the shoulder prospectively followed for fifteen years: study II-the evolution of dislocation arthropathy. J Shoulder Elbow Surg. 2006;15(3):279–89.

32. Hovelius L, Sandstrom B, Sundgren K, Saebö M. One hundred eighteen Bistow-Latarjet repairs for recurrent anterior dislocation of the shoulder prospectively followed for fifteen years: study I-clinical results. J Shoulder Elbow Surg. 2004;13(5):509–16.

33. Cole BJ, Warner JJ. Arthroscopic versus open Bankart repair for traumatic anterior shoulder instability. Clin Sports Med. 2000;19(1):19–48.

34. Jolles BM, Pelet S, Farron A. Traumatic recurrent anterior dislocation of the shoulder: two- to four-year follow-up of an anatomic open procedure. J Shoulder Elbow Surg. 2004;13(1):30–4.

35. Jorgensen U, Svend-Hansen H, Bak K, Pedersen I. Recurrent post-traumatic anterior shoulder dislocation-open versus arthroscopic repair. Knee Surg Sports Traumatol Arthrosc. 1999;7(2):118–24.

36. Millett PJ, Clavert P, Warner JJ. Open operative treatment for anterior shoulder instability: when and why? J Bone Joint Surg Am. 2005;87(2):419–32.

37. Mohtadi NG, Bitar IJ, Sasyniuk TM, Hollinshead RM, Harper WP. Arthroscopic versus open repair for traumatic anterior shoulder instability: a meta-analysis. Arthroscopy. 2005;21(6):652–8.

38. Ozbaydar M, Elhassan B, Diller D, Massimini D, Higgins LD, Warner JJ. Results of arthroscopic capsulolabral repair: Bankart lesion versus anterior labroligamentous periosteal sleeve avulsion lesion. Arthroscopy. 2008;24(11):1277–83.

39. Pulavarti RS, Symes TH, Rangan A. Surgical interventions for anterior shoulder instability in adults. Cochrane Database Syst Rev. 2009;4, CD005077.

40. Rouxel Y, Rolland E, Saillant G. Les récidives post-opératoires: résultats et reprises chirurgicales. Rev Chir Orthop Reparatrice Appar Mot. 2000;86 Suppl 1:137–47.

41. Walch G, Boileau P, Levigne C, Mandrino A, Neyret P, Donell S. Arthroscopic stabilization for recurrent anterior shoulder dislocation: results of 59 cases. Arthroscopy. 1995;11(2):173–9.

42. Harish S, Nagar A, Moro J, Pugh D, Rebello R, O'Neill J. Imaging findings in posterior instability of the shoulder. Skeletal Radiol. 2008;37(8):693–707.

43. Sanders TG, Tirman PF, Linares R, Feller JF, Richardson R. The glenolabral articular disruption lesion: MR arthrography with arthroscopic correlation. Am J Roentgenol. 1999;172(1):171–5.

44. Silfverskiold JP, Straehley DJ, Jones WW. Roentgenographic evaluation of suspected shoulder dislocation: a prospective study comparing the axillary view and the scapular 'Y' view. Orthopedics. 1990;13(1):63–9.

45. Rowe CR. The shoulder. New York: Churchill Livingstone; 1988.

46. Essadki B, Dumontier C, Sautet A, Apoil A. Posterior shoulder instability in athletes: surgical treatment with iliac bone block. A propos of 6 case reports. Rev Chir Orthop Reparatrice Appar Mot. 2000;86(8):765–72.

47. Neer CS. Shoulder reconstruction. Philadelphia: WB Saunders; 1990. p. 551.

48. Bradley JP, Tejwani SG. Arthroscopic management of posterior instability. Orthop Clin North Am. 2010;41(3):339–56.

49. Betz M, Traub S. Bilateral posterior shoulder dislocations following seizure. Int Emerg Med. 2007;2:63–5.

50. Hawkins RJ, Neer CS, Pianta RM, Mendoza FX. Locked posterior dislocation of the shoulder. J Bone Joint Surg Am. 1987;69(1):9–18.

51. Neer CS, Foster CR. Inferior capsular shift for involuntary inferior and multidirectional instability of the shoulder. A preliminary report. J Bone Joint Surg Am. 1980;62(6):897–908.

52. Pollock RG, Owens JM, Flatow EL, Bigliani LU. Operative results of the inferior capsular shift procedure for multidirectional instability of the shoulder. J Bone Joint Surg Am. 2000;82(7):919–28.

53. Walch G, Agostini JY, Levigne C, Nové-Josserand L. Recurrent anterior and multidirectional instability of the shoulder. Rev Chir Orthop Reparatrice Appar Mot. 1995;81(8):682–90.

54. Abrams JS, Bradley JP, Angelo RL, Burks R. Arthroscopic management of shoulder instabilities: anterior, posterior, and multidirectional. Instr Course Lect. 2010;59:141–55.

55. Hamada K, Fukuda H, Nakajima T, Yamada N. The inferior capsular shift operation for instability of the shoulder. Long-term results in 34 shoulders. J Bone Joint Surg Br. 1999;81(2):218–25.

56. Fuchs B, Jost B, Gerber C. Posterior-inferior capsular shift for the treatment of recurrent, voluntary posterior subluxation of the shoulder. J Bone Joint Surg Am. 2000;82(1):16–25.

57. Porcellini G, Paladini P, Campi F, Paganelli M. Shoulder instability and related rotator cuff tears: arthroscopic findings and treatment in patients aged 40 to 60 years. Arthroscopy. 2006;22(3):270–6.

58. Vandenbussche E. Les luxations invétérées de l'épaule. Conférences d'enseignement de la SOFCOT n°99. Paris: Elsevier Masson; 2010. p. 1–17.

59. Wall B, Nové-Josserand L, O'Connor DP, Edwards TB, Walch G. Reverse total shoulder arthroplasty: a review of results according to etiology. J Bone Joint Surg Am. 2007;89(7):1476–85.

60. Apaydin N, Shane Tubbs R, Loukas M, Duparc F. Review of the surgical anatomy of the axillary nerve and the anatomic basis of its iatrogenic and traumatic injury. Surg Radiol Anat. 2010;32:193–201.

61. Mallon WJ, Bassett FH, Goldner RD. Luxatio erecta: the inferior glenohumeral dislocation. J Orthop Trauma. 1990;4(1):19–24.

62. Samilson RL, Prieto V. Dislocation arthropathy of the shoulder. J Bone Joint Surg Am. 1983;65(4):456–60.

63. Simonet WT, Cofield RH. Prognosis in anterior shoulder dislocation. Am J Sports Med. 1984;12(1):19–24.

64. Tauber M, Resch H, Forstner R, Raffl M, Schauer J. Reasons for failure after surgical repair of anterior shoulder instability. J Shoulder Elbow Surg. 2004;13(3):279–85.

65. van der Zwaag HM, Brand R, Obermann WR, Rozing PM. Glenohumeral osteoarthrosis after Putti-Platt repair. J Shoulder Elbow Surg. 1999;8(3):252–8.

Recurrent Glenohumeral Instability

Mark Tauber and Peter Habermeyer

Contents

Keywords

Gleno-humeral instability: anterior • Inferior • Posterior and multidirectional labral lesions • Superior labral lesions (SLAP tears) • Glenoid rim bone lesions

General Introduction

Glenohumeral instability represents mainly a pathology of the young patient. An unstable shoulder creates discomfort, pain and restriction of daily living or sports activities. Additionally, glenohumeral instability seems to represent a major risk factor for development of osteoarthritis. An accurate evaluation of history and clinical examination is crucial to make the correct diagnosis. Uni-directional instabilities can often be the only symptom of multi-directional forms. Treatment of only the symptomatic direction is associated with a high risk of failure and recurrence. Objective assessment of the patient's activity and risk profile should determine the treatment algorithm. The surgical approach and technique is dependent from the underlying pathology. It should address in a sufficient manner soft tissue pathologies, bone loss or associated injuries of the rotator cuff or long head of biceps tendon. Incorrect diagnosis and inadequate surgical treatment results in an increased failure rate requiring revision surgery.

M. Tauber (✉) • P. Habermeyer
Section for Shoulder and Elbow Surgery, ATOS Clinic,
Munich, Germany
e-mail: tauber@atos-muenchen.de

G. Bentley (ed.), *European Surgical Orthopaedics and Traumatology*,
DOI 10.1007/978-3-642-34746-7_233, © EFORT 2014

Aetiology and Classification

Contemporaneously to the evolving science of shoulder pathologies, new classification systems of shoulder instability have been presented. Prerequisites for a classification system are simplicity, completeness, practicability, and high intra- and interobserver reliability. In addition to a diagnostic value, a therapeutical consequence should result for the physician. The different classification systems are based on various criteria as time (acute – chronic), aetiology (traumatic – atraumatic – habitual) or direction (unidirectional – multidirectional, anterior – posterior – inferior). From an aetiological aspect it is essential to distinguish traumatic from atraumatic instabilities. In addition, an accurate history must point out if the trauma was adequate or not. Traumatic instabilities are associated with typical intraarticular injuries as labrum lesions, capsular stretching or avulsion, ligament tears, impression fractures at the humeral head (Hill-Sachs or reversed Hill-Sachs-lesion), bony glenoid rim lesions, rotator cuff tears or SLAP-lesions.

The most widely used classification systems of shoulder instability are:

- The TUBS (traumatic, unidirectional, Bankart, and usually requiring surgery) and AMBRI (atraumatic, multidirectional, bilateral, rehabilitation, and occasionally requiring an inferior capsular shift) classification according to Matsen and Harryman [1]
- *Classification of the instability according to Gerber* [2]
  - Type I: chronic dislocation
  - Type II: unidirectional instability without hyperlaxity
  - Type III: unidirectional instability with multidirectional hyperlaxity
  - Type IV: multidirectional instability without hyperlaxity
  - Type V: multidirectional instability with hyperlaxity
  - Type VI: uni- or multidirectional voluntary dislocation

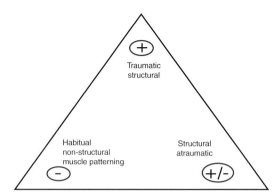

Fig. 1 Classification of shoulder instability according to Bailey [3]. Three main groups form the base of the classification (traumatic structural, atraumatic structural, habitual, non-structural, muscle patterning) with a fluid transition between them

- *Classification of the instability according to Bailey* [3] (Fig. 1)
  - Polar group I: traumatic structural (adequate trauma, often Bankart lesion, usually unidirectional, no muscular dysfunction)
  - Polar group II: atraumatic structural (no trauma, structural articular pathology, capsular dysfunction, no muscular dysfunction, sometimes bilateral)
  - Polar group III: habitual, non-structural, muscle patterning (no trauma, no structural articular damage, capsular dysfunction, muscle dysfunction, often bilateral)

Bony defects at the anterior glenoid rim can emerge from an acute or chronic setting. Acute glenoid fractures can be seen either as depression fractures with medialization of the fragment resulting in step formation at the articular surface or as avulsion fractures in terms of a bony capsulo-ligamentous detachment.

The most frequently used classification is:

- *Classification of bony anterior glenoid rim lesions according to Bigliani* [4]
  - Type I: the detached fragment is adjacent to the capsulo-ligament complex
  - Type II: the fragment is malunited medially at the glenoid neck (Fig. 2)
  - Type III: erosion of the glenoid rim
    Type IIIA: defect size < 25 %
    Type IIIB: defect size > 25 %

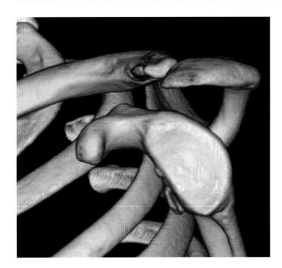

Fig. 2 To evaluate the size of the bony glenoid defect a computed tomography scan with a 3D reconstruction should be performed. On the en-face view the defect size can be measured setting the indication for a bone block augmentation procedure with a bone loss of 20 % of the antero-posterior diameter. Note the medialized, partially resorbed bone fragment at the anterior glenoid rim

A special entity of labral lesion is represented by the so called "SLAP" (superior labrum anterior to posterior) lesions, first described by Snyder et al. in 1990 [5]. Four types of lesions have been described:

- Type I: fraying of the superior labrum and the biceps anchor without detachment from the glenoid
- Type II: detachment of the superior labrum-biceps-complex from the glenoid
- Type III: bucket-handled tear of the labrum. The biceps anchor remains intact
- Type IV: longitudinal splitting of the labrum and the biceps tendon. The inferior part of the tear can dislocate into the articular rim

SLAP-II-lesions have been divided from arthroscopic observations into three subtypes [6]:

- II A: anterior
- II B: posterior
- II C: combined anterior-posterior

Maffet et al. [7]. extended this classification for further three types:

- Type V: extension of the SLAP-lesion to antero-inferior in terms of a combined Bankart-SLAP II – lesion

- Type VI: unstable labrum-flap
- Type VII: extension into the MGHL with weakening of its function

Relevant Applied Anatomy, Pathology and/or Basic Science, e.g., Biomechanics

Several factors are responsible for the potential instability of the glenohumeral joint. First, the bony dimensions of the articulating partners have to be mentioned with the large humeral head articulating with the small and shallow glenoid. Furthermore, stability is provided by the soft tissues including the capsulo-ligamentous structures, rotator cuff, scapular stabilizers, and the biceps tendon enabling a large range of motion at the same time [8–10]. Static stabilizers as the bony articulating structures, the glenohumeral joint capsule and its ligaments have to be distinguished from dynamic stabilizers as the rotator cuff and the biceps tendon. In patients with multidirectional instability (MDI) and posterior instability deficiency of the rotator interval represents a further key factor contributing to increased inferior and posterior translation [11]. Bony factors may influence glenohumeral stability as well. Glenoid hypoplasia or excessive glenoid retroversion represent important intrinsic aspects in posterior instability with an atraumatic history in most cases. Glenoid rim bone loss can be developmental or acquired. This can be either from an acute fracture or chronic erosion or rarely from hypoplasia.

In a cadaveric study, Itoi et al [12]. described a defect of 20 % of the glenoid length at the 6.00 o'clock position as a relevant bone loss resulting in antero-inferior gleno-humeral instability. For several years this defect size was the critical size representing the indication for bone reconstruction at the glenoid. Yamamoto et al. found that in recurrent glenohumeral instability the defect is not located antero-inferiorly, but at the 3.00 o'clock position [13] and as the critical size has to be seen a defect of 6 mm in the sagittal plane, which corresponds to 20 % of the glenoid length [14]. With this defect size the stability ratio decreases significantly from 32 % to 17 %.

In recent years the focus of research concentrated on glenoid bone loss. Several authors reported on bony defects of the anterior glenoid rim as one of the most relevant factors associated with recurrent instability after surgical stabilization [15–18]. Thus, it is crucial to detect significant glenoid bone loss preoperatively in patients with recurrent glenohumeral instability, in terms to recognize the need for a bone block procedure, which usually has to be performed as open procedure. This represents essential information for the surgeon, but for the patient as well.

In general, intraarticular capsulo-ligamentous lesions can occur at three different anatomical locations [19]:
- At the antero-inferior glenoid rim (Fig. 3a and b)
- Along the anterior capsule or gleno-humeral ligaments
- At their humeral insertion

Capsulo-ligamentous injuries (Fig. 4) in traumatic anterior gleno-humeral instability can be classified according to their morphologic differences into:
- The classic Bankart-lesion includes avulsion of the capsule-labral complex from the antero-inferior glenoid rim. Hereby, the concavity of the glenoid, which is determined for 50 % by the labrum, is reduced significantly and the MGHL and IGHL lose their origin resulting in anterior instability
- The Perthes lesion is defined by the subperiosteal avulsion of the AIGHL from the scapular neck. The labrum remains still in contact with the glenoid rim (extralabral lesion of the capsular origin)
- ALPSA (anterior labroligamentous periosteal sleeve avulsion)-lesion [20]: during the spontaneous healing process the labrum and the capsular origin can be slipped medially along the scapular neck by the intact periosteum and scar
- Interligamentous capsular tears are rare, because isolated capsular stretching occurs due to repetitive microtrauma
- The HAGL (humeral avulsion of glenohumeral ligaments)-lesion: avulsion of

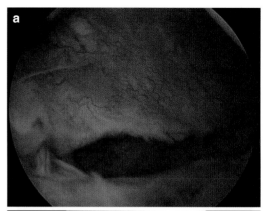
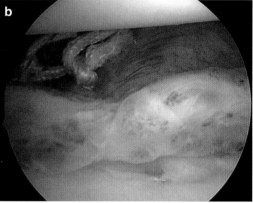

Fig. 3 (**a**) Arthroscopic view of a longitudinal capsule-ligamentous avulsion of the inferior gleno-humeral ligament from the labrum in a 20 year-old wrestler's left shoulder. (**b**) The inferior gleno-humeral ligament has been sutured by two mattress sutures to the glenoid rim and labrum. The gap between labrum and capsule/ligament is closed completely. Arthroscopic view with the patient in lateral decubitus position

the glenohumeral ligaments from their insertion at the humeral head. Variants are the bony HAGL with detachment of the IGHL together with a bony fragment, avulsion of the posterior IGHL (P-HAGL) in posterior dislocation and avulsion of the IGHL from the glenoid and humeral head (floating IGHL) [21]

Posterior shoulder instability is rare (about 5 % of cases of glenohumeral instability) and often occurs as part of MDI. In traumatic cases, posterior labral lesions can occur equivalently to anterior labrum tears and may be responsible for recurrent posterior shoulder instability. In most patients, posterior glenohumeral instability appears as a result

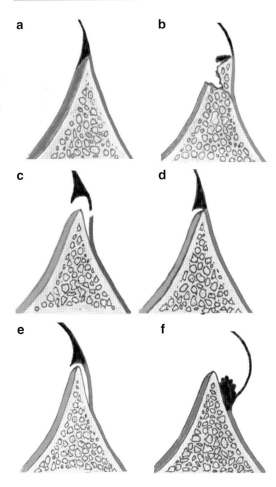

Fig. 4 Anterior rim morphology in glenohumeral instability. (**a**) Normal. (**b**) Bony Bankart lesion. (**c**) Bankart lesion involving the labrum and the capsule. (**d**) Bankart lesion with avulsion of only the labrum. The capsule is not detached from the labrum. (**e**) Perthes' lesion with subperiosteal avulsion of the AIGHL from the scapular neck. The labrum remains still in contact with the glenoid rim. (**f**) ALPSA lesion with the labrum and the capsular origin slipped medially along the scapular neck. The periosteum remains intact

the IGHL, especially in internal rotation and 90° of flexion (corresponding to the jerk test position).

To understand the entity of SLAP-lesions an appropriate knowledge of the anatomy of the superior labrum-biceps-complex is required. The superior labrum does not insert adjacently at the glenoid, but shows a meniscoid shape. Frequently, at the 12 o'clock position a small recessus between the superior labrum and the superior glenoid pole is present, which can lead to misdiagnosis in the MR-arthrography. This kind of insertion extends to the 4 o'clock position [23]. The superior labrum forms always a complex with the biceps tendon. The insertion point of the biceps at the superior labrum differs and can be postero-superior or at the superior glenoid tubercle [24, 25]. The vascular supply of the superior labrum-biceps-complex shows significantly less blood vessels than the inferior labrum-capsule-complex. Cooper et al [23]. observed periosteal and capsular vessels supporting the labrum in its entire circumference from the periphery, but reduced vascularity at the superior and antero-superior parts.

To avoid misdiagnoses two anatomical variants at the antero-superior labrum insertion have to be known:

- *Sublabral foramen* [26]: physiologic detachment of the antero-superior labrum from the 1 to 2 o'clock position without pathological character in contrast to the Andrews lesion [27] at the same position.
- *Buford-Complex* [28]: absence of the anterosuperior labrum from the 1 to 2 o'clock position and presence of a "cord-like" strong MGHL inserting at the bony glenoid rim or at the biceps anchor.

Diagnosis

History

A careful history is of utmost importance in patients presenting with glenohumeral instability. Information regarding the dominating symptoms (looseness, insecurity, or pain), onset, direction,

from repetitive microtrauma or from a traumatic impact to the anterior shoulder. Associated pathomorphological changes include capsulolabral detachment, capsular laxity, and rotator interval lesions. A special structural pathology represents the Kim lesion, which is an incomplete and concealed avulsion of the posteroinferior aspect of the labrum [22]. An effective contributor to posterior stability represents the posterior band of degree of instability, need for reduction, recurrence, and previous surgical treatment are provided. The presence of an adequate trauma suggests the intraarticular pathomorphological lesions, whereas in the absence of a trauma hyperlaxity, voluntary dislocation, scapular dyskinesia or connective tissue pathologies as Ehlers-Danlos or Marfan syndromes have to be considered. The activity profile of the patients with traumatic antero-inferior shoulder dislocation is directly related to the risk for recurrence. Young patients performing contact sports show a risk of recurrence gaining 90 % to 95 % [29].

Clinical Examination

The clinical evaluation of the shoulder must differentiate two entities: laxity and instability:

- Laxity represents the passive and usually physiological translation of the humeral head in every direction without symptoms of instability. Laxity is individual and physiological. Laxity diminishes with increasing age.
- Instability is defined as inability of the patient to center and to keep the humeral head centered into the glenoid cavity [30]. Usually, instability is symptomatic: the patient suffers a dislocation or subluxation with subjective instability or pain.

Examination of Shoulder Instability

Whereas an anterior instability has to be expected in abduction and external rotation, for a posterior instability flexion and internal rotation movements are typical. The unpleasant position is the best indication for the direction of the instability.

Tests to Evaluate Anterior Instability

- *Apprehension test*: [31] With the patient sitting or standing, the arm is brought in abduction and external rotation with pressure of the contralateral hand from a posterosuperior direction onto the proximal humerus. The test results positive,

if a reflectory muscle contracture is seen to prevent subluxation or dislocation or the patient refers subjective instability. The face of the patient has to be observed. Discomfort, insecurity, movements of compensation or insufficient abduction and external rotation are indicative for a positive test. Pain alone is no criterion for a positive test. The test is done in 60°, 90° and 120° of abduction. In 60° abduction the medium glenhumeral ligament (MGHL) is tested, in 90° of abduction the MGHL and inferior glenohumeral ligament (IGHL). Usually, a positive Apprehension test is associated with a traumatic Bankart-lesion [32]. The apprehension test can be performed in a lying position modified as fulcrum-, relocation- or surprise-test.

- *Fulcrum test*: with the patient in a supine position, the free hand of the examiner during the abduction and external rotation is set as hypomochlion under the proximal humerus. This increases the lever mechanism and allows the controlled provocation of the anterior subluxation resulting into subjective instability or pain.
- *Relocation test* [33]: With the patient supine the arm is abducted 90° and external rotated. This position provokes anterior subluxation with increasing muscle fatigue of the anterior stabilizing muscles and apprehension. Push by the examiner from an anteroinferior direction reduces the humeral head and reduces the pain and apprehension. External rotation is increased until a positive apprehension sign appears again. The positive relocation test is valid for diagnosis of an internal impingement, as well. In 79 % of the throwing athletes, the pain during the relocation test correlates with the contact between posterosuperior rotator cuff and posteriosuperior labrum, or partial rotator cuff tear and labral lesion [34].
- *Surprise(Release) test*: [35]: During one hand of the examiner brings the arm of the patient in abduction and external rotation, the other pushes against the humeral

head from anterior and stabilizes the glenohumeral joint. Releasing suddenly the anterior support, an intense apprehension can be provoked.

Tests to Evaluate Posterior Instability

- *Posterior Apprehension test*: in patients with posterior instability a corresponding posterior apprehension test with the patient supine is performed [31]
- *Jerk-test*: with the patient in a sitting position the shoulder girdle is stabilized with one hand from posterior. The other hand takes the elbow of the patient with shoulder flexion of 90°. Performing increasing internal rotation, adduction of the humerus and posterior compression a posterior drawer or subluxation can be provoked. With horizontal abduction the shoulder can be reduced ("clunk").

Examination of SLAP-Lesions

The clinical image of patients with a SLAP-lesion is complex. Usually, the patients are young and active and refer the initial symptoms during sports activities, mainly overhead sports. During normal routine and daily living activities these patients don't have complaints. The onset can be traumatic or slowly increasing over the time. Normally, the range of motion (ROM) is free, in throwing athletes an increased external rotation and reduced internal rotation at the dominant upper extremity can be observed. The isometric rotator cuff tests present normal without loss of strength.

Tests to Evaluate SLAP-Lesions

- *Biceps load test II* [36]: With the patient supine and flexion of the shoulder of 120° the arm is brought in full external rotation. The elbow is flexed 90°, the forearm in supination. The test is positive, when increasing active elbow flexion provokes pain or pain enhancement. For this test a sensitivity of 89.7 % and a specificity of 92.1 % has been reported.
- *Supine flexion resistance test* [37]: The patient is supine with the shoulder in maximal flexion.

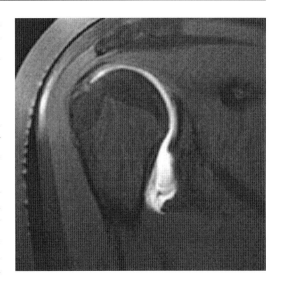

Fig. 5 MR-arthrography of a right shoulder 4 days after traumatic anterior dislocation. The paracoronar slices show the "J-sign", which is typical for a humeral avulsion of the inferior gleno-humeral ligament (HAGL lesion)

The patient is asked to extend the arm against the resistance of the examiner. Pain in the shoulder is predictive for a SLAP-lesion with a sensitivity of 92 %.

- Positive can be the impingement test according to Hawkins, the horizontal-adduction, O'Brien, Palm-up, Yergason, apprehension tests. All these tests don't have a sufficient sensitivity for clinical diagnosis of a SLAP-lesion [38].

Imaging

- Standard radiographs: true-a.p.-view in neutral rotation and in external rotation, Stryker-view, West-Point-view, Bernageau's view, Garth's apical-oblique profile view
- 3D-computed tomography (Fig. 2): assessment of glenoid defect (en-face view) [39–41] and version of the glenoid (glenoid dysplasia)
- MR-arthrography (evaluation of soft-tissue pathology): capsular volume, lesions of the capsuloligamentous complex, HAGL-lesion (Fig. 5), extension of Bankart-lesion, rotator cuff tears, rotator interval, SLAP-lesion

Indications for Surgery

Indications for Conservative Treatment

- Atraumatic etiology (Polar type II according to Bailey [3])
- Pathologic muscle patterning (Polar type III according to Bailey [3])
- Scapula dyskinesia
- Loose shoulder [42]
- Ehlers-Danlos syndrome
- Marfan syndrome
- Incompliance
- Psychiatric disease

Indications for Surgical Treatment

Glenohumeral Instability
- Chronic anterior instability with traumatic etiology and structural capsulo-labral-ligamentous pathologies
- Recurrent dislocation or subluxation with relevant anterior glenoid bone loss (>25 %)
- HAGL-/PHAGL-lesions
- Chronic posterior instability without laxity
- Chronic posterior instability with laxity but without pathologic muscle pattern and posterior glenoid bone loss
- Multidirectional instability after failure of conservative treatment for at least 6 months

SLAP-Lesions
The surgical strategies to treat SLAP-lesions depend on the type of lesion, the history (traumatic or microtraumatic repetitive) and from the activity and sports specific profile of the patient. Surgical repair of the SLAP-lesion has most success in patients with an acute traumatic injury and in low demand patients. Those patients with overuse symptoms, chronic microtraumatic lesions of throwing or overhead sports who want to return to their pre-injury sports are not candidates for refixation, but for tenodesis of the long head of the biceps tendon because of the much less predictable results [43].

Ide [44] and Kim [45] report on a return rate to previous sports in athletes in 60–70 % and 22 %, respectively. Out of these poor perspectives for athletes, Boileau et al [46]. proposed biceps tenodesis using an interference screw as an alternative procedure to treat SLAP-type-II lesions. The return rate to previous sports differed significantly in favour to the biceps tenodesis group (87 %), compared to the SLAP-repair group (40 %).

Following therapeutic strategies are recommended:
- Type I: debridement, electrothermical trimming
- Type II: reconstruction using
  II A: anchor and suture of MGHL
  II B: posterior anchor
  II C: anterior and posterior anchor with suture of MGHL

In microtraumatic cases: tenodesis of the long head of the biceps tendon:
- Type III: reconstruction or resection of the bucket-handle, if necessary tenodesis of the long head of the biceps tendon
- Type IV: reduction and reconstruction, if necessary resection or tenodesis of the long head of the biceps tendon

Pre-Operative Preparation and Planning

Complete imaging is a prerequisite to determine the necessity for bone grafting at the glenoid. For this purpose we recommend performance of a CT-scan with 3D-reconstruction. This information is decisive if stabilization surgery can be carried out arthroscopically or open, which has to be told to the patient preoperatively. In the case of free bone autografting, the patient has to be informed about risks and complications, as well as donor site morbidity at the iliac crest. [47, 48] Usually, the bone autograft is harvested from the ipsilateral side.

The procedure is performed under general anaesthesia combined with an interscalene nerve block (Winnie block). The beach chair position is the authors' preferred patient position

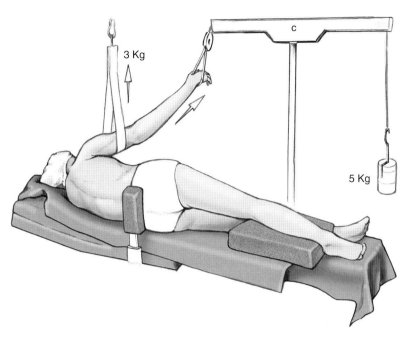

Fig. 6 Lateral decubitus position with antero-lateral arm traction. Note the padding of the lower extremities in order to avoid nerve damage and skin bruises (From Schulterchirurgie, 4. edition. Editor: Habermeyer P, Lichtenberg S, Magosch P. Elsevier, Munich, 2010)

3 Kg

5 Kg

for arthroscopic and open surgery at the anterior aspect of the glenohumeral joint. Procedures for posterior or multidirectional instability are carried out in the lateral decubitus position with the arm in antero-lateral traction (Fig. 6).

Operative Technique

Arthroscopic Bankart and Capsular Shift Procedures

- Mobilization of medialized labrum and ligament insertion (Fig. 7a)
- Proper decortication of glenoid neck
- Labrum reconstruction (the use of fewer than 4 suture anchors is risk for anterior shoulder stabilization failure) [49] (Fig. 7b and c)
- Postero-inferior capsular plication (Fig. 8a and b) via a posterior-inferior portal in cases with pathologic hyperabduction test according to Gagey
- Antero-inferior capsular shift: south–north/east-west [50]
- Closure of HAGL and R-HAGL lesions: side to side repair

- Closure of rotator interval in patients with passive external rotation of more than 85° (extensive laxitiy) [51]
- Remplissage: posterior capsulodesis and infraspinatus tenodesis in patients with isolated large Hill-Sachs defect and without bony Bankart defect [52]

Open Procedures

- Open Bankart repair
- Capsule T-shift according to Neer [53]

Bone Block Procedures

Arthroscopic [54]/Open Trillat Procedure

- Indication: glenoid defect < 20 % + capsular deficiency/capsular hyperlaxity
- Surgical principle: extra-articular coraco-biceps tenodesis/ligamentoplasty. The conjoined tendon is fixed above the subscapularis tendon at the level of the scapular neck using an interference screw. After the transfer, the conjoined tendon functions as a sling reinforcing the antero-inferior capsule-labral structures by lowering the subscapularis musculotendinous unit [50].

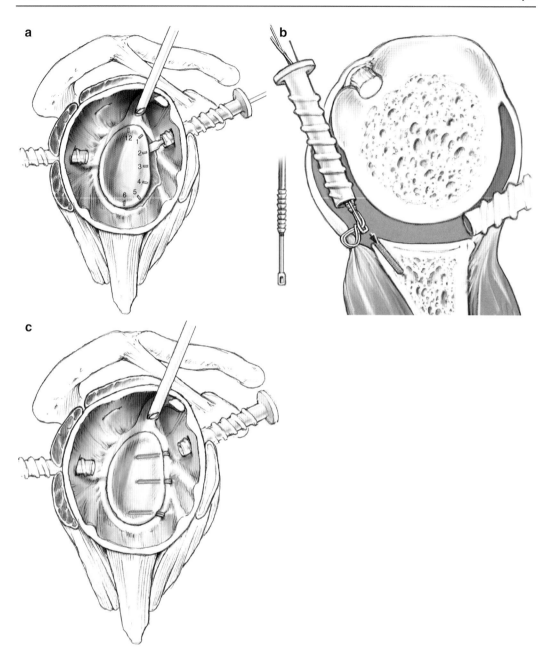

Fig. 7 (**a**) Graph showing the intraarticular position of the posterior, antero-superior and antero-inferior portals. Using a rasp the anterior capsule-labrum-complex is mobilized along the anterior glenoid rim. In cases of medialization towards the anterior glenoid neck visualization can be improved using the antero-superior portal for the scope. The glenoid neck has to be roughened by a burr to improve healing of the capsule-labrum complex to the glenoid rim (From Schulterchirurgie, 4. edition. Editor: Habermeyer P, Lichtenberg S, Magosch P. Elsevier, Munich, 2010). (**b**) The capsule and labrum are perforated with a double loaded suture wire using a curved suture needle. To fix the capsule-labrum complex to the glenoid rim knotless implants are used (From Schulterchirurgie, 4. edition. Editor: Habermeyer P, Lichtenberg S, Magosch P. Elsevier, Munich, 2010). (**c**) Final result showing anatomic capsule-labrum repair using three knotless anchors. To introduce the inferior anchor a transsubscapularis portal is recommended in order to gain the correct angle between implant and glenoid (From Schulterchirurgie, 4. edition. Editor: Habermeyer P, Lichtenberg S, Magosch P. Elsevier, Munich, 2010)

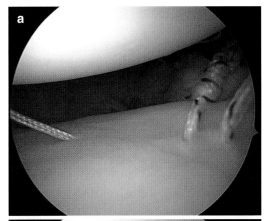

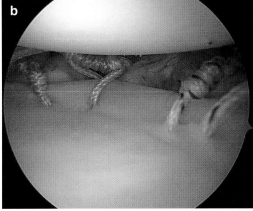

Fig. 8 (**a**) View from the antero-superior portal to the postero-inferior glenoid rim in a right shoulder with the patient in lateral decubitus position. Two plication sutures are already knot. One additional suture at the 6.30 position has sticked through the capsule and underneath the labrum. Note the wide postero-inferior capsular pouch in this patient with hyperlaxity. (**b**) Two additional sutures complete the postero-inferior plication. Note the tightened capsule with significantly reduced pouch

Arthroscopic [54]/Open Coracoid Transfer (Bristow-Latarjet Procedure)

- Surgical technique: transfer of the tip of the coracoid process through a subscapularis muscle split onto the level of the anterior glenoid surface.
- Principle: triple locking of the shoulder by
- Advantages of the coracoid transfer compared with the iliac crest autograft: – no morbidity of iliac crest harvesting; – vascularised bone graft; – a dynamic sling is created additionally to the bone block due to the

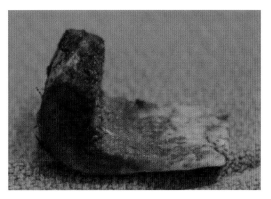

Fig. 9 J-Span. Bicortical bone graft from the iliac crest to restore the anterior glenoid bone stock. The dimensions of the bone graft are 20 × 15 × 7 mm (length × width × height)

lowering effect of the inferior part of the subscapularis by the conjoint tendon [50].

Arthroscopic [55]/Open Iliac Crest Autograft (Eden- Hybinette)

- Tricortical bone graft as an extra-articular platform combined with an anatomic labral and capsulo-ligamentous repair [56]
- Surgical technique [55, 56]:
  - Tricortical bone graft harvesting (1 cm by 2 cm) from the iliac crest
  - Glenoid preparation by the detachment of the anterior capsulo-ligamentous complex from the 2 o'clock to the 6 o'clock position.
  - Transfer of the bone graft: fixation of the bone graft using two cannulated screws at the anterior glenoid neck, aligned with the glenoid rim.
  - Refixation of the anterior capsulo-ligamentous complex.

Open J-Span Technique According to Resch [57]

- Surgical technique:
  - Bicortical bone graft harvesting (~20 mm by 10 mm) from the iliac crest (J-span) (Fig. 9)
  - "intraarticular" ostoetomy at the anterior scapular neck
  - "press fit" impaction of the J-span into the osteotomized anterior scapular neck until

the cancellous internal side of the short limb of the J-span is plane to the articular surface of the glenoid.

– Closure of the capsule over the impacted J-span.

Advantage

• no implantation of hardware
• Full and reliable graft integration
• Anatomic remodelling

Surgical Treatment of SLAP-Lesions

• SLAP-repair: arthroscopic technique using a posterior, anteroinferior and lateral transtendineous portal.
  – Debridement of frayed or ruptured labral tissue
  – Glenoid preparation using a burr
  – Using either two suture anchors or knotless anchors to fix the labrum anterior and posterior from the biceps anchor (even one possible suture through the biceps anchor itself)
  – Tenodesis of the long head of the biceps using a suprabicipital portal.
  – Tenotomy at the biceps anchor after fixation with a clamp through the suprabicipital portal
  – Extracorporal suture fixation
  – Tenodesis screw fixation in a drill hole at the entrance of the bicipital groove or knotless fixation using anchors

Post-Operative Care and Rehabilitation

Arthroscopic Bankart-Repair

The shoulder is immobilized for 3 weeks in 15° of abduction in a pillar. During this period only lymph drainage and isometric muscle exercises are allowed. Afterwards, passive mobilization within the pain limits is begun. Within the first 6 weeks, flexion and abduction are limited to 90° and external rotation to 0°. After free range of motion is achieved, muscle strengthening is increased including the rotator cuff, deltoid and periscapular muscles.

Simple sports activities as jogging or cycling on an ergometer are allowed after 8 weeks, cycling after 12 weeks, and all high impact, contact or overhead sports activities after 6 months.

In patients with atraumatic shoulder instability undergoing stabilization procedures the postoperative protocol doesn't differ from the previous anterior stabilization program. In patients with hyperlaxity we recommend to extend the immobilization period for 6 weeks.

The postoperative protocol for posterior instability restricts the internal rotation for the first 3 weeks to the neutral position. For further 3 weeks the internal rotation is limited to 30°, with slow increase after the sixth postoperative week. The time of return to sports activities is identical to anterior stabilization surgery.

SLAP – Repair

The shoulder is immobilised for 2 weeks using a Gilchrist bandage. Then passive shoulder motion is begun under a physiotherapist's guidance with limitation of the range of motion in abduction and flexion to 90° and 0° of external rotation for 6 weeks. For this time active exercising of the biceps has to be avoided. Afterwards regain of full range of motion, active exercises within the pain-free limits. Return to throwing or overhead activities is allowed after 4 months.

Most reports in literature describe a delayed postoperative course and some cases of postoperative shoulder stiffness [58, 59].

Complications

General complications of surgical interventions as haemorrhage, wound infection, vascular or nerve injuries or venous thrombosis/embolism are rare. More often complications result from inadequate preoperative diagnostics or insufficient technical performance of surgery.

The most frequent complications are:

- Untreated pathology
  - Underdiagnosed MDI
  - Underdiagnosed collagenosis
  - Underdiagnosed HAGL lesion
  - Underdiagnosed loose shoulder
  - Underdiagnosed pathologic muscle patterning
  - Significant bony defects
- Insufficient treatment of pathology
- Asymmetric capsular repair and overtightening (tightening of the capsule anteriorly and superiorly, untreating the inferior instability by violation of the inferior glenohumeral ligament and the inferior capsular pouch, which is resulting in a restriction of the external rotation but a positive sulcus sign) [60]
- Overcorrection
- Arthrofibrosis
- "Hardware" problems such as:
  - Suture anchor malpositioning
  - Suture anchor loosening
  - Knot impingement creating humeral head cartilage damage
  - Glenoid bone cyst formation around bioabsorbable implants
- Non-anatomic Bankart repair (medialization of the repair through fixing the labral tissue proximal or medial to the glenoid margin results in the loss of concavity, 46 %–100 % of failed instability procedures [61–64]
- Plexus-/nerve-lesions
- Infection
- Rotator cuff deficiency (esp. subscapularis 0.01–5 %) after open Bankart repair or Bristow/Latarjet procedure

Summary

Glenohumeral instability represents a complex pathology of the shoulder appearing mainly in the young people. For the physician is important to perform an accurate clinical evaluation after obtaining a detailed history. Additional imaging should complete the diagnostic process leading to the correct diagnosis allowing for the adequate therapy option which often is surgical. Surgery must address the underlying pathomorphological substrate and be performed technically correct. The presence of relevant glenoid bone defects usually requires open procedures. The postoperative protocol must be followed accurately and full return to sports activities, including risk sports, is possible after 6 months. The general complication rate is low. The failure rate depends on various factors including age, number of dislocations, number of anchors used, tissue quality, hyperlaxity, and grade of activity.

References

1. Matsen 3rd FA, Harryman 2nd DT, Sidles JA. Mechanics of glenohumeral instability. Clin Sports Med. 1991;10(4):783–8.
2. Gerber C, Nyffeler RW. Classification of glenohumeral joint instability. Clin Orthop Relat Res. 2002;400:65–76.
3. Jaggi A, Lambert S. Rehabilitation for shoulder instability. Br J Sports Med. 2010;44(5):333–40.
4. Bigliani LU, Newton PM, Steinmann SP, Connor PM, McLlveen SJ. Glenoid rim lesions associated with recurrent anterior dislocation of the shoulder. Am J Sports Med. 1998;26(1):41–5.
5. Snyder SJ, Karzel RP, Del Pizzo W, Ferkel RD, Friedman MJ. SLAP lesions of the shoulder. Arthroscopy. 1990;6(4):274–9.
6. Morgan CD, Burkhart SS, Palmeri M, Gillespie M. Type II SLAP lesions: three subtypes and their relationships to superior instability and rotator cuff tears. Arthroscopy. 1998;14(6):553–65.
7. Maffet MW, Gartsman GM, Moseley B. Superior labrum-biceps tendon complex lesions of the shoulder. Am J Sports Med. 1995;23(1):93–8.
8. Debski RE, Sakone M, Woo SL, Wong EK, Fu FH, Warner JJ. Contribution of the passive properties of the rotator cuff to glenohumeral stability during anterior-posterior loading. J Shoulder Elbow Surg. 1999;8(4):324–9.
9. Harryman 2nd DT, Sidles JA, Harris SL, Matsen 3rd FA. The role of the rotator interval capsule in passive motion and stability of the shoulder. J Bone Joint Surg Am. 1992;74(1):53–66.
10. Warner JJ, McMahon PJ. The role of the long head of the biceps brachii in superior stability of the

glenohumeral joint. J Bone Joint Surg Am. 1995;77(3):366–72.

11. Cole BJ, Rodeo SA, O'Brien SJ, Altchek D, Lee D, DiCarlo EF, et al. The anatomy and histology of the rotator interval capsule of the shoulder. Clin Orthop Relat Res. 2001;390:129–37.

12. Itoi E, Lee SB, Berglund LJ, Berge LL, An KN. The effect of a glenoid defect on anteroinferior stability of the shoulder after Bankart repair: a cadaveric study. J Bone Joint Surg Am. 2000;82(1):35–46.

13. Saito H, Itoi E, Sugaya H, Minagawa H, Yamamoto N, Tuoheti Y. Location of the glenoid defect in shoulders with recurrent anterior dislocation. Am J Sports Med. 2005;33(6):889–93.

14. Yamamoto N, Itoi E, Abe H, Kikuchi K, Seki N, Minagawa H, et al. Effect of an anterior glenoid defect on anterior shoulder stability: a cadaveric study. Am J Sports Med. 2009;37(5):949–54.

15. Kim SH, Ha KI, Jung MW, Lim MS, Kim YM, Park JH. Accelerated rehabilitation after arthroscopic Bankart repair for selected cases: a prospective randomized clinical study. Arthroscopy. 2003;19(7):722–31.

16. Tauber M, Resch H, Forstner R, Raffl M, Schauer J. Reasons for failure after surgical repair of anterior shoulder instability. J Shoulder Elbow Surg. 2004;13(3):279–85.

17. Burkhart SS, De Beer JF. Traumatic glenohumeral bone defects and their relationship to failure of arthroscopic Bankart repairs: significance of the inverted-pear glenoid and the humeral engaging Hill-Sachs lesion. Arthroscopy. 2000;16(7):677–94.

18. Lo IK, Parten PM, Burkhart SS. The inverted pear glenoid: an indicator of significant glenoid bone loss. Arthroscopy. 2004;20(2):169–74.

19. Bigliani LU, Pollock RG, Soslowsky LJ, Flatow EL, Pawluk RJ, Mow VC. Tensile properties of the inferior glenohumeral ligament. J Orthop Res. 1992;10(2):187–97.

20. Neviaser TJ. The anterior labroligamentous periosteal sleeve avulsion lesion: a cause of anterior instability of the shoulder. Arthroscopy. 1993;9(1):17–21.

21. Bui-Mansfield LT, Banks KP, Taylor DC. Humeral avulsion of the glenohumeral ligaments: the HAGL lesion. Am J Sports Med. 2007;35(11):1960–6.

22. Kim SH, Ha KI, Yoo JC, Noh KC. Kim's lesion: an incomplete and concealed avulsion of the posteroinferior labrum in posterior or multidirectional posteroinferior instability of the shoulder. Arthroscopy. 2004;20(7):712–20.

23. Cooper DE, Arnoczky SP, O'Brien SJ, Warren RF, DiCarlo E, Allen AA. Anatomy, histology, and vascularity of the glenoid labrum. An anatomical study. J Bone Joint Surg Am. 1992;74(1):46–52.

24. Habermeyer P, Kaiser E, Knappe M, Kreusser T, Wiedemann E. Functional anatomy and biomechanics of the long biceps tendon. Unfallchirurg. 1987; 90(7):319–29.

25. Pal GP, Bhatt RH, Patel VS. Relationship between the tendon of the long head of biceps brachii and the glenoidal labrum in humans. Anat Rec. 1991;229(2):278–80.

26. Rames RD, Morgan CD, Snyder SJ. Anatomical variations of the glenohumeral ligaments. Arthroscopy. 1991;7:1.

27. Andrews JR, Carson Jr WG, McLeod WD. Glenoid labrum tears related to the long head of the biceps. Am J Sports Med. 1985;13(5):337–41.

28. Williams MM, Snyder SJ, Buford Jr D. The Buford complex–the "cord-like" middle glenohumeral ligament and absent anterosuperior labrum complex: a normal anatomic capsulolabral variant. Arthroscopy. 1994;10(3):241–7.

29. Rowe CR, Sakellarides HT. Factors related to recurrences of anterior dislocations of the shoulder. Clin Orthop. 1961;20:40–8.

30. Matsen III FA, Thomas S, Rockwood CA. Glenohumeral instability. In: Rockwood CA, Matsen FA, editors. The shoulder. Philadelphia: Saunders; 1990. p. 526–32.

31. Rowe CR, Zarins B. Recurrent transient subluxation of the shoulder. J Bone Joint Surg Am. 1981;63(6):863–72.

32. Pappas AM, Zawacki RM, Sullivan TJ. Biomechanics of baseball pitching. A preliminary report. Am J Sports Med. 1985;13(4):216–22.

33. Jobe FW, Jobe CM, Kvitne RS. The shoulder in sports. In: Rockwood CA, Matsen FA, editors. The shoulder. Philadelphia: Saunders; 1990. p. 961–90.

34. Hamner DL, Pink MM, Jobe FW. A modification of the relocation test: arthroscopic findings associated with a positive test. J Shoulder Elbow Surg. 2000;9(4):263–7.

35. Gross ML, Distefano MC. Anterior release test. A new test for occult shoulder instability. Clin Orthop Relat Res. 1997;339:105–8.

36. Kim SH, Ha KI, Ahn JH, Choi HJ. Biceps load test II: A clinical test for SLAP lesions of the shoulder. Arthroscopy. 2001;17(2):160–4.

37. Ebinger N, Magosch P, Lichtenberg S, Habermeyer P. A new SLAP test: the supine flexion resistance test. Arthroscopy. 2008;24(5):500–5.

38. Parentis MA, Mohr KJ, ElAttrache NS. Disorders of the superior labrum: review and treatment guidelines. Clin Orthop Relat Res. 2002;400:77–87.

39. Sugaya H, Moriishi J, Dohi M, Kon Y, Tsuchiya A. Glenoid rim morphology in recurrent anterior glenohumeral instability. J Bone Joint Surg Am. 2003;85-A(5):878–84.

40. Itoi E, Lee SB, Amrami KK, Wenger DE, An KN. Quantitative assessment of classic anteroinferior bony Bankart lesions by radiography and computed tomography. Am J Sports Med. 2003;31(1):112–8.

41. Huysmans PE, Haen PS, Kidd M, Dhert WJ, Willems JW. The shape of the inferior part of the glenoid: a cadaveric study. J Shoulder Elbow Surg. 2006; 15(6):759–63.

42. Stehle J, Gohlke F. Complication management after unsuccessful operative shoulder stabilization. Orthopade. 2009;38(1):75–8. 80–2.

43. Gorantla K, Gill C, Wright RW. The outcome of type II SLAP repair: a systematic review. Arthroscopy. 2010;26(4):537–45.

44. Ide J, Maeda S, Takagi K. Sports activity after arthroscopic superior labral repair using suture anchors in overhead-throwing athletes. Am J Sports Med. 2005;33(4):507–14.

45. Kim SH, Ha KI, Choi HJ. Results of arthroscopic treatment of superior labral lesions. J Bone Joint Surg Am. 2002;84-A(6):981–5.

46. Boileau P, Parratte S, Chuinard C, Roussanne Y, Shia D, Bicknell R. Arthroscopic treatment of isolated type II SLAP lesions: biceps tenodesis as an alternative to reinsertion. Am J Sports Med. 2009;37(5):929–36.

47. Heneghan HM, McCabe JP. Use of autologous bone graft in anterior cervical decompression: morbidity & quality of life analysis. BMC Musculoskelet Disord. 2009;10:158.

48. Schaaf H, Lendeckel S, Howaldt HP, Streckbein P. Donor site morbidity after bone harvesting from the anterior iliac crest. Oral Surg Oral Med Oral Pathol Oral Radiol Endod. 2010;109(1):52–8.

49. Boileau P, Villalba M, Hery JY, Balg F, Ahrens P, Neyton L. Risk factors for recurrence of shoulder instability after arthroscopic Bankart repair. J Bone Joint Surg Am. 2006;88(8):1755–63.

50. Boileau P, Zumstein M, Old J, O'Shea K. Decision process for the treatment of anterior instability. In: Boileau P, editor. Shoulder concepts 2010. Montpellier: Sauramps Medical; 2010. p. 65–78.

51. Boileau P, Richou J, Lisai A, Chuinard C, Bicknell RT. The role of arthroscopy in revision of failed open anterior stabilization of the shoulder. Arthroscopy. 2009;25(10):1075–84.

52. O'Shea K, Vargas P, Pinedo M, Old J, Zumstein M, Boileau P. Arthroscopic Hill-Sachs Remplissage: does the capsulo-tenodesis really heal? In: Boileau P, editor. Shoulder concepts 2010. Montpellier: Sauramps Medical; 2010. p. 49–64.

53. Neer 2nd CS, Foster CR. Inferior capsular shift for involuntary inferior and multidirectional instability of the shoulder. A preliminary report. J Bone Joint Surg Am. 1980;62(6):897–908.

54. Lafosse L, Boyle S. Arthroscopic Latarjet procedure. J Shoulder Elbow Surg. 2010;19 Suppl 2:2–12.

55. Taverna E, Golano P, Pascale V, Battistella F. An arthroscopic bone graft procedure for treating anterior-inferior glenohumeral instability. Knee Surg Sports Traumatol Arthrosc. 2008;16(9):872–5.

56. Warner JJ, Gill TJ, O'Hollerhan JD, Pathare N, Millett PJ. Anatomical glenoid reconstruction for recurrent anterior glenohumeral instability with glenoid deficiency using an autogenous tricortical iliac crest bone graft. Am J Sports Med. 2006;34(2):205–12.

57. Auffarth A, Schauer J, Matis N, Kofler B, Hitzl W, Resch H. The J-bone graft for anatomical glenoid reconstruction in recurrent posttraumatic anterior shoulder dislocation. Am J Sports Med. 2008;36(4):638–47.

58. Brockmeier SF, Voos JE, Williams 3rd RJ, Altchek DW, Cordasco FA, Allen AA. Outcomes after arthroscopic repair of type-II SLAP lesions. J Bone Joint Surg Am. 2009;91(7):1595–603.

59. Yung PS, Fong DT, Kong MF, Lo CK, Fung KY, Ho EP, et al. Arthroscopic repair of isolated type II superior labrum anterior-posterior lesion. Knee Surg Sports Traumatol Arthrosc. 2008;16(12):1151–7.

60. Boone JL, Arciero RA. Management of failed instability surgery: how to get it right the next time. Orthop Clin North Am. 2010;41(3):367–79.

61. Levine WN, Arroyo JS, Pollock RG, Flatow EL, Bigliani LU. Open revision stabilization surgery for recurrent anterior glenohumeral instability. Am J Sports Med. 2000;28(2):156–60.

62. Zabinski SJ, Callaway GH, Cohen S, Warren RF. Revision shoulder stabilization: 2- to 10-year results. J Shoulder Elbow Surg. 1999;8(1):58–65.

63. Marquardt B, Garmann S, Schulte T, Witt KA, Steinbeck J, Potzl W. Outcome after failed traumatic anterior shoulder instability repair with and without surgical revision. J Shoulder Elbow Surg. 2007;16(6):742–7.

64. Kim SH, Ha KI, Kim YM. Arthroscopic revision Bankart repair: a prospective outcome study. Arthroscopy. 2002;18(5):469–82.

Open Capsuloplasty for Antero-Inferior and Multi-Directional Instability of the Shoulder

Pierre Hoffmeyer

Contents

Keywords

Antero-inferior and multi-directional instability • Bankart lesion • Bankart repair • Capsule to glenoid suture • Capsuloplasty • Complications • Cruciate repair • Glenoid neck preparation • Preparing humeral neck • Rehabilitation • Results • Shoulder • Subscapularis repair • Surgical indications • Surgical Technique

Indications for Surgery

Recurrent antero-inferior glenohumeral post-traumatic dislocation is the main indication for this operation. Some patients will have only a perceived subluxation of the shoulder with no real episode of dislocation. Balg and Boileau have devised a scoring system whereby it is possible to choose with some accuracy between open and closed (arthoscopic) surgical techniques. A distended capsule, whether of post-traumatic or congenital origin with or without a Bankart or Perthes' lesion and, an intact non-fractured glenoid rim, is the ideal situation indicating an open capsuloplasty [1–5, 8, 9, 11–15].

Technique

Positioning

Under general anaesthesia and in some cases with an additional scalene block, the patient is placed on the operating table in a semi-sitting

P. Hoffmeyer
University Hospitals of Geneva, Geneva, Switzerland
e-mail: Pierre.Hoffmeyer@hcuge.ch;
pierre.hoffmeyer@efort.org

G. Bentley (ed.), *European Surgical Orthopaedics and Traumatology*,
DOI 10.1007/978-3-642-34746-7_3, © EFORT 2014

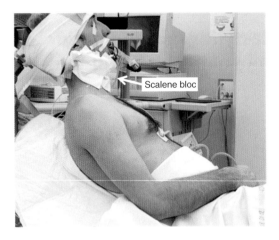

Scalene bloc

Fig. 1 Under General anaesthesia in "beach chair" position, the head secured, the shoulder well exposed at the front and the back, the unimpaired upper limb is ready to be prepared and draped

"beach chair" position. It is important that the table be slightly up-tilted so that the buttocks rest squarely in the seat of the table avoiding any tendency to downward slippage. The head is held securely in a head rest with a firm bandage providing secure fixation. The cervical spine is in neutral position without inclination, rotation, extension or flexion. Special care should be given to protecting the patient's eyes. It is important to verify the position of the contralateral upper extremity so as to avoid any untoward pressure areas.

The totality of the shoulder region from the supero-lateral torso and including the whole upper extremity should be left free. Some modular tables will allow removal of an upper cornerpiece therefore allowing access to all parts of the shoulder. The downside of this possibility is that the scapula tends to sag backwards somewhat. This may be counteracted by rolling the table slightly towards the opposite side. If this possibility does not exist a bolster may be used to prop up the scapula.

The upper limb may then be prepared and draped leaving the shoulder well exposed at the front and the back with the upper extremity fully accessible and mobility unimpaired (Fig. 1).

Examination Under Anaesthesia

Before proceeding with the procedure a thorough examination of the shoulder under anaesthesia must be carried out. Mobility must be assessed to ensure that it is full. A posterior drawer test must be carried out to assess the posterior laxity as well as a sulcus sign test to ascertain any evidence of inferior laxity. Direction of dislocation must be determined first by pushing anteriorly on the humeral head with the arm at the side in internal rotation, where it should dislocate easily if the diagnosis is correct. A grating sensation will indicate the presence of a cartilaginous defect or of a bony Bankart lesion [2]. With the arm in external rotation the anterior structures, i.e., the capsule and subscapularis tendon, are stretched taut and the shoulder will not dislocate. The degree of rotation needed to stabilize the shoulder will give a gross estimate as to the amount of capsular laxity.

Incision

It is important to draw the skin incision with a surgical pen before applying any type of plastic adhesive draping, iodine impregnated or otherwise, as this will deform the skin and its natural creases. Usually the incision is 6–7 cm in length, vertical, extending from the axillary skin crease to a point midway to the tip of the coracoid. In muscular patients the incision might have to be somewhat longer. It is important to undermine the skin in the avascular layer of the subcutaneous overlying the muscular fascia (Fig. 2).

Delto-Pectoral Interval

The delto-pectoral groove is then identified. In case of difficulty proceed superiorly while palpating the coracoid. At the divergence between deltoid and pectoralis it will usually be easy to find the groove and the cephalic vein. The vein should be separated from the pectoralis but left adherent to the deltoid. The deltoid fascia which extends around and under the anterior third of the deltoid should be carefully incised so as to give access to the subdeltoid and subacromial spaces. At this point some degree of abduction will be helpful. A retractor will then be placed underneath the deltoid which will tend to subluxate the humeral anteriorly stretching the underlying subscapularis and capsule. The conjoint tendon

appears and it is retracted medially with the pectoralis (Fig. 3a, b).

Interval Subscapularis-Supraspinatus

With the arm in external rotation and some adduction, the subscapularis tendon comes into view. The upper two-thirds of the subscapularis insertion onto the lesser tuberosity are tendinous while the lower third is muscular. The humeral head is palpated to identify the biceps tendon in its groove and the interval between subscapularis and supraspinatus. If this interval is deemed too wide i.e., more than 1 cm, it may be sutured closed at this point. Palpating the axillary nerve may be done at this time. To do so the index finger is passed under the conjoint tendons in front of the subscapularis with the arm in neutral or in slight internal rotation. The nerve is felt easily and it is surprisingly large and taught. Internal rotation will tighten the nerve along its course while external rotation will loosen it. Some authors also recommend palpating the musculocutaneous nerve that penetrates the coracobrachialis some 3–5 cm below the coracoid tip [7].

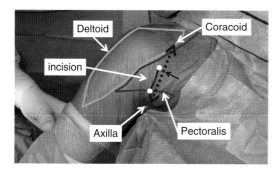

Fig. 2 The vertical incision (*solid black line*) follows an axillary fold and spans from the inferior border of the Pectoralis tendon (*outlined red*) to the mid-point (*arrow*) between the coracoid and the axilla (*Deltoid outlined orange*). The bony contours are always marked out with a surgical pen

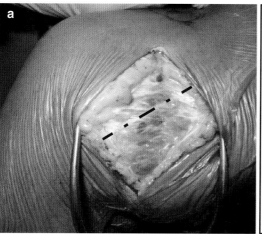

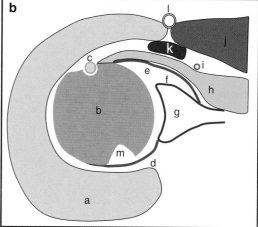

Fig. 3 (**a**) The subcutaneous skin is undermined so as to expose the Deltopectoral groove (*dotted line*). (**b**) Schematic shoulder: transverse plane: (*a*) Deltoid muscle, (*b*) Humeral head, (*c*) Biceps tendon and groove, (*d*) Posterior capsule, (*e*) Anterior distended capsule, (*f*) Anterior

glenoid neck and Bankart lesion area, (*g*) Glenoid, (*h*) Subscapularis muscle, (*i*) Axillary nerve, (*j*) Pectoralis muscle (*k*) Conjoint tendon (*l*) Cephalic vein, (*m*) Hill-Sachs lesion

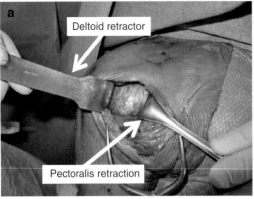
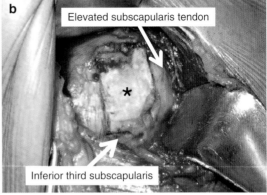

Fig. 4 (**a**) Deltoid separated from the Pectoralis leaving the cephalic vein laterally. (**b**) Subscapularis tendon elevated from the underlying capsule (*) with sharp dissection. Leave attached the inferior muscular third of the subscapularis insertion

Subscapularis

A subscapularis tendon flap extending medially is now created. This tendinous flap, about 2 cm wide, extends from just below the supraspinatus-subscapularis interval to just above the muscular distal third of the subscapularis insertion. Near the insertion on the lesser tuberosity the subscapularis and the capsule are intimately imbricated and therefore the subscapularis must be sharply dissected off the capsule. As a rule of thumb it is better to err towards a thicker capsule and a thinner subscapularis tendon (Fig. 4a, b).

As the tendon is dissected off medially, muscular fibres appear and it becomes easier to separate the actual tendon from the smooth capsule underneath. Stay sutures are then inserted to allow for immediate retraction and future re-fixation (Fig. 5a, b).

"T-eeing" the Capsule

The capsular surface is individualized with a soft tissue rasp such as a Cobb elevator or a Darrach rasp and a Hohmann retractor is placed on the anterior neck of the glenoid to provide good visualization. A smaller blunt retractor may be inserted inferiorly to protect the axillary nerve. Using a small blade the capsule is incised in "T" fashion. The vertical bar of the T starts below the interval and follows the neck

of humerus leaving 1 cm of capsule along its insertion stopping at the level of the insertion of the muscular part of subscapularis. The horizontal part of the T extends from the middle of the capsule laterally to the glenoid insertion. Stay sutures are placed on each of the two corners of the upper and lower triangular flaps. A Fukuda type retractor pushes the humeral head away so that it is possible to examine the articular surface of the glenoid. The capsular insertion of the inferior flap on the glenoid is inspected. When the capsular insertion on the glenoid is intact (=Absence of a Bankart lesion) the cruciate repair, as described below, can performed without further ado [11, 12] (Fig. 6a, b).

In the case of *multi-directional instability* it will be necessary to detach the humeral insertion of the capsule circumferentially all the way around the head to reach its equator while progressively delivering the humeral head into external rotation. This will produce a much larger inferior capsular flap which can then pulled up and sutured to the base of the superior flap [12, 13].

Bankart Lesion

Usually a soft tissue Bankart or Perthes lesion extending from 2 o'clock to 6 o'clock on a right glenoid and accompanied by some glenoid bony eburnation or cartilage damage, is encountered. The labrum is usually absent or damaged.

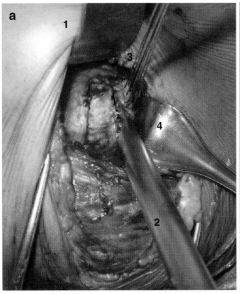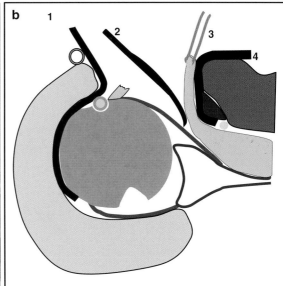

Fig. 5 (**a**) The Deltoid retractor (*1*) will cause a forward subluxation of the humeral head thereby tightening the anterior structures which eases the dissection of the subscapularis tendon off of the capsule, first by sharp dissection then with a Cobb elevator (*2*) and held by stay sutures (*3*). Conjoint tendon and pectoralis are retracted medially (*4*). (**b**) Using a Cobb elevator [2] to dissect the subscapularis off the capsule and put stay sutures in the subscapularis tendon

If a significant bony defect (involving more than 25 % of the glenoid surface) is found this would justify a bone block operation. Precise preoperative imaging will avoid this situation and identify other unsuspected lesions [2].

Glenoid Neck Preparation

In the case of a Bankart or Perthes lesion the glenoid neck should be decorticated to bleeding bone. Any loose or poorly-healed bone or cartilage fragment should be removed. High speed burrs should be avoided as this tends to cause heat and bone necrosis; use preferentially a sharp osteotome. Occasionally when the anterior glenoid neck is prepared venous bleeding occurs. Temporary packing will stop this oozing (Fig. 7a, b).

Bankart Sutures or Anchors

The next step consists in passing three to four transosseous sutures. Vicryl$^{©}$ number two is usually sufficient; the sutures should be long to allow for ease of tying and manipulation. Heavy, cutting, small diameter Mayo needles are made to pass through the pre-prepared holes using heavy towel clip type clamps. For ease of use and speedy intervention, many authors use bone anchors. Resorbable anchors tend to create osteolysis and metal anchors must be placed at the glenoid bone-cartilage angle and buried deeply so as not to damage the humeral head cartilage [6, 10]. Metallic anchors will interfere with any future MRI imaging (Fig. 8a, b).

Suturing the Capsule (Reverdin Needle) to the Glenoid

Once the Bankart sutures are in place they must be passed through the lower flap of the capsule. Both strands are passed in a U pattern. It is important that the sutures slide freely guaranteeing a tight knot. The sutures are then tied down securing the capsule firmly to the glenoid at the bone-cartilage junction and thus re-creating a labrum.

a

b

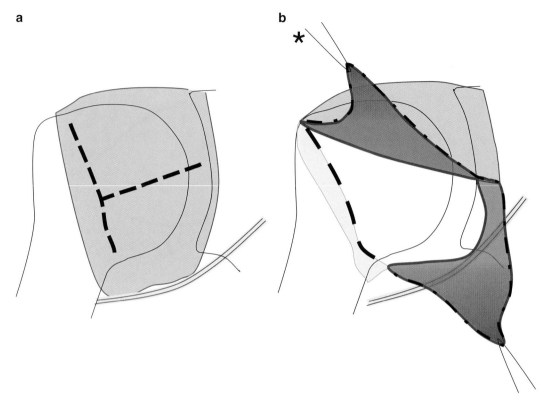

Fig. 6 (**a**) The capsule is incised using a lying down T incision (*dotted lines*). (**b**) The upper and lower flaps are unfolded allowing identification of the inferior half of the glenoid neck. Identify the axillary nerve that lies on the subscapularis and passes underneath the capsule

Because of the position of the sutures passing from the glenoid neck anterior cortex through the spongiosa and exiting on the cartilage surface the capsule comes automatically to the right place on the glenoid edge when it is tightened down. To pass the sutures through the capsule a Reverdin needle is most useful. The index finger is placed under the conjoint tendon protecting the surprisingly close axillary nerve (Fig. 9a, b).

Preparing the Humeral Neck

The capsular insertion groove on the humeral neck is abraded to bleeding bone. This is especially important in cases of *multi-directional instability* where the abrasion must go all around the humeral neck so as to obtain a bleeding surface favourable for strong adhesion of the re-inserted capsule. This may be done with a high speed burr but preferably with osteotomes and rongeurs to avoid overheating the spongiosa.

Cruciate Repair

The tip of the lower flap is then sutured as high as possible laterally at the level of the neck-capsule junction. At this point the arm should be in neutral rotation and slight abduction. More sutures are placed along the lateral border of the flap so as to secure it to the humeral neck. The upper flap is lowered and the tip is sutured as low as possible over the upper flap (Fig. 10a–c).

Suturing Subscapularis

Subscapularis is then sutured back to its original insertion site and any overtightening is avoided.

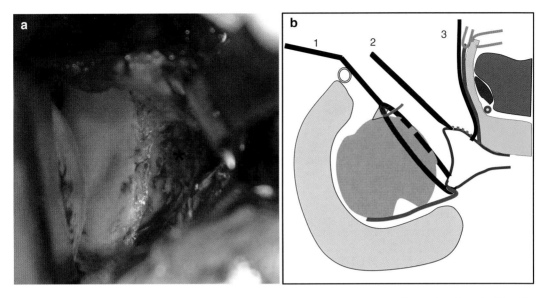

Fig. 7 (**a**) Major Bankart lesion with a bare glenoid neck (*) attesting to the avulsion of the glenohumeral ligament insertion and absent labrum. (**b**) Fukuda retractor (*1*) keeps the humeral head away allowing decortications with a sharp osteotome of the glenoid neck (*2*) while the capsule is retracted with a sharp-tipped Hohmann retractor (*3*)

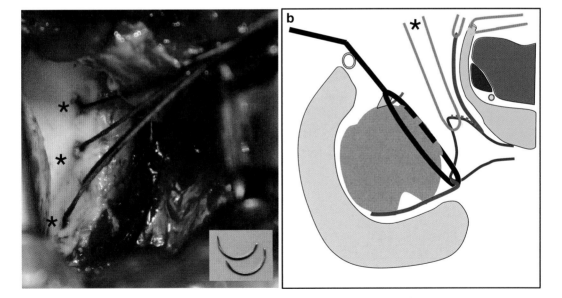

Fig. 8 (**a**) Transosseous glenoid sutures (*) using 2Vicryl© and passed with trocar point needles (*inset*). (**b**) Passage of transosseous sutures (*)

At this point the shoulder stability is tested with an anterior drawer manoeuvre in neutral or slight internal rotation with the arm at the side. There should be a solid resistance felt. Elevation to 100° should be free as well as external rotation up to 30°. If sutures tear during this manoeuvre the subscapularis needs to be lengthened and the flaps might need to be re-positioned. Usually

Passing the transglenoid sutures through the inferior flap

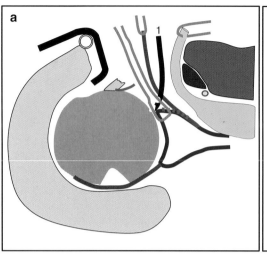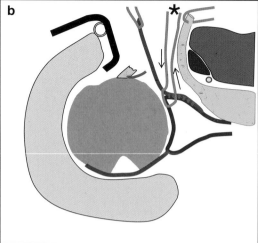

Fig. 9 (**a**) Transglenoid sutures are then passed through the inferior capsular flap using a Reverdin needle (*1*). (**b**) The sutures (*) must pass through the capsular flap and should slide freely to allow a tight knot. The axillary nerve must be protected during this phase

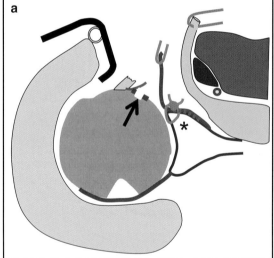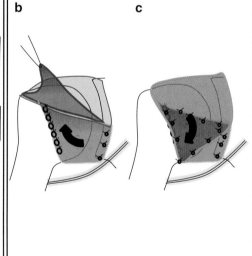

Fig. 10 (**a**) The capsule is tied down to the decorticated glenoid neck (*). The humeral capsular insertion groove is also decorticated (*arrow*) to enhance osseous capsular attachment. (**b**) The inferior flap is pulled up as high as possible and sutured in place on the remaining lateral capsule. (**c**) The superior flap is pulled down and sutured to the remaining lateral capsule and to the inferior flap

overtightening the structures is the problem, not undertightening (Fig. 11).

In the case of multi-directional instability it is sometimes necessary to add a posterior capsular shift.

Closure

Abundant rinsing is done with haemostasis as needed and the cephalic vein is inspected for injury; the deltopectoral interval can be closed

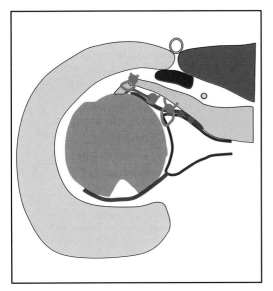

Fig. 11 Repair completed: The capsular flaps are doubled and the subscapularis is sutured back to its original insertion avoiding any overtightening

with loose sutures. The wound is then closed in the usual fashion using subcuticular sutures over a 24-h suction drain if felt necessary.

Recovery Room

In the recovery room the shoulder is tested for neurovascular integrity. Isometric contractions of the deltoid are routinely tested at that time. An AP Scout film is routinely performed. Overnight surveillance and pain control are routine although many Surgeons perform this intervention as an out-patient procedure.

Rehabilitation

For the first 3 weeks the patient is instructed to keep his arm in internal rotation in a sling. After 3 weeks the arm is freed and may be used for activities of daily living. At 6 weeks strengthening exercise are introduced along with some range-of-motion exercises. At 12 weeks the patient is allowed full use of the shoulder.

Contact sports or sports with a high probability of falling such as skiing are permitted after 1 year post-operatively.

For the patient with *multi-directional instability* a specific post-operative regimen is installed. The shoulder is maintained in neutral rotation with 20° of antepulsion and 20° of abduction. A "handshake" brace is installed in the recovery room and the patient is instructed to keep the brace for a period of 8 weeks. During this period of immobilisation, isometric exercises are recommended to keep the shoulder musculature toned. After removal of the brace range-of-motion exercises are started. All contact or "at-risk" sports activities are forbidden for the year following the operation.

Complications

The most common immediate complication is a haematoma which may need, in rare cases, aspiration or even revision. Adhesive capsulitis may develop in the post-operative phase but this is very uncommon. Infection is a rare complication also. Most organisms are involved but one should be especially aware of infections with propionibacterium acnes that is frequent around the shoulder. A prompt reaction, with a surgical wash-out of the operative wound along with the proper antibiotics chosen after an infectious diseases consultation, should effectively deal with the situation. Neurological problems may arise ranging from temporary axillary or musculocutaneous nerve palsy to a full blown permanent plexus injury. As a rule these lesions are due to neurapraxia or axonotmesis and tend to recover. A neurology consultation along with EMG studies is mandatory. In the case of neurotmesis or outright section of the nerve a reconstructive procedure may be necessary. Later the main complication is recurrence of the dislocation or the persistence of apprehension. In the years that follow glenohumeral arthrosis may set in. It is not clear whether the arthrosis is due to the initial dislocation with its concomitant cartilaginous damage or to the stabilising procedure.

Results

Recurrence rates vary in the literature between 0 % and 20 %. This depends on the exact technique, the length of follow-up and the completeness of the review process. Most authors agree that loss of range of motion is slight usually not more than 10° for external rotation. As for residual pain and stiffness neither is reported as occurring with any significant frequency. Many authors report a non-negligible percentage of remaining apprehension in the patients, up to 20 %. The exact cause is not determined, whether it is a mechanical phenomenon with subluxation or a deficit of proprioception. Up to 50 % of operated shoulders will be found to have some degree of arthritis when the x-rays are reviewed and classified according to Samilson. For the great majority of patients this does have any significant clinical repercussions [3, 4, 6, 8, 9, 11–15].

References

1. Balg F, Boileau P. The instability severity index score. J Bone Joint Surg Br. 2007;89(11):1470–7.
2. Bankart A. The pathology and treatment of recurrent dislocation of the shoulder. Br J Surg. 1938;26:23–9.
3. Bigliani LU, Kurzweil PR, Schwartzbach CC, Wolfe IN, Flatow EL. Inferior capsular shift procedure for anterior-inferior shoulder instability in athletes. Am J Sports Med. 1994;22(5):578–84.
4. Bonnevialle N, Mansat P. Selective capsular repair for the treatment of anterior-inferior shoulder instability: review of seventy-nine shoulders with seven years'
5. average follow-up. J Shoulder Elbow Surg. 2009;18(2):251–9.
6. Matsen FA, Lippitt S, Bertlesen A, Rockwood CA, Wirth MA. Glenohumeral instability. In: Rockwood CA, Matsen FA, Wirth MA, Lippitt SB, editors. The shoulder. 4th ed. Philadelphia: Saunders Elsevier; 2009. p. 616–75.
7. Ferretti A, De Carli A, Calderaro M, Conteduca F. Open capsulorrhaphy with suture anchors for recurrent anterior dislocation of the shoulder. Am J Sports Med. 1998;26(5):625–9.
8. Flatow EL, Bigliani LU. An anatomic study of the musculocutaneous nerve and its relationship to the coracoid process. Clin Orthop Relat Res. 1989;244:166–71.
9. Hamada K, Fukuda H, Nakajima T, Yamada N. The inferior capsular shift operation for instability of the shoulder. Long-term results in 34 shoulders. J Bone Joint Surg Br. 1999;81(2):218–25.
10. Hovelius LJ, Thorling J, Fredin H. Recurrent anterior dislocation of the shoulder. Results after the Bankart and Putti-Platt operations. J Bone Joint Surg Am. 1979;61(4):566–9.
11. Kartus J, Ejerhed L, Funck E, Köhler K, Sernert N, Karlsson J. Arthroscopic and open shoulder stabilization using absorbable implants. A clinical and radiographic comparison of two methods. Knee Surg Sports Traumatol Arthrosc. 1998;6(3):181–8.
12. Neer CS. Shoulder reconstruction. Philadelphia: W.B. Saunders; 1990.
13. Neer CS, Foster CR. Inferior capsular shift for involuntary inferior and multidirectional instability of the shoulder. A preliminary report. J Bone Joint Surg Am. 1980;62(6):897–908.
14. Pollock RG, Owens JM. Operative results of the inferior capsular shift procedure for multidirectional instability of the shoulder. J Bone Joint Surg Am. 2000;82-A(7):919–28.
15. Simonet WT, Cofield RH. Prognosis in anterior shoulder dislocation. Am J Sports Med. 1984;12(1):19–24.
16. Walch G. La luxation récidivante antérieure de l'épaule. Table ronde. Rev Chir Orthop Reparatrice Appar Mot. 1991;77 Suppl 1:177–91.

Shoulder Instability in Children and Adolescents

Jörn Kircher and Rüdiger Krauspe

Contents

J. Kircher (✉)
Shoulder and Elbow Surgery, Klinik Fleetinsel Hamburg,
Hamburg, Germany

Department of Orthopaedics, Medical Faculty,
Heinrich–Heine–University, Düsseldorf, Germany
e-mail: joern.kircher@med.uni-duesseldorf.de;
j-kircher@web.de

R. Krauspe
Department of Orthopedic Surgery, University Hospital of
Düsseldorf, Düsseldorf, Germany

Abstract

Shoulder instability is a common problem in Orthopaedic practice for children and adolescents. Dislocations under the age of 12 are rare. The group of adolescents and young adults, especially male, who are active in high risk sports have the highest reported recurrence rates.

There are no widely-accepted classification systems for shoulder instability of children and adolescents and the most commonly used systems are the same as for adults.

It needs to be emphasized that hyperlaxity and hypermobility are a frequent clinical condition in this age group which needs to be taken into consideration with regard to decision-making for therapy.

Every muscular dysbalance and disturbed scapulo-thoracic rhythm needs intensive conservative treatment whether the decision is made for surgery or not.

Arthroscopic stabilization is the treatment of choice for severe structural damages, especially substantial glenoid bone loss, which results in lower recurrence rates and better clinical function.

Keywords

Aetiology, Classification • Anatomy • Biomechanics • Complications • Diagnosis • Surgical Techniques • Pathology • Rehabilitation • Results • Shoulder instability-children, adolescents • Surgical indications

G. Bentley (ed.), *European Surgical Orthopaedics and Traumatology*,
DOI 10.1007/978-3-642-34746-7_63, © EFORT 2014

General Introduction

Shoulder instability is a common problem in the general population but is rare in children and young adolescents under the age of 12 [1, 2]. It accounts for 0.01 % of all injuries in this age group [3, 4] and for 2.5–4.7 % of all shoulder dislocations [5, 6].

Compared to adult shoulder dislocations there are many more atraumatic dislocations with an increasing number of traumatic cases with increasing age [5, 7–9].

The majority of reported cases (about 80 %) are classic Bankart-like lesions with only 50 % of classic Hill-Sachs lesions [1, 7, 10, 11].

Girls are generally younger than boys at the time of their first dislocation and are two times less affected [1].

Aetiology and Classification

The scapula develops by intramembranous ossification starting at eight centres or more which is complete at the time of delivery except for the glenoid, acromion, coracoid, medial margin and inferior angle [12].

The glenoid cavity shows a superior and inferior centre of ossification. The superior centre appears around the age of ten and fuses at the age of 15. At this time the inferior centre appears as a horseshoe-shaped epiphysis with a thinner central portion and a thicker peripheral rim. Injury to these ossification centres can lead to the development of bony abnormalities such as glenoid hypoplasia. The association with other disorders such as birth palsy, infection, muscular dystrophy, vitamin deficiency, arthrogryposis and others have been described [13–25].

A positive family history and ethnic origin have been reported [15, 22, 24, 26, 27].

There are three ossification centres at the proximal humerus which fuse at about the age of seven and fuse with the humeral shaft at the age of 14–18 [28].

Therefore a significant trauma is more likely to injure the open physes based on the epiphyseal anchoring of the joint capsule in very young individuals than to dislocate the shoulder [28].

In adolescents a significant trauma is associated with dislocation in up to 86 %. The most common activities and mechanisms, in descending order, are football, falls, basketball, wrestling, hockey, baseball or softball, swimming, and tennis [1, 29].

The extent of dislocation can be graded into apprehension, subluxation or dislocation. The direction of instability can be uni-directional (anterior, posterior, inferior and superior) or multi-directional. Shoulder instability can be congenital, acute or chronic (recurrent or fixed). According to the pathogenesis shoulder instability can be traumatic, due to repetitive microtrauma or non-traumatic.

There are three commonly-used classification systems which are similar to those for adult shoulder instability. Matsen et al. described two major forms of instability which are based on clinical findings and treatment:
- TUBS (traumatic, uni-directional, Bankart lesion, surgical repair) and
- AMBRII (atraumatic, multi-directional, bilateral, rehabilitation, inferior capsular shift, interval) [30, 31].

Gerber et al. differentiated shoulder instability into six sub-groups which can easily be used in clinical practice [32]:
I. Chronic dislocation
II. Uni-directional instability without hyperlaxity
III. Uni-directional instability with multi-directional hyperlaxity
IV. Multi-directional instability without hyperlaxity
V. Multi-directional instability with multi-directional hyperlaxity
VI. Uni- or multi-directional voluntary instability

Bayley et al. have introduced a more sophisticated model consisting of three major poles [33]:
- Polar type 1: traumatic, structural
- Polar type 2: atraumatic, structural
- Polar type 3: muscle patterning, non-structural

The form of instability can be assigned to one or more poles to a certain degree which in our opinion helps in defining each individual case but at the same time is less accurate and comparable to others. We suggest the use of the latter two classification systems and the addition of supplementary information based on the facts listed at the beginning of this section.

There is still a somewhat poorly-defined use of the terms instability, hyperlaxity and hypermobility. We prefer the term "laxity" to describe the amount of physiological glenohumeral translation and "hyperlaxity" as a condition with pathologically increased glenohumeral translation, usually involving the opposite shoulder also. Instability describes the inability to actively centre the joint and it is certainly pathological. Hypermobility is an increased range of motion of the joint along the physiological axes and alone represents a normal variant.

General joint hypermobility (GJH) has a prevalence of 8–39 % in children of school age [34–38]. Several studies show a decrease by increasing age and an increased frequency in Caucasians and females [39–44]. Juul-Kristensen et al. have shown that the presence of general joint hypermobility does not need to be associated with musculoskeletal pain and injuries but that children with GJH performed better in motor competence tests. This may be an explanation, that hypermobile children are often found in sports with a high demand for flexibility such as ballet, dancing, gymnastics and swimming [45–48]. In contrast to the findings of Juul-Kristensen in 8-year old school children there were increased frequencies of injuries observed for participants in elite sports [49, 50]. General joint hypermobility can be classified using the Beighton score and demarcated from the benign joint hypermobility syndrome (BJHS) by the Brighton criteria [41, 51–53].

Although the data about general joint hypermobility is sometimes conflicting, especially in drawing a line between normal and pathological conditions, it certainly needs to be taken into account in decision-making for the treatment of shoulder instability [44, 54–56].

Relevant Applied Anatomy, Pathology, Basic Science and Biomechanics

The glenohumeral joint is the most mobile joint of the human body with a complex synergetic inter-operation of several factors that provide sufficient stability.

There are several factors that influence the stability of the glenohumeral joint [57]:
- Static stabilizers
  - Bone/cartilage
    - Humerus
    - Glenoid
    - Scapula – Thorax
    - Coracoid
    - Acromion
    - Clavicle
  - Labrum
    - About 50 % increase of the contact area
    - About 60 % contribution to resistance against applied forces
    - SLAP complex with the biceps tendon origin [58, 59]
  - Glenohumeral ligaments
    - Superior glenohumeral ligament (SGHL) (stabilizing the biceps tendon at the pulley system)
    - Medium glenohumeral ligament (MGHL)
    - Inferior glenohumeral ligament (IGHL), anterior and posterior part
  - Long head of biceps tendon
- Dynamic stabilizers
  - Surrounding muscles
  - Compression-concavity mechanism of the rotator cuff
- The position of the scapula in relation to the humerus

As described in the former section "Aetiology and Classification" children and adolescents commonly present with a certain degree of hyperlaxity of the joints with a particular focus at the shoulder. This hyperlaxity usually is bilateral and decreases with increasing age. This condition is often combined with a varying degree of motor incompetence and a disturbed scapulo-thoracic rhythm. A physical rehabilitation programme with specific attention to these problems can often restore normal shoulder function but needs more time than commonly expected.

The reduced strength of the soft tissue static stabilizers of the glenohumeral joint compared to adults make bony injuries to the glenoid (bony Bankart lesion) and the humerus (Hill-Sachs lesion, Malgaigne or reversed Bankart lesion) less likely and less marked but on the other hand may be an important factor in the much higher recurrence rates [5, 6, 8, 60].

Diagnosis

The diagnosis is based on the history of present complaints, a thorough clinical investigation and diagnostic imaging.

It is important to define the mechanism of injury, if there was any trauma, the amount of displacement (complete dislocation vs. subluxation) and the circumstances of reduction (spontaneous, manipulation by the patient, manipulation by the doctor with or without anaesthesia) and the history of recurrence (how often, how much and under which circumstances). In younger children it can be difficult to obtain these data and the surgeon often has to rely on the parent's incomplete memorisation. During clinical examination the patient is assessed for any general abnormality (e.g. asymmetry, differences of appearance, circumference and length of the upper extremities and shoulder girdle, muscle atrophy, hyperlaxity, etc.).

The cervical spine is assessed for any signs of abnormality. The range of motion of the shoulder is assessed both actively and passively. The examiner should notice little differences vey carefully without trying to replicate tests and manoeuvres and save time and compliance of the child for the important issues.

The normal range of motion can have a high variability and the ability to anteriorly dislocate the joint by the examiner does not need to be pathological but can present as a normal variant [61–65]. Also an asymmetric amount of laxity per se does not need to be pathological or represent an unstable joint [61, 66]. The amount of normal inferior translation (sulcus test) remains controversial [57].

General hyperlaxity can checked by the Beighton criteria [51, 67]:
- Thumb apposition to the forearm with a palmar-flexed hand at both sides
- Hyperextension >90° of the fifth finger at both sides
- Hyperextension >10° of the knee joint at both sides
- Hyperextension >10° of the elbows at both sides
- Spine flexion with extended knees and palms on the floor

Hyperlaxity at the shoulder can be tested by the Gagey test (Fig. 1) and an increased external rotation in adduction (Fig. 2) and the sulcus test (Fig. 3).

The apprehension test (Fig. 4) should be performed very carefully, it can be positive with very small amounts of abduction and external rotation. As this test can be very uncomfortable for children it should be performed at the end of the clinical examination. This applies as well for the load and shift test and the sulcus sign (Fig. 5).

The clinical examination is accompanied by a series of basic radiographs, which should include a true anterior-posterior view, an outlet view and an axillary view (the Velpeau view may be used in painful shoulders or where there is inability to perform the necessary abduction).

In any case of a traumatic dislocation we recommend an accompanying MRI to rule out any osteochondral lesion [70–72]. If the clinical examination cannot be performed properly because of non-compliance of the child, a second attempt at a different time during clinic should be made, but sometimes an MRI is indicated based on the history of trauma and the parent's information alone.

Fig. 1 Hyperabduction test according to Gagey [68, 69]: glenohumeral abduction is performed at maximum level with a fixed scapula. A range of motion of more than 90–100° is considered to be positive

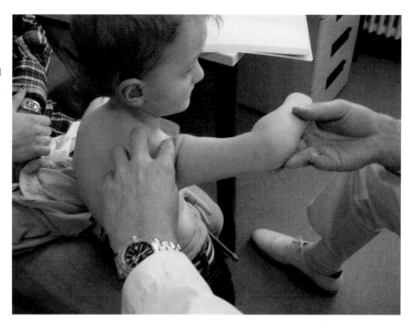

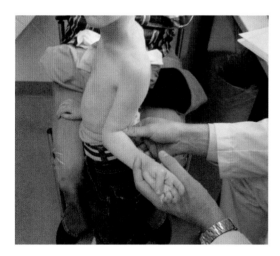

Fig. 2 External rotation of the arm in adduction of more than 90° is considered to be positive

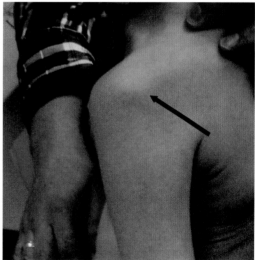

Fig. 3 Sulcus sign: Axial traction of the arm in adduction is graded in three grades. Note the acromion becomes obvious (*black arrow*) with inferior subluxation of the humeral head out of the glenoid fossa giving a positive sulcus sign

Indications for Surgery

There is no consensus about the management of primary shoulder dislocations in young individuals.

In cases of acute injuries with massive haematoma and any suspicion of an osteochondral lesion an arthroscopic evaluation is recommended by the authors. If osteochondral lesions are found, they should be addressed as necessary and of course any attempt should be made to maintain

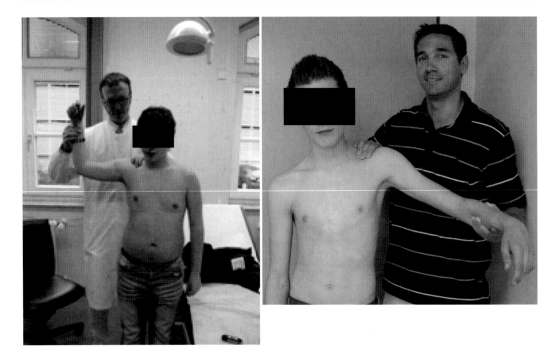

Fig. 4 Apprehension sign: External rotation of the 90° abducted arm and additional anterior push with the left hand causes discomfort and apprehension (*left*). This test can be positive in very early abduction and external rotation (*right*)

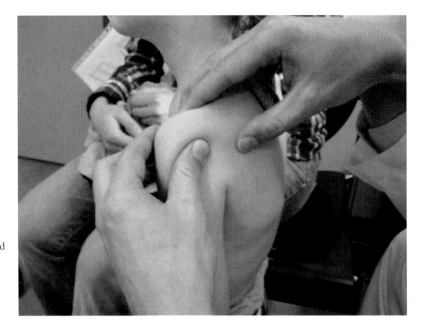

Fig. 5 Anterior drawer test: The left humeral head is pushed anteriorly (and posteriorly) with the left hand while the right hand fixes the scapula with the glenoid

the hyaline joint cartilage [73], but refixation of osteochondral fragments at the shoulder is technically challenging because of the size of the defect in relation to the joint and the angulations of the instruments in relation to the defect and often a resection and debridement is necessary.

Bony Bankart lesions in the early post-traumatic period usually can be anatomically repaired, as long as they are in contact with the labrum and the capsulo-ligamentous complex and not substantially retracted, using suture anchors. Figure 6a–d Conservative treatment is based on a period of immobilization. We usually use a customized Gilchrist sling (Fig. 7) for 2 weeks with early physiotherapy and passive mobilization in a phased rehabilitation protocol. The use of external rotation orthotic devices has become popular in adults but there are no reports about the use in children and adolescents [74–77].

Lawton et al. [1] reported the treatment and results in the largest study of 101 children and adolescents with an age below 16 years (mean age 13.2 years, range 4–16) from 1976 to 1999. Ten percent of the patients were below the age of ten. Girls were significantly younger compared to boys and atraumatic, voluntary dislocations and multi-directional instabilities were more frequent in younger individuals. 50 % of the patients did not have frank dislocations but subluxations. Trauma was associated with the first dislocation in 86 %.

67 % of the patients began physical therapy and 40 % eventually underwent surgery. Of the 28 operated shoulders, 18 (65.8 %) had participated in physical therapy before surgery. Bankart repairs with capsular shift were performed in 11 (39 %) of the surgical patients, Bristow procedures in 5 (18 %), Putti-Platt procedures in 3 (11 %), capsular shift in 3 (11 %), and Bankart repair alone (no capsular shift) in 1 (4 %). One patient had an arthroscopic anterior Bankart repair with capsular tightening.

Surgery was used less often among patients with voluntary instability compared with those without, a trend that approached statistical significance. Six initially conservatively-treated patients underwent secondary surgery at a different institution. Surgically-treated patients were significantly less likely to report symptoms at final follow-up. Among patients with >2 years of follow-up, 9 % had recurrent instability; of these, two had dislocations and the remaining four had subluxations. Both of the patients with dislocation had been treated with physical therapy alone at their institution. One (4 %) of the 28 surgically-treated patients with >2 years of follow-up had recurrent dislocations.

When stratified by treatment modality (surgical vs. physical therapy alone), surgically- treated patients were more likely to report moderate discomfort, which occurred in six (21 %) of the surgically-treated shoulders compared with one (2 %) of those treated with physical therapy alone. Otherwise, there were no significant differences in pain when patients were stratified by traumatic versus atraumatic onset, voluntary instability, and direction of instability. Age at first episode was not related to stability. To summarize the broad statistical information, the authors identified four groups of patient profiles:

- The first reflects a positive relationship between older boys with traumatic onset of their instability, absence of voluntary instability, treatment with surgery, and good outcomes both at clinical and survey follow-up.
- The second grouping shows that older girls with traumatic dislocation and voluntary instability had poorer outcomes independent of treatment.
- The third grouping represents a positive relationship between multiple dislocations, atraumatic onset, treatment with physical therapy and surgery, and favourable outcome. In other words, patients who had those features treated with physical therapy before surgery were more likely to be stable and less likely to report limitations than those with fewer characteristics.
- The fourth group reflects a relationship between early atraumatic instability, multiple dislocations, voluntary instability, and poor outcome after surgical treatment: patients with these features did not do as well with surgery in terms of stability and function at follow-up [1].

Jones et al. [29] retrospectively reviewed 32 consecutive arthroscopic Bankart repairs (ABR) in 30 paediatric patients with anterior shoulder instability mainly after trauma or sports activities (17 males and 13 females; average age 15.4 years, range 11–18; average follow-up 25.2 months). Sixteen shoulders failed initial non-operative therapy before, whereas surgical stabilization was the primary treatment in 16 shoulders for patients who were aiming to return to athletics. In the initial non-operative

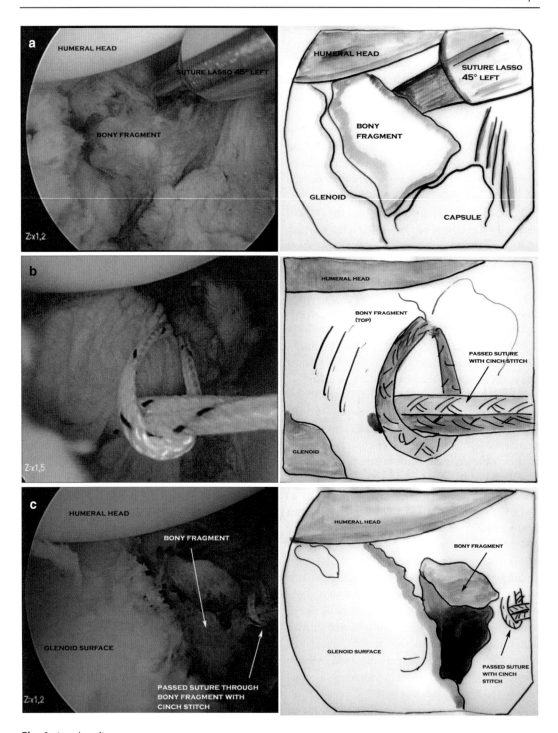

Fig. 6 (continued)

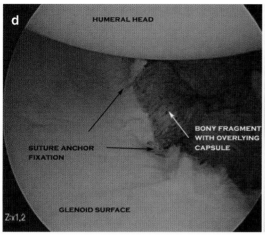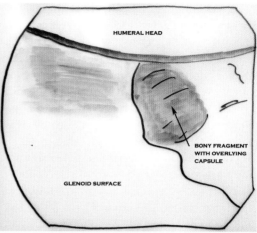

Fig. 6 Supero-lateral arthroscopic view of a left shoulder (right anterior, left posterior, top inferior). The bony Bankart fragment is pierced with a left curved suture lasso® (Arthrex, Naples, FL) (**a**). Note the drill hole at the glenoid edge on the left and an inferior fixation point already created. After retrograde passing of a non-absorbable suture with a cinch-stitch (**b**) the bony fragment is shifted upward and anteriorly into anatomic position (**c**). After fixation of the suture at the glenoid edge with a knotless resorbable suture anchor (3.5 mm Biopushlock®, Arthrex, Naples, FL) the inferior glenoid surface is anatomically restored (**d**). Note the absence of knots or sutures at the glenohumeral articulation to avoid cartilage damage

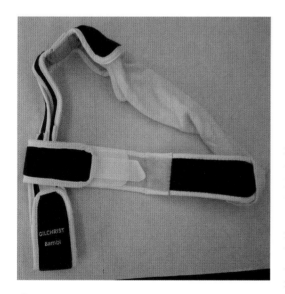

Fig. 7 Custom-made Gilchrist sling for very young individuals

group, the average SANE score was 92.2 and there were three shoulder re-dislocations in two patients (18.75 %). In the 16 shoulders treated with ABR as initial therapy, the average SANE score was 91.8, and there were two shoulder redislocations in two patients (12.5 %).

Hovelius reported about a recurrence rate of 47 % for patients with conservative treatment after primary shoulder dislocation in the age group of patients of 12–22 years after 2 years of follow-up [78]. By further sub-grouping into the ages of 12–14 and 15–19 years there were five males without recurrence, one with recurrence and three females without recurrence and two with a recurrences in the younger group. In the older group there were 22 males without recurrence, 23 with recurrence and five females without recurrence and five with recurrence. Patients with a tuberosity fracture, which were highest at the age 12–13 had a significantly better long-term prognosis regarding stability [79].

At the 10 year follow-up 63 % (initial conservative treatment with a sling only) and 70 % (immobilization with the arm tied with a bandage to the torso for 3–4 weeks) respectively of the 12–22 year old patients had at least one recurrence. A history of trivial trauma was found in 71 % and a history of violent trauma in 65 % of the patients with recurrent dislocation in the group 12–22 years at that time [80].

In the sub-group of patients at the age of 12–16 years 38 % had had operative treatment after 10 years compared with 37 % of the patients between 17 and 19 years. At the so-far final follow-up of the initial cohort of patients in 2003, 26 % of the patients overall showed a moderate to severe dislocation arthropathy (56 % if mild arthropathy was included; this has a predictive value of 60 % for progression into moderate to severe arthropathy during the next 15 years) [81]. Younger patients (<25 years) had less arthropathy than older ones. In the age group 12–16 30 % had mild arthropathy and 70 % no arthropathy. In the age group 17–19 there were about 20 % with moderate to severe arthropathy, about 30 % with mild arthropathy and about 50 % without arthropathy which is better than all other groups consisting of older patients. Overall, surgically stabilized shoulders were less likely to develop dislocation arthropathy. Shoulders that became stable over time had more arthropathy than solitary shoulders (one dislocation only). The authors conclude that the trauma of shoulder dislocation has long-time biological effects on the joint physiology.

There is a lot of information and conclusions to be drawn by this excellent longitudinal study but it does not answer all of our questions. We should keep in mind, that the study began more than 30 years ago in 1978 and all patients were initially treated conservatively. Since than, the evolution of surgical techniques especially the arthroscopic stabilization techniques has been tremendous. Therefore comparison of historical studies (Table 1) and their recurrence rates must be interpreted with caution.

Risk factors for recurrent dislocations in adults are a substantial bony defect of the glenoid >25 % [83–85], hyperlaxity [83] and the presence of a significant Hill-Sachs-lesion [83, 86]. This is probably true for children and adolescents too but has not been worked out so far.

Patients with a multi-directional instability do respond well to a specific course of shoulder-strengthening exercise [87] although a number of patients continue to have long-term symptoms [88].

In conclusion, there is good evidence for a conservative treatment approach in the first line for acute traumatic dislocations, except in some special circumstances, such as an osteochondral injury, additional severe ligamentous injury, locked dislocation or the inability to keep a centred glenohumeral joint. With modern arthroscopic stabilization techniques the Orthopaedic surgeon has an armamentarium that should allow an anatomical repair with minimal iatrogenic damage to the joints in most cases and we anticipate an increasing number of surgical interventions with favourable short and long-term success rates in the near future.

Pre-Operative Preparation and Planning

The pre-operative planning begins with the identification of additional problems associated with the apparent shoulder instability. This is based on a thorough clinical investigation and diagnostic imaging. The clinical examination should include both shoulders with the focus on the amount and direction of instability (see above "Aetiology and Classification" section).

There is a variety of tests, such as the apprehension test, re-location test according to Jobe, posterior and anterior drawer test according to Gerber-Ganz, load and shift test according to Silliman and Hawkins and tests for hyperlaxity such as the Gagey-test, sulcus sign and the increase external rotation in adduction [89] (Figs. 1–5). A special interest should be focussed on the scapulo-thoracic rhythm and signs of scapular dyskinesia [90–93].

A series of standard radiographs (see "Diagnosis" section) together with MRI scans not older than 3 months are the standard. The patient and the parents are informed about the planned procedure, the length of the hospital stay and the duration and modality of post-operative rehabilitation, e.g. duration of immobilization, the need for braces or orthoses, absences from school and sports participation etc. The operation should be carefully timed to fit into bank or school holidays if possible [94].

Table 1 Clinical results of therapeutic intervention (surgical an non-surgical) for shoulder instability in children and adolescents

Authors	Year	Number of individuals	Indication	Mean age (range)	Treatment	Follow-up period	Recurrence	Outcome	Complications
Rowe [5]	1956	n = 8		<10 years			100 %		
		n = 99		10–20 years			92 %		
		n = 107		<20			83 %		
		n = 488 (500 shoulders)	Shoulder dislocation (95 % anterior)	48 years (primary); 23 years (recurrent)		4.8 years	38 %		n = 27/500 (5.4 %) nerve injuries (no sub grouping for children)
Hovelius [79]	1983	n = 102	Primary dislocation	<22 years	Non-surgical	2 years	47 %		
Wagner [6]	1983	n = 9 (10 shoulders)	Traumatic anterior dislocation	13.5 year (12–16)	8/9 patients closed reduction and immobilization in sling	72 months (26–135)	8 %	6/8 underwent secondary stabilization (Magnuson-Stack, one Bristow proc.)	None
Marans [8]	1992	n = 21 (15 boys)	Traumatic anterior shoulder dislocation		n = 9 patients no immobilization, n = 12 immobilization 4–6 weeks; 62 % open stabilization (12 Putti-Platt, 1 Bristow)	6.5 years (1–13)	100 % (average time to redislocation 8 months)	Most of the operated patients returned to preinjury activity; non-operated shoulders without restriction of ROM, operated loss of ER 10–50°	
Postaccini [10]	2000	n = 33	Primary anterior dislocation (75 % traumatic); 86 %	12–17	n = 7 patients surgical repair (5 traumatic)	7.1 years	Traumatic primary dislocations	Mean constant score (CS) 75 % (65–96); operated	

(continued)

Table 1 (continued)

Authors	Year	Number of individuals	Indication	Mean age (range)	Treatment	Follow-up period	Recurrence	Outcome	Complications
			recurrent dislocations				age 14–17 92 %; atraumatic primary dislocations age 14–16 86 %	group 92 %; CS 71 % non-surgical	
Lawton [1]	2002	n = 101 (107 shoulders)	21 % multidirectional, 16 % voluntary; 62 % Hill-Sachs lesion	13.2 (4–16); 10 % < 10 years	n = 40 patients initial surgery, n = 2 secondary surgery; variety of techniques (Bankart repairs with capsular shift in 11 (39 %), Bristow procedures in 5 (18 %), Putti-Platt procedures in 3 (11 %), capsular shift in 3 (11 %), Bankart repair alone (no capsular shift) in 1 (4 %), one patient with arthroscopic anterior Bankart repair with capsular tightening)	Short-term FU 6–24 months; long-term FU 2–21 y	9 % recurrent instability; 2 dislocations (initially non-surgical)	59 % no instability symptoms, 31 % apprehension, 6 % subluxation, 3 % recurrent dislocation; 25 % instability symptoms after surgical treatment vs. 51 % non-surgical; surgical: more likely for self-rated improvement	
Deitch [60]	2003	n = 32		11–18	n = 16 operated	4 years (1–14)	0.75	Outcome scores similar for	

| Lefort [82] | 2004 | n = 29 | Traumatic anterior shoulder dislocation Voluntary dislocation; n = 15 posterior dislocations; uncertain laxity and multidirectional instability | 5–15 years | n = 8 with posterior capsulorrhaphy; n = 3 anterior capsulorrhaphy | 8 years (7–10) | No | patients for surgical and non-surgical patients n = 11 rehab without improvement after 8 months; all stable, ROM normal, sports resumed |
| Jones [29] | 2007 | n = 48 (30 reached for FU) | Failed conservative treatment for athletes; 27 traumatic dislocations during sports, 3 falls; 1 girls bilateral multidirectional instability | 11–18 years | Arthroscopic Bankart repair | 24 months | Primary surgery: 2/16 (12.5 %) redislocation (1 wrestler); secondary surgery: 3/16 (18.75 %) redislocation (2 hyperlax) | |

Operative Technique

We describe an arthroscopic technique for primary surgical stabilization which today is the standard of care at our institution. The patient is put in a lateral decubitus position with the affected arm pointing upwards and fixed in a lateral and axial arm extension of 3.5 kg and 1.5 kg respectively. The traction needs to be adjusted to the patients age and constitution and the amount of laxity of the shoulder. Prolonged shoulder traction can cause brachial plexus disturbance which usually spontaneously dissolves but should be avoided. A standard intra-articular pressure of 50 mmHg usually is sufficient throughout the procedure.

We suggest a watertight draping to avoid the patient being drenched which could lead to hypothermia and problems with electrical devices. This can be accomplished by the use of a well fixed rubber-like first layer and a second layer of heavy draping.

Bony landmarks (border of acromion with posterior corner, clavicle, ac-joint, coracoid process) are marked with a pen. We start with a posterior portal which usually is located more laterally and distally compared to standard posterior portals with respect to the changed position of the glenohumeral joint under arm traction. After a thorough inspection of the joint in all parts
- Superior: SLAP-complex, biceps tendon, supraspinatus and infraspinatus tendon
- Central: joint cartilage; anterior: anterior labrum, Malgaigne or reversed Hill-Sachs lesion, subscapularis tendon, glenohumeral ligaments, GLAD lesion
- Inferior: labrum, joint capsule, inferior glenohumeral ligaments; posterior: labrum, posterior inferior glenohumeral ligament, Hill-Sachs lesion, teres minor tendon
- Peripheral: joint capsule, HAGL lesion.

The decision for the kind of surgical therapy and the strategy in terms of the chronological order is then made.

We establish an antero-inferior portal and a twist-in cannula just above the subscapularis tendon with respect to the angulation to the glenoid surface for possible placement of suture anchors. A probe is introduced into the joint and every structure and compartment visualized and probed if necessary. Rotation of the humerus brings all aspects of the joint cartilage into the field of view and the amount of engagment of any Hill-Sachs-lesion is quantified. The amount of any anterior glenoid bony defects can be measured with the probe. The estimation of bone loss can be facilitated if the centre of the inferior glenoid surface is detected (so-called "bare spot", Tubercle of Assaki [95]) and the posterior radius is taken as a reference for the entire sphere of the inferior part of the pearl-shaped glenoid.

If an injury to the upper labrum and biceps anchor complex (SLAP lesion) is noted, we suggest starting with the SLAP-repair. An additional antero-lateral portal is created which usually lies close to the antero-lateral tip of the acromion entering the joint in the interval region between the supraspinatus and subscapularis tendon just above the long head of the biceps tendon (Fig. 8).

The superior glenoid rim is mobilized with a Bankart chisel and rasp or shaver and debrided down to bleeding bone to enhance fibroligamentous healing of the repaired labrum (Fig. 9). We prefer the use of absorbable knotless suture anchors at this location. The guiding instrument is placed at the upper glenoid rim just at the border to the cartilage and a bone tunnel is created with a drill with angulation into the good bone stock away from the joint surface. The superior labrum is pierced with a Suture-lasso (Arthrex, Naples, FL) or other devices and a partially-resorbable suture (Orthocord, Johnson & Johnson Medical, Norderstedt, Germany) is passed in a retrograde fashion as a loop. The free ends of the loop are grasped with a suture retriever and put through the loop resulting in a self-locking cinch-stitch around the labrum (Fig. 6b).

The suture end is passed in the eyelet of the anchor, the tip of the anchor device is put into the bone tunnel via the antero-lateral portal, and the suture is finally tensioned again and locked in the bone tunnel by the Biopushlock-anchor (Arthrex, Naples, FL).

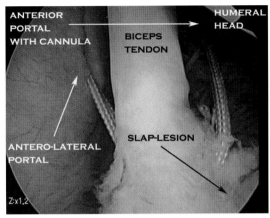
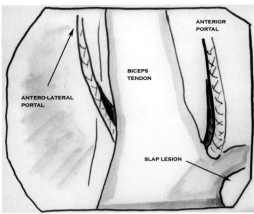

Fig. 8 Arthroscopic view from a posterior portal of a right shoulder. Note the antero-superior portal just above the biceps tendon and the SLAP complex for SLAP-repair and an anterior working and shuttle portal with transparent twist-in cannula

The sutures are cut as close as possible. The same procedure needs to be repeated anteriorly to the biceps anchor if the lesion extend further anteriorly with a second anchor. The bone tunnel then usually can be placed more easily from anteriorly. Care should be taken not to violate the rotator cuff with the used instruments by using the antero-lateral portal. The use of an additional cannula, which can be used as a tunnel through the subacromial space, can be helpful in special cases.

After a final check of the stability of the repair the arthroscope is switched to the antero-lateral portal by using two switching sticks (antero-lateral and posterior). After visualization is established another transparent twist-in cannula is inserted from posteriorly. The entire antero-inferior labrum can be assessed at this time (Fig. 11a, b). It needs to be pointed out, that the judgement of labrum lesions cannot be made from a solitary posterior portal alone, especially not for retracted tissue as described for ALPSA (anterior labrum periosteal sleeve avulsion) lesions. The entire antero-inferior capsulo-ligamentous complex is mobilized with the Bankart knife, meniscus punch and shaver until the glenoid neck becomes visible (Fig. 9a, b). The joint distension by the arthroscopy pump can be stopped at this time to check for completion of mobilization: if the capsulo-ligamentous complex spontaneously moves in an anatomical position with bleeding of the anterior glenoid neck surface a solid basis for the following re-fixation is achieved.

As described above, most of the lesions are Bankart lesions and anterior capsulo-ligamentous labrum repair is sufficient to stabilize the joint. We prefer double-loaded threaded absorbable suture anchors for this procedure. The guiding device is placed at the very edge of the glenoid rim (rather to the joint surface than away from it) and the bone tunnel is created through the anterior portal. By using the 3.5 mm BioFasttak anchor (Arthrex, Naples, FL) the cortex is punched and a thread is created. The suture anchor is threaded in and checked for stability by a powerful pull. We start placing the most inferior anchor first at the five-o'clock (or seven o'clock position for a left shoulder). Care should be taken to find the right angulation away from the joint surface and to avoid penetration out of the glenoid bone stock. This can be simulated by a switching stick before. If the right angulation cannot be achieved, the portals need to be adjusted. A deep 5-o'clock portal has been described with the advantage of better angulation but iatrogenic injury to the muscular part of the subscapularis is possible and therefore it is not routinely used by the authors [96].

The sutures are parked at the posterior portal and an additional suture anchor is placed at the

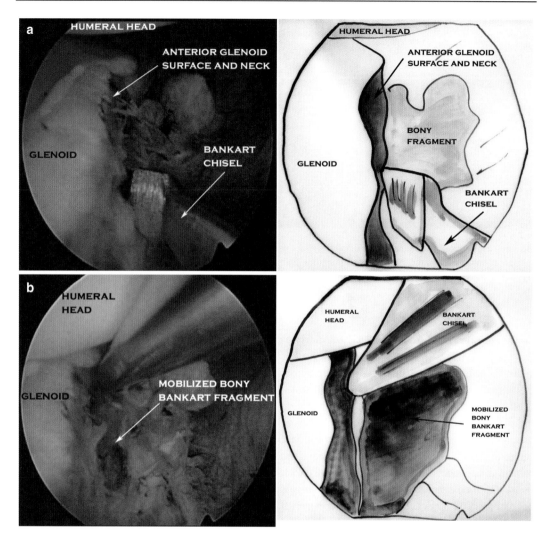

Fig. 9 Arthroscopic view from superior of a left shoulder with a bony Bankart lesion. The labrum with the bony fragment is mobilized using an arthroscopic Bankart knife (**a**) down to the inferior pole of the glenoid surface (6 o'clock) (**b**) until full separation and the ability to shift the capsule together with the fragment upward into an anatomic position

4-o'clock position in the same manner. The antero-inferior capsulo-ligamentous complex is pierced with the 45° Suture-lasso (Arthrex, Naples, FL) (left angulation for a left shoulder) from the antero-inferior portal and one of the dorsally parked sutures is passed through the capsulo-ligamentous complex in a retrograde fashion anteriorly. The associated suture-end is passed in a similar fashion leaving a sufficient soft tissue bridge to prevent pullout of the suture resulting in a mattress stitch. The second pair of suture ends can be put as a second mattress stitch in line with the first, as an interlocking stitch or in a modified Mason-Allen-technique (Fig. 10).

The individual stitch configuration depends on the surgeon's preferences and more on the quality of the soft tissues. The less mechanical strength the tissue provides the more the surgeon must think about the right stitch configuration. In cases of very poor tissue quality, self-locking loop-stitches can be used which takes more time and attention to place them (Fig. 11a–c). As a general rule there is

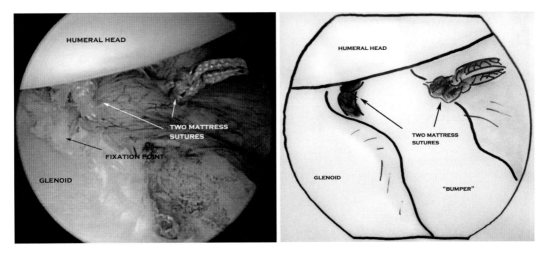

Fig. 10 Result after knot-tying of two retrograde shuttled non-absorbable sutures creating a new "bumper" by two mattress sutures

the need for an upward shift of the capsulo-ligamentous complex because of the retraction which is part of the pathology. The amount of shift needs to be adjusted to every individual case by the appropriate amount, which is based on the experience of the surgeon, and a well tensioned antero-inferior glenohumeral ligament. By using the 4-o'clock anchor first for placing the sutures the upward shift is facilitated and an additional shift and placement of the most inferior sutures are made much easier. The disadvantage of this technique is the nescessity for a careful suture management to avoid knotting.

The third anchor is placed at the 3-o'clock position in a similar fashion. As shifting of the capsulo-ligamentous complex already is accomplished, the placement of these sutures is easier. Care should be taken not to inadvertently grasp the medial glenohumeral ligament at this point which can lead to a reduced ROM post-operatively. In our opinion it is very rarely necessary to put suture anchors more cranial to that position. The additional closure of the rotator interval is reserved for exceptional cases because the contribution to stability is low and external rotation is frequently limited by that procedure [97–99].

After inspection of the result and thorough probing the operation can be finished at this time with photo and/or video documentation and removal of the instruments for antero-inferior uni-directional instability without hyperlaxity (Gerber type II). All cases with multi-directional instability and remarkable hyperlaxity may need an additional inferior or postero-inferior capsular shift to stabilize the joint.

For cases without injury to the labrum and an intact fibrous limbus we prefer the modified arthroscopic technique according to Snyder (Fig. 11a–c).

The amount of shift depends on the patient's age, the history of shoulder dislocation and the pre-operative clinical examination, especially the amount of hyperlaxity and/or hypermobility. There are no established landmarks to help the surgeon except the posterior inferior glenohumeral ligament and its amount of tension and the general additional stability achieved by placing sutures and anchors which more and more limits the ability to visualize the inferior aspects of the joint. The traction can be released to test for joint stability at this time but joint play is altered by the preceding surgery and distension. Care should be taken not to inadvertently injure the joint surface at this time with the arthroscope in the more and more narrow joint. The used suture material should be resorbable or partially resorbable to avoid mechanical irritation of the joint surface over time. Although we do believe in the longevity of our stabilizing procedures, a number of those

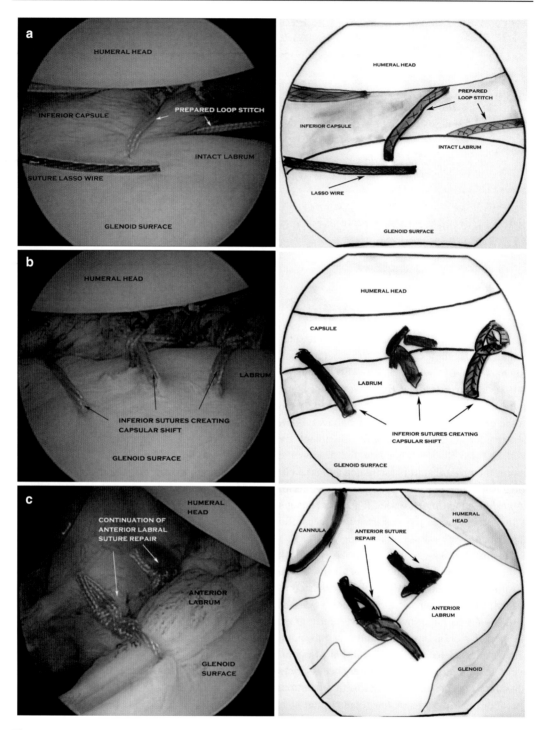

Fig. 11 Illustration of antero-inferior capsular shift for multi-directional instability with hyperlaxity. Arthroscopic view from superior of a right shoulder. Partially absorbable sutures (Orthocord®, Johnson & Johnson Medical, Norderstedt, Germany) are retrograded passed through the inferior capsule and the intact labrum using a 90° curved Suture lasso® (Arthrex, Naples, FL) with a modified loop stitch (**a**). After completion of the inferior capsular shift (**b**) the anterior labral suture repair and capsular shift is completed (**c**)

sutures may cut through the tissue or get loose by time which are sometimes found during revision surgery.

Post-Operative Care and Rehabilitation

The patient is rested in a Gilchrist sling for the first 2 days with early passive mobilization (pendulum self exercises, physiotherapy) starting at day one. We usually use an additional abduction splint for the first 3 weeks. During that time passive exercises are performed with limitation of 60° flexion and abduction and neutral external rotation. Lymph drainage can be added as necessary but manual therapy and joint mobilization techniques by the therapist are avoided. After 3 weeks the patient begins with active-assisted exercises in the pain-free interval with the same limitation for ROM. After 5 weeks ROM can be increased to 90° of flexion and abduction. After 6 weeks the patient can actively start to re-establish the full ROM in the pain-free interval. After full flexion is achieved external rotation becomes the focus of exercises. Water aerobics and aqua jogging are allowed and muscle training for the rotator cuff, the deltoid and the other stabilizers are started and can be combined with additional proprioceptive training and PNF (proprioceptive neuromuscular facilitation).

After 3 months the individual sport activity usually can be started again but should be discussed with the surgeon in each individual case.

Complications

Common surgical complications such as nerve and vessel injury or infection are very rare in this age group as well as in adults. Disturbance of sensation can be the cause of prolonged surgery under too much traction and should be avoided but fortunately usually spontaneously resolves after a couple of days.

Recurrence of instability remains the major concern and reaches the highest rates in adolescents and early adulthood (Table 1).

Summary

Shoulder instability is a common problem in children and adults. Surgical therapy very rarely is necessary under the age of 12 but becomes more frequent during adolescence. During that period the number of violent traumatic events increases and boys are more frequently affected than girls. Surgical stabilization results in higher amounts of long-term success in preventing redislocation. Hyperlaxity should always be taken into account in decision-making about surgical therapy. The indication for surgery treating multidirectional instabilities should be made with special care and a course of specific physiotherapy must be an important part of any treatment plans regardless the decision for surgical therapy.

References

1. Lawton RL, Choudhury S, Mansat P, Cofield RH, Stans AA. Pediatric shoulder instability: presentation, findings, treatment, and outcomes. J Pediatr Orthop. 2002;22(1):52–61.
2. Sanders JO, Cermak MB. Fractures, dislocations, and acquired problems of the shoulder in children. In: Rockwood CA, Matsen FA, Wirth MA, Lippitt SB, editors. The shoulder, vol. 2. Philadelphia: Saunders; 2004. p. 1349.
3. Kraus R, Pavlidis T, Dongowski N, Szalay G, Schnettler R. Children and adolescents with posttraumatic shoulder instability benefit from arthroscopic stabilization. Eur J Pediatr Surg. 2010;20(4):253–6.
4. Kraus R, Pavlidis T, Heiss C, Kilian O, Schnettler R. Arthroscopic treatment of post-traumatic shoulder instability in children and adolescents. Knee Surg Sports Traumatol Arthrosc. 2010;18(12):1738–41. doi: 10.1007/s00167-010-1092-6.
5. Rowe CR. Prognosis in dislocations of the shoulder. J Bone Joint Surg Am. 1956;38A(5):957–77.
6. Wagner KT. Adolescent traumatic dislocations of the shoulder with open epiphyses. J Pediatr Orthop. 1983;3(1):61–2.
7. Hovelius L. Anterior dislocation of the shoulder in teen-agers and young adults. Five-year prognosis. J Bone Joint Surg Am. 1987;69(3):393–9.
8. Marans HJ, Angel KR, Schemitsch EH, Wedge JH. The fate of traumatic anterior dislocation of the shoulder in children. J Bone Joint Surg Am. 1992;74(8):1242–4.

9. Rowe CR, Pierce DS, Clark JG. Voluntary dislocation of the shoulder. A preliminary report on a clinical, electromyographic, and psychiatric study of twenty-six patients. J Bone Joint Surg Am. 1973;55(3): 445–60.

10. Postacchini F, Gumina S, Cinotti G. Anterior shoulder dislocation in adolescents. J Shoulder Elbow Surg. 2000;9(6):470–4.

11. Hovelius L. The natural history of primary anterior dislocation of the shoulder in the young. J Orthop Sci. 1999;4(4):307–17.

12. Wirth MA. Hypoplasia of the glenoid. A review of sixteen patients. J Bone Joint Surg Am. 1993; 75(8):1175–84.

13. Chung SM, Nissenbaum MM. Congenital and developmental defects of the shoulder. Orthop Clin North Am. 1975;6(2):381–92.

14. Fairbank T. Dysplasia epiphysialis multiplex. Br J Surg. 1947;34(135):225–32.

15. Kozlowski K, Scougall J. Congenital bilateral glenoid hypoplasia: a report of four cases. Br J Radiol. 1987; 60(715):705–6.

16. Kozlowski K, Colavita N, Morris L, Little KE. Bilateral glenoid dysplasia (report of 8 cases). Australas Radiol. 1985;29(2):174–7.

17. McClure JG, Raney RB. Anomalies of the scapula. Clin Orthop Relat Res. 1975;110:22–31.

18. Wood VE, Marchinski L. Congenital anomalies of the shoulder. In: Rockwood CA, Matsen FA, Wirth MA, Lippitt SB, editors. The shoulder, vol. 1. Philadelphia: Saunders; 1990. p. 120–2.

19. Matsen FA, Rockwood CA, Wirth MA, Lippitt SB, Parsons M. Glenohumeral arthritis and its management. In: Rockwood CA, Matsen FA, Wirth MA, Lippitt SB, editors. The shoulder, vol. 2. Philadelphia: Saunders; 2004. p. 879–1007.

20. Sutro CJ. Dentated articular surface of the glenoid–an anomaly. Bull Hosp Joint Dis. 1967;28(2):104–8.

21. Scaglietti O. The obstetrical shoulder trauma. Surg Gynecol Obstet. 1938;66:868–77.

22. Samilson RL. Congenital and developmental anomalies of the shoulder girdle. Orthop Clin North Am. 1980;11(2):219–31.

23. Resnick D, Walter RD, Crudale AS. Bilateral dysplasia of the scapular neck. AJR Am J Roentgenol. 1982;139(2):387–9.

24. Pettersson H. Bilateral dysplasia of the neck of scapula and associated anomalies. Acta Radiol Diagn (Stockh). 1981;22(1):81–4.

25. Owen R. Bilateral glenoid hypoplasia; report of five cases. J Bone Joint Surg Br. 1953;35B(2):262–7.

26. Triquet J. Mono-epiphyseal dysplasia of the glenoid cavity of the scapula [DYSPLASIE MONO-EPIPHYSAIRE DE LA CAVITE GLENOIDE DE L'OMOPLATE]. Arch Fr Pediatr. 1980;37(10): 683–4.

27. Edelson JG. Localized glenoid hypoplasia. An anatomic variation of possible clinical significance. Clin Orthop Relat Res. 1995;321:189–95.

28. Curtis Jr RJ. Operative management of children's fractures of the shoulder region. Orthop Clin North Am. 1990;21(2):315–24.

29. Jones KJ, Wiesel B, Ganley TJ, Wells L. Functional outcomes of early arthroscopic bankart repair in adolescents aged 11 to 18 years. J Pediatr Orthop. 2007;27(2):209–13.

30. Matsen FA, Thomas SC, Rockwood Jr CA. Anterior glenohumeral instability. Philadelphia: WB Saunders; 1990. p. 526–622.

31. Wahl CJ, Warren RF, Altchek DW. Shoulder artrhroscopy. In: Rockwood CA, Matsen FA, Wirth MA, Lippitt SB, editors. The shoulder, vol. 1. Philadelphia: Saunders; 2004. p. 283–354.

32. Gerber C. Observations on the classification of instability. In: Warner JJP, Iannotti C, Gerber C, editors. Complex and revision problems in shoulder surgery. Philadelphia: Lippincott-Raven; 1997. p. 9–18.

33. Bayley I. The classification of shoulder instability-new light through old windows. In: Habermeyer P, Magosch P, editors. 16th congress of the European Society for surgery of the shoulder and the elbow. Budapest: Bálványossy; 2002.

34. Juul-Kristensen B, Kristensen JH, Frausing B, Jensen DV, Rogind H, Remvig L. Motor competence and physical activity in 8-year-old school children with generalized joint hypermobility. Pediatrics. 2009;124(5):1380–7.

35. Forleo LH, Hilario MO, Peixoto AL, Naspitz C, Goldenberg J. Articular hypermobility in school children in Sao Paulo, Brazil. J Rheumatol. 1993; 20(5):916–7.

36. Rikken-Bultman DG, Wellink L, van Dongen PW. Hypermobility in two Dutch school populations. Eur J Obstet Gynecol Reprod Biol. 1997;73(2): 189–92.

37. Decoster LC, Vailas JC, Lindsay RH, Williams GR. Prevalence and features of joint hypermobility among adolescent athletes. Arch Pediatr Adolesc Med. 1997;151(10):989–92.

38. Larsson LG, Baum J, Mudholkar GS, Srivastava DK. Hypermobility: prevalence and features in a Swedish population. Br J Rheumatol. 1993;32(2):116–9.

39. Jansson A, Saartok T, Werner S, Renstrom P. General joint laxity in 1845 Swedish school children of different ages: age- and gender-specific distributions. Acta Paediatr. 2004;93(9):1202–6.

40. Remvig L, Jensen DV, Ward RC. Epidemiology of general joint hypermobility and basis for the proposed criteria for benign joint hypermobility syndrome: review of the literature. J Rheumatol. 2007;34(4): 804–9.

41. Beighton P, Solomon L, Soskolne CL. Articular mobility in an African population. Ann Rheum Dis. 1973;32(5):413–8.

42. Hakim AJ, Cherkas LF, Grahame R, Spector TD, MacGregor AJ. The genetic epidemiology of joint hypermobility: a population study of female twins. Arthritis Rheum. 2004;50(8):2640–4.

43. Child AH. Joint hypermobility syndrome: inherited disorder of collagen synthesis. J Rheumatol. 1986; 13(2):239–43.

44. Bensahel H, Souchet P, Pennecot GF, Mazda K. The unstable patella in children. J Pediatr Orthop B. 2000;9(4):265–70.

45. Gannon LM, Bird HA. The quantification of joint laxity in dancers and gymnasts. J Sports Sci. 1999;17(9):743–50.

46. Grahame R, Jenkins JM. Joint hypermobility – asset or liability? A study of joint mobility in ballet dancers. Ann Rheum Dis. 1972;31(2):109–11.

47. Briggs J, McCormack M, Hakim AJ, Grahame R. Injury and joint hypermobility syndrome in ballet dancers – a 5-year follow-up. Rheumatology (Oxford). 2009;48(12):1613–4.

48. McCormack M, Briggs J, Hakim A, Grahame R. Joint laxity and the benign joint hypermobility syndrome in student and professional ballet dancers. J Rheumatol. 2004;31(1):173–8.

49. Smith R, Damodaran AK, Swaminathan S, Campbell R, Barnsley L. Hypermobility and sports injuries in junior netball players. Br J Sports Med. 2005;39(9): 628–31.

50. Klemp P, Stevens JE, Isaacs S. A hypermobility study in ballet dancers. J Rheumatol. 1984;11(5): 692–6.

51. Grahame R, Bird HA, Child A. The revised (Brighton 1998) criteria for the diagnosis of benign joint hypermobility syndrome (BJHS). J Rheumatol. 2000; 27(7):1777–9.

52. Beighton P, De Paepe A, Steinmann B, Tsipouras P, Wenstrup RJ. Ehlers-Danlos syndromes: revised nosology, Villefranche, 1997. Ehlers-Danlos National Foundation (USA) and Ehlers-Danlos Support Group (UK). Am J Med Genet. 1998;77(1):31–7.

53. Juul-Kristensen B, Rogind H, Jensen DV, Remvig L. Inter-examiner reproducibility of tests and criteria for generalized joint hypermobility and benign joint hypermobility syndrome. Rheumatology (Oxford). 2007;46(12):1835–41.

54. Carter C, Sweetnam R. Familial joint laxity and recurrent dislocation of the patella. J Bone Joint Surg Br. 1958;40B(4):664–7.

55. Carter C, Sweetnam R. Recurrent dislocation of the patella and of the shoulder. Their association with familial joint laxity. J Bone Joint Surg Br. 1960;42-R:721–7.

56. Adib N, Davies K, Grahame R, Woo P, Murray KJ. Joint hypermobility syndrome in childhood. A not so benign multisystem disorder? Rheumatology (Oxford). 2005;44(6):744–50.

57. Bahk M, Keyurapan E, Tasaki A, Sauers EL, McFarland EG. Laxity testing of the shoulder: a review. Am J Sports Med. 2007;35(1):131–44.

58. Patzer T, Lichtenberg S, Kircher J, Magosch P, Habermeyer P. Influence of SLAP lesions on chondral lesions of the glenohumeral joint. Knee Surg Sports Traumatol Arthrosc. 2010;18(7):982–7.

59. Patzer T. A comparative biomechanical study on the effect of SLAP lesion of the shoulder on the development of a glenohumeral chondral lesion [Vergleichende biomechanische Untersuchung zum Einfluss der SLAP-Läsion der Schulter auf die Entstehung einer glenohumeralen Chondralläsion]. Sport Orthop Traumatol. 2008;24(3):178–80.

60. Deitch J, Mehlman CT, Foad SL, Obbehat A, Mallory M. Traumatic anterior shoulder dislocation in adolescents. Am J Sports Med. 2003;31(5):758–63.

61. Lintner SA, Levy A, Kenter K, Speer KP. Glenohumeral translation in the asymptomatic athlete's shoulder and its relationship to other clinically measurable anthropometric variables. Am J Sports Med. 1996;24(6):716–20.

62. McFarland EG, Hsu CY, Neira C, O'Neil O. Internal impingement of the shoulder: a clinical and arthroscopic analysis. J Shoulder Elbow Surg. 1999;8(5):458–60.

63. Harryman 2nd DT, Sidles JA, Harris SL, Matsen 3rd FA. The role of the rotator interval capsule in passive motion and stability of the shoulder. J Bone Joint Surg Am. 1992;74(1):53–66.

64. Douglas TH, John AS, Scott LH, Frederick AM. Laxity of the normal glenohumeral joint: a quantitative in vivo assessment. J Shoulder Elbow Surg/Am Shoulder Elbow Surg. 1992;1(2):66–76.

65. Emery RJ, Ho EK, Leong JC. The shoulder girdle in ankylosing spondylitis. J Bone Joint Surg Am. 1991;73(10):1526–31.

66. Ellenbecker TS, Mattalino AJ, Elam E, Caplinger R. Quantification of anterior translation of the humeral head in the throwing shoulder. Manual assessment versus stress radiography. Am J Sports Med. 2000;28(2):161–7.

67. Beighton P, Grahame R, Bird H. Joint instability: methods of measuring and epidemiology. Orthopade. 1984;13(1):19–24.

68. Molina V, Pouliart N, Gagey O. Quantitation of ligament laxity in anterior shoulder instability: an experimental cadaver model. Surg Radiol Anat. 2004;26(5):349–54.

69. Gagey O, Bonfait H, Gillot C, Mazas F. The mechanics of shoulder elevation. Role of the coracohumeral ligament. Rev Chir Orthop Reparatrice Appar Mot. 1985;71 (Suppl 2):105–7.

70. Elser F. Glenohumeral joint preservation: current options for managing articular cartilage lesions in young, active patients. Arthroscopy. 2010;26(5): 685–96.

71. Accadbled F. Arthroscopic surgery in children. Orthop Traumatol Surg Res. 2010;96(4):447–55.

72. Choi YS, Potter HG, Scher DM. A shearing osteochondral fracture of the humeral head following an anterior shoulder dislocation in a child. HSS J. 2005;1(1):100–2.

73. Hoshino CM, Thomas BM. Late repair of an osteochondral fracture of the patella. Orthopedics. 2010;270–3. doi: 10.3928/01477447-20100225-25.

74. Scheibel M. How long should acute anterior dislocations of the shoulder be immobilized in external rotation? Am J Sports Med. 2009;37(7):1309–16.

75. Yamamoto N, Sano H, Itoi E. Conservative treatment of first-time shoulder dislocation with the arm in external rotation. J Shoulder Elbow Surg. 2010;19(2 Suppl):98–103.

76. Itoi E, Hatakeyama Y, Sato T, Kido T, Minagawa H, Yamamoto N, Wakabayashi I, Nozaka K. Immobilization in external rotation after shoulder dislocation reduces the risk of recurrence. A randomized controlled trial. J Bone Joint Surg Am. 2007; 89(10):2124–31.

77. Yamamoto N, Itoi E, Abe H, Minagawa H, Seki N, Shimada Y, Okada K. Contact between the glenoid and the humeral head in abduction, external rotation, and horizontal extension: a new concept of glenoid track. J Shoulder Elbow Surg. 2007;16(5):649–56.

78. Hovelius L, Lind B, Thorling J. Primary dislocation of the shoulder. Factors affecting the two-year prognosis. Clin Orthop Relat Res. 1983;176:181–5.

79. Hovelius L, Eriksson K, Fredin H, Hagberg G, Hussenius A, Lind B, Thorling J, Weckstrom J. Recurrences after initial dislocation of the shoulder. Results of a prospective study of treatment. J Bone Joint Surg Am. 1983;65(3):343–9.

80. Hovelius L, Augustini BG, Fredin H, Johansson O, Norlin R, Thorling J. Primary anterior dislocation of the shoulder in young patients. A ten-year prospective study. J Bone Joint Surg Am. 1996;78(11):1677–84.

81. Hovelius L, Saeboe M. Neer Award 2008: arthropathy after primary anterior shoulder dislocation–223 shoulders prospectively followed up for twenty-five years. J Shoulder Elbow Surg. 2009;18(3):339–47.

82. Lefort G, Pfliger F, Mal-Lawane M, Belouadah M, Daoud S. Capsular shift for voluntary dislocation of the shoulder: results in children. Rev Chir Orthop Reparatrice Appar Mot. 2004;90(7):607–12.

83. Boileau P, Villalba M, Hery JY, Balg F, Ahrens P, Neyton L. Risk factors for recurrence of shoulder instability after arthroscopic Bankart repair. J Bone Joint Surg Am. 2006;88(8):1755–63.

84. Kim TK, Queale WS, Cosgarea AJ, McFarland EG. Clinical features of the different types of SLAP lesions: an analysis of one hundred and thirty-nine cases. J Bone Joint Surg Am. 2003;85A(1):66–71.

85. Burkhart SS. Articular arc length mismatch as a cause of failed Bankart repair. Arthroscopy. 2000;16(7): 740–4.

86. Burkhart SS. Traumatic glenohumeral bone defects and their relationship to failure of arthroscopic Bankart repairs: significance of the inverted-pear glenoid and the humeral engaging Hill-Sachs lesion. Arthroscopy. 2000;16(7):677–94.

87. Ide J, Maeda S, Yamaga M, Morisawa K, Takagi K. Shoulder-strengthening exercise with an orthosis for multidirectional shoulder instability: quantitative evaluation of rotational shoulder strength before and after the exercise program. J Shoulder Elbow Surg. 2003;12(4):342–5.

88. Misamore GW, Sallay PI, Didelot W. A longitudinal study of patients with multidirectional instability of the shoulder with seven- to ten-year follow-up. J Shoulder Elbow Surg. 2005;14(5):466–70.

89. Buckup K. Clinical tests for the musculosceletal system. Examinations – signs – phenomena. Stuttgart/ New York: Thieme; 2004.

90. Pluim BM, van Cingel RE, Kibler WB. Shoulder to shoulder: stabilising instability, re-establishing rhythm, and rescuing the rotators! Br J Sports Med. 2010;44(5):299.

91. Burkhart SS, Morgan CD, Kibler WB. The disabled throwing shoulder: spectrum of pathology Part III: the SICK scapula, scapular dyskinesis, the kinetic chain, and rehabilitation. Arthroscopy. 2003;19(6): 641–61.

92. Kibler WB, McMullen J. Scapular dyskinesis and its relation to shoulder pain. J Am Acad Orthop Surg. 2003;11(2):142–51.

93. Kibler WB. The role of the scapula in athletic shoulder function. Am J Sports Med. 1998;26(2):325–37.

94. Trentacosta NE, Vitale MA, Ahmad CS. The effects of timing of pediatric knee ligament surgery on short-term academic performance in school-aged athletes. Am J Sports Med. 2009;37(9):1684–91.

95. De Wilde LF, Berghs BM, Audenaert E, Sys G, Van Maele GO, Barbaix E. About the variability of the shape of the glenoid cavity. Surg Radiol Anat. 2004;26(1):54–9.

96. Imhoff AB, Ansah P, Tischer T, Reiter C, Bartl C, Hench M, Spang JT, Vogt S. Arthroscopic repair of anterior-inferior glenohumeral instability using a portal at the 5:30-o'clock position: analysis of the effects of age, fixation method, and concomitant shoulder injury on surgical outcomes. Am J Sports Med. 2010;38(9):1795–803.

97. Mologne TS. The addition of rotator interval closure after arthroscopic repair of either anterior or posterior shoulder instability: effect on glenohumeral translation and range of motion. Am J Sports Med. 2008;36(6):1123–31.

98. Provencher MT. An analysis of the rotator interval in patients with anterior, posterior, and multidirectional shoulder instability. Arthroscopy. 2008;24(8): 921–9.

99. Provencher MT. The use of rotator interval closure in the arthroscopic treatment of posterior shoulder instability. Arthroscopy. 2009;25(1):109–10.

Frozen Shoulder

Tim Bunker and Chris Smith

Contents

T. Bunker (✉) • C. Smith
Princess Elizabeth Orthopaedic Centre, Exeter, UK
e-mail: Tim.bunker@exetershoulderclinic.co.uk

Keywords

Clinical features • Frozen • Shoulder • Incidence • Investigations-arthrography, arthroscopy, surgical features • Natural history • Pathology and cytogenics • Terminology • Treatment-steroids, physiotherapy, manipulation, arthroscopic release

Introduction

Until recently Frozen shoulder has been an Orthopaedic enigma. It is only in the last decade that the histopathology has been described and this has unlocked the pathway towards successful surgical treatment. However although the Orthopaedic surgical profession now understands much more about this disease, this evidence has not trickled down to primary care physicians and allied health professionals, let alone the world-wide-web and, at the end of the chain, the patients. Although we now understand a lot about the natural history of this condition, it's associations, the arthroscopic appearance of the shoulder, the histopathology, molecular biology, genetics and evidence-based treatments there are still many things that we do not understand. For instance what is the trigger that leads to the cascade of inflammation and then fibrosis of the joint? Why should it occur in late middle life, but not in the young, nor the old? Why should it be associated with diabetes and Dupuytren's contractures? Why do some respond well to treatment, but not others? There is a great need for on-going research into this condition.

Terminology

All agree that this is a condition that presents with pain and stiffness in the shoulder. The pain is unremitting true shoulder pain, excruciating when the shoulder is jerked, and severe enough to awaken the patient at night, and often many times at night. Stiffness gradually appears, after the onset of the pain, such that in the early stages before the stiffness has become apparent the condition can be confused with impingement, calcific tendonitis and rotator cuff tears. The stiffness causes global passive limitation to joint movement with a firm end-point to movement. Rotation might be stiffer than elevation, the key being external rotation less than 50 % of the unaffected side. The condition can be mimicked by calcific tendonitis, the late stages of cuff tearing and arthritis, but the radiographs are normal in frozen shoulder and abnormal in all the conditions that mimic it.

2009 was the 75th anniversary of the introduction by Codman of the term "frozen shoulder". Frozen shoulder is termed "adhesive capsulitis" in the United States of America, although it turns out to have no adhesive nor adhesions. The French call it "capsulite retractile", although, in fact, the capsule turns out to be contracted rather than retracted. The Germans call it "Steiffschulter", which is honest, but perhaps too basic, and the Japanese call it "fifty-year old shoulder". Over the last 20 years a large body of research has built up that allows us to understand and treat this common, enigmatic, protracted, painful and disabling condition. Perhaps it is now time to reflect on the progress that has been made over the last two decades into understanding and successfully treating this disease.

Prevalence

The condition is less common than the oft-quoted figure of 2 % of the population. This figure was arrived at 40 years ago when shoulder disease was ill-understood and frozen shoulder was used as a "dustbin diagnosis" for any stiff and painful shoulder. When Hazelman performed arthrograms of 36 patients diagnosed as frozen shoulder 40 years ago, eleven had complete tears of the rotator cuff. So of that study 30 % were proven misdiagnosed, and probably 50 % were actually overdiagnosed. Studies in the UK 30 years ago showed that only 50 % of patients referred as having frozen shoulder actually had visual/tactile evidence of the disease (50 % overdiagnosed), and studies from Canada 20 years ago showed that only 37 of 150 patients referred with the diagnosis of frozen shoulder actually had the proper diagnosis (76 % overdiagnosed). It is doubtful that primary care physicians and allied health professionals do any better today! The author's repeated studies on frozen shoulder (all verified by arthroscopy) show that it only accounts for 5 % of shoulder disease, and since shoulder disease affects, at most, 15 % of the population then it would be reasonable to suggest that the real incidence of capsular contracture is about 0.75 % of the population.

Frozen shoulder is said to be more common in females. A recent meta-analysis quotes 25 papers on frozen shoulder that studied 935 patients where 58 % were female. However most of the recent studies with arthroscopic control showed a ratio of 1;1 male to female, and it was the more historic papers that showed a higher preponderance of female patients.

Natural History

The disease follows a distinct course, starting with pain and night awakening. "Jerk pain" is never mentioned in the text-books, but if you enquire many patients will describe a jerk to the contracted shoulder bringing tears to the eyes. The painful phase merges into the stiffening phase. Finally there is a phase of resolution in all but 10 % of patients. The course of the disease is very variable, but follows a Gaussian distribution, some recovering quickly, some very slowly and 10 % very, very slowly, if ever.

Codman stated "*even the most protracted cases recover with or without treatment in about two years*". Once again this statement has been handed down from author to author without any questioning of the evidence. This has led to the commonly held and false view that this is a benign condition that resolves completely. Many eminent surgeons who have researched this disease have pleaded that complete resolution is not inevitable, but their pleas have fallen upon deaf ears. Simmonds stated "complete recovery is not my experience" and DePalma stated' it is erroneous to believe that in all instances restoration of function is attained'. Shaffer et al. [71] in the most detailed follow-up study in the literature found that at 7 years 50 % had mild pain, stiffness or both. They found that 60 % has measurable restriction of passive mobility and they concluded "this made us question whether this is a benign self-resolving condition". Griggs et al. confirmed these findings and stated that "even amongst the patients who were satisfied, a substantial number were not pain free"; 10 % had mild pain at rest, and 27 % had mild or moderate pain with activity. 40 % of the satisfied patients had abnormal shoulder function. Our own studies at 2–5 years showed that although 86 % had an improvement in their level of pain, this did not mean that they had no pain. Only 53 % had no pain, 33 % had an occasional pain and 14 % had marked residual pain. These findings have been confirmed by the largest ever study from Oxford on 273 patients followed for up to 20 years. Using the Oxford Shoulder Score they demonstrated that 41 % of their patients had mild to moderate persistent symptoms at 7 years and 6 % had severe ongoing symptoms with pain and functional loss.

Associations

Many other diseases have been linked to shoulder contracture, yet only two, diabetes and Dupuytren's disease withstand scientific scrutiny. A recent controlled study showed that 29 % of patients with a contracted shoulder had diabetes and that this was significantly elevated over the control population. This same study showed that the prevalence of thyroid disease in the patients with contracted shoulders was 13 %,

but this proved to be the same as the control group. Our own study of 100 arthroscopically-proven frozen shoulder patients has demonstrated a significantly higher incidence of diabetics (24 %) compared to an age- and sex-matched control group. Another recent study showed that the prevalence of diabetes in patients with frozen shoulder was 32.9 %. Care must be taken in interpreting studies of type I diabetics, for some studies look at young patients with an average age of 30, when frozen shoulder rarely presents until the magic age of 50. Even in the 30 year-old diabetics 10 % already had a contracted shoulder.

The link with Dupuytren's disease is robust. Meulengracht and Schwarz found evidence of Dupuytren's disease in 18 % of their patients with frozen shoulder. Schaer found that 25 % of their patients with frozen shoulder had Dupuytren's contracture. We studied a group of 56 patients with contracted shoulder and found evidence of Dupuytren's disease, often in a minor form such as pits and nodules, in 52 % of our patients. This "terrible triad" of contracted shoulder, Dupuytren's contracture and diabetes pervades this whole area of scientific enquiry.

Thyroid disease, high cholesterol and cardiac disease have been said to be associated with frozen shoulder but we found that the incidence was similar to an age- and sex-matched control group. This probably means that thyroid disease, high cholesterol and cardiac disease are found in 50 year-old people, but are not associated with frozen shoulder.

Symptoms and Signs

Codman was an extremely astute clinician, and a keen observer, so he was able to define this condition very precisely. He stated that these patients have 12 features in common. *"The condition comes on slowly; pain is felt near the insertion of deltoid; inability to sleep on the affected side; painful and incomplete elevation and external rotation; restriction of both spasmodic and adherent type; atrophy of the spinati; little local tenderness; X-rays negative except for*

Table 1 Codman's 12 criteria for frozen shoulder

1. The condition comes on slowly;
2. The pain is felt near the insertion of deltoid;
3. There is inability to sleep on the affected side;
4. There is painful and incomplete elevation
5. and external rotation;
6. There is restriction of both spasmodic
7. and adherent type;
8. There is atrophy of the spinati;
9. There is little local tenderness;
10. X-rays are negative except for bony atrophy;
11. The pain was very trying to every one of them;
12. But they were all able to continue their daily habits and routines.

bony atrophy; the pain was very trying to every one of them; but they were all able to continue their daily habits and routines." (Table 1).

Unfortunately, he did not go on to analyse each of these 12 symptoms and signs in detail, as he did when discussing the 18 features of rotator cuff tear, for, had he done so, he could well have solved the enigma forthwith.

One of the frustrations of frozen shoulder is that it shares many features with those far more common shoulder disorders, impingement, partial-thickness and full-thickness rotator cuff tears. In particular, its onset, the site of pain, awakening at night, restricted elevation and muscle spasm are all found in rotator cuff disease; although I would disagree with Codman about wasting, for this is rarely seen in frozen shoulder, whilst it is commonly seen in cuff disease. This has led to frozen shoulder being a diagnosis of exclusion. So, let us look critically at three aspects of Codman's definition, for they hold the key to the condition.

The Condition Comes on Slowly

This does not get us far, for there are many disorders of the shoulder such as impingement, which are far more common, and also come on slowly. Codman had noticed that "they usually give a story of slight trauma or overuse".

This association with minor trauma is well known to all Orthopaedic surgeons who, for instance, always caution patients with a Colles' fracture to keep the shoulder moving lest they develop a frozen shoulder. Surgery may be another initiating factor, for instance breast surgery, and it had been thought that it was the immobilization, which led to the development of the frozen shoulder, but you will see, as our story unravels, it is more likely the molecular response to the injury or surgery that is responsible.

Painful and Incomplete External Rotation

We now come to the first distinguishing feature of frozen shoulder, which is limitation of external rotation. There are only four shoulder conditions that restrict external rotation;

Arthritis, locked posterior dislocation, the late stage of a massive cuff tear and frozen shoulder. All of these have specific radiographic changes. Arthritis shows diminution of joint space, inferior osteophytes, sclerosis and occasional cysts; locked posterior dislocation shows a "light bulb sign" on the anteroposterior film and posterior dislocation on the axillary view; massive cuff tear shows upward subluxation of the head with a break in Shenton's line of the shoulder and irregularity of the greater tuberosity; whilst frozen shoulder shows an entirely normal radiographic appearance of the shoulder.

Limitation of the Spasmodic and Mildly Adherent Type

Terminology has changed and we would now state "limitation of active and passive movement". The key to the puzzle is the limitation of passive movement that, in the shoulder, can only be caused by two things: firstly, irregularity of the joint surface, as is found in arthritis and locked dislocation; and secondly, contracture of the ligaments that bind the humerus to the glenoid. Certainly, if you are going to be pedantic there are some rare muscular conditions, such as deltoid contracture (a handful of cases in the world literature), which also cause restricted passive movement, but in pragmatic terms, if the radiograph is normal and the joint shows passive restriction, then this can only be caused by contracture of the ligaments. The ligaments contract in the late stages of massive rotator cuff tears and in frozen shoulder. Therefore frozen shoulder is caused by contracture of the ligaments of the shoulder capsule. Indeed, as our story unfolds, you will see that this is, in fact, the case. So Codman actually had the solution within his grasp, and if only he had realized this and called the condition "Contracted shoulder", instead of frozen shoulder, three generations of Orthopaedic surgeons would have been spared from puzzling over this elusive condition.

Investigation

Radiology

Radiographs, as we have said, are normal in frozen shoulder. However the arthrogram is pathognomonic. Neviaser performed arthrograms on the shoulders of patients with frozen shoulder and showed that the capsule of the shoulder is contracted. The joint has a diminished volume, there is absent filling of the infraglenoid recess, and the subscapular recess and bicipital tunnel are obliterated in frozen shoulder. It is rare to do arthrograms these days unless as part of an MRA (MR arthrogram).

Magnetic resonance imaging (MRI) has not shed much further light on the condition. Emig et al. described thickening of the joint capsule and synovium in frozen shoulder. Tamai et al. 4 have described a technique of gadolinium-enhanced dynamic MRI, which has shown an increased blood flow to the synovium of the shoulder in frozen shoulder.

Ultrasound can show thickening of the coracohumeral ligament and increased blood flow on Doppler ultrasound. However the worst pathological changes occur under the coracoid process, and ultrasound can not see through bone.

Arthroscopy

There have now been numerous studies that have detailed the arthroscopic findings in frozen shoulder. In the early stages the major finding is angiogenesis, or new blood vessel formation (Fig. 1). This can be quite spectacular with fan- shaped areas of blood vessel formation, vascular fronts, petechial haemorrhages and even glomeruli. Within the infraglenoid recess the vessels line up in a radial fashion that we term the "lava flow". Granulation tissue that is red, highly vascular, with a villous or fronded appearance of the synovium occurs in the rotator interval area. Angiogenesis occurs on the adjacent glenoid labrum, as well as around the base of the long head of the biceps tendon. The granulation tissue may extend on to the top surface of the subscapularis tendon, and on to the anterior edge of the supraspinatus tendon. It is interesting that angiogenesis is a feature of diabetes for frozen shoulder is common in diabetics.

In the late stages the angiogenesis diminishes. The joint is less red, but thick bands of scar tissue can be found obliterating the normal structure of the capsule. The superior gleno-humeral ligament becomes thickened, obliterating the rotator interval. Scar can cover the top edge of subscapularis, and we term this the "involucrum". Occasionally long head of biceps can be scarred to the cuff. The middle gleno-humeral ligament is thickened, as indeed is the whole of the capsule.

The joint surface is usually normal. There are no intra-articular adhesions in this condition, a fact that has been documented in eight recent arthroscopic studies on frozen shoulder.

The joint volume is reduced, making insertion of the arthroscope and navigation around the contracted joint difficult. As was found arthrographically, the infraglenoid recess is contracted, and the synovium is moderately inflamed in this area as well.

Fig. 1 Angiogenesis seen arthroscopically in frozen shoulder

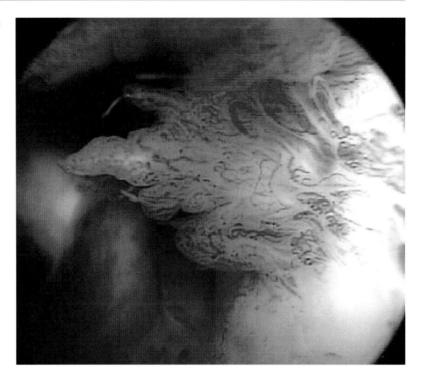

Blood Tests

The full blood count, white cell count and ESR are all normal in this condition. CRP may be elevated in the early stages. Calcium, phosphate, serum globulins and bone alkaline phosphatase are all normal. Cholesterol and triglycerides may be elevated in frozen shoulder but clearly this is not a specific test. However, what is interesting is that cholesterol and triglycerides may also be elevated in that other contractile disease, Dupuytren's contracture, one of many associations shared by these two contractile diseases.

Surgical Findings

Codman was probably the first to surgically explore the frozen shoulder. He stated, "I used to give ether and open the (subacromial) bursa. The appearance of the floor of the bursa was always the same - a congestion over the supraspinatus tendon on the base of the bursa like that of a bloodshot eye. Adhesions were often found. The congestion was in the synovia,

not in the tendon below it." He does not state whether he ever opened the shoulder joint itself. Neviaser reported on ten patients with frozen shoulder upon whom he had operated. He approached the shoulder using a deltopectoral approach, incising subscapularis vertically to give a good view of the capsule.

The capsule he found to be thickened, adherent to the humeral head and, when it was released, it was found to be under such tension that it sprung apart and could not be re-approximated. Although he never mentioned the word contracture, his description speaks for itself. Simmonds described the rotator cuff as "looking like a vascular, leathery hood with no obvious demarcation between the tendons." We now term the demarcation between the tendons the "rotator interval". The rotator interval is the triangle formed between supraspinatus and subscapularis, the base being the coracoid process. Normally, the capsule here is quite thin, being strengthened by the superior glenohumeral ligament, and also by the coracohumeral ligament, which runs from the base of the coracoid process to the biceps sulcus, the area between the lesser and greater tuberosities of the humerus. This, remember, is the area that appears so abnormal at arthroscopy, being obliterated with granulation tissue. DePalma stated that "The coracohumeral ligament is converted into a tough inelastic band of fibrous tissue spanning the interval between the coracoid process and the tuberosities of the humerus. It acts as a powerful checkrein ... division of the coracohumeral ligament allows early restoration of scapulohumeral movement". This is truly the most elegant description of a contracture of the coracohumeral ligament. DePalma was clearly a hairsbreadth away from resolving the enigma of frozen shoulder when he got distracted by the long head of biceps, and concluded that tethering of biceps was the cause of frozen shoulder.

Lundberg exposed the shoulder in 20 patients with frozen shoulder. He noted peri-articular inflammatory changes, especially at the insertion of the cuff on to the greater tuberosity. In six patients, he performed an arthrotomy and found thickening of the capsule and no intra-articular adhesions. Neer stated, "The senior author has found that in pathological conditions such as frozen shoulder, old fractures, or arthritis, the coracohumeral ligament may become shortened, and may have to be released at surgical reconstruction to restore external rotation."

Ozaki surgically explored 17 patients with recalcitrant chronic frozen shoulder and stated, "At operation, the major cause of the restricted glenohumeral movement was found to be contracture of the coracohumeral ligament and rotator interval. Release of the contracted structures relieved pain and restored motion of the shoulder in all patients."

In a consecutive series of 25 patients with severe frozen shoulder, which had failed to resolve with manipulation, we found a consistent abnormality of the coracohumeral ligament and rotator interval area. This area of the capsule was abnormal, thickened and vascular. There seems to be new vessel formation (much like Codman's bloodshot eye). The thickening prevented easy determination of the edges of the rotator interval (Simmonds, no obvious demarcation). When the shoulder was forced into external rotation the contracted coracohumeral ligament became taught and stood out as a palpable thickening (DePalma's checkrein), often as thick as the surgeon's little finger. When the tissue was incised it bled, often forcefully, and was found to be very adherent (Neviaser's adherence) to the underlying long head of biceps, and the incision was accompanied by release of the passive restraint to glenohumeral external rotation (as stated by Neer and Ozaki). Surgical release gave us the ability to inspect the tissue histologically.

Pathology of Frozen Shoulder

In 1995 we examined the tissue excised from the rotator interval area of twelve consecutive patients with severe frozen shoulder. Macroscopically, the tissue was an inextensible nodular fleshy band. Histological examination of the tissue showed a background matrix of dense collagen, arranged in nodules and laminae (Fig. 2). The cell population was moderate to high.

The samples were prepared for immunocytochemistry to demonstrate precisely what type of cell was present. This staining showed that the cells were fibroblasts (Fig. 3), with some transformation to the contractile fibroblast that has been termed the "myofibroblast". The samples showed that the tissue was particularly vascular. As for inflammatory cells, none was present within the thick collagen of the contracture itself, but some were present both in the synovium and around blood vessels. Such an appearance, of a dense collagen matrix, populated by fibroblasts and myofibroblasts, can be found in healing scar tissue and in contracture. This appearance is very similar to the palmar contracture of Dupuytren's disease.

Historically Neviaser examined his tissue microscopically and found considerable or extensive fibrosis in 6 of 10 cases. Simmonds reported dense collagen fibres, increased vascularity and the presence of fibroblasts. DePalma found fibrosis, increased vascularity, thickening of the synovial membrane and cellular infiltration. Despite the evidence of fibrosis, all three authors concluded that the changes represented low-grade inflammation.

Fig. 2 Pathology shows
bands and nodules of
type III collagen

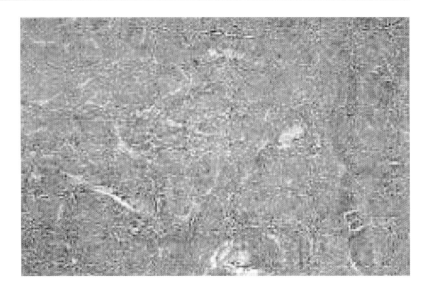

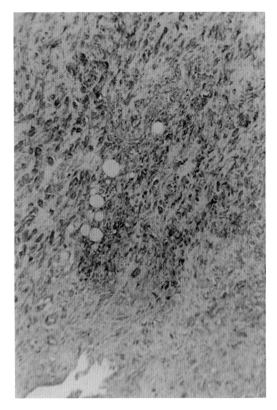

Fig. 3 Vimentin stains for fibroblasts

appearance of this contracture with palmar contracture, although he attributed the idea to his pathologist Norden. Kay and Slater also noted the resemblance between the histology of shoulder joint capsule in frozen shoulder and the palmar contracture of Dupuytren. Ozaki noted fibrosis in their tissue, and Hannifin et al. found diffuse capsular fibroplasia, thickening and contracture.

In the modern era, further to our immunocytochemical studies, Killian's group have confirmed the presence of fibroblasts laying down collagen within the capsule. They performed electron microscopic studies showing that the collagen structure was grossly abnormal with thickened fibrils in the frozen shoulder group. Carr's group from Oxford confirmed the presence of fibroblasts laying down collagen. Like us they found some inflammatory cells, but they have also shown the presence of mast cells and postulate that these cells may be modulating some inflammatory process that triggers the fibroblastic response.

The Basic Science of Healing and Contracture

Lundberg reported a compact, dense capsule with an increase of cells that were fibroblasts; he was the first to mention the similarity of the

The healing process is divided into three phases: an early inflammatory phase; a repair phase with the formation of granulation tissue; and finally scar formation, maturation and contracture.

Contracture may be physiological, when the healing wound contracts to pull the wound edges into apposition, or it may be pathological, where there is an imbalance between scar formation and remodelling, resulting in abnormal scarring and contracture. It is the late stages of healing, the formation of granulation tissue, scar formation, contracture and remodelling that hold the key to understanding the molecular biology of frozen shoulder.

Fibroblasts are controlled by certain cytokines. Cytokines are peptide molecules that act as cell messengers. They control many aspects of cell migration and growth, acting in minute concentrations by binding to receptors on the target cell. Cytokines regulate fibroblast chemotaxis, fibroblast proliferation and collagen synthesis.

Because the fibroblast appears to be the key cell in frozen shoulder, we elected to measure cytokine and growth factor levels in 17 consecutive patients with severe frozen shoulder? The reverse transcription polymerase chain reaction (PCR) method was used to measure the levels of cytokines and growth factors in tissue biopsied from these patients with frozen shoulder. The tissue showed an over-expression of a number of cell-signalling molecules. The intensity of signal for the fibrogenic growth factors such as transforming growth factor (TGF) beta, platelet-derived growth factor (PDGF) alpha, and fibroblast growth factor (FGF) was elevated and was higher than the pro-inflammatory cytokines such as interleukin 1 and tumour necrosis factor (TNF), although there was a high level of interleukin 6. This work has been elegantly confirmed by Colville's group who took joint fluid from patients with capsular contracture and found that this tissue caused a 5000 % increase in in-vitro fibroblast proliferation compared with control groups. These elevated cytokine levels in frozen shoulder have also been demonstrated by Rodeo, Hannafin and Warren using monoclonal antibody techniques. They found TGF-beta and PDGF to be elevated, and suggested that these cytokines may act as a persistent stimulus causing capsular fibrosis and the development of frozen shoulder.

Hamada, in Japan, has found increased levels of vascular endothelial growth factor (VEGF) in stiff shoulders that may account for the angiogenesis that is seen at arthroscopy. Ryu et al. demonstrated strong expression of VEGF and angiogenesis in diabetic frozen shoulders. Killian et al. showed an increase in alpha-1(I) mRNA transcription in both frozen shoulder and Dupuytren's contracture. Since Insulin-like growth factor is known to stimulate fibrosis in connective tissue they measured the serum IGF-1 and IGF-1 receptor levels but found them to be similar in contracted shoulder and control capsule.

Patients with palmar contracture also have elevated levels of cytokines and growth factors, which, although not identical to those changes found in frozen shoulder, show a higher intensity for the fibrogenic growth factors than the inflammatory ones.

Of course, when we look at the development of contractures, we have to examine not only the factors that may act as a persistent stimulus to scar formation, but we must also look at the opposite side of the equation, the failure of remodelling. The remodeling of the extracellular collagen matrix is undertaken by a family of enzymes that used to be called collagenases, but now go by the glorious name of the matrix metalloproteinases (MMPs). MMPs share five basic attributes: they degrade the extracellular matrix, they contain zinc, they are secreted in a latent pro-form, they are inhibited by tissue inhibitors (TIMPs), and they share common amino-acid sequences.

We decided to examine the levels of MMPs and TIMPs in frozen shoulder, once again using the reverse transcription PCR technique. We found a strong expression of MMPs in frozen-shoulder tissue, particularly MMP2. However, we found an even greater expression of their natural inhibitor TIMP

This leads us to speculate as to whether there may not be a failure to remodel in frozen shoulder due to persistent high levels of T1MP.

A broad-spectrum TIMP has been synthesized (Marimastat®, British Biotech Ltd, Oxford, UK) and a remarkable study has been carried out with it. Twelve patients with inoperable gastric carcinoma were enrolled into a study to see whether TIMP could slow down the progression of their disease by inhibiting MMPs (which are found to be elevated in gastric carcinoma), thereby preventing the dissemination of the tumour through the extracellular matrix and naturally encasing the tumour in scar tissue. Of the 12 patients treated, six developed bilateral frozen shoulder within 4 months of starting treatment and three also developed palmar contractures. This remarkable in-vivo experiment would appear to confirm our thoughts on the role of TIMP in the formation of frozen shoulder. There have been a number of case reports of shoulder contracture occurring during treatment of HIV-positive patients on protease inhibitors such as Indinavir.

The Cytogenetics of Frozen Shoulder

Clonal chromosomal abnormalities have been discovered in a variety of contractile diseases. In particular trisomy 7 and 8 have been found in Dupuytren's disease, and multiple clonal chromosomal abnormalities in Peyronie's disease. We therefore elected to see if there were any clonal chromosomal abnormalities in frozen shoulder. We took capsular tissue from ten consecutive patients with frozen shoulder, cultured the cells in tissue culture and then performed metaphase arrest, and performed in-situ G banding to look for abnormal karyotypes. To our surprise, we found clonal chromosomal abnormalities in frozen shoulder. These abnormalities were trisomy of chromosomes 7 and 8.

A twin study examining 865 pairs of heterozygous and 963 pairs of homozygous twins estimated a heritability of 42 % for frozen shoulder and stated that genetic factors are implicated in the aetiology of frozen shoulder.

Our own study of 100 arthroscopically-proven frozen shoulder patients revealed that 16 % of patients with a sibling, had at least one sibling who had suffered from frozen shoulder and was significantly higher than that of a sex- and age-matched control group.

So where does all this science take us? We can now say that the symptoms and signs of frozen shoulder make us postulate that this is a contractile disease. This is confirmed by arthrography, by MRI, by arthroscopy, by its associations with palmar contracture, by surgical exploration, by histology, and by immunocytochemistry. In frozen shoulder, fibrogenic growth factors are dominant, remodelling is prevented by high levels of TIMP, and treating cancer sufferers with TIMP causes both frozen shoulder and palmar contracture. Finally, both frozen shoulder and palmar contracture demonstrate clonal chromosomal abnormalities with duplication of the same chromosomes.

Treatment of Frozen Shoulder

Do patients want to be treated? They certainly do. The pain of capsular contracture (frozen shoulder) is severe, night pain is worse, night awakening is universal, sleep deprivation is constant, and these symptoms persist for months and months on end. Many doctors say that there is no point treating frozen shoulder for it gets better in 18 months to 2 years. This is patronizing in the extreme. How would you react to a being told that your severe pain and night awakening was not worth treating for it would get better in 2 years? This is akin to a woman in labour being told that there was no need for pain relief because the pain would go once the baby was delivered!

What do patients desire of treatment? They want the pain to disappear. They want the pain to go NOW. If not now they want the pain to go AS SOON AS POSSIBLE. They want to be able to sleep. They want to be able to sleep tonight, and it would be a bonus if their movement could return, at least to a functional level.

Finally, do we have a treatment that can deliver immediate and long-lasting freedom from pain, return of a normal sleep pattern, and a functional range of movement? The short answer is yes, not for everyone, not always immediately, but for the majority arthroscopic release can deliver this package. Before discussing arthroscopic release we should examine the evidence behind other forms of treatment.

Steroid Therapy

Steroids have been shown in four randomised prospective controlled studies to have no benefit over home exercises. However all four papers can be severely criticised as they studied painful stiff shoulders, in other words primary and secondary frozen shoulder so many of the patients would have had other shoulder disease. One of these papers included arthrograms of the study group and 11 of 36 had cuff tears, yet were kept in the study! This is a recurring criticism of so many papers on capsular contracture; the diagnosis is wrong. A recent randomised double-blind study of a 3-week course of oral Prednisolone showed no significant difference between the active and placebo arms of the study at 6 weeks and 3 months.

Physiotharapy

The best paper on physiotherapy is that of Diercks et al. that showed that intensive physiotherapy prolonged the natural history of the disease from 15 months to 24 months and achieved a lower Constant Score of 76 compared to 87 in the control group who did home exercises. Once again we must stress that what the patients want is not for their disease to be prolonged from 15 to 24 months, but for it to end TODAY.

Manipulation Under Anaesthetic

Manipulation under anaesthetic has been used historically by many Orthopaedic surgeons, and is still used by some today. However, it has had a chequered career. Professor Sir John Charnley, before he became famous for his hip replacement, was intrigued by frozen shoulder. He published a paper on his personal results of manipulation of frozen shoulders in 1959. Before performing the study, he sent a questionnaire to his colleagues in the British Orthopaedic Association, asking for their views on manipulation of frozen shoulder. Seventy per cent said they would never perform a manipulation, as all would eventually get better, and some could be harmed. Lesser men would have been put off by such a reply, but not Charnley. In a consecutive series of 35 patients he found that he did no harm, pain was eased by manipulation, and, however long the duration of the disease, most were free of symptoms by 10 weeks.

Andersen, Sjobjerg and Sneppen have shown that 79 % of patients with frozen shoulder are relieved of their pain, and 75 % regain a near normal range of movement after manipulation. We have arthroscoped patients before and after manipulation to discover exactly what is happening. Essentially, what we found was that elevation, or abduction, tears the capsule from the neck of the humerus, releasing the inferior capsule, and this occurs with relative ease. It is much harder to free rotation, but forced external rotation tears the coracohumeral ligament. This is an extra-articular ligament, so what is seen arthroscopically is haemorrhage in the rotator interval. Often, the coracohumeral ligament is so contracted that it will not tear and the patient is left with limitation of external rotation. Loew has shown that manipulation is not without complications.

Arthroscopic Release

Arthroscopic release, in the hands of the expert shoulder surgeon, has transformed the management of capsular contracture (Fig. 4). Many of the studies can be criticised for purporting to show the results of treating capsular contracture when the index group was actually made up of any stiff shoulder including fractures, cuff disease and post-surgical stiff shoulders and then pooling the results. For instance one paper started with 1720 stiff shoulders of which only 11 had an arthroscopic release for primary adhesive capsulitis. Four articles are worthy of study. Ogilvie-Harris et al. [57] compared the results of manipulation versus arthroscopic release. Although both groups gained the same substantial

Fig. 4 Arthroscopic
release of frozen shoulder

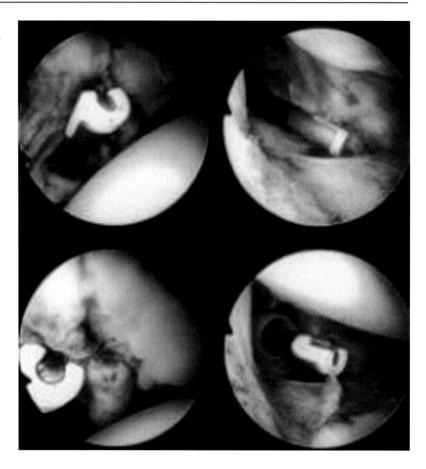

improvement in range of motion the arthroscopic group had significantly better pain relief and function, to the extent that twice as many were graded excellent. The following year J.P. Warner [80] showed a 49° increase in elevation, 42° increase in external rotation and improvement in Constant Scores from 13 to 77/100. Harryman and Matsen published a year later [39] and demonstrated fantastic results. The range of motion went from 41 % of the opposite side to 78 % *on the first postoperative day* and 93 % at the end of the study. Before surgery 6 % could sleep and after 73 %. They were the first to show the dramatic speed of recovery following treatment, which is the very thing that patients want. Berghs et al. [4] confirmed this with a dramatic improvement on day one post- surgery in 36 % and 88 % improvement within 2 weeks. Pain improved from 3.6/15 to 12.6/15 and the partial Constant

Scores from 20/75 to 62/75. There were no complications in three of these studies, but one transient axillary neurapraxia in the Harryman study. Arthroscopic release appears to show great promise for it delivers what the patient wants; relief of pain, undisturbed nights and improved function TODAY, or if not today THIS WEEK, in the majority of people, with minimally invasive, keyhole day-case surgery.

However it is not a panacea, for it appears that 10 % of patients fail to improve whatever treatment is used. This group can be predicted to a certain extent. Those who fall into this worse group are men, diabetics, those with marked Dupuytren's disease, bilateral disease, severe contractures and those with failed previous treatment.

Arthroscopic release gives a good improvement in forward elevation, and external rotation, but internal rotation can be disappointing.

Several authors have seen whether this can be improved by posterior release but Snow and Funk showed no significant difference in range of motion with the addition of a posterior release. Against this Pouliart and Gagey have described variations in the superior capsule-ligamentous complex, and explain that the ramifications of this limits internal rotation reach in contracture, and that the release needs to be extended postero-superiorly.

We have recently published our results from arthroscopic capsular release in over 100 patients, by far the largest series in the world literature to date. 98 % of patients would recommend the surgery to a friend in a similar situation. The mean post-operative Oxford shoulder score was 41 with an average improvement of 24 points. 70 % had regained full forward flexion, but only 45 % had achieved full external rotation. The mean time for pain relief was 16 days, although 10 % of patients felt their pain had never been resolved. All but 11 % could now sleep through the night and took on average 12 days to achieve this. 16 % of patients complained that the stiffness returned after an initial period of success. Only one complication was encountered, a superficial wound infection.

Summary

Frozen shoulder is a contracture of the shoulder joint capsule. Although the disease causes a global contracture of the shoulder joint, it appears maximal in the rotator interval area, and particularly around the coracohumeral ligament. The contracture can be visualized by arthrography and arthroscopy, and the capsule is seen to be thickened and vascular on MRI. Surgical exploration confirms the capsular contracture, and the fact that it is maximal around the coracohumeral ligament.

Histology shows that this contracture is made of a dense collagen matrix, which shows a high degree of cellularity, and the cells are fibroblasts and myofibroblasts. Fibroblasts are under the control of fibrogenic cytokines and growth factors, which are found to be elevated in patients with frozen shoulder. Remodelling may be slow in frozen shoulder due to high levels of TIMP. In an unusual study, frozen shoulder has been shown to be produced by administering TIMP to humans. Arthroscopic release now gives an effective, rapidly-working, day-case minimally-invasive treatment for this condition. Understanding the nature of frozen shoulder allows us to apply effective treatments to the condition, and opens the doors to the possibility of manipulating the course of the disease, so that patients who develop this common, disabling, painful and protracted condition may, in the future, enjoy effective early resolution of their disease.

References

1. Andersen NH, Sojbjerg JO, Johannsen HV, Sneppen O. Frozen shoulder: arthroscopy and manipulation under general anesthesia and early passive motion. J Shoulder Elbow Surg. 1998;7(3):218–22.
2. Aslan S, Celiker R. Comparison of the efficacy of local corticosteroid injection and physiotherapy for the treatment of adhesive capsulitis. Rheumatol Int. 2001;21(1):20–3.
3. Beaufils P, Prevot T, Boyer N, et al. Arthroscopic release of the glenohumeral joint in shoulder stiffness: a review of 26 cases. French Society for Arthroscopy. Arthroscopy. 1999;15:49–55.
4. Berghs BM, Sole-Molins X, Bunker TD. Arthroscopic release of adhesive capsulitis. J Shoulder Elbow Surg. 2004;13(2):180–5.
5. Buckbinder R, et al. Short course prednisolone for adhesive capsulitis. Ann Rheum Dis. 2004;63(11):1460–9.
6. Bulgen D, Binder A, Hazelman B, Park J. Immunological studies in frozen shoulder. J Rheumatol. 1982;9:893–8.
7. Bunker TD. Time for a new name for frozen shoulder. British Med J. 1985;290:1233–1234.
8. Bunker TD. Frozen shoulder; unravelling the enigma. Annals R College Surg Engl. 1997;79:210–213.
9. Bunker TD, Anthony PP. The pathology of frozen shoulder. J Bone Joint Surg. 1995;77B:677–83.
10. Bunker TD, Reilly J, Baird K, Hamblen DL. Expression of growth factors, cytokines and matrix metalloproteinases in frozen shoulder. J Bone Joint Surg (B). 2000;82-B:768–73.
11. Bunker TD, Esler CNA. Frozen shoulder and lipids. J Bone Joint Surg. 1995;77B:684–6.
12. Bunker TD, Lagae K, DeFerm A. Arthroscopy and manipulation in frozen shoulder. J Bone Joint Surg. 1994;76(B)(Supp 1):53.

13. Bunker TD. Frozen Shoulder. In: Norris T, editor. Orthopaedic knowledge update: shoulder and elbow. IL: American Academy Orthopaedic Surgery; 1997.

14. Bunker TD. Frozen Shoulder. In: Bunker TD, Schranz PJ, editors. Clinical challenges in orthopaedic; the shoulder. Oxford: Isis; 1998.

15. Callinan N, McPherson S, Cleaveland S. Effectiveness of hydroplasty and therapeutic exercise for treatment of frozen shoulder. J Hand Ther. 2003;16(3):219–24.

16. Carrette S, Moffet H, Tardif J, et al. Intraarticular corticosteroids in the treatment of adhesive capsulitis: a placebo controlled trial. Arthritis Rheum. 2003;48(3):829–38.

17. Castelleran G, Ricci M, Vedovi E, et al. Manipulation and arthroscopy under general anaesthesia and early rehabilitative treatment for frozen shoulders. Arch Phys Med Rehabil. 2004;85(8):1236–40.

18. Chambler AF, Carr A. The role of surgery in frozen shoulder. J Bone Joint Surg Br. 2003; 85(6):789–95.

19. Codman EA, editor. Tendinitis of the short rotators. In: Ruptures of the supraspinatus tendon and other lesions in or about the subacromial bursa. Boston: Thomas Todd; 1934. p. 216–24.

20. Colville J. Analysis of FGF in joint fluid from patients with frozen shoulder. Annual Meeting BESS, Newport; 2004.

21. DeGreef I, Steeno P, DeSmet L. Summary of risk factors in females with Dupuytren's disease. Acta Orthop Belgl; 2008.

22. DePalma AF. Loss of scapulohumeral motion (frozen shoulder). Annals of Surg. 1952;135(2): 194–204.

23. DePonti A, Vigano M, Taverna E, Sansone V. Adhesive capsulitis of the shoulder in HIV positive patients. J Shoulder Elbow Surg. 2006;15(2):188–90.

24. Diwan DB, Murrell GA. An evaluation of the effects of the extent of capsular release. Arthroscopy. 2005;21(9):1105–13.

25. Dodenhoff RM, Levy O, Wilson A, Copeland SA. Manipulation under anaesthesia for primary treatment of frozen shoulder. J Shoulder Elbow Surg. 2000;9:23–6.

26. Edwards T, Carr A, Pathology of frozen shoulder. In: Annual scientific meeting SECEC 2005, Rome.

27. Emig EW, Schweizer ME, Karasick D, Lubowitz J. Adhesive capsulitis of the shoulder: MRI diagnosis. Am J Radiol. 1995;164:1457–9.

28. Esch JC. Arthroscopic treatment of resistant primary frozen shoulder (abstract). J Shoulder Elbow Surg. 1994;3:S71.

29. Feldman A, Bunker TD, Delmege D. Clonal chromosomal abnormalities in frozen shoulder. Shoulder and Elbow; 2009. Submitted.

30. Gam AN, Schydlowski P, Rossel P, et al. Treatment of frozen shoulder with distension. Scand J Rheumatol. 1998;27(6):425–30.

31. Gerber C, Espinosa N, Perren TG. Arthroscopic treatment of shoulder stiffness. Clin Orthop. 2001;390:119–28.

32. Griggs S, Ahn A, Green A. Idiopathic adhesive capsulitis. A prospective functional outcome study of nonoperative treatment. J Bone Joint Surg Am. 2000;82-A(10):1398–407.

33. Hakim A, Cherkas L, Spector T, Macgregor A. Twin studies of frozen shoulder. Rheumatology. 2003;42(6):739–42.

34. Handa A, Goto M, Hamada K. Vascular endothelial growth factor 121 and 165 in the subacromial bursa are involved in shoulder joint contracture in type II diabetics with rotator cuff disease. J Orthop Res. 2003;21(6):1138–44.

35. Hand CA. Long term follow up of outcome of patients with frozen shoulder. In: Annual Scientific meeting BESS, Cambridge 2005.

36. Hand C, Clipsman K, Rees J, Carr A. The long term outcome of frozen shoulder. J Shoulder Elbow Surg. 2008;17(2):231–6.

37. Hand C, Athanason N, Matthews T, Carr A. Pathology of frozen shoulder. J Bone Joint Surg. 2007; 89(B):928–32.

38. Hannafin JA, DiCarlo EF, Wickiewicz TL. Adhesive capsulitis: capsular fibroplasia of the shoulder joint. J Shoulder Elbow Surg. 1994;3(1):S5.

39. Harryman II DT, Matsen III FA, Sidles JA. Arthroscopic management of refractory shoulder stiffness. Arthroscopy. 1997;13:133–47.

40. Holloway GB, Schenk T, Williams GR, Ramsey ML, Iannotti JP. Arthroscopic capsular release for the treatment of refractory postoperative or post-fracture shoulder stiffness. J Bone Joint Surg Am. 2001;83:1682–7.

41. Hsu SY, Chan KM. Arthroscopic distension in the management of frozen shoulder. Int Orthop. 1991;15:79–83.

42. Hutchinson JW, Tierny JM, Parsons SL, Davies TR. Dupuytren's disease and frozen shoulder induced by treatment with a matrix metalloproteinase inhibitor. J Bone Joint Surg. 1998;80(B):907–8.

43. Jacobs L, Barton M, Wallace W, et al. Intra-articular distension and steroids in the management of capsulitis of the shoulder. BMJ. 1991;302:1498–501.

44. Janda DH, Hawkins RJ. Shoulder manipulation in patients with adhesive capsulitis and diabetes mellitus. J Shoulder Elbow Surg. 1993;2:36–8.

45. Jerosch J. 360 degrees arthroscopic capsular release in patients with adhesive capsulitis of the glenohumeral joint – indication, surgical technique, results. Knee Surg Sports Traumatol Arthrosc. 2001;9:178–86.

46. Jerosch J, Filler TJ, Peuker ET. Which joint position puts the axillary nerve at lowest risk when performing ACR in patients with adhesive capsulitis? Knee Surg Sports Traumatol Arthrosc. 2002;10(2):126–9.

47. Killian O, Kriegsman J, Berghauser K, et al. Die frozen shoulder. Der Chirurg. 2001;72:1303–08.

48. Killian O, Pfeil U, Wenisch S, et al. Enhanced alpha-1 mRNA expression in frozen shoulder and Dupuytren's disease. Eur J Med Res. 2007;12(12):585–90.

49. Klinger HM, Otte S, Baums MH, Haerer T. Early arthroscopic release in refractory shoulder stiffness. Arch Orthop trauma Surg. 2002;122(4):200–3.

50. Loew M, Heichel TO, Lehner B. Intraarticular lesions in primary frozen shoulder after manipulation under general anaesthetia. J Shoulder Elbow Surg. 2005;14(1):16–21.

51. Lundberg BJ. The frozen shoulder. Acta Orthop Scand. 1969;119:1–59.

52. Massoud SN, Pearse EO, Levy O. Operative management of the frozen shoulder in patients with diabetes. J Shoulder Elbow Surg. 2002;11(6):609.

53. Milgrom C, Novack V, Weil Y, Jaber S. Risk factors for idiopathic frozen shoulder. Isr Med Assoc J. 2008;10(5):591–5.

54. Neviaser JS. Adhesive capsulitis of the shoulder. J Bone Joint Surg. 1945;27:211–21.

55. Nicholson GP. Arthroscopic capsular release for stiff shoulders: effect of etiology on outcomes. Arthroscopy. 2003;19(1):40–9.

56. Ogilvie-Harris D, Myerthall S. The diabetic frozen shoulder: arthroscopic release. Arthroscopy. 1997;13:1–8.

57. Ogilvie-Harris D, Biggs D, Fitsialos D, Mackay M. The resistant frozen shoulder. Clin Orthop Relat Res. 1995;319:238–48.

58. Ogilvie Harris DJ. The present state of shoulder arthroscopy. In: Bunker TD, Schranz PJ, editors. Clinical challenges in orthopaedic; the shoulder. Oxford: Isis; 1998.

59. Omari A, Bunker TD. Open surgical release for frozen shoulder: surgical findings and results of the release. J Shoulder Elbow Surg. 2001;10:353–7.

60. Ozaki J, Nakagawa Y, Sakurai G, Tamai S. Recalcitrant chronic adhesive capsulitis of the shoulder. Role of contracture of the coracohumeral ligament and rotator interval in pathogenesis and treatment. J Bone Joint Surg Am. 1989;71:1511–5.

61. Pearsall AW, Holovacs TF, Speer KP. The intraarticular component of the subscapularis tendon: anatomic and histological correlation in reference to surgical release in patients with frozen-shoulder syndrome. Arthroscopy. 2000;16:236–42.

62. Pearsall AW, Osbahr DC, Speer KP. An arthroscopic technique for treating patients with frozen shoulder. Arthroscopy. 1999;15:2–11.

63. Piotte F, Gravel D, Moffet H, et al. Effects of repeated distension arthrographies in idiopathic adhesive capsulitis. Am J Phys Med Rehabil. 2004;83(7):537–46.

64. Pollock RG, Duralde XA, Flatow EL, Bigliani LU. The use of artroscopy in the treatment of resistant frozen shoulder. Clin Orthop. 1994;304:30–36.

65. Pouliart N, Somers K, Gagey O. Variations in the superior capsuloligamentous complex. J Shoulder Elbow Surg. 2007;16(6):821–36.

66. Price MR, Tillett ED, Acland RD, Nettleton GS. Determining the relationship of the axillary nerve to the shoulder joint capsule from an arthroscopic perspective. J Bone Joint Surg Am. 2004;86A (10):2135–42.

67. Rodeo S, Hannafin J, Tom J, Warren R, Wieckicz T. Immunolocalisation of cytokines and their receptors in frozen shoulder. J Orthop Res. 1997;15:427–36.

68. Ryans I, Montgomery A, Galway R, et al. A randomized controlled trial of intraarticular triamcinalone in shoulder capsulitis. Rheumatology. 2005;44(4):529–35.

69. Ryu J, et al. Expression of VEGF and angiogenesis in diabetic frozen shoulders. J Shoulder Elbow Surg. 2006;15(6):676–85.

70. Segmuller HE, Taylor DE, Hogan CS, Saies AD, Hayes MG. Arthroscopic treatment of adhesive capsulitis. J Shoulder Elbow Surg. 1995;4:403–8.

71. Shaffer B, Tibone JE, Kerlan RK. Frozen shoulder. A long-term follow-up. J Bone Joint Surg Am. 1992;74:738–46.

72. Simmonds FA. Shoulder pain. With particular reference to the "frozen" shoulder. J Bone Joint Surg Br. 1949;31:426–32.

73. Smith CD, Bunker TD. Patient reported outcome and speed of recovery after arthroscopic capsular release for insidious onset frozen shoulder. (Submitted to JSES)

74. Smith CD, Bunker TD. The associations of frozen shoulder; myths or reality? (Submitted to JSES)

75. Smith SP, Deveraj VS, Bunker TD. The association between frozen shoulder and Dupuytren's disease. J Shoulder Elbow Surg. 2001;10:149–51.

76. Snow M, Boutros I, Funk L. Posterior arthroscopic capsular release in frozen shoulder. Arthroscopy. 2009;25(1):19–23.

77. Tamai K, Yamato M. Abnormal synovium in frozen shoulder: a preliminary report with dynamic magnetic resonance imaging. J Shoulder Elbow Surgery. 1997;6:534–43.

78. Uitvligt G, Detrisac DA, Johnson LL, Austin MD, Johnson C. Arthroscopic observations before and after manipulation of frozen shoulder. Arthroscopy. 1993;9(2):181–185.

79. Vad VB, Sakalkae D, Warren RF. The role of capsular distension in adhesive capsulitis. Arch Phys Med Rehabil. 2005;84(9):1290–2.

80. Warner JJP, Allen A, Marks PH, Wong P. Arthroscopic release for chronic, refractory adhesive capsulitis of the shoulder. J Bone Joint Surg Am. 1996;78:1808–16.

81. Warner JJP. Frozen shoulder: diagnosis and management. J Am Acad Orthop Surg. 1997;5(3):130–40.

82. Wiley AM. Arthroscopic appearance of frozen shoulder. Arthroscopy. 1991;7:138–43.

83. Zanotti RM, Kuhn JE. Arthroscopic capsular release for the stiff shoulder. Description of technique and anatomic considerations. Am J Sports Med. 1997;25(3):294–8.

Shoulder Arthrodesis

Jean-Luc Jouve, Gerard Bollini, R. Legre,
C. Guardia, E. Choufani, J. Demakakos, and B. Blondel

Contents

J.-L. Jouve (✉) • G. Bollini • C. Guardia • E. Choufani
Orthopedic Pediatric Department, Timone Children
Hospital, Marseille, France
e-mail: jean-luc.jouve@ap-hm.fr;
gerard.bollini@ap-hm.fr

R. Legre
Plastic and Reconstructive Surgery Department,
Conception Hospital, Marseille, France

J. Demakakos
Hospital for Joint Diseases, New York University,
New York, NY, USA

B. Blondel
Orthopedic Pediatric Department, Timone Children
Hospital, Marseille, France

Hospital for Joint Diseases, New York University,
New York, NY, USA

G. Bentley (ed.), *European Surgical Orthopaedics and Traumatology*,
DOI 10.1007/978-3-642-34746-7_234, © EFORT 2014

Abstract

In recent years, surgical indications for performing a shoulder arthrodesis have continuously decreased. Nowadays, such a procedure is reserved to specific pathological conditions like severe sequelae from brachial plexus palsy by Chammas et al. (J Bone Joint Surg Br 86(5):692–695, 2004), repeated failures after shoulder arthroplasty by Scalise et al. (J Bone Joint Surg Am 91(Suppl 2 Pt 1):30–7, 2009), high energy trauma with complex fractures or more frequently, malignant tumor of the humeral upper extremity by Viehweger et al. (Rev Chir Orthop Reparatrice Appar Mot 91(6):523–9, 2005).

The main difficulty in shoulder arthrodesis is to obtain the best position for fusion in order to achieve the best functional outcome. While surfaces for fusion between the upper humeral extremity and the scapula are limited, a rigorous arthrodesis technique is necessary, especially when using a free vascularized transplant. In most of the cases, internal osteosynthesis will be necessary and pre-bent custom-made plates can therefore be very useful. Such devices will use the supraspinous fossa as the upper fixation and will give adequate angulation for management of fusion position in the coronal and sagittal planes however, control of the rotation remains the trickiest aspect of the procedure [Rühmann et al. (Orthopade 33(9):1061–80, 2004); Safran et al. (J Am Acad Orthop Surg 14(3):145–53, 2006)].

When following a strict and appropriate technique, shoulder arthrodesis leads to satisfactory functional outcomes in complex reconstruction procedures. This is particularly useful in situations where the rotator cuff and deltoid are inefficient, resulting in unsatisfactory outcomes of shoulder arthroplasty in these cases [Clare et al. (J Bone Joint Surg Am A(4):593–600, 2001; Cofield et al. (J Bone Joint Surg Am 61(5):668–77, 1979].

Keywords

Arthrodesis • Bone tumour • Brachial palsy • Shoulder

General Introduction

Shoulder arthrodesis or gleno-humeral arthrodesis is a demanding surgery with decreasing indications according to outcomes achieved with shoulder arthroplasty. However, it remains a must-know technique in various salvage situations such as tumoral resection. Functional outcomes will depend on the quality and the positioning of the gleno-humeral fusion.

Aetiology and Classification

Gleno-humeral arthrodesis consists in a surgical bony fusion between the upper extremity of humeral bone and the scapula.

Relevant Applied Anatomy, Biomechanics

Two conditions must be taken into account: arthrodesis positioning and quality of the fusion [10, 11].

Arthrodesis Positioning

After fusion, residual mobility will occur in the scapulo-thoracic joint. Therefore, arthrodesis positioning must be planned in three dimensions:
- In the coronal plane, abduction must be fixed in order to allow the best range of motion for the patient and preserving the possibility to stay in anatomical position. The most common accepted position is abduction around 30° to the vertical but, such angle is very difficult to evaluate during the surgical procedure. According to our experience, it is easier to take into account the angle between the lateral side of the scapula and the humeral diaphysis in the coronal plane (Fig. 1). The value of this angle is around 60° and attention must be paid not to increase this angle in order to avoid pain during adduction movement by tensioning of the superior fibers of the trapezius muscle.

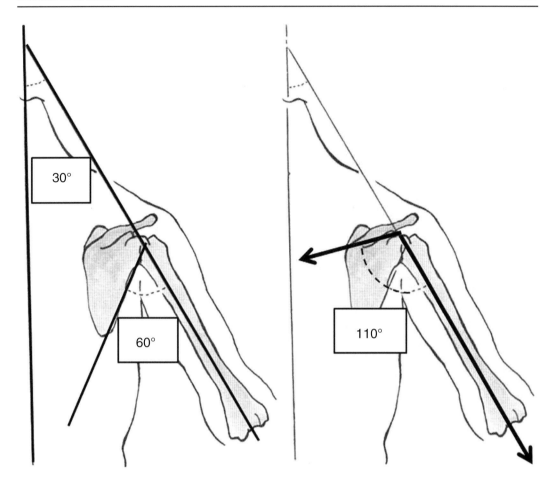

Fig. 1 Positioning of the shoulder arthrodesis in the coronal plane. (**a**) Humerus axis should draw a 30° angle towards the vertical. This angle is corresponding to an angle of 60° between the scapula lateral side and the humerus (**b**) With this position there is a 110° angle between supraspinous fossa and the humeral diaphysis

Of note, an angle of 60° between the lateral side of the scapula and the humeral diaphysis is equivalent to a 110° angle between supraspinous fossa and humeral diaphysis.

- Considering sagittal plane, humeral diaphysis must draw an angle around 20°–30° towards the vertical. In prone position during surgery, we take into account the lateral side of the scapula and to give an orientation around 30°–40° in order to achieve this goal (Fig. 2).
- Some authors have reported that the resection of the distal part of the clavicle could lead to a 20° increase in abduction but we do not have experience on this complication.
- Restoring the appropriate rotation in the fusion is the most critical point. It must be well fixed in order to allow the patient a range of motion from the face to the perineum area. In cases of wrong positioning, these movements will be restrained and will have a strong impact on the patient disability level. We are referencing the horizontal plane passing through the elbow when the arm has the desired flexion and abduction for the arthrodesis. In this situation and when the elbow is flexed, the hand will take the direction of the opposite shoulder with an angle around 20°–25° which will give the patient the necessary range of motion (Fig. 3).

In order to facilitate the surgical procedure, in our institution we use a custom-made 110° angulated plate that gives the theoretical ideal

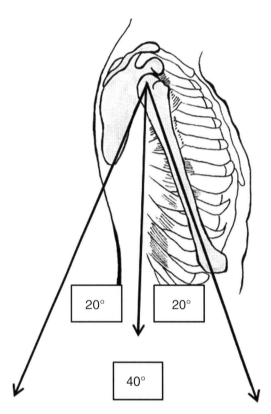

Fig. 2 Positioning of the shoulder arthrodesis in the sagittal plane. Humerus axis should draw a 20°–30° angle towards the vertical. It is also possible to use as a reference a 40° angle between the scapula lateral side and the humeral diaphysis

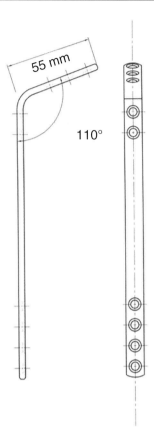

Fig. 4 Example of a custom-made osteosynthesis plate designed for supraspinous fossa fixation. Plate is designed with an 110° angle corresponding to the theoretical ideal angle between supraspinous fossa and humeral diaphysis. The size of the horizontal part of the plate is around 55 mm, allowing insertion of three vertical screws in the supraspinous fossa

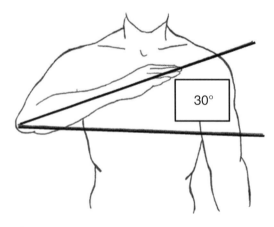

Fig. 3 Positioning of the shoulder arthrodesis in rotation. When taking as a reference the elbow horizontal plane the shoulder arthrodesis is positioned in both sagittal and coronal planes, forearm must draw a 20°–30° angle in the direction of the opposite shoulder

abduction. The proximal part of the plate is locked on the supraspinous fossa while the distal part is locked on the humeral diaphysis after setting of the rotation in order to give the best compromise between flexion and rotation (Fig. 4).

Articular Fixation

Fusion of the gleno-humeral arthrodesis can be difficult regarding the small bony surfaces available, the forces applied by the arm, and the difficulty of fixation on the scapula [6]. Once proper alignment of bone elements is achieved, surface of contact on the glenoid

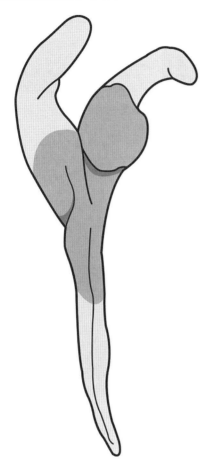

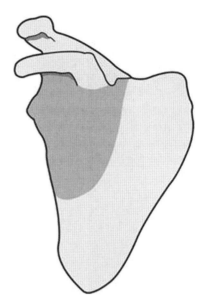

Fig. 6 Coronal view of the scapula. *Grey* part represents the site for best screw fixation. Starting from the supra epinous fossa, three screws sized 35–50 mm can be inserted on a 55 mm long surface towards the distal scapula

Fig. 5 Sagittal view of the scapula. *Grey* part represents the site for bone fixation using 35–50 mm screws inserted from the supraspinous fossa

humeral diaphysis) in order to oppose the forces applied on the arthrodesis by the arm [4, 10, 11].

Diagnosis, Surgical Indications

cavity is 35 mm × 20 mm while the thickness of the scapular neck is evaluated around 15 mm. Considering practical surgical aspects, when a screw is inserted perpendicular to the glenoid cavity, satisfactory bone anchorage is possible on the first 35 mm before getting out of the bone (Fig. 5). The scapular spine is therefore the most reliable site for bone anchorage and when a screw is inserted from the bottom of the supraspinous fossa in the scapular spine, a solid anchorage is possible for 40–50 mm before getting out of the bone (Fig. 6).

Various authors have emphasized the necessity to ensure a bone fixation as far away from the gleno-humeral arthrodesis as possible (i.e., on the medial part of the scapular spine and on the distal

Shoulder arthrodesis is currently a rare intervention with specific indications regarding to various progress in shoulder surgery such as, rotator cuff repair or shoulder arthroplasty.

Reasons to perform a shoulder arthrodesis are now mainly restricted to situations where shoulder locomotor structures (deltoid muscle and rotator cuff) cannot assume their functions due to palsy or a tumoral resection. Less frequently, it can be a salvage procedure in case of recurrent shoulder arthroplasty, high degenerative lesions or post-trauma cases.

- Shoulder palsy sequela [1]:
  In these cases, shoulder arthroplasty is a part of the global management of brachial plexus palsy, in association with nerves grafts and muscular transfers. Surgical indication is associated with best outcomes when there

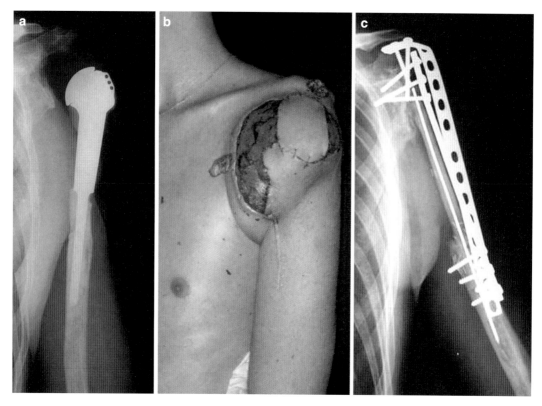

Fig. 7 (**a**) Indication for shoulder arthrodesis. In this clinical example, multiples septic conditions occurred during evolution of shoulder arthroplasty. (**b**) A failure a latissimus dorsi flap was responsible for an exposure of the shoulder arthroplasty. (**c**) A shoulder arthrodesis was performed using a vascularized fibular graft. At 18 years follow up the patient is teaching sea scooter in a beach hotel resort

is an unstable shoulder with a preserved active elbow flexion.

• Shoulder arthrodesis after recurrent surgical failures:

In most of these cases, the patients present major sequelae due to arthroplasty failure and/or infectious conditions (Fig. 7). Post-trauma cases such as chronic dislocation or open lesions with bone loss and soft tissues injuries can also be considered for arthrodesis due to the impossibility for arthroplasty.

• Tumoral resection:

It is in our experience the most common case, as the upper extremity of the humeral bone is the second most frequent site for primary bone tumors. Pathological lesions can be malignant (osteosarcoma, Ewing tumor or chondrosarcoma), but can also be benign with a high extensive ability (Giant Cell tumor) [9, 13].

Performing a shoulder arthrodesis in these cases is tricky considering the large bone loss and the necessity to achieve satisfactory stability.

In this chapter, we will mainly focus on the technique of shoulder arthrodesis for bone tumors. In these cases, reconstruction must be done after tumoral resection that will not only include the upper humeral bone extremity but also sometimes the glenoid cavity and scapula. During this surgery, the axillary nerve is always removed with the tumor, leading to an inefficient deltoid. Meanwhile, the rotator cuff is removed. All these resections erase active shoulder function leading to two remaining options: a reversed prosthesis with a loose shoulder or an arthrodesis with active mobility. According to the fact that mobility in the scapula-humeral joint is reduced, it is therefore crucial to plan a good positioning for the arthrodesis (Fig. 8).

Pre-Operative Preparation and Planning

When indication for arthrodesis is decided, planning will take care of the reconstruction strategy and the bone fixation. An arthroscopic technic has been described but we have no experience with these indications [7].

In daily practice, three types of fixation are described:

- Internal osteosynthesis associated with a compressive external fixator (Fig. 9).

  Various authors have reported results associated with a primary external fixation followed by an internal osteosynthesis using two or three screws [4]. The primary concern is the limited quality of bone fixation in the scapula leading to a fragile construct and risk for bone fracture related to external fixation on a poor quality bone. For malignant tumors, this strategy is not usable due to the risks for patients under frequent chemotherapy and aplasia.

- Internal osteosynthesis using an acromio-humeral plate (Fig. 10).

  This technique described by Muller is using a pre-bended plate fixed on the scapular spine, the acromion and the upper humeral extremity [3, 8]. The plate must be "soft" in order to bend according to the patient anatomy. Due to poor bone fixation quality and to avoid rotator disorders, Muller and Cofield have proposed to add a second posterior plate. One of the most common problems is related to the fact that this plate is just under the skin leading to frequent soft tissues disorders and potential infection in patients with previously altered skin.

- Internal osteosynthesis using a fixation in the supraspinous fossa (Fig. 11). We consider this the best technique for three reasons [5, 9, 13]:

  - Osteosynthesis is deep, in the fossa, leading to few possibilities for hardware exposure, decreasing infectious risks.

- Bone fixation is using vertical bicortical screws with an increased stability.
- The use of a custom made pre-bended 110° plate allows an automatic positioning of abduction in the coronal plane and also helps in the other planes (Fig. 4).

Operative Technique

According to the recent evolution for shoulder arthrodesis, we will only describe the internal osteosynthesis using a supraspinous fossa fixation in this chapter. The custom made pre-bended plate allows its use for palsy sequelae or reconstruction after tumoral resection.

Patient Positioning and Surgical Approach

Position on the surgical table is related to the surgical indication. For paralytic shoulder, a sitting position can be used as well as lateral decubitus. Patients undergoing a tumoral resection will be installed in a prone position with a cushion between the scapula and the spine (Fig. 12). Approach will be made using a deltopectoral incision. Length of incision will be adapted to the planned resection and can be enlarged towards the scapular spine and internally, after passing anteriorly to the coracoid process. Specific attention must be paid to draping in order to include the supraspinous fossa in the operative field for further resection, reconstruction and arthrodesis (Fig. 13).

Approach of the gleno-humeral joint will depend on the etiology:

- For paralytic shoulder, the deltoid's incision is done longitudinally in its medium part and the axillary pedicle is ligatured. This part is normally easy due to muscular atrophy. Deltoid is then detached from the acromion and the supraspinous fossa is exposed through the superior part of the trapezius. The supraspinatus muscle is subsequently removed using a rugine.

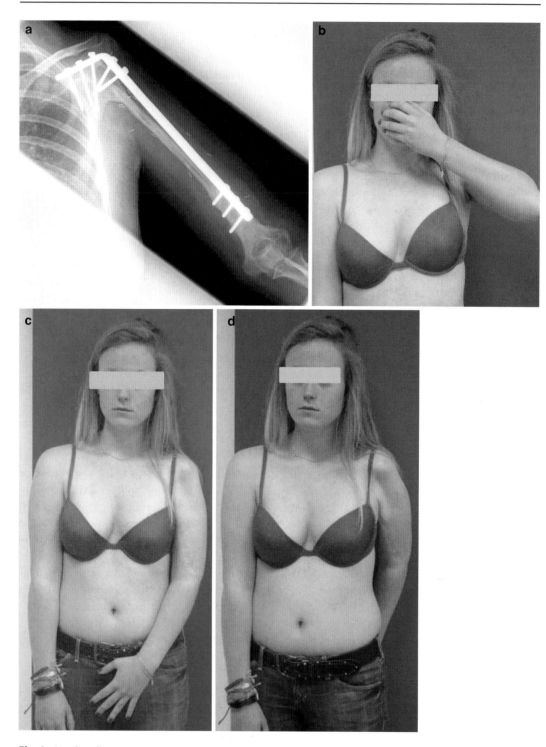

Fig. 8 (continued)

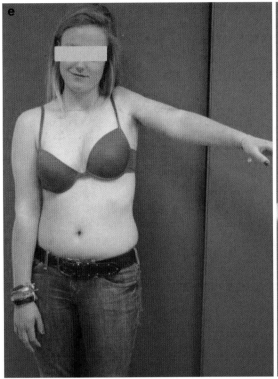

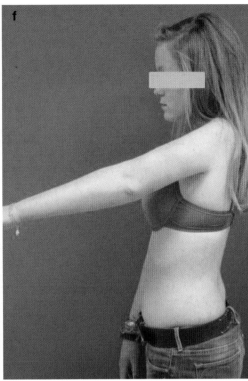

Fig. 8 (**a**) Functional recovery after shoulder arthrodesis in a 16 year-old patient diagnosed with an Ewing sarcoma the upper humeral extremity. Previous resection was including axillary nerve, rotator cuff and 21 cm of the upper humeral extremity. (**b, c, d, e, f**) At 4-years follow-up the patient was able to return to her previous studies and became hair-cutter

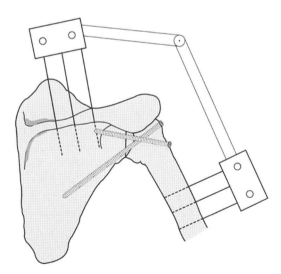

Fig. 9 Shoulder arthrodesis using an external fixator eventually in association with internal osteosynthesis

- During tumoral resection, a delto-pectoral incision approach is done and the supraspinous fossa is exposed in the same method.

It is fundamental to have access to the lateral scapula border and we commonly expose the anterior side of the scapula in order to get sufficient access and control of this area. This step is useful for positioning the arthrodesis but also to verify screws effraction on the anterior side of the scapula and to avoid excessive length.

Articular Preparing and Osteosynthesis

For paralytic shoulder, articular surface abrasion is done using an osteotome or a saw and confrontation of the bone part must be perfect. In order to

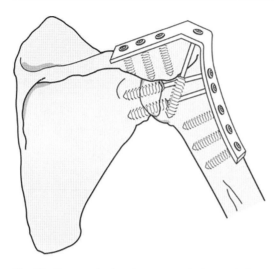

Fig. 10 Osteosynthesis using an acromio-humeral plate. Majors inconvenient of this technique are represented by residual pain and conflict between osteosynthesis plate and sub-cutaneous tissues (with potential exposure in front of the acromion)

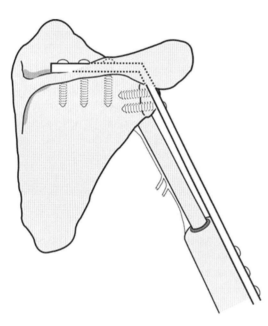

Fig. 11 Osteosynthesis using a plate with supraspinous fossa fixation. Main interest of the 110° pre-bend plate is the possibility to insert two screws in the glenoid cavity and three in the supraspinous fossa. This technique is preferentially used in case of large bone loss with free-vascularized fibular graft reconstruction

limit the risk of having the plate just under the skin, mostly around the great tubercle, the lateral part of the humerus can be drilled.

On the other hand, when dealing with tumoral resection, we are using a free vascularized fibular transplant. A hole is therefore drilled on the inferior part of the glenoid cavity and is used for transplant fixation. After dissection of the fibular periosteum, the transplant is locked in the hole while the periosteum is sutured to the scapular neck in order to facilitate bone consolidation. On the distal part, a tunnel measuring around 2 cm is drilled in the remaining humeral diaphysis in order to affix the fibular transplant inside. This part is also associated with a periosteum suture for consolidation purposes (Fig. 11).

During the next step, the custom-made osteosynthesis plate is fixed. By its angulation at 110°, abduction control is automatic (Fig. 4). Then using an angle of 40° in the sagittal plane between scapular pillar and the plate allows for control in the sagittal plane. Three screws are therefore inserted in the supraspinous fossa in direction of the anterior side of the scapula. The drill and the screws are inserted with exposure of the supraspinous fossa between the clavicle and the acromion. Deep retractors can be necessary to provide a correct exposure. In order to ensure a maximal fixation, the screws must be bicortical (around 35–50 mm) and pass at least 2 mm through the anterior cortex of the scapula.

Two more screws are then inserted horizontally through the scapular glenoid towards the neck giving a triangular fixation with the previous screws (Fig. 14).

Further steps correspond to the distal fixation of the plate to the humerus. At this time, control of the rotation must be done and properly planned. A rotation of 25° measured with a 90° elbow flexion will allow the patient to move the forearm from the mouth to the perineum area. The final step consists of inserting distal screws in the humerus after final positioning verification.

For paralytic shoulder, horizontal screws will be inserted at the end, after rotation positioning and distal fixation since the

Fig. 12 Patients undergoing a tumoral resection are installed in a prone position with a cushion between the scapula and the spine. A tourniquet is installed on the lower limb considering the vascular fibular graft dissection

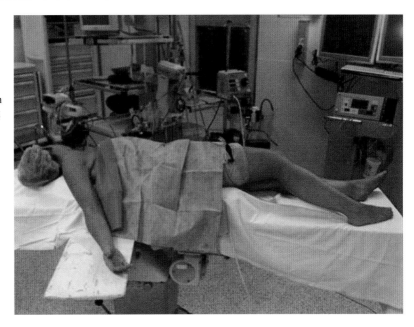

screws will go through both the humeral head and glenoid cavity.

Wound closure is done using habitual technique, but attention must be paid to bend down the coracoids process and the acromial angle after weakening them in order to avoid skin conflict.

Post-Operative Course

Immediate post-operative immobilization is prescribed using an abduction cushion. Then according to the clinical context, further immobilization is done using the 45° abduction cushion or a thoraco-brachial plaster cast for 8 weeks. This period is systematic for us as it is very difficult to obtain reliable consolidation proofs on x-rays examinations.

Post-Operative Care and Rehabilitation

Rehabilitation is fundamental in order to achieve best outcomes after shoulder arthrodesis. During the first 8 weeks, physiotherapy is started for the

hand, fingers and elbow. Articular range of motion must be preserved but the scapula-thoracic joint must not be used.

As it is hard to establish clear consolidation criteria, after immediate postoperative x-ray, we used to ask for a second control at 8 weeks postoperatively. When a fibular transplant has been used, presence of periosteum apposition around the scapula-humeral junction and absence of osteolysis around the screws are comforting factors. At this time scapula-thoracic physiotherapy can start in order to develop compensatory mobility and satisfactory functional outcomes. After starting with passive mobilization and elevation/abduction movements, active work is started a second time. Muscular reinforcement is a key parameter for favorable outcomes and is strongly recommended after a few months in order to improve mobility. The majority of results improve with time and global mobility can be evaluated around 180° in the three planes (70° abduction, 50° internal rotation, while external rotation is fixed around 0°).

When the arthrodesis is consolidated with good positioning and the patient is

Fig. 13 (**a**) Draping must include cervical region, upper limb and lower limb. (**b**) Approach will be made using a deltopectoral incision. Length of incision will be adapted to the planned resection and can be enlarged towards the scapular spine and internally, after passing anteriorly to the coracoid process. Specific attention must be paid to draping in order to include the supraspinous fossa in the operative field for further resection, reconstruction and arthrodesis

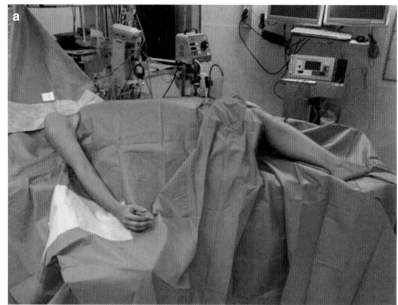

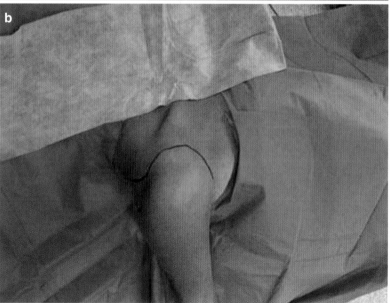

following an appropriate physiotherapy program, functional rehabilitation can be perfect (Fig. 8).

In our experience, 15 shoulder arthrodesis procedures have been done using this technique (13 for tumoral reconstruction) and among these patients one is a surgeon, two are hair-cutter and all the patients who healed with their tumoral disease have been back to work.

Complications

Pseudoarthrodesis

This condition corresponds to a lack of consolidation. With improvement of osteosynthesis techniques, this complication is less frequent nowadays and out of our series of 15 patients,

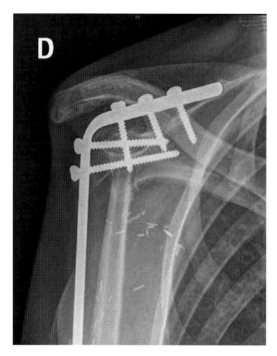

Fig. 14 Example of reconstruction using a free-vascularized fibular graft in a 15 year-old patient diagnosed with a Ewing sarcoma of the humeral upper extremity. At 6 months follow up the periosteal flap improves the consolidation on the mild part of the scapula

only one showed an absence of consolidation of the upper extremity of the fibular graft. A second procedure with iliac cortico-spongious bone graft at the junction between the scapula and the fibular graft was done with a favorable outcome. Of note, presence of a thin and well-tolerated pseudoarthrodesis is possible. If the patient is not complaining or if successive x-ray controls do not show degradation, a second procedure is not mandatory.

Humeral Fractures

They are a characteristic of paralytic etiologies. Most of the time it occurs at the level of a screw or external fixator pin on a porotic bone. In these cases, due to the consequent traumatic malpositioning of the arthrodesis, a conservative treatment is not indicated and a second surgery is necessary.

Post-Operative Chronic Pain

They can be related to two different causes:
- In most of the cases, such pain phenomenon is related to neurological disorder, mainly for plexus palsy and they are not related to the arthrodesis technique.
- Sometimes they are related to the surgery by an excessive abduction responsible for a painful traction on the supra-scapular nerve or a painful traction on thoraco-scapular muscles.

After acromio-humeral arthrodesis, pain is also frequent and mostly related with soft tissues conflict with the osteosynthesis or the acromion.

Aesthetic Complications

During tumoral resection and reconstruction procedures, using a supraspinous fossa plate osteosynthesis is helpful. However, this technique can also be associated with a shortening and an inesthetic shoulder deformation. It is possible in a second procedure to fill the soft-tissues defect with a custom-made silicone implant. In our experience, we recommend this surgery a minimum of 2 years after the initial one (Fig. 15).

Summary

During the last 20 years, surgical indications for shoulder arthrodesis have continuously decreased. They are now reserved for the management of brachial plexus palsy sequelae and after tumoral resection. Less frequently it can be done after recurrent failures of shoulder arthroplasty or high energy complex trauma of the shoulder.

Two main challenges are associated with this surgery. First is to ensure perfect positioning of the arthrodesis as it will be correlated with functional outcomes. Second is to ensure a good quality fusion with small bone contact surfaces. This technique must therefore be precise and provide a satisfactory stability.

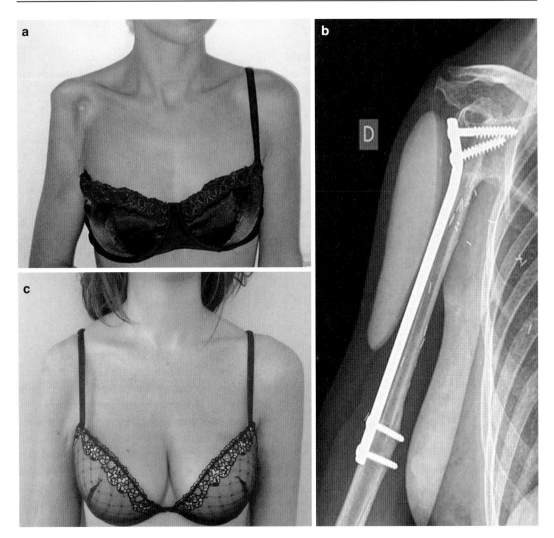

Fig. 15 Mid-term cosmetic revision after shoulder reconstruction procedure. (**a**) Results of shoulder arthrodesis in an 18 year-old patient diagnosed with a malignant tumor of the upper extremity of the humerus. The patient presents the characteristic aspect after vascularized bone reconstruction. There is a large defect under the acromion and a prominent coracoid process. (**b**) Insertion of a custom-made silicone prosthesis in order to fill the shoulder cavity after resection. (**c**) Cosmetic results 5 years after insertion of the silicone prosthesis and 10 years after initial resection-reconstruction procedure

Three different kinds of procedures are described in the literature, internal osteosynthesis with external fixation, acromio-humeral internal osteosynthesis or internal osteosynthesis using the supraspinous fossa as a fixation point.

Patients that will undergo a shoulder arthrodesis often have had several previous surgeries or will have postoperative chemotherapy after tumoral resection. These situations can lead to soft-tissue disorders as well as poor quality bone anchorage.

In our institution we use a custom-made osteosynthesis plate with a proximal fixation in the supraspinous fossa. The pre-bended plate provides an automatic positioning of the abduction. Fives screws with triangulation directions can be inserted in the scapula (three in the supraspinous fossa and two horizontal in the glenoid cavity) for optimized fixation.

This technique gives a stable osteosynthesis in order to compensate a late bone consolidation and a rehabilitation program during the immediate post-operative course. Physiotherapy is fundamental in order to provide muscular reinforcement and better functional outcomes than a loose shoulder.

References

1. Chammas M, Goubier JN, Coulet B, Reckendorf GM, Picot MC, Allieu Y. Glenohumeral arthrodesis in upper and total brachial plexus palsy. A comparison of functional results. J Bone Joint Surg Br. 2004;86(5):692–5.
2. Clare DJ, Wirth MA, Groh GI, Rockwood Jr CA. Shoulder arthrodesis. J Bone Joint Surg Am. 2001;83-A(4):593–600.
3. Cofield RH, Briggs BT. Glenohumeral arthrodesis. Operative and long-term functional results. J Bone Joint Surg Am. 1979;61(5):668–77.
4. Johnson CA, Healy WL, Brooker Jr AF, Krackow KA. External fixation shoulder arthrodesis. Clin Orthop Relat Res. 1986;211:219–23.
5. Klonz A, Habermeyer P. Arthrodesis of the shoulder. A new and soft-tissue-sparing technique with a deep locking plate in the supraspinatus fossa. Unfallchirurg. 2007;110(10):891–5.
6. Miller BS, Harper WP, Gillies RM, Sonnabend DH, Walsh WR. Biomechanical analysis of five fixation techniques used in glenohumeral arthrodesis. ANZ J Surg. 2003;73(12):1015–7.
7. Morgan CD, Casscells CD. Arthroscopic-assisted glenohumeral arthrodesis. Arthroscopy. 1992;8(2):262–6.
8. Richards RR, Sherman RM, Hudson AR, Waddell JP. Shoulder arthrodesis using a pelvic-reconstruction plate. A report of eleven cases. J Bone Joint Surg Am. 1988;70(3):416–21.
9. Rose PS, Shin AY, Bishop AT, Moran SL, Sim FH. Vascularized free fibula transfer for oncologic reconstruction of the humerus. Clin Orthop Relat Res. 2005;438:80–4.
10. Rühmann O, Schmolke S, Bohnsack M, Kirsch L, Wirth CJ. Shoulder arthrodesis. Indications, techniques, results, complications. Orthopade. 2004;33(9):1061–80 (quiz 1081-).
11. Safran O, Iannotti JP. Arthrodesis of the shoulder. J Am Acad Orthop Surg. 2006;14(3):145–53.
12. Scalise JJ, Iannotti JP. Glenohumeral arthrodesis after failed prosthetic shoulder arthroplasty. Surgical technique. J Bone Joint Surg Am. 2009;91(Suppl 2 Pt 1):30–7.
13. Viehweger E, Gonzalez JF, Launay F, Legre R, Jouve JL, Bollini G. Shoulder arthrodesis with vascularized fibular graft after tumor resection of the proximal humerus. Rev Chir Orthop Reparatrice Appar Mot. 2005;91(6):523–9.

Resurfacing Arthroplasty of the Shoulder

Stephen A. Copeland and Jai G. Relwani

Contents

Abstract

The design of the surface replacement arthroplasty has evolved over the past 20 years. From cemented prostheses such as the SCAN, to cementless prosthesis such as the Copeland, the basic concept and design of the surface replacement favouring maximal bone preservation has remained constant. The indications and surgical technique have been refined over this period. The indications are similar to those in degenerative conditions, but its use is contra-indicated in fresh fractures. The prosthesis can be used as a hemi-arthroplasty or a total shoulder replacement. The surface replacement prosthesis has demonstrated clinical results at least equal to those of conventional stemmed prostheses. The indications, surgical technique and results of surface replacement shoulder arthroplasty are presented.

Keywords

Complications • Copeland results • Future designs and techniques • History • Problem replacements • Re-surfacing arthroplasty • Rehabilitation • Results • Shoulder • Surgical indications • Surgical Techniques

S.A. Copeland (✉)
The Reading Shoulder Surgery Unit, Capio Reading Hospital, Reading, UK
e-mail: stephen.copeland@btinternet.com

J.G. Relwani
East Kent University Hospital, Ashford, Kent, UK

History and Scope of the Problem

Zippel in Germany implanted two surface replacements that were fixed by a trans-osseous screw [1] but no follow-up is recorded for these cases. Steffee and Moore in the United States were implanting a small hip-resurfacing prosthesis into the shoulder [2] and, in Sweden, in greater numbers, a surface replacement SCAN (Scandinavian) cup was being used as a cemented surface replacement [3].

Development of the Copeland Cementless Surface Replacement Arthroplasty (CSRA) began in 1979. The prosthesis was first used clinically in 1986. From 1993 the entire bony surface of the glenoid and humeral components have been hydroxyapatite- coated so that the initial mechanical fix is transformed into a biological fixation with bony in-growth to the hydroxyapatite coating.

Simple instruments allow anatomical placement of the humeral head by identifying the center of the sphere. Once this point has been identified, the prosthesis can be positioned to replicate the original anatomical bearing surface including version, offset, and angulation. With current advances in technology, it is possible to determine this centre with extreme accuracy, using computer-assisted navigation techniques, thereby increasing the precision of prosthesis placement.

The potential advantages of a cementless surface replacement include:

1. Anatomical siting of head, restoring anatomical variations of version, offset, and angulation in each individual patient.
2. No intra-medullary canal reaming or cementation, making it a less traumatic and safer procedure in an elderly patient, with a smaller risk of fat embolus or hypotension.
3. There is no problem if the intra-medullary canal has already been filled with cement, the stem of an elbow replacement, or fracture fixation devices. If there is a mal-union at the proximal end of the humeral with secondary osteoarthritis, the mal-union can be left undisturbed, the tuberosities intact, and just the humeral articulation is resurfaced.
4. Unlike stemmed prosthesis, there is no stress riser effect that could result in a shaft fracture at the tip of the prosthesis.

5. It can be used in congenital abnormalities of the humerus that would not allow the passage of standard intra-medullary stemmed prostheses.
6. Revision surgery to a stemmed prosthesis or arthrodesis can be performed easily as there is no loss of bone stock and no cement to retrieve from within the humeral shaft.

Indications/Contra-Indications

Primary and secondary arthritis of the shoulder is the commonest indication. The prosthesis has also been used successfully for rheumatoid and other inflammatory arthritides [3–7], avascular necrosis, cuff tear arthropathy, instability arthropathy, post- trauma arthritis, post-infective arthritis, and arthritis secondary to glenoid dysplasia and dysplasia of the epiphysis. It is not intended for use in fresh fractures.

The results of surface replacement, as in any other shoulder replacement, depend on the indications and diagnosis. The best results are achieved in osteoarthritis with an intact cuff, and the worst results in cuff tear arthropathy and post-traumatic arthritis [8]. The surface replacement arthroplasty can even be used in circumstances of moderate to severe erosion of the humeral head, in conjunction with bone graft. If there is more than 60 % contact between the undersurface of the trial prosthesis and humeral head, after it has been milled, then it would be suitable for surface replacement, that is, up to 40 % of the humeral head may be replaced by bone graft.

The contra-indications for surface replacement arthroplasty are active infection, bone loss of the humeral head exceeding 40 % of the surface, and acute fractures.

92 % of our cases requiring shoulder arthroplasty receive a surface replacement. We feel that surface replacement should be the standard replacement of choice for all cases, unless specifically contra-indicated; the question now is not when to use a surface replacement, but what are the limited residual indications for a stemmed implant.

Surgical Technique

Anaesthesia

This operation can be performed under general and/or regional anaesthesia, according to local preferences. We favour a light total intravenous anaesthetic together with an inter-scalene block for effective analgesia.

Position

The patient is placed in the "beach-chair" position with a sandbag underneath the medial scapular border to thrust the shoulder forward. An arm board is attached to the table at the level of the elbow to support the forearm. Drape the arm free to allow full movement at the shoulder and confirm that it can be adequately extended and adducted.

Approach

Either a standard anterior deltopectoral approach or the antero-superior approach as described by Neviaser [9] and Mackenzie [10] can be used to insert the prosthesis. The advantages of the Mackenzie incision include a smaller and neater scar, easier and more direct access via the rotator interval to the glenoid, and better access to the posterior and superior rotator cuff for reconstruction. It also allows for excision arthroplasty of the acromio-clavicular joint and acromioplasty if these are indicated. The acromio-clavicular joint excision can be a useful source of bone graft.

The antero-superior approach leads onto the rotator cuff. If the cuff is intact or there is a repairable tear, then perform an anterior acromioplasty with partial resection of the coraco-acromial ligament. Leave the coracoacromial arch undisturbed if the rotator cuff is extensively torn or non-functional. If pre-operative radiographs have shown arthritic changes of the acromio-clavicular joint and symptoms suggest this is a site of pain, then perform an excision arthroplasty at this stage. This further improves the surgical exposure. We excise the acromio-clavicular joint in almost all patients with osteoarthritis as they usually do not have adequate pre-operative range of motion to demonstrate symptoms arising from this joint. At least 80° of forward flexion is required to induce pain at this site, and once range of movement has been restored, this joint can become irritable and impede function of the shoulder. Identify the rotator interval at the base of the coracoid. Release the coracohumeral ligament to gain external rotation. Incise longitudinally along the line of the long head of biceps and the rotator interval to define the insertion of the subscapularis. Detach the subscapularis with an osteoperiosteal flap from the medial border of the biceps groove. Deliver the head of the humerus through the wound by extending and adducting the shoulder. If the long head of biceps is intact, displace it posteriorly over the humeral head.

Humeral Preparation

The key landmark for determining the ideal position of the humeral component is the line-of-junction of the head and the anatomical neck of the humerus. Demonstrate this by removing osteophytes around the neck. Place the humeral drill guide over the head with its free edge parallel to the junction of the anatomical neck and the humeral head (Fig. 1).

The humeral drill guide should be central on the humeral head and parallel to the anatomical neck line; this reproduces the patient's own version, inclination, and offset. Using the centred drill guide, drive a guide-wire through the centre of the head and into the lateral humeral cortex for firm purchase. Remove the guide jig and visually check that the guide-wire is in the centre of the head (Fig. 2). If the guide-wire does not look centred, then it should be re-positioned.

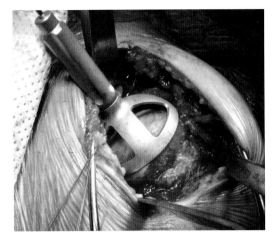

Fig. 1 Sizing and alignment using the centralising jig to insert the guide-wire

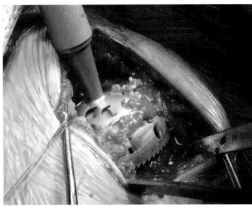

Fig. 3 Reaming of the humeral surface until bone is seen exiting the fenestrations in the reamer

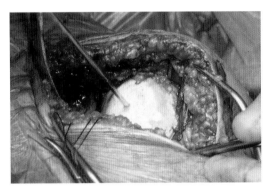

Fig. 2 Central position of the guide-wire in the head confirmed

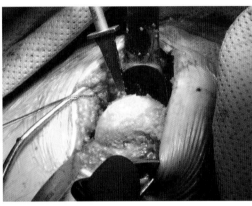

Fig. 4 The stem cutter is then used over the guide-wire to create a hole for the stem of the prosthesis

With the guide-wire central in the humeral head, choose the size of the humeral guide that closest matches the size of the humeral head. If the head falls between guide sizes, it is better to undersize as this allows you to correct to a larger size later.

The appropriate cannulated humeral surface reamer is then passed over the guide-wire. Whilst the reamer is rotating, light pressure is applied on the humeral head to engage the cutting teeth. This should be continued until reamings are seen exiting from all the holes in the shaper (Fig. 3). Ideally all remnants of articular and fibro-cartilage should be removed, but preserve as much subchondral bone as possible to support the prosthesis. The reamer has a safety mechanism to prevent over-reaming and removing too much bone. Save all the reamings scavenged from the humeral head for later bone grafting. Remove any residual osteophytes from the circumference of the neck.

Once the appropriate humeral size is decided, use the corresponding sized stem-cutter over the guide-wire and drill down to, but not beyond, the shoulder of the cutter to remove the correct amount of bone for the central stem hole (Fig. 4). The cutter and guide-wire are then removed.

Insert the trial component. If only a hemi-arthroplasty is to be done, test the stability of the humeral component and the range of movement. Consider appropriate soft-tissue releases and balancing at this stage. If a hemi-arthroplasty is to be performed, the glenoid still needs to be prepared at this stage as described below.

Glenoid Preparation

Leave the trial humeral component in situ to protect the prepared humeral head. Retract the humeral head postero-inferiorly with a Murphy skid or Fukuda retractor. The decision concerning glenoid replacement is made at this stage. Pre-operative imaging using an axillary view radiograph and C.T. may be helpful in this regard. If glenoid replacement is **not** intended, it is our routine practice to drill multiple holes in the glenoid with a 2 mm guide-wire, or create a micro-fracture with a chondral pick just penetrating the hard osteochondral surface of the bone to induce bleeding and some fibro-cartilaginous regeneration. If the glenoid requires replacement, it is carried out using the appropriate technique which we have described earlier [11] and is beyond the scope of this chapter.

Humeral Replacement

Now return your attention to the humerus. Remove the trial component and create multiple drill holes, using a 2 mm drill, through the sclerotic subchondral bone to improve bone reactivity. Place the rest of the bone graft mix inside the definitive humeral component (Fig. 5). Apply the prosthesis onto the prepared humeral head (Fig. 6). Using the impactor, apply two or three sharp blows with the mallet to seat the component fully. Wash away any excess bone, then reduce the joint and test again for stability.

Closure

If the centre of rotation has been lateralized, then subscapularis may need relative

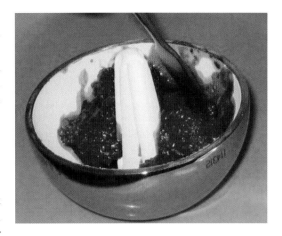

Fig. 5 The Copeland Mark III prosthesis (hydroxyapatite coated) containing autologous bone graft and blood paste prior to insertion

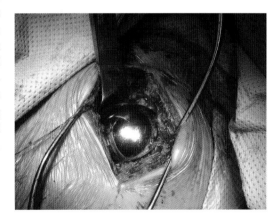

Fig. 6 Surface replacement in situ prior to reduction

lengthening by either a stepwise cut in the tendon or by medialization of the insertion of the tendon. Close only the lateral part of the rotator interval. Now repair any rotator cuff tear if possible. Capsulotomy or sutures may be required at this stage to balance the reduction. Ensure a firm repair of deltoid to the acromion using transosseous sutures if necessary. Close the subcutaneous fat with interrupted absorbable sutures, and insert a subcuticular running stitch.

Apply a sterile dressing and place the patient into a sling with a body belt.

Surgical pearls	Confirm that patient position allows arm to extend and adduct adequately on table
	Have a low threshold for an acromioplasty and AC joint excision
	Expose the junction of the head and anatomical neck adequately, this step is crucial and requires removal of all osteophytes on the humerus
	Accurately identify the centre of the humeral head before proceeding
	If in doubt about the size, downsize
	Preserve as much of the bone reamings in the patient's blood as possible, to augment any bone loss in the humeral head. Up to 40 % bone loss can be reconstituted during a surface replacement
	Remember to perform soft tissue release/balancing as necessary
	Drill the glenoid surface to stimulate bleeding and fibrocartilage regeneration
	Carefully reconstruct the soft tissues, including deltoid repair during closure
Surgical Pitfalls	Do not be too aggressive with the acromioplasty and AC joint excision in cases with poor or irreparable rotator cuff. Consider using the deltopectoral approach in these cases
	Do not use the prosthesis in cases of fracture or if bone loss from the head is > 40 %.

Post-Operative Restrictions and Rehabilitation

Only passive movement is allowed for the first 48 h, then passive assisted movements for 5 days. Begin active movements at 1 week if pain allows, and discard the sling at 3 weeks. Retrict external rotation for 3 weeks to protect the subscapularis repair. Encourage the patient to stretch and strengthen for many months as improvement will continue up to 18 months post-operatively.

Follow-Up

Patients are discharged home when comfortable and safe, typically 48 h post-operatively. They are reviewed in clinic at 3 weeks, 3 months and 12 months and yearly thereafter. Radiographs are obtained post-operatively, at 3 months, 12 months, and yearly thereafter (Fig. 7).

Results of Surface Replacement

Zippel in Germany implanted two surface replacements that were fixed by a transosseous screw [1] but no follow-up is recorded for these cases.

Good clinical early results have been obtained with cups developed by Steffee and Moore [2], and by Jonsson et al. [3]. Rydholm and Sjögen [7] from Sweden reported the results of the 'SCAN cup' in 1993 and 2003. Rydholm [5] performed 84 SCAN cups, a hemi-spherical cemented cup, in 70 patients, and 72 cups in 59 patients were followed for 4.2 years (range, 1.5–9.9 years). The clinical results obtained showed 94 % of the patients being pleased regarding pain relief and 82 % reporting improved shoulder mobility. Shoulder function was significantly improved. Radiographs were analyzed regarding the position of the cup, proximal migration of the humerus, and glenoid attrition during the follow-up period. Change of the distance between the superior margin of the cup and the greater tuberosity and/or change of inclination of the prosthesis were regarded as signs of prosthetic loosening. With that definition, 25 % of the cups were found to be loose at follow up. Prosthetic loosening, however, had no bearing on the clinical result. Progressive proximal migration of the humerus in 38 % of the shoulders and central attrition of the glenoid in 22 % of the shoulders did not show any relationship to gain of mobility, pain relief, or functional ability. Note that no central fixation peg was used for this cup. Long term follow-up at 13 years included 54 cups in 46 patients (13 patients deceased, no revisions). Six cups had been revised 10 years (range, 5–16 years) after the index operation (4 – persistent pain, 1 – stiffness, and 1 – prosthetic loosening). Pain at rest on a 100-mm visual analogue scale was 15 mm (range, 0–62 mm) and

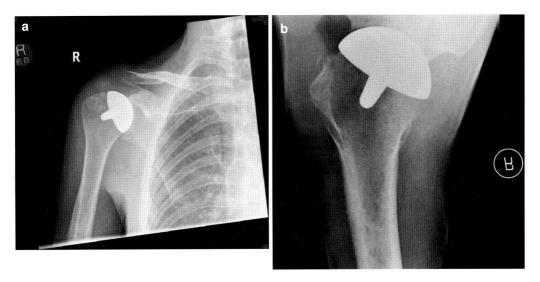

Fig. 7 Radiographs of the Copeland cementless resurfacing arthroplasty (pre- and post-operative)

pain on motion was 32 mm (range, 0–85 mm). Twenty-six (50 %) could comb their hair (compared with 56 % at first follow-up), 32 (62 %) could wash their opposite axilla (90 % at first follow-up), and 31 (60 %) could reach behind (77 % at first follow-up).

Alund et al. [12] reported on 40 shoulder surface replacements for rheumatoid disease using the SCAN prosthesis. They reported 1 revision to total shoulder replacement, and 39 shoulders were followed up for a mean of 4.4 years (0.9–6.5 years). The median Constant score was 30 (15–79), mean proximal migration of the humerus 5.5 (SD 5.2) mm and mean glenoid erosion 2.6 (SD 1.7) mm. Proximal migration and glenoid erosion did not correlate with shoulder function or pain. Radiographic signs of loosening (changes in cup inclination combined with changes in cup distance above the greater tuberosity) occurred in 25 % of the shoulders. At follow-up, 26 (65 %) patients were satisfied with the procedure, despite poor shoulder function and radiographic deterioration.

Fink et al. [13] prospectively evaluated 45 Durom Cups in 39 patients (30 women, 9 men) with rheumatoid disease. The average follow-up was 45.1 ± 11.6 months with a minimum of 36 months. Fifteen shoulders had an intact

cuff (group A), 18 had a partial tearing or a repaired rotator cuff (group B), and 12 shoulders a massive cuff tear (group C). In group A rheumatic shoulders, the Constant Score increased from 21.5 ± 9.6 points pre-operatively to 66.1 ± 9.8 points at 36 months post-operatively; in shoulders of group B, from 19.6 ± 9.7 points pre-operatively to 64.9 ± 9.6 points at 36 months post-operatively; and in shoulders of group C, from 17.5 ± 8.7 points to 56.9 ± 9.8 points at the latest follow-up examination. All shoulders were pain-free at the latest examination. No complications, component loosening or changes of cup position were observed.

Copeland Mark I and II Prosthesis Results

The Copeland surface replacement prosthesis has developed from the original Mark I version that was first implanted in 1986 to the current Mark III version first implanted in 1993. The Mark 1 prosthesis was fixed with a central smooth round peg and a screw passed from the lateral side of the humeral screw into the prosthesis to act as an anti-rotation bar. This was used clinically on 19 patients. We realized that the fixation was adequate with the impaction peg alone. The screw was unnecessary and we worried that if the prosthesis was to loosen, the toggling of this anti-rotation bar might dissociate or disrupt the tuberosities, presenting a difficult reconstruction problem. Therefore the use of the screw was discarded at an early stage, with a modified peg design to improve the press-fit.

Between 1990 and 1993, 103 Mark-II prostheses were inserted into 94 patients (nine bilateral) [8]. The indications included osteoarthritis, rheumatoid arthritis, avascular necrosis, instability arthropathy, post-traumatic arthropathy and cuff arthropathy. The mean follow-up was 6.8 years [5–10]. The best results were achieved in primary osteoarthritis, with Constant scores of 93.7 % for total shoulder replacement and 73.5 % for hemiarthroplasty. The poorest results were encountered in patients with arthropathy of the cuff, instability arthropathy and other causes such as arthropathy secondary to septic arthritis, with adjusted Constant scores of 61.3 %, 62.7 % and 58.7 %, respectively. Of the 88 humeral implants available for radiological review, 61 (69.3 %) showed no evidence of radiolucency, nor did 21 (35.6 %) of the 59 glenoid prostheses. Three were definitely loose, and eight shoulders required revision (7.7 %), two (1.9 %) for primary loosening. The results of this series are comparable with those for stemmed prostheses with a similar follow-up and case mix [14–19].

Mark III Prosthesis Results

From 1993, the entire non-articular surface (implant – bone interface) of the glenoid and humeral components has been hydroxyapatite-coated. The initial mechanical press-fit is thus followed later by a biological fix with bony ingrowths due to the hydroxyapatite coating. This is the current Mark III design.

Between September 1993 and August 2002, 209 shoulders underwent surface replacement arthroplasty at our unit using the Mark III prosthesis with hydroxyapatite coating. Clinical and radiological outcome was assessed at an average duration of follow-up of 4.4 years. No evidence of radiolucency was seen in any humeral implant. Thomas et al. [6] reported a 6.3 % incidence of lucencies in their series using the Mark III implant. Asymptomatic non-progressive lucency of less than 2 mm was seen in seven of the twenty-nine glenoid components inserted, which did not require further treatment.

Six shoulders (2.8 %) required revision surgery (one mal-position of glenoid, two instability and three painful arthroplasties). Using the Kaplan- Meier analysis, the probability that the implant would survive to the start of the tenth year after surgery was estimated to be 96.4 %. The results of Mark III Copeland Shoulder Replacement Arthroplasty are comparable to conventional stemmed prostheses. There was no difference between hemi-arthroplasty and total shoulder arthroplasty in terms of functional outcome. No hemi-arthroplasty has been revised for component loosening.

The table below summarises the hitherto published results of surface replacement prostheses (Table 1).

Complications

1. Aseptic loosening – 5.1 % (pre hydroxyapatite coating), 0 % post HA coating (Mark III).
2. Deep Infection – 0.7 %.
3. Myositis Ossificans – 0.7 %.

The revision rate at 5–10 years of using the Mark II design has been 5.9 %. The indications were:

1. Instability following total shoulder resurfacing arthroplasty for instability arthropathy in two patients.
2. One peri-prosthetic fracture (surgical neck) after a fall. This was treated in a collar and cuff sling for 6 weeks and healed uneventfully.
3. One disassociation of the polyethylene glenoid from the metal part of the glenoid component (obviated by immediate design change).
4. One glenoid loosening following a fall.

Table 1 Table comparing the published results of surface replacement prostheses.

Author	Copeland/Levy [8]	Thomas [6]	Alund [12]	Rydholm U [5]	Fink [13]
Implant	Copeland Mark II (pre-HA coating)	Copeland Mark III	SCAN	SCAN	Durom
Indication	Mixed	Mixed	Rheumatoid	Rheumatoid	Rheumatoid
No. of replacements	103	48	39	72	45
Average age at surgery (years)	64.3	70	55	51	62.7
Follow-up (months)	60–120 (mean 80)	24–63 (mean 34.2)	24–72 (mean 52)	50–95 (mean 50)	45.1 +/− 11
Mean preop constant score	15.4	16.4	NA	NA	19.5
Mean postop constant score	52.4	54	30	Not available but 92 % of patients satisfied with pain improvement	62.6
Preop VAS	NA	NA	80 (median)		NA
Postop VAS	NA	NA	16 (median)	15–32 (mean)	NA
Radiologic lucent/lytic lines	5.1 % (Pre-HA coating)	6.3 %	20 %	25 %	0 %
Overall patients satisfied	93.9 %	NA	83 %	92 %	94 %

5. Two aseptic loosenings – one involved both humerus and glenoid, and one glenoid only.

Revision surgery was greatly simplified having originally implanted a Cementless surface replacement. At the time of revision of a surface replacement arthroplasty, the only bone lost was the bone that would have been removed had a stemmed prosthesis been used at the first operation. There was no need to remove a cemented stemmed prosthesis, which is associated with loss of bone stock, perforation, and fracture of the humeral shaft. The preservation of bone facilitated revision to a stemmed prosthesis or to glenohumeral arthrodesis.

The current Mark III design has had no cases of radiological lucent lines or loosening with its hydroxyapatite coating. The revision rate of the Mark III design is 2.8 %, with a predicted survival probability of 96.4 % at 10 years using Kaplan Meier analysis.

The Problem Surface Replacement

The patient returning with a painful or non-functioning surface replacement immediately leads one to suspect glenoid wear as the cause of pain and to consider a revision shoulder replacement as the solution. However, several causes of the painful shoulder arthroplasty should first be considered [20].

The commonest cause is residual subacromial impingement which presents with a good range of movement but a positive impingement arc abolished by injection of local anaesthetic into the subacromial space. This is resolved by an arthroscopic subacromial decompression. Biceps disorders give rise to anterior pain, and may require a tenodesis or tenotomy. Cuff rupture can occur which requires re-exploration and cuff repair or

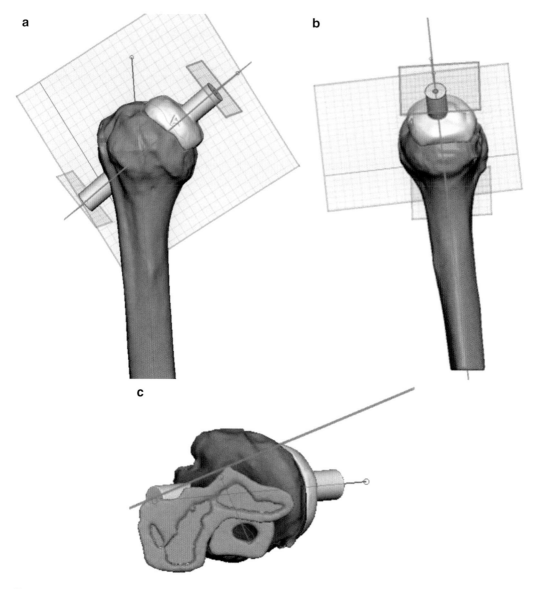

Fig. 8 (**a**, **b**, **c**) Signature Guide templating for patient-specific Copeland Replacement

conversion to reverse geometry prosthesis if the cuff is irreparable. A previously arthritic acromioclavicular joint can become symptomatic following increased glenohumeral movement after a surface replacement, and we recommend and routinely excise the AC joint during the primary procedure to avoid this problem in the post-operative period. Capsular fibrosis is a diagnosis to be considered once all other causes are eliminated. This can be treated by an arthroscopic capsular release. Last but not the least, the diagnosis of infection must always be kept in mind. If all else fails to relieve the pain, the glenohumeral joint is injected with local anaesthetic to try and determine whether the glenohumeral articulation is the source of pain. This then requires a revision to a total shoulder arthroplasty.

Summary and Conclusions

Surface replacement of the shoulder has been proven to be at least as successful as stemmed implants in the treatment of shoulder arthritis. The hydroxyapatite coating has been a major advance in reducing lucent lines and loosening. The bone-preserving nature of the implant allows it to be used in a most situations, including cases of deformity. If complications do occur, then they can be more easily treated, and the results of surface hemi-arthroplasty appear to be better than stemmed hemi-arthroplasty. The geometry and mechanics of the shoulder joint are now much better understood. It is no longer justifiable to continue with intramedullary (either cementless or cemented) fixation in a straightforward arthritic problem.

Future Considerations

Future prostheses for the shoulder are likely to be of the bone-preserving nature. As materials improve, wear will hopefully become less of a problem. Modern technology allows for more accurate pre-operative planning. Computer assistance during surgery could translate this planning to a practical solution to optimise implant position and soft tissue balancing, which ultimately with improved materials should increase longevity of the prosthesis and improve function after shoulder arthroplasty [21]. We have performed the first 'Signature' computer-assisted Copeland surface arthroplasty to optimise the three-dimensional positioning of the implant. The centre of the humeral head (in three axes) is identified by a logarithm with data obtained using high resolution CT scan and MR scans, and a patient-specific custom disposable jig is then created to anatomically site the guide-wire, and size the implant (Fig. 8a–c). This has allowed accurate recreation of the functional anatomy in the individual. The next challenge facing us will probably be that of regenerating the surface!

References

1. Zippel J. Dislocation-proof shoulder prosthesis model BME. Z Orthop Ihre Grenzgeb. 1975;113(4): 454–7.
2. Steffee AD, Moore RW. Hemi-resurfacing arthroplasty of the rheumatoid shoulder. Contemp Orthop. 1984;9:51–9.
3. Jonsson E, Egund N, Kelly I, Rydholm U, Lidgren L. Cup arthroplasty of the rheumatoid shoulder. Acta Orthop Scand. 1986;57(6):542–6.
4. Levy O, Funk L, Sforza G, Copeland SA. Copeland surface replacement arthroplasty of the shoulder in rheumatoid arthritis. J Bone Joint Surg Am. 2004;86-A(3):512–8.
5. Rydholm UMD. Humeral head resurfacing in the rheumatoid shoulder. Tech Orthop. 2003;18(3):267–71.
6. Thomas SR, Wilson AJ, Chambler A, Harding I, Thomas M. Outcome of Copeland surface replacement shoulder arthroplasty. J Shoulder Elbow Surg. 2005;14(5):485–91.
7. Rydholm U, Sjögren J. Surface replacement of the humeral head in the rheumatoid shoulder. J Shoulder Elbow Surg. 1993;2:286–95.
8. Levy O, Copeland SA. Cementless surface replacement arthroplasty of the shoulder. 5- to 10-year results with the Copeland Mark-2 prosthesis. J Bone Joint Surg Br. 2001;83(2):213–21.
9. Neviaser RJ, Neviaser TJ. Lesions of musculotendinous cuff of shoulder: diagnosis and management. Instr Course Lect. 1981;30:239–57.
10. Mackenzie DB. The antero superior exposure of a total shoulder replacement. Arthop Traumatol. 1993;2:71–7.
11. Copeland SAF, Levy OM, Brownlow HCF. Resurfacing arthroplasty of the shoulder. Tech Shoulder Elb Surg. 2003;4(4):199–210.
12. Alund M, Hoe-Hansen C, Tillander B, Heden BA, Norlin R. Outcome after cup hemiarthroplasty in the rheumatoid shoulder: a retrospective evaluation of 39 patients followed for 2–6 years. Acta Orthop Scand. 2000;71(2):180–4.
13. Fink B, Singer J, Lamla U, Ruther W. Surface replacement of the humeral head in rheumatoid arthritis. Arch Orthop Trauma Surg. 2004;124(6):366–73.
14. Neer CS, Watson KC, Stanton FJ. Recent experience in total shoulder replacement. J Bone Joint Surg Am. 1982;64(3):319–37.
15. Barrett WP, Franklin JL, Jackins SE, Wyss CR, Matsen III FA. Total shoulder arthroplasty. J Bone Joint Surg Am. 1987;69(6):865–72.
16. Torchia ME, Cofield RH, Settergren CR. Total shoulder arthroplasty with the Neer prosthesis: long-term results. J Shoulder Elbow Surg. 1997;6(6):495–505.

17. Cofield RH. Total shoulder arthroplasty with the Neer prosthesis. J Bone Joint Surg Am. 1984;66(6):899–906.

18. Gartsman GM, Russell JA, Gaenslen E. Modular shoulder arthroplasty. J Shoulder Elbow Surg. 1997;6(4):333–9.

19. Boileau P, Walch G. The three-dimensional geometry of the proximal humerus. Implications for surgical technique and prosthetic design. J Bone Joint Surg Br. 1997;79(5):857–65.

20. Tytherleigh-Strong GM, Levy O, Sforza G, Copeland SA. The role of arthroscopy for the problem shoulder arthroplasty. J Shoulder Elbow Surg. 2002;11(3):230–4.

21. Relwani J, Sivaprakasam M. Principles of computer assisted shoulder arthroplasty and the signature shoulder replacement. ICSES. 2010; Instructional course abstracts IC5.4, p. 16.

Treatment of Proximal Humerus Fractures by Plate Osteosynthesis

David Limb

Contents

Abstract

Plate fixation for fractures of the proximal humerus is the most reliable technique for obtaining secure fixation of multi-fragmentary injuries. Although the security of fixation has further improved with the introduction of locking plates, the complication rate remains high. This is in part due to the nature of the injury itself, with the attendant risk of avascular necrosis and peri-articular tissue stiffness, but also due to the difficulties of applying correct surgical technique. Despite improved plate designs, the requirement to obtain fixation in good subchondral bone leaves a high risk of intra-articular penetration by screws and this is one contributor to the relatively high rate of re-operation. This chapter describes current surgical technique for plate fixation of proximal humeral fractures, illustrated by perhaps the most common method of locking plate fixation through a deltopectoral approach.

Keywords

Anatomy, Pathology and Biomechanics • Bone plate • Complications • Fixation • Fracture • Locking plate • Operative Technique • Osteosynthesis • Pre-operative planning and imaging • Reduction • Rehabilitation • Shoulder • Surgical indications

D. Limb
Chapel Allerton Hospital, Leeds, UK
e-mail: d.limb@leeds.ac.uk

G. Bentley (ed.), *European Surgical Orthopaedics and Traumatology*,
DOI 10.1007/978-3-642-34746-7_59, © EFORT 2014

General Introduction

In treating fractures of the proximal humerus the surgeon is faced with some difficult choices. Perhaps the most important of these is the one that has to be made in the face of conflicting or inadequate evidence – should the patient be offered surgery or will non-operative treatment be adequate? Historically we know that non-operative management has good reported outcomes, certainly for minimally-displaced fractures, but even apparently innocuous injuries can give rise to prolonged stiffness. Stable fixation may allow earlier and faster rehabilitation, and perhaps minimise stiffness, but the evidence from randomised trials is lacking. It is also the case that non-operative treatment for significantly displaced fractures, multi-part fractures and those associated with dislocation, is associated with poor functional results. However the surgical management of these injuries is also unproved and we still await trials with sufficient power to establish the role of surgical fixation.

The second problem is what fixation method to use? Percutaneous methods may minimise soft tissue injury and carry less risk to the vascularity of the humeral head, but by their nature do not always give sufficient stability to allow aggressive early motion. Rehabilitation is facilitated if strong fixation of the fragments is obtained using plates or nails, but there is inevitably a greater insult to the blood supply. In reality the technique a surgeon selects will also depend on his/her own experience and training and will be influenced by a range of patient – related factors. This chapter will therefore present plate fixation as one method of managing proximal humeral fractures and it is probably the most popular current method. However, most shoulder surgeons would include all alternative methods of fixation described in this text in their repertoire, tailoring the choice to their own skills and experience, their assessment of the patient and the patient's own choice and their interpretation of the literature, which shapes the final decision.

Aetiology and Classification

The surgical anatomy of the shoulder has been described elsewhere. Most proximal humeral fractures occur as a result of a fall from standing height and there are several contributory factors to the pattern of injury observed. The energy of injury refers to the energy dissipated in creating the fracture and, in general, the higher the energy dissipated the more fracture lines exist and the greater is the displacement of fracture fragments. The actual pattern of injury observed depends on the direction of force application, whether this pushes the humeral head into the glenoid, up into the acromion or translates it to the glenoid rim or even into a position of dislocation. Furthermore the pull of the strong rotator cuff tendons (or lack of it in the presence of a cuff tear) will nave an influence, as will the degree of osteoporosis.

A number of classification systems have been proposed for proximal humeral fractures and none stands up to rigorous testing in terms of inter- and intra-observer agreement [1, 2]. Each has its own unique attributes and problems – for example the AO classification [3] is quite granular and may be useful for research, but is quite difficult to use on a day-to-day basis, as it is not intuitive. However, these classification systems are very useful in communication and in helping the surgeon shape his/her thoughts when assessing a fracture. The Neer classification system in particular has become part of the common language of trauma surgery [4]. This system simplifies the anatomy of the proximal humerus into functional units between which fracture lines tend to pass – a concept proposed by Codman [5] and more recently developed by Hertel with the 'Lego brick' model [6].

These classification systems describe the proximal humerus as four separate 'parts' that can be dis-assembled by injury. The parts are the shaft of the humerus, the articular part of the humeral head, the greater tuberosity and the lesser tuberosity. This is useful conceptually, as the two tuberosities carry the attachments of the rotator cuff, which normally stabilises the articular part of the humeral head in the socket and creates a stable fulcrum for movement of the humeral shaft. It is therefore clear to see that any significant disruption of any one of these 'parts' will have a marked effect on shoulder function. Furthermore it becomes apparent that the best chance of restoring normal function will be with treatment that maintains or restores these four 'parts' into their correct relationship with each other.

If a classification system is used that considers the proximal humerus as four parts this does not, of course, enable accurate description of all fracture patterns. Neer added two further factors to his classification system to enable description of injuries that have a prognosis that is more compromised – the presence or absence of associated glenohumeral dislocation (which disrupts capsular attachments, compromises blood supply and has a higher risk of non-union and avascular necrosis) and the occurrence of a 'head split' – a displaced fracture of the articular surface of the humeral head itself. This not only carries a risk of arthritis if not anatomically reduced, but also has a significant effect on the blood supply to one or more of the articular head segments, leading Neer to suggest that the appropriate treatment was humeral head replacement in all cases. However the valgus impacted fracture (Fig. 1) has a much more favourable prognosis than its classification, according to Neer, would suggest [7, 8]. Note that the subdivision into fracture sub-types requires that the fracture is displaced by at least 1 cm or rotated by 45°, according to Neer's system – most proximal humeral fracture patterns involve displacements that are less than this and only those parts meeting these criteria should be counted as separate parts. Thus the majority of shoulder fractures are in fact one part fractures, even though fracture lines may involve the surgical neck or tuberosities, and have a good prognosis and are suitable for non-operative management.

The most obvious fallacy with classification systems that rely on the description of four parts is that there is an assumption that fracture lines occur at the junction between the four parts. This description is usually appropriate for fractures

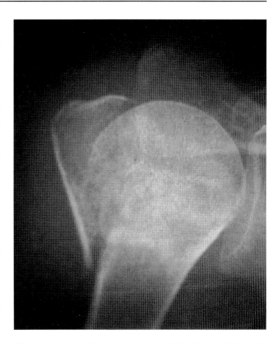

Fig. 1 A valgus impacted fracture. The 'medial hinge' is intact, giving this fracture pattern more mechanical stability and a lower risk of avascular necrosis

between the humeral head segment and the shaft, and indeed between the tuberosities and the humeral head. However the fracture lines rarely pass directly between the lesser and greater tuberosity as this is the location of the bicipital groove, which has a floor of dense cortical bone and a reinforced roof across the groove, connecting the greater and lesser tuberosities. Thus fracture lines tend to pass lateral to the bicipital groove, or on both sides with the segment of bone containing the groove separating as a unique fragment – the 'shield' [9]. Whilst this might not affect decision-making it can affect surgery, as the approach to the fracture for reduction is usually through the fracture lines and stabilisation of the separate fragments will be required when definitive fixation is undertaken.

An appreciation of the overall pattern of disruption is therefore communicated by classification, but the imaging of each injury has to be studied carefully in preparing the surgical tactic, as the anatomy of the fracture can vary significantly even between fractures that are classified into the same group.

Relevant Applied Anatomy, Pathology and Biomechanics

The relevant anatomy of the proximal humerus is described by the above classification systems; the shaft, humeral head, greater- and lesser tuberosities often being considered as the four main 'parts' upon which these systems are based. This concept has not simply been developed for anatomical convenience however. The pattern of fractures has a large part to play in determining the long-term outcome, as each of the 'parts' described above is not only structurally important but is integral to the normal biomechanical environment of the shoulder and in the pattern of blood flow around the shoulder.

In addressing shoulder fractures some simple anatomical facts must be borne in mind. For instance, the humeral head is retroverted such that it faces the glenoid fossa when the humerus is in neutral rotation. We are used to looking at AP radiographs of the shoulder showing a plate on the lateral cortex of the proximal humerus. However these films are taken also with the humerus turned so that the forearm faces forwards, so that humeral rotation is neutral. In reconstructing the shoulder therefore the patient must not be positioned with the arm across the chest, as this internally rotates the shaft by almost 90° – if a plate is fixed laterally with the arm across the chest then a gross internal rotation deformity will result and external rotation will not return. The arm should be free so that the forearm can be pointed forwards, bringing the humerus into neutral rotation. In this position screws should be directed about 30° posterior to the coronal plane, in the line of the retroverted humeral head articulating with the glenoid. It is also important to restore the length of the humerus as shortening will weaken deltoid and inhibit rehabilitation.

The humeral head articulates with the glenoid and any violation of this relationship, by dislocation or intra-articular injury, will clearly disrupt glenohumeral joint function. Likewise anything that impacts or tilts the humeral head will affect the length-tension relationships in the rotator cuff muscles, the deltoid and in the other scapulohumeral and axohumeral muscles that cross the joint. After fracture the shoulder may function well with a degree of mal-union, but it cannot function normally if the head and shaft are not restored to their normal length, alignment and rotation (see chapter on ▶ "Biomechanics of the Shoulder"). Fortunately even moderately large deficits in range or strength can be absorbed by the compensatory mechanisms within the articulations of the ipsilateral upper limb and by transfer to the opposite upper limb, so function may be maintained.

The functions of the rotator cuff are described elsewhere in this text. If the greater and/or lesser tuberosities are separated from the humeral head and shaft they will displace by the pull of the cuff muscles and a significant functional deficit will occur. Care should be taken on radiographs to identify such fractures and to treat accordingly. Minimally displaced fractures can displace with time, so repeated radiographs are required during rehabilitation. On the AP view a greater tuberosity fragment attached to supraspinatus may be seen displaced into the acromiohumeral space, where it is obvious. However a larger fragment with infraspinatus attached (particularly if there was a pre-existing supraspinatus tear – not uncommon over the age of 65) will displace posteriorly and can be missed on the AP view. Axial views are mandatory and may be the only plain images on which displaced lesser- and greater tuberosity fragments are visible. The functional effects of a displaced tuberosity may be much more significant that a cuff tear de-functioning a similarly-sized area of tuberosity, as the bone fragment itself will malunite and physically block rotation through the subacromial space or against the margin of the glenoid, depending on the direction of displacement.

Blood Supply

The blood supply to the humeral head is derived normally from the nutrient artery, via the shaft. This is clearly interrupted in fractures of the surgical neck. A supply also enters through the rotator cuff insertion, but also at the capsular insertion. The anterior two-third of the humeral head is supplied by the anterior circumflex humeral artery, which sends an ascending branch to the anterior capsule adjacent to the bicipital groove [10]. Note however that this is a common site of fracture and this significant blood vessel may be injured by the fracture itself. Worse still, perhaps, it is vulnerable to injury at surgery if dissection is carried out in the region of the biceps tendon or if plates are applied in this area.

Medially there are several branches, which enter at the capsule insertion, and this has implications for one particular fracture pattern – the valgus impacted fracture. It has long been noted that although 4-part fractures, according to the Neer classification, have a significant risk of avascular necrosis, those with minimal displacement of the 'medial hinge' [6] – the junction between head and shaft medially – do not share this poor prognosis. Thus, valgus impacted fractures can be carefully reduced and fixed with the expectation of a much lower risk of late complications. However this relies on the surgeon avoiding dissection or significant displacing forces on the intact hinge, which would interrupt the supply. Such fractures are therefore ideal for percutaneous methods of reduction and fixation or plate fixation after reducing the fracture by careful elevation of the head using access through fracture lines.

Biomechanics

The biomechanics of the implants that can be used to fix proximal humerus fractures also deserves brief mention. Although plate fixation has been practiced for years, it was recognised that if the fracture itself was unstable then displacement could, and frequently did, occur after fixation with conventional screws and plates, as the screws could toggle in the plate-holes and offered no resistance to relative movement between fracture fragments unless the fragments were compressed together, which is not usually possible in multi-fragmentary fractures typical of osteoporotic injuries. The situation was improved by the introduction of specific blade-plates for use in the

shoulder, which are fixed-angle devices that can be shown on testing to significantly resist fracture displacement. Unfortunately the complication rate was found to be high [11] and impaction of the blade into the head of an unstable 3 or 4 part fracture was itself apt to cause displacement of previously minimally-displaced tuberosity fragments. Locking plates were developed and these provide stable fixation [12] and have similar biomechanical properties to blade-plates but are inserted in a manner that is much easier to control, with a hold that includes bone from a greater proportion of the head than a blade can reach. Although blades do engage in the strongest, central bone in the humeral head, multiple screws or pins can take advantage of the strong bone that is distributed around the entire humeral head in a subchondral location [13]. For now, angular stable locking plates are the implant of choice when plate fixation is selected for the fixation of shoulder fractures but, as will be seen, they are not without complications themselves.

Diagnosis

Diagnosis in trauma cases is usually straightforward, with a history of an impact to the shoulder or transmitted through the arm followed by severe pain and dysfunction. There is tenderness proximally and, with fractures involving the surgical neck in particular, there may be fracture crepitus. Radiographs in at least two planes are mandatory and will be discussed further when pre-operative planning is considered. Radiographs in two planes will significantly increase the chances of identifying dislocations and displacement of fractured tuberosities. However, thorough clinical assessment will be needed to identify other aspects of the injury that can influence management. Thus a careful assessment of the skin condition, and any open wound, should be followed by a documented assessment of the neurovascular status. Fracture-dislocations in particular can be associated with nerve and vessel injuries, including brachial plexus injuries. In very high energy injuries, particularly those involving an associated clavicle fracture, a chest radiograph will have been taken and should be reviewed to ensure the scapulae are equidistant from the spine – an increase in the distance between medial border of the scapula and the spine is seen in scapulothoracic dissociation, which carries a very high risk of arterial injury and brachial plexus avulsion; fixation of the proximal humerus may be an important part of reconstruction. Low energy injuries may reflect underlying osteoporosis, but other causes of pathological fracture may have to be sought and excluded.

Indications for Surgery

The indications for surgical fixation of proximal humeral fractures have not been clearly defined. Furthermore the suitability of one method of fixation over another has not been subjected to sufficiently rigorous scientific inquiry to be able to define where plate fixation has clear advantages over percutaneous methods, intramedullary fixation and indeed whether a locking plate will give better results than a (usually cheaper) non-locking option.

That being said, it is a fundamental concept in the management of fractures by internal fixation that earlier mobilisation and function are encouraged. In practice, therefore, the internal fixation of proximal humeral fractures is carried out when the patient and surgeon agree that the risks of treatment are outweighed by the potential benefits in restoring proximal humeral anatomy and allowing early active use.

Thus plate fixation is usually considered to be indicated when there is a displaced fracture of the proximal humerus that can be reduced to an anatomic or near-anatomical state, be held there by devices that are sufficiently robust to allow early physiological loading without incurring a very high risk of avascular necrosis of the whole, or part, of the humeral head. 3- and 4-part fractures are therefore commonly treated by fixation. Similar fracture configurations associated with dislocation, or head-splitting fractures, are more likely to be considered for humeral head replacement, particularly in the elderly.

Two-part fractures involving the surgical neck are more likely to be treated by internal fixation if there is significant medial displacement of the shaft, particularly if contact between shaft and head is lost completely. No benefit has been shown for internal fixation of any of these fractures in the very elderly and infirm, particularly if they are incapable of following a fairly rigorous rehabilitation regime after surgery.

Two-part fractures involving the surgical neck are ideal fractures for fixation using intramedullary devices, though it has to be borne in mind that locking nails and locking plates may be a very expensive option for a fracture that may heal well without surgery, or with simpler devices such as percutaneous wires or straightforward non-locking plates and screws.

The question of intervention thresholds with respect to fracture displacement has not been clearly answered and in any event has to be considered taking in all patient-related as well as injury-related factors. However we know that varus deformity of more than 20° is not tolerated well [14, 15] and it is generally accepted that greater tuberosity displacement of more than 5 mm carries a high risk of functional impairment.

Pre-Operative Preparation and Planning

Imaging is important in deciding whether or not to fix a fracture, as well as in deciding which methods of fixation may be appropriate. It is then important in planning surgery, once the decision has been made to treat by internal fixation using a plate. The same images serve both purposes.

Plain radiographs in at least two planes are essential. The standard trauma series for the shoulder includes AP, scapular lateral and axillary views. However all of the necessary information is usually available on the AP and axillary views alone (Fig. 2) and many units limit radiation exposure in the acute setting to these two projections. A single AP view is inadequate and poses a particular risk for missing a posterior dislocation, with or without a fracture.

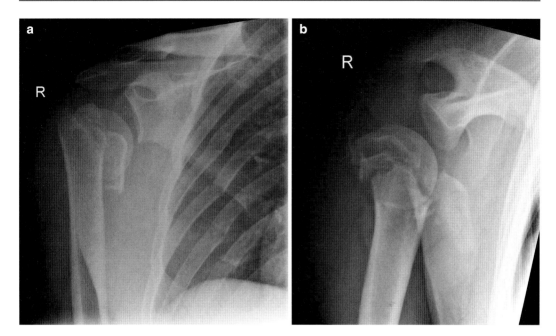

Fig. 2 AP and axial views contain most of the information needed to plan surgical treatment for proximal humeral fractures, though supplementary scans, especially CT with multi-planar reconstruction, can be invaluable

Many units will also supplement plain radiographs with 3D imaging, most usefully CT with multi-planar or 3D reconstruction. Whilst the latter has the potential to give the surgeon the best concept of the size and displacement of the main fracture fragments, it also has some drawbacks. At present the rendering software that is used to reconstruct 2-dimensional slices into a representation of a solid form relies on smoothing software to take off steps and sharp edges between layers. In doing so it can render undisplaced or minimally-displaced fracture lines invisible. 3D reconstructions should always therefore be read in conjunction with 2D slices. However, 3D reconstructions are invaluable in the visualisation of complex fracture patterns and in planning the most appropriate approach and fixation construct for such injuries.

Imaging therefore confirms the number of fracture lines and therefore the number of main fracture fragments. It indicates which fragments are displaced and to what degree. This not only allows fractures to be categorised for communication and research purposes, for example with Neer's classification, but also permits the surgical tactic to be planned.

The vast majority of fractures can be approached and fixed through a deltopectoral approach. However this approach is disadvantageous when the greater tuberosity, under the influence of the attached infraspinatus and supraspinatus, is displaced posterior to the humeral head and in a medial direction, towards the glenoid margin. If imaging does suggest that reduction manoeuvres behind the humeral head may be necessary then a lateral deltoid split can be performed, as originally described for the management of posterior fracture dislocations, though originally felt to be limited to an operative window above the axillary nerve [16]. However, more recently it has been demonstrated that the axillary nerve can be identified and windows created above and below the nerve for access [17]. A plate can therefore be inserted into the superior incision and can be slid under the nerve and down the lateral shaft. A separate window below the nerve can be used to insert distal screws in the plate. This approach places the plate more laterally on the shaft than a deltopectoral approach

Fig. 3 Theatre set-up. The surgeon should have access to the operative site with a clear view of the image intensifier screen. The intensifier itself should be positioned to allow imaging without interference with the surgical access

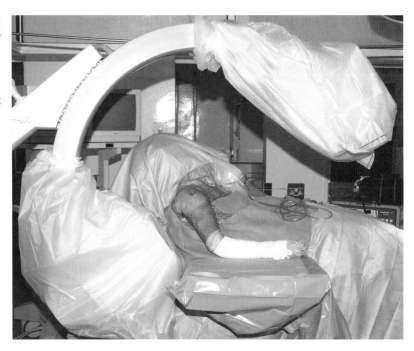

and, if a long plate is used, detachment of the deltoid insertion becomes necessary. However, the deltoid tendon is in continuity with the lateral intermuscular septum and there do not appear to be any significant functional consequences of subperiosteal release of the anterior deltoid insertion to allow plate fixation. It should be borne in mind that whatever approach is used, it should be suitable for re-use at a future time. A recent systematic review of the treatment of 3- and 4-part fractures with locking plates revealed a re-operation rate of 13.7 % [18].

Surgery will entail reduction manoeuvres that must be carried out with minimal disturbance of the soft tissue envelope, and any remaining attachments of tendon, capsule and fascia to fracture fragments must be preserved in order to preserve the blood supply. Consequently an image intensifier becomes essential and arrangements must be made for the relevant equipment and staff to be available. Theatre set-up must also be planned to accommodate the intensifier and allow a clear line of vision between the surgeon and the image screen (Fig. 3).

The incidence of infection is low. However, the axillary sweat glands are a reservoir for Proprionobacter spp. and this can be very difficult to isolate from specimens taken in cases of suspected infection and may need longer incubation than the 48 h commonly employed in clinical laboratories. Proprionobacter acnes remains the commonest organism causing infection of shoulder replacements and after rotator cuff surgery and should be considered if infection develops after plate fixation [19, 20]. Local antibiotic prophylaxis guidelines should be adhered to and these should take into account the potential infecting organisms.

Operative Technique

Regardless of whether a deltopectoral or deltoid-splitting approach is used the patient is best prepared in a "beach-chair" position with the arm draped free to allow manipulation and rotation of the humeral shaft via the forearm (if it is not also injured). The arm can be rested on a side table and, by adjusting the height of this to abduct the arm slightly, tension in the deltoid can be relieved to facilitate retraction and exposure of the proximal humerus (Fig. 4). This chapter will describe fixation using the deltopectoral approach, which has the advantage

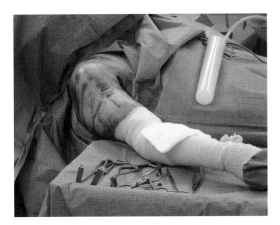

Fig. 4 The arm is rested on a table so that it can be manipulated to facilitate reduction. Raising the table and abducting the arm both relieve tension in the deltoid, improving access

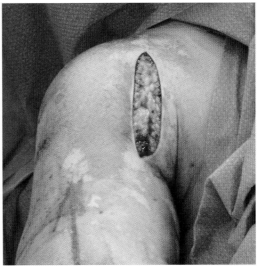

Fig. 5 The incision extends from the lateral margin of the coracoid towards the upper medial part of the arm, lateral to the axillary fold

of being a general utility incision for the shoulder and can be used for almost any future shoulder surgery the patient may need.

The skin incision should be sufficient without being unnecessarily long. The incision will usually start at the lateral edge of the coracoid process, but this depends partly on the locking plate being used as this dictates how high on the lateral humerus it will sit. The incision then passes down to the top of the anterior axillary crease and can continue in the deltopectoral interval for as long as is necessary to obtain sufficient length of plate beyond the fracture (Fig. 5). For complex fractures a bridge-plate technique may be used, in which case a smaller proximal incision is made to allow reduction and fixation of the head and tuberosities, the plate being slid in contact with bone distally where it can be exposed through a separate incision, beyond the zone of bone injury, to secure distal fixation.

After making the skin incision the deltopectoral interval is opened. The cephalic vein can be retracted medially or laterally – lateral retraction puts the vein under more tension with retraction and it is more likely to be injured when using drills and screwdrivers. However medial retraction often results in avulsion of short tributaries from the deltoid, which can be difficult to control except by tying off and sacrificing the vein. There is no significant morbidity if the cephalic vein is lost,

whichever method is chosen. A self-retaining retractor is inserted to separate the deltoid and pectoralis major.

The surgeon is then confronted by swollen, bruised tissue quite unlike the expected appearance gleaned from anatomy texts and most manufacturer's surgical technique guides. The thoracobrachial fascia extends laterally from the conjoined tendon and contains blood and oedema from the fracture site, obscuring any view of the subscapularis tendon and proximal humerus (Fig. 6). The fascia is opened along the lateral edge of the conjoined tendon and can be excised with the underlying oedematous areolar tissue to expose the lesser tuberosity and attached subscapularis (Fig. 7).

Hereafter the procedure depends on the fracture configuration but consists of two steps – reduction of the fracture fragments and stabilisation with an internal fixation device.

Reduction

The rotator cuff, biceps tendon and its roofed tunnel, pectoralis major and deltoid insertions all bind and restrain elements of the fracture so

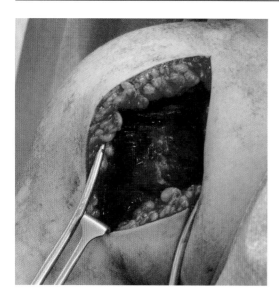

Fig. 6 The deltopectoral interval is opened and the thoracobrachial fascia is encountered. This is usually oedematous and bruised, obscuring vision of the underlying subscapularis and tuberosities

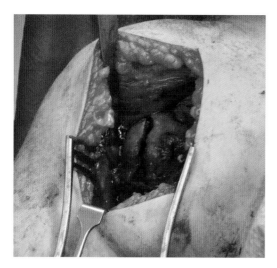

Fig. 7 After excising thoracobrachial fascia the tuberosities and fracture lines that are not obscured by cuff attachments come into view

visualisation requires image intensification. Any soft tissue attachments should be preserved, even if release would facilitate direct visualisation of the reduction. The various fragments should therefore be mechanically controlled so that they can be brought together with the correct length, alignment and rotation before fixation. With two-part fractures this is relatively simple in theory (though often surprisingly tricky in practice, especially if the bone is osteoporotic and fragmented). The shaft can be controlled by gripping the arm and manually positioning it under the head to bring the fracture surfaces together. Difficulty can arise if there has been significant displacement at the time of injury, which can leave soft tissue, including the long head of biceps tendon, caught in the fracture over bone spikes and blocking reduction.

For multi-fragmentary fractures it is usually necessary to obtain some sort of hold on each fragment so that all fragments can be independently rotated, pulled and pushed to secure reduction. If the humeral head still has an attached tuberosity this can be controlled either by a stout wire through the tuberosity, which can be used as a joystick, or by taking a bite of the rotator cuff at its insertion into the tuberosity with strong suture material (No. 5 braided polyester, for example). For separated tuberosity fragments the latter technique is best, as wires tend to split the shell of bone attached to a separated tuberosity.

The most critical suture is that which is most difficult to place – that controlling the greater tuberosity from posterior displacement under the influence of infraspinatus. If the greater tuberosity is displaced behind the humeral head this can be difficult to reach through a deltopectoral approach and consideration may have been given to using a lateral deltoid split. However the suture can be positioned by using a 'piggy-back' technique. A stout suture is placed in the supraspinatus and is used to pull the greater tuberosity forwards. This exposes a more posterior segment of the cuff, in which a second stout suture is placed. The first is removed, then the second is used to pull the cuff forwards again. Stepwise the cuff, and its attached bony fragments, is brought into view until eventually a suture can be placed behind the greater tuberosity, and can be used to apply traction to reduce and fix the tuberosity.

For 3- and 4-part fractures stout sutures, for example No. 5 braided polyester as described

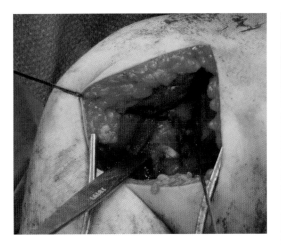

Fig. 8 Reducing the fracture – the lesser tuberosity has been reduced and fixed to the head with a temporary wire whilst a braided suture through the posterior cuff insertion is being used to control the greater tuberosity. An elevator passes through the neck fracture site and is being used to elevate the humeral head

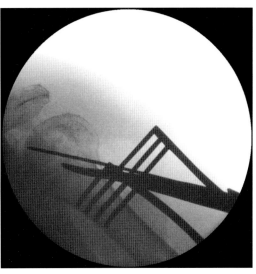

Fig. 9 Image intensifier view of the humeral head being elevated into the coracoacromial arch to obtain fracture reduction

above, should be passed through the cuff where it inserts into each bony fragment. Once the tuberosity fragments are controlled in this way the head should be reduced. This is achieved by passing an elevator of some sort (the author uses the periosteal elevator from a small fragment set) through the fracture site and into contact with the fracture surface of the humeral head (Fig. 8). The head can then be pushed up into the coracoacromial arch whilst the arm is pulled down, using image intensification (Fig. 9) to check that the force is being applied in the correct place to reduce the head (for example, pushing up on the lateral part of the fracture surface of a valgus head). Once the head is reduced in relation to the glenoid fossa the tuberosities can be pulled out to restore their positions around the head – if the head is correctly reduced the tuberosities can lock around it and a surprisingly stable fracture reduction may be obtained. At this point further consideration can be given to temporary stabilisation with K wires through the tuberosities into the reduced head. Sometimes it is possible to take the suture that is passing through the posterior part of the cuff around the front and take a bite of the subscapularis insertion. This can then be tied as a tension band

connecting the greater to lesser tuberosities around the head (indeed, one form of minimally-invasive surgery does just this, then secures the greater tuberosity to the shaft with another suture giving a reduction that can be maintained without further implants, though it is not capable of withstanding physiological loads until union begins). If a suture is tied as a lateral tension band in this way, it will come to lie under the plate and care will have to be taken to avoid damaging the suture when drilling holes for screws. If the plate is applied first, then the sutures pre-placed in the rotator cuff insertions can be passed through purpose-made holes designed into most modern locking implants to stabilise the tuberosities.

If there is a void beneath the humeral head, consideration should be given at this stage to filling this to improve initial stability. It is not known whether this makes any difference to the risk of loss of reduction in the longer term. The void can be filled with bone graft or bone graft substitutes (which avoid the problem of donor site morbidity, particularly in fragility fractures where donor bone may also be of poor structural quality). Other authors have used structural support beneath the humeral head, either in the form of fibular strut graft [21], bone cement or

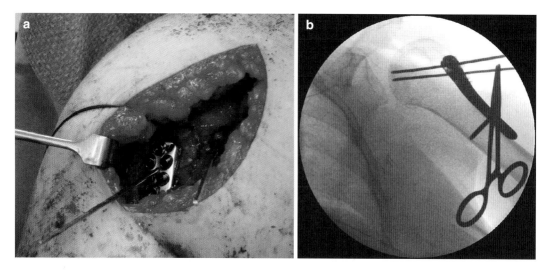

Fig. 10 After provisional reduction a plate is applied with an initial wire or screw through the plate (**a**) to allow screening in two planes to check correct plate positioning (**b**)

substitutes [22] or metallic implants specifically designed to support the humeral head and resist the tendency to tip into varus or valgus.

Once the tuberosities and head are stabilised in this way the 3- or 4-part fracture has been converted to a 2-part fracture and all that remains is to reduce the shaft beneath the head/tuberosity construct and stabilise this with a plate.

Fixation

Whilst locking plates have the advantages that come with a fixed-angle design, this also means that the first screw in the construct fixes the position of the plate in relation to the humerus. If this is incorrect, the locking screws will not evenly distribute through the head but will group towards the front or back of the head, making some screw holes unusable. It is good practice, therefore, to select the plate position and insert a single, central screw (or wire (Fig. 10a, b), if the plate is designed to allow wires to be passed on a fixed trajectory through the plate) and to screen the device in both AP and axillary planes before completing the fixation.

The shaft may be medially displaced and, if reduction of the head fragments has not been straightforward, one may not be keen to manipulate the shaft forcefully to lateralise the shaft. In these circumstances consider placing the plate in its correct height in relation to the head then drilling and measuring for a non-locking screw passing through the plate into the medially-displaced shaft. If the displacement is not too great, tightening the screw will pull the shaft to the plate, bringing it back under the head. The screw will then be too long, but can be changed or removed once the remaining screws have been placed in the proximal humerus and the shaft.

The placement of locking screws or pegs into the head fragment should fix the relationship between the head and shaft (Fig. 11a, b). If the screws pass through the tuberosity fragments then these too will be stabilised. However, a laterally-placed plate will not, in many cases, allow screws passing through the plate to stabilise the lesser tuberosity or a separated posterior greater tuberosity fragment. For this reason many locking plate systems allow heavy sutures or wires to be passed through holes in the plate – this allows the No 5 braided sutures that have been used to reduce the fracture to maintain the reduction by incorporation into the fixation device. Securing the tuberosities is a critical step and migration of

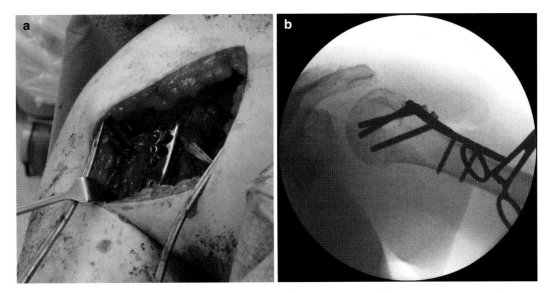

Fig. 11 After confirming plate position the remaining screws and/or pegs are inserted (**a**) and checked (**b**)

the tuberosities results in significant impairment of the outcome. Tenuous fixation relying on one or two of the screws catching the edge of the tuberosity fragments is simply not acceptable.

If locking screws are not used great care has to be taken to minimise forces on the screws that might allow the head fragment to rotate, as this will allow the screws to toggle in the plate and the head will tilt into varus or valgus (usually returning towards the displacement that was reduced before fixation). The most effective way of neutralising these forces is to obtain anatomical reduction of the head and tuberosities when good bone stock is present – if there has been impaction or comminution, stability may require reconstitution of the defect as described above. With locking plate systems, however, these defects will often fill in without the need for graft.

The placement of screws should take advantage of the best bone for fixation and this is inevitably in the subchonral region of the head. Holes for screws should be drilled up to the subchondral plate but drilling into the joint should be avoided, not least because it facilitates screw penetration into the joint if there is any error in measurement or if the head settles down onto the fixation device during rehabilitation.

For the same reasons careful measurement is required. Blunt pegs, rather than screws, can be used in the humeral head. These allow the head to sit on an array of pegs but they do not have sharp tips, theoretically reducing the risk of screw cut-out and head penetration (Fig. 12).

Once the locking screws have been placed into the head, which itself has already been secured to the shaft with one screw, all that remains is for the remaining screws to be placed in the plate as it lies on the shaft. If there is metaphyseal comminution a larger plate may have been selected to bridge the area, otherwise a plate with three bicortical screws below the head is generally sufficient. With modern systems these screws may be locked, improving the performance of the fixation in osteoporotic bone. Images are checked in two planes, as the most common complication of most locking plate systems is penetration of the humeral head by screws [23].

Thereafter the wound is washed out, taking care not to disturb any bone graft. If graft has not been used by this stage, there is one more opportunity to consider inserting it before the wound is closed. Otherwise the deltopectoral groove is allowed to fall back together, a drain is inserted if desired and the fat and skin layers are closed.

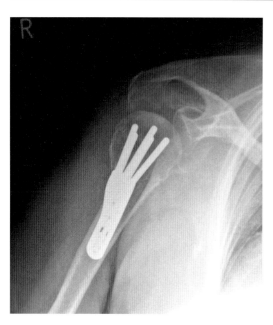

Fig. 12 After fixation check films are taken – in this case a system has been used that supports the humeral head on a series of blunt pegs. Alternatively screws may be used in the humeral head segment

Post-Operative Care and Rehabilitation

Open reduction and internal fixation is carried out to restore the mechanics of the shoulder so that ultimately a normal, or near-normal, outcome is possible. When plate fixation is selected, rather than minimally-invasive or minimal fixation methods, the second aim is to allow early physiological loading to accelerate rehabilitation. Thus, early range of movement exercises and the promotion of early function are desirable. Patients may be fitted with a sling for comfort, and movements may be delayed long enough to ensure that wound healing has commenced (therefore could be delayed if there is any wound discharge), but in general the rehabilitation programme can commence as soon as the patient has recovered from anaesthesia.

There is a wide range of opinion on exactly how rehabilitation care should be delivered after shoulder surgery, and this article will only touch on the guiding principles. The first of these is that few health care systems can afford for reliance to be placed on a third party for delivering the rehabilitation programme. Whilst physiotherapists may assess, advise, progress and facilitate the programme, the onus is on the patient to get the shoulder working again using the rehabilitation programme outlined to them, as this is a job that can occupy several hours a day. Indeed this should be impressed on patients before surgery, as a beautifully-fixed fracture, that is rested in a sling and all painful activity avoided permanently, will become a useless shoulder.

Rehabilitation programmes attend to pain, range of movement, strength and finally functional restoration of correct neuromuscular control. Most studies show that early rehabilitation gives the best results [24]. As the elderly population are primarily affected attention should be paid to secondary prevention, not only in the detection and treatment of osteoporosis, but also in falls prevention with rehabilitation of balance and neuromuscular control mechanisms. A sling may be used for pain relief – a collar-and-cuff may allow gravity assistance with the maintenance of alignment in non-operatively treated fractures, though this is only true when the patient is upright. Many one-part fractures are sufficiently stable that movement can begin immediately – often gentle, unloaded swinging movements such as pendular exercises. The same is true for operatively-fixed fractures and the aim of plate fixation is to allow immediate motion to reduce the duration and extent of stiffness: few shoulder fractures, even after anatomical reduction and fixation, will regain absolutely normal range of movement.

No hard and fast guidelines can be made about the speed of progress through rehabilitation as this depends in part on the security of fixation achieved at surgery. Even in osteoporotic bone one is usually confident that the head-shaft fixation is good enough to allow gentle active motion immediately. Tuberosity fixation that is dependant on sutures may bring an element of caution to the resumption of loaded use of the muscles attached to the relevant tuberosity or passive stretch of the same to increase range of movement. However, progressive increase in the application of physiological loading to fixed fractures is needed to stimulate union and in the vast majority of cases one should be able to resume active assisted treatment aimed at the resumption of full range by 3 weeks after surgery and the commencement of loaded activities by 6 weeks.

Complications

The overall complication rate of shoulder fracture fixation with locking plates is high [18, 25], and although fixation systems are becoming more reliable they are also encouraging surgeons to attempt fixation of fractures that would previously have been treated by hemiarthroplasty or by nonoperative means. There is therefore no indication that, as our experience of treating these complex injuries increases, the complication rate is decreasing.

Complications can be related to anaesthesia and, although this is a matter for the anaesthetist to discuss with the surgeon, one should be aware that pneumothorax can acutely compromise respiration but diaphragmatic paralysis can threaten those with pre-existing chest disease. The C4/5 roots are targeted with interscalene blocks for shoulder surgery and many will remember the aide memoire 'C345 keeps the diaphragm alive'. An interscalene block can therefore easily impair diaphragmatic function, which for most patients is easily accommodated by their respiratory reserve. Fortunately this reverses when the block wears off, but this could mean 24 h of respiratory difficulty for those with poor pre-operative lung function. Pneumothorax is a much rarer complication, and is becoming rarer with more widespread use of ultrasound to direct needle insertion and anaesthetic infiltration. Overall, however, interscalene blocks have proved to be very safe [26].

The risks of neurovascular injury in the injured limb are particularly high if there is a dislocation. The axillary nerve is also at risk with deltoid splitting approaches, though recent literature indicates the risk can be significantly minimised if the nerve is properly identified and protected, working through windows above and below the nerve. The "beach-chair" position does result in a small risk of air embolus if division of the cephalic vein is not recognised.

The tissues around the shoulder are very vascular and this mitigates against a high infection risk. However the reported infection rate after fracture fixation is still of the order of 1 % and, as noted above, Proprionobacterium acnes is not uncommon as a causative organism and can be difficult to detect [19, 20].

The most common complications in recent literature relate to the biology of the injury and the mechanics of the fixation. Even with modern locking plates and careful dissection, avoiding soft tissue stripping, the rate of avascular necrosis is significant, the incidence depending on the fracture pattern. If 2- part fractures are discounted, rates of 9 % for avascular necrosis are typical [14]. Decision-making at the time of surgery based on the presence or absence of apparent ischaemia is not reliable, as this has not been shown to be related to the likelihood of future necrosis [27].

However, the rate of screw perforation into the glenohumeral joint is higher still, either occurring at the time of initial surgery or later, if displacement or avascular necrosis of the head occur. In two large multi-centre trials the rate of primary screw perforation was reported to be 14 % [28, 29], and secondary perforation in 8 %. Secondary displacement of fractures after locked-plate fixation is much more common when the initial fracture is displaced into varus compared to when the initial displacement is valgus – 79 % versus 19 % in one study [15].

The true risk-benefit ratio for internal fixation (of any kind) of the proximal humerus is not known. Although many published studies have failed to show dramatic benefits the quality of available studies is not high. This creates significant problems in interpretation as most surgeons agree that a well- motivated, active patient is an ideal candidate for surgery but the inclusion criteria for many studies are based on radiological criteria and the absence of mental insufficiency. Furthermore, publication bias confounds matters further – a moderate benefit from surgery in a poorly constructed trial is unlikely to be published but very poor results, even in a poorly-constructed study, may be published. Randomised trials are on-going and the most recent suggest moderate benefit even in elderly patients, but at the cost of a reoperation rate of almost one in three [25].

Summary

Plate fixation remains the most versatile method of fixing fractures of the proximal humerus, as it can be employed from cases of simple surgical neck fracture with displacement through to complex 3- and 4- part fractures and fracture-dislocations. However the evidence about which fractures should be treated by internal fixation is poor. In the very elderly with poor quality bone and a mental state that does not allow them to co-operate with a rehabilitation regime there is little doubt that the results of surgical treatment are no better than non-operative management. Likewise there is little doubt that the open proximal humeral fracture with axillary artery division needs emergency stabilisation. It is making decisions between these extremes that poses questions to the surgeon that may be impossible to answer with our current knowledge base.

References

1. Siebennrock KA, Gerber C. The reproducibility of classification of fractures of the proximal end of the humerus. J Bone Joint Surg Am. 1993;75(A):1751–5.
2. Sidor ML, Zuckerman JD, Lyon T. The Neer classification system for proximal humeral fractures. An assessment of the interobserver reliability and intraobserver reproducibility. J Bone Joint Surg Am. 1993;75(A):1745–50.
3. Jakob RP, Ganz R. Proximale humerusfrakturen. Helv Chir Acta. 1981;48:595–610.
4. Neer CS. Four-segment classification of proximal humerus fractures. Instr Course Lect. 1975;24:160–8.
5. Codman EA. The shoulder: rupture of the supraspinatus tendon and other lesions in or about the subacromial bursa. Boston: Thomas Todd; 1934.
6. Hertel R, Hempfing M, Stiehler M, Leunig M. Predictors of humeral head ischaemia after intracapsular

7. fracture of the proximal humerus. J Shoulder Elbow Surg. 2004;13(4):427–33.
7. Jakob RP, Miniachi A, Anson PS, et al. Four-part valgus-impacted fractures of the proximal humerus. J Bone Joint Surg Br. 1991;73B:295–8.
8. Resch H, Povacz P, Frohlich R, et al. Percutaneous fixation of three- and four-part fractures of the proximal humerus. J Bone Joint Surg Br. 1997;79B(2): 295–300.
9. Edelson G, Kelly I, Vigder F, Reis ND. A three-dimensional classification for fractures of the proximal humerus. J Bone Joint Surg Br. 2004;86B(3): 413–25.
10. Gerber C, Schneeberger AG, Vinh TS. The arterial vascularisation of the humeral head. An anatomical study. J Bone Joint Surg Am. 1990;72(10): 1486–94.
11. Meier RA, Messmer P, Regazzoni P, Rothfischer W, Gross T. Unexpected high complication rate following internal fixation of unstable proximal humerus fractures with an angled blade plate. J Orthop Trauma. 2006;20(4):253–60.
12. Chudik SC, Weinhold P, Dahners LE. Fixed-angle plate fixation in simulated fractures of the proximal humerus: a biomechanical study of a new device. J Shoulder Elbow Surg. 2003;12(6):578–88.
13. Liew AS, Johnson JA, Patterson SD, King GJ, Chess DG. Effect of screw placement on fixation in the humeral head. J Shoulder Elbow Surg. 2000;9(5): 423–6.
14. Solberg BD, Moon CN, Franco DP, Paiement GD. Surgical treatment of three and four-part proximal humeral fractures. J Bone Joint Surg Am. 2009; 91A(7):1689–97.
15. Solberg BD, Moon CN, Franco DP, Paiement GD. Locked plating of 3- and 4-part proximal humerus fractures in older patients: the effect of initial fracture pattern on outcome. J Orthop Trauma. 2009;23(2): 113–9.
16. Stableforth PG, Sarangi PP. Posterior fracture-dislocation of the shoulder. A superior subacromial approach for open reduction. J Bone Joint Surg Br. 1992;74B(4):579–84.
17. Gardner MJ, Griffith MH, Dines JS, Briggs SM, Weiland AJ, Lorich DG. The extended anterolateral acromion approach allows minimally invasive access to the proximal humerus. Clin Orthop. 2005;434: 123–9.
18. Thanasas C, Kontakis G, Angoules A, Limb D, Giannoudis P. Treatment of proximal humerus fractures with locking plates: a systematic review. J Shoulder Elbow Surg. 2009;18(6):837–44.
19. Levy PY, Fenollar F, Syein A, et al. Proprionobacterium acnes postoperative shoulder arthritis: an emerging clinical entity. Clin Infect Dis. 2008;46:1884.
20. Sperling JW, Kozak TKW, Hanssen AD, Cofield RH. Infection after shoulder arthroplasty. Clin Orthop Relat Res. 2001;382:206–16.

21. Gardner MJ, Boraiah S, Helfet DL, Lorich DG. Indirect medial reduction and strut support of proximal humerus fractures using an endosteal implant. J Orthop Trauma. 2008;22(3):195–200.

22. Kwon BK, Goertzen DJ, O'Brien PJ, Broekhuyse HM, Oxland TR. Biomechanical evaluation of proximal humeral fracture fixation supplemented with calcium phosphate cement. J Bone Joint Surgery Am. 2002;84A(6):951–61.

23. Konrad G, Bayer J, Hepp B, et al. Open reduction and internal fixation of proximal humeral fractures with the use of the locking proximal humerus plate. Sugical technique. J Bone Joint Surg Am. 2010; 92A(Supp 1, pt 1):85–95.

24. Hodgson S, Iannotti JP, Evans PJ. Proximal humerus fracture rehabilitation. Clin Orthop Relat Res. 2006; 442:131–8.

25. Olerud P, Ahrengart L, Ponzer S, et al. Internal fixation versus nonoperative treatment of displaced 3-part proximal humeral fractures in elderly patients: a randomized controlled trial. J Shoulder Elbow Surg. 2011;20:747–55.

26. Borgeat A, Ekatodramis G, Kalberer F, Benz C. Acute and nonacute complications associated with interscalene block and shoulder surgery: a prospective study. Anesthesiology. 2001;95(4):875–80.

27. Bastian JD, Hertel R. Initial post-fracture humeral head ischemia does not predict development of necrosis. J Shoulder Elbow Surg. 2008;17(1):2–8.

28. Brunner F, Sommer C, Bahrs C, et al. Open reduction and internal fixation of proximal humerus fractures using a proximal humeral locked plate: a prospective multicenter analysis. J Orthop Trauma. 2009;23(3): 163–72.

29. Sudkamp N, Bayer J, Hepp P, et al. Open reduction and internal fixation of proximal humeral fractures with use of the locking proximal humerus plate. Results of a prospective, multicenter, observational study. J Bone Joint Surg Am. 2009;91A(6):1320–8.

Intramedullary Nail Fixation
of the Proximal Humerus

Carlos Torrens

Contents

Abstract

Despite multiple published treatment options proximal humeral fractures remain difficult to manage. When considering treatment options the most important factor to be considered is the osteoporosis nature of the vast majority of these fractures. Most of poor outcomes and complications of surgically-treated proximal humeral fractures are related to osteoporosis. Simple techniques avoiding rigid constructions with hard material are preferred to deal with these elderly-population fractures. Understanding the forces of cuff tendons attached to the fragments is crucial to reduce the fractures properly and also to plan the best osteosynthesis option. Tuberosities must be anatomically reduced and fixed to re-establish shoulder function. In such an elderly population sutures passed through the cuff attachments seem to be the best option to manage tuberosity fixation. When significant displacement between the head complex and the humeral shaft is associated, endomedullary support has to be provided to ensure stability of the tuberosity reconstruction, especially in two- and three-part fractures. Modified Ender's nail have proved to give enough dynamic stability to obtain consolidation whilst avoiding rigid constructions. A supplementary hole to pass sutures has to be made at the top of the Ender nail to be able to deeply introduce the nail into the humeral head to avoid nail protrusion in the subacromial space. Few complications are to

C. Torrens
Orthopedic Department, Hospital Universitario del Mar de Barcelona, Barcelona, Spain
e-mail: Ctorrens@parcdesalutmar.cat

G. Bentley (ed.), *European Surgical Orthopaedics and Traumatology*,
DOI 10.1007/978-3-642-34746-7_60, © EFORT 2014

be expected using this simple technique and most of the elderly proximal humeral fractures can be successfully managed by osteosutures alone or associated with Ender's nails when there is significant displacement of the humeral head and the diaphysis.

Keywords

Anatomy • Complications • Diagnosis • Epidemiology • Humerus-proximal fractures • Intramedullary nailing • Locked plates and hemi-arthroplasty • Operative Techniques • Rehabilitation • Surgical indications

Introduction - Epidemiology

Most of the proximal humeral fractures have to be considered osteoporotic fractures with a -uni-modal distribution in older men and women [1]. Women are likely to present with a proximal humeral fracture three times more frequently than men and the average age of women sustaining a proximal humeral fracture is significantly older than that in men (70 years-old in women versus 56 years-old in men) [2]. Proximal humeral fractures are the third most frequent fracture in elderly people after hip and Colles' fractures and are exponentially increasing. Palvanen et al. have published that the total number of Finnish adults 60 years and older hospitalized with a proximal humeral fracture rose during their study period from 208 in 1970 to 1120 in 2002. The overall incidence of these fractures also increased 63 %, and the mean age of patients with proximal humeral fractures also increased from 72 years old (1970) to 77 years old (2002), concluding that if these trends continue, the current number of fractures in the elderly will triple during the next three decades [3]. The vast majority of fractures are produced by falls from a standing height (87 %), while sports injuries and road accidents constitute a small number of proximal humeral fractures (8 %) and represent the younger population (33 years-old for sport injuries and 46 years-old for road accidents) whose fracture patterns and treatment considerations are not representative of

the common osteoporotic proximal humeral fracture [2]. An increase in the rate of falls, independent of the average rate, may be associated with a higher risk of humeral fractures [4]. Fall-related risk factors include previous falls, diabetes mellitus, difficulty walking in dim light, seizure medication use, depression, almost always using a hearing aid and left-handedness [5]. Conversely, patients who present with a proximal humeral fracture are much fitter than those who present with proximal femoral fractures, and pre-fracture functional status studies reveal that nine-tenths live at home [2]. When planning treatment options, this situation has to be taken into account to preserve pre-operative functional status.

Although the majority of the proximal humeral fractures are considered to be non-displaced that does not avoid the fact that mortality after shoulder fracture is considered to be higher than that of the general population immediately after the fracture and that this tendency is maintained until 5 years after fracture when mortality is not significantly different from the mortality of the general population [6]. Even more, at the age of 60 years-old, a previous shoulder fracture is associated with an immediate risk of hip, forearm or spine fracture that is significantly higher than that of the age and sex-matched population [7]. Any time surgical treatment is to be considered the osteoporotic condition has to be taken into account to avoid pitfalls and complications related to the use of materials and strategies designed to deal with hard non-osteoporotic bone.

Most proximal humeral fractures can be properly managed conservatively, obtaining reasonable good functional results, as has already been published, even in severely-displaced fractures [25]. Patients presenting complex humeral fractures and willing to obtain better functional outcome than reported with conservative management are candidates for surgical treatment. Fractures with significant displacement between the cephalic complex and diaphysis are at risk of non-union and also constitute an indication for surgical treatment.

Applied Anatomy

The displacement of the fragments of proximal humeral fractures follows the attachments of the rotator cuff tendons. Understanding of the forces present in the fracture pattern is mandatory to obtain reduction of the fracture.

When the humeral head is disconnected from the diaphysis, the pectoral muscles internally translate the proximal humeral shaft while the humeral head remains in place. Some release of the pectoralis major tendon can be done to more easily obtain good reduction of the fragments.

In the valgus impacted three-part fracture of the greater tuberosity, the humeral head is displaced into a valgus position pushing out the greater tuberosity. Because the valgus position of the humeral head, the greater tuberosity looks upwardly migrated. A closer analysis of the fracture pattern shows that the greater tuberosity remains in place but has no room to be reduced. Just elevating the humeral head and restoring the cephalo-diaphysis angle creates enough room to properly reduce the greater tuberosity.

When there is disconnection of the cephalic complex of the diaphysis and there is also a greater tuberosity fracture, the greater tuberosity typically migrates posteriorly because of the infraspinatus attachment while the rest of the humeral head is internally rotated following the subscapularis attachment. Gentle traction of the greater tuberosity together with external rotation of the humeral head is needed to obtain good reduction.

Before attempting to reduce any proximal humeral fracture is extremely useful to determine precisely the fragments taking part in the fracture and the direction of the forces that support these fragments because of the muscle attachments.

Diagnosis

Traditionally, proximal humeral fractures have been studied by the so called "trauma series" including a true antero-posterior view, lateral projection in the scapular plane and axillary view as described by Neer [9]. In acute fractures good axillary views are not always easy to obtain because of the pain induced by arm mobilization and because most of these x-rays are done in the emergency room. Recently, the axillary view has been progressively substituted by CT studies. It has been proved that CT scans provide clinically useful information for the treatment of complex proximal humeral fractures when radiographs provide inadequate information [10]. The rationale may be to obtain from each projection what can be obtained instead of trying to allocate an image to a rigid classification system. The antero-posterior view clearly defines the relationship between humeral head and humeral shaft and some articular and greater tuberosity fractures, but fails to inform about the posterior displacement of the greater tuberosity fragment and gives little information about the lesser tuberosity. Multiple radiographic views are needed to evaluate displacement of the greater tuberosity appropriately [11]. Lateral projection provides good information about anterior or posterior dislocation and the relationship between humeral head and humeral shaft but gives unclear information of the position of the tuberosities. CT scan is helpful in the analysis of greater and lesser tuberosity fracture pattern as well as displacement and gives information on the quality of subchondral bone of the humeral head.

Recently, different sequential image analysis systems have been proposed to rationally analyze the fracture patterns and obtain a better understanding of the fracture itself by answering simple questions [12–14].

Indications for Surgery

Recent studies demonstrate that even displaced proximal humeral fractures can be successfully treated conservatively in a selected elderly population [8]. Any time the patient has limited functional expectations or is not willing to undergo a strong rehabilitation program after surgery, conservative treatment must be considered. If non-operative treatment is decided upon in impacted proximal humeral fractures, early mobilization seems to be safe and more effective for quickly restoring the physical capability of the injured arm, although differences tend to disappear at 6 months follow-up [15].

The risk of development of avascular necrosis of the humeral head has routinely been advocated when considering surgery. Avascular necrosis rate depends on the fracture pattern, the treatment applied and the follow-up accomplished, and has been reported from 20 % to 90 %. Despite the fact that anatomical studies suggest that some fracture patterns strongly correlate with blood supply disruption of the humeral head [16, 17], Hertel et al. in a series of 100 intracapsular fractures of the proximal humerus treated by open surgery, defined that the most relevant predictors of ischaemia were:

1. The length of the dorso-medial metaphyseal extension (shorter than 8 mm in all ischaemic heads),
2. The integrity of the medial hinge (also previously described by Resch et al. [18]), the basic fracture type determined with the binary description system with an anatomic neck component, also stating that besides the disruption of the medial hinge, all other directions of fracture displacement did not strongly correlate to the vascular status [12]. Later on, the same group published the longer follow-up of those patients considered to be at risk of developing necrosis of the humeral head, and surprisingly 8 of the 10 initially ischaemic humeral heads did not collapse over time indicating that re-vascularization may occur and 4 of the 30 initially perfused heads developed avascular necrosis with an unclear explanation for that phenomena [19]. For all these reasons there is no strong recommendation for any surgery to prevent avascular necrosis of the humeral head.

Pseudoarthrosis development in proximal humeral fractures is rare. Court-Brown found a prevalence of proximal humeral non-union of 1.1 %, although a higher percentage is to be expected (8 %) if metaphyseal comminution is present and even more (10 %) if there is between 33 % and 100 % translation of the surgical neck [20]. It seems reasonable to consider surgical treatment in fit patients with significant displacement between the humeral head and the diaphysis where consolidation of the fracture can be compromised.

Elderly patients sustaining a proximal humeral fracture can be initially allocated into two groups:

1. The first one including elderly fit patients in good mental condition and willing to restore their previous functional level.
2. The second includes elderly unfit patients in fair mental condition and non-motivated to follow rehabilitations programmes.

In the second group, almost all proximal humeral fractures can be properly managed in a conservative way since non-operative treatment has been proven to obtain good pain relief and a functional level good enough for this selected population [8]. In the first group, pros. and cons. of surgical treatment have to be discussed with the patient taking into account that surgery may almost only be indicated in patients willing to gain good function. The Surgeon also has to be aware that elderly people may mostly use their arms in a below-shoulder level but that active external rotation is present in almost every single daily activity and must be preserved. Patients also have to be aware that acute treatment of proximal humeral fractures conservatively is relatively easy and gives good results whereas surgical treatment is complex and with limited results.

In summary, surgical treatment has to be considered when, after sharing with the patient the pros. and cons. of conservative treatment, the patient demands better functional outcome than that offered by conservative treatment. Surgical treatment also has to be planned when there is reasonable risk of non-union of the fracture.

Intramedullary nailing of the proximal humerus is specially indicated in fractures with significant displacement between the humeral head and the diaphysis where axial stabilization is required to support osteosutures passed through tuberosity fragments.

Pre-Operative Preparation and Planning

Despite the increased age of patients suffering proximal humeral fractures they are usually fit and present few associated medical disorders. Anyway any medical disorder present at the time of the fracture must be corrected previously to surgery.

The patient must be informed of the functional limits expected and associated with the fracture pattern as well as of the treatment considered. The patient also has to be aware of the post-operative care to plan any home help required until shoulder is functionally recovered.

X-ray and CT exam are required for every fracture planned for surgery. The number and displacement of the fragments must be recorded and strategy of reduction and fixation has to be planned. Comminution of the fragments and osteoporosis also has to be considered when deciding treatment options.

Despite outcomes published of different techniques, surgeons must consider their own skill with different techniques and choose the one they are more familiar with.

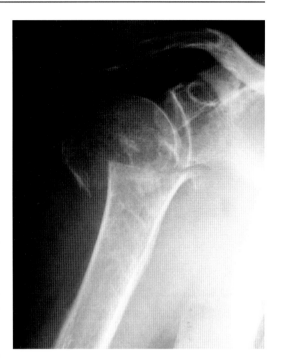

Fig. 1 AP X-ray view of a two-part surgical neck fracture of the humerus

Operative Technique

The patient is placed in the "beach-chair" position with the arm free. The preferred approach is the deltopectoral to be able to correct any tuberosity displacement and also because it causes no deltoid damages. The axillary nerve is routinely identified under the conjoined tendon. Retractors are placed beneath the humeral shaft and the humeral head to retract the deltoid muscle. Special care is given to the tuberosity fragments as they may be extremely fragile and porotic. In simple two-part surgical neck fractures (Fig. 1), a traction suture is placed through the supraspinatus junction to manage the cephalic part of the fracture and another non-absorbable suture is placed through two drilled holes in the diaphysis (Fig. 2). Sometimes pectoralis partial release is done to facilitate humeral shaft reduction. Once proper reduction has been tested, the first Ender nail is introduced

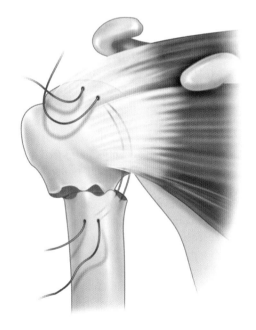

Fig. 2 Traction sutures passed through the supraspinatus tendon junction and through the subscapularis tendon to allow management and reduction of the fragments

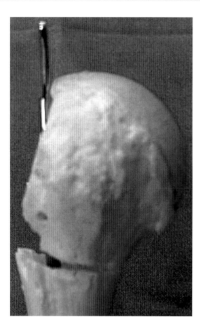

Fig. 3 Insertion of the first Ender's nail at the junction of the greater tuberosity and the humeral head cartilage

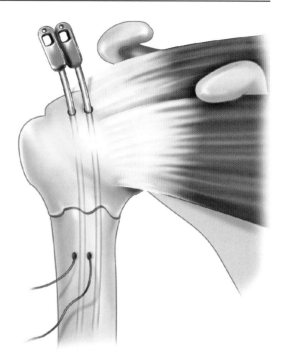

Fig. 4 Reduction of the fracture and stabilization with the aid of a second Ender's nail

through the junction of the greater tuberosity and the humeral head cartilage limit (Fig. 3). As the Ender nail is being pushed down the diaphysis the fracture is gently reduced. Direct view of the Ender nail progression into the diaphysis is used so there is no need of fluoroscopic control of nailing. To obtain better rotatory stability a second Ender nail is introduced 0.5 cm apart from the first (Fig. 4). The suture used for diaphysis traction is passed through the pre-manufactured small holes at the top of the Ender nails before they are deeply introduced in the humeral head in an eight-band figure (Figs. 5 and 6). The suture placed in the supraspinatus is then removed and the wound is closed leaving one deep suction drain (Fig. 7).

In the case of a three-part greater tuberosity fracture with significant displacement of the humeral head and the diaphysis the same approach is developed but the first step of surgery consists of reducing and securing the greater tuberosity to the humeral head (Fig. 8). For this purpose two non-absorbable sutures are placed at the junction of the cuff attachment to the greater tuberosity. Another suture is placed through the

subscapularis tendon to externally rotate the humeral head that has been moved to internal rotation because the subscapularis un-balanced traction (Fig. 9). Once the humeral head has been externally rotated the greater tuberosity is gently pulled to be reduced properly. The two sutures previously passed through the greater tuberosity are used to secure it to the lesser tuberosity through pre-drilled holes taking care not to produce a biceps tenodesis (Fig. 10). After that, the fracture can be considered as a two-part surgical neck fracture and can be managed as previously described (Fig. 11).

Post-Operative Care and Rehabilitation

After surgery the arm is fixed in an internal position with a sling-type immobilization and the drain is removed at 24 h. The patient's discharge from the Hospital is commonly on the second day after surgery and simple instructions are given to

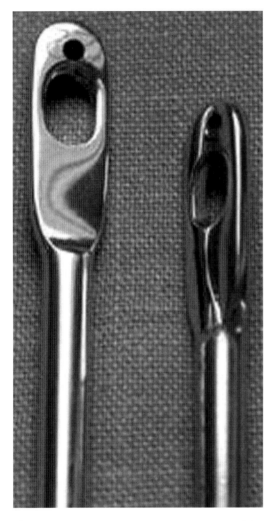

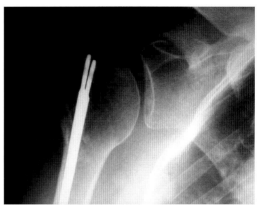

Fig. 7 AP X-ray at follow-up showing fracture consolidation

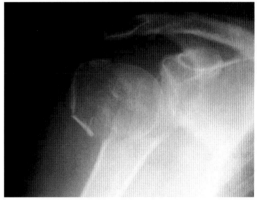

Fig. 5 Upper part of the Ender's nail with the pre-drilled small hole to pass the sutures and allow deep impaction of the nail into the humeral head

Fig. 8 AP X-ray view of a three-part greater tuberosity fracture with displacement of the humeral shaft and the cephalic complex

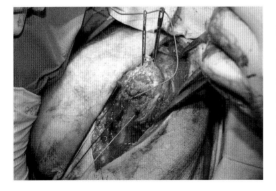

Fig. 6 Diaphysis suture passed through the holes at the top of the Ender's nails in an "eight-band" fashion

start rehabilitation of the hand and the elbow. After 3 weeks the sling is removed and the patient starts with assisted forward elevation with the aid of a pulley and is allowed to use the arm for self-care tasks such as dressing or eating. Once 120° of passive forward elevation are reached internal rotation exercises are added. This commonly occurs in the second or third week after immobilization is removed. One or two weeks later, when internal rotation reaches the L3 vertebra, external rotation exercises are added. Abduction exercises are avoided during the

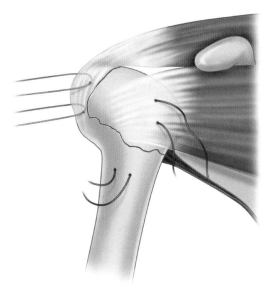

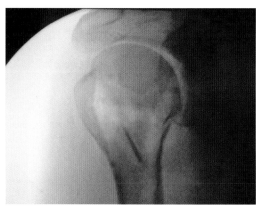

Fig. 11 Post-operative AP X-ray view showing correct reduction of the fracture with the aid of osteosutures

Fig. 9 Traction sutures passed through the greater tuberosity at the supraspinatus tendon junction, through the subscapularis tendon and through the humeral shaft to allow proper reduction

The vast majority of patients can do this simple rehabilitation program on their own at home and just a few cases require specially- trained people to assist them in specific centres.

Complications

Many different surgical treatments have been proposed for the management of severely-displaced proximal humeral fractures, including osteosutures [20], Ender's-nails together with osteosutures [21], plate fixation [22], extramedullary pinning [23] and intramedullary nailing [24]. All of them achieve reasonable functional results and also in most of the cases a pain-free shoulder. The commonest complications include loss of reduction, need for a second operation to remove metal implants, avascular necrosis of the humeral head, stiffness and infection at different rates depending on the populations selected, the fracture pattern and the treatment choice.

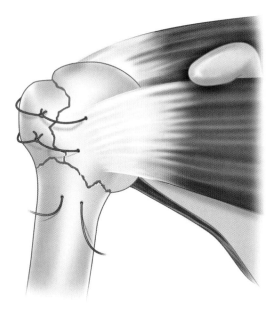

Fig. 10 Reduction of the fracture and suture of the greater tuberosity to the lesser tuberosity transforming the fracture into a two-part surgical neck fracture

Locked Plates and Hemi-Arthroplasty

entire rehabilitation program. Most of the time strengthening is not necessary as this selected elderly population may have pain with such programmes.

Recently-developed locked plates have changed the treatment map of proximal humeral fractures and their use has spread widely over the recent years. Specially developed to obtain strong fixation in osteoporotic bone, locked plates were expected to improve on older designs. Early published results are not so encouraging and numerous complications have also been reported. Fankhauser et al. reported in a series of 29 fractures at a follow-up of 1 year a final mean Constant Score result of 74.6, and despite early mobilization, there was a slow functional recovery of the patients evaluated at 1.5, 3, 6 and 12 months. Age and complexity of the fracture also influenced the end-result [25]. Koukakis et al. in a small series of 20 patients also obtained a mean final Constant Score of 76.1 % in a relatively young population with a mean age of 61.7 years [26]. Moonot et al. have reported in a series of 32 patients with a mean age of 59.9 years-old a mean final Constant Score of 66.5 in a short follow-up of 11 months [27]. Handschin et al. in a series of 31 patients presented a mean final adjusted Constant Score of 80 % and compared the results with an historic control group of 60 patients operated for the same fracture types using two one-third tubular plates and found no differences in complication rate, return to work and functional outcome. Differences were noted in the total cost, being of 684 Euros for angular-stable plates and of 158 for the one-third tubular plate [28]. On the other hand, several complications have been published associated to the use of locked plates. Egol et al. reported in a serie of 51 patients the development of 16 complications in 12 patients, including screw penetration, necrosis, non union, infection and early failure of the implant [29]. Owsley et al in a series of 53 patients reported, in 36 % of the patients, the presence of radiographic complications, including 23 % of screw cut-outs, 25 % of varus displacement and 4 % of aseptic necrosis. They also reported 13 % of revision surgery, and showed that complications tended to affect elderly people. being significant in patients older than 60 years [30].

Neer reported in 1970 early results of prosthetic replacement in severely-displaced proximal humeral fractures, and although his excellent results have never been reached again, hemiarthroplasty still remains as the treatment of choice in those more complex fractures [31]. Antuña et al. have reported the results of 57 patients with a long follow-up (minimum of 5 years) treated with a shoulder hemiarthroplasty for acute fractures of the proximal humerus with a mean age of 66 years. There were 27 patients satisfied and 30 unsatisfied. 16 % referred moderate or severe pain and range of motion averaged 100° for anterior elevation (20°–180°) and 30° for external rotation (0°–90°). They concluded that hemi-arthroplasty gives good pain relief but unpredictable functional result [32]. Looking closer to the results presented, the average movement may not be representative of the general status due to the wide range observed, with patients moving from 20° to 180° of anterior elevation. Grönhagen et al. also found, in a series of 46 patients a mean Constant score of 42 but ranging from 11 to 83 in primary hemi-arthroplasty for comminuted proximal humerus fractures. Constant score decreased significantly in 24 prostheses that had migrated superiorly [33].

Boileau et al. in a series of 66 patients tried to find out the reasons for poor outcomes after hemiarthroplasty. There were 27 % of initially badly-positioned tuberosities and 23 % of tuberosity detachments and migration. Final tuberosity malposition was observed in 50 % of the patients and correlated with unsatisfactory result, superior migration of the prosthesis, stiffness or weakness and persistent pain. The factors associated with failure of tuberosity osteosynthesis were poor initial position of the prosthesis, poor position of the greater tuberosity and women over age of 75 years [34]. Poor initial positioning of the prosthesis is related to the lack of landmarks in acute fractures with distorted anatomy. Different attempts have been done to find anatomical references to properly position prosthesis in acute fractures. The bicipital groove has been considered helpful reproduce accurate retroversion [35, 36] while others believe that a significant internal rotation occurs along the course of the bicipital groove (15.9°) that has clinical implications if it is used as a landmark for humeral head replacement in acute fractures [37]. Recently the upper insertion of the pectoralis major has been proposed as a landmark for proper restoration of the humeral height [38–40] as well as to determine retroversion of the humeral head. It has been stated that placing the humeral head at 5.6 cm from the upper pectoralis major insertion and locating the posterior prosthesis fin 1.06 cm posterior to the upper pectoralis insertion will result in anatomical height and version restoration.

Due to the unpredictable functional outcome of hemi-arthroplasty in complex humeral fractures, reversed designs have increasingly become part of the therapeutic choice. Avoiding the need for cuff function by improving the deltoid, the reverse prosthesis was thought to be the solution for such these osteoporotic commi-nuted fractures. Once again recent results are not so encouraging as expected and in a series of 43 patients with a short mean follow-up of 22 months, the mean active elevation was of 97° (35°–160°) and mean external rotation was 30° (0°–80°). The mean Constant Score was 44 (16–69). Peri-prosthetic calcification was observed in 90 % of the patients, displacement of the tuberosities in 53 % and a scapular notch in 25 % [41]. However, complex fractures will be in the future more often treated with the reverse system because it provides more predictable res-toration of function specially if tuberosities are preserved and reattached.

Specific complications related to the use of Ender nails is upper migration of the Ender nail to the subacromial space causing impinge-ment and subsequent pain and loose of function. This complication can be avoided by including a tension band suture from the diaphysis to the pre-drilled proximal hole on the Ender nail. In cases where there is loose reduction of the frac-ture and collapse of the fracture, the nails may also protrude to the subacromial space causing pain. In such this circumstance, the nails may have to be removed to allow a pain-free rehabil-itation program.

Our personal series includes 38 patients (30 female and 8 male), with a mean age of 72 years with a mean follow-up of 7,5 years and comprising 8 two-part surgical neck fractures, 25 three-part greater tuberosity fractures and 5 four-part fractures. Final Constant score reached 70,1 with most of the patients free of pain and able to do activities of daily living and with a mean for-ward elevation of 117°. After radiological analy-sis four cases were considered to have incomplete reduction after surgery and in eight cases a secondary displacement was noted at the final radiological exam. Two cases of avascular necro-sis of the humeral head developed in two four-part fractures but no further surgery was required because the patients experienced functional reduction with no pain and were old enough not to wish to for improved function through a surgical procedure. Just in two cases the Ender's nails needed to be removed because of subacromial impingement in 2 three-part fractures that suffered secondary displacement. Removal of the Ender's nails was done at 3 and 4 months after surgery because of pain and limited rehabilitation outcome. After removal, the patients remained pain-free and had improved function without significant differences with the rest of the series at final follow-up (unpublished data).

Summary

The total number and complexity of humeral fractures is increasing, as is the age of presenta-tion. When planning treatment strategies the oste-oporotic nature of these fractures has always to be considered. In selected elderly populations with limited expectations conservative treatment may be an effective option for almost all the fracture patterns. Surgical treatment is indicated when painful pseudoarthrosis is expected to develop and also when, after sharing with the patient pros. and cons. of surgical versus conservative management of the fracture the patient asks for a better functional outcome. When there is severe displacement between the cephalic part and the diaphysis endomedullary nailing may be consid-ered in two-part surgical neck and three-part greater tuberosity fractures. Modified Ender's nail provide stability enough to facilitate consol-idation of these fractures. An eight-figure osteo-suture passed through the added holes at the top of the Ender's nails avoids proximal migration of the nails to the subacromial space. In three-part fractures reduction and fixation of the tuberosity through osteo-sutures is required prior to nailing the fracture. After a 3-week immobilization period most of the patients can follow a simple at-home rehabilitation programme and end-up with a pain-free functional shoulder.

References

1. Court-Brown CM, Caesar B. Epidemiology of adult fractures: a review. Injury. 2006;37:691–7.
2. Court-Brown CM, Garg A, McQueen MM. The epidemiology of proximal humeral fractures. Acta Orthop Scand. 2001;72:365–71.
3. Palvanen M, Kannus P, Niemi S, Parkkari J. Update in the epidemiology of proximal humeral fractures. Cin Orthop. 2006;442:87–92.
4. Schwartz AV, Nevitt MC, Brown BW, Kelsey JL. Increased falling as a risk factor for fracture among older women. Am J Epidemiol. 2005;161:180–5.
5. Chu SP, Kelsey JL, Keegan THM, Sternfeld B, Prill M, Quesenberry CP, Sidney S. Risk factors for proximal humeral fracture. Am J Epidemiol. 2004;160:360–7.
6. Johnell O, Kanis JA, Odén A, Sernbo I, Redlund-Johnell I, Petterson C, De Laet C, Jönsson B. Mortality after osteoporotic fractures. Osteoporos Int. 2004;15:38–42.
7. Johnell O, Kanis JA, Odén A, Sernbo I, Redlund-Johnell I, Petterson C, De Laet C, Jönsson B. Fracture risk following an osteoporotic fracture. Osteoporos Int. 2004;15:175–9.
8. Edelson G, Safuri H, Salami J, Vigder F, Militianu D. Natural history of complex fractures of the proximal humerus using a three-dimensional classification system. J Shoulder Elbow Surg. 2008;17:399–409.
9. Neer II CS. Displaced proximal humeral fractures. Part I. Classification and evaluation. J Bone Joint Surg [Am]. 1970;52:1077–89.
10. Castagno AA, Shuman WP, Kilcoyne RF, Haynor DR, Morris ME, Matsen FA. Complex fractures of the proximal humerus: role of CT in the treatment. Radiology. 1987;165:759–62.
11. Parsons BO, Klepps SJ, Miller S, Bird J, Gladstone J, Flatow E. Reliability and reproducibility of radiographs of greater tuberosity displacement. A cadaveric study. J Bone Joint Surg [Am]. 2005;87:58–65.
12. Hertel R, Hempfing A, Stiehler M, Leuning M. Predictors of humeral head ischemia after intracapsular fracture of the proximal humerus. J Shoulder Elbow Surg. 2004;13:427–33.
13. Shrader MW, Sanchez-Sotelo J, Sperling JW, Rowland CM, Cofield R. Understanding proximal humerus fractures: image analysis, classification, and treatment. J Shoulder Elbow Surg. 2005;14:497–505.
14. Mora JM, Sanchez A, Vila J, Cañete E, Gamez F. Proposed protocol for reading images of humeral head fractures. Clin Orthop. 2006;448:225–33.
15. Lefevre-Colau MM, Babinet A, Fayad F, Fermanian J, Anract P, Roren A, Kansao J, Revel M, Poiraudeau S.

16. Gerber C, Schneeberger AG, Vinh JS. The arterial vascularization of the humeral head. An anatomical study. J Bone Joint Surg [Am]. 1990;72:1486–94.
17. Brooks CH, Revell WJ, Heatley FW. Vascularity of the humeral head after proximal humeral fractures. J Bone Joint Surg Br. 1993;75:132–6.
18. Resch H, Beck E, Bayley I. Reconstruction of the valgus-impacted humeral head fracture. J Shoulder Elbow Surg. 1995;4:73–80.
19. Bastian JD, Hertel R. Initial post-fracture humeral ischemia does not predict development of necrosis. J Shoulder Elbow Surg. 2008;17:2–8.
20. Court-Brown CM, McQueen MM. Nonunions of the proximal humerus: their prevalence and functional outcome. J Trauma. 2008;64:1517–21.
21. Dimakopoulos P, Panagopoulos A, Kasimatis G. Transosseous suture fixation of proximal humeral fractures. J Bone Joint Surg Am. 2007;89:1700–9.
22. Cuomo F, Flatow EL, Maday MG, Miller SR, McIlveen SJ, Bigliani LU. Open reduction and internal fixation of two- and three-part displaced surgical neck fractures of the proximal humerus. J Shoulder Elbow Surg. 1992;1:287–95.
23. Esser RD. Treatment of three- and four-part fractures of the proximal humerus with a modified cloverleaf plate. J Orthop Trauma. 1994;8:15–22.
24. Lin J, Hou S-M, Hang Y-S. Locked nailing for displaced surgical neck fractures of the humerus. J Trauma. 1998;45:1051–7.
25. Fankhauser F, Boldin C, Schippinger G, Haunschmid C, Szyszkowitz R. A new locking plate for unestable fractures of the proximal humerus. Clin Orthop. 2005;430:176–81.
26. Koukakis A, Apostolou CD, Taneja T, Korres DS, Amini A. Fixation of proximal humerus fractures using the Philos plate. Clin Orthop. 2006;442:116–20.
27. Moonot P, Ashwood N, Hamlet M. Early results for treatment of three- and four-part fractures of the proximal humerus using the Philos plate system. J Bone Joint Surg Br. 2007;89:1206–9.
28. Handschin AE, Cardell M, Contaldo C, Trentz O, Wanner GA. Functional results of angular-stable plate fixation in displaced proximal humeral fractures. Injury. 2008;39:306–13.
29. Egol KA, Ong CC, Walsh M, Jazrawi LM, Tejwani NC, Zuckerman JD. Early complications in proximal humerus fractures (OTA types 11) treated with locked plates. J Orthop Trauma. 2008;22:159–64.
30. Owsley KC, Gorczyca JT. Displacement/Screw cutout after open reduction and locked plate fixation of humeral fractures. J Bone Joint Surg Am. 2008;90:233–40.
31. Neer II CS. Displaced proximal humeral fractures. Part II. Treatment of three-part and four-part displacement. J Bone Joint Surg [Am]. 1970;52:1090–103.

32. Antuña SA, Sperling JW, Cofield RH. Shoulder hemiarthroplasty for acute fractures of the proximal humerus: a minimum five-year follow-up. J Shoulder Elbow Surg. 2008;17:202–9.

33. Grönhagen CM, Abbaszadegan H, Révay SA, Adolphson PY. Medium-term results after primary hemiarthroplasty for comminute proximal humerus fractures: a study of 46 patients followed up for an average of 4.4 years. J Shoulder Elbow Surg. 2007;16:766–73.

34. Boileau P, Krishnan SG, Tinsi L, Walch G, Coste JS, Mole D. Tuberosity malposition and migration: reasons for poor outcomes after hemiarthroplasty for displaced fractures of the proximal humerus. J Shoulder Elbow Surg. 2002;11:401–12.

35. Hempfing A, Leunig M, Ballmer FT, Hertel R. Surgical landmarks to determine humeral head retrotorsion for hemiarthroplasty in fractures. J Shoulder Elbow Surg. 2001;10:460–3.

36. Angibaud L, Zuckerman JD, Flurin PH, Roche C, Wright T. Reconstructing proximal humeral fractures using the bicipital groove as a landmark. Clin Orthop. 2007;458:168–74.

37. Itamura J, Dietrick T, Roidis N, Shean C, Tibone J. Analysis of the bicipital groove as a landmark for humeral head replacement. J Shoulder Elbow Surg. 2002;11:322–6.

38. Murachovsky J, Ikemoto RY, Nascimento LGP, Fujiki EN, Milani C, Warner JJP. Pectoralis major tendon reference (PMT): a new method for accurate restoration of humeral length with hemiarthroplasty for fracture. J Shoulder Elbow Surg. 2006;15:675–8.

39. Greiner SH, Kääb MJ, Kröning I, Scheibel M, Perka C. Reconstruction of humeral length and centering of the prosthetic head in hemiarthroplasty for proximal humeral fractures. J Shoulder Elbow Surg. 2008;17:709–14.

40. Torrens C, Corrales M, Melendo E, Solano A, Rodríguez-Baeza A, Caceres E. Pectoralis major tendon as a reference for restoring humeral length and retroversion with hemiarthroplasty for fracture. J Shoulder Elbow Surg. 2008;17:947–50.

41. Bufquin T, Hersan A, Hubert L, Massin P. Reverse shoulder arthroplasty for the treatment of three- and four-part fractures of the proximal humerus in the elderly. J Bone Joint Surg Br. 2007;89:516–20.

Fractures of the Proximal Humerus Treated by Plate Fixation

Pierre Hoffmeyer

Contents

Abstract

Treatment of displaced fractures of the proximal humerus in the fit and active patient remains a challenge. Accurate imaging is essential first with plain x-rays and with three-dimensional imaging. Knowledge of the vascular anatomy of the humeral head is mandatory to understand the consequences of the fracture pattern. When surgery is contemplated, positioning of the patient must allow a quasi-circumferential approach to the shoulder. The deltopectoral approach is the most popular but lesser invasive transdeltoid approaches are coming into vogue. Plates with locking screws afford great stability and ease of use. However the basics of biomechanics must not be forgotten, namely the presence of a medial buttress. Ignoring the principles will need to failure. Rehabilitation must be tailored to each patient but gentle early motion is encouraged in all cases. Complications of the technique are reviewed.

Keywords

Deltopectoral approach • locking plates • proximal humerus fractures • rehabilitation • surgical technique • transdeltoid approach • delto-pectoral approach • three and four part fractures • two-part fractures

P. Hoffmeyer
University Hospitals of Geneva, Geneva, Switzerland
e-mail: Pierre.Hoffmeyer@hcuge.ch;
pierre.hoffmeyer@efort.org

G. Bentley (ed.), *European Surgical Orthopaedics and Traumatology*,
DOI 10.1007/978-3-642-34746-7_6, © EFORT 2014

Introduction

Fractures of the proximal humerus present a major clinical problem and the techniques of fixation including nailing, percutaneous pinning, osteosuture and plating have evolved over time [1–22]. Plate fixation for proximal humerus fractures has gained in popularity with the advent of new locking plates that afford greater stability and are easier to apply than standard plates because of the immediate stability they provide [19, 23–35]. Clearly the ultimate prognosis of a fracture of the proximal humerus depends largely on the vascular status of the proximal humerus and the more specifically on the location of the main fracture line [8, 36–38] (Fig. 1). With a high fracture line an interruption of the vascular supply is likely. If the fracture line is lower the chances of necrosis become lower (Fig. 2).

Indications

The indications for plating are determined by the fracture pattern, essentially displaced two- and three-part fractures, as determined by Codman and Neer and refined by other authors using advanced imaging techniques such as 3D CT [2, 39–44]. Displaced head-split fractures not amenable to reduction should be treated with other means such as hemi- or total arthroplasty whether anatomic or inverted. Clearly to determine the indication an accurate diagnosis is necessary and this is only possible with well executed x-rays, if possible of digital quality, that need to be perpendicular to the glenohumeral joint in the frontal anteroposterior plane and in the transverse axial plane (Fig. 3). CT and 3D CT images may also be of assistance in the understanding of complex fractures [39, 45–47].

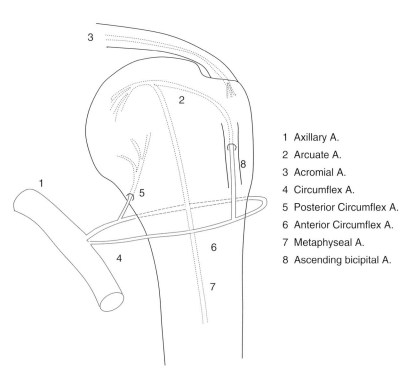

1 Axillary A.
2 Arcuate A.
3 Acromial A.
4 Circumflex A.
5 Posterior Circumflex A.
6 Anterior Circumflex A.
7 Metaphyseal A.
8 Ascending bicipital A.

Fig. 1 Vascularisation of the humeral head

Fig. 2 Fracture line determines the risk of necrosis. (**a**) High fracture line (*arrow*) with high risk of necrosis. (**b**) Low fracture line (*arrow*) with a lesser risk of necrosis

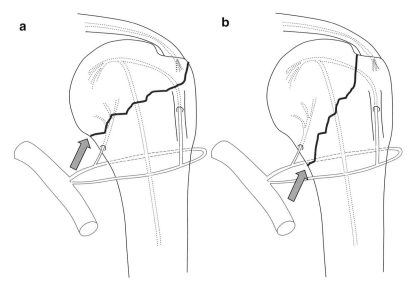

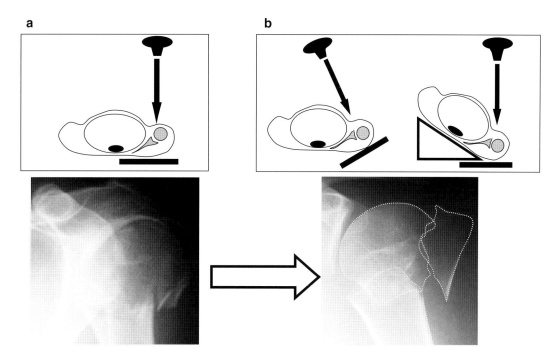

Fig. 3 Accurate radiological assessment is necessary. (**a**) AP perpendicular to the coronal plane is unsatisfactory. (**b**) Strict AP view perpendicular to the scapular plane is necessary for diagnosis

Surgical Technique

Patient Positioning

Under general anaesthesia and in some cases with an additional scalene block, the patient is placed on the operating table in a semi-sitting "beach-chair" position. It is important that the table be slightly up-tilted so that the buttocks rest squarely in the seat of the table avoiding any tendency to downward slippage. The head is held securely in a head rest with a firm bandage providing secure fixation. The cervical spine is in neutral position without inclination, rotation, extension or flexion. Special care should be given to protecting the patient's eyes. It is important to verify the position of the contralateral upper extremity so as to avoid pressure areas [24, 28] (Fig. 4).

The totality of the shoulder region from the superolateral torso and including the whole upper extremity should be left free. Some modular tables will allow removal of an upper corner piece therefore allowing access to all parts of the shoulder. The downside of this possibility is that the scapula tends to sag backwards somewhat. This may be counteracted by slightly rolling the table contralaterally. If this possibility does not exist a bolster may be used to prop-up the scapula. Care is taken to ensure that the shoulder may be thoroughly explored with a C-arm fluoroscope. Modern smaller C-arms are extremely manoeuvrable. Test the images obtained before definitive draping and adjust so as to obtain AP and axial views of the glenohumeral joint [24, 28] (Fig. 5).

Pain management modalities must be discussed with the anaesthetist. In some cases a scalene block may be indicated. In acute cases where nerve damage is possible this is best avoided. Routine single dose intravenous prophylaxis with an appropriate antibiotic administered before the incision, usually 20 min, is recommended [48].

Surgical Approaches

Trans-Deltoid Approach

This approach is appropriate for a displaced tuberosity fracture. Some authors use this approach as their standard for fractures of the proximal humerus [27, 29, 34]. The vertical incision of 5–7 cm starts from the acromion at the junction between the anterior and the middle third of the deltoid. After undermining the subcutaneous tissue the acromion, the acromioclavicular joint, clavicle and deltoid muscle are recognized. The anterior and mid-deltoid portions are then split through an often identifiable tendinous streak using a cold knife or electrocautery. This separation should not exceed 5 cm distal to the acromion and the axillary nerve should be identified either by palpation or visualization. Neer [49] recommended placing a suture at the end of the muscle slit to avoid unnecessary propagation. If absolutely necessary the deltoid may be economically released from the acromion in T fashion. The subacromial bursa is then opened and the surprisingly wide separation of the fracture lines will come into view. Traction sutures inserted through the supra- and infra-spinatus tendons will aid in reduction. Once the fracture is reduced, the plate is slipped along the bone and screws are inserted. The distal screws may be inserted through separate cutaneous incisions underneath the passage of the axillary nerve [27, 29]. The imager intensifier is used to control the fracture reduction. Remember that the vision is limited using this approach and that the utmost care in placing the implant must be exerted. The most frequent complications of this approach are malreduction of the fracture, malposition of the plate and injury to the axillary nerve with denervation of the anterior deltoid as a result (Fig. 6).

Fig. 4 Patient positioning.
The patient is in semi-
sitting position and the head
is in the neutral position
fixed in a headrest. The
shoulder and upper
extremity is free so as to
allow image intensifier use.
A scalene block may be
used to provide post-
anesthesia pain control

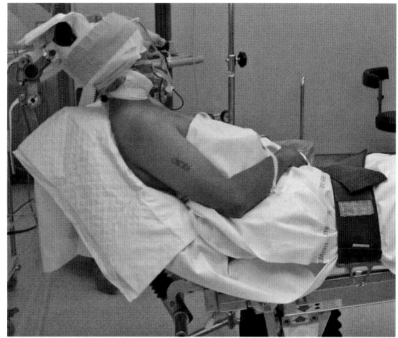

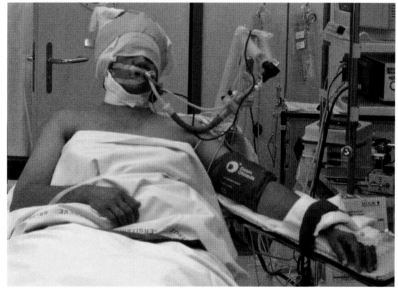

Fig. 4 Patient positioning. The patient is in semi-sitting position and the head is in the neutral position fixed in a headrest. The shoulder and upper extremity is free so as to allow image intensifier use. A scalene block may be used to provide post-anesthesia pain control

Delto-Pectoral Approach

The delto-pectoral approach is the favoured approach for proximal humerus fractures. It is a utilitarian and extensile approach both proximally and distally that respects the anatomy of the shoulder [28, 49]. For proximal humeral fractures a straight or oblique 10–15 cm incision is the best choice starting at the junction of the mid- and lateral third of the clavicle, passing over the coracoid and

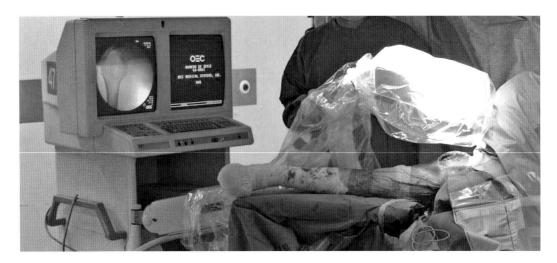

Fig. 5 In a semi-sitting position, the arm is placed on a Mayo stand in abduction to relax the deltoid. Intra-operatively the image-intensifier allows control of the reduction manoeuvres

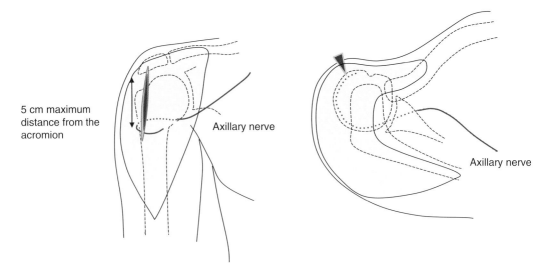

5 cm maximum distance from the acromion

Axillary nerve

Axillary nerve

Fig. 6 Trans-deltoid approach. The cutaneous incision is straight going down from the acromion at the junction of the anterior and middle third of the deltoid. Separation of the deltoid fibres should not exceed a point 5 cm. distal to the acromion to protect the axillary nerve

ending distally near the insertion of the deltoid. Subcutaneous tissues are undermined and the delto-pectoral interval must be clearly identified. Haematoma and swelling may render this difficult so that it may be necessary to find the interval high up between the pectoralis and the deltoid proximally at their clavicular insertion. The cephalic vein is preserved and left either laterally along the deltoid or medially. The deltoid fascia is incised to allow palpation of the axillary nerve on the underside of the anterior deltoid by running a finger around the proximal humeral metaphysis [3, 9]. The pectoralis muscle is retracted medially while the deltoid is retracted laterally (Fig. 7). Abduction will facilitate deltoid retraction and exposure. The conjoint tendon is then retracted medially to identify the subscapularis muscle and its tendon. At this time it is wise to find the axillary nerve coursing on the anterior surface of the subscapularis muscle so as to protect it [50].

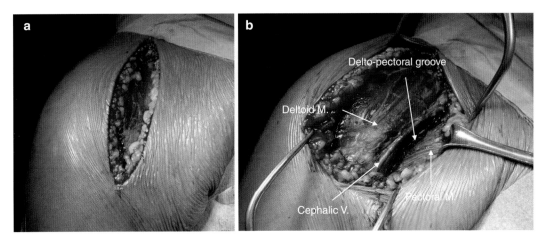

Fig. 7 Delto-pectoral approach: (**a**) The skin incision begins at the junction of the proximal and lateral thirds of the clavicle, passes over the coracoid and stops over the direction of pectoralis major. (**b**) The subcutaneous tissue is undermined in order to visualize the delto-pectoral groove. Proximally the vein can be found where it plunges into the brachial vein in the triangle between deltoid and pectoralis insertion origins

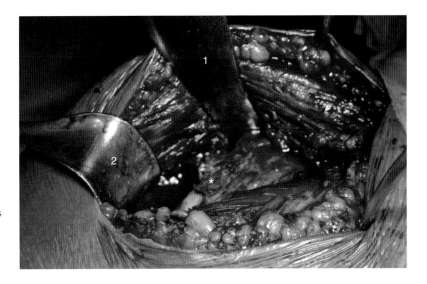

Fig. 8 Exposing the fracture. A blunt curved Hohmann retractor (1) is placed in the subacromial space and a wide Richardson retractor pulls away the deltoid (2) with the arm in abduction, allowing exposure of the fracture site (*)

Beware of the musculocutaneous nerve that penetrates the coracobrachialis at a mean distance of 5 cm from the tip of the coracoid [28, 49]. The tendon of the long biceps is a precious landmark and if damaged should not be sectioned for tenodesis until the fracture is properly reduced and the implants are in place [3]. The trajectory of the tendon must be straight and lie squarely in the groove. This will guide the reduction as the groove can generally be identified in the majority of fractures. Furthermore, the structures medial to the long biceps tendon make up the lesser tuberosity and subscapularis complex while the structures lateral to the long biceps are the greater tuberosity and supra- and infraspinatus [3, 9, 28]. To augment the exposure, the coraco-acromial ligament may be incised and the distal insertion of the deltoid may be released on the humerus. Rarely the anterior deltoid may be released from the clavicle. In this case the incision of the muscle insertion must be on top of the clavicle to leave a tendinous band for reinsertion [3] (Fig. 8).

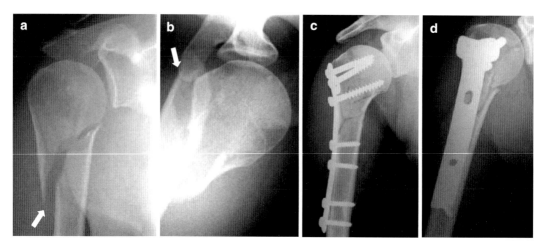

Fig. 9 Two part fracture (**a, b**) with a long spiral (*arrows*). (**c, d**) Fixation with a long T-plate

Standard Plates

There are many different types of plates including standard plates. They all have in common the possibility of inserting multiple screws into the humeral head. Some are T-shaped, others are cloverleaf or racket-shaped [6, 7, 20, 51]. These implants can be used through delto-pectoral or trans-deltoid approaches (Fig. 9). Biomechanically all plates are placed on the lateral cortex to produce a tension band effect. For best function and results a medial buttress and a valgus reduction must be obtained. If no medial buttress is present the implants will fatigue and ultimately fracture [28, 30, 31, 34, 35]. It should also be noted that in the osteoporotic bone multiple screws of a small diameter (3.5 mm) are more efficient than a large diameter screw (6.5 mm) [8, 27, 28, 31].

Anatomical Plates with Divergent Locked Screws

The trend is towards anatomically designed plates with engineered screw holes able to lock angularly stable and diverging screws These locking screw holes impose a direction to the screws although the latest models allow a greater latitude in the choice of angles.

This angular stability with diverging screws is an advantage for the stabilization of osteoporotic fractures [19, 23–35].

Blade-Plates

For indications where a high degree of stability is required, 90° angled blade-plates for the proximal humerus provide rigid fixation and allow interfragmentary compression. These implants are useful in certain situations such as non-unions or for fixing osteotomies after a malunion [52].

Fractures of the Anatomical Neck (Two Fragments)

This is a rare lesion often associated with a dislocation or a subluxation of the cephalic fragment. This pattern is most often encountered in high energy trauma in the young. Reduction is performed through a delto-pectoral approach and an arthrotomy through the rotator interval will permit visualization of the displaced fragment. Once anatomical reduction is obtained a plate may be used for fixation, preferably a plate with locked screws to obtain a rigid fixation of this intra-articular fragment. Prognosis is dismal however with a high rate of post-traumatic necrosis of the cephalic fragment [53].

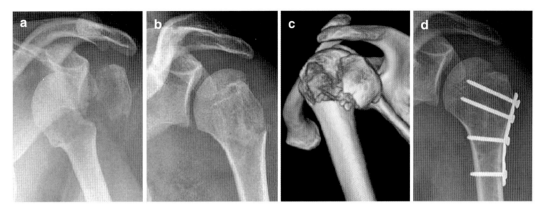

Fig. 10 Plate fixation with a third tubular plate. Glenohumeral dislocation and tuberosity fracture (**a**) After closed reduction a posterior displacement of the greater tuberosity (**b, c**) Reduction and fixation of the greater tuberosity with a third tubular plate (**d**)

Isolated Fractures of the Greater Tuberosity (Two Fragments)

Fractures of the greater tuberosity with posterior and superior displacement are typically associated with antero-inferior dislocations of the shoulder. These fractures are in fact completed Hill-Sachs fracture impactions. Surgical intervention is considered with a displacement of the tuberosities greater than 3 mm in young active patients. Up to 1 cm of displacement may be tolerated in less active elderly patients [49]. A trans-deltoid approach may be used. Once the fracture is reduced, a plate with locking screws may be used to stabilize the fragment. To ensure adequate fixation sutures however are passed through the supraspinatus, infraspinatus and subscapularis tendons and secured to the plate [54] (Fig. 10).

Fractures of the Surgical Neck (Two Fragments)

Fractures of the surgical neck tend to be unstable because of the actions of the rotator cuff muscles, the teres minor and major muscles, the deltoid and the pectoralis [23, 25, 32]. With an angularly displaced fracture ($>30°$) surgical stabilization is necessary. These fractures may be displaced into valgus or varus and the fixation technique will vary.

Valgus Displacement

If a plate is used, a standard 1/3 or 1/2 tubular plate may be inserted using either a delto-pectoral or a trans-deltoid approach. The plate is placed without any attempt at contouring. A screw inserted distally to the fracture line is gradually tightened thus bringing the plate in close contact with the cortex. In case of a valgus displacement reduction is obtained automatically. Care must be taken that the proximal fragment is well aligned in the sagittal plane and that no excessive flexion or extension remain [8] (Fig. 11).

Varus Displacement

In case of varus displacement it is imperative to reduce the proximal fragment so as to obtain a satisfactory alignment both in the frontal and in the sagittal planes. A Steinmann pin fixed into the humeral head may be useful as a "joystick" to obtain the reduction. Sutures are also passed through the supraspinatus, subscapularis and infraspinatus tendons. These may also be useful in reducing the varus displaced proximal humerus. Once the proximal fragment is well seated on the metaphysis and after ascertaining that the reduction is clinically acceptable, using an image intensifier if necessary, a plate with locking screws is used to secure the fixation.

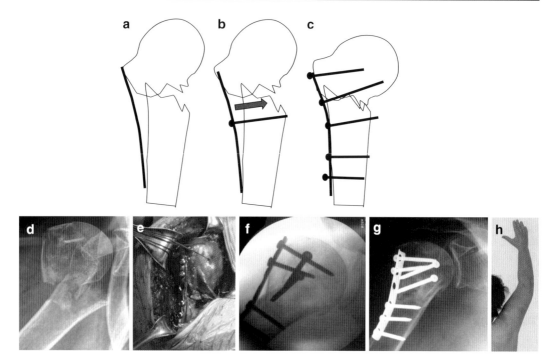

Fig. 11 Three-part fracture in valgus. (**a, b, c**) In this situation the spring properties of a semi- or third tubular plate may be used to reduce a displaced fracture. After a delto-pectoral approach, the plate is applied on the diaphysis and gradual tightening of a screw placed distally to the fracture line will bring about the reduction. It is important not to pre-bend the plate. (**d, e, f**) In this example two extra screws are used to fix a non-displaced lesser tuberosity fragment. (**g, h**) Healed fracture and functional result at 1 year

The cuff tendon sutures are tied to the plate using empty screw holes or specific holes in the plate (Fig. 12) [18, 28].

Three and Four Fragment Fractures

For a displaced three or four fragment fracture in a young active individual osteosynthesis with a rigid fixation and accurate reduction is always the first choice. For elderly less active patients a less rigid fixation using heavy suture material may be sufficient. No matter the fixation technique it is important to restore the anatomical relationships as only this will guarantee the best chances for recovering a functional articulation [4, 28].

These fractures when displaced should be reduced and fixed and the surgical approach may be delto-pectoral or trans-deltoid. The author's preference is the delto-pectoral approach which allows a good visualization of the fracture lines and adequate control of the fracture fragments for the purpose of obtaining a satisfactory reduction. Priority is given to tuberosity placement. If too high it will impinge against the acromion and damage the cuff, whilst if too low there will be undue tension on the rotator cuff tendons. Ideally the greater tuberosity should lie 10 mm under the humeral head [1, 3, 8, 28, 32, 34, 35].

After the standard delto-pectoral approach the fracture fragments must be identified. Stay sutures are placed in the tendons at the tendino-osseous junction of the fractured tuberosities. These sutures placed in the tendons along with a 2.5 mm Steinmann fixed in the cephalic fragment as a joystick will allow manipulation of the fragments. The medial fracture line at the head-metaphysis junction identified with the image intensifier is a landmark that will aid in adequately reducing the cephalic fragment on the metaphysis. A solid medial buttress is essential in

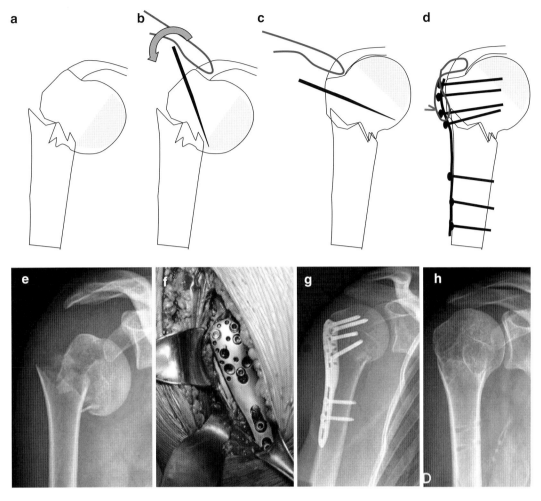

Fig. 12 Two-part fracture in varus. (**a, b, c, d**) After a delto-pectoral approach a Steinmann pin is inserted into the cephalic fragment and used as a joystick, a plate is applied for fixation. (**e, f**) Clinical case: Displaced two-part fracture fixed with a locking plate. Once reduced a locking plate is applied. (**g, h**) Result after fracture healing and hardware removal

ensuring a stable construct. Inspection of the articular surface may necessitate an arthrotomy through the rotator interval if the view afforded by lifting the tuberosity fragment is not sufficient. A pin fixing temporarily the cephalic fragment on the metaphysis is sometimes necessary. Rarely a bone graft is needed which may be inserted between the metaphysis and the cephalic fragment to maintain the head in good position. The tuberosities are then coaxed and manipulated into a reduced position around the cephalic fragment and fixed using the previously-inserted transtendinous sutures. The tuberosity fragment usually has a pointed triangular point which will fit into the metaphyseal mirror triangular fracture line. The position and alignment of the biceps tendon is a good witness as to the quality of the reduction. After the biceps tendon has been ascertained to be in good position, if its integrity is in doubt, a tenodesis may be needed [28, 33].

The transtendinous traction sutures may be then passed through holes in the locking screw-plate. The plate needs to be positioned on the metaphysis avoid the bicipital groove. Care must be taken that the plate is not too high or impingement on the acromion will occur.

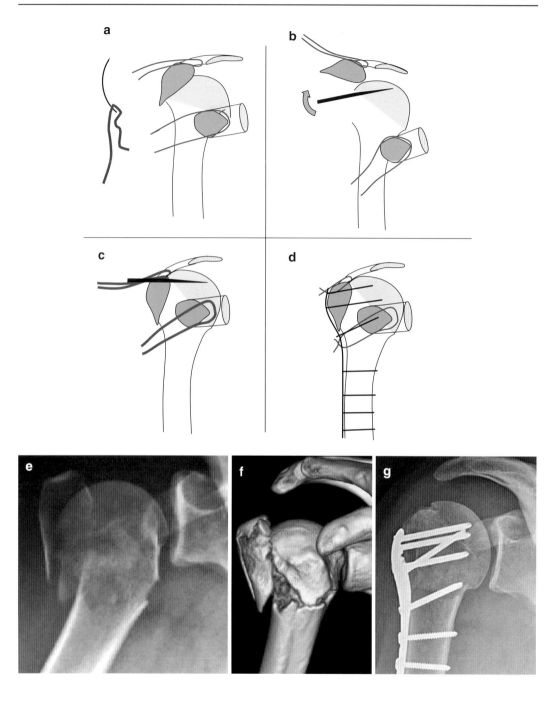

Fig. 13 Three-part fracture. (**a, b, c, d**) Transtendinous sutures are placed followed by reduction of the humeral head using a joystick manoeuvre with a Steinmann pin. Once the reduction achieved the locking plate is applied and sutures are tied onto the plate. (**e, f, g**) Clinical case: Three-part fracture fixed with a locking plate

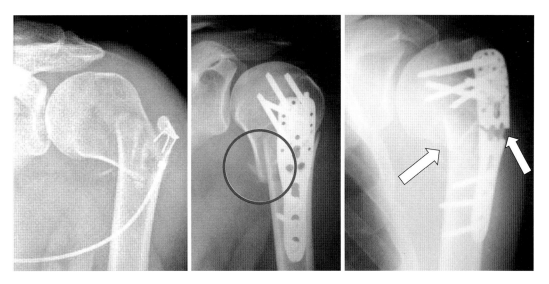

Fig. 14 Lack of a mechanically sound medial buttress (*Circle*) such as in this two- part fracture will lead to fracture collapse into varus and plate breakage

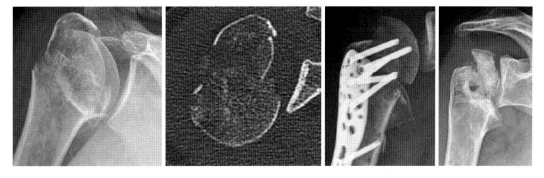

Fig. 15 Complications of plating. A fracture-dislocation with a head split in a 25 years-old woman. Attempt at plating leads to failure with collapse and severe necrosis

The image intensifier will control the reduction and position of the plate. The 3.5 mm screws are then inserted beginning with a screw in the middle of the plate and proceeding to insert the proximal cephalic screws. Length must be carefully gauged to avoid protrusion, more than 35 mm of length is unusual. Once the screw is inserted the transtendinous sutures should be tied on the plate. An image intensifier check will ascertain that the fracture is well reduced, that a good medial buttress has been achieved and that the screws are of the right length. The last screws are inserted into the cephalic fragment and locked into the plate.

For Titanium implants always use the torque-limiting device on the screwdriver when indicated by the manufacturer so as to avoid a so-called "cold" welding effect, rendering future hardware removal almost impossible without destroying the screw head. The lesser tuberosity may be fixed with screws outside the plate but as a rule transtendinous sutures tied down to the plate will afford an adequate fixation [28, 33].

Before closure, a last image intensifier check, taking the shoulder through a range of motion will verify that no screws are intra-articular and that the reduction is adequate (Fig. 13).

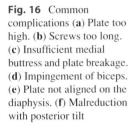

Fig. 16 Common complications (**a**) Plate too high. (**b**) Screws too long. (**c**) Insufficient medial buttress and plate breakage. (**d**) Impingement of biceps. (**e**) Plate not aligned on the diaphysis. (**f**) Malreduction with posterior tilt

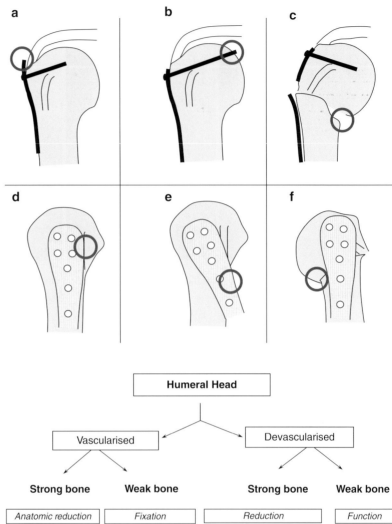

Fig. 17 Algorithm for managing displaced proximal humeral fractures

Complications

Complications are many and the literature is rich in articles and reports detailing the types of complications most frequently encountered [26, 27, 34, 35]. A strong medial buttress must be present if varus displacement and plate breakage are to be avoided (Fig. 14). The indication must be well determined. Certain head-split fracture-dislocations are not amenable to reduction and fixation and even if that were the case necrotic collapse is inevitable (Fig. 15). The main complications related to technique are described in Fig. 15. A plate too high will lead to impingement. Screws that are too long will damage the articular surfaces and lead to pain, as a general rule avoid screws longer than 35 mm in the humeral head. Lack of a strong medial buttress will lead to fracture collapse in varus. The plate should not impinge on the biceps if it is left in place. The plate should be placed on the diaphysis and not obliquely as this is potentially an unstable situation. Frequently a malreduction, where the proximal fragment remains tilted posteriorly, is encountered. This will lead to reduced motion and possibly residual pain (Fig. 16).

As a general rule plates should be used according to the algorithm below. The best indication is a displaced fracture occurring in strong bone with a pattern that preserves the vascularity of the articular cephalic fragment (Fig. 17).

Rehabilitation

As a rule the shoulder should be mobilized as early as possible (Rehabilitation will pass through three phases -I-II-III). During phase I the accent is placed on passive assisted mobilization in some cases under scalene bloc. The shoulder should be mobilized in elevation in the plane of the scapula by the physiotherapist and the patient is encouraged to mobilize himself the injured shoulder using his uninjured arm. The exercises should be performed supine and then later in the sitting position. Exercising in the water in an adapted pool under supervision should be started as soon as possible. In some cases a watertight film may be applied to the operative wound even before suture removal, thus allowing the patient to exercise in water with his wound kept dry. This phase should last for the first 6 weeks post-operatively, the aim being to achieve the best possible range of motion. Phase II starts at 6 weeks and active movements are encouraged along with strengthening exercise. At this time slings and shoulder immobilizers are stopped. The goal is to obtain a full range of motion. Starting at week 10, phase III stats. with strengthening and stretching exercises that are recommended and encouraged. After 3 months, formal physiotherapy is discontinued and the patient is encouraged to use his shoulder as normally as possible [11, 49, 53].

References

1. Bigliani LU. Treatment of two- and three-part fractures of the proximal humerus. AAOS Instr Course Lect. 1989;38:231–44.
2. Codman EA. The Shoulder. Malabar: Krieger; 1984. p. 319.
3. Cofield RH. Comminuted fractures of the proximal humerus. Clin Orthop. 1988;230:49–57.
4. Court-Brown CM, Garg A, McQueen MM. The translated two-part fracture of the proximal humerus. Epidemiology and outcome in the older patient. J Bone Joint Surg Br. 2001;83:799–804.
5. Duparc J, Largier A. Fracture-dislocations of the upper end of the humerus (French). Rev Chir Orthop Reparatrice Appar Mot. 1976;62:91–110.
6. Ehlinger M, Gicquel P, Clavert P, Bonnomet F, Kempf J-F. A new implant for proximal humeral fracture: experimental study of the basket plate (French). Rev Chir Orthop Reparatrice Appar Mot. 2004;90:16–25.
7. Esser RD. Treatment of three- and four-part fractures of the proximal humerus with a modified cloverleaf plate. J Orthop Trauma. 1994;8:15–22.
8. Hertel R. Fractures of the proximal humerus in osteoporotic bone. Osteoporos Int. 2005;16(Suppl 2):S65–72.
9. Hoffmeyer P. The operative management of displaced fractures of the proximal humerus. J Bone Joint Surg Br. 2002;84:469–80.
10. Ko JY, Yamamoto R. Surgical treatment of complex fracture of the proximal humerus. Clin Orthop. 1996;327:225–37.
11. Koval KJ, Gallagher MA, Marsicano JG, Cuomo F, McShinawy A, Zuckerman JD. Functional outcome after minimally displaced fractures of the proximal part of the humerus. J Bone Joint Surg Am. 1997;79:203–7.
12. Mittlmeier TWF, Stedtfeld H-W, Ewert A, Beck M, Frosch B, Gradl G. Stabilization of proximal humeral fractures with an angular and sliding stable anterograde locking nail (Targon PH). J Bone Joint Surg Am. 2003;85:136–46.
13. Mouradian WH. Displaced proximal humeral fractures. Seven years' experience with a modified Zickel supracondylar device. Clin Orthop. 1986;212:209–18.
14. Park MC, Murthi AM, Roth NS, Blaine TA, Levine WN, Bigliani LU. Two-part and three-part fractures of the proximal humerus treated with suture fixation. J Orthop Trauma. 2003;17:319–25.
15. Resch H, Pocacz P, Frölich R, Wambacher M. Percutaneous fixation of three and four-part fractures of the proximal humerus. J Bone Joint Surg Br. 1997;79:295–300.
16. Robinson CM, Page RS. Severely impacted valgus proximal humeral fractures. Results of operative treatment. J Bone Joint Surg Am. 2003;85:1647–55.
17. Rowles DJ, McGrory JE. Percutaneous pinning of the proximal part of the humerus. An anatomic study. J Bone Joint Surg Am. 2001;83:1695–9.
18. Schlegel TF, Hawkins RJ. Displaced proximal humeral fractures: evaluation and treatment. J Am Acad Orthop Surg. 1994;12:54–78.
19. Siegel HJ, Lopez-Ben R, Mann JP, Ponce B. Pathological fractures of the proximal humerus treated with a proximal humeral locking plate and bone cement. J Bone Joint Surg Br. 2010;92:707–12.
20. Wanner GA, Wanner-Schmid E, Romero J, Hersche O, von Smekal A, Trentz O, Ertel W. Internal fixation of displaced proximal humeral fractures with two one-third tubular plates. J Trauma. 2003;54:536–44.

21. Wijgman AJ, Roolker W, Patt TW, Raaymakers EL, Marti RK. Open reduction and internal fixation of three and four-part fractures of the proximal part of the humerus. J Bone Joint Surg Am. 2002;84:1919–25.

22. Zyto K, Ahrengart L, Sperber A, Tornkvist H. Treatment of displaced proximal humeral fractures in elderly patients. J Bone Joint Surg Br. 1997;79:412–7.

23. Agudelo J, Schürmann M, Stahel P, Helwig P, Morgan SJ, Zechel W, Bahrs C, Parekh A, Ziran B, Williams A, Smith W. Analysis of efficacy and failure in proximal humerus fractures treated with locking plates. J Orthop Trauma. 2007;21:676–81.

24. Badman BL, Mighell M. Fixed-angle locked plating of two-, three-, and four-part proximal humerus fractures. J Am Acad Orthop Surg. 2008;16:294–302.

25. Chudik SC, Weinhold P, Dahners LE. Fixed-angle plate fixation in simulated fractures of the proximal humerus: a biomechanical study of a new device. J Shoulder Elbow Surg. 2003;12:578–88.

26. Clavert P, Adam P, Bevort A, Bonnomet F, Kempf JF. Pitfalls and complications with locking plate for proximal humerus fracture. J Shoulder Elbow Surg. 2010;19:489–94.

27. Helwig P, Bahrs C, Epple B, Oehm J, Eingartner C, Weise K. Does fixed-angle plate osteosynthesis solve the problems of a fractured proximal humerus? A prospective series of 87 patients. Acta Orthop. 2009;80:92–6.

28. Konrad G, Bayer J, Hepp P, Voigt C, Oestern H, Kääb M, Luo C, Plecko M, Wendt K, Köstler W, Südkamp N. Open reduction and internal fixation of proximal humeral fractures with use of the locking proximal humerus plate: surgical technique. J Bone Joint Surg Am. 2010;92:85–95.

29. Laflamme GY, Rouleau DM, Berry GK, Beaumont PH, Reindl R, Harvey EJ. Percutaneous humeral plating of fractures of the proximal humerus: results of a prospective multicenter clinical trial. J Orthop Trauma. 2008;22(3):153–8.

30. Lescheid J, Zdero R, Shah S, Kuzyk PR, Schemitsch EH. The biomechanics of locked plating for repairing proximal humerus fractures with or without medial cortical support. J Trauma. 2010;69:1235–42.

31. Lever JP, Aksenov SA, Zdero R, Ahn H, McKee MD, Schemitsch EH. Biomechanical analysis of plate osteosynthesis systems for proximal humerus fractures. J Orthop Trauma. 2008;22:23–9.

32. Lungershausen W, Bach O, Lorenz CO. Locking plate osteosynthesis for fractures of the proximal humerus. Zentralbl Chir. 2003;128:28–33.

33. Ricchetti ET, DeMola PM, Roman D, Abboud JA. The use of precontoured humeral locking plates in the management of displaced proximal humerus fracture. J Am Acad Orthop Surg. 2009;17:582–90.

34. Sproul RC, Iyengara JJ, Devcica Z, Feeley BT. A systematic review of locking plate fixation of proximal humerus fractures. Injury. 2010. doi:10.1016/j.Injury.2010.11.058.

35. Südkamp N, Bayer J, Hepp P, Voigt C, Oestern H, Kääb M, Luo C, Plecko M, Wendt K, Köstler W, Konrad G. Open reduction and internal fixation of proximal humeral fractures with use of the locking proximal humerus plate. Results of a prospective, multicenter, observational study. J Bone Joint Surg Am. 2009;91:1320–8.

36. Gerber C, Hersche O, Berberat C. The clinical relevance of posttraumatic avascular necrosis of the humeral head. J Shoulder Elbow Surg. 1998;7:586–90.

37. Gerber C, Schneeberger AG, Vinh TS. The arterial vascularzation of the humeral head. An anatomical study. J Bone Joint Surg Am. 1990;72:1486–94.

38. Laing PG. The arterial supply of the adult humerus. J Bone Joint Surg Am. 1956;38:1105–16.

39. Jurik AG, Albrechtsen J. The use of computed tomography with two- and three-dimensional reconstructions in the diagnosis of three- and four-part fractures of the proximal humerus. Clin Radiol. 1994;49:800–4.

40. Muller ME, Nazarian S, Koch P. Classification A.O. des fractures. Berlin: Springer; 1987.

41. Neer II CS. Displaced proximal humeral fractures. I. Classification and evaluation. J Bone Joint Surg Am. 1970;52:1077–89.

42. Neer CS. Four segment classification of proximal humeral fractures: purpose and reliable use. J Shoulder Elbow Surg. 2002;11:389–400.

43. Sidor ML, Zuckerman JD, Lyon T, Koval K, Cuomo F, Schoenberg N. The Neer classification system for proximal humeral fractures. An assessment of interobserver reliability and intraobserver reproducibility. J Bone Joint Surg Am. 1993;75:1745–50.

44. Siebenrock KA, Gerber CH. The reproducibility of classification of dractures of the proximal end of the humerus. J Bone Joint Surg Am. 1992;75:1751–5.

45. Bahrs C, Rolauffs B, Südkamp NP, Schmal H, Eingartner C, Dietz K, Pereira PL, Weise K, Lingenfelter E, Helwig P. Indications for computed tomography (CT-) diagnostics in proximal humeral fractures: a comparative study of plain radiography and computed tomography. BMC Musculoskelet Disord. 2009;2:10–33.

46. Bernstein J, Adler LM, Blank JE, Dalsey RM, Williams GR, Iannotti JP. Evaluation of the Neer system of classification of proximal humeral fractures with computerized tomographic scans and plain radiographs. J Bone Joint Surg Am. 1996;78:1371–5.

47. Edelson G, Kelly I, Vigder F, Reis ND. A three-dimensional classification for fractures of the proximal humerus. J Bone Joint Surg Br. 2004;86:413–25.

48. Culebras X, Van Gessel E, Hoffmeyer P, Gamulin Z. Clonidine combined with a long acting local anesthetic does prolong postoperative analgesia after brachial plexus block but does induce hemodynamic changes. Anesth Analg. 2001;92:199–204.

49. Neer CS. Shoulder reconstruction. Philadelphia: W.B. Saunders; 1990. p. 363–401.

50. Flatow EL, Bigliani LU. Tips of the trade. Locating and protecting the axillary nerve in shoulder surgery. The tug test. Orthop Rev. 1992;21:503–5.

51. Bahrs C, Oehm J, Rolauffs B, Eingartner C, Weise K, Dietz K, Helwig P. T-plate osteosynthesis–an obsolete osteosynthesis procedure for proximal humeral fractures? Middle-term clinical and radiological results (In German). Z Orthop Unfall. 2007;145:186–94.

52. Jupiter JB, Mullaji AB. Blade plate fixation of proximal humeral non-unions. Injury. 1994;25:301–3.

53. Hodgson SA, Mawson SJ, Stanley D. Rehabilitation after two-part fractures of the neck of the humerus. J Bone Joint Surg Br. 2003;85:419–22.

54. Gruson KI, Ruchelsman DE, Tejwani NC. Isolated tuberosity fractures of the proximal humeral: current concepts. Injury. 2008;39(3):284–98.

Hemi-Arthroplasty for Fractures of the Proximal Humerus

Tony Corner and Panagiotis D. Gikas

Contents

Abstract

Complex fractures of the proximal humerus are some of the most common and difficult fractures to treat. Treatment options include benign neglect, internal fixation or arthroplasty. A hemiarthroplasty for a complex proximal humeral fracture is a challenging procedure even in the experienced shoulder surgeon's hands.

This chapter aims to explain the operative technique and tips to aid the surgeon perform the procedure safely and successfully, avoiding complications. A review of published outcomes of hemiarthroplasty for proximal humeral fractures is presented as well as possible complications and available rehabilitation protocols for the patient post-operatively.

Keywords

Fracture • Hemiarthroplasty • Humerus • Proximal

General Introduction

Complex fractures of the proximal humerus are some of the most difficult fractures to treat. Codman was the first surgeon to help us understand the patho-anatomy of these fractures and appreciate the mechanics and constituent parts of the fracture with respect to the head, tuberosities and shaft [1]. Charles Neer originally reported high failure rates for open reduction and internal fixation of three-part and four-part fractures of

T. Corner (✉)
West Hertfordshire Hospitals NHS Trust, Watford and St. Albans Hospitals, Watford, UK

P.D. Gikas
The London Sarcoma Service, Royal National Orthopaedic Hospital, Stanmore, Middlesex, UK

West Hertfordshire Hospitals NHS Trust, Watford and St. Albans Hospitals, Watford, UK
e-mail: panosgikas@me.com

G. Bentley (ed.), *European Surgical Orthopaedics and Traumatology*,
DOI 10.1007/978-3-642-34746-7_225, © EFORT 2014

the proximal humerus in the 1950's. He therefore proposed treating these fractures with a hemiarthroplasty. The first arthroplasty designed by Neer was a monoblock prosthesis and in 1953 he reported the first use of such a prosthesis in the treatment of a proximal humerus fracture as part of a fracture dislocation [2, 3].

Since this first generation monoblock design there have been numerous advances in shoulder hemiarthroplasty design with new modular implants allowing adjustable head neck angles, variable offset and methods of tuberosity fixation. Although developments have been made in arthroplasty technology and instrumentation, excellent equipment cannot compensate for poor surgical technique. Arthroplasty for proximal humerus fracture is one of the most technically demanding operations to perform correctly and achieve a satisfactory outcome for the patient. This chapter aims to guide the surgeon perform a shoulder hemiarthroplasty safely and effectively for complex fractures of the proximal humerus.

Aetiology and Classification

In 1934, Codman [1] described fractures of the proximal humerus and classified them as occurring in the head, shaft, or greater or lesser tuberosity. He indicated that surgical treatment is needed if these fractures are displaced. In 1970, Neer [2] described a classification system of displaced proximal humeral fractures that clarified and expanded on the earlier work of Codman.

In the Neer classification, one fragment or part is the humeral shaft, so the simplest displaced fracture is called a "two-part" fracture. The classification includes two-part fractures; three-part fractures; four- part fractures; and fracture-dislocations, including head-splitting fractures.

According to Neer [2–4], displacement of a fracture fragment by more than a centimeter or angulation of more than 45° is considered significant. The Neer Classification is summarized as follows:

- Minimally displaced one part *fracture*
- No segment displaced >1 cm or angulated >45°

- Two part *fracture* of anatomical neck, articular segment displaced
- High risk of AVN
- Two part *fracture* of the surgical neck with shaft displacement
- Two part greater tuberosity displacement
- Two part lesser tuberosity displacement
- Three part displacements: one tuberosity remains attached to the head
- Greater tuberosity displacement
- Lesser tuberosity displacement
- Four part *fractures*, *fracture* dislocation and head splitting *fractures*: articular segment displaced, out of contact with glenoid, no soft tissue attachment, no tuberosity contact.

In Hertel's Binary or Lego description system (Fig. 1) for proximal *humerus fractures* five basic fracture planes are identified:

1. Between the greater tuberosity and the head
2. Between the greater tuberosity and the shaft
3. Between the lesser tuberosity and the head
4. Between the lesser tuberosity and the shaft
5. Between the lesser tuberosity and the greater tuberosity Figure

This leads to 12 basic *fracture* patterns:

Six possible *fractures* dividing the *humerus* into two fragments,

Five possible *fractures* dividing the *humerus* into three fragments,

Single *fracture* pattern dividing the *humerus* into four fragments

The AO classification (Fig. 2), which is less frequently used than the Neer and Codman classification systems, emphasizes determination of whether vascularity to the articular fragment is significantly compromised. Type A is an extra-articular unifocal fracture that involves one of the tuberosities with or without a concomitant metaphyseal fracture. Type B is an extra-articular bifocal fracture or fracture-dislocation with tuberosity and metaphyseal involvement. Type C is a fracture or fracture-dislocation of the articular surface; this type is considered the most severe because the vascular supply is thought to be at the greatest risk of injury, thereby making the humeral head susceptible to the development of osteonecrosis.

Fig. 1 Hertel's Binary or Lego description system

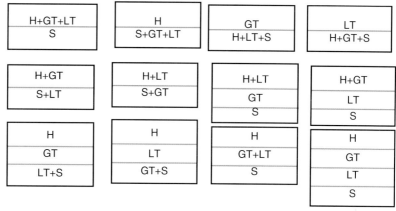

H= HEAD HUMERUS, GT= GREATER TUBEROSITY,
LT= LESSER TUBEROSITY, S=SHAFT HUMERUS

In the preoperative evaluation of patients with proximal humeral fractures, we routinely obtain an anteroposterior and an axillary (if patient can tolerate postioning of their arm for the radiograph) or scapular lateral radiograph [2]. Sometimes it is difficult to see the exact position of the fracture fragments, or the patient may be difficult to position. Kristiansen et al. [5] found wide interobserver variation in the classification of proximal humeral fractures when only plain radiographs were used. Accuracy of assessment improved with more experience in the use of the Neer classification. CT scan can be useful in these difficult cases where the amount of displacement or rotation of fragments is difficult to determine on plain radiographs. Although additional imaging is routinely used to further characterize these fractures, Sjödén et al. [12] demonstrated that the addition of CT and three-dimensional imaging did not improve interobserver reproducibility of either the Neer or AO classification system (see below). Majed and colleagues found only slight to moderate interobserver agreement between four senior shoulder surgeons classifying complex humeral fractures on CT scans with the Neer, AO, Codman-Hertel and prototype classification by Resch (see [33]). The highest interobserver reliability was for the Codman-Hertel classification system.

Specific cases in which the plain films may underestimate displacement include greater or lesser tuberosity fractures, impression fractures of the humeral head, head-splitting fractures, or loose bodies in the shoulder joint. In those instances CT can be helpful in showing the abnormality.

Relevant Applied Anatomy and Physiology

The shoulder has the greatest range of motion of any articulation in the body; this is due to the shallow glenoid fossa that is only 25 % of the size of the humeral head and the fact that the major contributor to stability is not bone, but a soft tissue envelope composed of muscle, capsule and ligaments.

The proximal humerus can be divided into four osseous segments that have different deforming muscular forces:
- The humeral head
- The lesser tuberosity; displaced medially by the subscapularis
- The greater tuberosity; displaced superiorly and posteriorly by the supraspinatus and external rotators
- The humeral shaft; displaced medially by the pectoralis magor

The major blood supply to the proximal humerus is by the anterior and posterior humeral circumflex arteries. The arcuate artery is a continuation of the ascending branch of the anterior humeral circumflex. It enters the bicipital groove and supplies most of the humeral head.

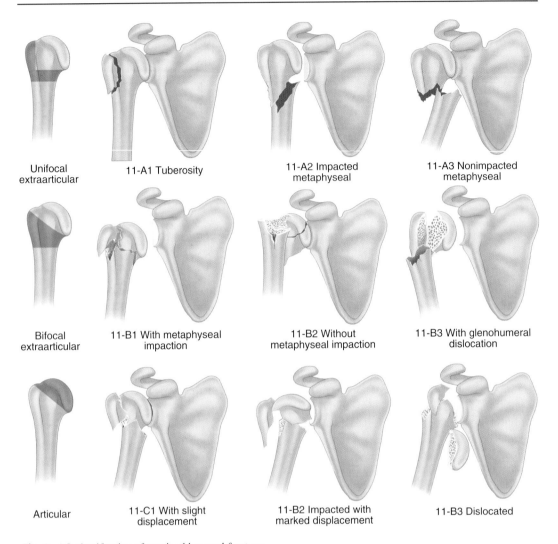

Unifocal extraarticular	11-A1 Tuberosity	11-A2 Impacted metaphyseal	11-A3 Nonimpacted metaphyseal
Bifocal extraarticular	11-B1 With metaphyseal impaction	11-B2 Without metaphyseal impaction	11-B3 With glenohumeral dislocation
Articular	11-C1 With slight displacement	11-B2 Impacted with marked displacement	11-B3 Dislocated

Fig. 2 AO classification of proximal humeral fractures

Small contributions to the supply of the humeral head arise from the posterior circumflex humeral. Fractures of the anatomic neck are uncommon but they have a poor prognosis due to the precarious blood supply to the humeral head.

Preservation of proximal humerus vascularity is important when distinguishing between valgus impacted and varus angulated three- and four-part proximal humerus fractures. The valgus impacted fracture is characterized by intact medial soft tissues, which can potentially preserve the blood supply to the humeral head. Acceptable results have been achieved with reduction and percutaneous pinning or plate osteosynthesis in patients with these fractures [8]. In the markedly displaced four-part proximal humerus fracture with significant varus malalignment, disruption of the medial soft-tissue envelope can potentially compromise perfusion to the humeral head.

The axillary nerve courses just anteroinferior to the glenohumeral joint, traversing the quandrangular space. It is at particular risk for traction injury owing to its relative rigid fixation at the posterior cord and deltoid as well as its proximity to the inferior capsule where it is susceptible to injury during anterior fracture dis-location. The incidence of neurologic injuries associated with proximal humerus fractures is high (59 % for nondisplaced fractures, but as high as 82 % if the fracture was displaced, according to Visser et al.). Fortunately, nerve recovery is usually expected and only a small percentage of fractures result in permanent nerve damage.

Hertel has identified certain anatomical fea-tures that can help identify those fractures at risk of avascular necrosis:

Good predictors of ischemia:

Length of metaphyseal head extension (accuracy 0.84 for calcar segments <8 mm)

Integrity of the *medial* hinge (accuracy 0.79 for disrupted hinge)

Basic *fracture* pattern (accuracy 0.7 for *fractures* comprising the anatomic neck)

Poor predictors of ischemia

Angular displacement of the head (accuracy 0.62 for angulations over 45 deg)

Extent of displacement of the tuberosities (dis-placement over 10 mm: accuracy 0.61)

Gleno-humeral dislocation (accuracy 0.49)

Head-split components (accuracy 0.49)

By combination of the above criteria: ana-tomic neck, short calcar, disrupted medial hinge, are associated with a positive predictive value for AVN of up to 97 % according to Hertel's study. However, Hertel later published a study evaluating the occurrence of avascular necrosis in intracpsular fractures of the humerus treated with internal fixation. Hertel found that eight of ten heads that were initially ischaemic did not go on to develop avascular necrosis indi-cating that revascularization may occur if ade-quate reduction and stable conditions are obtained (see [34]).

Diagnosis

The diagnosis of a proximal humeral fracture may be suspected based on the history of a traumatic injury and the clinical examination. Significant bruising and swelling, especially notable further down the arm rather than locally over the shoulder girdle itself, is often present. Plain radiographs are sufficient to make the diagnosis of proximal humeral fracture. To further delineate the fracture lines and position of fracture fragments then a CT scan may be obtained as discussed earlier.

Indications for Surgery

Hemiarthroplasty of the proximal humerus is indicated for most patients with four part frac-tures, displaced three part fractures, fracture dis-locations and also fractures involving a severe head split.

Charles Neer reported [15] 96 % failure of fixation with open reduction and internal fixation of four part fractures however those treated with a hemiarthroplasty had satisfactory or excellent results. In Neer's paper as many as 90 % of cases developed avascular necrosis however more recent studies [16–18] report much more encour-aging results for fixation of four part proximal humeral fractures rather than hemiarthroplasty. Not all patients with avascular necrosis of the head following internal fixation do poorly and in fact Gerber et al. [19] showed that patients who developed avascular necrosis but had anatomic healing of their tuberosities post-fixation had out-comes comparable to those of patients treated with hemiarthroplasty for complex proximal humerus fractures.

Following Neer's original report showing 100 % satisfaction with hemiarthroplasty follow-ing four part proximal humerus fractures, no other surgeon in recent times has been able to replicate these excellent results. Overall most patients experience satisfactory pain relief but their functional outcome can be unpredictable and unsatisfactory to the patient. In younger active patients with good bone quality it is advis-able to attempt open reduction and internal fixa-tion for complex proximal humerus fractures however hemiarthroplasty in older, lower demand patients with complex proximal humeral fractures remains an acceptable treatment modality.

Osteoporosis is not a contraindication to hemiarthroplasty for proximal humerus fractures. Some surgeons may argue that primary open reduction and internal fixation should be advised first as one can always resort to an arthroplasty as a secondary salvage procedure. However, performing an arthroplasty for failed internal fixation is very difficult and is also associated with worse outcomes [20, 21].

Contraindications to hemiarthroplasty are significant medical co-morbidities, which preclude the patient undergoing surgery. In younger patients with good bone stock every effort should be made to perform bone-preserving surgery with internal fixation.

Pre-Operative Preparation and Planning

Complex fractures of the proximal humerus can be associated with significant soft tissue injury and oedema. It may be advisable to allow the surrounding soft tissues to settle for 6–10 days prior to traumatising the tissues further by performing a hemiarthroplasty for a fracture. However, some surgeons prefer to perform surgery as soon as possible so that the patients can commence their recovery.

It is essential that the surgeon is familiar with the hemiarthroplasty implant technique being used in the operation.

As discussed earlier a CT scan may be obtained to identify the fracture fragments and plan surgery accurately [6, 7].

Operative Technique

Rather than considering a hemiarthroplasty for a complex proximal humeral fracture as a humeral head replacement arthroplasty it would be better for the surgeon to consider the operation as an osteosynthesis of the displaced tuberosities with replacement of the humeral head. The position and healing of the tuberosities around a correctly positioned arthroplasty with accurate restoration of height and retroversion is of paramount importance for a successful outcome. The overriding principal of treating these fractures with a hemiarthroplasty is to restore the patient's anatomy. To achieve a satisfactory result it is crucial to restore accurate humeral length, humeral version and achieve stable fixation of the tuberosities to each other and to the shaft/prosthesis.

Surgery is usually performed under a general anaesthetic with an interscalene block, which is used to ensure satisfactory post-operative pain relief. Pre-operative intravenous antibiotics are given to the patient after induction of anaesthesia. The patient is positioned safely in a beach chair position (Fig. 3). The skin is prepared and draped appropriately allowing adequate exposure to the shoulder girdle. An adhesive impervious sheet is also applied over the skin and drape to further "shut off" the patient's axilla. This is to minimise any potential contamination to the surgeon's gloves by the axillary skin during surgery.

The deltopectoral approach is used with an incision commencing superior to the coracoid and extending diagonally down to an inch lateral to the anterior axillary skin fold. The fascia over the deltopectoral groove is incised and the cephalic vein retracted laterally with the deltoid muscle and the pectoralis major medially. A Kolbel shoulder retractor with adjustable blades is introduced underneath the anterior deltoid and deep to the conjoint tendon following digital identification of the musculocutaneous nerve deep to the conjoint tendon. A Homan retractor is placed superiorly over the coracoacromial ligament and retracted superiorly. The fracture fragments are identified and the surgeon must take care to avoid any injury to the axillary nerve which passes the under surface of the subscapularis tendon. The long head of biceps is identified and a tenotomy performed. A stay suture is inserted into the biceps tendon which will later be incorporated into a soft tissue tenodesis.

Alternatively a deltoid split approach ,may be used but it is imperative that the axillary nerve is clearly identified and protected.

In a four part fracture the fracture line between the lesser and greater tuberosities is invariably

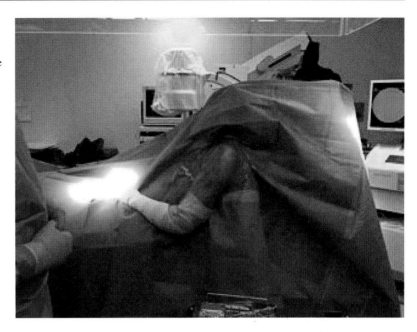

Fig. 3 The patient is positioned in the beach chair position and the left arm is draped free with the shoulder girdle exposed and covered in an impervious sheet

5–6 mms lateral to the bicipital groove. Stay sutures are inserted into the tendo-osseous junction of the subscapularis tendon and lesser tuberosity and also posteriorly at the tendo-osseous junction of the supraspinatus and infraspinatus tendons inserting onto the greater tuberosity fragment. Care must be taken not to inadvertently crush the tuberosities with instruments such as Kocher's, particularly in elderly patients with osteoporotic bone. After stay sutures are placed through the tendo-osseous junctions of the lesser and greater tuberosities the split through the anterior section of the supraspinatus which runs in line with the fracture between the tuberosities is identified and extended medially in the line of the rotator cuff fibres to allow greater exposure and access to the humeral head fragment.

Once the tuberosity fragments are mobilised the humeral head can be extracted. Any soft tissue attachments to the tuberosities should be preserved. If the humeral head is dislocated, for example in an anterior fracture dislocation, then great care should be taken when extracting the head as it will be lying in intimate proximity to the axillary vessels and brachial plexus. After the head is resected the tuberosities can be gently retracted apart and the remnant of the long head

of biceps completely resected. The glenoid articular surface should be inspected to exclude any concomitant pathology. Any associated glenoid fracture should be treated at this point. If the patient has concomitant glenoid arthrosis then a glenoid replacement arthroplasty should also be performed.

The excised humeral head is then sized with the trial implants of the arthroplasty (Fig. 4). If the patient's humeral head is in between trial sizes then the smaller arthroplasty head should be used and "over stuffing" the shoulder joint with a large head should be avoided.

The excised native humeral head will be used later for the acquisition of cancellous bone graft when repairing the tuberosities to the fracture arthroplasty stem.

Often there is a segment of the medial calcar which remains attached to the excised humeral head and this length should be measured as it will be used later to help guide the position and height of the arthroplasty stem and head offset (Fig. 5).

The metaphysis of the shaft should be exposed by extending, adducting and externally rotating the humerus and then pushing the humerus superiorly to deliver it through the surgical wound. The humeral shaft is prepared and rasped. The following surgical principals are of crucial

Fig. 4 The size of the excised humeral head is measured against a trial head from the arthroplasty implant system

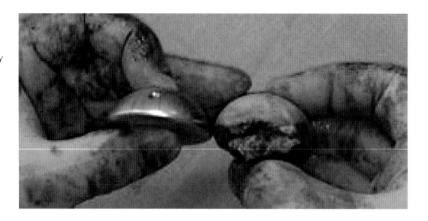

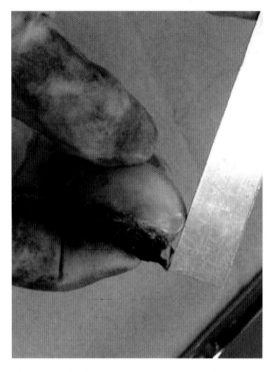

Fig. 5 A ruler is used to measure the length of calcar which is still attached to the excised humeral head

importance when selecting the appropriate size and position of implants. The correct humeral length must be restored and therefore the arthroplasty must be inserted and held at the appropriate height. The surgeon must also judge the correct humeral version in which to implant the prosthesis. This is obviously difficult in the case of fracture, contrary to surgery for articular

degeneration, as the anatomical landmarks are distorted. There is a variety of techniques available to the operating surgeon to achieve the correct implant height and retroversion (Fig. 6). By measuring the length of medial calcar which was fractured with the humeral head the operating surgeon can use this as a reference distance that the hemiarthroplasty head should be from the tip of the remaining medial calcar on the shaft of the humerus. This is a reliable technique to help the surgeon recreate the anatomical arc of the medial calcar. If this technique is used the distance usually measures approximately 5–7 mms unless there is significant metaphyseal comminution associated with a fracture.

A further option is to reduce the greater tuberosity fracture fragment back to an anatomical position in relation to the humeral shaft and using the superior margin of the greater tuberosity as a landmark to judge the correct height of the superior margin of the arthroplasty humeral head (Fig. 7). The anatomical study by Iannotti et al concluded that the top of the greater tuberosity sits 8 ± 3.5 mm below the top of the humeral articular surface [24]. Therefore if the fractured greater tuberosity is held in an anatomically correct position in relation to the humeral shaft then the height of the implant can be judged correctly.

Some surgeons prefer to take full-length AP humeral radiographs of both the injured arm and the contralateral humerus to measure the appropriate humeral lengths and use an intraoperative ruler to judge the appropriate height for the hemiarthroplasty.

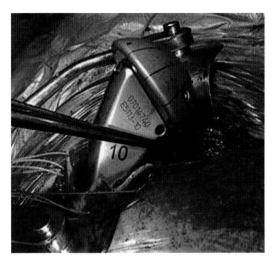

Fig. 6 A trial stem has been inserted to the humerus. If the stem is at the correct height and the head in the correct position then the distance from the tip of the remaining calcar and medial edge of the implant should be the same distance as the measurement of the section of calcar attached to the excised head. Also, if the implant is in the correct position then an imaginary line continuing the contour of the humeral medial calcar should meet the medial tip of the head implant

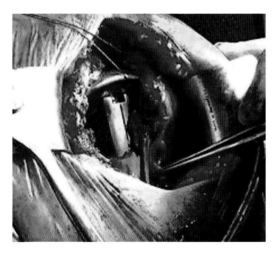

Fig. 7 The greater tuberosity is reduced to an anatomical position and the height of the implant can be correctly estimated

A further reference point to judge the correct head height is to reference from the pectoralis major tendon insertion. Torrens et al reported that anatomical height restoration could be achieved by placing the tangent of the humeral head 5.6 cm above the upper insertion of the pectoralis major tendon [23]. In the same study the authors reported that correct retro version could be achieved by placing the posterior fin of the prosthesis 1.06 cm from the pectoralis major insertion.

Intraoperative fluoroscopy can occasionally be useful in gauging the correct height of the humeral implant.

It is of crucial importance to the long-term outcome of the surgery that the correct humeral height is achieved for the implant. If the prosthesis is inserted in a position, which is too low this will cause a lack of tension in the deltoid muscle and inadequate space for fixation of the tuberosities under the implant head. If the implant is too high then it will not be possible to reduce the tuberosities over the implant to the correct anatomical position.

To achieve the correct humeral head retroversion either the bicipital groove can be used as a reference point or the transepicondylar axis. It is important not to excessively retrovert the implant as this can lead to poor function and even posterior dislocation. If the posterior fin of the humeral stem is implanted 8 mm lateral to the bicipital groove, with the distance measured along the lateral cortex of the shaft, then this will place the humeral implant in the correct version [25]. However, the cadaveric study by Balg and Boileau demonstrates that there is variability in the orientation of the biceps groove at the anatomical neck and surgical neck. As there is great variation in groove orientation and the position for lateral fin placement at the surgical neck has not been documented the authors caution the surgeon regarding the use of the groove as a reliable landmark for calculating retroversion in shoulder replacement surgery for fractures (see [35]).

Usually the surgeon would aim to put the implant in approximately 25° of retroversion, which is the average retroversion of the humeral head [26] (Fig. 8). However, we know from previous anatomical studies that the patient's native retroversion could vary from 10° to 45° [27, 28]. By aiming for 25° of retroversion this will also

Fig. 8 A retrotorsion bar is attached to either the humeral rasp or trial stem and the goniometer attached to the bar is referenced against the axis of the forearm to determine the degree of retroverion of the rasp of implant

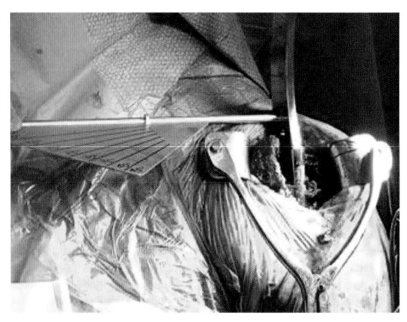

avoid undue tension on the greater tuberosity repair with the arm internally rotated. The inter-epicondylar axis at the distal humerus can also be used as a guide to judge accurate retroversion. A trial stem is inserted to the humeral shaft and a goniometer attached to the prosthetic stem via a retrotorsion bar is used to measure the correct retroversion in relation to the inter-epicondylar axis and forearm axis.

Following preparation of the humeral canal a cement restrictor is inserted into the humeral shaft at the appropriate distance to prevent extrusion of any cement distally in the humeral shaft. The trial stem is again reinserted to ensure that the cement restrictor is distal enough in the shaft to allow satisfactory placement of the humeral stem. Modern modular implants allow the offset of the humeral head to be adjusted and this allows the surgeon to ensure that the inferior tip of the head is in line with the medial calcar and the superior tip of the head is at the correct height above the superior tip of the greater tuberosity, as mentioned earlier.

The modular prosthesis is constructed and prepared for implantation.

The suture or wires that are to be used to reattach the tuberosities are inserted via the supraspinatus tendo-osseous junction or greater tuberosity fragment. These wires or sutures should ideally be placed prior to insertion of the humeral implant as access to this area of the greater tuberosity tendo-osseous junction is much easier prior to implant insertion. To prepare for later fixation of the tuberosities, two 2 mm drill holes should be placed in the proximal humerus both medial and lateral to the bicipital groove 5 mm distal to the fracture line at the surgical neck. This should be done prior to implantation of the prosthesis and high tensile sutures are now passed in a horizontal mattress fashion through the holes for later tension band suture fixation to the rotator cuff and tuberosities.

The humeral stem is cemented using standard third generation technique and the surgeon should take care that the prosthesis is inserted in the correct retroversion and height. Excess cement around the collar of the implant should be removed. Cementing of the prosthesis affords the surgeon greater control in establishing accurate height of the implant.

Cancellous bone graft is harvested from the native humeral head, which can then be implanted around the proximal stem of the implant to help encourage fixation of the tuberosity fragments to the implant.

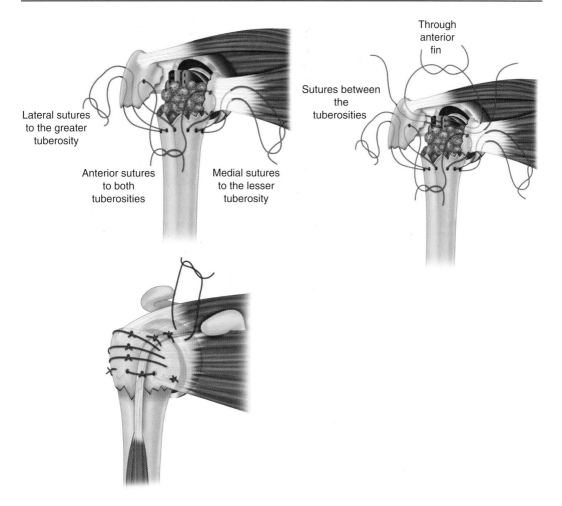

Through anterior fin

Sutures between the tuberosities

Lateral sutures to the greater tuberosity

Anterior sutures to both tuberosities

Medial sutures to the lesser tuberosity

Fig. 9 Suture fixation of tuberosities to the implant

The method of suture fixation of the tuberosities to the implant varies with the prosthesis being used (Fig. 9). Some implants have two holes in the proximal stem, which allow either a high tensile suture or a 1 mm steel wire to be used to reattach the tuberosities. With the humeral head implanted but still in an anteriorly dislocated position the cables or sutures are passed through the corresponding holes of the stem or medial to the stem neck and then through the lesser tuberosity anteriorly. The head can now be reduced to the glenoid and the tuberosities can be repaired in place around the humeral stem. Any void under the tuberosities should be filled with cancellous bone harvested from the native humeral head. The sutures passed earlier through the drill holes in the shaft can then be used to perform a tension band suture technique with one being tied as a loop anteriorly through the subscapularis tendo-osseous junction and two sutures through the posterosuperior rotator cuff tendo-osseous junction. The sutures from the tuberosities to the shaft are tied first followed by the tuberosity-to-tuberosity sutures.

When fixing the tuberosities over-reduction should be avoided. Over-reduction of the lesser tuberosity will restrict external rotation whereas over-reduction of the greater tuberosity will limit internal rotation. If the prosthesis is in the correct position with respect to height and retroversion then it should not be difficult to reduce the tuberosities into a satisfactory

Fig. 10 Final view of the tuberosities sutured in place. At the base of the wound some of the drill holes for the sutures can be seen. The tuberosities have been reduced to an anatomical position and not under- or over-reduced. Knots can be seen from the sutures linking the tuberosities and humeral stem and further sutures, tied in a figure of 8 fashion, from the humeral metaphysis drill holes to the rotator cuff tendons

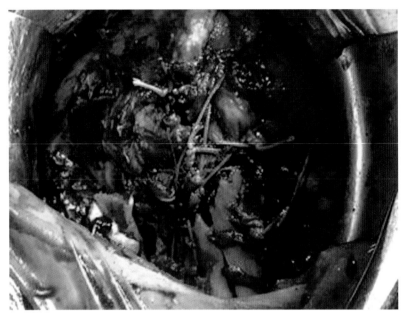

position (Fig. 10). If the surgeon is finding it difficult to reduce the tuberosities adequately then this should be a warning to the surgeon that the prosthesis may not be in the correct anatomical position.

Successful healing of the tuberosities in the correct position is of great importance for the success of the hemiarthroplasty and this depends on accurate prosthetic implantation and also on a fixation technique adequate to withstand early passive motion of the shoulder. Once the tuberosities are repaired then the shoulder is mobilised through a full range of motion to ensure adequate stable fixation of the tuberosities without micro motion.

The split through the leading edge of supraspinatus in line with the fracture is repaired with the arm externally rotated 20°.

At the end of the procedure the biceps tendon is sutured to the pectoralis major fascia with non-absorbable sutures to perform a soft tissue tenodesis.

Following sufficient irrigation and haemostasis, a redivac drain is placed deep to the deltoid and the wound closed in layers. The arm is protected in a sling. The drain is removed 24 h post surgery.

Post-Operative Care and Rehabilitation

Sutures should be removed at 2 weeks following surgery and patients will often require their sling for the first 6 weeks post-surgery.

Patients should be warned preoperatively that it can take up to a year to achieve their maximum functional potential following the hemiarthroplasty and this recovery may be longer if there is a concomitant nerve injury secondary to the initial fracture.

The post-operative rehabilitation is divided into three phases. The patient's arm is initially immobilised in a sling with the arm in internal rotation. Immediate passive motion is commenced the day after surgery and under the supervision of the physiotherapists passive active assisted exercises are allowed during the first 6 weeks. If at 6 weeks postoperatively a check x-ray shows that the tuberosities are uniting in a satisfactory position then the patient can start active range of movement exercises. As some patients may have very osteoporotic tuberosities then each patient should ideally have an individualised rehabilitation protocol, which the surgeon can decide based on the patient's bone quality, the intraoperative range of motion, adequacy of the tuberosity fixation and expected patient compliance. In the third phase of rehabilitation resistance exercises, for example using therabands, can be commenced at 12 weeks following surgery. The three-phase system of rehabilitation was devised by Hughes and Neer [29].

Complications

Complications following hemiarthroplasty for complex proximal humeral fractures include the standard complications following any surgery. Haematoma formation and deep infection are a significant risk. Kontakis et al. [9] showed a deep infection rate of 0.64 % and a superficial infection rate of 1.55 %. A further complication specific to this procedure is proximal migration of the head, which was seen in 6.8 % of patients. Arguably the leading complication following a hemiarthroplasty for proximal humeral fractures relates to the tuberosities. The tuberosities may fail to unite, displace or even suffer osteolysis, "the vanishing tuberosities." Boileau et al. in 2002 reported factors associated with failure of tuberosity osteosynthesis [30]. Women over 75 years of age have poorer results and a worse outcome was also noted with excessive humeral retroversion of over 40°, a prosthesis over 10 mm above the tuberosities or a greater tuberosity over 5 mm above the humeral head. Overall the worst association was found with a high, retroverted head with a low greater tuberosity forming an "unhappy triad" leading to posterior migration of the greater tuberosity and a subsequent poor result.

In Boileau's series lengthening the humerus more than 10 mm correlated with a tuberosity detachment and subsequent proximal migration of the prosthesis under the coracoacromial arch. This may indeed be from a non-union of the greater tuberosity at the humeral diaphysis or from a subsequent rotator cuff tear secondary to the tension. Shortening of the humerus was much better tolerated clinically. Humeral shortening of 2 cm or more is required before deltoid power and function is adversely affected [30, 32].

Tanner and Cofield identified greater tuberosity displacement as the most common complication following this type of surgery. Complications were more frequent with fracture dislocations and chronic fractures [31].

Outcomes

Functional results following hemiarthroplasty surgery for proximal humerus fractures have been unpredictable although an arthroplasty usually gives adequate pain relief. As a consequence open reduction and internal fixation is the preferred treatment of choice for younger patients with three and four part proximal humerus fractures so that the young patient's natural bone stock is preserved.

Hemiarthroplasty serves as a viable option for pain relief in persons with displaced four-part proximal humerus fracture; however, the affected shoulder rarely returns to its baseline level of function, specifically baseline range of motion. Kontakis et al. [9] reported the outcomes of early management of proximal humerus fractures with hemiarthroplasty in a total of 808 patients (810 hemiarthroplasties). At a mean follow-up of 3.7 years, mean active forward elevation was 105.7°, mean abduction was 92.4°, and external rotation was 30.4°. These results are similar to those of other reports [10, 11]. Kontakis et al. [9] identified the Constant score for a total of 560 patients in eight studies; the mean Constant score in patients who underwent replacement of a proximal humerus prosthesis was 56.6 out of 100 (range, 11–98).

In recent years there has been a trend in Europe to treat these complicated injuries in older patients with a reverse geometry arthroplasty on the theoretical basis that the patients will achieve a greater functional outcome compared to a standard hemiarthroplasty, as a reverse arthroplasty is not reliant on the tuberosities and rotator cuff for function. Bufquin et al [13] prospectively studied a cohort of 43 patients with three- or four-part proximal humerus fractures treated with RTSA. At an average 22-month follow-up, mean active forward elevation and external rotation with the arm in abduction were 97° and 30°, respectively. The mean Constant score was 44. The authors concluded that adequate clinical results could be achieved with RTSA in patients with three- or four part fractures, despite loss of reduction of the tuberosities. Gallinet et al [14] retrospectively studied a series of 40 patients with complex three- or four-part proximal humerus fractures who underwent either hemiarthroplasty or RTSA. Twenty-one patients underwent hemiarthroplasty with a standard cemented stem, and 19 underwent RTSA using a reverse prosthesis with a cemented stem. Constant scores, active abduction, and forward elevation were higher in the RTSA group compared with the hemiarthroplasty group. However, external rotation was greater in the hemiarthroplasty group (13.5° vs. 9°). In the hemiarthroplasty group, radiographs showed failed tuberosity healing in 3 of 17 patients (18 %). In the RTSA group, 15 of 16 patients (94 %) demonstrated radiographic evidence of scapular notching; however, no cases of glenosphere loosening were reported.

Arguably the most difficult thing to achieve for a standard anatomical hemiarthroplasty for fracture is well healed tuberosities in an anatomical location that allow the patient to achieve excellent active range of movement of their shoulder post-surgery. Many authors have stressed the importance of meticulous stable suture fixation of the tuberosities [22]. Boileau et al found that factors associated with failure of tuberosity osteosynthesis included poor initial position of the prosthesis in particular excessive height or retroversion, poor position of the greater tuberosity and women over the age of 75 who may have osteopenic bone (see [36]).

Summary

The successful surgical management of complex proximal humerus fractures is a challenge even for the most experienced shoulder surgeon. This chapter has outlined the principles and techniques used to perform a hemiarthroplsty for fracture of the proximal humerus. Tuberosity union in an

anatomical position, restoration of humeral height and correct retroversion are some of the challenges that must be conquered to achieve successful outcomes following hemiarthroplasty.

Prosthetic humeral head replacement has been shown to be effective in providing good pain relief, however, the affected extremity will not reach pre-injury levels of function. Hemiarthroplasty for complex proximal humeral fractures is a useful treatment option, however, in younger patients with good bone stock osteosynthesis should be the preferred treatment of choice.

References

1. Codman EA. Rupture of the supraspinatus tendon and other lesions in or about the subacromial bursa. In: Codman EA, editor. The shoulder. New York: G. Miller; 1934.
2. Neer CS. Indications for replacement of the proximal humeral articulation. Am J Surg. 1955;89:901–7.
3. Neer CS, Brown TH, McLaughlin HL. Fracture of the neck of the humerus with dislocation of the head fragment. Am J Surg. 1953;85:252–8.
4. Neer CS. Displaced proximal humeral fractures. Part I: classification and evaluation. J Bone Joint Surg Am. 1970;52A:1077–89.
5. Kristiansen B, Andersen LS, Olsen CA, Vasmarken JE. The Neer classification of fractures of the proximal humerus: an assessment of interobserver variation. Skeletal Radiol. 1988;17:420–2.
6. Castagno AA, Shuman WP, Kilcoyno AF, Haynor OR, Moms ME, Matson FA. Complex fractures of the proximal humerus: role of CT in treatment. Radiology. 1987;165:759–62.
7. Hertel R, Hempfing A, Stiehler M, Leunig M. JSES. Predictors of humeral head ischemia after intracapsular fracture of the proximal humerus. 2004;13:427–33.
8. Jakob RP, Miniaci A, Anson PS, Jaberg H, Osterwalder A, Ganz R. Four-part valgus impacted fractures of the proximal humerus. J Bone Joint Surg Br. 1991;73(2):295–8.
9. Kontakis G, Koutras C, Tosounidis T, Giannoudis P. Early management of proximal humeral fractures with hemiarthroplasty: a systematic review. J Bone Joint Surg Br. 2008;90(11):1407–13.
10. Naranja Jr RJ, Iannotti JP. Displaced three- and four-part proximal humerus fractures: evaluation and management. J Am Acad Orthop Surg. 2000;8(6):373–82.
11. Goldman RT, Koval KJ, Cuomo F, Gallagher MA, Zuckerman JD. Functional outcome after humeral head replacement for acute three- and four- part

proximal humeral fractures. J Shoulder Elbow Surg. 1995;4(2):81–6.

12. Sjödén GO, Movin T, Aspelin P, Güntner P, Shalabi A. 3D-radiographic analysis does not improve the Neer and AO classifications of proximal humeral fractures. Acta Orthop Scand. 1999;70(4):325–8.

13. Bufquin T, Hersan A, Hubert L, Massin P. Reverse shoulder arthroplasty for the treatment of three- and four-part fractures of the proximal humerus in the elderly: a prospective review of 43 cases with a short-term follow-up. J Bone Joint Surg Br. 2007;89(4):516–20.

14. Gallinet D, Clappaz P, Garbuio P, Tropet Y, Obert L. Three or four parts complex proximal humerus fractures: hemiarthroplasty versus reverse prosthesis. A comparative study of 40 cases. Orthop Traumatol Surg Res. 2009;95(1):48–55.

15. Neer CS. Indications for replacement of the proximal humeral articulation. Am J Surg. 1955;89:901–7.

16. Lee CK, Hansen HR. Post-traumatic avascular necrosisof the humeral head in displaced proximal humeral fractures. J Trauma. 1981;21:788–91.

17. Esser RD. Treatment of three and four part fractures of the proximal humerus with a modified cloverleaf plate. J Orthop Trauma. 1994;8:15–22.

18. Darder A, Sanchis V, Gastaldi E, et al. Four-part displaced proximal humeral fractures: operative treatments using Kirschner wires and a tension band. J Orthop Trauma. 1993;7:497–505.

19. Gerber C, Hersche O, Berberat C. The clinical relevance of post traumatic a vascular necrosis of the humeral head. J Shoulder Elbow Surg. 1998;7:586–90.

20. Tanner MW, Cofield RH. Prosthetic arthroplasty for fractures and fracture-dislocations of the proximal humerus. Clin Orthop. 1983;179:116–28.

21. Norris TR, Green A, McGuigan FX. Late prosthetic shoulder arthroplasty for displaced proximal humeral fractures. J Shoulder Elbow Surg. 1995;4(4):271–80.

22. Zuckermann JD, Cuomo F, Coval KJ. Proximal humeral replacement for complex fractures indications and surgical technique. Instr Course Lecture. 1997;46:7–14.

23. Torrens C, Corrales M, Melendo E, Solano A, Rodriquez-Baeza A, Careres E. The pectoralis major tendon as a reference for restoring humeral length and retroversion with hemiarthroplasty for fracture. J Shoulder Elbow Surg. 2008;17(6):947–50.

24. Iannotti JP, Gabriel JP, Schneck SL, Evans BG, Misra S. The normal glenohumeral relationships. An anatomical study of one hundred and forty shoulders. J Bone Joint Surg Am. 1992;74(4):491–500.

25. Hempfing A, Leunig M, Ballmer FT, Hertel R. Surgical landmarks to determine humeral head retrotorsion or hemiarthroplasty in fractures. J Shoulder Elbow Surg. 2001;10(5):460–3.

26. Hertel R, Knothe U, Ballmer FT. Geometry of the proximal humerus and implications for prosthetic design. J Shoulder Elbow Surg. 2002;11(4):331–8.

27. Boileau P, Bicknell RT, Mazzoleni N, Walch G, Urien JP. CT scan method accurately assesses humeral head retroversion. Clin Orthop Relat Res. 2008;466(3):661–9.

28. Hernigou P, Duparc F, Hernigou A. Determining humeral retroversion with computed tomography. J Bone Joint Surg Am. 2002;84(10):1753–62.

29. Hughes M, Neer CS. Glenohumeral joint replacement and postoperative rehabilitation. Phys Ther. 1975;55:850–8.

30. Boileau P, Krishnan SG, Tinsi L, Walch G, Coste JS, Mole D. Tuberosity malposition and migration: reasons for poor outcomes after hemiarthroplasty for displaced fractures of the proximal humerus. J Shoulder Elbow Surg. 2002;11(5):401–12.

31. Tanner MW, Cofield RH. Prosthetic arthroplasty for fractures and fracture dislocations of the proximal humerus. Colin Orthop Relat Res. 1983;179:116–28.

32. Neer CS, Kirby RM. Revision of humeral head and total shoulder arthroplasties. Clin Orthop Relat Res. 1982;170:189–95.

33. Majed A, Macleod I, Bull AM, Zyto K, Resch H, Hertel R, Reilly P, Emery RJ. Proximal humeral fracture classification systems revisited. J Shoulder Elbow Surg. 2011;20(7):1125–32.

34. Bastian JD, Hertel R. Initial post-fracture humeral head ischaemia does not predict development of necrosis. J Shoulder Elbow Surg. 2008;17(1):2–8.

35. Balg F, Boulianne M, Boileau P. Bicipital groove orientation: considerations for the retroversion of a prosthesis in fractures of the proximal humerus. J Shoulder Elbow Surg. 2006;15(2):195–8.

36. Boileau P, Krishnan SG, Tinsi L, Walch G, Coste JS, Mole D. Tuberosity malposition and migration: reasons for poor outcomes after hemiarthroplasty for displaced fractures of the proximal humerus. J Shoulder Elbow Surg. 2002;11(5):401–12.

Humeral Shaft Fractures - Principles of Management

Deborah Higgs

Contents

Abstract

Humeral shaft fractures account for approximately 3 % of all fractures. Vascular injury in association with humeral shaft fractures occurs in only a small percentage of cases. Most humeral shaft fractures can be managed non-operatively with expected good or excellent results. Both patient and fracture characteristics need to be considered when deciding the most appropriate treatment option.

Keywords

Anatomy • Classification • Complications-radial nerve and vascular • Diagnosis • Humeral shaft fractures • Mechanisms • Non-operative bracing • Surgical indications

Anatomy

The humeral shaft extends from the surgical neck proximally to the condyles distally. Proximally it has a cylindrical shape in cross-section and the cortex is thin. It is conical in its middle section where the cortex is very thick and the medulla narrow. In the distal third the humerus becomes more flattened in the coronal plane giving it a trapezoidal shape. The medulla ends just above the olecranon fossa.

The humeral head is just proximal to, and in line with the distal end of the canal. The upper arm is completely covered with muscle apart from the medial and lateral epicondyles.

D. Higgs
Royal National Orthopaedic Hospital, Stanmore, Middlesex, UK
e-mail: dhiggs@doctors.org.uk

G. Bentley (ed.), *European Surgical Orthopaedics and Traumatology*,
DOI 10.1007/978-3-642-34746-7_250, © EFORT 2014

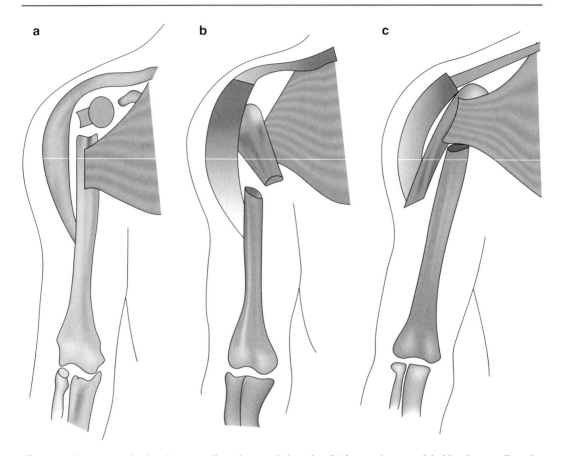

Fig. 1 (**a**) Fracture proximal to the pectoralis major muscle insertion (**b**) fracture between deltoid and pectoralis major insertions (**c**) fracture distal to deltoid

The muscles are divided into flexor and extensor compartments, separated by medial and lateral intermuscular septa. The flexor(anterior) compartment contains biceps, brachialis and coracobrachialis. The extensor(posterior) compartment contains triceps. If the fracture is situated between the rotator cuff and the pectoralis major muscle, the humeral head will be abducted and internally rotated. If the fracture is between the pectoralis muscle and the insertion of deltoid, the proximal fragment will be adducted and the distal fragment laterally displaced. In fractures distal to the deltoid insertion, the proximal fragment will be abducted. In fractures proximal to the brachioradialis and extensor muscles, the distal fragment will be rotated laterally (Fig. 1).

The brachial artery (and vein) lie well medial to the shaft proximally and is superficial throughout its course in the upper arm. In the lower arm the artery lies anteromedially on the brachialis muscle. The median nerve crosses in front of the artery from lateral to medial in the cubital fossa (Fig. 2).

The ulnar nerve lies medial to the brachial artery as it exits the axilla, and at the junctions of the middle and distal thirds of the upper arm perforates the medial intermuscular septum to run on the posterior aspect of the medial epicondyle (Fig. 3).

The radial nerve lies posterior to the origin of the brachial artery crossing the subscapularis muscle and teres major tendon. It passes obliquely distally (from medial to lateral) in the spiral groove directly on the posterior aspect of the shaft of the humerus with the profunda brachii artery. It perforates the lateral intermuscular septum at the junction of the middle and distal thirds of the humerus from posterior to anterior

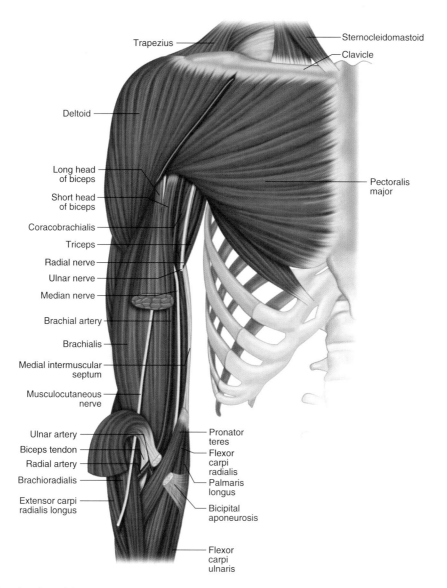

Fig. 2 Anterior view of the upper arm

compartments. Here the nerve is less mobile and is vulnerable when fragments displace. It continues distally between the brachialis medially and the brachioradialis and extensor carpi radialis muscles laterally.

The axillary nerve, which is initially posterior to the axillary artery, crosses the subscapularis then continues posteriorly traversing the quadrilateral space. It winds around the surgical neck with the posterior circumflex artery about 5–6 cm below the acromion.

The musculocutaneous nerve passes through the muscle belly of the coracobrachialis and runs between biceps and brachialis.

Mechanism of Injury

Typically humeral shaft fractures occur as a result of a simple fall, often in the older patient, or as a result of motor vehicle accidents. Sporting injuries and fractures following a direct blow are

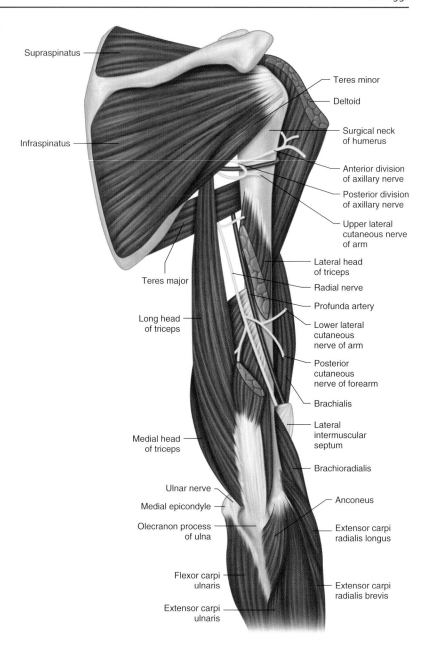

Fig. 3 Posterior view of the upper arm

comparatively rare. Pure compressive forces result in proximal or distal humerus fractures; torsional forces in spiral fractures; bending forces in transverse fractures. Combined bending and torsion results in an oblique fracture, often with a butterfly fragment. The typical oblique distal shaft fracture described by Holstein and Lewis (1963) [8] is associated with arm wrestling. Higher energy injuries result in a greater degree of comminution and soft tissue injury.

Pathological fractures from metastatic bone disease and myeloma are an important subgroup. A review of 249 humeral shaft fractures by McQueen [21] showed a bi-modal distribution: with peaks in the third and seventh decades with the division at 50 years of age. In the under-50-year group, 70 % of fractures occurred in men with over two-thirds the result of moderate to severe trauma. In the over- 50-year group 73 % were in women with nearly 80 % of fractures resulting from a simple fall. This epidemiological information differs from other data published. Mast et al. [9], in a retrospective study of 240 fractures of the humeral shaft in a level-1 trauma centre, found that 60 % occurred in the under-30-year age group, with a fairly even distribution of injury within the shaft 17 % of the fractures were the result of gunshot wounds. Rose et al. [14] reviewed 586 humeral fractures of which 116 (20 %) were of the shaft. They noted a bi-modal distribution for the latter injuries with a peak in the under-30-year and over-30-year age groups. Nearly 70 % of the fractures occurred in the former group, and were a result of severe trauma with just over half being sustained in men.

Classification

Traditionally diaphyseal fractures of the humerus have been classified depending on:
1. Fracture location – proximal, middle, or distal third of the humeral shaft;
2. The fracture pattern – transverse, oblique, spiral, segmental, or comminuted;
3. Bone quality – normal or pathological;
4. Associated soft tissue injury – open or closed;
5. Associated neurovascular injury.

Currently as with all diaphyseal fractures, the major classification for humeral shaft fractures is the AO classification. This classification combines the position of the fracture in the diaphysis with the fracture morphology. It divides humeral diaphyseal fractures into three basic types: A, B and C:

Type A fractures are simple fractures without any degree of comminution.

Type B fractures are wedge fractures associated with intact or fragmented butterfly fragments.

Type C fractures are complex fractures with significant comminution or a segmental component. Each AO fracture type is divided into three groups and each group into three

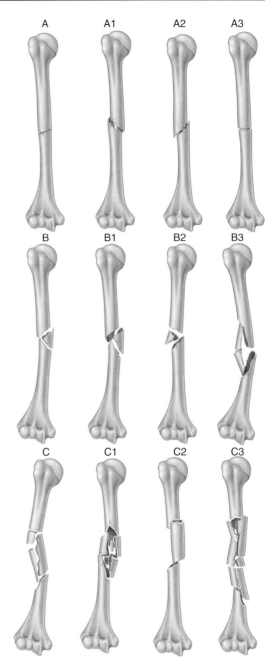

Fig. 4 AO classification of humeral shaft fractures

sub-groups depending on fracture pattern. In their series McQueen [21] reported over 60 % of humeral shaft fractures occurred in the middle segment of the shaft of the humerus and over 60 % were AO type A (Fig. 4).

The principal disadvantage with the AO classification is that the state of the soft tissues is not taken into account.

For open fractures of the humerus, as with open fractures elsewhere in the skeleton, the commonly used Gustilo [5, 6] and Tscherne [11] classifications can be used.

In the series from Edinburgh [21] less than 10 % of the fractures were reported as open; with a bi-modal age distribution with a peak in the third decade as a result of moderate to severe injury in men and a larger peak in the seventh decade after a simple fall in women.

Diagnosis

The mechanism of injury is important. With high energy injuries it is particularly important to assess for associated injuries. Compliance with conservative treatment needs to be assessed. In cases of pathological fractures the primary diagnosis and the presence of other metastatic lesions should be considered when planning treatment.

Examination

The upper arm should be examined for swelling, bruising, and deformity. The entire upper limb should be examined for vascular and neurological changes, especially the radial nerve. Soft tissue abrasions need to be differentiated from open fractures. Examination of the shoulder and elbow can be difficult in the presence of a humeral shaft fracture but they should be assessed for injury and stiffness secondary to arthrosis.

X-rays are obtained in two planes, anteroposterior and lateral. The elbow and shoulder joint should be included on each view. This is to assess for intra-articular fracture extension, dislocations and pre-existing arthrosis. It is important not to rotate the arm through the fracture site. CT scans and MRI scans are rarely indicated. In pathological fractures additional studies such as MRI, CT or technetium bone scans are likely to be necessary prior to planning treatment.

Initial Management

Initial splinting of humeral shaft fractures can be difficult. A collar and cuff allowing the arm to hang dependent provides provisional splinting. The best pain-relieving splint is provided by a U-slab of plaster of paris applied to the outer aspect of the arm from the acromion around the elbow, held in 90° of flexion and continued along the inner aspect of the arm to the axilla. The plaster is applied to the arm over vellband and held in place by crepe bandage. The radial nerve should be assessed before and after application of the cast. If radial nerve function is normal before and abnormal after application of the cast then open exploration of the radial nerve with internal fixation of the fracture should be performed.

Methods of Treatment

The goal of treatment is to obtain union with acceptable alignment to allow the patient to return to their previous level of function.

The decision whether to treat a humeral shaft fracture operatively or non-operatively requires an understanding of the relevant anatomy and the fracture pattern.

The majority of humeral shaft fractures can be managed conservatively. Moderate angulation (less than 20° anterior and 30° varus angulation), rotation, and shortening (less than 3 cm) are well tolerated. Mast et al. [9], in their retrospective study of 240 humeral shaft fractures showed that in 100 patients treated non-operatively there were five non-unions and 15 delayed unions with 96 % incidence of excellent or satisfactory results.

Non-Operative Management

There are many options for non-operative treatment including U-slabs and hanging casts. Many surgeons now use humeral functional bracing. This was described by Sarmiento in 1977 [17] and effects fracture reduction through soft tissue compression. The original casts have given way to functional braces. These braces have Velcro straps which can be tightened as swelling decreases. Proximally the brace approaches the acromion laterally and the axilla medially encircling the upper arm. Distally the brace does not cover the medial and lateral epicondyles to allow free elbow movement. Sarmiento and others have reported excellent results with their use. In a review of 85 extra-articular comminuted distal-third humeral shaft fractures Sarmiento reported only one pseudarthrosis and one asymptomatic mal-union. The average time to union was 10 weeks. All cases of radial nerve palsy resolved during treatment. Zargorski et al. [22] reported a series of 233 humeral shaft fractures treated with a pre-fabricated humeral brace. Of 170 patients available for follow-up 98 % (167) had united with an average time to union of 9.5 weeks for closed fractures and 13.6 weeks for open fractures. 95 % (158) had an excellent functional result (Fig. 5).

A functional brace can be applied acutely or 1–2 weeks after application of a U-slab. Many surgeons choose the latter option. A radiograph after brace application is advisable to check the fracture position. Radial nerve function should be assessed before and after application of the brace. The patient is followed at weekly intervals with radiographs for the first 3–4 weeks. The brace is worn for a minimum of 8 weeks.

There can however be problems associated with bracing. The straps have to be tightened as swelling decreases to ensure a firm fit. There is an incidence of skin problems and shoulder stiffness. Obese patients and certain fracture patterns, such as transverse fractures at the level of the deltoid insertion or segmental fractures, are more difficult to treat in a brace. Zagorski et al. [22] identified three patients with significant varus angulation all of whom were obese women whose ipsilateral breast had acted as a fulcrum around which the fracture had angulated. Use of a sling may also result in varus angulation (Fig. 6).

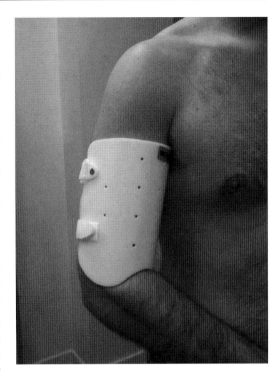

Fig. 5 Pre-fabricated functional humeral brace

Operative Management

There are absolute and relative indications for surgical stabilization.

Absolute indications:

Polytrauma
Open fractures
Bilateral humeral shaft fractures
Pathological fracture
Floating elbow
Vascular injury
Radial nerve injury after closed reduction
Non-union

Relative indications:

Long spiral fractures
Transverse fractures
Brachial plexus injuries
Inability to maintain reduction
Obese patients

The patient's age, fracture pattern, associated injuries, co-morbidity, and ability to comply with treatment must be considered.

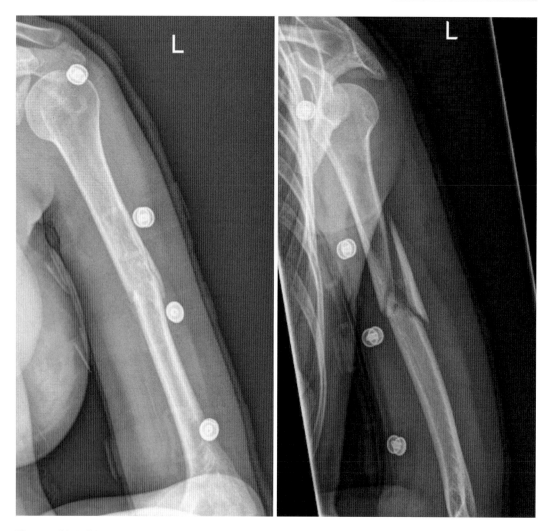

Fig. 6 Mid-shaft humeral fracture in a 31-year-old female sustained in a motor vehicle accident. Radiograph taken with arm in a functional brace

Vascular Injury

Fractures of the humeral shaft are rarely associated with vascular injury. Mechanisms of brachial artery injury include penetrating trauma, entrapment between fracture fragments and secondary occlusion due to swelling. Fractures complicated by vascular injury are an Orthopaedic emergency. Stabilisation of the fracture is required to protect the vascular repair and minimise further soft tissue injury. Whether the humerus is stabilised prior to or after the vascular repair depends on the ischaemia time and is a decision made by the vascular and Orthopaedic surgeon.

Nerve Injury

Radial nerve injuries have been associated with up to 11 % of humeral shaft fractures [19]. The site of the fracture is important. Despite the Holstein- Lewis fracture (distal-third, oblique fracture) being associated with a radial nerve palsy, middle-third humeral shaft fractures are

Fig. 7 Radiographs taken 8 months post-injury showing a united fracture

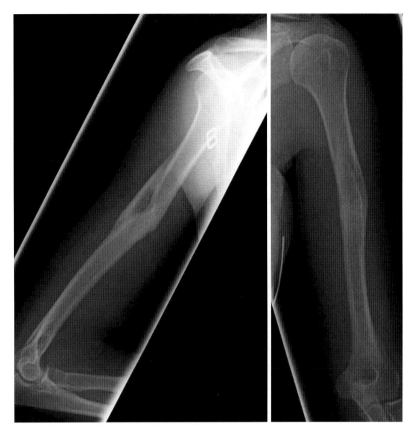

the most common for radial nerve involvement. In this area up to 30 % of fractures may show radial nerve involvement. Most lesions take the form of a neuropraxia, or rarely axonotmesis, with a reported 90 % resolving within 3–4 months.

Indications for early operative exploration of the radial nerve include radial nerve palsies associated with an open fracture, penetrating trauma, and secondary nerve palsies post-fracture reduction.

However management of a primary radial nerve palsy associated with a closed humeral shaft fracture remains controversial. Those who advocate non-operative treatment state that 80–90 % of lesions will resolve spontaneously and that surgical exploration does not always lead to satisfactory results. Postacchini and Morace [12] reported on 42 cases treated non-operatively or with early or late exploration of the radial nerve. They concluded that the decision to perform an early or late exploration of the nerve should be based on four criteria:

1. Level of the fracture,
2. Degree of fracture displacement,
3. Nature of the soft tissue injury,
4. Degree of neurologic deficit.

Other authors recommend surgical exploration 3 or 4 months after injury if there is no sign of neurological recovery, and no later than 6 months [19].

Open Fracture

The same management principles should be applied to open fractures of the humeral shaft as for any open long-bone fracture. The wound should be covered with a sterile dressing, the arm splinted, appropriate antibiotics and tetanus prophylaxis administered. The fracture and soft tissue injury should be treated surgically. The open wound should be extended beyond the zone of injury and all necrotic and devitalised tissue excised and the wound irrigated. The fracture should be stabilized to prevent further soft tissue injury. Those with extensive soft tissue injury require a second-look debridement at 48 h.

Pathological Fracture

The humeral shaft is a relatively common site for metastatic disease. Operative stabilisation is recommended for these fractures for pain relief and ease of nursing. Several authors [18] have recommended the use of polymethylmethacrylate to aid fixation in cases of large bony defects caused by tumour.

Summary

The primary aim of treatment should be to restore function. The surgeon should be aware of the advantages and disadvantages of all treatment options available. The fracture configuration, the associated soft tissue injury and the patient as a whole, all need to be taken into consideration when choosing the most appropriate treatment option.

References

1. Amillo S, Barrios RH, Martinez-Peric R, Losada JI. Surgical treatment of the radial nerve lesions associated with fractures of the humerus. J Orthop Tr. 1993;7:211–5.
2. Balfour GW, Mooney V, Ashby ME. Diaphyseal fractures of the humerus treated with a ready made fracture brace. J Bone Joint Surg Am. 1982;64:11–3.
3. Dabezies EJ, Banta CJ, Murphy CP, d'Ambrosia RD. Plate fixation of the humeral shaft for acute fractures, with and without radial nerve injuries. J Orthop Trauma. 1992;6:10–3.
4. Foster RJ, Swiontkowski MF, Bach AW, Sack JT. Radial nerve palsy caused by open humeral shaft fractures. J Hand Surg. 1993;18:121–4.
5. Gustilo RB, Anderson JT. Prevention of infection in the treatment of one thousand and twenty-five open fractures of long bones: retro- spective and prospective analysis. J Bone Joint Surg Am. 1976;58-A:453–8.
6. Gustilo RB, Mendoza RM, Williams DN. Problems in the management of type III (severe) open fractures: a new classification of type III open fractures. J Trauma. 1984;24:742–6.
7. Heim D, Herkert F, Hess P, Regazzoni P. Surgical treatment of humeral shaft fractures: the Basel experience. J Trauma. 1993;35:226–32.
8. Holstein A, Lewis GB. Fractures of the humerus with radial-nerve paralysis. J Bone Joint Surg Am. 1963;45:1382–8.
9. Mast JW, Spiegel PG, Harvey Jr JP, Harrison C. Fractures of the humeral shaft: a retrospective study of 240 adult fractures. Clin Orthop. 1975;112:254–62.
10. Müller ME, Nazarian S, Koch P, Schatzker J. The comprehensive classification of fractures of long bones. Berlin: Springer; 1990.
11. Oesterne H-J, Tscherne H. Pathophysiology and classification of soft tissue injuries associated with fractures. In: Tscherne H, Gotzen L, editors. Fractures with soft tissue injuries. Berlin: Springer; 1984. p. 1–9.
12. Pollock FH, Drake D, Bovill EG, Day L, Trafton PG. Treatment of radial neuropathy associated with fractures of the humerus. J Bone Joint Surg Am. 1981;63-A:239–43.
12. Postacchini F, Morace G. Fractures of the humerus associated with paralysis of the radial nerve. Ital J Orthop Traumatol. 1988;14:455–64.
13. Rose SH, Melton LJ, Morrey BF, Ilstrup DM, Riggs BL. Epidemiologic features of humeral fractures. Clin Orthop. 1982;168:24–30.
14. Samardzic M, Grujicic D, Milinkovic ZB. Radial nerve lesions associated with fractures of the humeral shaft. Injury. 1990;21:220–2.
15. Sarmiento A, Horowitch A, Aboulafia A, Vangsness Jr C. Functional bracing for comminuted extra-articular fractures of the distal third of the humerus. J Bone Joint Surg Br. 1990;72:283–7.
16. Sarmiento A, Kinman PB, Galvin EG, Schmitt RH, Phillips JG. Functional bracing of fractures of the shaft of the humerus. J Bone Joint Surg Am. 1977;59:596–601.
17. Schatzker J, Ha'Eri EB. Methylmethacrylate as an adjunct in the internal fixation of pathologic fractures. Can J Surg. 1979;22:179.
18. Shao YC, Harwood P, Grotz MRW, Limb D, Giannoudis PV. Radial nerve palsy associated with fractures of the shaft of the humerus. A systematic review. J Bone Joint Surg Br. 2005;87:1647–52.
19. Sonneveld GJ, Patka P, Van Mourik JC, Broere G. Treatment of fractures of the shaft of the humerus accompanied by paralysis of the radial nerve. Injury. 1987;18:404–6.
20. Tytherleigh-Strong G, Walls N, McQueen MM. The epidemiology of humeral shaft fractures. J Bone Joint Surg Br. 1998;80-B:249–53.
21. Zagorski JB, Latta LL, Zych GA, Finnieston AR. Diaphyseal fractures of the humerus: treatment with prefabricated braces. J Bone Joint Surg Am. 1988;70:607–10.
22. Zagorski JB, Zych GA, Latta LL, McCollough NC. Modern concepts in functional fracture bracing: the upper limb. In: Instructional course lectures, vol. 36. Park ridge, IL: American academy of Orthopaedic surgeons; 1987. p. 377–401.